THERAPEUTIC TARGETS
IN AIRWAY INFLAMMATION

LUNG BIOLOGY IN HEALTH AND DISEASE

Executive Editor

Claude Lenfant
Director, National Heart, Lung, and Blood Institute
National Institutes of Health
Bethesda, Maryland

ADDITIONAL VOLUMES IN PREPARATION

The opinions expressed in these volumes do not necessarily represent the views of the National Institutes of Health.

THERAPEUTIC TARGETS IN AIRWAY INFLAMMATION

Edited by
N. Tony Eissa
David P. Huston
Baylor College of Medicine
Houston, Texas, U.S.A.

MARCEL DEKKER, INC. NEW YORK · BASEL

Library of Congress Cataloging-in-Publication Data
A catalog record for this book is available from the Library of Congress.

ISBN: 0–8247–0956-X

This book is printed on acid-free paper.

Headquarters
Marcel Dekker, Inc.
270 Madison Avenue, New York, NY 10016
tel: 212–696–9000; fax: 212–685–4540

Eastern Hemisphere Distribution
Marcel Dekker AG
Hutgasse 4, Postfach 812, CH-4001 Basel, Switzerland
tel: 41–61–260–6300; fax: 41–61–260–6333

World Wide Web
http://www.dekker.com

The publisher offers discounts on this book when ordered in bulk quantities. For more information, write to Special Sales/Professional Marketing at the headquarters address above.

PRINTED IN THE UNITED STATES OF AMERICA

To the memory of my parents, who taught me right from wrong.

NTE

To my trainees, for their thirst for knowledge and efforts to educate me.

DPH

INTRODUCTION

Today, inflammation is largely recognized as a cardinal feature of many, perhaps even all, chronic diseases. Intense research has focused on the inflammatory processes and pathways in such conditions, and it has been well established that these pathways are many and varied, and sometimes characteristic of the particular organ or tissue that is affected.

For example, researchers have demonstrated a role for inflammation in atherosclerosis that will undoubtedly be shown to be completely different from the pathway that leads to asthma. Yet, in both cases, we witness remodeling as a consequence of inflammation.

Consider two diseases that affect the lung, asthma and COPD. We know that inflammation is essential to the development of asthma but, as well, there is recent and very convincing evidence that inflammation plays a role in the occurrence of COPD. However, it is clear that the pathologies of asthma and COPD are very different and, furthermore, that corticosteroids reduce inflammation in asthma but not in COPD. Why? Evidently there are no simple answers to these seemingly simple questions, but this example reinforces the complexity of the inflammatory pathway.

To further complicate the issue, more than one pathway may cause the same disease; such is the case in asthma. Over the last two decades, the increase in prevalence of asthma—and the discovery of its complexity and of the inflammatory pathways causing it— has stimulated the research and clinical communities to conduct intensive work that has led to important and promising observations and discoveries.

Volume 15 of the Lung Biology in Health and Disease series of monographs, published in 1980, discussed inflammation of the airways only specifically. In volume 19, published in 1983, inflammation became the central theme of the volume. Subsequently, a landmark discussion of inflammation and its multiple pathways was presented in volume 54, published in 1991.

Today, 12 years later, the Lung Biology in Health and Disease series is proud to present this volume, which is truly a giant step in the march toward understanding inflammation, its multiple pathways, and how therapeutic approaches are strategized. The sheer number of chapters (44) and the number of contributors (more than 100) provides assurance that the editors, Drs. Eissa and Huston, sought to cover all aspects of inflammation. They term the contributors the "dream team." This book may indeed help the readership to fulfill the dream of their patients, to receive better and better treatment!

I am grateful to the editors and the "dream team" for the opportunity to present this excellent volume.

Claude Lenfant, M.D.
Bethesda, Maryland, U.S.A.

PREFACE

Asthma has many etiological aspects and should be treated according to the various causes that bring it about . . . , the success of relieving the patient from asthma depends largely on an intimate knowledge of the total patient . . . , the physician should not treat the disease but the patient who is suffering from it . . . , I have no magic cure to report.

—Moshe ben Maimon (1135–1204)

These words of wisdom, uttered almost a thousand years ago, still ring true today. Moshe ben Maimon, a physician, philosopher, and rabbi, practiced in Cairo in the court of Saladin, Sultan of Egypt, whose nephew suffered from asthma. The prince, who lived in Alexandria, found he could tide over an asthmatic attack more quickly by going to Cairo. Maimon attributed this favorable response to the cleaner environment in Cairo as opposed to the contaminated air of Alexandria. He emphasized understanding the patient and the balance between him and his environment (1).

This lack of balance has been linked to asthma over centuries and across civilizations. The ancient Egyptians used the hieroglyphics to mean asthma several millennia ago. The lizard was used as a reference to the wheezing noise a chameleon makes when it deflates its lungs in anger (2). Chinese healers understood that xiao-chuan, or "wheezy breathing," was a symptom of imbalance in the life force. The ancient Greco-Roman physicians' treatment for "gasping" was tailor-made for an individual's unique balance of the four "humors": yellow bile, black bile, blood, and phlegm. Native Americans recognized the effect of the environment on the disease and designated the rain god Tláloc as the god of asthma (3). It seems educational to recall these earlier perspectives on asthma at a time when an increase in both asthma incidence and its severity has reached epidemic proportions. One cannot help wondering what sort of imbalance is propagating this epidemic and, more importantly, what specific therapies can target this imbalance. Over the last two decades, airway inflammation has become recognized as a cornerstone in asthma pathogenesis. In a philosophical sense, inflammation can be recognized as a sort of imbalance between the host and its environment. However, inflammation or imbalance encompasses many underlying pathways and mechanisms. If we are to make a serious leap—one that is badly needed—in our understanding and treatment of asthma, we have to dissect the wide variety of complex pathways that contribute to airway inflammation. Only by doing so can we identify potential therapeutic targets. This book attempts to meet this challenge. It should not be perceived not as a prescription for asthma, but rather as a springboard from which future asthma medicine will evolve.

In producing this book, we have assembled a group of physicians and scientists who are considered leaders in their respective fields. The list of contributors is truly a "dream team" of asthma experts. In spite of the length of the book, justified by the vast subject matter, we chose not to divide it into parts because biological processes often defy our arbitrary classification. Instead, we have organized it into rather invisible domains. The emphasis in the early chapters is on the pathophysiology of the disease. Throughout the book, as different mediators are discussed, clear links to therapeutic targets are envisioned. The latter chapters emphasize therapeutic strategies that are in a more advanced stage of development. The book is a state-of-the-art assessment of our understanding of the biology and therapeutic targets in airway inflammation.

We would like to thank all of the authors for contributing their time and expertise and, quite often, their prepublication data, which were vital for the book's success. We are also indebted to Dr. Claude Lenfant for his unwavering enthusiasm and support during the production of this book.

N. Tony Eissa
David P. Huston

REFERENCES

1. The Medical Writings of Moses Maimonides, *Treatise on Asthma*. Muntner S, ed. Philadelphia: Lippincott, 1963.
2. *The Healing Hand: Man and Wound in the Ancient World*. Majno G, ed. Cambridge, MA: Harvard University Press, 1975.
3. Breath of Life, www.nlm.nih.gov/hmd/breath/breathhome.html.

CONTRIBUTORS

Roberto Adachi, M.D.   Assistant Professor, Baylor College of Medicine, and Pulmonary and Critical Care Medicine, Houston VA Medical Center, Houston, Texas, U.S.A.

Anurag Agrawal, M.D.   Postdoctoral Fellow, Baylor College of Medicine, Houston, Texas, U.S.A.

Rafeul Alam, M.D., Ph.D.   Professor and Director, Division of Allergy and Immunology, National Jewish Medical and Research Center, Denver, Colorado, U.S.A.

F. Runa Ali, M.B., B.S.   Department of Allergy and Clinical Immunology, National Heart and Lung Institute, Faculty of Medicine, Imperial College, and Royal Brompton Hospital, London, England

Jacques Banchereau, Ph.D.   Director, Baylor Institute for Immunology Research, Dallas, Texas, U.S.A.

Arnob Banerjee, M.D., Ph.D.   Integrated Program, College of Physicians and Surgeons, Columbia University, New York, New York, U.S.A.

Suman K. Banerjee, M.D., Ph.D.   Senior Research Associate, Department of Biochemistry and Molecular Biology, University of Texas–Houston Medical School, Houston, Texas, U.S.A.

Peter J. Barnes, D.M., D.Sc., F.R.C.P.   Department of Thoracic Medicine, National Heart and Lung Institute, Faculty of Medicine, Imperial College, London, England

Michael R. Blackburn, Ph.D.   Assistant Professor, Department of Biochemistry and Molecular Biology, University of Texas–Houston Medical School, Houston, Texas, U.S.A.

Eugene R. Bleecker, M.D.   Professor and Director, Pulmonary Medicine, and Co-Director, Center for Human Genomics, Wake Forest University School of Medicine, Winston-Salem, North Carolina, U.S.A.

Bruce S. Bochner, M.D.   Professor, Department of Medicine, Johns Hopkins University School of Medicine, Baltimore, Maryland, U.S.A.

Jean Bousquet, M.D.   Hôpital Arnaud de Villeneuve, Montpellier, France

David H. Broide, M.B., Ch.B.   Professor, Department of Medicine, University of California, San Diego, La Jolla, California, U.S.A.

Paula J. Busse, M.D.   Department of Clinical Immunology, Mount Sinai Hospital, New York, New York, U.S.A.

William W. Busse, M.D.   Charles E. Reed Professor of Medicine, Department of Medicine, University of Wisconsin, Madison, Wisconsin, U.S.A.

George H. Caughey, M.D.   Professor of Medicine, Cardiovascular Research Institute and Department of Medicine, University of California at San Francisco, San Francisco, California, U.S.A.

David M. Center, M.D.   Gordon and Ruth Snyder Professor of Pulmonary Medicine and Chief, Department of Pulmonary and Critical Care, Boston University School of Medicine, Boston, Massachusetts, U.S.A.

Arjun B. Chatterjee, M.D.   Center for Human Genomics, Wake Forest University School of Medicine, Winston-Salem, North Carolina, U.S.A.

Augustine M. K. Choi, M.D.   Professor, Department of Medicine, University of Pittsburgh, Pittsburgh, Pennsylvania, U.S.A.

James R. Copeland, M.D., Ph.D. Critical Care Medicine Department, Warren G. Magnuson Clinical Center, National Institutes of Health, Bethesda, Maryland, U.S.A.

David B. Corry, M.D. Department of Medicine, Biology of Inflammation Center, Baylor College of Medicine, Houston, Texas, U.S.A.

Carroll E. Cross, M.D. Professor, Division of Pulmonary and Critical Care Medicine, Department of Medicine, University of California, Davis, Sacramento, California, U.S.A.

William W. Cruikshank, Ph.D. Professor, Department of Pulmonary and Critical Care Medicine, Boston University School of Medicine, Boston, Massachusetts, U.S.A.

Rosemarie H. DeKruyff, Ph.D. Professor, Division of Immunology and Allergy, Department of Pediatrics, Stanford University, Stanford, California, U.S.A.

Pascal Demoly Hôpital Arnaud de Villeneuve, Montpellier, France

George T. De Sanctis, Ph.D., F.C.C.P. Head, Department of Respiratory Pharmacology/Pathology, Aventis Pharmaceuticals, Bridgewater, New Jersey, U.S.A.

Burton F. Dickey, M.D. Professor and Chairman, Department of Pulmonary Medicine, M. D. Anderson Cancer Center; Professor of Medicine and Molecular Physiology and Biophysics, Baylor College of Medicine; and Houston VA Medical Center, Houston, Texas, U.S.A.

Claire M. Doerschuk, M.D. Professor, Department of Pediatrics and Biomedical Engineering, Case Western Reserve University, Cleveland, Ohio, U.S.A.

Jeffrey M. Drazen, M.D. Parker B. Francis Professor of Medicine, Department of Pulmonary and Critical Care, Brigham and Women's Hospital and Harvard Medical School, Boston, Massachusetts, U.S.A.

Jason P. Eiserich, Ph.D. Assistant Professor, Division of Nephrology, Department of Internal Medicine, University of California, Davis, Sacramento, California, U.S.A.

N. Tony Eissa, M.D. Associate Professor, Department of Medicine, Baylor College of Medicine, Houston, Texas, U.S.A.

Serpil C. Erzurum, M.D. Director, Lung Biology Program, Departments of Pulmonary and Critical Care and Cancer Biology, Lerner Research Institute, Cleveland Clinic Foundation, Cleveland, Ohio, U.S.A.

Christopher Evans, Ph.D. Postdoctoral Fellow, Baylor College of Medicine, Houston, Texas, U.S.A.

John V. Fahy, M.D. University of California, San Francisco, San Francisco, California, U.S.A.

Kenneth C. Fang, M.D. Assistant Professor, Department of Medicine, University of California at San Francisco, San Francisco, California, U.S.A.

John L. Faul, M.D. Assistant Professor, Department of Medicine, Stanford University School of Medicine, Stanford, California, U.S.A.

Richard A. Flavell, Ph.D., F.R.C. Professor/Investigator, Section of Immunobiology, Howard Hughes Medical Institute, Yale University School of Medicine, New Haven, Connecticut, U.S.A.

Paul S. Foster, Ph.D. Division of Molecular Bioscience, John Curtin School of Medical Research, Australian National University, Canberra, Australia

Stephen J. Galli, M.D. Professor and Chair, Department of Pathology, Stanford University School of Medicine, Stanford, California, U.S.A.

Benjamin Gaston, M.D. Department of Pediatrics, University of Virginia Health System, Charlottesville, Virginia, U.S.A.

Craig Gerard, M.D., Ph.D. Department of Pediatrics, Harvard Medical School, Boston, Massachusetts, U.S.A.

Norma P. Gerard, Ph.D. Professor of Medicine, Harvard Medical School, Boston, Massachusetts, U.S.A.

Mark T. Gladwin, M.D. Senior Investigator, Critical Care Medicine Department, Warren G. Magnuson Clinical Center, National Institutes of Health, Bethesda, Maryland, U.S.A.

Tannishia M. Goggans Research Technologist, Departments of Pulmonary and Critical Care and Cancer Biology, Lerner Research Institute, Cleveland Clinic Foundation, Cleveland, Ohio, U.S.A.

Michael E. Greenberg, Ph.D. Research Associate, Department of Cell Biology, Cleveland Clinic Foundation, Cleveland, Ohio, U.S.A.

El-Bdaoui Haddad, Ph.D. Section Leader, Department of Respiratory Pharmacology, Aventis Pharmaceuticals, Bridgewater, New Jersey, U.S.A.

Miera B. Harris, M.D., Ph.D. Integrated Program, College of Physicians and Surgeons, Columbia University, New York, New York, U.S.A.

Stanley L. Hazen, M.D., Ph.D. Professor, Department of Cell Biology, Cleveland Clinic Foundation, Cleveland, Ohio, U.S.A.

Josephine Hjoberg Brigham and Women's Hospital and Harvard Medical School, Boston, Massachusetts, U.S.A.

Stephen T. Holgate, M.D., D.Sc., F.R.C.Path., F.I.Biol., FmedSci. MRC Clinical Professor, Inflammation and Repair Division, Department of Respiratory, Cell and Molecular Biology, University of Southampton, Southampton, England

Michael J. Holtzman, M.D. Pulmonary and Critical Care Medicine, Department of Medicine, Washington University School of Medicine, St. Louis, Missouri, U.S.A.

Timothy D. Howard, Ph.D. Assistant Professor, Department of Pediatrics, Center for Human Genomics, Wake Forest University School of Medicine, Winston-Salem, North Carolina, U.S.A.

Jennifer C. Huang Research Fellow, Howard Hughes Medical Institute, Department of Medicine, Biology of Inflammation Center, Baylor College of Medicine, Houston, Texas, U.S.A.

John Hunt, M.D. University of Virginia Health System, Charlottesville, Virginia, U.S.A.

David P. Huston, M.D. Cullen Professor of Immunology, Department of Medicine and Immunology, and Director, Biology of Inflammation Center, Baylor College of Medicine, Houston, Texas, U.S.A.

Christopher L. Karp, M.D. Professor and Director, Division of Molecular Immunology, Department of Pediatrics, Cincinnati Children's Hospital Medical Center, Cincinnati, Ohio, U.S.A.

A. Barry Kay, M.D., Ph.D. Department of Allergy and Clinical Immunology, National Heart and Lung Institute, Faculty of Medicine, Imperial College, and Royal Brompton Hospital, London, England

Farrah Kheradmand, M.D. Assistant Professor, Department of Medicine, Biology of Inflammation Center, Baylor College of Medicine, Houston, Texas, U.S.A.

Brian J. Knoll, Ph.D. Associate Professor, Department of Pharmacological and Pharmaceutical Sciences, University of Houston, Houston, Texas, U.S.A.

Jörg Köhl, M.D.   Professor, Division of Molecular Immunology, Department of Pediatrics, Cincinnati Children's Hospital Medical Center, Cincinnati, Ohio, U.S.A.

Pawel J. Kolodziejski, M.D.   Department of Medicine, Baylor College of Medicine, Houston, Texas, U.S.A.

Mark Larché, Ph.D.   Department of Allergy and Clinical Immunology, National Heart and Lung Institute, Faculty of Medicine, Imperial College, and Royal Brompton Hospital, London, England

Aili L. Lazaar, M.D.   Assistant Professor, Pulmonary, Allergy and Critical Care Division, Department of Medicine, University of Pennsylvania Medical Center, Philadelphia, Pennsylvania, U.S.A.

Frédéric F. Little, M.D.   Division of Pulmonary, Allergy, and Critical Care Medicine, Boston University School of Medicine, Boston, Massachusetts, U.S.A.

Margarita Martinez-Moczygemba, Ph.D.   Assistant Professor, Department of Medicine, Biology of Inflammation Center, Baylor College of Medicine, Houston, Texas, U.S.A.

Harvey E. Marshall   Duke University Medical Center, Durham, North Carolina, U.S.A.

Robert H. Moore, M.D.   Assistant Professor, Departments of Pediatrics and Molecular Physiology and Biophysics, Baylor College of Medicine, Houston, Texas, U.S.A.

Brian Morrissey, M.D.   Division of Pulmonary and Critical Care Medicine, Department of Internal Medicine, University of California, Davis, Sacramento, California, U.S.A.

Anthony P. Nguyen   Research Associate, Department of Immunology, Biology of Inflammation Center, Baylor College of Medicine, Houston, Texas, U.S.A.

Rupesh Nigam, M.D.   Baylor College of Medicine, Houston, Texas, U.S.A.

Lyle J. Palmer   Brigham and Women's Hospital and Harvard Medical School, Boston, Massachusetts, U.S.A.

A. Karolina Palucka   Baylor Institute for Immunology Research, Dallas, Texas, U.S.A.

Reynold A. Panettieri, Jr., M.D.   Robert L. Maycock and David A. Cooper Professor of Medicine, Pulmonary, Allergy, and Critical Care Division, Department of Medicine, University of Pennsylvania Medical Center, Philadelphia, Pennsylvania, U.S.A.

John F. Parkinson, Ph.D.   Senior Scientist, Department of Research, Berlex Biosciences, Richmond, California, U.S.A.

Marc Peters-Golden, M.D.   Professor, Division of Pulmonary and Critical Care Medicine, Department of Internal Medicine, University of Michigan Health System, Ann Arbor, Michigan, U.S.A.

Loretta G. Que   Duke University Medical Center, Durham, North Carolina, U.S.A.

Eyal Raz, M.D.   Professor, Department of Medicine, University of California, San Diego, La Jolla, California, U.S.A.

Anthony E. Redington, M.D.   Senior Lecturer, Academic Department of Medicine, University of Hull, Hull, England

Kirtee Rishi   Department of Medicine, Baylor College of Medicine, Houston, Texas, U.S.A.

Marc E. Rothenberg, M.D., Ph.D.   Director and Endowed Professor, Division of Allergy and Immunology, Department of Pediatrics, Cincinnati Children's Hospital Medical Center, Cincinnati, Ohio, U.S.A.

Paul Rothman, M.D.   Professor, Departments of Medicine and Microbiology, College of Physicians and Surgeons, Columbia University, New York, New York, U.S.A.

Jigme M. Sethi, M.D.   Assistant Professor, Department of Medicine, University of Pittsburgh, Pittsburgh, Pennsylvania, U.S.A.

James H. Shelhamer, M.D.   Critical Care Medicine Department, Warren G. Magnuson Clinical Center, National Institutes of Health, Bethesda, Maryland, U.S.A.

Eric S. Silverman   Brigham and Women's Hospital, Harvard Medical School, and Harvard School of Public Health, Boston, Massachusetts, U.S.A.

Jonathan S. Stamler   Duke University Medical Center, Durham, North Carolina, U.S.A.

Kelan Tantisira   Brigham and Women's Hospital and Harvard Medical School, Boston, Massachusetts, U.S.A.

Ulla-Angela Temann, Ph.D.   Section of Immunobiology, Howard Hughes Medical Institute, Yale University School of Medicine, New Haven, Connecticut, U.S.A.

Dale T. Umetsu, M.D., Ph.D.   Professor, Division of Immunology and Allergy, Department of Pediatrics, Stanford University, Stanford, California, U.S.A.

Albert van der Vliet, Ph.D.   Associate Professor, Department of Pathology, University of Vermont, Burlington, Vermont, U.S.A.

Antonio M. Vignola   Istituto di Fisiopatologia Respiratoria, Palermo, Italy

David M. Walter, Ph.D.   Research Scientist, Neurobiology Unit, Roche Bioscience, Palo Alto, California, U.S.A.

Michael J. Walter, M.D.   Pulmonary and Critical Care Medicine, Department of Medicine, Washington University School of Medicine, St. Louis, Missouri, U.S.A.

Scott T. Weiss, M.D.   Associate Physician, Brigham and Women's Hospital and Harvard Medical School, Boston, Massachusetts, U.S.A.

Francis Whalen, M.D.   Senior Fellow, Department of Medicine, University of Pittsburgh, Pittsburgh, Pennsylvania

Marsha Wills-Karp, Ph.D.   Professor and Director, Division of Immunobiology, Department of Pediatrics, Cincinnati Children's Hospital Medical Center, Cincinnati, Ohio, U.S.A.

Weiling Xu, M.D.   Research Associate, Departments of Pulmonary and Critical Care and Cancer Biology, Lerner Research Institute, Cleveland Clinic Foundation, Cleveland, Ohio, U.S.A.

Nives Zimmermann, M.D.   Assistant Professor, Division of Allergy and Immunology, Department of Pediatrics, Cincinnati Children's Hospital Medical Center, Cincinnati, Ohio, U.S.A.

CONTENTS

THERAPEUTIC TARGETS
IN AIRWAY INFLAMMATION

1

Pathophysiology of Airway Inflammation in Asthma

PAULA J. BUSSE

Mount Sinai Hospital
New York, New York, U.S.A.

WILLIAM W. BUSSE

University of Wisconsin
Madison, Wisconsin, U.S.A.

I. Introduction

Asthma is a chronic disease of the airways that in most cases has its inception in early childhood with physiological hallmarks of increased airway inflammation, bronchial hyperresponsiveness, and airflow obstruction that is largely reversible. Clinically, asthmatic patients have symptoms of coughing (especially at night), shortness of breath, chest tightness, and wheezing. The diagnosis of asthma is made by these clinical symptoms and is confirmed by the demonstration of reversible airflow obstruction.

The airway hyperresponsiveness in asthma is, in part, considered to be secondary to airway inflammation, which is the result of a complex orchestration of many inflammatory cells (mast cells, eosinophils, T lymphocytes, neutrophils, and macrophages) whose activities are coordinated by the release of proteins such as cytokines and chemokines. The release of mediators from these cells may also cause airway narrowing, mucus production, vascular edema, and injury to the airways, which in turn lead to many of the common features of the asthmatic response. Finally, these inflammatory processes may eventually result in permanent changes (i.e., "remodeling") in the airways of asthmatic patients (Fig. 1).

For many years asthma was considered to be solely a genetic disorder, and the genes associated with asthma are being identified. However, equally important

1

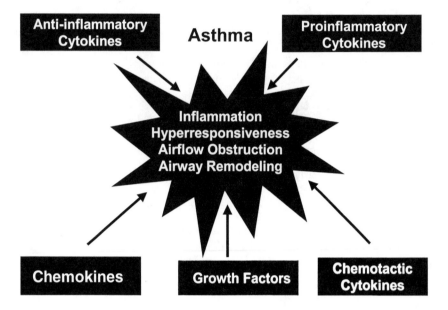

Figure 1 Factors influencing the development of asthma and leading to the characteristic features of the disease: inflammation, airflow obstruction, and hyperresponsiveness.

in the etiology of asthma are environmental factors. The development of asthma likely depends on the interaction of these two forces, and this belief is comprised within the "gene-by-environment" hypothesis.

II. Epidemiology

The prevalence of asthma has increased greatly in the past two decades. The Centers for Disease Control and Prevention (CDC) documented that between 1980 and 2000, asthma cases in the United States, in children and adults, have more than doubled, from 6.8 to 17.3 million (1,2). This increase in asthma cases has not been uniformly distributed in the world's population or geography. Rates of asthma tend to be highest in African American and Hispanic children who live in large inner cities, such as New York City, Baltimore, Los Angeles, Philadelphia, and Chicago (3–6). Explanations for these "pockets" of asthma are many, including an increased exposure to secondhand cigarette smoke, indoor allergens (i.e., cockroaches, mice, and dust mites), lack of follow-up medical care, and diminished access to appropriate medical therapy.

The growing prevalence of asthma extends beyond the United States and is a worldwide epidemic (7,8). There are common themes emerging to explain the rise in asthma outside the United States. English-speaking and western countries tend to have the highest prevalence and fastest growth rates of asthma. In contrast, Vietnam,

Finland, Taiwan, and New Guinea are among the areas of the world with the lowest prevalence of asthma, whereas Scotland, Australia, and New Zealand have markedly higher rates (9). The areas of the world with higher asthma rates are considered to be more "westernized." In addition, asthma rates are higher in urbanized areas. In Zimbabwe, for example, the prevalence of asthma has been shown to be greater in an urban area than in a rural one (10). These epidemiological observations have given insight into the mechanisms of asthma.

III. Natural History of Asthma

A. Infancy to Early Adulthood

Although asthma may present at any age, it typically begins in early childhood. It is estimated that half of all asthmatic patients are diagnosed by 3 years of age, and 80% by 6 years of age. Young children usually begin to experience episodes of coughing, difficulty breathing, or wheezing after an upper respiratory infection or moderate exertion. For some individuals, these episodes are transient and do not persist, but for others, these are early symptoms of asthma. Some asthmatic patients develop their disease later in life, which is less common and probably has different pathophysiological mechanisms (Fig. 2).

Several prospective cohort studies (either clinic-based or population-based cohorts) followed children through early adulthood with objective measurements of

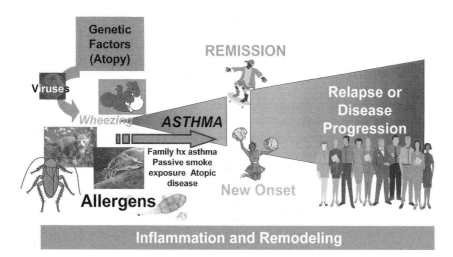

Figure 2 Natural history of asthma. For most patients, asthma begins in early life. An initial event associated with early wheezing may include a viral respiratory infection. This is followed by sensitization to environmental allergens. The events associated with allergic sensitization and allergic inflammation in the airways can include bronchial remodeling. (From Robert Lemanske.)

lung function, skin-prick testing, and environmental exposure. In one sample, 482 asthmatic children, ages 8–12 years, who were referred to a pediatric pulmonary outpatient clinic were followed to a mean age of 24.7 years. This study demonstrated, among many other findings, that the childhood FEV_1 was predictive of adult FEV_1, and that the childhood degree of bronchial responsiveness strongly correlated to bronchial responsiveness in adulthood (11). Melbourne, British, and Tasmanian population-based cohorts led to similar conclusions after tracking children with asthma until their mid-30s (12–14). The finding of these studies strongly suggests that children with persistent episodes of wheezing, and a greater severity of asthma, were almost twice as likely to have persistent wheezing or asthma as adults. In addition, the Melbourne and Tasmanian studies demonstrate that the measurement of lung function in early childhood predicted persistence of asthma into adulthood (i.e., those children with low levels of lung function early in life were more likely to have wheezing as adults) (14,15).

These cohort studies examine the possible effect of asthma upon the decline of lung function. The Melbourne study demonstrates that the rate of decline of lung function among children without asthma, and with different severities of asthma, did not differ appreciably with time. However, children with more severe asthma had an initial lower lung function as measured by FEV_1/FVC (15). Other studies suggest that lung function in asthma declines after the age of 35 years and that some individuals may experience approximately twice the rate of decline in FEV_1 compared with nonasthmatics (16). The rate of decline in lung function is compounded by smoking (17).

Besides a low FEV_1 and a high degree of airway hyperresponsiveness in childhood, several other factors correlate with the persistence of asthma in adulthood: these patients are more likely to be female, have higher rates of atopy, and have experienced significant exposure to cigarette smoke, typically primary.

B. Adulthood Asthma

If a patient's asthma does not go into remission in later childhood, it is less likely that he or she will experience a remission later in life. Burrows and colleagues found that in adults over 65 years of age only 20% experienced a remission and that these patients tended to have mild disease (18). Panhuysen et al. followed 181 adult asthma patients (mean age 24 years) over a 25-year period and found that 11% attained remission as defined by an absence of pulmonary symptoms, bronchial hyperresponsiveness, and $FEV_1 > 90\%$ predicted. Thus, the absence of asthma after the 25-year observation period was associated with better lung function at the initial visit, a shorter period without treatment prior to the first visit, less initial airway responsiveness, and a lower serum IgE. This group was unable to demonstrate that gender or atopy (as defined as one or more positive prick skin tests) relates to asthma outcome and bronchial hyperresponsiveness (BHR) in adult patients (19).

Panhuysen et al.'s study also demonstrated that the majority of the asthmatic patients who were "persistent" in adulthood also showed a decrease in postbronchodilator FEV_1 over time, suggesting increased irreversible airflow obstruction (19).

It has been hypothesized that despite appropriate therapy, some adult patients may develop irreversible airflow obstruction from asthma (20), and this may be intrinsic to asthma itself. In a Danish population, Lange and colleagues (21) followed FEV_1 measurements over a 15-year time interval. They found a decline of 38 mL/y in adults with asthma compared with 22 mL/y in those without asthma, a trend seen in both genders and compounded by smoking. Peat et al. followed 92 asthmatic patients and 186 normal subjects for 18 years and found a 50 mL/y loss of FEV_1 compared to 35 mL/y in the normal subjects (22). Reed found that in a population of patients over the age of 65 years, that there was no correlation between FEV_1 and duration of the disease as known by symptoms (23). Ulrik et al. (24) found that patients with so-called intrinsic asthma had a lesser decline in FEV_1 over a 10-year period than did extrinsic asthmatics (50 mL/y vs. 23 mL/y. This work suggests that atopy may have an adverse effect on lung decline. Overall, these results demonstrate that, unlike asthma in children, asthma in adults may produce more significant changes in airway function over time, one feature of which is an enhanced loss of lung function.

IV. Genetic and Environmental Factors Involved in the Pathogenesis of Asthma

A. Introduction and Hygiene Hypothesis

For many years, the genetic make-up of an individual was felt to be the most important risk factor for developing asthma. Today, however, it is known that the development of asthma involves not only the inheritance of specific genes, but also environmental factors (Fig. 3). The concept that the environment plays a significant role in the development of allergic diseases, notably asthma, is evolving and provides potential explanations for its increasing prevalence and pathophysiology.

The theory that the "westernization" of our society affects the development of the immune system has been labeled the "hygiene hypothesis." The basis of this hypothesis centers on work done in mice, in which their T lymphocytes are broken down into Th1 and Th2 subtypes based upon the specific cytokine profile that they produce. Type 1 helper T cells (Th1) produce interleukin-2 (IL-2) and interferons (IFN-γ and IFN-β), which are associated with viral immunity and delayed-type hypersensitivity reactions (i.e., tuberculosis). Type 2 helper T cells (Th2) produce IL-4, -5, -6, -9, and -13, which mediate allergic inflammation. In addition, Th1-type cytokines will generally inhibit the production of Th2-type cytokines. IL-3, tumor necrosis factor (TNF-α), and granulocyte-macrophage colony-stimulating factor (GM-CSF) are produced by both Th1 and Th2 T lymphocytes (25). T lymphocytes that secrete both Th1 and Th2 cytokines are termed Th0 (26). In addition, a recently discovered subtype of T lymphocytes, Th3, is believed to play a role in oral tolerance and other regulatory functions (27) (Table 1).

The theory behind the hygiene hypothesis is that there is reciprocal balance between the Th1 and Th2 arms of the immune system, which may be influenced by certain environmental factors. Advances in medicine such as an increased use

At-Risk Population

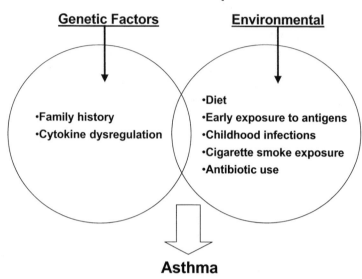

Figure 3   Asthma is felt to represent a "gene-by-environment" interaction. Genetic factors may include a cytokine dysregulation with a shift to proinflammatory mediator production. Environmental factors can determine whether the genetic factors are allowed to express themselves and lead to the development of airway disease and asthma.

Table 1   Th1 and Th2 Cytokines: Their Potential Role in Allergic Diseases and Asthma

	Th1	Th2
Functions	Delayed-type hypersensitivity	Atopy
	Viral infections	Parasitic infections
Cytokines	IL-2	Il-4
	TNF-α	IL-5
	γ-IFN	IL-13
	IL-3	IL-3
	IL-10	IL-2
Factors favoring phenotype	Rural environment	Use of antibiotics, vaccines
	Large family size	Early sensitization to indoor antigens
	Tuberculosis	antigens
	Day care	Urban environment

of antibiotics and vaccinations and decreased congestion of living quarters lessens the likelihood of developing early childhood infections or severity, thereby swaying the developing immune system toward the Th2-like arm (28). (The Th1-like arm has been connected with the defense against many childhood infections.) The following observational studies support this hypothesis; infections with measles (29); hepatitis A (30) and tuberculosis (31,32) produce lower rates of atopy in these individuals. However, these observations have not always been replicated, insofar as a recently published work demonstrates that children and adolescents with a history of naturally occurring measles have *greater* rates of atopic disease (33). The most likely explanation for these discrepancies is that the development of asthma is a combination of both genetic and environmental factors and that their interaction is influenced by many factors.

B. The Intrauterine Environment

Since the development of asthma usually takes place early in life, it is not surprising that the intrauterine environment plays a role in the pathogenesis of allergic disease and asthma. Previous data suggest that pregnancy may be associated with the deviation of the maternal immune system towards the Th2 cytokine pattern, which may prevent the rejection of the fetus (33). Certain Th1 cytokines, in particular IFN-γ, could directly damage the placenta or activate cytotoxic activity, which causes fetal injuries. Therefore, the Th2-like environment may protect the fetus from rejection and allow the developing immune system of the unborn child to grow in an "allergic" environment. Some research suggests evidence for a "favorable" Th2-like immune status in fetal development by observations that mothers who are atopic may tend to have more children than nonatopic mothers, as the pregnancies of the former are more viable (34). Additional evidence also suggests that the fetus may have a low but significant and specific immune response to either foods and and/or inhalant allergens to which the mother has been exposed. Studies have demonstrated that cord blood T-cells proliferate in vitro when exposed to ovalbumin, β-lactoglobulin (BLG), house dust mite, cat, and pollen allergens (35–37). The cord cells that respond to these antigens have been demonstrated to be fetal in origin and not maternal (38). As the immune system needs to be "primed" in order to respond by T-cell proliferation to allergic antigens, prior exposure is both necessary and critical. Therefore, these findings in the neonatal period further suggest that antigens to which the mother is exposed may influence her fetus. This early exposure, in combination with the surrounding Th2-like environment, may be required for the development of atopy in an at-risk infant.

C. Presence of Other Atopic Diseases and Family History of Atopy

Asthma often accompanies other atopic diseases. It has been estimated that approximately 50% of the asthma phenotype can be accounted for by the coexistence of atopy (39). Although this suggests that factors other than atopic history (i.e., the environment) are risk factors for the development of asthma, it also underscores the strong role that atopy plays in the development of asthma. For example, Martinez et al. (40) examined the influence of a maternal history of atopy on persistent asthma in childhood. In this prospective cohort, they were able to demonstrate that children who wheeze before the age of 3 years and have persistent wheezing at 6 years of age were more likely to have been born to mothers with a history of asthma, have elevated serum IgE levels, and have diminished lung functions at 3 years of age. On the other hand, children who had transient wheezing before the age of 3 years, but not after 6 years, were more likely to have a normal serum IgE level, negative skin-prick test responses, diminished lung functions only at 1 year of age, and to have been born to a mother without a history of asthma, but who smoked.

Studies have demonstrated that atopic diseases may emerge progressively from infancy through early childhood, termed the "atopic march." Infants develop sensitivity to an antigen, which leads to the development of a series of atopic diseases, such as atopic dermatitis, allergic rhinitis, and eventually to asthma. The presence of eczema in infancy is a strong indicator of childhood wheezing (41). In addition, an elevated serum IgE to hen's egg proteins is a good predictor of subsequent sensitization to aeroallergens and the development of allergic airway symptoms, including asthma (42).

D. Early Exposure to Antigens

It is well recognized that early exposure to both outdoor (pollens, molds) and, perhaps more importantly, indoor (house dust mite, cockroach, cat and dog hair, indoor molds) antigens is strongly associated with developing sensitization to them. The relationship, however, between sensitization and the eventual development of asthma is less clear. Studies demonstrate that early exposure to the house dust mite, *Dermatophagoides spp.*, leads both to sensitization and to increased rates of asthma in atopic individuals (43). Similar findings were noted in nonatopic individuals exposed to greater concentrations of the dust mite (44). More recent data by one of these groups, however, and others suggest that although early exposure to indoor allergens is important for sensitization, it may not be directly linked to development of airway hyperresponsiveness, as previously believed (45). In fact, some work demonstrates that early exposure to certain animals (i.e., house pets) may actually *prevent* asthma (46). This phenomenon has also been noted in children growing up on a farm (47). Mechanistically, this protective effect is felt to be secondary to the bacterial endotoxins produced by these farm livestock, which in turn produce IL-12 or IL-18, causing downregulation of Th2-like cells (48). As will be noted later in this chapter, however, endotoxin exposure may not be protective against atopy and may actually contribute to its development.

E. Viral Infections

Epidemiological studies demonstrate that lower respiratory infections in infancy or early childhood may lead to wheezing and, in some, to asthma. Between 30 and 60% of children wheeze with respiratory infections in the first 5 years of life (49). However, only approximately 20% of these children who wheeze with these infections will develop persistent wheezing or asthma. The virus usually implicated in this relationship is respiratory syncytial virus (RSV), although other viruses that have been implicated include parainfluenza virus (PIV), adenovirus, coronavirus, and influenza virus (50). By age 3, almost 80% of children have been exposed to RSV strains, therefore it is relatively uncommon for an adult to acquire such an infection. How RSV produces wheezing in some children and the development of asthma in a subset of them is unclear, but there are several hypotheses. Lower respiratory infection with RSV may cause airway injury and remodeling and, as a consequence, affect lung development, predisposing the child to asthma. Although viruses typically are controlled by CD8+ T cells, RSV protein can induce a Th2-like cytokine response (51,52) and promote allergic sensitization in animals (53). Why some children develop more severe reactions is not clear.

Although not well documented, a family history of atopy may predispose an infant to wheeze after RSV and to eventually develop asthma. Rooney and Williams evaluated the hospital records of infants hospitalized for bronchiolitis prior to 18 months of age and found that those infants who had recurrent wheezing had a family history of asthma and allergic diseases (54). These children with atopic histories and more persistent wheezing may have a different response to the RSV, such as greater change in eosinophils, transient IgE increases, and increased eosinophilic cationic protein (ECP) (55–57). In addition, T-cell responses to the viral antigen may be different in patients with atopy, and infection with RSV may lead to allergen sensitization. Animal models showed that allergen sensitization could potentiate the physiological and structural changes induced by bronchiolitis (58). In addition, in a study done by Sigurs et al., it was reported that infants hospitalized early in life with wheezing from RSV were more likely to have allergen-specific IgE (32% vs. 9%) and asthma (23% vs. 1%) by the age of 3 years, particularly if there was a family history of allergy (59). Other studies have found consistent results (60).

F. Bacterial Infection

Recent work has suggested that bacterial infections, especially ones produced by the atypical bacteria *Chlamydia pneumoniae*, may produce new-onset asthma in adulthood or exacerbation of preexisting asthma. Reports that antibiotic treatment improved symptoms in moderate persistent (61,62) and steroid-dependent asthma (63) suggested a linkage between this atypical bacteria and asthma. The mechanisms of *C. pneumoniae*-induced asthma exacerbation and asthma pathogenesis have been speculated to be similar to those of viral onset asthma. Like RSV, *C. pneumoniae* can infect the bronchial tree to produce ciliary dysfunction (64) and epithelial damage (65). In addition, several *Chlamydia* species produce inflammatory cytokines both in vitro and in vivo (66,67). IgE against *C. pneumoniae* can develop after infection in children (68) whose asthma has been exacerbated by this infection, as well as with adult-onset asthmatics (69). Some of the heat-shock proteins in *Chlamydia* may induce changes in the lung parenchyma leading to asthma (69–71).

G. Tobacco Smoke

Despite measures to curb tobacco smoking, environmental tobacco smoke (ETS) remains a major health concern. Whether ETS is causally related to the development of asthma in children and infants is controversial (72–75), but there is support for such a relationship. Studies have provided evidence the ETS adversely affects lung growth and development, leading to wheezing or to lower respiratory viral infections. Martinez et al. demonstrated an increased risk for early transient wheezing that was more strongly correlated to a history of maternal cigarette smoking than to atopy, although the risk of persistent wheezing was more strongly correlated with maternal atopy and infant elevated serum IgE (40). The relative risk of asthma in children born to mothers who smoked has been reported to be 1.2–2.6 (76). The pooled odds ratio for asthma prevalence from 14 case-control studies was 1.37 if either parent smoked (75) for atopic history; children of mothers who smoked 10 or more cigarettes per day were 2.5 times more likely to have asthma than were children of mothers who did not smoke or who smoked fewer than 10 cigarettes per day (77).

Mechanisms of ETS producing increased risk of asthma are most likely multifactorial, and there may be differences depending on whether the child was exposed in utero or after birth. ETS most likely causes airway changes that predispose infants to developing lower viral infections, which in turn may produce asthma. It has been suggested that in utero, especially prior to the middle of the third trimester, tobacco smoke exposure produces the greatest alterations in lung development (78). It has also been suggested, based upon studies of rodents exposed to tobacco smoke during the in utero period, that newborns have increased bronchial reactivity (79). It is unlikely that ETS produces allergic sensitization leading to asthma, as has been demonstrated by meta-analysis (74), because cigarette smoke is an irritant and not an allergen. However, children of smoking parents have increased peripheral blood eosinophils (80). Thus, ETS may cause nonspecific changes in the airways, including eosinophilia and hyperresponsiveness, that may contribute to asthma pathogenesis.

Few studies have evaluated the potential for ETS to be a cause of adult-onset asthma. The results of these studies are somewhat difficult to interpret because they have potential for recall bias, accuracy of assessing the cigarette exposure in the workplace, and a selection bias. Greer and colleagues noted that ETS increased the risk 1.45 times over a 10-year period during which patients developed asthma at a mean age of 56.5 years (81). Additionally, Flodin et al. demonstrated a similar odds ratio for exposure for passive smoking at work in relation to a diagnosis of asthma (82).

H. Air Pollution and Diesel Exhaust Fuel

Reliance upon motor vehicles and industrial production has resulted in increased atmospheric diesel exhaust particles (DEPs) and ozone. Whether DEPs and other air pollutants produce asthma remains controversial. Studies of the German reunification have not demonstrated that air pollution results in increases in asthma (83). However, other studies have shown that closures of a steel mill resulted in decreases of asthma admissions for preschool children (84) and that experimental exposure of humans to this particulate matter provokes inflammatory responses in the airways of nonasthmatics (85). Discrepancies among studies may exist due to different compositions of particulate matter and whether patients have established asthma. There has been speculation as to how DEPs may result in an increase in atopy and asthma prevalence. They can induce IgE production (86) and, when inhaled with other antigens, can direct T lymphocytes toward a Th2 pattern (87). DEPs may also inhibit IFN-γ production, enhancing the IL-4 response. Finally, DEPs potentially promote sensitization by enhancing antigen presentation (88). Most of the literature suggests that ozone exposure does not cause asthma, but instead exacerbates preexisting asthma in a dose-dependent fashion. Initial studies demonstrated that low ozone concentrations did not typically produce bronchoconstriction (89), but using a higher inhaled dose of ozone, Kreit et al. demonstrated that there was increased airway resistance and larger decrements in FEV_1 and FEV_1/FVC with ozone exposure (90). In addition, exercise appears to further confound the effect of ozone on asthma exacerbations. When a group of asthmatic individuals performed light exercise under ozone exposure, there was a larger FEV_1 fall and more bronchoconstriction than in patients without asthma exposed to a similar duration and concentration of ozone (91). Investigation of normal subjects exposed to ozone shows transient levels of bronchial hyperresponsiveness and airway inflammation (similar to asthma), but not permanent airway damage typically seen in asthma (92,93).

I. Endotoxin

Endotoxins are soluble portions of lipopoly saccharide (LPS) found on the outer membrane of gram-negative bacteria. As previously mentioned, early exposure to endotoxin may have different outcomes. Some have shown that it may prevent the development of asthma (94,95), but others have suggested that it may cause bronchial hyperresponsiveness and asthma (96). There are several potential mechanisms by which endotoxin may enhance the development of asthma. Endotoxin increases inflammation of the airways by stimulating alveolar macrophages and type II epithelial cells to produce multiple cytokines, chemokines, and adhesion molecules. Specifically, endotoxin enhances the production of IL-8 (a chemotactic factor and cytokine that recruits neutrophils to the airways) and upregulates ICAM-1 (97). Endotoxin also inhibits apoptosis, prolonging the survival of the inflammatory cells in the airways (98). Endotoxin can increase IgE-mediated histamine release from mast cells and basophils (99,100). However, the net effect of endotoxin on the predisposition to asthma most likely depends upon its exposure dose, as well as the age and genetic background of the individual.

J. Diet/Breast-Feeding

Both breast-feeding of the infant and early dietary influences are likely important in the development of asthma, yet controversial, as there are many confounding factors in the research. Several studies have pointed to an important relationship between breast-feeding/early diet and the development of atopy in the infant. Although the relationship between breast-feeding (versus cow's milk) and prevention of atopic diseases has recently become of great interest, this question was originally addressed over 60 years ago. Grulee and Sanford demonstrated that eczema was reduced sevenfold in infants breast-fed as compared to infants fed with boiled cow's milk in a group of nearly 20,000 infants (101). Recent studies have shown that respiratory allergy was significantly reduced in a group of 150 infants followed until 17 years of age, grouping them into the following categories of breast-feeding: (1) less than 1 month, (2) 1–6 months, and (3) prolonged (6 months). This relationship was not affected by a family history of atopy (102). There are additional studies conferring a positive protective effect of breast-feeding versus early introduction of cow's milk formula against the development of asthma. There is research as well that disputes this relationship (103,104). One recent study cited that if the maternal serum IgE is high, breast-feeding will actually lead to increased serum IgE of the infant with prolonged breast-feeding, which may be a significant prognostic factor for the development of asthma (105).

The mechanisms to explain protective or detrimental effects of breast-feeding versus early introduction of cow's milk are multiple, including transfer of polyunsaturated fatty acids in human milk (106), cytokines in breast milk, and prevention of infection by passive transfer of IgA antibody. Dietary intervention may also influence gut flora, in turn influencing the development of atopy. Infants with a low prevalence of allergy at the age of one year in Estonia and Sweden were more likely to have lactobacilli and eubacteria in their gut, whereas infants with *Clostridium difficile* were more likely to have allergy (107,108). At 2 years of age, nonatopic children were more likely to have lactobacilli and bifidobacteria than atopic children, who had higher counts of coliform bacteria (109). In addition, products of lactobacilli-degraded casein proteins from cow's milk have been shown to stimulate lymphocyte proliferation, inhibit IL-4 production, and enhance IFN-γ production (110). In mice fed lactobacilli, spleen cells were predominantly Th1 cytokines such as IFN-γ and IL-2 (111).

K. Genetic Factors

Although environmental factors play a strong role in the pathogenesis of asthma, so do certain genetic factors. Unlike many other chronic diseases, the study of the genetics of asthma is difficult, as it is not a single disease entity with a common presentation or triggers, nor is it a single-gene disorder. Asthma may have many different phenotypes including atopic asthma—exercise-induced, occupational, and drug-induced (including aspirin)—that may be attributable to different genotypes. Furthermore, asthmatic patients have different levels of disease severity and hyperresponsiveness (i.e., "brittle" or steroid-dependent vs. mild intermittent), and these factors may also be linked to entirely different genetic loci.

The concept of asthma as a genetic disease arose from observations that asthma and atopic diseases tend to cluster in families (112). In addition, twin studies demonstrate that there is a higher concordance for an atopic phenotype in monozygotic (MZ) twins, who share 100% of their genes, versus dizygotic (DZ) twins, who share 50% of their genetic material. In a large survey of 7000 twin pairs, concordance rates for asthma, eczema, and hay fever were all higher for MZ than for DZ twins (113). This phenomenon has also been demonstrated for several markers of asthma severity and atopy including bronchial hyperresponsiveness, serum IgE, and skin-prick testing results (114,115). Interestingly, studies conducted on twins who were raised apart demonstrated that, whether raised together or separately, MZ twins have a higher rate of asthma, emphasizing the importance of genetics in asthma pathogenesis (116,117).

Linkage analysis with functional cloning and association analysis for mutations of "candidate" genes have identified several genetic loci of asthma. Both of these methods have identified specific chromosomal regions that are associated not only with certain phenotypes of asthma, but also with different cytokines, growth cell factors, IgE production, and receptors, e.g., the β-adrenergic receptor.

Results of Linkage Studies

Chromosomal regions that are frequently linked to asthma include 5q, 6p, 11q, 12q, 13q, 14q, 16p, and 19q (118). However, as the human genome has been mapped, additional sites are been identified, including 1, 2q, 3, 9, and 17, although their phenotypic linkage is still unknown. Linkage to the 5q region is particularly important in asthma severity. Work in the early 1990s demonstrated the linkage between chromosome 5q31–33 and total serum IgE concentration (119). This relationship has been noted in several populations, including Amish (120) and Dutch (121). Marsh et al. (120) also showed a relationship between this chromosome and several cytokine genes, including IL-3, -4, -5, and IL-13, and the GM-CSF gene. Chromosome 5q has also been linked to bronchial responsiveness (119) and the β_2-adrenergic receptor.

Chromosome 11 has been associated with variants in the high-affinity receptor for IgE (FcεRIβ chain) (122,123). Chromosome 12 has shown linkage to bronchial hyperresponsiveness and total IgE levels in Afro-Caribbean and Amish populations (124). In addition, IFN-γ, nitric oxide synthase (NOS-1), and mast cell growth factor have mapped to this region (125). Two studies have shown linkage between 16p and specific IgE (126) and positive skin-prick tests (127).

Results of Candidate Gene Association Studies

These studies have demonstrated different polymorphisms of specific genetic loci important in asthma. In vivo, IL-4 plays a major role in allergic disease as it mediates the Ig isotype switching from IgM to IgE (128). Work has suggested that a polymorphism with a C-to-T exchange, at position 590 upstream from the open reading frame of the IL-4 gene (C-590T), is associated with greater transcription activity and elevated levels of IgE in asthmatic families (129). Recent work documents that this C-to-T sequence variant in the IL-4 gene promoter was associated with a small but significant decrease in FEV_1 in Caucasian asthmatic patients (130). Some groups have contested this finding (131). A polymorphism on the IL-4 receptor subunit, a substitution of guanine for arginine at nucleotide 1902, causing a change from glutamine to arginine at position 576 (R576), was also demonstrated to be strongly associated with atopy (132). Another group also demonstrated that R576 was significantly increased in individuals with asthma, and its presence correlated with asthma severity

(133). However, some work suggests that the phenotype of this allele may be dependent upon ethnicity as no association was found in a Japanese population (134).

Candidate gene studies have identified point mutations on the β_2-adrenergic receptor that affect the airways responsiveness to β agonists, but are not necessarily a risk factor for asthma. A point mutation at arginine (Arg) 16 (which normally functions to bind agonist and transmit the signal across the cell membrane to the guanine nucleotide-binding protein) to a glycine substitution has been found in more severe asthma (135). This consequence may be secondary to an increased agonist-promoted down regulation of receptor expression (136). In addition, the point mutation at Arg 16 has been found in patients with greater nocturnal symptoms of asthma (137). A substitution of glutamic acid for glutamine at position 27 on the β_2-adrenergic receptor may make the receptor more resistant to β agonist down regulation and has been shown to be associated with less severe airway hyperresponsiveness (138). In addition, work has found that those individuals with Arg 16 homozygous have an increased odds ratio of developing asthma if they smoke, which is correlated in a dose-responsive fashion (139).

Research on these point mutations of the β_2-adrenergic receptor has identified that these changes may also cause varied responses to albuterol treatment and may differ between certain racial groups. Israel et al. demonstrated that subjects homologous for the Arg at position 16, and who used albuterol regularly, demonstrated a small but significant decline in morning peak expiratory flows (PEFs) as compared to those individuals who used albuterol only on an as-needed basis (140). Interestingly, the Gln 27 allele may be more common in African Americans than in Caucasians (141). In addition, there is most likely a linkage between genetic and racial diversity (142).

V.   Cellular Inflammation in Asthma

A.   General Comments

Early postmortem studies first suggested that asthma was an inflammatory disease (143). Autopsies revealed that patients who died from status asthmaticus had overinflated airways, felt to be secondary to multiple mucous plugs, desquamated epithelium, infiltration of macrophages, and products of activated eosinophils. These postmortem findings also demonstrated smooth muscle hypertrophy and hyperplasia, thickening of the basement membrane, goblet cell hyperplasia, and eosinophilic infiltration of the bronchial wall (143,144). However, the concept of asthma as an inflammatory disease did not fully come into acceptance until the use of bronchoscopy and biopsy in patients with mild asthma (145–147).

Inflammation in chronic asthma is complex and involves interplay between multiple inflammatory cells including eosinophils, mast cells, T lymphocytes, macrophages, epithelial cells, fibroblasts and bronchial smooth muscle and their capacity to release pro-inflammatory mediators, and cytokines. These cellular products can produce changes in the respiratory epithelium, smooth muscle contraction, and bronchial hyperresponsivness (148,149). Even mild, stable asthma is likely to have ongo-

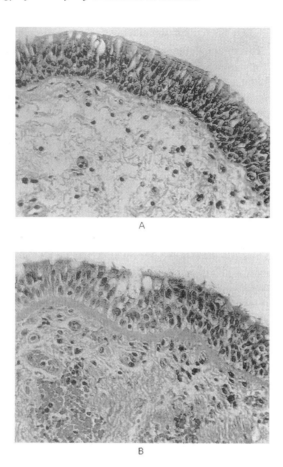

Figure 4 Specimen of bronchial mucosa from a subject without asthma (A) and a patient with mild asthma (B) (Trichrome ×40). In the subject without asthma, the epithelium is intact; there is no thickening of the subbasement membrane, and there is no cellular infiltrate. In contrast, in the patient with mild asthma, there is evidence of goblet-cell hyperplasia in the epithelial-cell lining. The subbasement membrane is thickened with collagen deposition in the submucosal area, and there is a cellular infiltrate. (Photographs courtesy of Nizar N. Jarjour, M.D., University of Wisconsin; see Ref. 334.)

ing and persistent airway inflammation (150). Thus, chronic allergic inflammation is a feature of asthma (Fig. 4).

B. Mast Cells

Mast cells are derived from bone marrow precursor cells expressing the surface CD34+ antigen, but do not mature until they reach tissue, express the c-kit and the high-affinity IgE-binding receptors, and are exposed to stem-cell factor (SCF) and

IL-3 (151). Human mast cells are classified into two subtypes, mucosal (MC-$_T$) and connective tissue (MC-$_{TC}$), based upon the mediators they release, and not upon their location, as their name may imply. Both subtypes contain tryptase, heparin, and chondroitin sulfates A and E, but only MC-$_{TCs}$ have chymase. MC-$_{TCs}$ are typically located in the skin, nasal mucosa, heart, intestinal submucosa, and conjunctiva and are important in fibrotic reactions and angiogenesis (152,153), whereas MC-$_{Ts}$ are distributed in the small intestinal mucosa, alveolar wall, and bronchi/bronchioles, and play a central role in immune system and host defense reactions (154).

Release of mast cell mediators upon degranualtion produces many of the characteristic symptoms of asthma and is pivotal in initiating the inflammatory cascade in asthma (Fig. 5). The mast cell is host to many preformed (i.e., histamine, tryptase, heparin, proteases) and immediately synthesized (lipid mediators, cytokines) mediators. Histamine release produces many of the "trademark" symptoms of asthma by binding to its receptors—H$_1$, H$_2$, and H$_3$. In asthma, the H$_1$ receptors located on blood vessels, airway smooth muscle cells, and nerves play a key role, and their activation results in inositol phospholipid hydrolysis, producing smooth muscle contraction, vascular leakage with resulting airway edema, and stimulation of cough receptors and sensation of pruritis. Heparin and chondroitin sulfate E are the main proteoglycans in the mast cell. Their main functions are not clearly established, but are felt to bind histamine to prevent swelling of the granules in the mast cell, as well as binding to precursors of proteases to convert them to their active forms. Tryptase can be of two subtypes: α- or β-tryptase. β-Tryptase is the predominant form stored in secretory granules and is released during degranulation, whereas α-protrypase is secreted constitutively (155). The biological role of tryptase has been demonstrated to have multiple effects including generation of anaphylatoxin C3a

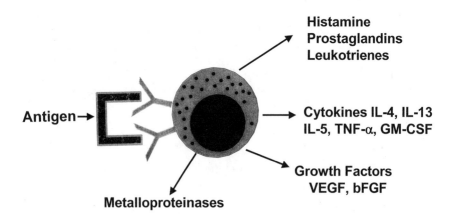

Figure 5 Mast cell involvement in asthma includes the generation of vasoactive amines (histamine), proinflammatory cytokines, growth factors, and metalloproteinases. The array of these mediators, and their action, indicates the multiple steps at which mast cells can contribute to asthma.

from C3 (156) enhancement of the contractile effects of histamine on airway smooth muscle, release of fibronectin from connective tissue (157), and epithelial cell proliferation and production of IL-8 (158), among other functions. Upon activation, mast cells also produce immunoregulatory cytokines: Th1-like (IFN-γ, IL-12) and Th2-like (IL-4, -5, -13) (159–163).

Elevated levels of histamine (164), β-tryptase (165), PGD_2 (166), and LTC_4 (167) in bronchoalveolar lavage (BAL) fluid of asthmatics first suggested the role of the mast cell in asthma. Detection of these mediators as early as 12 minutes after antigen challenge in atopic asthmatics and in some nonatopic asthmatics suggested a model for inflammation in asthma in which the mast cell may play a critical role in initiation, termed the "early asthmatic reaction" (EAR). This correlates well with clinical symptoms of asthma in which many atopic and nonatopic asthmatics, approximately 10–20 minutes after allergen challenge, experience a decrease in FEV_1 and expression of symptoms, which disappears after 2 hours. However, many of these patients will have a return of asthmatic symptoms and a reduction of FEV_1 4–6 hours later. This is termed the "late asthmatic response" (LAR).

FcϵR$_I$, the high-affinity IgE receptor, although not specific for mast cells, plays a critical role in its function in the EAR model in asthma. It binds preformed IgE molecules, the "allergic antibody," which, when attached to their specific antigen, leads to cross-linking of these receptors. This activates the mast cell to release preformed mediators such as histamine and tryptase and begin synthesis of other mediators including arachidonic acid metabolites, cytokines, and growth factors (168). The role of the mast cell in the LAR is less well understood, but is most likely related to activation and recruitment of other inflammatory cells to the airways produced by release of its mediators. The mast cell itself is not felt to play as critical a role as it did during the EAR. The fall in tryptase with increased concentrations of histamine, PGD_2, and LTC_4 collected from BAL fluid (BALF) 4–6 hours after challenge is felt to be secondary to basophils and eosinophils, and not the mast cell (169). In addition, BAL studies 4–6 hours after antigen challenge show eosinophilia (170), which is consistent with airway biopsies done at the same time (171). In addition, basophils that are usually not present have been collected in low numbers from BALF during this LAR phase (172).

There is some controversy as to whether the *total* numbers of airway mast cells are significantly increased in the lungs of asthmatics, but most researchers have demonstrated that they are not (173,174). Instead, the increase in mast cells found in the airway epithelial layer (175), bronchial brushings (176), induced sputum (177), and BALF (178) in asthmatics is most likely the result of migration of the airway mast cell. In addition, the "migration" of the mast cell to the bronchial epithelial tissue also occurs in stable asthmatics (179). BALF samples from stable asthmatics compared to normal controls have also demonstrated increased numbers of mast cells (150,165). Mast cells in the airways of asthmatics also appear to be undergoing constant activation, even in stable asthmatics.

The mast cell has also been suggested to play a role in nonatopic asthma. Humbert and colleages showed an increase in cells expressing FcϵR$_I$ in both atopic and nonatopic individuals (180). In addition, occupational asthma pathophysiology may depend upon the mast cell; in toluene diisocyanate (TDI), the number of mast cells is increased compared to normal controls with evidence of degranulation (181). The role of the mast cell in exercise-induced asthma is not entirely clear, but some have suggested that changes in the osmolarity of airway secretions from airway drying may degranulate mast cells. Furthermore, there has been some suggestion of the mast cell degranulating with exposure to respiratory viruses as well as nonsteroidal anti-inflammatory drugs.

Although there is much evidence for the importance of the mast cell in many phenotypes of asthma, there is also evidence for mast cell–independent pathways in asthma pathophysiology. Recent trials of a monoclonal antibody preparation of IgE in asthmatics indicated not only a decrease in the use of rescue medication and steroid treatments (182), but also a suppression of the late phase reaction to antigen inhalation challenge (183). Because the role of the mast cell in LAR is not entirely clear, this finding suggests that there may be a mast cell–independent IgE pathway in asthma. One possible explanation may be that the IgE binding to its low-affinity receptor, CD23, may be more important than felt for asthma pathophysiology. CD23 is found on B cells and facilitates their antigen presentation to T lymphocytes (184). In addition, medications that are "mast cell"–stabilizing, such as sodium cromoglycate or nedocromil sodium, have little effect on the EAR of asthma, as one may hypothesize based upon the model. In addition, these medications only control the LAR in about 20–30% of adult asthmatic patients, although children respond better (185).

Further evidence for mast cell–independent mechanisms of asthma come from mice models. Mice models of asthma are created by intraperitoneal injection of ovalbumin (OVA) at specified time intervals and later given airway challenges to OVA-producing airway reactivity. However, in mast cell–deficient mice, depending on how the mouse is given initial sensitization to OVA—either with or without adjuvant—they will not or will demonstrate airway hyperreactivity and eosinophilia, respectively (186). This suggests that the mast cell may or may not be important in asthma. In addition, mast cell–deficient asthma mice models develop lung eosinophilia in response to antigen provocation (187).

C. T Lymphocytes

T lymphocytes have emerged as the principal effector cells in asthma (188,189) that coordinate many of the actions of other inflammatory cells in the airways through the release of cytokines and chemokines. They are broadly classified into two distinct subsets according to specific surface markers: those expressing the CD4 antigen are typically involved in humoral immunity, whereas those with the CD8 antigen are involved in cell-mediated responses, such as viral infections and regulation of tumor-infected cells.

There is convincing evidence that lymphocytes are critical for the development of asthma and are found in the airways of asthmatic subjects with differing disease severity (143,190,191). Their numbers are also increased when compared to normal controls matched for age, sex, smoking history, lung function, and airway size (192).

The number of T lymphocytes may be correlated to disease severity and is increased in patients with fatal asthma (193). The severity of asthma is also reflected by the activation state of the lymphocyte (194). Exacerbations of chronic asthma show presence of surface markers of activation, including CD25 + (IL-2 receptor) from lymphocytes recovered in peripheral blood (195), BAL fluid, and bronchial biopsies (196).

A balance toward the Th2-like subtype most likely favors development of asthma in certain individuals. In concept, it seems logical that Th2-like cytokines are important for the development of inflammation in the asthmatic airways, as they produce several key effects, including enhanced recruitment and survival of eosinophils. The role of cytokines in asthma will be further addressed in other chapters. The function and contribution of lymphocytes in asthma is multifactorial and centers on their ability to secrete cytokines. Activated T cells are a source of IL-4 and IL-13. These two cytokines are important as they can induce the activated B cell to produce IgE to a specific antigen. These two cytokines can also enhance expression of cellular adhesion markers, in particular vascular cell adhesion molecule (VCAM-1), which will promote eosinophil recruitment to the airways.

Several groups have found increases in Th2-like cytokines in asthmatic airways. After allergen challenge, IL-5 sputum is elevated (197). Bronchial biopsies in asthma have significantly increased mRNA for IL-5 compared to normal controls and correlates with the number of CD25 + cells (activated T lymphocytes), EG2 + (activated eosinophils), and total eosinophil count (198). The presence of mRNA to IL-5 also correlates to asthma severity (199). Furthermore, cells from asthmatic BAL fluid contain more mRNA for IL-3, -4, -5, and GM-CSF as compared to normal controls (200), and these levels of cytokine mRNA correlate with disease severity (194). In addition, after allergen challenge, many allergen-specific T cells in bronchial biopsy or BAL fluid are of the Th2-like type (201). Treatment with glucocorticoids and a reduction in asthmatic symptoms correlates with the suppression of BAL cells expressing IL-4 and IL-5 and increases those expressing IFN-γ (194). Corrigan et al. (202) demonstrated similar results in patients treated with steroids. A predilection for Th2-like cells is not limited to atopic asthmatics. Bronchial biopsies from patients with both symptomatic allergic asthma and nonallergic asthma contain increased concentrations of mRNA for IL-4 and IL-5 (203).

The Th1/Th2 imbalance is not a strict dogma in asthma pathogenesis. Although IFN-γ downregulates IgE synthesis and promotes uncommitted T lymphocytes to the Th1-like phenotype, in vivo studies have not unanimously supported that these patients have fewer asthma symptoms. IFN-γ was elevated in the serum of patients with severe asthma during an exacerbation (204), in supernatants from cultures of unstimulated and stimulated BAL fluid cells (205), and in lavage fluid after allergen challenge (206). Therefore, asthma may not be solely a CD4 + T-cell–driven disease. Although most T lymphocytes involved in asthma exacerbations have the cell CD4 surface marker (202), some groups have suggested that CD8 + T cells also are associated with the pathology of asthma deaths (207). CD8 + cells may also be a source for cytokines IL-4 and IL-5 in asthmatic airways (208) (Fig. 6).

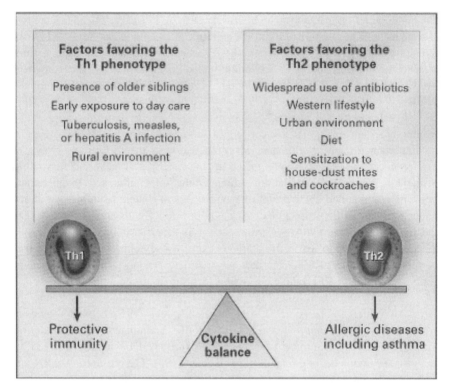

Figure 6   The importance of establishing a balance between Th1-type and Th2-type cytokine responses. Numerous factors, including alterations in number or type of infections early in life, the widespread use of antibiotics, adoption of the western lifestyle, and repeated exposure to allergens, may affect the balance between Th1-type and Th2-type cytokine responses and increase the likelihood that the immune response will be dominated by Th2 cells and thus will ultimately lead to the expression of allergic disease such as asthma. (See Ref. 334.)

The increase in airway lymphocytes, in particular CD4 + cells, represents a combination of cellular recruitment of peripheral cells to the airways and increased activation of resident airway cells. The numbers of CD4 + T cells increase in BAL 48 hours after antigen challenge and remain elevated at 98 hours (209). Gerblich et al. demonstrated that this reduction in CD4 + cells in the periphery correlated with an increase in these cells in the BAL after antigen challenge (210). This concept has not been consistently confirmed by others (171,211,212). The fact that anti-IgE treatment attenuates this particular T-lymphocyte component of the reaction to antigen suggests mast-cell dependent mechanisms. For example, it has been demonstrated that mast cell–deficient mice can develop asthma, whereas CD4 + T-cell–, IL-4–, STAT-6– (transcription factor needed for IgE production), or IL-5–deficient mice cannot (213,214). How IgE interacts without mast-cell involvement in asthma is not defined but may be through the low-affinity receptors for IgE, CD23, present on B lymphocytes, monocytes, and eosinophils. Activation of CD23 has been demonstrated to increase antigen presentation to, and activation of, T lymphocytes, which in turn increase their cytokine production (184,215). The importance of CD23 is further seen in OA-sensitized mice models of asthma with CD23 overexpression, in which treatment with anti-CD23 abolished eosinophilia and normalized bronchial hyperactivity (216).

D. Eosinophils

Eosinophils are also derived from undifferentiated bone-marrow hematopoietic cells expressing surface CD34 antigen marker and mature in specific organ tissue under the presence of IL-5 (217). They have a unique morphology and are characterized by their bilobed nuclei and multiple cytoplasmic membrane–bound granules that have great avidity for the acidic dye eosin.

For many years, the primary function of the eosinophil was felt to be antiparasitic, although Huber and Koessler had first suggested in 1922 that it may be involved in asthma. The eosinophil's role in asthma was, however, largely ignored until the last two decades. Additional functions of this cell, including the ability to initiate tissue injury and remodeling, present antigens, and to defend against viruses, have revived enthusiasm for the eosinophil's role in asthma (218,219). Additionally, studies of peripheral venous blood samples, bronchial fluid lavages, and bronchial biopsies have consistently demonstrated that eosinophils are increased in asthma and that their numbers relate to features of asthma severity (220). Eosinophilia is seen in asthma of varying severity and etiology, nonatopic asthma (221–224), and occupational asthma (225). Asthmatic airways have increased eosinophilia even when disease is clinically "silent" (226). Bronchial biopsies of children may also demonstrate eosinophilia before asthma is clinically expressed (233).

Eosinophils increase in the airway tissue and lavage after allergen challenge and during acute exacerbations. Eosinophils typically increase in the 24 hours after allergen challenge, correspond to the late allergic phase reaction, and can remain elevated up to 96 hours post challenge in BAL fluid (209,228). Mechanisms to explain the increase in eosinophil recruitment to the lungs are complex and involve selective interactions with adhesion markers and release of specific chemotactic factors. The interactions between VLA-4 on eosinophils and VCAM-1 on endothelial cells have an important role in their recruitment to the airways and allow for selective recruitment of eosinophils versus neutrophils followed antigen challenge (Fig. 7). In addition, production of bone-marrow eosinophil precursors 24 hours after allergen exposure (coinciding with the late asthmatic response) is associated with an increase in IL-5 receptor α subunit (IL-5Rα) on these cells, suggesting that this interaction "prepares" this cell to respond to IL-5 activation (229). The factors that stimulate the bone marrow to cause these changes in eosinophils are not well understood.

In addition, there is enhanced survival of the airway eosinophils in asthma. Apoptosis, or programmed cell death, is intended to limit tissue inflammation and injury (230). The number of apoptotic eosinophils is significantly reduced in the

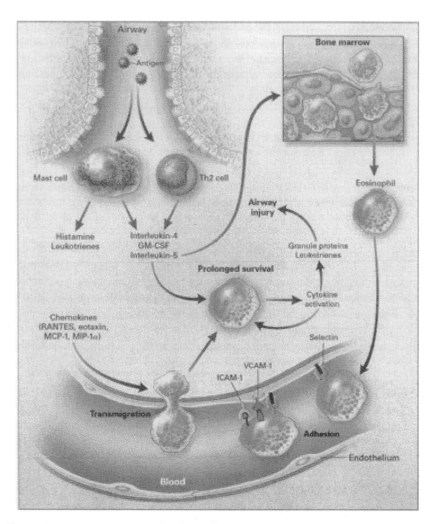

Figure 7 The role of eosinophils in allergic inflammation. Inhaled antigen activates mast cells and Th2 cells in the airway. They in turn induce the production of mediators of inflammation (such as histamine and leukotrienes) and cytokines including interleukin-4 and interleukin-5. Interleukin-5 travels to the bone marrow and causes terminal differentiation of eosinophils. Circulating eosinophils enter the area of allergic inflammation and begin migrating to the lung by rolling, through interactions with selectins, and eventually adhering to endothelium through the binding of integrins to members of the immunoglobulin superfamily of adhesion proteins: vascular-cell adhesion molecule 1 (VCAM-1) and intercellular adhesion molecule 1 (ICAM-1). As the eosinophils enter the matrix of the airway through the influence of various chemokines and cytokines, their survival is prolonged by interleukin-5 and granulocyte-macrophage colony-stimulating factor (GM-CSF). On activation, the eosinophil releases inflammatory mediators such as leukotrienes and granule proteins to injure airway tissues. In addition, eosinophils can generate GM-CSF to prolong and potentiate their survival and contribution to persistent airway inflammation. MCP-1 denotes monocyte chemotactic protein, and MIP-1α macrophage inflammatory protein. (See Ref. 334.)

bronchial mucosa of asthmatic subjects when compared with normal subjects, and these values are inversely correlated with the clinical severity of asthma (231). The presence of increased IL-5 prevents eosinophil apoptosis. IL-5, produced by T lymphocytes, differentiates and enhances survival of eosinophils within tissues, as well as inducing maturation, proliferation, and possibly release of eosinophil precursors from the bone marrow, thereby playing an important role in eosinophil biology (232,233).

The ability of the eosinophil to produce changes in the airways found in asthma relates to its ability to produce mediators and store several proteins in their granules. Transmission electron micrography reveals that there are several types of granules in the eosinophil (234). The secondary granules are the most numerous and contain the four principal basic proteins: major basic protein (MBP), eosinophilic cationic protein (ECP), eosinophil peroxidase (EPO), and eosinophil-derived neurotoxin (EDN). MBP was first believed to function as a parasitic toxin. Although MBP may function as an antiparasitic mechanism, it also produces many of the deleterious effects on the airway tissue seen in asthma. MBP has been found in high concentrations and deposited adjacent to areas of desquamated epithelium in asthmatic airways (235,236) and in primates can increase sensitivity to methacholine in a dose-related fashion (237). MBP has also been suggested to act as an allosteric inhibitor of muscarinic M2 receptors, which results in enhanced vagally mediated bronchoconstriction (238). EPO plays an important role in combining with hydrogen peroxide to catalyze the oxidation of halides (bromide, chloride, and iodine) and produce reactive hyphalous acids with potent bactericidal and fungal activities and also injury to airway tissues. Both EDN and ECP have toxic effects against helminthes larvae, can inhibit T-lymphocyte proliferation by unconfirmed mechanisms, and have the ability to produce ataxia and paralysis and degeneration of white matter of the cerebellum, pons, and spinal cord (239). ECP has been suggested to have many different forms based upon posttranslational modifications that lead to different variants of toxicity. The eosinophil also contains other primary granules that lack the crystalloid-containing material that the secondary granules contain. These primary granules may contain Charcot-Leyden crystal protein. In addition, there are dense small granules that are positive for enzymes such as acid phosphatase and arylsulfatase. Eosinophils release the contents of their granules via several different mechanisms. These include exocytosis, necrotic release (in which the eosinophilic membrane disintegrates and intact membrane-bound granules are released into the surrounding tissues), and finally piecemeal degranulation.

When eosinophils are activated by cytokines, e.g., IL-5, they become "primed" to produce cytotoxic proteins, lipid mediators, and cytokines (240). Eosinophils contain the enzyme phospholipase A_2 (PLA_2), which upon activation produces leukotrienes including LTB_4, LTC_4, and platelet-activating factor (PAF) (240). Eosinophils produce many cytokines, a role originally ascribed primarily to lymphocytes and other monocytes, including IL-1, -2, -3, -5, -6, -10, and -16 (241–243). However, unlike lymphocytes, eosinophils can *store* cytokines, including GM-CSF, IL-2, -4, -5, and TNF-γ, in their granules for extended periods of time. Whether they release all of these cytokines upon activation is not fully defined. The concentration of these cytokines released by eosinophils is equivalent to or less than those produced by lymphocytes. Eosinophils also produce the growth factors TGF-α, PDGF-β, GM-CSF and chemokines, including macrophage inflammatory protein (MIP)-1α and RANTES (244).

Eosinophilic inflammation is associated with markers of airway remodeling such as increased levels of transforming growth factor-beta (TGF-β) expression and a thickened basement membrane (245). Furthermore, markets of eosinophilic activation and participation in asthma, such as MBP, IL-5, and eotaxin, are elevated in asthma (246). Eosinophils may also contribute to airway hyperresponsiveness via interactions with parasympathetic nerves and acetylcholine release (247).

Despite the evidence of eosinophilia in asthma and its functions, which may explain, in part, changes in the asthmatic airways, its role in asthma has recently come under some question. In a recent clinical trial evaluating the effect of a monoclonal antibody against IL-5 in patients with mild atopic asthma, peripheral eosinophilia count was decreased for up to 16 weeks after a single dose and sputum eosinophilia up to 4 weeks (248). This treatment had no effect on the development of the immediate and late phase responses to inhaled antigen. This study with anti-IL-5 has caused the research community to reexamine precisely how, and under what conditions, eosinophils affect asthma and what changes in airway function are regulated by this cell.

E. Epithelial Cells

The role of the bronchial epithelium in asthma extends beyond that of a protective barrier to the external environment. Epithelial layers regulate fluid transport in the airways and contribute to regulation of mucus secretion, modulate airway smooth muscle tone, produce growth factors and cytokines, and present antigens. Mucosal biopsies in asthma demonstrate several important changes in the bronchial epithelium. These changes have been noted even in asthmatic subjects whose disease may be mild or in "clinical remission." In addition, the epithelial damage seen in the asthmatic epithelium can be correlated with bronchial hyperreactivity, as asthmatic subjects tend to shed more epithelial cells into BAL fluid and sputum than controls (249,250). Autopsy studis of patients with a history of asthma confirm that injury, or in some cases destruction, of the epithelial barrier is a common feature in asthma (251). Changes typically noted in the mucosal tissue include increased deposition of collagen, inflammatory cell infiltration, and thickening of the reticular lamina. These changes are proposed to occur as part of the regeneration from damage to this layer and may thus contribute to airway remodeling. In addition, tissue from asthma subjects usually has a greater loss of columnar cells, perhaps as a consequence of environmental factors (252). Thickening of the sub-basement membrane is a characteristic feature of chronic asthma and is believed to be secondary to collagen deposition below the lamina reticularis (146,253). It has also been suggested that the asthmatic airways may exhibit an altered response to inflammatory injury, thus resulting in greater injury (254).

Epithelial cells may be stimulated by multiple factors: allergens (255), proteases (158), oxidants (256), and respiratory viruses (257). These cells can then release a variety of proinflammatory mediators including 15-HETE, prostaglandin E_2 (PGE_2), fibronectin, and endothelin (258). Epithelial cells also express adhesion molecules (259), endothelin (260), nitric oxide synthase, and cytokines (261) following activation. Cytokines released by epithelial cells include IL-8, IL-6, IL-1β, TNF-α, IL-11, IL-10, IL-16, IL-18, GM-CSF (262,263), and, more recently, IL-5 (264) and IL-13 (265).

Increased expression of the epidermal growth factor receptor (EGFR, c-erbB1) in asthmatic airways is potentially important in asthma pathogenesis. In normal airway epithelium, EGFR serves a central role in epithelial function (266), and acute lung injury produces its ligands, which upon binding stimulate gene transcription for proteins that promote cellular growth (254,267). In asthma there may be an overexpression of EGFR, in both damaged and nondamaged airway epithelium, that correlates with the sub-basement membrane thickness (268). This may be secondary to a failure to downregulate EGFR expression, or a counterregulatory mechanism by TGF-β, which activates intracellular proteins that translocate to the nucleus and initiate transcription of genes to cause growth arrest (254). Thus, current evidence indicates that the epithelium is an active participant in the injury-repair process that occurs in asthma, and these changes can directly alter function, promote airflow obstruction, and enhance bronchial hyperresponsiveness.

F. Basophils

Although basophils and mast cells contain many similar mediators, receptors on their cell surface, i.e., high-affinity IgE receptor (269,270) and IgG receptor FcγR$_{II}$ (CD32), and stain positively with metachromatic staining, these two cells have different functions and patterns of growth. Basophils differentiate and mature in the bone marrow, afterwards surviving in the vascular compartment or peripheral circulation, whereas the mast cells mature and remain in tissue. The basophil is more similar to the eosinophil. They are both derived from a common progenitor cell under the presence of cytokines TGF-β, GM-CSF, IL-3, and IL-5 (271–273). Both respond to growth factors IL-3, IL-5, and GM-CSF for differentiation and have the capacity to produce MBP (273).

The basophil also has preformed mediators (histamine, proteoglycans, kallikrein, neutrophil chemotactic factor) and the ability to make many mediators (LTC_4, LTD_4, LTE_4, PAF, and cytokines IL-4, -8, -13, and MIP-1α). It is involved both in the early and late phase reactions to inhaled antigen, as evidenced from studies of antigen challenge in which PGD_2 and tryptase diminish 24 hours after an antigen challenge, whereas histamine and LTD_4 persist (172,274,275). In addition, basophils have been recognized in the bronchial biopsy in the late phase of the asthmatic response to antigen (276).

Basophils have on their cell surface several cytokine receptors, IL-1 through IL-5, chemokine receptors, CCR1-3, IL-8, and multiple complement receptors for 1, 3, 4, and 5a, as well as multiple adhesion molecules including VLA-4 and -5,

LFA-1, selectins, and ICAM-1, -2, and -3. These receptors are important for cell growth and migration into the tissues by complement fragment C5a, for example (277), and IL-8 and growth factors IL-3, IL-5, and GM-CSF (278).

The exact role of the basophil in asthma is not clearly understood. It has been detected in the sputum of more than 50% of individuals with perennial asthma (279) and is occasionally increased in the BAL fluid of atopic asthmatic subjects as compared to controls (280). Given its presence with late phase reactions and its profile of mediators, especially LTC4, it is likely to contribute to inflammation.

G. Neutrophils

Neutrophilic polymorphonuclear leukocytes originate from myeloid precursor cells in the bone marrow, and their primary role is defense against bacterial infections through release of proteases, hydrolases, microbicidal proteins (including myeloperoxidase), and enzymes stored in heterogeneous granules. They are one of the first cells recruited to the site of infected or injured tissues in response to the release of cytokines, namely TNF-α and IL-1. The participation of the neutrophil in asthma was first suggested by animal studies and later confirmed in humans, although its specific involvement in asthma pathogenesis is not fully elucidated.

Some studies have demonstrated neutrophils within airway parenchyma after allergen challenge in asthma (148,194,281). However, other studies have shown that asthmatic subjects will respond to inhaled antigen with an increase in airway neutrophils (171,282). One possible explanation to these different observations is that although neutrophil numbers are not necessarily increased in the airways, they may become activated cyclooxygenase, 15-lipoxygenase, and neutrophil release products of myeloperoxidase as have been seen in asthma (283). It is more likely that the neutrophil plays an important role in certain "subtypes" of asthma. Neutrophil accumulation frequently is a hallmark of patients who die suddenly from asthma (284,285) or in severe asthma as noted in the airways of corticosteroid-dependent asthmatic subjects (286). The increase in neutrophils in severe asthma may be secondary to an increase in IL-8 and neutrophil elastase (287). Neutrophils may also be important in occupational asthma and exercise-induced asthma (288) and nocturnal asthma (289). Finally, the neutrophil is the predominant cell found during virus-induced exacerbations of asthma.

H. Macrophages

Alveolar macrophages (AM) make up the majority of airway cell types in both normal and asthmatic subjects (290). Their location in the alveoli and distal airspaces, cytokine and growth factor production, and an ability to process and present antigens make them a critical cell in the airways and in the development and regulation of inflammation. Although their role in asthma has not been studied as extensively as the eosinophil or T lymphocyte, they nonetheless are likely to play a critical role in the pathogenesis of asthma.

Evidence for a role for AM in asthma comes from a number of observations. AMs are recruited to the airways after antigen challenge (172). The low-affinity receptor for IgE (CD23) has been found on AM cells of asthmatic subjects (291), and its function has been hypothesized to increase the ability of this cell to present antigens more efficiently. Binding of CD23 with its ligand, IgE, also results in cytokine production and release. Monocytes and macrophages have the ability to produce IL-1, TNF-α, IL-6, IL-8, IL-10, and GM-CSF (292–294). IL-1 is particularly important in asthma as it activates lymphocytes, induces mucus secretion (295), and primes mast cells for enhanced mediator release. Macrophages produce TGF-β, which is central to airway remodeling, and it stimulates fibroblasts to produce fibronectin and collagen, which create thickening of the airways (296). Thus, it is likely that these cells are involved both in the acute asthmatic reaction and in persistent inflammation and remodeling.

VI. Recruitment of Inflammatory Cells to Airways

Although there may be an increase in the numbers of resident inflammatory cells in the airways of asthmatic subjects, many of these cells are also recruited to the airways at the time of antigen exposure (Fig. 8). The mechanisms responsible for the extravasation of leukocytes through the endothelial barriers and into the lung mucosa and parenchyma are complex and will be covered in greater detail in later chapters. Briefly, however, these processes involve activation of specific cellular

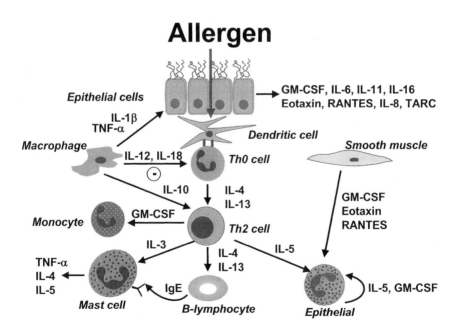

Figure 8 Interactions between resident and inflammatory cells and cytokines in the airways. (See Ref. 262.)

proteins, such as cell-adhesion molecules (CAMs), on the surface of inflammatory cells and endothelial cells. Binding of these CAMs allows the leukocytes to "roll" along the endothelial border and "stick," and eventually diapedesis across the membrane into the airway and lung occurs.

CAMs are classified into three main types—selectins, integrins, and immunoglobulin superfamilies, based upon their cellular distribution and structural characteristics. Selectins are found on endothelial cells (P-selectin and E-selectin) and leukocytes (L-selectin) and are transmembrane glycoproteins. P-selectin and L-selectin are constitutively produced, but E-selectin must be synthesized de novo by induction from cytokines, lipopolysaccharides, and other inflammatory mediators. Binding of the L-selectin to the P- and E-selectin results in a "loose" adhesion and rolling of the inflammatory cell. As the leukocytes become "primed" by the presence of cytokines, lipid mediators, and chemokines, they begin to increase production of intergrins on their surface. Intergrins are noncovalently linked heterodimers of large alpha and smaller beta chains. The main integrins that are important in leukocyte-endothelial cell interations are leukocytes function–associated antigen-1 (LFA-1), Mac-1, and p150,95 (CD11c/CD18) of the β2 subfamily and VLA-4, mucosal addressin cell adhesion molecule-1 (MAdCAM-1), integrins of the β1 subfamily. VLA-4 plays a critical role in the recruitment of eosinophils and lymphocytes. Integrins allow for "firmer" binding of the leukocytes to the endothelial surface as they bind to the last type of CAMs, the immunoglobulin superfamilies. The process of crossing through the endothelial barrier to the lung parenchyma involved "loosening" of these CAMs and the presence of specific chemoattractants.

VII. Models and Orchestration of Airway Inflammation

The airway response to inhaled antigen is conceptually divided into both early and late phase responses. The early asthmatic or allergic reaction typically presents within minutes of antigen exposure and is clinically associated with acute shortness of breath, wheezing, cough, and chest-tightness. Maximal airway obstruction is usually achieved within 20–30 minutes of exposure to antigen (297). This early reaction has been attributed to mast cell activation and release of its mediators including histamine, prostanoids, and leukotrienes and their direct action on airway smooth muscle. However, that the mast cell is the primary effector cell in the development of the early asthmatic reaction is not entirely clear, as mast-cell–deficient mice also have an immediate reaction to inhaled antigen. (298). At a cellular level in the airways, the release of these mast cell products produces a variety of physiological changes: vasculature dilation, leakage of the vascular bed, activation of cough neural pathways, and smooth muscle constriction.

The early asthmatic response also appears to prime the airways for the late phase allergic reaction (LPR). The LPR presents 4–10 hours after antigen inhalation and is characterized clinically by a return of symptoms seen at the early response

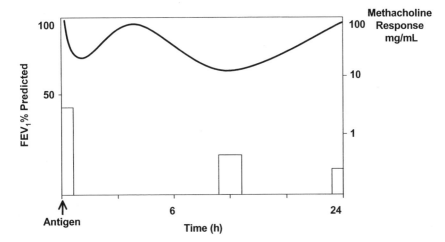

Figure 9 The airway response to inhaled antigen with the development of an immediate and late response (6 hours after antigen challenge). Associated with this response to antigen is an increase in airway responsiveness, as indicated by enhanced airway sensitivity to methacholine.

and airflow obstruction (Fig. 9). Early cellular activation of mast cells and release of its mediators promote cell adhesion on the airway vascular to facilitate recruitment of other inflammatory cells, notably T lymphocytes, eosinophils, and basophils, most likely through cytokine action, to the airways where these cells are activated and thus lead to airway inflammation and airflow obstruction. These cellular events are maximal 24 hours after allergen challenge and then return to baseline levels, but this often requires up to 7 days (299). The late phase reaction to inhaled antigen has been used as a model to study and characterize the allergic inflammatory events that might occur in asthma.

VIII. Airway Hyperresponsiveness in Asthma

Airway hyperresponsiveness is a central feature of asthma. Although airway hyperresponsiveness is not specific to asthma, all symptomatic asthma patients demonstrate bronchial hyperresponsiveness. A variety of stimuli can be used to enhance existing airway hyperresponsiveness in asthma, including inhaled allergens, viral respiratory infections, emotional stress, and occupational exposures including low molecular weight chemicals or acids and ozone. In addition, links between the upper and lower airway suggest that sinus infections, or symptomatic allergic rhinitis, will also increase bronchial hyperresponsiveness. Finally, gastroesophageal reflux disease (GERD) has been noted to increase airway hyperresponsiveness. The exact mechanisms underlying increased airway hyperresponsiveness in the airways of asthmatic patients are unknown, but likely include inflammation, effect mediators released, and airway smooth muscle abnormalities.

IX. Patterns of Airway Injury in Asthma

A. Persistent Inflammation

Although airway inflammation is a recognized pathological pattern in asthma, it is less well defined what regulates this persistent inflammatory reaction or what happens to inflammation in the airways when a patient's asthma is well controlled or in a "remission." Several more studies have demonstrated that despite the absence of symptoms, spirometric abnormalities and bronchial hyperresponsivness (BHR) to methacholine (MCh) or cold air challenge (300,301), elevated levels of exhaled nitric oxide (eNO) and responsiveness to inhaled MCh and adenosine-5'-monophosphate (AMP) still persist (302). However, how these markers of inflammation, including nonspecific BHR or circulating inflammatory cells like the eosinophils, relate to the actual pathological changes seen in the airways is not totally clear (303–305). Recent work, however, on a small subset of asthmatic subjects who were defined as in "asthma remission" (i.e., not needing medications and without symptoms for a mean of 5 years) demonstrated significantly elevated levels of eosinophils, T cells, mast cells, and IL-5 in the airway mucosa compared to normal control patients. In addition, there was significant airway remodeling in adolescents with a history of asthma (306). Thus, one of the important areas for future investigation will be the study of phases of inflammations and how these transitions are regulated and modulated.

B. Airway Remodeling

Although asthma is considered a disease of reversible obstruction, there is increasing evidence that, over time, inflammation may lead to permanent changes in the airway tissue and produce fixed airway obstruction or remodeling. The specific pathological changes that occur in the airway and the mechanisms of their appearance and whether early therapeutic interventions will affect these outcomes are not defined, nor is it clear which patients are at risk for "remodeling." This topic will be covered extensively in later chapters.

X. Special Topics in Asthma

A. Steroid Resistance

As the morbidity and mortality of asthma have increased over the past decades, it has been suggested that these changes are attributable to factors that make asthma difficult to treat. The concept of steroid-resistant asthma was developed over 30 years ago when it was noticed that several patients did not clinically respond to high doses of intravenous cortisol. In a nonrandomized comparison-control study, patients with asthma resistant to steroid treatment demonstrated decreased eosinopenic responses to corticosteroids (307). The diagnosis of steroid-resistant asthma is not a simple procedure. One first has to exclude the possibility that the person does not have asthma, for example, that the patient does not have vocal chord dysfunction or other fixed lesions of the trachea or chronic obstructive pulmonary disease (COPD). It is also necessary to consider other potential risk factors of asthma such as sinusitis or GERD, which may modify the response to corticosteroids. It is also necessary to establish that offending agents, such as pets, have been removed from the environment and that medication compliance is good. If these factors have been addressed and maintained for at least 6 months, then the diagnosis of steroid-resistant asthma can be critically entertained (308).

There have been several potential explanations as to why a patient may not respond to steroids. Glucocorticoids typically work by freely penetrating the plasma membrane of cells to bind to the glucocorticoid receptors (GCR), which results in the exposure of a DNA-binding site. This complex then translocated to the nucleus, where it forms a dimer that binds to DNA at glucocorticoid response elements (GRE) in the 5′-upstream promoter regions of steroid-responsive genes. This interaction can lead to either increased or repressed gene transcription. In particular, interaction with transcription factors AP-1 and NF-κB may lead to decreased repression on the promoter sequence (309). In steroid-resistant asthma, it is proposed that enhanced generation of cytokines, such as IL-2 and IL-4, will interfere with this intracellular response and lessen the actions of corticosteroids.

B. Viral Exacerbation of Asthma

Respiratory viruses may also play a role in exacerbating preexisting asthma in both children and adults (310–312). Of the respiratory viruses associated with asthma exacerbation, rhinovirus (RV) is the most common provoker. Up to 80–85% of wheezing episodes in children (312) and in approximately half of the asthma exacerbations in adults are associated with RV infection (313). It is of particular interest how an upper viral antigen can trigger lower airway symptoms, although it is unclear how much of this virus enters the lower airway.

The exact mechanisms of virus-induced asthma are not fully elucidated, but studies using experimental inoculation with viruses, such as RV 16, have allowed studies to better define how the RV antigen can induce inflammation of the lower airways and thus exacerbate asthma. Viral infections may induce distinct changes in the lower airways to account for an increase in airway hyperactivity, reduced peak flow, and impaired response to β-agonists. Cheung et al. inoculated 14 subjects with mild asthma with either RV16 or placebo and discovered that the RV infection increased the maximal contractile response to inhaled methacholine for up to 15 days after the acute infection (314). Using bronchoscopy and airway segmental antigen challenge, it has also been demonstrated that a RV infection increases release of histamine to antigen in the lower airway and augments the recruitment both of total leukocytes and eosinophils into the airways 48 hours after allergen challenge (315,316). These changes were only noted in atopic subjects and not in normal nonallergic controls. In addition, bronchoalveolar lavage secretions have demonstrated RV RNA from volunteers after experimental inoculation with RV16 (317), suggesting that the virus can, and does, enter the lower airways. In addition, enhanced increased submucosal lymphocytes and epithelial eosinophils have been associated with RV interaction (318).

Unlike respiratory syncytial virus (RSV), RV infections rarely cause epithelial damage of the airways. However, the epithelial cells are the site of RV replication and, as such, are most likely to be the primary areas for inflammatory cytokine production. In addition, in vitro work has demonstrated that RV particles may also directly infect airway smooth muscle cells and submucosal gland cells (319,320). This may explain how viral infection could directly affect muscle cell responsiveness and airway secretion. It appears that once RV infection occurs and enters the lower airways, epithelial cell activation and replication follows. As it enters the epithelial cell, NF-κB is present, which then leads to increased cytokine and chemokine production and release (321–323), including GM-CSF, IL-6, IL-8, RANTES, and IL-11. In addition, adhesion molecule expression may also be increased. Thus, the stage is set for propagation of the underlying inflammatory response.

As a result of cytokine, chemokine, and adhesion molecule production, additional inflammatory cells are recruited to the airways. One of the most important cells recruited to the airways is the neutrophil. Neutrophils are the main cells found in nasal and lower airway secretions during acute viral infections (324,325). IL-8 is a major chemoattractant factor for neutrophils, and its levels are increased in nasal secretions during acute rhinovirus infection and parallel cold symptoms (326). The increase in neutrophils correlates with cold-induced changes in airway hyperresponsiveness (326). Airway neutrophils, after activation, possibly by viral particles, release inflammatory mediators such as superoxide and proteases, which are potent secretagogues for airway submucosal glands (327). The early stages of airway inflammation during a RV infection may result in nonspecific airway inflammation and later airflow obstruction. In addition, it is likely that airway monocytes and macrophages are involved in this early inflammation. Macrophages also bind RV particles and then secrete cytokines that have antiviral activity such as IFN-α as well as proinflammatory potential (328).

Besides recruitment of neutrophils, eosinophils are recruited to the airways with respiratory viral infections, resulting in allergen response. The mechanism most likely involves release of the inflammatory cytokines and chemokines from endothelial as well as other resident airway cells. RANTES is a major attractant for eosinophils. Eosinophils can further existing inflammation, and there is now evidence that they may have some component of antiviral activity. Eosinophil cationic protein, a granule protein released on eosinophil activation, has RNase activity and can inhibit replication of some respiratory viruses such as RSV (329). Other cytokines can contribute to eosinophil recruitment to the airways, including GM-CSF. Eosinophil granule proteins in respiratory secretions of infants and children with wheezing from rhinovirus infections has been demonstrated (330,331).

Lymphocytes play a key role in antiviral inflammation, which, in turn, may also contribute to inflammation in asthma. Viruses can indirectly activate lymphocytes by either an innate or an adaptive immune response. The RV particle binds to its receptor, ICAM-1 or LDLr, found on antigen-presenting cells. This binding appears to activate the innate response and generate IFN-α, IL-12, and/or IL-18, which in turn activate lymphocytes and generate IFN-γ secretion by T cells and natural killer cells. Antigen presentation may also activate virus-specific T-cell responses, which usually takes 7–10 days after exposure to the virus and represents an adaptive immune response (332). These T-cell–specific cells help to clear viruses from the airways (333), but may also produce inflammation.

XI. Conclusion

Our knowledge about the pathogenesis of asthma is continually expanding. We know that asthma is a disease of airway inflammation, which contributes to several of the clinical characteristics of asthma. In addition, airway inflammation explains many of the physiological changes in asthmatic airways, i.e., bronchial hyperresponsiveness and airflow obstruction, and in the long term may produce chronic changes in the bronchus and lung parenchyma. The development of airway inflammation in asthma is the result of both genetic and environmental factors. This gene-by-environment hypothesis helps explain why the prevalence of asthma is increasing in westernized countries and inner cities. With this and the additional knowledge about the cellular pathways in asthma it is hoped that the basic mechanism of the disease can be further defined and, as a consequence, improved treatment established.

References

1. Weiss ST. Epidemiology and heterogeneity of asthma. Ann Allergy Asthma 2001; 87(suppl):5–8.
2. Overview of Allergic Diseases. The Allergy Report, vol. 1. Milwaukee, WI. The American Academy of Allergy, Asthma and Immunology, Inc., 2000:1–97.
3. Carr W, Zeitel L, Weiss K. Variations in asthma hospitalizations and deaths in New York City. Am J Public Health 1992; 82:59–65.
4. Gottlieb DJ, Beiser AS, O'Connor GT. Poverty, race, and medication use are correlates of asthma hospitalization rates. A small area analysis in Boston. Chest 1995; 108: 28–35.
5. Lang DM, Polansky M. Patterns of asthma mortality in Philadelphia from 1969 to 1991. N Engl J Med 1994; 331:1542–1546.
6. Targonski PV, Persky VW, Orris P, Addington W. Trends in asthma mortality among African Americans and Whites in Chicago, 1968 through 1991. Am J Public Health 1994; 84:1830–1833.
7. Anderson HR. Is the prevalence of asthma changing? Arch Dis Child 1989; 64: 172–175.
8. Anderson HR, Butland BK, Strachan DP. Trends in prevalence and severity of childhood asthma. BMJ 1994; 308:1600–1604.
9. Beasley R, Crane J, Lai C, Pearce N. Prevalence and etiology of asthma. J Allergy Clin Immunol 2000; 105:S466–472.

10. Keeley DJ, Neill P, Gallivan S. Comparison of the prevalence of reversible airways obstruction in rural and urban Zimbabwean children. Thorax 1991; 46:549–553.
11. Roorda RJ, Gerritsen J, van Aalderen WMC, Schouten JP, Veltman JC, Weiss ST, Know K. Follow-up of asthma from childhood to adulthood. J Allergy Clin Immunol 1994; 93:575–584.
12. Oswald H, Phelan PD, Lanigan A, Hibbert M, Bowes, G, Olinsky A. Outcome of childhood asthma in mid-adult life. BMJ 1994; 309:95–96.
13. Strachan DP, Butland BK, Anderson HR. Incidence and prognosis of asthma and wheezing illness from early childhood to age 33 in a national British cohort. BMJ 1996; 312:1195–1199.
14. Jenkins MA, Hopper JL, Bowes G, Carlin JB, Flander LB, Giles GG. Factors in childhood as predictors of asthma in adult life. BMJ 1994; 309:90–93.
15. Oswald H, Phelan PD, Lanigan A, Hibbert N, Carlin JB, Bowes G, Olinsky A. Childhood asthma and lung function in mid-adult life. Pediatr Pulmonol 1997; 23:14–20.
16. Peat JK, Woolcock AJ, Cullen K. Rate of decline of lung function in subjects with asthma. Eur J Respir Dis 1987; 70:171–179.
17. Burrows B, Bloom JW, Traver GA, Cline MG. The course and prognosis of different forms of chronic airways obstruction in a sample from the general population. N Engl J Med 1987; 317:1309–1314.
18. Burrows B, Barbee RA, Cline MG, Kundson RJ, Lebowitz MD. Characteristics of asthma among elderly adults in a sample of the general population. Chest 1991; 100: 935–942.
19. Panhuysen CIM, Vonk JM, Koeter GH, Schouten JP, van Altena R, Bleecker ER, Postma DS. Adult patients may outgrow their asthma: a 25-year follow-up study. Am J Respir Crit Care Med 1997; 155:1267–1272.
20. Backman KS, Greenberger PA, Patterson R. Airways obstruction in patients with long-term asthma consistent with "irreversible asthma." Chest 1997; 112:1234–1240.
21. Lange P, Parner J, Vestbo J, Schnohr P, Jensen G. A 15-year follow-up study of ventilatory function in adults with asthma. N Engl J Med 1998; 339:1194–2000.
22. Peat JK, Woolcock AJ, Cullen K. Rate of decline of lung function in subjects with asthma. Eur J Respir Dis 1987; 70:171–179.
23. Reed CE. The natural history of asthma in adults: the problem of irreversibility. J Allergy Clin Immunol 1999; 103:539–547.
24. Ulrik CS, Backer V, Dirksen A. A 10-year follow-up of 180 adults with bronchial asthma: factors important for the decline in lung function. Thorax 1992; 47:14–18.
25. Mosmann TR, Coffman RL. Heterogeneity of cytokine secretion patterns and functions of helper T cells. Adv Immunol 1989; 46:111–147.
26. Firestein GS, Roeder WD, Laxer JA, Townsend KS, Weaver CT, Hom JT, Linton J, Torbett BE, Glasebrook AL. A new murine CD4+ T cell subset with an unrestricted cytokine profile. J Immunol 1989; 143:518–525.
27. Mosmann TR, Sad S. The expanding universe of T-cell subsets: Th1, Th2 and more. Immunol Today 1996; 17:138–146.
28. Strachan DP. Hay fever, hygiene, and household size. BMJ 1989; 299(6710): 1259–1260.
29. Shaheen SO, Aaby P, Hall AJ, Barker DJ, Heyes CB, Shiell AW, Goudiaby A. Measles and atopy in Guinea-Bissau. Lancet 1996; 347:1792–1796.
30. Matricardi PM, Rosmini F, Ferrigno L, Nisini R, Rapicetta M, Chionne P, Stroffolini T, Pasquini P, D'Amelio R. Cross sectional retrospective study of prevalence of atopy

among Italian military students with antibodies against hepatitis A virus. BMJ 1997; 314(7086):999–1003.

31. Shirakawa T, Enomoto T, Shimazu S, Hopkin JM. The inverse association between tuberculin responses and atopic disorder. Science 1997; 275(5296):77–79.

32. von Herzen L, Klaukka T, Mattila H, Haahtela T. J Allergy Clin Immunol 1999; 104: 1211–1214.

33. Paunio M, Heinonen OP, Virtanen M, Leinikki P, Patja A, Peltola H. Measles history and atopic diseases: a population-based cross-sectional study. JAMA 2000; 283: 343–346.

34. Wegmann TG, Lin H, Guilbert L, Mosmann TR. Bidirectional cytokine interactions in the maternal-fetal relationship: Is successful pregnancy a TH2 phenomenon? Immunol Today 1993; 14:353–356.

35. Nilsson L, Kjellman NI, Lofman O, Bjorksten B. Parity among atopic and non-atopic mothers. Pediatr Allergy Immunol 1997; 8:134–137.

36. Warner JA, Miles EA, Jones AC, Quint DJ, Colwell BM, Warner JO. Is deficiency of interferon gamma production by allergen triggered cord blood cells a predictor of atopic eczema? Clin Expl Allergy 1994; 24:423–430.

37. Prescott SL, Macaubas C, Smallacombe T, Holt BJ, Sly PD, Holt PG. Development of allergen-specific T-cell memory in atopic and normal children. Lancet 1999; 353: 196–200.

38. Prescott SL, Macaubas C, Holt BJ, Smallacombe TB, Loh R, Sly PD, Holt PG. Transplacental priming of the human immune system to environmental allergens: universal skewing of initial T cell responses toward the Th2 cytokine profile. J Immunol 1998; 160:4730–4737.

39. Pearce N, Pekkanen J, Beasley R. How much asthma is really attributable to atopy? Thorax 1999; 54:268–272.

40. Martinez FD, Wright AL, Taussig LM, Holberg CJ, Halonen M, Morgan WJ. Asthma and wheezing in the first six years of life. N Engl J Med 1995; 332:133–138.

41. Bergmann RL, Edenharter G, Bergmann KE, Forster J, Bauer CP, Wahn V, Zepp F, Wahn U. Atopic dermatitis in early infancy predicts allergic airway disease at 5 years. Clin Exp Allergy 1998; 28:965–970.

42. Nickel R, Kulig M, Forster J, Bermann R, Bauer CP, Lau S, Guggenmoos-Holzmann, Wahn U. Sensitization to hen's egg at the age of 12 months is predictive of allergic sensitization to common indoor and outdoor allergens at the age of three years. J Allergy Clin Immunol 1997; 99:613–617.

43. Sporik R, Holgate ST, Platts-Mills TA, Cogswell JJ. Exposure to house-dust mite allergen (Der P I) and the development of asthma in childhood. A prospective study. N Engl J Med 1990; 323:520–527.

44. Kuehr J, Frischer T, Meinert R, Barth R, Forster J, Schraub S, Urbanek R, Karmaus W. Mite allergen exposure is a risk for the increase of specific sensitization. J Allergy Clin Immunol 1994; 94:44–52.

45. Lau S, Illi S, Sommerfeld C, Niggemann B, Bergmann R, von Mutius E, Wahn U. Early exposure to house-dust mite and cat allergens and development of childhood asthma: a cohort study. Multicentre Allergy Study Group. Lancet 2000; 356: 1392–1397.

46. Hesselmar B, Aberg N, Aberg B, Eriksson B, Bjorksten B. Does early exposure to cat or dog protect against later allergy development? Clin Exp Allergy 1999; 29: 611–617.

47. Riedler J, Braun-Fahrlander C, Eder W, Schreuer M, Waser M, Maisch S, Carr D, Schierly R, Nowak D, von Mutis E; ALEX Study Team. Exposure to farming in early life and development of asthma and allergy: a cross-sectional survey. Lancet 2001; 358:1129–1133.

48. Braun-Fahrlander C, Gassner M, Grize L, Neu U, Sennhauser FH, Varonier HS, Vuille JC, Wuthrich B. Prevalence of hay fever and allergic sensitization in farmer's children and their peers living in the same rural community. Clin Exp Allergy 1999; 29:28–34.

49. Tager IB, Hanrahan JP, Toreson TD, Castile RG, Brown RW, Weiss ST, Speizer FE. Lung function, pre- and post-natal smoke exposure, and wheezing in the first year of life. Am Rev Respir Dis 1993; 147:811–817.

50. Johnson SL. The role of viral and atypical bacterial pathogens in asthma pathogenesis. Pediatr Pulmonol 1999; S18:141–143.

51. Jackson M, Scott R. Different patterns of cytokine induction in cultures of respiratory syncytial (RS) virus-specific human T-H cell lines following stimulation with RS virus and RS virus proteins. J Med Virol 1996; 49:161–169.

52. Alwan WH, Record FM, Openshaw PJM. Phenotypic and functional characterization of T cell lines specific for individual respiratory syncytial virus proteins. J Immunol 1993; 150:5211–5218.

53. Suzuki S, Suzuki T, Yamamoto N, Matsumoto Y, Shirai A, Okbubo T. Influenza A virus infection increases IgE production and airway responsiveness in aerosolized antigen-exposed mice. J Allergy Clin Immunol 1998; 102:732–740.

54. Rooney JC, Williams HE. The relationship between proven viral bronchioloititis and subsequent wheezing. J Pediatr 1971; 79:744–747.

55. Koller DY, Wojnarowski, Herner KR, Weinlander G, Raderer M, Eichler I, Frishcer T. High levels of eosinophillc cationic protein in wheezing infants predict the development of asthma. J Allergy Clin Immunol 1997; 99:752–756.

56. Reijonen TM, Korppi M, Kleemola S, Savolainen K, Kuikka L, Mononen I, Remes K. Nasopharyngeal eosinophil cationic protein in bronchiolitis—relation to viral findings and subsequent wheezing. Pediatr Pulmonol 1997; 24:35–41.

57. Martinez FD, Stern DA, Wright AL, Taussig LM, Halonen M. Differential immune responses to acute lower respiratory illness in early life and subsequent development of persistent wheezing and asthma. J Allergy Clin Immunol 1998; 102:915–920.

58. Robinson PJ, Hegele RG, Schellenberg RR. Allergic sensitization increases airway reactivity in guinea pigs with respiratory syncytial virus bronchiolitis. J Allergy Clin Immunol 1997; 100:492–498.

59. Sigurs N, Bjarnason R, Sigurbersson R, et al. Asthma and immunoglobulin E antibodies after respiratory syncytial virus bronchiolitis: a prospective cohort study with matched controls. Pediatrics 1995; 95:500–505.

60. Noble V, Murray M, Webb MS, Alexander J, Swarbrick AS, Milner AD. Respiratory status and allergy nine to ten years after acute bronchiolitis. Arch Dis Child 1997; 76: 315–319.

61. Hahn DL. Treatment of *Chlamydia pneumoniae* infection in adult asthma: a before-after trial. J Fam Pract 1995; 41:345–351.

62. Emre U, Roblin PM, Gelling M, Dumornay W, Rao M, Hammerslag MR, Schacter J. The association of *Chlamydia pneumoniae* infection and reactive airway disease in children. Arch Pediatr Adol Med 1994; 148:727–732.

63. Hahn D, Bukstein D, Luskin A, Zeitz H. Evidence for *Chlamydia pneumoniae* infection in steroid-dependent asthma. Ann Allergy Asthma Immunol 1998; 80:45–49.

64. Shemer-Avni Y, Lieberman D. *Chlamydia pneumoniae*-induced ciliostasis in ciliated bronchial epithelial cells. J Infect Dis 1995; 171:1274–1278.
65. Kishimoto T, Nakajima M, Nakagawa Y, Hino J, Watanabe M, Nakahama C, Okimoto N, Yagi S, Soejima R. A case of pneumonia caused by *Chlamydia pneumoniae*, strain TWAR. J Jpn Assoc Infect Dis 1990; 64:510–515.
66. Redecke V, Dalhoff K, Bohnet S, Bohnet S, Braun J, Maass M. Interaction of *Chlamydia pneumoniae* and human alveolar macrophages: infection and inflammatory response. Am J Respir Cell Mol Biol 1998; 19:721–727.
67. Leinonen M. Pathogenetic mechanisms and epidemiology of *Chlamydia penumoniae*. Eur Heart J 1993; 14(suppl K):56–71.
68. Emre U, Sokolovkaya N, Roblin P, Schachter J, Hamerschag MR. Detection of *Chlamydia pneumoniae*-IgE in children with reactive airway disease. J Infect Dis 1995; 172:265–267.
69. Peeling RW, Hahn D, Dillon E. *Chlamydia pneumoniae* infection and adult-onset asthma. Proceedings of the Third Meeting of the European Society for Chlamydia Research, Vienna, Austria, Società Editrice Esculapio, Bologna, 1996, p. 228 [abstr].
70. Vignola AM, Chanerz P, Polla BS, Vic P, Godard P, Bosquet J. Increased expression of heat shock protein 70 on airway cells in asthma and chronic bronchitis. Am J Respir Cell Mol Biol 1995; 13:683–691.
71. Hahn, DF. *Chlaymdia pneumoniae*, asthma, and COPD: what is the evidence? Ann Allergy Asthma Immunol 1999; 83:271–292.
72. Tager IB, Ngo L, Hanrahan JP. Maternal smoking during pregnancy. Effects on lung function during the first 18 months of life. Am J Respir Crit Care Med 1995; 152: 977–983.
73. Stick SM, Burton PR, Gurrin L, Sly PD, LeSouef PN. Effects of maternal smoking during pregnancy and a family history of asthma on respiratory function in newborn infants. Lancet 1996; 348:1060–1064.
74. Strachan DP, Cook DG. Health effects of passive smoking. 5. Parental smoking and allergic sensitisation in children. Thorax 1998; 53:117–123.
75. Strachan DP, Cook DG. Health effects of passive smoking. 6. Parental smoking and childhood asthma: longitudinal and case-control studies. Thorax 1998; 53:204–212.
76. Willners S, Svenonius E, Skarping G. Passive smoking and childhood asthma: urinary cotinine levels in children with asthma and in referents. Allergy 1991; 46:330–334.
77. Martinez FD, Cline M, Burrows B. Increased incidence of asthma in children of smoking mothers. Pediatrics 1992; 89:21–26.
78. Hoo AF, Henschen M, Dezateux C, Coteloe K, Stocks J. Respiratory function among preterm infants whose mother smoked during pregnancy. Am J Respir Crit Care Med 1998; 158:700–705.
79. Joad JP. Perinantal exposure to aged and diluted sidestream cigarette smoke produces airway hyperresponsivness in older rat. Toxicol Appl Pharmacol 1999; 155:253–260.
80. Ronchetti R, Marcri F, Ciofetta G, Indinnimeo L, Cutrera R, Bonci E, Antognoni G, Martinez FD. Increased serum IgE and increased prevalence of eosinophila in 9-year-old children of smoking parents. J Allergy Clin Immunol 1990; 86:400–407.
81. Greer JR, Abbey DE, Burchette RJ. Asthma related to occupational and ambient air pollutants in nonsmokers. J Occup Med 1993; 35:909–915.
82. Flodin U, Jonsson P, Ziegler J, Axelson O. An epidemiologic study of bronchial asthma and smoking. Epidemiology 1995; 6:503–505.
83. von Mutius E, Martinez FD, Fritzsch C, Nicolai T, Roell G, Thiemann HH. Prevalence of asthma and atopy in two areas of West and East Germany. Am J Respir Crit Care Med 1994; 149:358–364.

84. Ransom MR, Pope CA. Elementary school absences and PM10 pollution in Utah Valley. Environ Res 1992; 58:204–219.
85. Ghio A, Devlin RB. Inflammatory lung injury after bronchial instillation of air pollution particles. Am J Respir Crit Care Med 2001; 64:704–708.
86. Diaz-Sanchez D, Dotson AR, Takenaka H, Saxon A. Diesel exhaust particles induce local IgE production in vivo and alter the pattern of IgE messenger RNA isoforms. J Clin Invest 1994; 94:1417–1425.
87. Diaz-Sanchez A, Tsien A, Fleming J, Saxon A. Combined diesel exhaust particulate and ragweed allergen challenge markedly enhances human in vivo nasal ragweed-specific IgE and skews cytokine production to a T helper cell 2-type pattern. J Immunol 1997; 158:2406–2413.
88. Don Porto Carero A, Hoet PH, Nemery B, Schoeters G. Increased HLA-DR expression after exposure of human monocytic cells to air particulates. Clin Exp Allergy 2002; 32:296–300.
89. Silverman, F. Asthma and respiratory irritants (ozone). Environ Health Perspect 1979; 29:131–136.
90. Kreit JW, Gross KB, Moore TB, Lorenzen TJ, D'Arcy J, Eschenbacher WL. Ozone-induced changes in pulmonary function and bronchial responsiveness in asthmatics. J Appl Physiol 1989; 66:217–222.
91. Horstman DH, Ball BA, Brown J, Gerrity T. Folinsbee LJ. Comparison of pulmonary responses of asthmatic and nonasthmatic subjects performing light exercise while exposed to a low level of ozone. Toxicol Ind Health 1995; 11:369–385.
92. Tattersfield AE. Air pollution: brown skies research. Thorax 1996; 51:13–22.
93. Balmes JR. The role of ozone exposure in the epidemiology of asthma. Environ Health Perspect 1993; 101(suppl 4):219–224.
94. von Mutius E, Braun-Fahrlander C, Schierl R, Riedler J, Ehlermann S, Maisch S, Waser M, Nowak D. Exposure to endotoxin or other bacterial components might protect against the development of atopy. Clin Exp Allergy 2000; 30:1230–1234.
95. Martinez FD, Holt PG. Role of microbial burden in aetiology of allergy and asthma. Lancet 1999; 354:S1112–1115.
96. Park J, Gold DE, Spiegelman DA, Burge HA, Milton DK. House dust endotoxin and wheeze in the first year of life. Am J Respir Crit Care Med 2001; 163:322–328.
97. Kamochi F, Kim YB, Sawh S, Sanders JM, Sarembock I, Green S, Young JS, Ley K, Fu SM, Rose CE Jr. P-selectin and ICAM-1 mediate endotoxin-induced neutrophil recruitment and injury to the lung and liver. Am J Physiol 1999; 277:L310–319.
98. Nolan B, Duffy A, Paquin L, De M, Collette H, Graziano CM, Bankey P. Mitogen-activated protein kinases signal inhibition of apoptosis in lipopolysaccharide-stimulated neutrophils. Surgery 1999; 126:406–412.
99. Clementsen P, Milman N, Kilian M, Fomsgaard A, Baek L, Norn S. Endotoxin from Haemophilus influenzae enhances IgE-mediated and non-immunological histamine release. Allergy 1990; 45:10–17.
100. Norn S, Skov PS, Jensen C, Jarlov JO, Espersen F. Histamine release induced by bacteria. A new mechanism in asthma? Agents Actions 1987; 20:29–34.
101. Grulee CG, Sanford HN. The influence of breast and artificial feeding on infantile eczema. J Pediatr 1930; 9:223–225.
102. Saarenin UM, Kajosaari M. Breastfeeding as prophylaxis against atopic disease: prospective follow-up study until 17 years old. Lancet 1995; 346:1065–1069.

103. Poysa L, Korppi M, Remes K, Juntunen-Backman K. Atopy in childhood and diet in infancy. A nine-year follow-up study. I. Clinical manifestations. Allergy Proc 1991; 12:107–111.

104. Savilahti E, Tainio VM, Samenpera L Siimes MA, Perheentupa J. Prolonged exclusive breast feeding and heredity as determinants in infantile atopy. Arch Dis Child 1987; 62:269–273.

105. Wright AL, Sherrill D. Holberg CJ, Halonen M, Martinez FD. Breast-feeding, maternal IgE, and total serum IgE in childhood. J Allergy Clin Immunol 1999; 104:589–594.

106. Duchen T, Yu G, Bjorksten B. Atopic sensitization during the first year of life in relation to long chain polyunsaturated fatty acid levels in human milk. Pediatr Res 1998; 44:478–484.

107. Braback L, Breborowicz A, Julge K, Knutsson A, Riikjarv MA, Vasar M, Bjorksten B. Risk factors for respiratory symptoms and atopic sensitisation in the Baltic area. Arch Dis Child 1995; 72:487–493.

108. Sepp E, Julge K, Vasar M, Naaber P, Bjorksten B, Mikelsaar M. Intestinal microflora of Estonian and Swedish infants. Acta Paediatr 1997; 86:956–961.

109. Bjorkstein B, Naaber P, Sepp E, Mikelsaar M. The intestinal microflora in allergic Estonian and Swedish 2-year-old children. Clin Exp Allergy 1999; 29:342–346.

110. Shida K, Makino K, Morishita A, Takamizawa K, Hachimura S, Ametani A, Sato T, Kumagai T, Habu S, Kaminogawa S. *Lactobacillus casei* inhibits antigen-induced IgE secretion through regulation of cytokine production in murin splenocyte cultures. Int Arch Allergy Immunol 1998; 115:278–287.

111. Matsuzaki T, Yamazaki R, Hasimoto S, Yokokura T. The effect of oral feeding of *Lactobacillus casei* strain Shirota on immunoglobulin E production in mice. J Dairy Sci 1998; 81:48–53.

112. Gerrard JY, Ko CG, Vickers P, Gerrard CD. The familial incidence of allergic disease. Ann Allergy 1976; 36:10–15.

113. Edford-Lubs ML. Allergy in 7000 twins. Acta Allergol 1971; 26:249–285.

114. Wuthrich B, Baumann RA, Fries RA, Schnyder UW. Total and specific IgE (RAST) in atopic twins. Clin Allergy 1981; 11:147–154.

115. Hopp RJ, Bewtra AK, Biven R, Nair NM, Townley RG. Bronchial reactivity pattern in non asthmatic parents of asthmatics. Ann Allergy 1988; 61:184–186.

116. Hanson B, McGue M, Roitman-Johnson B, Segal NL, Bouchard TJ Jr, Blumenthal MN. Atopic disease and immunoglobulin E in twins reared apart and together. Am J Hum Genet 1991; 48:873–879.

117. Skadhauge LR, Christensen K, Kyvik KO, Sissgaard T. Genetic and environmental influence on asthma; a population-based study of 11,688 Danish twin pairs. Eur Respir J 1999; 13:8–14.

118. Holgate ST. Genetic and environmental interaction in allergy and asthma. J Allergy Clin Immunol 1999; 104:1139–1146.

119. Postma DS, Bleecker ER, Amelung PJ, Holroyd K, Xu J, Panhusen CIM, Meyers D, Levitt RC. Genetic susceptibility to asthma-bronchial hyperresponsiveness coinherited with a major gene for atopy. N Engl J Med 1995; 333:894–900.

120. Marsh DG, Neely JD, Breazeale DR, Ghosh B, Freidhoff L, Ehrlich-Kautzky E, Schous C, Krishnaswamy G, Beaty TH. Linkage analysis of IL-4 and other chromosome 5q31.1 markers and total serum IgE concentrations. Science 1994; 264:1152–1156.

121. Meyers DA, Postma DS, Panhuysen CI, Xu J, Amelung PJ, Levitt RC, Bleecker ER. Evidence for a locus regulating total serum IgE levels mapping to chromosome 5. Genomics 1994; 23:464–470.

122. Cookson WO. C. M, Sharp PA, Faux JA, Hopkin JM. Linkage between immunoglobulin E responses underlying asthma and rhinitis and chromosome 11q. Lancet 1989; 1: 1292–1295.

123. Moffatt MF, Sharp PA, Faux JA, Young RP, Cookson WO, Hopkin JM. Factors confounding genetic linkage between atopy and chromosome 11q. Clin Exp Allergy 1992; 22:1046–1051.

124. Barnes KC, Neely ND, Duffy DL, Freidhoff LR, Breazeale DR, Schou C, Naidu RP, Levett PN, Ranult B, Kucherlapati R, Ionzzinos, Ehrlich E, Beaty TH, Marsh DG. Linkage of asthma and total serum IgE concentration to markers on chromosome 12q: evidence from Afro-Caribbean and Caucasian population. Genomics 1996; 37: 41–50.

125. Wiesch DG, Meyers DA, Bleecker ER. Genetics of asthma. J Allergy Clin Immunol 1999; 104:895–901.

126. Deichmann KA, Heinzmann A, Forster J, Dischenger S, Mehl C Brueggenolte E, Hildebrandt F, Moseler M, Kuehr J. Linkage and allelic association of atopy and markers flanking the IL-4 receptor gene. Clin Exp Allergy 1998; 28:151–155.

127. Ober C, Tselenko A, Willadsen SA, Newman D, Daniel R, Wu X, Andal J, Hoki D, Schneider D, True K, Schou C, Parry R, Cox N. Genomewide screen for atopy susceptibility alleles in the Hutterites. Clin Exp Allergy 1999; 4 (suppl):11–15.

128. Gauchat JF, Lebman DA, Coffman RL, Gascan H, de Vries JE. Structure and expression of germline epsilon transcripts in human B cells induced by interleukin 4 to switch to IgE production. J Exp Med 1990; 172:463–473.

129. Borish L, Mascali JJ, Klinnert M, Leppert LJ, Rosenwasser LJ. SSC polmorphisms in interleukin genes. Hum Mol Genet 1995; 4:974.

130. Burchard E, Silverman E, Rosenwasser LJ, Borish L, Yandava C, Pillari A, Weiss S, Hasday J, Lilly CM, Ford JG, Drazen JM. Association between a sequence varient in the IL-4 gene promoter and FEV1 in asthma. Am J Respir Crit Care Med 1999; 160: 919–922.

131. Walley J, Cookson WO. Investigation of an interleukin-4 promoter polymorphism for associations with asthma and atopy. J Med Genet 1996; 33:689–692.

132. Hershey GK, Friedrich MF, Esswein LA, Thoma ML, Chatila TA. The association of atopy with a gain-of-function mutation in the α subunit of the interleukin-4 receptor. N Engl J Med 1997; 337:1720–1725.

133. Rosa-Rosa L, Zimmermann N, Bernstein J, Rothenberg ME, Hershey GK. K. The R576 interleukin-4 receptor alpha allele correlates with asthma severity. J Allergy Clin Immunol 1999; 104:1008–1014.

134. Noguchi E, Shibaski M, Arnami T, Takeda K Tokouchi Y, Kobaysahi K, Imoto N, Nakahara S, Matusui A, Hamaguchi H. Lack of association of atopy/asthma and the interleukin-4 receptor α gene in Japanese. Clin Exp Allergy 1999; 29:228–233.

135. Reihsaus EM, Innis M, MacIntyre N, Liggett SB. Mutations in the gene encoding for the β2-adrenergic receptor in normal and asthmatic subjects. Am J Respir Cell Mol Biol 1993; 8:334–339.

136. Green SA, Turki J, Innis M, Liggett SB. Amino-terminal polymorphisms of the human β2-adrenergic receptor impart distinct agonists-promoted regulatory properties. Biochemistry 1994; 33:9414–9419.

137. Turki J, Pak J, Green A, Martin RJ, Liggett SB. Genetic polymorphisms of the β2-adrenergic receptor in nocturnal and nonnocturnal asthma. J Clin Invest 1995; 95: 1635–1641.

138. Hall IP, Wheatley A, Wilding P, Liggett SB. Association of Glu 27 β2-adrenergic polymorphism with lower airway reactivity in asthma subjects. Lancet 1995; 345: 1213–1214.

139. Wang Z, Chen C, Niu T, Wu D, Yang J, Wang B, Fang Z, Yandava CN, Drazen JM, Weiss ST, Xu X. Association of asthma with beta (2)-adrenergic receptor gene polymorphism and cigarette smoking. Am J Respir Crit Care Med 2001; 163: 1404–1409.

140. Israel E, Drazen JM, Liggett SB, et al. Effect of polymorphism of the beta (2)-adrenergic receptor on response to regular use of albuterol in asthma. Int Arch Allergy Immunol 2001; 124:183–186.

141. Weir TD, Mallek, Sandford AJ, Bai TR, Awadh N, Fitzgerald JM, Cockcroft D, James A, Liggett SB, Pare PD. B2-adrenergic receptor haplotypes in mild, moderate and fatal/near fatal asthma. Am J Respir Crit Care Med 1998; 158:787–791.

142. Collaborative Study of the Genetics of Asthma. A genome-wide search for asthma susceptibility loci in ethnically diverse populations. Nat Genet 1997; 15:389–397.

143. Dunhill MS. The pathology of asthma, with special reference to changes in the bronchial mucosa. J Clin Pathol 1960; 13:27–33.

144. Dunhill MS, Massarella GR, Anderson JA. A comparison of the quantitative anatomy of the bronchi in normal subjects, in status asthmaticus, in chronic bronchitis and in emphysema. Thorax 1969; 24:176–179.

145. Laitinen LA, Heino M, Laitenen A, Kava T, Haahtela T. Damage of the airway epithelium and bronchial reactivity in patients with asthma. Am Rev Respir Dis 1985; 131: 599–606.

146. Beasley R, Roch WR, Roberts JA, Holgate ST. Cellular events in the bronchi in mild asthma and after provocation. Am Rev Respir Dis 1989; 139:806–817.

147. Roche WR, Beasley R, Williams JH, Holgate ST. Subepithelial fibrosis in the bronchi of asthmatics. Lancet 1989; 1:520–524.

148. Bentley AM, Meng Q, Robinson DS, Hamid Q, Kay AB, Durham SR. Increases in activated T lymphocytes, eosinophils, and cytokine mRNA expression for interleukin-5 and granulocyte/macrophage colony-stimulating factor in bronchial biopsies after allergen inhalation challenge in atopic asthmatics. Am J Respir Cell Mol Biol 1993; 8:35–42.

149. Frew AJ, St-Pierre J, Teran LM, Trefilieff A, Madden J, Peroni D, Bodey KM, Walls AF, Howarth PH, Carroll MP, Holgate ST. Cellular and mediator responses twenty-four hours after local endobronchial allergen challenge of asthmatic airways. J Allergy Clin Immunol 1996; 98:133–143.

150. Kirby JG, Hargreave FE, Gleich GJ, O'Byrne PM. Brochoalveolar cell profiles of asthmatic and nonasthmatic subjects. Am Rev Resp Dis 1987; 136:379–383.

151. Galli SJ. Complexity and redundancy in the pathogenesis of asthma: reassessing the roles of mast cells and T cells. J Exp Med 1997; 186:343–347.

152. Marks RM, Roche WR, Czerniecki M, Penny Y, Nelson DS. Mast-cell granules cause proliferation of human microvascular endothelial cells. Lab Invest 1986; 55:289–294.

153. Sorbo J, Jakobsson A, Norrby K. Mast-cell histamine is angiogenic through receptors for histamine 1 and histamine 2. Int J Exp Pathol 1994; 75:43–50.

154. Irani AM, Bradford TR, Kepley CL, Schechter NM, Schwartz LB. Detection of MCT and MCTC types of human mast cells by immunohistochemistry using new monoclonal anti-tryptase and anti-chymase antibodies. J Histochem Cytochem 1989; 37: 1509–1515.
155. Schwartz LB, Sakia K, Bradford TR, Ren S, Zweiman B, Worobec AS, Metcalfe DD. The alpha form of human tryptase is the predominant type present in blood at baseline in normal subjects and is elevated in those subjects with systemic mastocytosis. J Clin Invest 1995; 96:2702–2710.
156. Schwartz LB, Kawahara MS, Hugli TE, Vik D, Fearon DT, Austen KF. Generation of C3a anaphylatoxin from human C3 by human mast cell tryptase. J Immunol 1983; 130:1891–1895.
157. Lohi J, Harvima I, Keski-Oja J, Pericellular substrates of human mast cell tryptase: 72,000 dalton gelatinase and fibronectin. J Cell Biochem 1992; 50:337–349.
158. Cairns JA, Walls AF. Mast cell tryptase is a mitogen for epithelial cells. Stimulation of IL-8 production and intercellular adhesion molecule-1 expression. J Immunol 1996; 156:275–283.
159. Bradding P. Human mast cell cytokines. Clin Exp Allergy 1996; 26:13–19.
160. Burd PR, Thompson WC, Max EE, Mills FC. Activated mast cells produce interleukin-13. J Exp Med 1995; 181:1373–1380.
161. Gordon JR, Burd PR, Galli SJ. Mast cells as a source of multifunctional cyokines. Immunol Today 1990; 11:458–464.
162. Bradding P, Roberts JA, Britten KM, Montefort S, Djukanovic R, Mueller R, Heusser CH, Howarth PH, Holgate ST. Interleukin-4, -5, and -6 and tumor necrosis factor-α in normal and asthmatic airways: evidence for the human mast cell as a source of these cytokines. Am J Respir Cell Mol Biol 1994; 10:471–480.
163. Ying S, Durham SR, Corrigan CJ, Hamid Q, Kay AB. Phenotype of cells expressing mRNA for Th-2 type (interleukin-4 and interleukin-5) and Th-1 type (interleukin-2 and interferon-γ) cytokines in brochoalveolar lavage and bronchial biopsies from atopic asthmatic and normal control subjects. Am J Respir Cell Mol Biol 1995; 12:477–487.
164. Casale TB, Wood D, Richerson HB, Zehr B, Zavala D, Humminghake GW. Direct evidence of a role for mast cells in the pathogenesis of antigen-induced bronchoconstriction. J Clin Invest 1987; 80:1507–1511.
165. Wenzel SE, Fowler AA. 3d, Schwartz LB. Activation of pulmonary mast cells by bronchoalveolar allergen challenge. In vivo release of histamine and tryptase in atopic subjects with and without asthma. Am Rev Respir Dis 1988; 137:1002–1008.
166. Liu MC, Bleecker ER, Lichtenstein LM, Kagey-Sobotka A, Niv Y, McLemore TL, Dermutt S, Proud D, Hubbard WC. Evidence for elevated levels of histamine, prostaglandin D2, and other bronchoconstricting prostaglandins in the airways of subjects with mild asthma. Am Rev Respir Dis 1990; 142:126–132.
167. Wardlaw AJ, Hay H, Cromwell O, Collins JV, Kay AB. Leukotrienes, LTC4 and LTB4, in bronchoalveolar lavage in bronchial asthma and other respiratory diseases. J Allergy Clin Immunol 1989; 84:19–26.
168. Lane SJ, Lee TH. Mast cell effector mechanisms. J Allergy Clin Immunol 1996; 98: S67–S72.
169. Sedgwick JB, Calhoun WJ, Gleich GJ, et al. Localized airway eosinophil response to bronchial segmental antigen challenge. Am Rev Respir Dis 1990; 141:A93.
170. Metzger WJ, Zavala D, Richerson HB, Moseley P, Iwamota P, Monick M, Sjoerdsma K, Hunninghake GW. Local allegen challenge and bronchalveolar lavage of allergic

asthmatic lungs. Description of the model and local airway inflammation. Am Rev Respir Dis 1987; 135:433–440.

171. Montefort S, Gratziou C, Goulding D, Polosa R, Haskard DO, Howarth PH, Holgate ST, Caroll MP. Bronchial biopsy evidence for leukocyte infiltration and upregulation of leukocyte-endothelial cell adhesion molecules 6 hours after local allergen challenge of sensitized asthmatic airways. J Clin Invest 1994; 93:1411–1421.

172. Liu MC, Hubbard WC, Proud D, Stealey BA, Galli SJ, Kagey-Sobotka A, Bleecker ER, Lichenstein LM. Immediate and late inflammatory responses to ragweed antigen challenge of the peripheral airways in allergic asthmatics. Cellular, mediator, and permeability changes. Am Rev Respir Dis 1991; 144:51–58.

173. Djukanovic R, Wilson JW, Britten KM, Wilson SJ, Walls AF, Roche WR, Howarth PH, Holgate ST. Quantitation of mast cells and eosinophils in the bronchial mucosa of symptomatic atopic asthmatics and healthy control subjects using immunohistochmeistry. Am Rev Respir Dis 1990; 142:863–871.

174. Bradley BL, Azzawi M, Jacoson M, Assoufi B, Collins JV, Irani AM, Schwartz LB, Durham SR, Jeffery PK, Kay AB. Eosinophils, T-lymphocytes, mast cells, neutrophils, and macrophages in bronchial biopsy specimens from atopic subjects with asthma: comparison with biopsy specimens from atopic subjects without asthma and normal control subjects and relationship to bronchial hyperresponsinvess. J Allergy Clin Immunol 1991; 88:661–674.

175. Pesci A, Foresi A, Bertorelli G, Chetta A, Oliveri D, Oliveri D. Histochemical characteristics and degranulation of mast cells in epithelium and lamina propria of bronchial biopsies from asthmatic and normal subjects. Am Rev Respir Dis 1993; 147:684–689.

176. Gibson PG, Allen CJ, Yang JP, Wong BJ, Dolovich J, Denburg J, Hargreave FE. Intraepithelial mast cells in allergic and nonallergic asthma: assessment using bronchial brushings. Am Rev Respir Dis 1993; 148:80–86.

177. Pin I, Gibson PG, Kolendowicz R, Girgis-Gabardo A, Denburg JA, Hargreave FE, Dolovich J. Use of induced sputum cell counts to investigate airway inflammation in asthma. Thorax 1992; 47:25–29.

178. Tomioka M, Ida S, Shindoh Y, Ishihara T, Takishima T. Mast cells in bronchoalveolar lumen of patients with bronchial asthma. Am Rev Respir Dis 1984; 129:1000–1005.

179. Bradding P, Roberts JA, Britten KM, Montefort S, Djukanovic R, Mueller R, Heusser CH, Howarth PH, Holgate ST. Am J Respir Cell Mol Biol 1994; 10:471–480.

180. Humbert M, Grant JA, Taborda-Barata L, Durham SR, Pfister R, Menz G, Barkans J, Ying S, Kay AB. High-affinity IgE receptor (FcepsilonRI)-bearing cells in bronchial biopsies from atopic and nonatopic asthma. Am J Respir Crit Care Med 1996; 153: 1931–1937.

181. Saetta M, Di Stefano A, Maestrelli P, De Marzo N, Milani GF, Pivirotto F, Mapp CE, Fabbri LM. Airway mucosal inflammation in occupational asthma induced by toluene diisocyanate. Am Rev Respir Dis 1992; 145:160–168.

182. Milgrom H, Fick RB, Su JQ, Reimann JD, Bush RK, Watrous ML, Metzger WJ. Treatment of allergic asthma with monoclonal anti-IgE antibody. N Engl J Med 1999; 341:1966–1973.

183. Fahy JV, Fleming HE, Wong HH, Liu JT, Su JQ, Reimann J, Fick RB Jr, Boushey HA. The effect on an anti-IgE monoclonal antibody on the early- and late-phase responses to

allergen inhalation in asthmatic subjects. Am J Respir Crit Care Med 1997; 155: 1828–1834.

184. Kehry MR, Yamashita LC. Low-affinity IgE receptor (CD23) function on mouse B cells: role in IgE-dependent antigen focusing. Proc Natl Acad Sci USA 1989; 86: 7556–7560.

185. Holgate ST. Epithelial damage and response. Clin Exp Allergy 2000; 30(suppl 1): 28–32.

186. Williams C, Galli SJ. Mast cells can amplify airway reactivity and features of chronic inflammation in an asthma model of mice. J Exp Med 2000; 192:455–462.

187. Brusselle GG, Kips JC, Tavernier JH, van der Heyden JG, Cuvelier CA, Pauwels RA, Bluethmann H. Attenuation of allergic airway inflammation in IL-4 deficient mice. Clin Exp Allergy 1994; 24:73–80.

188. Robinson DS, Bentley AM, Hartnell A, Kay AB, Durham SR. Activated memory T helper cells in bronchoalveolar lavage fluid from patients with atopic asthma: relation to asthma symptoms, lung function, and bronchial responsiveness. Thorax 1993; 48: 26–32.

189. Kon OM, Kay AB. T cells and chronic asthma. Int Arch Allergy Immunol 1999; 118: 133–135.

190. Wardlaw AJ, Dunnette S, Gleich GJ, Collins JV, Kay AB. Eosinophils and mast cells in brochoalveolar lavage in mild asthma: relationship to bronchial hyperactivity. Am Rev Respir Dis 1988; 137:62–69.

191. Jeffery PK, Wardlaw AJ, Nelson FC, Collins JV, Kay AB. Bronchial biopsies in asthma: an ultrastructural, quantitative study and correlation with hyperactivity. Am Rev Respir Dis 1989; 140:1745–1753.

192. Hamid Q, Song Y, Kotsimbos TC, Minshall E, Bai TR, Hegele RG, Hogg JC. Inflammation of small airways in asthma. J Allergy Clin Immunol 1997; 100:44–51.

193. Azzawi M, Johnston PW, Majumdar S, Kay AB, Jeffery PK. T lymphocytes and activated eosinophils in airway mucosa in fatal asthma and cystic fibrosis. Am Rev Respir Dis 1992; 145:1477–1482.

194. Robinson DS, Ying S, Bentley AM, Meng Q, North J, Durham SR, Kay AB, Hamid Q. Relationships among numbers of bronchoalveolar lavage cells expressing messenger ribonucleic acid for cytokines, asthma symptoms, and airway methacholine responsiveness in atopic asthma. J Allergy Clin Immunol 1993; 92:397–403.

195. Corrigan CJ, Hartnell A, Kay AB. T lymphocyte activation in acute severe asthma. Lancet 1988; 1:1129–1132.

196. Hamid Q, Barkans J, Robinson DS, Durham SR, Kay AB. Co-expression of CD25 and CD3 in atopic allergy and asthma. Immunology 1992; 75:659–663.

197. Keatings VM, Keatings VM, O'Connor BJ, Wright LG, Huston DP, Corrigan CJ, Barnes PJ. Late response to allergen is associated with increased concentrations of tumor necrosis factor-α and IL-5 in induced sputum. J Allergy Clin Immunol 1997; 99:693–698.

198. Hamid Q, Azzawi M, Ying S, Moqbel R, Wardlaw AJ, Corrigan CJ, Bradley B, Durham SR, Collins JV, Jeffery PK, et al. Expression of mRNA for interleukin-5 in mucosal bronchial biopsies from asthma. J Clin Invest 1991; 87:1541–1546.

199. Hamid Q, Azzawi M, Ying S, Moqbel R, Wardlaw AJ, Corrigan CJ, Bradley B, Durham SR, Collins JV, Jeffery PK, et al. Interleukin-5 mRNA in mucosal bronchial biopsies from asthmatic subjects. Int Arch Allergy Appl Immunol 1991; 94(1–4): 169–170.

200. Robinson DS, Hamid Q, Ying S, Tsiscopoulos A, Barkans J, Bentley AM, Corrigan C, Durham SR, Kay AB. Predominant TH2-like bronchoalveolar T-lymphocyte population in atopic asthma. N Engl J Med 1992; 326:298–304.

201. Del Prete GF, De Carli M, D'Elios MM, Maestrelli P, Ricci M, Fabbri L, Romagnani S. Allergen exposure induces the activation of allergen-specific Th2 cells in the airway mucosa of patients with allergic respiratory disorders. Eur J Immunol 1993; 23: 1445–1449.

202. Corrigan CJ, Hamid Q, North J, Barkans J, Moqbel R, Durham S, Gemou-Engesaeth V, Kay AB. Peripheral blood CD4 but not CD8 T-lymphocytes in patients with esacerbation of asthma transcribe and translate messenger RNA encoding cytokines which prolong eosinophil survival in the context of a Th2-type pattern: effect of glucocorticoid therapy. Am J Respir Cell Mol Biol 1995; 12:567–578.

203. Humbert M, Durham SR, Ying S, Kimmitt P, Barkans J, Assoufi B, Pfister R, Menz G, Robinson DS, Kay AB, Corrigan CJ. IL-4 and IL-5 mRNA and protein in bronchial biopsies from patients with atopic and nonatopic asthma: evidence against "intrinsic" asthma being a distinct immunopathologic entity. Am J Respir Crit Care Med 1996; 1545:1497–1504.

204. Corrigan CJ, Kay AB. CD4 T-lymphocyte activation in: relation to disease severity and atopic status. Am Rev Respir Dis 1990; 141:970–977.

205. Cembrzynska-Nowak M, Szklarz E, Inglot AD, Teodorczyk-Injeyan JA. Elevated release of tumor necrosis factor-alpha and interferon-gamma by bronchoalveolar leukocytes from patients with bronchial asthma. Am Rev Respir Dis 1993; 1472: 291–295.

206. Calhoun WJ, Reed CE, Moest DR, Stevens CA. Enhanced superoxide production by alveolar macrophages and air-space cells, airway inflammation and alveolar macrophage density changes after segmental antigen bronchoprovocation in allergic subjects. Am Rev Respir Dis 1992; 145:317–325.

207. O'Sullivan S, Cormican L, Faul JL, Ichinohe S, Johnston SL, Burke CM, Poulter LW. Activated, cytotoxic CD8 + T lymphocytes contribute to the pathology of asthma death. Am J Respir Crit Care Med 2001; 164:560–564.

208. Coyle A, Erard F, Bertrand C, Walti S, Pircher H, Le Gros G. Virus-specific CD8 + cells can switch to interleukin-5 production and induce airway eosinophilia. J Exp Med 1995; 181:1229–1233.

209. Metzger WJ, Zavala D, Richerson HB, Moseley P, Iwmota P, Monick M, et al. Local allergen challenge and bronchoalveolar lavage of allergic asthmatic lungs: description of the modle and local airway inflammation. Am Rev Respir Dis 1987; 135:433–440.

210. Gerblich AA, Salik H, Schuyler MR. Dynamic T-cell changes in peripheral blood and bronchoalveolar lavage after antigen bronchoprovocation in asthmatics. Am Rev Respir Dis 1991; 143:533–537.

211. Gratziou C, Carroll M, Montefort S, Teran L, Howarth PH, Holgate ST. Inflammatory and T-cell profile of asthmatic airways 6 hours after local allergen provocation. Am J Respir Crit Care Med 1996; 153:515–520.

212. Frew AJ. Cloning T cells from sites of allergic inflammation [editorial; comment]. Clin Exp Allergy 1999; 29:1155–1157.

213. Ricci M, Matucci A, Rossi O. New advances in the pathogenesis and therapy of bronchial asthma. Ann Ital Med Int 1998; 13:93–119.

214. Ray A, Cohn L. Th2 cells and GATA-3 in asthma: new insights into the regulation of airway inflammation. J Clin Invest 1999; 104:985–993.

215. Pirron U, Schlunck T, Prinz JC, Rieber EB. P. IgE-dependent antigen focusing by human B lymphocytes is mediated by the low affinity receptor for IgE. Eur J Immunol 1990; 20:1547–1551.

216. Haczku A, Takeda K, Hamelmann E, Loader J, Joetham A, Redai I, Irvin CG, Lee JJ, Kikutani H, Conrad D, Gelfand EW. CD23 exhibits negative regulatory effects on allergic sensitization and airway hyperresponsiveness. Am J Respir Crit Care Med 2000; 161:952–960.

217. Shalit M, Sekhsaria S, Malech HL. Modulation of growth and differentiation of eosinophils from human peripheral blood CD34 + cells by IL-5 and other growth factors. Cell Immunol 1995; 1601:50–57.

218. Weller PF. The immunobiology of eosinophils. N Engl J Med 1991; 324:1110–1118.

219. Lacy P, Weller PF, Moqbel R. Special report. A report from the International Eosinophil Society: Eosinophils in a tug of war. J Allergy Clin Immunol 2001; 108:895–900.

220. Bousquet J, Chanez P, Lacoste JY, Barneon G, Ghavanian N, Enander I, Venge P, Ahlstedt S, Simony-Lafontaine J, Godard P, et al. Eosinophilic inflammation in asthma. N Engl J Med 1990; 323:1033–10399.

221. Church MK, Levi-Schaffer F. The human mast cell. J Allergy Clin Immunol 1997; 99:155–160.

222. Rossi GL, Olivieri D. Does the mast cell still have a key role in asthma? Chest 1997; 112:523–529.

223. Bentley AM, Menz G, Storz C, Robinson DS, Bradley B, Jeffery PK, Durham SR, Kay AB. Identification of T lymphocytes, macrophages, and activated eosinophils in the bronchial mucosa in intrinsic asthma. Relationship to symptoms and bronchial responsiveness. Am Rev Respir Dis 1992; 146:500–506.

224. Oehling AG Jr, Walker C, Virchow JC, Blaser K. Correlation between blood eosinophils, T-helper cell activity markers and pulmonary function in patients with allergic and intrinsic asthma. J Investig Allergol Clin Immunol 1992; 2:295–299.

225. Bentley AM, Maestrelli P, Saetta M, Fabbri LM, Robinson DS, Bradley BL, Jeffery PK, Durham SR, Kay AB. Activated T-lymphocytes and eosinophils in the bronchial mucosa in isocyanate-induced asthma. J Allergy Clin Immunol 1992; 89: 821–829.

226. Azzawi M, Bradley B, Jeffery PK, Frew AJ, Wardlaw AJ, Knowles G, Assouti B, Collins JV. Identification of Activated T Lymphocytes and Eosinophils in bronchial biopsies in stable atopic asthma. Am Rev Respir Dis 1990; 142:1407–1413.

227. Warner JA, Marquet C, Rao R, Roche WR, Pohunek P. Inflammatory mechanisms in childhood asthma. Clin Exp Allergy 1998; 28(5 suppl):71–75.

228. Aalbers R, Kauffman HF, Vrugt E, Koeter GH, de Monchy JG. Allergen-induced recruitment of inflammatory cells in lavage 3 and 24 hours after challenge in allergic asthmatic lungs. Chest 1993; 103:1178–1184.

229. Sehmi R, Wood LJ, Watson R, Foley R, Hamid Q, O'Byrne PM, Denburg JA. Allergen-induced increases in IL-5 receptor alpha-subunit expression on bone marrow-derived CD34 + cells from asthmatic subjects: a novel marker of progenitor cell commitment towards eosinophilic differentiation. J Clin Invest 1997; 100:2466–2475.

230. Haslett C, Savill JS, Whyte MK, Stern M, Dransfield I, Meager LC. Granulocyte apoptosis and the control of inflammation. Phil Trans R Soc Lond B Biol Sci 1994; 345:327–333.

231. Vignola AM, Chanez P, Chiappara G, Siena L, Merendino A, Reina C, Gagliardo R, Profita M, Bousquet J, Bonsignore G. Evaluation of apoptosis of eosinophils, macro-

phages, and T lymphocytes in mucosal biopsy specimens of patients with asthma and chronic bronchitis. J Allergy Clin Immunol 1999; 103:563–573.

232. Minshall EM, Schleimer R, Cameron L, Minnicozzi M, Egan RW, Gutierrez-Ramos JC, Eidelman DH, Hamid Q. Interleukin-5 expression in the bone marrow of sensitized Balb/c mice after allergen challenge. Am J Respir Crit Care Med 1998; 158:951–957.

233. Denburg JA, Sehmi R, Saito H, Pil-Seob J, Inman MD, O'Byrne PM. Systemic aspects of allergic disease: bone marrow responses. J Allergy Clin Immunol 2000; 106: S242–S246.

234. Dvorak AM, Furitsu T, Letourneau L, Ishizaka T, Ackerman SJ. Mature eosinophils stimulated to develop in human cord blood mononuclear cell-cultures supplemented with recombinant human interleukin-5. Part I. Piecemeal degranulation of specific granules and distribution of Charcot-Leyden crystal protein. Am J Pathol 1991; 138: 69–82.

235. Filley WV, Holley KE, Kephart GM, Gleich GJ. Identification by immunofluorence of eosinophil granule major basic protein in lung tissues of patients with bronchial asthma. Lancet 1982; 2:11–16.

236. Frigas E, Loegering DA, Sollegy GO, Farrow GM, Gleich GJ. Elevated levels of the eosinophil granule major basic protein in the sputum of patients with bronchial asthma. Mayo Clin Proc 1981; 56:345–353.

237. Gundel RH, Letts LG, Gleich GJ. Human eosinophil major basic protein induces airway constriction and airway hyperresponsiveness in primates. J Clin Invest 1991; 87: 1470–1473.

238. Jacoby DB, Gleich GJ, Fryer AD. Human eosinophil major basic protein is an endogenous allosteric antagonist at the inhibitory muscarinic M2 receptor. J Clin Invest 1993; 91:1314–1318.

239. Durack, Sumi SM, Klebanoff SJ. Neurotoxicity of human eosinophils. Proc Natl Acad Sci USA 1979; 76:1443–1447.

240. Busse WW, Nagata M, Sedwick JB. Characteristics of airway eosinophils. Eur Respir J Suppl 1996; 22:132S–135S.

241. Boyce JA. The pathobiology of eosinophilic inflammation. Allergy Asthma Proc 1997; 5:293–300.

242. Kay AB, Barata L, Meng Q, Durham SR, Ying S, Eosinophils and eosinophil-associated cytokines in allergic inflammation. Int Arch Allergy Immunol 1997; 113(1–3): 196–199.

243. Lim KG, Wan HC, Bozza PT, Resnick MB, Wong DT, Cruikshank WW, Kornfeld H, Center DM, Weller PF. Human eosinophils elaborate the lymphocyte chemoattractants. IL-16 (lymphocyte chemoattractant factor) and RANTES. J Immunol 1996; 156: 2566–2570.

244. Hamann KJ, Douglas I, Moqbel R. Eosinophil mediators. In: Busse WW, Holgate ST, eds. Asthma and Rhinitis. 2d ed. London: Blackwell Science, Ltd, 2000:394–428.

245. Wenzel SE, Schwartz LB, Langmack EL, Halliday JL, Trudeau JB, Gibbs RL, Chu HW. Evidence that severe asthma can be divided pathologically into two inflammatory subypes with distinct physiologic and clinical characteristics. Am J Respir Crit Care Med 1999; 160:100–1008.

246. Moqbel R, Barkans J, Bradley BL, Durham SR, Kay AB. Application of monoclonal antibodies against major basic protein (BMK-13) and eosinophil cationic protein (EG1 and EG2) for quantifying eosinophils in bronchial biopsies from atopic asthma. Clin Exp Allergy 1992; 22:265–273.

247. Jacoby DB, Costello RM, Fryer AD. Eosinophil recruitment to the airway nerves. J Allergy Clin Immunol 2001; 107:211–218.
248. Leckie MJ, ten Brinke A, Khan J, Diamant Z, O'Connor BJ, Walls CM, Mathur AK, Cowley HC, Chung KF, Djukanovic R, Hansel TT, Holgate ST, Sterk PJ, Barnes PJ. Effects of an interleukin-5 blocking monoclonal antibody on eosinophils, airway hyperresponsiveness, and the late asthmatic response. Lancet 2000; 356:2144–2148.
249. Naylor B. The shedding of the mucosa of the bronchial tree in asthma. Thorax 1962; 17:69–72.
250. Woltmann G, Ward RJ, Symon RA, Rew DA, Pavord ID, Wardlaw AJ. Objective quantitative analysis of eosinophils and bronchial epithelial cells in induced sputum by laser scanning cytometry. Thorax 1999; 54:124–130.
251. James AL, Carroll N. The pathology of fatal asthma. In: Holgate ST, Busse WW, editors. Inflammatory Mechanisms in Asthma. New York: Marcel Dekker; 1998: 1–26.
252. Williams SL, West M, Lackie PM. Morphometry of airway epithelial cells in asthma. Respir Med 1998; 92:A30.
253. Roche WR, Beasley R, Williams JH, Holgate ST. Subepithelial fibrosis in the bronchi of asthmatics. Lancet 1989; 1:520–524.
254. Holgate ST, Davies D, Lackie P, Wilson SJ, Puddicombe SM, Lordan JL. Epithelial-mesenchymal interactions in the pathogenesis of asthma. J Allergy Clin Immunol 2000; 105:193–204.
255. King C, Brennan S, Thompson PJ, Stewart GA. Dust mite allergens induce cytokine release from cultured epithelium. J Immunol 1998; 161:1645–1651.
256. Yamaga M, Sikizawa K, Masuda T, Morikawa M, Sawai T, Saski H. Oxidants affect permeability and repair of the cultured human trachea. Am J Physiol 1995; 268: L284–293.
257. Papi A, Johnston SL. Respiratory epithelial cell expression of vascular cell adhesion molecule-1 and its up-regulation by rhinovirus infection via NF-kB and GATA transcription factors. J Biol Chem 1999; 274:30041–30051.
258. Campbell AM, Chanez P, Vignola AM, Bousquet J, Couret I, Michel FB, Godard P. Functional characteristics of bronchial epithelium obtained by brushings from asthmatic and normal subjects. Am Rev Respir Dis 1993; 147:529–534.
259. Vignola AM, Campbell AM, Chanez P, Bousquet J, Paul-Lacoste P, Michel FB, Godard P. HLA-DR and ICAM-1 expression on bronchial epithelial cells in asthma and chronic bronchitis. Am Rev Respir Dis 1993; 148:689–694.
260. Springall DR, Howarth PH, Counihan H, Djuanovic R, Holgate ST, Polak JM. Endothelin immunoreactivity of airway epithelium in asthmatic patients. Lancet 1991; 337: 697–701.
261. Sousa AR, Lams BE, Pfister R, Christie PE, Schmitz M, Lee TH. Expression of interluekin-5 and granulocyte-macrophage colony-stimulating factor in aspirin-sensitive and non-aspirin-sensitive asthmatic airways. Am J Respir Crit Care Med 1997; 156:1384–1389.
262. Chung KF, Barnes PF. Cytokines in asthma. Thorax 1999; 54:825–857.
263. Knobil K, Jacoby DB. Mediator functions of epithelial cells. In: Holgate ST, Busse WW, eds. Inflammatory Mechanisms in Asthma. New York: Marcel Dekker; 1998: 469–495.
264. Salvi S, Semper A, Blomberg A, Holloway J, Jaffar Z, Papi A, Teran L, Polosa R, Kelly F, Sandstrom T, Holgate S, Frew A. Interleukin-5 production by human airway epithelial cells. Am J Respir Cell Mol Biol 1999; 20:984–991.

265. Popadopoulous NG, Stanciu LA, Papi A, Holgate ST, Johnston SL. A defective type I response to rhinovirus in atopic asthma. Thorax 2002; 57:328–332.
266. Hackel PO, Zwick E, Prenzel N, Ullrich A. Epidermal growth factor receptors: critical mediators of multiple receptor pathways. Curr Opin Cell Biol 1999; 11:184–189.
267. Davies DE, Polosa R, Puddicombe SM, Richter A, Holgate ST. The epidermal growth factor receptor and its ligand family: their potential role in repair and remodelling in asthma. Allergy 1999; 54:771–783.
268. Puddicombe SM, Polosa R, Richter A, Krishna MT, Howarth PH, Holgate ST, Davies DE. Involvement of the epidermal growth factor receptor in epithelial repair in asthma. FASEBJ 2000; 14:1362–1374.
269. Parmentier S, Kaplan C, Catimel B, McGregor GL. New families of adhesion molecules play a vital role in platelet function. Immunol Today 1990; 11:225–227.
270. Chihara J, Fukuda K, Yasuba H, Kishigami N, Sugihara R, Kubo H, Nakajima S. Platelet factor 4 enhances eosinophil IgG and IgE Fc receptor and has eosinophil chemotactic activity. Am Rev Respir Dis 1988; 137:421A.
271. Denburg JA. Differentiation of human basophils and mast cells. Chem Immunol 1995; 61:49–71.
272. Tsuda T, Wong D, Dolovich J, Bienenstock J, Marshall J, Denburg JA. Synergistic effects of nerve growth factor and granulocyte-macrophage colony-stimulating factor on human basophilic cell differentiation. Blood 1991; 77:971–979.
273. Denburg JA, Silver JE, Abrams JS. Interleukin-5 is a human basophilopoietin: induction of histamine content and basophilic differentation of HL-60 cells and of peripheral blood basophil-eosinophil progenitors. Blood 1991; 77:1462–1468.
274. Bascom R, Wachs M, Naclerio RM, Pipkorn U, Galli SJ, Lichtenstein LM. Basophilic influx occurs after nasal antigen challenge: effects to topical corticosteriod pretreatment. J Allergy Clin Immunol 1988; 81:580–589.
275. Charlesworth EN, Kagey-Sobotka A, Schleimer RP, Normal PS, Lichenstein LM. Predisone inhibits the appearance of inflammatory mediators and the influx of eosinophils and basophils associated with the cutaneous late-phase response to allergen. J Immunol 1999; 146:671–676.
276. Macfarlane AJ, Kon OM, Smith SJ, Zeibecoglou K, Khan LN, Barata LT, McEuen AR, Buckley MG, Walls AF, Meng Q, Humbert M, Barnes NC, Robinson DS, Ying S, Kay AB. Basophils, eosinophils, and mast cells in atopic and nonatopic asthma and in late-phase allergic reactions in the lung and skin. J Allergy Clin Immunol 2000; 105:99–107.
277. Lett-Brown MA, Boetcher DA, Leonard EJ. Chemotactic responses of normal human basophils to C5a and to lymphocytes-derived chemotactic factor. J Immunol 1976; 117:246–252.
278. Tanimoto Y, Takahashi K, Kimura I. Effects of cytokines on human basophil chemotaxis. Clin Exp Allergy 1992; 11:1020–1025.
279. Foresi A, Leone C, Pelucchi A, Mastropasqua B, Chetta A, D'Ippolito R, Marazzini L, Olivieri D. Eosinophils, mast cells, and basophils in induced sputum from patients with seasonal allergic rhinitis and perennial asthma: relationship to methacholine responsiveness. J Allergy Clin Immunol 1997; 100:58–64.
280. Heaney LG, Cross LJ, Ennis M. Histamine release from bronchoalveolar lavage cells from asthmatic subjects after allergen challenge and relationship to the late asthmatic response. Clin Exp Allergy 1998; 28:196–204.

281. Rossi GA, Crimi E, Lantero S, Gianiorio P, Oddera S, Crimi P, Brusasco V. Late-phase asthmatic reaction to inhaled allergen is associated with early recruitment of eosinophils in the airways. Am Rev Respir Dis 1991; 144:379–383.

282. Metzger WJ, Hunninghake GW, Richerson HB. Late asthmatic responses: inquiry into mechanisms and significance. Clin Rev Allergy 1985; 3:145–165.

283. Keatings VM, Barnes PJ. Granulocyte activated markers in induced sputum: comparison between chronic obstructive pulmonary disease, asthma, and normal subjects. Am J Respi Crit Care Med 1997; 155:449–453.

284. Carroll N, Carello S, Cooke C, James A. Airway structure and inflammatory cells in fatal attacks of asthma. Eur Respir J 1996; 9:709–715.

285. Sur S, Crotty TB, Kephart GM, Hyma BA, Colby TV, Reed CE, Hunt LW, Gleich GJ. Sudden-onset fatal asthma. A distinct entity with few eosinophils and relatively more neutrophils in the airway submucosa? Am Rev Respir Dis 1993; 148:713–719.

286. Wenzel SE, Szefler SJ, Leung DY, Sloan SI, Rex MD, Martin RJ. Bronchoscopic evaluation of severe asthma. Persistent inflammation associated with high dose glucocorticoids. Am J Respir Crit Care Med 1997; 156:737–743.

287. Fahy JV, Kim KW, Liu J, Boushey HA. Prominent neutrophilic inflammation in sputum from subjects with asthma exacerbation. J Allergy Clin Immunol 1995; 954:843–852.

288. O'Byrne PM. Leukotriene bronchoconstriction induced by allergen and exercise. Am J Respir Crit Care Med 2000; 161:S68–72.

289. Martin RJ, Cicutto LC, Smith HR, Ballard RD, Szefler SJ. Airway inflammation in nocturnal asthma. Am Rev Respir Dis 1991; 143:351–357.

290. Calhoun WJ, Bush RK. Enhanced reactive oxygen species metabolism of airspace cells and airway inflammation following antigen challenge in human asthma. J Allergy Clin Immunol 1990; 86:306–313.

291. Melewicz FM, Kline LE, Cohen AB, Spiegelberg HL. Characterization of Fc receptors for IgE on human alveolar macrophages. Clin Exp Immunol 1982; 49:364–370.

292. Gosset P, Tsicopoulos A, Wallaert B, Vannimenus C, Joseph M, Tonnel AB, Capron A. Increased secretion of tumor necrosis factor alpha and interleukin-6 by alveolar macrophages consecutive to the development of the late asthmatic reaction. J Allergy Clin Immunol 1991; 88:561–571.

293. Broide DH, Lotz M, Cuomo AJ, Coburn DA, Federman EC, Wasserman SI. Cytokines in symptomatic asthma airways. J Allergy Clin Immunol 1992; 89:958–967.

294. Borish L, Mascali JJ, Rosenwasser LJ. IgE-dependent cytokine production by human peripheral blood mononuclear phagocytes. J Immunol 1991; 146:63–67.

295. Cohen SG, Evans R 3rd. Asthma, allergy and immunotherapy; a historical review: Part I. Allergy Proc 1991; 6:407–415.

296. Mautino G, Henriquet C, Gougat C, Le Cam A, Dayer JM, Bousquet J, Capony F. Increased expression of tissue inhibitor of metalloproteinase-1 and loss of correlation with matrix metalloproteinase-9 by macrophages in asthma. Lab Invest 1999; 1:39–47.

297. Weersink EJ, Postma DS. Nocturnal asthma: not a separate disease entity. Respir Med 1994; 88:483–491.

298. Venkayya R, Lam M, Willkom M, Grunig G, Corry DB, Erle DJ. The Th2 lymphocyte products IL-4 and IL-13 rapidly induce airway hyperresponsiveness through direct effects on resident airway cells. Am J Respir Cell Mol Biol 2002; 26:202–208.

299. Gibson PG, Manning PJ, O'Byrne PM, Girgis-Gabardo A, Dolovich J, Denburg JA, Hargreave FE. Allergen-induced asthmatic responses: relationship between increases

in airway responsivness and increases in circulating eosinophils, basophils and their progenitors. Am Rev Respir Dis 1991; 143:331–335.

300. Kerrebijn KF, Fioole AC, van Bentveld RD. Lung function in asthmatic children after year of more without symptoms or treatment. BMJ 1978; 1(6117):886–888.

301. Gruber W, Eber E, Steinbrugger B, Modl M, Weinhandl E, Zach MS. Atopy, lung function and bronchial responsiveness in symptom-free paediatric asthma patients. Eur Respir J 1997; 10:1041–1045.

302. Van den Toorn LM, Prins JB, Overbeek SE, Hoogsteden HC, de Jongste JC. Adolescents in clinical remission of atopic asthma have elevated exhaled nitric oxide levels and bronchial hyperresponsiveness. Am J Respir Crit Care Med 2000; 162: 953–957.

303. Bousquet J, Corrigan CJ, Venge P. Peripheral blood markers: evaluation of inflammation in asthma. Eur Respir J Suppl 1998; 26:42S–48S.

304. Crimi E, Spanevello A, Neri M, Ind PW, Rossi GA, Brunasco V. Dissociation between airway inflammation and airway hyperresponsiveness in allergic asthma. Am J Respir Crit Care Med 1998; 157:4–9.

305. Möller GM, Overbeek SE, van Helden-Meeuwsen CG, Hoogsteden HC, Bogaard JM. Eosinophils in the bronchial mucosa in relation to methacholine dose-response curves in atopic asthma. J Appl Physiol 1999; 86:1352–1356.

306. Van Den Toorn LM, Overbeek SE, De Jongste JC, Leman K, Hoogsteden HC, Prins J-B. Airway inflammation is present during clinical remission of atopic asthma. Am J Respir Crit Care Med 2001; 164:2107–2113.

307. Schwartz H, Lowell F, Melby J. Steroid resistence in bronchial asthma. Ann Intern Med 1968; 69:493–499.

308. Woolcock AJ. Corticosteroid-resistant asthma. Am J Respir Crit Care Med 1996; 154: S45–48.

309. Barnes PJ. Mechanisms of action of glucocorticoids in asthma. Am J Respir Crit Care Med 1996; 154:S21–27.

310. Folkerts G, Busse WW, Nijkamp FP, Sorkness R, Gern JE. State of the art: virus-induced airway hyperresponsivness and asthma. Am J Respir Crit Care Med 1998; 157:1708–1720.

311. Pattemore PK, Johnston SL, Bardin PG. Viruses as precipitants of asthma symptoms, I: epidemiology. Clin Exp Allergy 1992; 22:325–336.

312. Johnston SL, Pattemore PK, Sanderson G, Pattemore PK, Sanderson G, Smith S, Lampe F, Josephs L, Symington P, O'Toole S, Myint SH, Tyrrell DA, et al. Community study of role of viral infections in exacerbations of asthma in 9–11 year old children. BMJ 1995; 310:1225–1229.

313. Nicholson KG, Kent J, Ireland DC. Respiratory viruses and exacerbations of asthma in adults. BMJ 1993; 307:982–986.

314. Cheung D, Dick EC, Timmers MC, de Klerk EP, Spaan WJ, Stert PJ. Rhinovirus inhalation causes long-lasting excessive airway narrowing in response to methacholine in asthmatic subjects in vivo. Am J Respir Crit Care Med 1995; 152:1490–1496.

315. Calhoun WJ, Swenson CA, Dick EC, Schwartz LB, Lemanske RF Jr, Busse WW. Experimental rhinovirus 16 infection potentiates histamine release after antigen bronchoprovocation in allergic subjects. Am Rev Respir Dis 1991; 144:1267–1273.

316. Calhoun WJ, Dick EC, Schwartz LB, Busse WW. A common cold virus, rhinovirus 16, potentiates airway inflammation after segmental antigen bronchoprovocation in allergic subjects. J Clin Invest 1994; 94:2200–2208.

317. Gern JE, Galagan DM, Jarjour NN, Dick EC, Busse WW. Detection of rhinovirus RNA in lower airway cells during experimentally-induced infection. Am J Respir Crit Care Med 1997; 155:1159–1161.

318. Fraenkel DJ, Bardin PG, Sanderson G, Lampe F, Johnston SL, Holgate ST. Lower airways inflammation during rhinovirus colds in normal and in asthmatic subjects. Am J Respir Crit Care Med 1995; 151:879–886.

319. Hakonarson H, Makeri N, Carter C, Hokinka RL, Campbell D, Grunstein MM. Mechanism of rhinovirus-induced changes in airway smooth muscle responsiveness. J Clin Invest 1998; 102:1732–1741.

320. Yamaya M, Sekizawa K, Suzuki T, Yamada N, Furukawa M, Ishizuka S, Nakayama K, Terajima M, Numazaki Y, Sasaki H. Infection of human respiratory submucosal glands with rhinovirus: effects on cytokine and ICAM-1 production. Am J Physiol 1999; 277:L362–371.

321. Zhu Z, Tang W, Ray A, Wu Y, Einarsson O, Landry ML, Gwaltney J Jr, Elias JA. Rhinovirus stimulation of interleukin-6 in vivo and in vitro. Evidence for nuclear factor kappa B-dependent transcriptional activation. J Clin Invest 1996; 97:421–430.

322. Zhu Z, Tang W, Gwaltney JMJ, Wu Y, Elias JA. Rhinovirus stimulation of interleukin-8 in vivo and in vitro: role of NF-κB. Am J Physiol 1997; 273:L814–824.

323. Jamaluddin M, Casola A, Garofalo RP, Han Y, Elliott T, Ogra PL, Brasier AR. The major component of IkappaBalpha proteolysis occurs independently of the proteasome pathway in respiratory syncytial virus-infected pulmonary epithelial cells. J Virol 1998; 72:4849–4857.

324. Grünberg K, Timmers MC, Smits HH, de Klerk EP, Dick EC, Spaan WJ, Hiemstra PS, Sterk PJ. Effect of experimental rhinovirus 16 colds on airway hyperresponsiveness to histamine and interleukin-8 in nasal lavage in asthmatic subjects in vivo. Clin Exp Allergy 1997; 27:36–45.

325. Winther B, Farr B, Thoner RB, Hendley JO, Gwaltney JM Jr, Mygind N. Histopathologic examination and enumeration of polymorphonuclear leukocytes in the nasal mucosa during experimental rhinovirus colds. Acta Otolaryngol (Stockh) 1984; 413 (suppl):19–24.

326. Everard ML, Swarbrick A, Wrightman M, McIntyre J, Dunkley C, James PD, Sewell HF, Milner AD. Analysis of cells obtained by bronchial lavage of infants with respiratory syncytial virus infection. Arch Dis Child 1994; 71:428–432.

327. Schuster A, Fahy JV, Ueki K, Nadel JA. Cystic fibrosis sputum induces a secretory response from airway gland serous cells that can be prevented by neutrophil protease inhibitors. Eur Respir J 1995; 8:10–14.

328. Hayden FG, Albrecht JK, Kaiser DL, Gwaltney JM Jr. Prevention of natural colds by contact prophylaxis with intranasal alpha 2-interferon. N Engl J Med 1986; 314:71–75.

329. Domachowske JB, Dyer KD, Bonville CA, Rosenberg HF. Recombinant human eosinophil-derived neurotoxin/RNase 2 functions as an effective antiviral agent against respiratory syncytial virus. J Infect Dis 1998; 177:1458–1464.

330. Grünberg K, Smits HH, Timeers MC, de Klerk EP, Dolhain RJ, Dick EC, Hiemstra PS, Sterk PJ. Experimental rhinovirus 16 infection: effects on cell differentials and soluble markers in sputum in asthmatic subjects. Am J Respir Crit Care Med 1997; 156:609–616.

331. Garofalo R, Kimpen JLL, Welliever RC, Ogra PL. Eosinophil degranulation in the respiratory tract during naturally acquired respiratory syncytial virus infection. J Pediatr 1992; 120:28–32.

332. Gern JE, Vrtis R, Kelly EAB, Dick EC, Busse WW. Rhinovirus produces non specific activation of lymphocytes through a monocyte-dependent mechanism. J Immunol 1996; 157:1605–1612.
333. Topham DJ, Tripp RA, Sarawar DR, Sangster MY, Doherty PC. Immune CD4(+) T cells promote the clearance of influenza virus from major histocompatibility complex class II -/- respiratory epithelium. J Virol 1996; 70:1288–1291.
334. Busse WW, Lemanske RF, Jr. Asthma. N Engl J Med 2001; 344:350–362.

2

Primary Human Lung Cells in the Evaluation of Airway Inflammation

TANNISHIA M. GOGGANS and SERPIL C. ERZURUM

Cleveland Clinic Foundation
Cleveland, Ohio, U.S.A.

I. Airway Epithelial Cells Obtained by Bronchoscopy

Human airway epithelial cells may be obtained from the trachea and bronchi during bronchoscopy of individuals by endobronchial biopsy or brushing of the airway surface. Endobronchial biopsies provide information on airway epithelial architecture and cell types in vivo (Fig. 1), are especially useful for localization of mRNA or protein expression by in situ hybridization or immunostaining respectively, but are less useful for in vitro studies. Cultures derived from biopsies occur by outgrowth of cells and are hampered by the presence of nonepithelial cells and limited growth (1). Bronchial cells may also be obtained by gently gliding a cytology brush over the airway surface. Relatively large numbers of cells may be sampled from the airway surface by repetitive brushing during bronchoscopy (2). In general, brushing the airway is less traumatic than endobronchial biopsies and is a convenient method to obtain epithelial cells for use in molecular analyses and especially in cell culture.

A. Differentials and Quantitation of Epithelial Cells

The airway is comprised of four major types of epithelial cells: ciliated, basal, secretory, and undifferentiated. Bronchial brushing provides a representative sample of the four major types of epithelial cells (Fig. 1). Differential cell counts performed

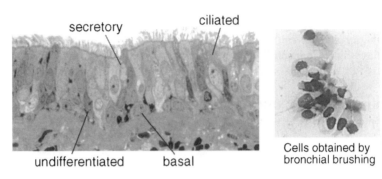

secretory   ciliated

undifferentiated   basal

Cells obtained by
bronchial brushing

Figure 1   Endobronchial biopsy from a healthy human airway (left panel). Arrows indicate the four major types of epithelial cells: ciliated, basal, secretory, and undifferentiated. Cells obtained by bronchial brushing at bronchoscopy are primarily airway epithelial cells (right panel). (All magnifications ×400.)

by experienced pathologists are reproducible with no significant interobserver variation (3). The normal airway epithelial bronchial brushing sample is composed of epithelial cells predominantly, with less than 3% inflammatory cells. The predominant inflammatory cell usually recovered by brushing is the lymphocyte, followed by the macrophage. Bronchial brushing from individuals with airway disease may have alterations in cell differentials. In individuals with asthma, epithelial cells are still the predominant cell type, but inflammatory cells may vary depending upon atopy and exposure to allergens. Cigarette-smoking individuals have increased numbers of secretory epithelial cells, but inflammatory cell numbers similar to those of healthy control nonsmokers (4). In cystic fibrosis (CF), the percentage of cells recovered by bronchial brushing is equally divided between epithelial and neutrophils (3).

It is often important to be able to accurately determine the number of epithelial cells in a particular sample, e.g., in order to estimate gene expression in epithelial cells. However, freshly isolated epithelial cells obtained by brushing include intact islands of cells, single intact cells, broken cells, debris, and mucus (3). This morphological heterogeneity makes accurate total cell counting difficult. To circumvent this hurdle, the number of cells in a cell lysate sample can be determined by quantifying the number of the repetitive DNA sequence *Alu* compared to a standard curve of human genomic DNA. To accomplish this, cell lysates and purified human genomic DNA are denatured, bound to a nylon membrane using a slot blotter, cross-linked to the membrane by ultraviolet irradiation, and evaluated by hybridization with ^{32}P-labeled *Alu* sequence DNA-specific probe. Quantification of signal can be done by the use of a Phosphoimager or by densitometry. The amount of DNA in the sample is determined by comparison to the standard curve. Since human cells contain approximately 7.2 pg of DNA per cell, the number of cells can be estimated from the amount of DNA in the sample (2,5–7). In general, 1–1.5 × 10^6 cells are obtained per each bronchial brush of the healthy human airway (2).

B. Analyses of Freshly Obtained Airway Epithelial Cells

Once human airway epithelial cells (HAEC) are obtained by bronchial brushing, they may be used immediately for evaluation of gene expression and function. Since alteration of gene expression can occur when cells are removed from the body, it is important that cells obtained by bronchial brushing be processed promptly. Upon lysis of cells, released RNases and proteases degrade RNA and proteins, respectively. Cells should be lysed, therefore, in "a protective buffer" appropriate for their intended use. Cells destined for RNA analysis should be handled in an RNase-free environment and lysed in a buffer containing guanidium thiocyanate, a powerful inactivator of RNases. Cells processed for protein analysis need to be lysed in the presence of antiproteases. An alternative approach is to freeze cells as a pellet to be thawed in a specific buffer depending on the intended use. The latter approach, however, carries a risk of degradation if samples are accidentally thawed.

Evaluation of amino acids, proteins, eicosanoids, and RNA in HAEC can yield useful information regarding the pathogenesis of lung diseases (8–13). Sufficient cells are obtained by bronchial brush to perform chromatography for specific amino acids, Western analyses for protein levels, or enzyme activity measures (8–11). Expression of mRNA may be determined using Northern analyses and/or polymerase chain reaction (PCR) techniques. For example, expression of nitric oxide synthase II, the enzyme that synthesizes nitric oxide, has been evaluated in healthy controls and asthmatics using Northern analyses (9).

C. In Vitro Studies of Airway Epithelial Cells

Cells may be studied to define changes following their removal to an ex vivo environment or in response to a controlled specific stimulus. This can be done by maintaining the cells in culture while performing the desired studies. HAEC from healthy control individuals may be maintained in culture under conditions that maintain cell growth and differentiation. Cells are grown on collagen-coated dishes in specialized serum-free media available from a number of sources (Biofluids, BRFF, Clonetics) (8). Cell cultures of bronchial brush samples lead to pure epithelial monolayer cultures (Fig. 2). In most culture systems, HAEC do not maintain a ciliary structure and do not produce or secrete mucins. However, redifferentiation into ciliated or mucin-secreting phenotypes is possible (14,15). Primary airway epithelial cells grown on a collagen substrate, on top of a permeant filter with the medium placed beneath the cells and only a humidified air environment above, result in well-differentiated epithelial cells essentially identical in structure and function to airway epithelium in situ (14,15).

The epithelial nature of cultured HAEC is confirmed by morphology and positive reactions to anticytokeratins, which are epithelial cell specific (8). Nontransformed HAEC are limited to ± 25 population doublings, a culture span of about 1 month, and a maximum of 5 passages (1). HAEC in culture have provided a powerful experimental system to study airway biology in response to environmental pollutants, cytokines, and inflammatory mediators (11,14,17–20). Recently, HAEC have also been used for investigation of intracellular signaling pathways by electrophoretic

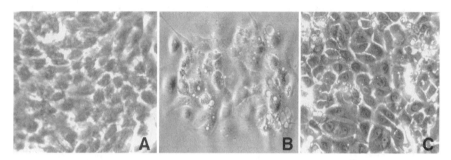

Figure 2   Culture of airway epithelial cells obtained from explanted lung at transplantation. Epithelial cells are placed onto precoated cell culture dishes. (A) Upon initial plating, sheets of epithelial cells attach, but maintain cilia and ciliary beating. (B) Following several days of culture, cells begin to change in morphology. (C) Finally, after several weeks of culture under media, cells become confluent with a uniform appearance. (Phase contrast, magnification ×40.)

mobility shift assays (9). Transfection of primary cells is less efficient than transformed or immortal cell lines, but up to 5% of HAEC may be transfected using the liposome system.

II.   Study of Human Airway Cells Obtained from Explanted Lungs

Hypotheses to be tested at the molecular and cellular level in human respiratory epitheliums may be only feasible with large numbers of cells. Direct access to large numbers of primary airway cells of diseased or control lungs is possible due to increasingly active clinical programs in lung transplantation. Lung tissue for experiments may be obtained from explanted diseased lungs. Nondiseased control lungs are also available as donor lungs not used in transplantation or lung tissue from autopsy of trauma individuals. Freshly obtained explant lung is dissected and segments of trachea are isolated. Fat and connective tissue are removed as much as possible and trachea segments washed with Hank's balanced salt solution (HBSS) several times to remove all blood and connective tissue followed by incubation in 0.1% protease solution with penicillin, streptomycin, and fungizone at 4°C overnight. Protease is neutralized with heat-inactivated fetal calf serum and the trachea segments incubated briefly in HBSS containing 10 mM EDTA at 37°C. For lungs infected or chronically colonized by bacteria, e.g., cystic fibrosis lungs, other antibiotics may be necessary during incubation steps, including ciprofloxacin and tobramycin (21). Subsequently, the epithelial side of the trachea is carefully scraped with a sterile cell lifter to retrieve all cells. Cells are also collected from all previous washes/supernatants and seeded on 100 cm plates, which are precoated with coating media containing collagen (vitrogen), bovine serum albumin, and fibronectin, in serum-free specialized media (from Biofluids, BRFF, or Clonetics) with antibiotic and antimycotic to prevent bacteria contamination. Using this technique upwards of 5×10^8 cells may be obtained depending on the size of the trachea/bronchus that was isolated. Doubling time and culture characteristics are similar to those obtained for cells obtained bronchoscopically.

III. Inflammatory Cells and Epithelial Lining Fluid Obtained by Bronchoalveolar Lavage

Bronchoalveolar lavage (BAL) is an invaluable means of evaluating inflammatory and immune processes in the airways. Lavage recovers cells resident in the bronchoalveolar space, which can be used for a variety of morphological and functional studies after separation from fluid by simple centrifugation (20,22,23). A sample of cells is evaluated by light microscopy for total cell number, differential cell count, cell morphology, and the presence of any abnormal substances. In normal subjects, lavage yields macrophages (>95%), lymphocytes (<5%), and fewer than 1% neutrophils, eosinophils and/or basophils (22,23) (Fig. 3). High lymphocyte count is frequently found in hypersensitivity pneumonitis and sarcoidosis. Elevated numbers of neutrophils are common in CF, idiopathic pulmonary fibrosis, connective tissue disorders, and adult respiratory distress syndrome.

Specific types of cells can be isolated from lavage fluids for further characterization, using an array of techniques depending on the cells needed. These techniques include adherence to plastic, band-density-gradient centrifugation, and the use of

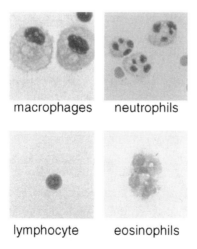

macrophages   neutrophils

lymphocyte   eosinophils

Figure 3 Cells from bronchoalveolar lavage of the lung. Macrophages are the predominant cell type usually obtained by lavage, followed by lymphocytes, and very small numbers of neutrophils or eosinophils.

cell-specific antibodies immobilized on the surface of superparamagnetic microspheres. This allows for further subdivision of cell populations, e.g., separation of lymphocytes into B cells and T cells and further categorization of T cells into CD4+ and CD8+ T cells. Inflammatory cells from BAL can also be evaluated for gene expression at the mRNA or protein level, the presence of a specific DNA sequence, or for activation of intracellular signaling pathways. Evaluation of amino acids, proteins, metals, cytokines, and other mediators in BAL can yield useful information regarding the inflammatory status of the lung (10,13,22–25). Analysis of BAL fluid are usually expressed relative to the volume of epithelial lining fluid (ELF), which is estimated by comparing concentrations of urea in samples of lavage fluid and plasma obtained simultaneously (26).

IV. Conclusions

Advances in molecular biology techniques together with immortalized lung cell lines and genetically altered animals have revealed exciting new information regarding pathogenesis of airway inflammation. However, direct study of lung cells is still necessary to put basic scientific findings into the physiologically relevant context of airway biology in health and disease. The ability to obtain and culture primary human lung cells is a powerful methodology that allows direct evaluation of molecular and cellular events in the healthy and diseased human lung.

Acknowledgments

The authors thank J. Drazba and J. Lang for assistance with cell photography and artwork.

References

1. Jorissen M, Schueren BVD, Berghe HVD, Cassiman JJ. Contribution of in vitro culture methods for respiratory epithelial cells to the study of the physiology of the respiratory tract. Eur Respir J 1991; 4:210–217.
2. Erzurum SC, Danel C, Chu CS, Trapnell BC, Crystal RG. In vivo antioxidant gene expression in human airway epithelium of normal individuals exposed to 100% O_2. J Appl Physiol 1993; 75:1256–1262.
3. Danel C, Erzurum SC, McElvaney NG, Crystal RG. Quantitative assessment of the epithelial and inflammatory cell populations in large airways of normals and individuals with cystic fibrosis. Am J Respir Crit Care Med 1996; 153:362–368.
4. Riise GC, Larsson S, Andersson BA. A bronchoscopic brush biopsy study of large airway mucosal pathology in smokers with chronic bronchitis and in healthy nonsmokers. Eur Respir J 1992; 5:382–386.
5. DeRaeve HR, Thunnissen FBJM, Guo FH, Lewis M, Kavuru M, Secic M, Thomassen MJ, Erzurum SC. Decreased superoxide dismutase activity in asthmatic airway epithelium: correction by inhaled corticosteroid in vivo. Am J Physiol 1997; 272:L148–L154.

6. Trapnell BC, Chu CS, Pääkkö PK, Banks TC, Yoshimura K, Ferrans VJ, Chernick MS, Crystal RG. Expression of the cystic fibrosis transmembrane conductance regulator gene in the respiratory tract of normal individuals and individuals with cystic fibrosis. Proc Natl Acad Sci USA 1991; 88:6565–6569.

7. Eissa NT, Chu CS, Danel C, Crystal RG. Evaluationof the respiratory epithelium of normals and individuals with cystic fibrosis for the presence of adenovirus E1a sequences relevant to the use of E1a⁻ adenovirus vectors for gene therapy for the respiratory manifestations of cystic fibrosis. Hum Gene Ther 1994; 5:1105–1114.

8. Guo FH, Uetani K, Haque J, Williams BRG, Dweik RA, Thunnisen F, Calhoun W, Erzurum SC. Interferon γ and interleukin-4 stimulate prolonged expression of inducible nitric oxide synthase in human airway epithelium through synthesis of soluble mediators. J Clin Invest 1997; 100:829–838.

9. Guo FH, Comhair SAA, Zheng S, Dweik RA, Eissa NT, Thomassen MJ, Calhoun W, Erzurum SC. Molecular mechanisms of increased nitric oxide (NO) in asthma: evidence for transcriptional and post-translational regulation of NO synthesis. J Immunol 2000; 164:5970–5980.

10. Comhair SAA, Bhathena PR, Dweik RA, Kavuru MS, Erzurum SC. Rapid loss of superoxide dismutase activity during antigen-induced asthmatic response. Lancet 2000; 355:624.

11. Comhair SAA, Thomassen MJ, Erzurum SC. Differential induction of extracellular glutathione peroxidase and nitric oxide synthase 2 in airways of healthy individuals exposed to 100% O_2 or cigarette smoke. Am J Respir Cell Mol Biol 2000; 23:350–354.

12. Guo FH, DeRaeve H, Rice TW, Stuehr D, Thunnissen FB. J. M, Erzurum SC. Continuous NO synthesis by inducible nitric oxide synthase in normal human airways in vivo. Proc Natl Acad Sci USA 1995; 92:7809–7813.

13. Melloni B, Lefebvre MA, Bonnaud F, Vergnenegre A, Grossin L, Rigaud M, Cantin A. Antioxidant activity in bronchoalveolar lavage fluid from patients with lung cancer. Am J Respir Crit Care Med 1996; 154:1706–1711.

14. Krunkosky TM, Fischer BM, Martin LD, Jones N, Akley NJ, Adler KB. Effects of TNF-alpha on expression of ICAM-1 in human airway epithelial cells in vitro: signaling pathways controlling surface and gene expression. Am J Respir Cell Mol Biol 2000; 22:685–692.

15. Adler KB, Li Y. Airway epithelium and mucus. Intracellular signling pathways for gene expression and secretion. Am J Respir Cell Mol Biol 2001; 25:397–400.

16. Comhair SAA, Bhathena PR, Farver C, Thunnissen FB. J. M, Erzurum SC. Extracellular glutathione peroxidase induction in asthmatic lungs: evidence for redox regulation of expression in human airway epithelial cells. FASEB J 2001; 15:70–78.

17. Wu W, Samet JM, Ghio AJ, Devlin RB. Activation of the EGF receptor signaling pathway in airway epithelial cells exposed to Utah Valley PM. Am J Physiol Lung Cell Mol Physiol 2001; 281:L483–489.

18. Prahalad AK, Inmon J, Dailey LA, Madden MC, Ghio AJ, Gallagher JE. Air pollution particles mediated oxidative DNA base damage in a cell free system and in human airway epithelial cells in relation to particulate metal content and bioreactivity. Chem Res Toxicol 2001; 14:879–887.

19. Fischer BM, Voynow JA. Neutrophil elastase induces MUC5AC gene expression in airway epithelium via a pathway involving reactive oxygen species. Am J Respir Cell Mol Biol 2002; 26:447–452.

20. Eissa NT, Erzurum SC. Flexible bronchoscopy in molecular biology. Clin Chest Medicine 2001; 22:343–353.

21. Randell SH, Walstad DL, Schwab UE, Grubb BR, Yankaskas JR. Isolation and culture of airway epithelial cells from chronically infected human lungs. In Vitro Cell Dev Biol 2001; 37:480–489.
22. Saltini C, Hance AJ, Ferrans VJ, Basset F, Bitterman PB, Crystal RG. Accurate quantification of cells recovered by bronchoalveolar lavage. Am Rev Respir Dis 1984; 130: 650–658.
23. Smith SF, Guz A, Winning AJ, Cooke NT, Burton GH, Tetley D. Comparison of human lung surface protein profiles from the central and peripheral airways sampled using two regional lavage techniques. Eur Respir J 1998; 1:792–800.
24. Comhair SAA, Lewis MJ, Bhathena PR, Hammel JP, Erzurum SC. Increased glutathione and glutathione peroxidase in lungs of individuals with chronic beryllium disease. Am J Respir Crit Care Med 1999; 159:1824–1829.
25. Gutteridge JMC, Mumby S, Quinlan GJ, Chung KF, Evans TW. Prooxidant iron is present in human pulmonary epithelial clining fluid: implications for oxidative stress in the lung. Biochem Biophys Res Comm 1996; 220:1024–1027.
26. Rennard SI, Basset G, Lecossier D, O'Donnell KM, Pinkston P, Martin PG, Crystal RG. Estimation of volume of epithelial lining fluid recovered by lavage using urea as marker of dilution. J Appl Physiol 1986; 60:532–538.

3

Airway pH Homeostasis in Asthma and Other Inflammatory Lung Diseases

JOHN HUNT and BENJAMIN GASTON

University of Virginia Health System
Charlottesville, Virginia, U.S.A.

I. Introduction

The addition or removal of protons (hydrogen ions)—rapid chemical reactions—modify the physical properties of macromolecules and alter the kinetics of nonenzymatic reactions. pH homeostasis is critically regulated in human organ systems to physiological advantage, although certain organs tolerate wider fluctuations in pH than others. For example, acidity is used in innate antimicrobial defense (1,2) in the stomach, where the gastric mucosa is protected from acid injury by barrier-forming and buffer-enhancing macromolecules (3), while blood pH requires such strict regulation that deviation by one pH unit results in death.

In the lung, as in the stomach, acids have an antimicrobial role. For example, low pH is critical to the function of lysosomes in phagocytic cells such as alveolar macrophages (4) and lytic granules of cytotoxic lymphocytes (5). However, the airway mucosa is very sensitive to acid injury (6–9). The airway is thought to protect itself from acid injury by forming pH-buffering glycoproteins and secretory bicarbonate (HCO_3^-)(6,10–13). Precise pH homeostatic mechanisms are poorly understood, in part because direct measurements are difficult to make. Recently there has been renewed interest in the role of airway pH in innate immunity and pathology. This chapter will review our current understanding of airway pH and propose future directions for research.

II. A Brief Overview of Proton Chemistry

Proton concentrations are presented, by convention, as the negative log of the H^+ concentration, or pH. A pH of 7 therefore represents a hydrogen ion concentration of 100 nanomolar (1×10^{-7}), a pH of 6 being 1 micromolar (1×10^{-6}), etc. Although protons are mixed with hydronium ions (H_3O^+) and other higher-order complexes of H_2O, we will refer to them as simple "protons" in solution. The concentration of these species is measured in the aggregate by proton-selective electrodes, colorimetric indicator dyes, and solid-state polymers.

Though a solution with a pH of 5 has, by definition, a 10 μM $[H^+]$, a greater number of protons may be available for reactions. For example, protons can be bound or released from buffering compounds in large numbers. Thus, the number of available protons in a solution of a strong acid, such as hydrochloric acid, is less than that in a weak acid, such as acetic acid, at the same pH. This is because the concentration of acetic acid needed to achieve a pH of 5 is much greater than that of hydrochloric acid. This represents the concept of titratable acidity: it is the available inventory of bound and free protons that is important, not just the number of free protons in solution at a given moment.

Bases behave similarly. Ammonia (NH_3; pKa = 9.4 at room temperature) will alkalinize water by removing protons from H_2O to form ammonium ion (NH_4^+). As protons are consumed by reaction with NH_3, hydroxide anion (OH^-) is released. With a complex mixture of basic and acidic solutes, the pH of the solution at equilibrium will depend on the concentrations and pKa of all the solutes.

The carbonic acid (H_2CO_3) buffer system is of particular interest in pulmonary physiology. Buffers maintain pH stability best within a log order of the relevant pKa. Thus, the NH_3/NH_4^+ buffer system functions best around pH 9.4. The H_2CO_3 buffer system (including its components HCO_3^- and CO_2) is the most important buffer in human blood, helping to maintain the pH at 7.4. However, the two protons of H_2CO_3 have pKa of 6.1 and 10.3—seemingly making them unsuitable to buffer at pH 7.4. The human being senses the concentrations of CO_2 and protons and modifies its behavior (by changing respiration rate or renal ammonia, phosphate, or bicarbonate excretion) to maintain pH at 7.4. If it were not for this sensing of—and physiological response to—a shift in the components of this buffer system in the blood, H_2CO_3 would be a poor buffer despite its high concentrations. Indeed, the so-called bicarbonate buffer system has limited ability to buffer added base. The utility of H_2CO_3 as a buffer in an organ that does not sense and respond to its component concentrations is minimal.

III. pH of the Healthy Airway

Measurement of airway pH in vivo—particularly in humans—has proved difficult. For example, even direct measurement by bronchoscopy is suspect because topical application of local anesthetics during the procedure is acidifying (14), and contamination of the measurement channel with oral secretions is common. Percutaneous transcricoid 24-hour tracheal pH monitoring in humans has revealed a mean baseline pH of 7.1 (15), although these patients had asthma and gastroesophageal reflux disease. One case report of an inadvertent passage of an esophageal pH electrode into the left mainstem bronchus of a presumed nonasthmatic elderly patient revealed values in the range of 7.8 throughout a 24-hour period, never falling below 7(16). Other endobronchial pH measurements have varied from as low as 6.2 to above 8 (17,18). Airway mapping by Guerrin revealed pH in trachea and bronchi of subjects who may have had lung disease to be near 7.0 (19). Measurements of secretions suctioned from the normal tracheo-bronchial tree of 126 subjects revealed geometric mean pH of 7.73 ± 0.54 (20). These data are very similar to pH of exhaled breath condensates from healthy subjects (7.65 ± 0.20) (21). The ex vivo tracheal pH of ferrets measured by pH probe is ~7.0 (22). The in vivo tracheal pH of rats has been shown to be 7.42–7.57 (23), in rabbits 7.7 (24), and in cows 7.67–8.27 (8).

IV. Airway pH in Disease

A. Asthma

Several studies have found that exhaled breath condensate pH is low in asthma (21,25,26), suggesting an abnormality in acid-base balance in the airway. Of note, condensates taken during acute asthma exacerbations were markedly acidic (mean 5.2 ± 0.21, but as low as 4.3; 3 log orders lower than normal) and normalized with corticosteroid therapy (Fig. 1). Values did not reflect an effect of hyperventilation (unpublished observations), salivary contamination, or collection system composition (27). In all of these studies, samples were deaerated, a process that removes carbon dioxide and alkalinizes the condensate. Acidification of condensate is consistent with the observations that (1) the pH of the nasal secretions is acidic during allergic and viral rhinitis, but slightly alkaline in bacterial rhinitis (28); (2) asthmatic sputum has been reported to be acidic (29,30); and (3) bronchoalveolar lavage fluid from guinea pigs following antigen challenge is substantially more acidic than is that from control animals (S. Sanjar, personal communication, 2000). Acidification in patients with stable, moderate asthma, particularly those treated with corticosteroids, and mild asthma also occurs, but is substantially less dramatic (25). The mechanisms by which this acidification may occur are discussed below.

B. Cystic Fibrosis

Because the cystic fibrosis transmembrane regulator (CFTR), which allows anions to enter the airway lumen, can regulate HCO_3^- efflux (11,31), a defect in airway alkalization has been proposed. Few in vivo data exist, but it has been reported that expectorated mucous pH in cystic fibrosis is low (32). However, in the CFTR knockout mouse model, airway pH does not differ from controls (33). Differentiation between chronic disease and acute exacerbations have not been explored. This is an area of active research.

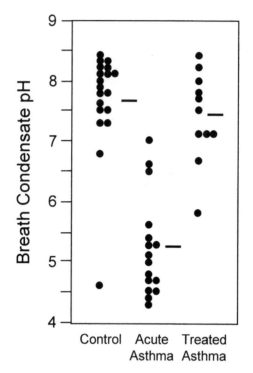

Figure 1 Exhaled breath condensate is acidified in acute asthma. Asthmatic subjects were studied on admission to the hospital for acute bronchospasm. Control subjects had no history of asthma and were free of respiratory symptoms. All subjects breathed orally through one-way valves and a 0.3 μm filter into a clean, dry condensing chamber. Condensate was deaerated for 10 min in Argon and the pH was measured under anaerobic conditions. This test was highly reproducible (average coefficient of variation 3.3%). Mean acute asthmatic pH (5.23 ± 0.21) was over 2 log lower than controls (7.65 ± 0.20) on admission and approached normal following treatment with systemic glucocorticoid therapy (7.4 ± 0.23; $p < 0.001$). (From Ref. 21.)

C. Chronic Obstructive Pulmonary Disease

Breath condensate pH of patients with chronic obstructive pulmonary disease (COPD) exacerbations is mildly acidic (mean pH 6.25) and rises steadily to near normal levels (mean pH 7.45) during 5 days of intense therapy (including antibiotics) (25,34).

D. Respiratory Failure/Pneumonia

The pH of respiratory mucus in critically ill intubated patients is 0.2–0.5 log order lower in patients with radiological evidence of pneumonia than in patients simply colonized with the same bacteria (35), with return to nonpneumonia levels with clinical recovery.

V. Effects of Acidification of the Airway

The potential toxicities of airway acidification are modeled by asthma. The pathophysiological features of asthma include inflammation, bronchial hyperreactivity, reversible airway obstruction, and mucus overproduction. Each of these features could result from airway acidosis: through augmented necrosis of inflammatory cells—particularly eosinophils—with release of cytotoxic mediators (36,37), enhanced toxicities of reactive nitrogen and oxygen species (38,39), decreased ciliary beating (40) (Fig. 2), increased mucus viscosity and conversion from sol to gel (8,41), acidity-induced epithelial dysfunction and sloughing (8), and augmentation

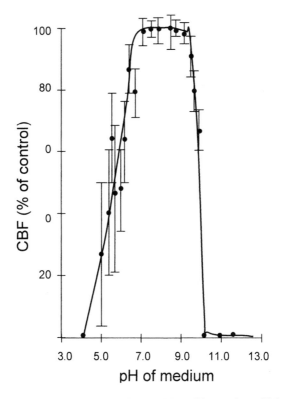

Figure 2 Effect of pH of medium on ciliary activity of human bronchial explants. Ciliary beat frequency (CBF) was measured at 37°C. The bars indicate standard deviation, and the line connecting the experimental datum points indicates the experimental trend. (From Ref. 40.)

of neurogenic bronchoconstriction and cough (42,43). Additionally, each of these toxicities may aggravate CF, COPD, bacterial pneumonia, and respiratory failure.

VI. Eosinophil-Mediated Toxicity

Peripheral blood eosinophils in cell culture medium at physiological pH generally undergo apoptosis within 96 hours. It is presumed that apoptotic eosinophils in vivo are rapidly recognized and consumed by phagocytic macrophages in what amounts to an anti-inflammatory process (44). We have noted that eosinophils are relatively intolerant of acidic conditions. After a 48-hour incubation at pH 5.2, isolated eosinophils undergo necrosis (21) with concomitant release of their proinflammatory granule products. An acidic environment would favor eosinophil necrosis, injuring the airway through release of cytotoxic mediators. Indeed, elevated levels of eosinophil degranulation products in sputum occur in association with natural acid fog exposure (9). In contrast, even mildly acidic pH (7.0) markedly attenuates eotaxin binding to eosinophil CCR3, with a resultant decrease in chemotaxis (45). This seemingly anti-inflammatory effect may partially contribute to the relative lack of eosinophils in comparison to neutrophils seen in severe asthma (46) and COPD, where data suggest that airway pH may be low.

VII. Nitrogen Oxide Chemistry

Airway acidosis has antimicrobial effects mediated through protonation reactions involving reactive nitrogen and oxygen species. Nitrite (NO_2^-), which is abundant in the airway (47,48), forms nitrous acid (HNO_2, pKa = 3.4) in acidic conditions. Nitric oxide (NO) is evolved from HNO_2 in a reaction that in part mediates the antimicrobial effects of gastric and urinary acidification (49). Consistent with this chemistry, acidification of the airway should deplete NO_2^- levels while increasing expired NO, and these alterations are indeed seen during acute asthma (21). Nitric oxide rapidly reacts with superoxide to form peroxynitrite anion ($OONO^-$). At even mildly acidic pH, however, $OONO^-$ is protonated to form the highly reactive species peroxynitrous acid ($OONOH$; pKa = 6.8), which can spontaneously decompose to relatively innocuous nitrate (NO_3^-)(39), or in the presence of molecular targets lead to rapid and potentially cytotoxic oxidation and nitration reactions. In fact, NO levels in the airways of patients with exacerbations of asthma are high (50), and evidence of oxidative and nitrative stress is abundant (51–54).

VIII. Oxidative Chemistry

In addition to nitrogen oxide–mediated injury, low pH favors the oxidative injury characteristic of the asthmatic airway (55–57). For example, acidification may favor formation of the most toxic of all radicals, hydroxyl, by two mechanisms. First, it favors H_2O_2 formation (58,59) by LeChatelier's principle:

$$2 O_2^- + 2 H^+ \rightarrow H_2O_2 + O_2$$

Hydroxyl formation from H_2O_2, in turn, is favored in an acidic environment because free iron is released from protein stores at pH less than or equal to 6 (60); the free iron catalyzes Fenton chemistry:

$$Fe^{+2} + H_2O_2 \rightarrow Fe^{+3} + OH^- + OH^\bullet$$
$$Fe^{+3} + O_2^- \rightarrow Fe^{+2} + O_2$$

In asthma, increased superoxide formation (57), together with loss of airway superoxide dismutase activity (61), may enhance the effect of airway acidification in favoring this cytotoxic chemistry.

IX. Mucociliary Clearance

Ciliary beat frequency in human bronchial explants is optimal at a pH between 7.0 and 9.0 and is variably inhibited when the surrounding fluid is acidified (40,62) (Fig. 2). Proximal bronchial cilia poorly tolerate a pH below 7. Cilia from more distal bronchioles show near-normal ciliary beat frequency at pH values as low as 5 (62), but the epithelium itself is highly dysfunctional, with cells tending to slough from the airway wall with prolonged exposure (24 hours) at pH 6.7, an effect that inhibits overall mucociliary clearance (8).

Additionally, there are pH-dependent changes in the viscoelastic properties of respiratory mucus. Mucus is minimally viscous at pH is 7.4 and increases in viscosity with either alkalinization or acidification (63). Furthermore, these viscosity effects are more pronounced if the mucus is already acid-saturated (i.e., negligible residual buffer capacity) as has been reported to occur in asthma (63).

X. Bronchoconstriction, Cough, and Asthma Risk

Acidic air pollution is a risk factor for bronchitis and asthma in several studies from different parts of the world (64–70). Experimental studies of acid fogs, however, have produced conflicting results. Lowry et al. report that only at pH of 2.6 are there notable effects of acidic aerosol on cough frequency in normal humans (71). Of note, this study used normal saline solutions with low titratable proton content. On the other hand, citric acid solutions have been used for decades to induce cough and to test the utility of antitussive compounds (72). The utility of citric acid to induce cough may result from the present of high numbers of titratable protons because of the relatively high pKa of its multiple acidic hydrogen ions (3,13,47,64). Indeed, Fine et al. have shown clearly that titratable acidity, not simply pH, is a relevant factor eliciting bronchoconstriction during acid inhalation challenges (73). Thus, regardless of the precise pH, sulfuric acid aerosols in the occupational exposure range (74–77) and acetic acid exposure (78) both result in changes in pulmonary function and/or respiratory symptomatology. Remarkably, recommendations exist to treat chlorine gas exposure (which essentially functions as an acid insult) with

NaHCO$_3$ inhalation (79–81). In this regard, NaHCO$_3$ aerosol given by nebulizer improves pulmonary function in patients with acute exacerbations of asthma (82,83) and has beneficial effect in producing bronchodilatation in stable asthma (Hunt and Gaston, unpublished observation).

XI. Other Effects

Airway chemoreceptors may also respond to a fall in pH by releasing neuropeptides. Indeed, protons activate ion channels to stimulate sensory nerves, sharing a common mode of action with capsaicin (43). Further, acidic challenge may (1) activate outwardly rectifying epithelial chloride channels, as has been demonstrated in the fetal lung (84), a process expected to increase secretion volume; (2) induce nitric oxide synthase (85); and (3) lead to induction of certain stress proteins (86).

XII. Mechanisms of pH Control in the Airway

A. Secretion of Acids

Several processes present an acid load to the airway. There are high levels of CO$_2$ in the distal airway. Lamellar bodies are acidified by H$^+$ channels and V-ATPases before being discharged into the alveolar space (87). Similarly, airway inflammatory cell granules can contribute to the acid load. Eosinophil ectocytic granules maintain a low pH (5.1) by means of a V-ATPase, and this acidification appears necessary for degranulation to occur (88). Likewise, macrophage lysosomes (89) and cytotoxic lymphocyte lytic granules maintain low pH (4.8–5.5)(5,90). Macrophages have a cytosolic membrane H$^+$ V-ATPase that serves to acidify paracellular space, allowing the extracellular activity of lysosomal acid hydrolases (91). Although the significance is uncertain, it may be of interest that several of these acidification mechanisms are inhibited by nitric oxide or related species in certain systems (92,93). Some airway epithelial cells also have a Na$^+$/H$^+$ exchange mechanism that excretes protons into the extracellular space (94), and there is evidence for tracheal proton secretion through Na$^+$/H$^+$ exchange in sheep (95).

We have recently identified the presence of an unsuspected acid in high concentrations in the exhaled breath of asthma patients during acute exacerbations of their disease. Acetic acid in equilibrium with its conjugate base acetate (pKa = 4.6) was detected in the majority of asthmatic patients (median 8.5, range 0–24.5 μg/ mL, $n = 11$) and concentrations correlated well with pH ($r^2 = 0.46$, $p < 0.001$). In contrast, acetic acid was undetectable in 16 of 18 controls (96). The source of the acetic acid remains obscure.

B. Secretion of Bases

Secretion of HCO$_3{}^-$ could serve to neutralize protons in airway lining fluid with release of CO$_2$ into the exhaled air. In this regard, anion exchange proteins in human airway epithelial cells permit HCO$_3{}^-$ secretion into the airway lumen (97). Further, the CFTR permits HCO_3^- efflux (31,98,99) and may contribute to Golgi apparatus pH control with implications for posttranslational modifications of proteins and *Pseudomonas* pathogenicity (100). Conduction for HCO_3^- is 10-fold less than for Cl^-, but, with a steeper gradient, its absence has been proposed to acidify the CF ALF (11). Of note, acetylcholine enhances apical HCO_3^- secretion along with water (101), and inhibitors of HCO_3^- secretion, in turn, decrease water secretion (13). Unfortunately, precise measurements of airway lining fluid HCO_3^- concentrations are not available in diseased lung and are uncertain even in healthy lung. Further, there is as yet no evidence that HCO_3^- secretion increases in response to local airway acidosis.

Ammonia (NH_3, pKa = 9.4) is an additional base present in the airway (26,102,103) that can readily diffuse through membranes. We have shown that during acute exacerbations of asthma, the quantity of exhaled NH_3 is low compared to healthy controls (26) (Fig. 3). One source of airway NH_3 is glutaminase, which catalyzes the breakdown of glutamine to glutamate and NH_3. In the proximal renal epithelium, this enzyme is upregulated in response to metabolic acidosis, making NH_3 available to neutralize excreted protons, thus preventing excessive acidification

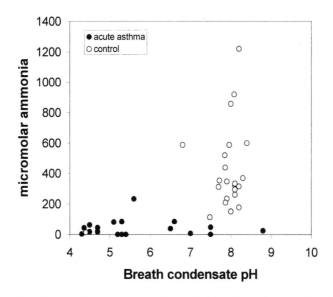

Figure 3 pH and ammonia concentration in exhaled breath condensate of patients during acute exacerbations of asthma are low. Exhaled breath condensate was collected from patients admitted to the hospital or seen in the emergency department with acute exacerbations of asthma or from healthy volunteers. Ammonia was measured spectrophotometrically. The median ammonia concentration in asthmatic subjects (30; range, 0–233; $n = 18$, age 23 ± 2.5 years) was 10-fold lower than in controls (327; range, 14–1220; age 24 ± 2.4 years) by Mann-Whitney rank-sum testing ($p < 0.001$). Of note is that a deficiency of ammonia is necessary but not sufficient for acidification of the breath condensate. (From Ref. 26.)

of the urine (104,105). Upregulation appears to occur through the acid-enhanced expression of an mRNA-stabilizing protein that binds to glutaminase message (106).

Glutaminase is expressed and active in airway epithelial cells, in vitro and in vivo. As in the kidney, expression of glutaminase by airway epithelial cells in culture is increased by acidic stress, and the resulting increase in NH_3 produced by these cells neutralizes the acid loads and preserves cell viability (26). As respiratory NH_3 has a well-described role neutralizing exogenous acidic aerosols (107,108), effectively limiting adverse effects of inhaled acidic fog (109), it should not be surprising that NH_3 also serves to neutralize endogenously formed acids. Intriguingly, glutaminase expression can be downregulated by proinflammatory cytokines (110) and may be upregulated by corticosteroids (111), both effects having potential relevance to asthma.

Mucus glycoproteins and albumin are also likely to be critically important macromolecular buffers for airway acid (41). There are individual variations in the ability of sputum to buffer added protons, with sputum from chronic asthmatic subjects reported to both have a lower pH (as low as 5.3)(29) and less ability to buffer added protons than sputum from control subjects. The acid saturation of this mucus increases its viscosity and allows access of acid to the airway epithelium (63).

XIII. Proposed Antimicrobial Role of Airway Acidification

A *Mycobacterium tuberculosis* gene product protecting against the bactericidal effects of NO_2 (112) allows survival at neutral but not acidic pH (113). Toxicity of HNO_2 results in part from its reactive decomposition to nitric oxide (NO), which inhibits mycobacterial growth(114). This NO production is expected to occur in acidic conditions (115,116) such as the stomach or inflamed airway environment (21). Additionally, hydrogen peroxide (H_2O_2), which is elevated in the airways of asthma patients(117), acts synergistically with HNO_2 to kill gram-negative organisms (118). A decline in airway pH would also favor formation of OONOH (119,120), a species involved in macrophage-mediated *Mycoplasma* killing(121). Taken together, these observations suggest that mild airway acidification may serve as a titratable host defense mechanism—one that takes advantage of the pKa of weak endogenous acids to defend the airway against airborne pathogens.

Of note, NH_3 promotes the growth in the respiratory tract both of mycobacterial species (120) and *Mycoplasma* (121,122)—likely through augmented substrate supply—as well as inhibition of lysosome-phagosome fusion in macrophages (123,124). It is therefore tempting to speculate that the asthmatic phenotype—in which airway NH_3 production is decreased and pH falls—is designed to protect the airway from invading NH_3-requiring organisms while promoting the formation of reactive nitrogen species specifically toxic to the pathogens. In this regard, it is important to note that (1) airway pH falls most dramatically during virally induced asthma exacerbations and can be triggered to fall by an experimental rhinovirus infection in humans

(125) and (2) Th1 cytokines inhibit airway epithelial glutaminase, permitting a fall in pH (26). Therefore, a fall in airway pH and ammonia levels, though injurious to the asthmatic airway, may be regarded as a Th1-cytokine–stimulated host defense mechanism that has a potentially important role in protecting the airway from infection by tuberculosis, viruses, and other pathogens.

Additional protective effects of low pH may involve the activation of innate antimicrobial effector molecules. For example, calcitermin is a peptide recently reported to be present in the airway lining fluid that targets gram-negative bacteria and has enhanced activity at pH 5.4 (126).

XIV. Conclusion

pH is a critical determinant in several biochemical processes relevant to airways disease. Emerging evidence suggests that airway pH is (1) abnormally low in a variety of lung disorders, most notably including acute exacerbations of asthma, and (2) carefully regulated—both to prevent cytotoxicity and to enhance host defense—by a variety of airway proteins, including glutaminase. Airway physiologists, biochemists, and a broad spectrum of other investigators will need increasingly to account for airway pH and its determinants as information accumulates, both about normal values and about variations characteristic of disease states. This "fresh look" at airway chemistry has the potential to stimulate the development of new therapies for asthma and other inflammatory lung diseases.

Acknowledgments

Supported by NHLBI: HL 59337 (BG), HL69170 (BG and JH), and NIH: HD01421-02 (JH); Henry B. Wallace Foundation (BG); GlaxoSmithKline (BG and JH); American Academy of Allergy, Asthma and Immunology Education and Research Trust (JH). JH is a Parker B. Francis Fellow in Pulmonary Research.

References

1. Armbrecht U, Bosaeus I, Gillberg R, Seeberg S, Stockbruegger R. Hydrogen (H_2) breath test and gastric bacteria in acid-secreting subjects and in achlorhydric and post-gastrectomy patients before and after antimicrobial treatment. Scand J Gastroenterol 1985; 20(7):805–813.
2. Xu J, Xu X, Verstraete W. The bactericidal effect and chemical reactions of acidified nitrite under conditions simulating the stomach. J Appl Microbiol 2001; 90(4): 523–529.
3. Werther JL. The gastric mucosal barrier. Mt Sinai J Med 2000; 67(1):41–53.
4. Schneider B, Gross R, Haas A. Phagosome acidification has opposite effects on intracellular survival of *Bordetella pertussis* and *B. bronchiseptica*. Infect Immun 2000; 68(12):7039–7048.

5. Kataoka T, Takaku K, Magae J, Shinohara N, Takayama H, Kondo S, Nagai K. Acidification is essential for maintaining the structure and function of lytic granules of CTL. Effect of concanamycin A, an inhibitor of vacuolar type $H(+)$-ATPase, on CTL—mediated cytotoxicity. J Immunol 1994; 153(9):3938–3947.

6. Effros RM, Jacobs ER, Schapira RM, Biller J. Response of the lungs to aspiration. Am J Med 2000; 108(suppl 4a):15S–19S.

7. Aris R, Christian D, Sheppard D, Balmes JR. Acid fog-induced bronchoconstriction. The role of hydroxymethanesulfonic acid. Am Rev Respir Dis 1990; 141(3):546–551.

8. Holma B, Lindegren M, Andersen JM. pH effects on ciliomotility and morphology of respiratory mucosa. Arch Environ Health 1977; 32(5):216–226.

9. Honma S, Tanaka H, Teramoto S, Igarashi T, Abe S. Effects of naturally-occurring acid fog on inflammatory mediators in airway and pulmonary functions in asthmatic patients. Respir Med 2000; 94(10):935–942.

10. Poulsen JH, Fischer H, Illek B, Machen TE. Bicarbonate conductance and pH regulatory capability of cystic fibrosis transmembrane conductance regulator. Proc Natl Acad Sci USA 1994; 91(12):5340–5344.

11. Choi JY, Muallem D, Kiselyov K, Lee MG, Thomas PJ, Muallem S. Aberrant CFTR-dependent HCO_3-transport in mutations associated with cystic fibrosis. Nature 2001; 410(6824):94–97.

12. Smith JJ, Welsh MJ. cAMP stimulates bicarbonate secretion across normal, but not cystic fibrosis airway epithelia. J Clin Invest 1992; 89(4):1148–1153.

13. Trout L, Gatzy JT, Ballard ST. Acetylcholine-induced liquid secretion by bronchial epithelium: role of Cl^- and HCO_3^- transport. Am J Physiol 1998; 275(6 Pt 1): L1095–1099.

14. Jack CIA, Tran J, Donnelly RJ, Hind CRK, Evans CC. Endo-bronchial pH measurements in anaesthetised subjects. Thorax 1991; 46:751P.

15. Jack CI, Calverley PM, Donnelly RJ, Tran J, Russell G, Hind CR, Evans CC. Simultaneous tracheal and oesophageal pH measurements in asthmatic patients with gastro-oesophageal reflux. Thorax 1995; 50(2):201–204.

16. Patel PH, Thomas E, Willis M, Roark E. Inadvertent bronchial pH monitoring [letter]. Gastrointest Endosc 1987; 33(6):465.

17. Donnelly RJ, Berrisford RG, Jack CI, Tran JA, Evans CC. Simultaneous tracheal and esophageal pH monitoring: investigating reflux-associated asthma. Ann Thorac Surg 1993; 56(5):1029–1033; discussion 1034.

18. Jack CI, Walshaw MJ, Tran J, Hind CR, Evans CC. Twenty-four-hour tracheal pH monitoring—a simple and non-hazardous investigation. Respir Med 1994; 88(6): 441–444.

19. Guerrin F, Voisin C, Macquet V, Robin RA, Lequien P. Apport de la pH metrie bronchique *in situ*. Prog Respir Res 1971; 6:372–383.

20. Metheny NA, Stewart BJ, Smith L, Yan H, Diebold M, Clouse RE. pH and concentration of bilirubin in feeding tube aspirates as predictors of tube placement. Nurs Res 1999; 48(4):189–197.

21. Hunt JF, Fang K, Malik R, Snyder A, Malhotra N, Platts-Mills TA, Gaston B. Endogenous airway acidification. Implications for asthma pathophysiology. Am J Respir Crit Care Med 2000; 161(3 Pt 1):694–699.

22. Kyle H, Ward JP, Widdicombe JG. Control of pH of airway surface liquid of the ferret trachea in vitro. J Appl Physiol 1990; 68(1):135–140.

23. Gatto LA. pH of mucus in rat trachea. J Appl Physiol 1981; 50(6):1224–1226.

24. Gatto LA. pH of mucus in rabbit trachea: cholinergic stimulation and block. Lung 1985; 163(2):109–115.

25. Kostikas K, Papatheodorou G, Ganas K, Psathakis K, Panagou P, Loukides S. pH in expired breath condensate of patients with inflammatory airway diseases. Am J Respir Crit Care Med 2002; 165:1364–1370.

26. Hunt JF, Erwin E, Palmer L, Vaughan J, Malhotra N, Platts-Mills TA. E. Expression and activity of pH-regulatory glutaminase in the human airway epithelium. Am J Respir Crit Care Med 2001; 165:101–107.

27. Hunt J, Gaston B. Endogenous airway acidification. (Response to letter). Am J Respir Crit Care Med 2001; 163(1):293–294.

28. Small PA. Rapid diagnostic method for distinguishing allergies and infections. US patent 5,910,421, 1999.

29. Ryley HC, Brogan TD. Variation in the composition of sputum in chronic chest diseases. Br J Exp Pathol 1968; 49(6):625–633.

30. Shimura S, Sasaki T, Sasaki H, Takishima T. Chemical properties of bronchorrhea sputum in bronchial asthma. Chest 1988; 94(6):1211–1215.

31. Ballard ST, Trout L, Bebok Z, Sorscher EJ, Crews A. CFTR involvement in chloride, bicarbonate, and liquid secretion by airway submucosal glands. Am J Physiol 1999; 277(4 Pt 1):L694–699.

32. Kwart H, Moseley WW, Katz M. The chemical characterization of human tracheobronchial secretion: a possible clue to the origin of fibrocystic mucus. Ann NY Acad Sci 1963; 106(2):709–721.

33. Jayaraman S, Song Y, Vetrivel L, Shankar L, Verkman AS. Noninvasive in vivo fluorescence measurement of airway-surface liquid depth, salt concentration, and pH. J Clin Invest 2001; 107(3):317–324.

34. Antczak A, Gorski P. Endogenous airway acidification and oxidant overload in infectious exacerbation of COPD. Am J Respir Crit Care Med 2001; 163(5):A725.

35. Karnad DR, Mhaisekar DG, Moralwar KV. Respiratory mucus pH in tracheostomized intensive care unit patients: effects of colonization and pneumonia. Crit Care Med 1990; 18(7):699–701.

36. Hunt J, Fang K, Platts-Mills T, Gaston B. Nitrogen oxide redox balance in asthma (abstr). Am J Respir Crit Care Med 1999; 159(3):A860.

37. Walsh GM. Human eosinophils: their accumulation, activation and fate. Br J Haematol 1997; 97(4):701–709.

38. Gaston B, Stamler JS. Nitrogen oxides. In: Crystal RG, ed. The Lung: Scientific Foundations. 2d ed. Philadelphia: Lippincott-Raven, 1997:239–253.

39. Crow JP, Spruell C, Chen J, Gunn C, Ischiropoulos H, Tsai M, Smith CD, Radi R, Koppenol WH, Beckman JS. On the pH-dependent yield of hydroxyl radical products from peroxynitrite. Free Radic Biol Med 1994; 16(3):331–338.

40. Luk CK, Dulfano MJ. Effect of pH, viscosity and ionic-strength changes on ciliary beating frequency of human bronchial explants. Clin Sci 1983; 64(4):449–451.

41. Holma B, Hegg PO. pH- and protein-dependent buffer capacity and viscosity of respiratory mucus. Their interrelationships and influence on health. Sci Total Environ 1989; 84:71–82.

42. Ricciardolo FLM, Rado V, Fabbri LM, Sterk PJ, Di Maria GU, Geppetti P. Bronchoconstriction induced by citric acid inhalation in guinea pigs: role of tachykinins, bradykinin, and nitric oxide. Am J Respir Crit Care Med 1999; 159(2):557–562.

43. Bevan S, Geppetti P. Protons: small stimulants of capsaicin-sensitive sensory nerves. Trends Neurosci 1994; 17(12):509–512.

44. Stern M, Meagher L, Savill J, Haslett C. Apoptosis in human eosinophils. Programmed cell death in the eosinophil leads to phagocytosis by macrophages and is modulated by IL-5. J Immunol 1992; 148(11):3543–3549.
45. Dairaghi DJ, Oldham ER, Bacon KB, Schall TJ. Chemokine receptor CCR3 function is highly dependent on local pH and ionic strength. J Biol Chem 1997; 272(45): 28206–28209.
46. Wenzel SE, Szefler SJ, Leung DY, Sloan SI, Rex MD, Martin RJ. Bronchoscopic evaluation of severe asthma. Persistent inflammation associated with high dose glucocorticoids. Am J Respir Crit Care Med 1997; 156(3 Pt 1):737–743.
47. Gaston B, Reilly J, Drazen JM, Fackler J, Ramdev P, Arnelle D, Mullins ME, Sugarbaker DJ, Chee C, Singel DJ. Endogenous nitrogen oxides and bronchodilator S-nitrosothiols in human airways. Proc Natl Acad Sci USA 1993; 90(23):10957–10961.
48. Hunt J, Byrns RE, Ignarro LJ, Gaston B. Condensed expirate nitrite as a home marker for acute asthma [letter]. Lancet 1995; 346(8984):1235–1236.
49. Weitzberg E, Lundberg JO. Nonenzymatic nitric oxide production in humans. Nitric Oxide 1998; 2(1):1–7.
50. Al-Ali MK, Howarth PH. Exhaled nitric oxide levels in exacerbations of asthma, chronic obstructive pulmonary disease and pneumonia. Saudi Med J 2001; 22(3): 249–253.
51. Dohlman AW, Black HR, Royall JA. Expired breath hydrogen peroxide is a marker of acute airway inflammation in pediatric patients with asthma. Am Rev Respir Dis 1993; 148(4 Pt 1):955–960.
52. Saleh D, Ernst P, Lim S, Barnes PJ, Giaid A. Increased formation of the potent oxidant peroxynitrite in the airways of asthmatic patients is associated with induction of nitric oxide synthase: effect of inhaled glucocorticoid. FASEB J 1998; 12(11):929–937.
53. Hanazawa T, Kharitonov SA, Barnes PJ. Increased nitrotyrosine in exhaled breath condensate of patients with asthma. Am J Respir Crit Care Med 2000; 162(4 Pt 1): 1273–1276.
54. Kaminsky DA, Mitchell J, Carroll N, James A, Soultanakis R, Janssen Y. Nitrotyrosine formation in the airways and lung parenchyma of patients with asthma. J Allergy Clin Immunol 1999; 104(4 Pt 1):747–754.
55. Rahman I, Morrison D, Donaldson K, MacNee W. Systemic oxidative stress in asthma, COPD, and smokers. Am J Respir Crit Care Med 1996; 154(4 Pt 1):1055–1060.
56. Wu W, Samoszuk MK, Comhair SA, Thomassen MJ, Farver CF, Dweik RA, Kavuru MS, Erzurum SC, Hazen SL. Eosinophils generate brominating oxidants in allergen-induced asthma. J Clin Invest 2000; 105(10):1455–1463.
57. Calhoun WJ, Reed HE, Moest DR, Stevens CA. Enhanced superoxide production by alveolar macrophages and air-space cells, airway inflammation, and alveolar macrophage density changes after segmental antigen bronchoprovocation in allergic subjects. Am Rev Respir Dis 1992; 145(2 Pt 1):317–325.
58. Hodgson EK, Fridovich I. The interaction of bovine erythrocyte superoxide dismutase with hydrogen peroxide: inactivation of the enzyme. Biochemistry 1975; 14(24): 5294–5299.
59. Tyrell RM. UVA (320–380 nm) radiation as an oxidative stress. In: Sies H, ed. In Oxidative Stress: Oxidants and Antioxidants. London: Academic Press, 1991:57–84.
60. Schraufstätter D, Cochrane CG. Oxidants: types, sources and mechanisms of injury. In: Crystal RG, ed. The Lung: Scientific Foundations. Philadelphia: Lippincott-Reven, 1997:2251–2269.

61. De Raeve HR, Thunnissen FB, Kaneko FT, Guo FH, Lewis M, Kavuru MS, Secic M, Thomassen MJ, Erzurum SC. Decreased Cu,Zn-SOD activity in asthmatic airway epithelium: correction by inhaled corticosteroid in vivo. Am J Physiol 1997; 272(1 Pt 1):L148–154.

62. Clary-Meinesz C, Mouroux J, Cosson J, Huitorel P, Blaive B. Influence of external pH on ciliary beat frequency in human bronchi and bronchioles. Eur Respir J 1998; 11(2):330–333.

63. Holma B. Influence of buffer capacity and pH-dependent rheological properties of respiratory mucus on health effects due to acidic pollution. Sci Total Environ 1985; 41(2):101–123.

64. Tanaka H, Honma S, Nishi M, Igarashi T, Teramoto S, Nishio F, Abe S. Acid fog and hospital visits for asthma: an epidemiological study. Eur Respir J 1998; 11(6): 1301–1306.

65. Kopferschmitt-Kubler MC, Blaumeiser-Kapps M, Millet M, Wortham H, Mirabel P, Nobelis P, Pauli G. [Study by questionnaire of the influence of weather conditions, particularly fog, on the symptomatology of asthmatic subjects]. Rev Mal Respir 1996; 13(4):421–427.

66. Thurston GD, Ito K, Hayes CG, Bates DV, Lippmann M. Respiratory hospital admissions and summertime haze air pollution in Toronto, Ontario: consideration of the role of acid aerosols. Environ Res 1994; 65(2):271–290.

67. Linn WS, Avol EL, Anderson KR, Shamoo DA, Peng RC, Hackney JD. Effect of droplet size on respiratory responses to inhaled sulfuric acid in normal and asthmatic volunteers. Am Rev Respir Dis 1989; 140(1): 161–166.

68. Raizenne ME, Burnett RT, Stern B, Franklin CA, Spengler JD. Acute lung function responses to ambient acid aerosol exposures in children. Environ Health Perspect 1989; 79:179–185.

69. Dockery DW, Cunningham J, Damokosh AI, Neas LM, Spengler JD, Koutrakis P, Ware JH, Raizenne M, Speizer FE. Health effects of acid aerosols on North American children: respiratory symptoms. Environ Health Perspect 1996; 104(5):500–505.

70. Neas LM, Dockery DW, Koutrakis P, Tollerud DJ, Speizer FE. The association of ambient air pollution with twice daily peak expiratory flow rate measurements in children. Am J Epidemiol 1995; 141(2):111–122.

71. Lowry RH, Wood AM, Higenbottam TW. Effects of pH and osmolarity on aerosol-induced cough in normal volunteers. Clin Sci (Colch) 1988; 74(4):373–376.

72. Winther FO. Experimentally induced cough in man by citric acid aerosol. An evaluation of a method. Acta Pharmacol Toxicol 1970; 28(2):108–212.

73. Fine JM, Gordon T, Thompson JE, Sheppard D. The role of titratable acidity in acid aerosol-induced bronchoconstriction. Am Rev Respir Dis 1987; 135(4):826–830.

74. Avol EL, Linn WS, Whynot JD, Anderson KR, Shamoo DA, Valencia LM, Little DE, Hackney JD. Respiratory dose-response study of normal and asthmatic volunteers exposed to sulfuric acid aerosol in the sub-micrometer size range. Toxicol Ind Health 1988; 4(2):173–184.

75. Balmes JR, Fine JM, Christian D, Gordon T, Sheppard D. Acidity potentiates bronchoconstriction induced by hypoosmolar aerosols. Am Rev Respir Dis 1988; 138(1): 35–39.

76. Koenig JQ, Covert DS, Pierson WE. Effects of inhalation of acidic compounds on pulmonary function in allergic adolescent subjects. Environ Health Perspect 1989; 79: 173–178.

77. Balmes JR, Fine JM, Gordon T, Sheppard D. Potential bronchoconstrictor stimuli in acid fog. Environ Health Perspect 1989; 79:163–166.

78. Zuskin E, Mustajbegovic J, Schachter EN, Pavicic D, Budak A. A follow-up study of respiratory function in workers exposed to acid aerosols in a food-processing industry. Int Arch Occup Environ Health 1997; 70(6):413–418.

79. Bosse GM. Nebulized sodium bicarbonate in the treatment of chlorine gas inhalation. J Toxicol Clin Toxicol 1994; 32(3):233–241.

80. Douidar SM. Nebulized sodium bicarbonate in acute chlorine inhalation. Pediatr Emerg Care 1997; 13(6):406–407.

81. Vinsel PJ. Treatment of acute chlorine gas inhalation with nebulized sodium bicarbonate. J Emerg Med 1990; 8(3):327–329.

82. Ahmed T, Ali JM, al-Sharif AF. Effect of alkali nebulization on bronchoconstriction in acute bronchial asthma. Respir Med 1993; 87(3):235–236.

83. Ahmed T, Iskandrani A, Uddin MN. Sodium bicarbonate solution nebulization in the treatment of acute severe asthma. Am J Ther 2000; 7(5):325–327.

84. Blaisdell CJ, Edmonds RD, Wang XT, Guggino S, Zeitlin PL. pH-regulated chloride secretion in fetal lung epithelia. Am J Physiol Lung Cell Mol Physiol 2000; 278(6): L1248–1255.

85. Baud L, Bellocq A, Philippe C, Fouqueray B. [Low extracellular pH has a role in the induction of NO synthase type 2 in macrophages]. Bull Acad Natl Med 1997; 181(2): 247–258; discussion 259–260.

86. Cohen DS, Palmer E, Welch WJ, Sheppard D. The response of guinea pig airway epithelial cells and alveolar macrophages to environmental stress. Am J Respir Cell Mol Biol 1991; 5(2):133–143.

87. Wadsworth SJ, Spitzer AR, Chander A. Ionic regulation of proton chemical (pH) and electrical gradients in lung lamellar bodies. Am J Physiol 1997; 273(2 Pt 1):L427–436.

88. Kurashima K, Numata M, Yachie A, Sai Y, Ishizaka N, Fujimura M, Matsuda T, Ohkuma S. The role of vacuolar H(+)-ATPase in the control of intragranular pH and exocytosis in eosinophils. Lab Invest 1996; 75(5):689–698.

89. Jabado N, Jankowski A, Dougaparsad S, Picard V, Grinstein S, Gros P. Natural resistance to intracellular infections: natural resistance-associated macrophage protein 1 (Nramp1) functions as a pH-dependent manganese transporter at the phagosomal membrane. J Exp Med 2000; 192(9):1237–1248.

90. Burkhardt JK, Hester S, Lapham CK, Argon Y. The lytic granules of natural killer cells are dual-function organelles combining secretory and pre-lysosomal compartments. J Cell Biol 1990; 111(6 Pt 1):2327–2340.

91. Tapper H, Sundler R. Cytosolic pH regulation in mouse macrophages. Proton extrusion by plasma-membrane-localized H(+)-ATPase. Biochem J 1992; 281(Pt 1):245–250.

92. Forgac M. The vacuolar H^+-ATPase of clathrin-coated vesicles is reversibly inhibited by S-nitrosoglutathione. J Biol Chem 1999; 274(3):1301–1305.

93. Tojo A, Guzman NJ, Garg LC, Tisher CC, Madsen KM. Nitric oxide inhibits bafilomycin-sensitive H(+)-ATPase activity in rat cortical collecting duct. Am J Physiol 1994; 267(4 Pt 2):F509–515.

94. Paradiso AM. ATP-activated basolateral Na^+/H^+ exchange in human normal and cystic fibrosis airway epithelium. Am J Physiol 1997; 273(1 Pt 1):L148–158.

95. Acevedo M, Steele LW. Na(+)-H^+ exchanger in isolated epithelial tracheal cells from sheep. Involvement in tracheal proton secretion. Exp Physiol 1993; 78(3):383–394.

96. Vaughan JW, Gaston B, MacDonald T, Erwin E, Malhotra N, Zaman K, Platts-Mills TAE, Hunt J. Acetic acid contributes to exhaled breath condensate acidity in asthma (abstr). Eur Respir J 2001; 18(suppl 33):P3083.

97. Dudeja PK, Hafez N, Tyagi S, Gailey CA, Toofanfard M, Alrefai WA, Nazir TM, Ramaswamy K, Al-Bazzaz FJ. Expression of the Na^+/H^+ and Cl^-/HCO^-_3 exchanger isoforms in proximal and distal human airways. Am J Physiol 1999; 276(6 Pt 1): L971–978.

98. Wheat VJ, Shumaker H, Burnham C, Shull GE, Yankaskas JR, Soleimani M. CFTR induces the expression of DRA along with $Cl(-)/HCO(3)(-)$ exchange activity in tracheal epithelial cells. Am J Physiol Cell Physiol 2000; 279(1):C62–71.

99. Devor DC, Singh AK, Lambert LC, DeLuca A, Frizzell RA, Bridges RJ. Bicarbonate and chloride secretion in Calu-3 human airway epithelial cells. J Gen Physiol 1999; 113(5):743–760.

100. Poschet JF, Boucher JC, Tatterson L, Skidmore J, Van Dyke RW, Deretic V. Molecular basis for defective glycosylation and *Pseudomonas* pathogenesis in cystic fibrosis lung. Proc Natl Acad Sci USA 2001; 98(24):13972–13977.

101. Inglis SK, Corboz MR, Taylor AE, Ballard ST. Regulation of ion transport across porcine distal bronchi. Am J Physiol 1996; 270(2 Pt 1):L289–297.

102. Larson TV, Covert DS, Frank R, Charlson RJ. Ammonia in the human airways: neutralization of inspired acid sulfate aerosols. Science 1977; 197(4299):161–163.

103. Ament W, Huizenga JR, Kort E, van der Mark TW, Grevink RG, Verkerke GJ. Respiratory ammonia output and blood ammonia concentration during incremental exercise. Int J Sports Med 1999; 20(2):71–77.

104. Welbourne TC, Phromphetcharat V. Renal glutamine metabolism and hydrogen ion homeostasis. In: Haussinger D, Sies H, eds. Glutamine Metabolism in Mammalian Tissues. New York: Springer-Verlag, 1984:161–177.

105. Laterza OF, Hansen WR, Taylor L, Curthoys NP. Identification of an mRNA-binding protein and the specific elements that may mediate the pH-responsive induction of renal glutaminase mRNA. J Biol Chem 1997; 272(36):22481–22488.

106. Laterza OF, Curthoys NP. Effect of acidosis on the properties of the glutaminase mRNA pH-response element binding protein. J Am Soc Nephrol 2000; 11(9):1583–1588.

107. Sarangapani R, Wexler AS. Growth and neutralization of sulfate aerosols in human airways. J Appl Physiol 1996; 81(1):480–490.

108. Chen LC, Fang CP, Qu QS, Fine JM, Schlesinger RB. A novel system for the in vitro exposure of pulmonary cells to acid sulfate aerosols. Fundam Appl Toxicol 1993; 20(2):170–176.

109. Utell MJ, Frampton MW, Morrow PE. Air pollution and asthma: clinical studies with sulfuric acid aerosols. Allergy Proc 1991; 12(6):385–388.

110. Sarantos P, Abouhamze A, Abcouwer S, Chakrabarti R, Copeland EM, Souba WW. Cytokines decrease glutaminase expression in human fibroblasts. Surgery 1994; 116(2): 276–283; discussion 283–284.

111. Sarantos P, Abouhamze Z, Copeland EM, Souba WW. Glucocorticoids regulate glutaminase gene expression in human intestinal epithelial cells. J Surg Res 1994; 57(1): 227–231.

112. Ehrt S, Shiloh MU, Ruan J, Choi M, Gunzburg S, Nathan C, Xie Q, Riley LW. A novel antioxidant gene from *Mycobacterium tuberculosis*. J Exp Med 1997; 186(11): 1885–1896.

113. Crowle AJ, Dahl R, Ross E, May MH. Evidence that vesicles containing living, virulent *Mycobacterium tuberculosis* or *Mycobacterium avium* in cultured human macrophages are not acidic. Infect Immun 1991; 59(5):1823–1831.

114. Long R, Light B, Talbot JA. Mycobacteriocidal action of exogenous nitric oxide. Antimicrob Agents Chemother 1999; 43(2):403–405.

115. Modin A, Bjorne H, Herulf M, Alving K, Weitzberg E, Lundberg JO. Nitrite-derived
     nitric oxide: a possible mediator of "acidic-metabolic" vasodilation. Acta Physiol Scand
     2001; 171(1):9–16.
116. Nelson BV, Sears S, Woods J, Ling CY, Hunt J, Clapper LM, Gaston B. Expired nitric
     oxide as a marker for childhood asthma. J Pediatr 1997; 130(3):423–427.
117. Antczak A, Nowak D, Shariati B, Krol M, Piasecka G, Kurmanowska Z. Increased
     hydrogen peroxide and thiobarbituric acid-reactive products in expired breath conden-
     sate of asthmatic patients. Eur Respir J 1997; 10(6):1235–1241.
118. Klebanoff SJ. Reactive nitrogen intermediates and antimicrobial activity: role of nitrite.
     Free Radic Biol Med 1993; 14(4):351–360.
119. Koppenol WH, Moreno JJ, Pryor WA, Ischiropoulos H, Beckman JS. Peroxynitrite,
     a cloaked oxidant formed by nitric oxide and superoxide. Chem Res Toxicol 1992;
     5(6):834–842.
120. Pryor WA, Squadrito GL. The chemistry of peroxynitrite: a product from the reaction
     of nitric oxide with superoxide. Am J Physiol 1995; 268(5 Pt 1):L699–722.
121. Hickman-Davis J, Gibbs-Erwin J, Lindsey JR, Matalon S. Surfactant protein A me-
     diates mycoplasmacidal activity of alveolar macrophages by production of peroxyni-
     trite. Proc Natl Acad Sci USA 1999; 96(9):4953–4958.
122. Schoeb TR, Davidson MK, Lindsey JR. Intracage ammonia promotes growth of *Myco-
     plasma pulmonis* in the respiratory tract of rats. Infect Immun 1982; 38(1):212–217.
123. Gordon AH, Hart PD, Young MR. Ammonia inhibits phagosome-lysosome fusion in
     macrophages. Nature 1980; 286(5768):79–80.
124. Dudchik G. [Glutaminase activity and intensity of glutamine metabolism in the lungs
     and lymph nodes in tuberculosis]. Probl Tuberk 1970; 48(7):54–58.
125. Hunt J, Gaston B, Zambrano J, Rakes G, Snyder A, Heymann P, Platts-Mills TAE.
     Condensed breath exhalate pH falls during experimental rhinovirus 16 infection in
     asthmatic subjects (abst). Am J Respir Crit Care Med 2000; 161(3):A104.
126. Cole AM, Kim Y, Tahk S, Hong T, Weis P, Waring AJ, Ganz T. Calcitermin, a
     novel antimicrobial peptide isolated from human airway secretions. FEBS Lett 2001;
     504(1–2):5–10.

4

Monitoring of Exhaled Breath to Assess Airway Inflammation in Asthma

PETER J. BARNES

National Heart and Lung Institute
Imperial College
London, England

I. Introduction

Traditionally asthma control has been monitored by symptoms and lung function measurements, particularly peak expiratory flow. Airway inflammation underlies asthma symptoms but is difficult to measure directly as this involves invasive procedures, such as bronchial biopsy and bronchoalveolar lavage. More recently, the less invasive procedure of sputum induction has been introduced (1). This is more acceptable to patients, but some patients find it unacceptable, and it is not possible to obtain adequate samples from other patients. It is also difficult to apply in young children. The procedure of sputum induction with hypertonic saline itself induces airway inflammation, so cannot be repeated frequently (2,3). This has led to a search for less invasive ways to measure airway inflammation in order to assess adequate control with anti-inflammatory treatments, to predict loss of asthma control, and to assess the response to novel anti-inflammatory treatments. Several markers in exhaled breath have now been explored (4), including:

1. *Exhaled gases*
   Nitric oxide
   Carbon monoxide
   Hydrocarbons (ethane and pentane)

2. *Exhaled breath condensate*
        Reactive oxygen and nitrogen species
        Inflammatory mediators
        Cytokines

This chapter discusses how these markers in exhaled breath have been used to assess airway inflammation and its control in asthma. This is a rapidly advancing field with the potential for enormous clinical impact. It provides new opportunities to explore the underlying inflammatory process in asthma, particularly in severe disease and in young children in whom it has been difficult to evaluate airway inflammation using traditional techniques. Noninvasive monitoring also allows repeated measurements to be made, thus allowing detailed studies of the kinetic effects of anti-inflammatory drugs.

II. Exhaled Nitric Oxide

Exhaled nitric oxide (NO) is the most extensively studied exhaled marker, and there is increasing support for its clinical use in monitoring of asthma control (5).

A. Increased Exhaled NO in Asthma

Asthmatic patients who are not treated with anti-inflammatory drugs show an increase in exhaled NO concentrations compared with normal control subjects (6,7). Exhaled NO is not affected by changes in airway caliber, but is increased during the late phase response to inhaled allergen (8). Exhaled NO also increases during asthma exacerbations (9). There is a correlation between exhaled NO and sputum eosinophils and airway hyperresponsiveness (10–12). This suggests that exhaled NO may be useful in monitoring the inflammatory process in patients with asthma.

Exhaled NO can also be measured in children, including infants, and may therefore be of particular importance in monitoring asthmatic inflammation in young children, in whom it is not possible to assess airway inflammation using more invasive procedures (13).

B. Effects of Corticosteroids

Treatment with oral or inhaled corticosteroids reduces exhaled NO concentrations (14,15), and the reduction in exhaled NO is related to the dose of corticosteroids (16). When the exhaled NO is partitioned using different exhaled flow rates, inhaled corticosteroids reduce the fraction of exhaled NO derived from the airways compared to the lung parenchyma (17). This inhibitory effect of corticosteroids is likely to be explained by the fact that inflammatory mediators in asthma, particularly proinflammatory cytokines, induce an inducible isoform of NO synthase (iNOS or NOS2),

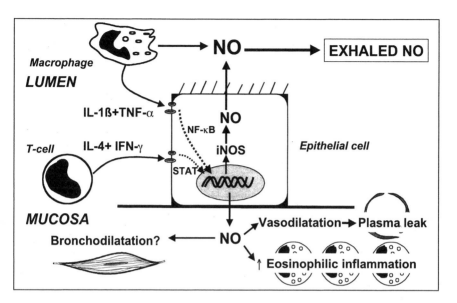

Figure 1 Generation of exhaled nitric oxide (NO) in asthma. NO is generated via the induction of inducible NO synthase (iNOS) after activation of transcription factors, such as nuclear factor-κB (NF-κB) and signal transduction activated transcription factors (STAT), which are themselves activated by cytokines such as interleukin-1 (IL-1) and interferon-γ (IFN-γ).

leading to the increased production of NO, which is detected in the breath (Fig. 1). Corticosteroids suppress inflammation by switching off multiple inflammatory genes, including genes for cytokines that induce iNOS and thereby reverse the induction of iNOS. In mice and rodents corticosteroids also directly inhibit the expression of iNOS, but this is not the case in human cells, probably because the promoter region of human iNOS differs and is regulated by different transcription factors (18). This suggests that the effect of corticosteroids is not a direct effect on iNOS but reflects the suppression of the inflammatory process by corticosteroids. Thus, exhaled NO may be a useful noninvasive way to monitor the effects of anti-inflammatory treatments in asthma. Exhaled NO may be a particularly useful measurement in children, and inhaled corticosteroids have been shown to reduce exhaled NO as in adults (19).

C. Effects of Other Drugs

Apart from corticosteroids, the effects of several other antiasthma drugs have been studied in asthma (20) (Table 1). Neither short- nor long-acting inhaled β_2-agonists reduce exhaled NO, consistent with the fact that β_2-agonists do not have direct anti-inflammatory effects (21). This shows that the measurement of exhaled NO is independent of airway function and therefore may be useful in monitoring inflamma-

Table 1 Effect of Drugs on Exhaled Nitric
Oxide

Drug	Effect
Corticosteroids	↓↓↓
β_2-Agonists	No effect
Antileukotrienes	↓
Theophylline	No effect
NO synthase inhibitors	↓↓

tion, despite treatment with inhaled bronchodilators. This may be of particular value in monitoring asthma treatment with combination inhalers, such as fluticasone/salmeterol and formoterol/budesonide, where it may be difficult to be certain about suppression of inflammation with concomitant administration of a long-acting bronchodilator (22). The antileukotriene montelukast has a weak inhibitory effect on exhaled NO compared to inhaled corticosteroids, consistent with its much weaker anti-inflammatory actions (23). Theophylline has no effect on exhaled NO (24).

Exhaled NO may be useful in assessing the anti-inflammatory effects of new classes of drugs that are not in clinical trial for asthma, including anti-IgE, phosphodiesterase-4 inhibitors, and cytokine modulators (25,26). Exhaled NO provides a simple noninvasive method that can easily be incorporated into large clinical trials and does not require complicated technical assessment. The measurement of exhaled NO has been standardized, so that measurements are identical between different laboratories (27,28). This means that the measurement is suited to multicenter trials that are often needed in the clinical assessment of new asthma treatments. Exhaled NO may also be useful in monitoring the effects of new treatments on airway inflammation in children with asthma, and particularly in infants where little is known about the effects of antiasthma therapies.

D. Exhaled NO to Measure Asthma Control

In patients who are well controlled with inhaled corticosteroids, exhaled NO levels are similar to those in normal subjects. This presumably reflects control of exhaled NO by inhaled corticosteroid treatment. However, in patients with severe asthma, who require high doses of inhaled corticosteroids and oral steroids, there may be an increase in exhaled NO that may reflect the relative resistance to corticosteroids seen in these patients (29,30). In patients who are stabilized on inhaled corticosteroids when the dose of inhaled corticosteroids is reduced, there is an increase in exhaled NO which precedes the increase in symptoms and fall in lung function (31). This was confirmed in a more detailed study in which reduction of the dose of inhaled corticosteroids led to an increase in exhaled NO before the increase in symptoms and fall in lung function. Exhaled NO also increased before an increase in sputum eosinophils (32). This suggests that exhaled NO may be an early warning sign for loss of asthma control, and this may allow patients to increase their controller medication in order to prevent the development of an exacerbation (33). Exhaled NO levels correlate with other markers of asthma control, such as symptoms, lung function, and use of rescue bronchodilators (34). Longitudinal studies in asthma have demonstrated that a rise in exhaled NO appears to be a reliable indicator of loss of asthma control (35).

Measurement of exhaled NO in the clinic may also be used to monitor compliance with inhaled corticosteroids therapy, as high levels in patients who are prescribed inhaled corticosteroids usually indicate a failure to take the medication (which is very common).

III. Exhaled Carbon Monoxide

Patient with asthma have increased levels of carbon monoxide (CO) in the breath (36,37). This is likely to be derived from increased expression and activation of the enzyme heme oxygenase-1 (HO-1), which is activated by cellular stress, including inflammation and oxidative stress. Many airway cells express HO-1 in human airways, including epithelial cells, macrophages, and inflammatory cells (38). Human airway epithelial cells express HO-1 with increased production of CO after exposure to inflammatory cytokines and oxidative stress in vitro (39) (Fig. 2). Macrophages in induced sputum from patients with asthma show increased expression of HO-1 compared to normal macrophages (37).

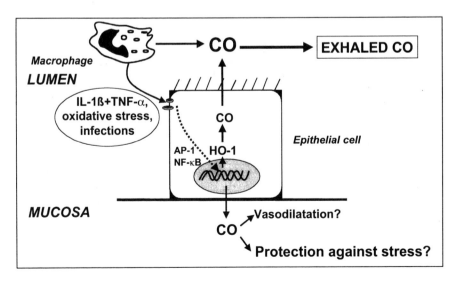

Figure 2 Generation of exhaled carbon monoxide (CO) in asthma. CO is generated from heme oxygenase-1 (HO-1), which is activated by transcription factors nuclear factor-κB (NF-κB) and activator protein-1 (AP-1).

Exhaled CO levels are also increased in exacerbations of asthma (40) and after allergen challenge (41). This suggests that exhaled CO may also be useful as a noninvasive marker of asthma. In children with asthma, exhaled CO is increased only in those with symptomatic asthma, whereas exhaled NO was increased in all children whether they were symptomatic or not (42).

A disadvantage of exhaled CO is that the values of asthmatics overlap with those of normal subjects, and environmental CO and cigarette smoke may interfere with measurements. It is less sensitive than exhaled NO to the effects of corticosteroids and so may not be useful in detecting loss of asthma control. Exhaled CO appears to reflect both inflammation and oxidative stress, whereas exhaled NO is more directly related to inflammation. The poor discrimination between asthmatics and normal subjects in exhaled CO measurements makes it of no value as a noninvasive marker to monitor drug effects. However, it does measure oxidative stress and is more elevated in severe asthma where oxidative stress is higher. It might be more useful where oxidative stress in asthma is the major target of therapy. In other diseases, such as cystic fibrosis, the levels of exhaled CO are much higher, particularly following exacerbations, and so this marker may be more useful in these situations (43–45).

IV. Exhaled Hydrocarbons

Pentane and ethane are formed by lipid peroxidation of cell membranes as a result of oxidative stress. Both may be detected in the breath by gas chromatography (46) and mass spectrometry. Exhaled pentane is increased during exacerbation of asthma (47). Exhaled ethane is elevated in asthma and is correlated with disease severity. There is a correlation between exhaled ethane and CO, at least in cystic fibrosis where the levels are very high (48).

While these are good markers of oxidative stress, they are difficult to measure in clinical practice at present. Gas chromatography and mass spectrometry are very expensive and time consuming, but in the future it is possible that ethane could be measured using other techniques. It may then prove to be a suitable marker for studying the effects of antioxidants in asthma.

V. Exhaled Breath Condensate

Exhaled breath condensate contains several markers of inflammation and oxidative stress (4,49) (Table 2). The technique is simple to perform and is completely noninvasive. The collected condensate may be stored for later analysis, but the technique cannot give an immediate readout. However, this technique might prove to be very useful in assessing the effects of anti-inflammatory treatments and particularly of inhibitors of mediators that are detectable in exhaled breath condensate.

A. Markers of Oxidative Stress

Exhaled hydrogen peroxide (H_2O_2) levels are increased in adults and children with asthma, particularly those with severe disease (50–53), and is correlated with airway

Table 2 Inflammatory Markers in Exhaled
Breath Condensate

Markers of oxidative and nitrative stress
  Hydrogen peroxide
  8-Isoprostane
  Thiobarbituric acid
  Nitrite/nitrate
  3-Nitrotyrosine
  S-Nitrosothiols
Inflammatory mediators
  Leukotriene B_4
  Cysteinyl-leukotrienes
  Prostaglandins
  Histamine
  Adenosine
  Interleukin-4
  Interleukin-6
  Interleukin-8
  Interferon-γ
  Hydrogen ions (pH)

---

hyperresponsiveness (54). The concentrations of H_2O_2 in exhaled condensate are reduced in asthmatic patients after treatment with inhaled corticosteroids (55). However, this marker is relatively unstable and there is a large variability.

8-Isoprostane is a more stable marker of oxidative stress that is formed nonenzymatically by oxidation of arachidonic acid. Levels of 8-isoprostane are increased in exhaled condensate of asthmatic patients and are correlated with disease severity (56). 8-Isoprostane may be well suited to assessment of oxidative stress in asthma and could be used to assess the effects of antioxidant therapies.

B. Markers of Nitrative Stress

Elevated levels of nitrite and nitrate are detectable in exhaled breath of patients with asthma (57,58). Nitrosothiols, formed from an interaction of NO with thiol groups on cysteine residues of proteins such as glutathione, are also elevated in asthma (59,60). The interaction of NO with superoxide anions formed from oxidative stress results in the formation of peroxynitrite, which is unstable but interacts with tyrosine residues in proteins to form stable 3-nitrotyrosine. 3-Nitrotyrosine levels are increased in exhaled breath of patients with asthma (61), and there is evidence of 3-nitrotyrosine immunoreactivity in the airways of asthmatic patients and in cells of induced sputum (62,63). It is likely that increased 3-nitrotyrosine levels in the breath may occur during exacerbations of asthma when oxidative stress increases.

C. Inflammatory Mediators

Several mediators of inflammation have been detected in the breath of patients with asthma. There is an increase in the levels of leukotriene B_4 and cysteinyl-leukotrienes (61). Several other mediators, including prostaglandins, histamine, and adenosine, may also be detectable in the breath (64). Even cytokines may be detectable in exhaled breath condensate, and in children with asthma there is an increase in the concentrations of interleukin-4 (IL-4) and a decrease in interferon-γ (IFN-γ) compared to normal children (65). Acidification of exhaled breath condensate (low pH) may also indicate acute inflammation in patients with asthma (66).

D. Use in Drug Discovery

Exhaled breath condensate is a simple, entirely noninvasive procedure that can be used in all patients with asthma, including children and patients with severe disease. It may be used repeatedly, thus allowing kinetic studies. The measurement of specific mediators and biomarkers means that it may be used to explore the effects of specific inhibitors, such as 5-lipoxygenase inhibitors, as well as anti-inflammatory effects.

VI. Exhaled Temperature

Increased blood flow during inflammation produces a local increase in heat or "calor," one of the classical signs of inflammation. This is reflected by a faster rise in the temperature of exhaled breath in patients with asthma compared to normal individuals (67). A β_2-agonist increases the temperature rise in normal subjects, presumably via its vasodilator action, whereas it has no effect in asthmatic patients as airway vessels may be already maximally dilated. These findings are consistent with the measurements of bronchial blood flow using an inhaled soluble gas dimethyl ether (68).

VII. Future Directions

There is increasing recognition that noninvasive markers may be used to monitor inflammation in asthmatic airways and that increased levels are able to detect deterioration of asthma control. As exemplified by exhaled NO, these markers may be early detectors of deterioration in asthma. While exhaled NO analyzers are currently expensive, it is likely that over the next few years they will become smaller and less expensive, so that they will be used more widely in medical practice. Eventually it may be possible to develop analyzers that are small enough for patients to use at home in the same way that they now use peak flow meters to monitor asthma control. Other markers, such as exhaled hydrocarbons, may also be more easily detectable in the future. Measurement of mediators in the breath is easy, and it may be possible in the future to develop detector systems that are rapid and semiquantitative to detect increase in key mediators. Exhaled breath measurements may also be useful in monitoring the effects of novel therapies for asthma, both in short-term clinical studies and in long-term clinical trials.

References

1. Parameswaran K, Pizzichini E, Pizzichini MM, Hussack P, Efthimiadis A, Hargreave FE. Clinical judgement of airway inflammation versus sputum cell counts in patients with asthma. Eur Respir J 2000; 15:486–490.
2. Nightingale JA, Rogers DF, Barnes PJ. Effect of repeated sputum induction on cell counts in normal volunteers. Thorax 1998; 53:87–90.
3. Magnussen H, Holz O. Monitoring airway inflammation in asthma by induced sputum. Eur Respir J 1999; 13:5–7.
4. Kharitonov SA, Barnes PJ. Exhaled markers of pulmonary disease. Am J Respir Crit Care Med 2001; 163:1693–1772.
5. Kharitonov SA, Barnes PJ. Clinical aspects of exhaled nitric oxide. Eur Respir J 2000; 16:781–792.
6. Persson MG, Zetterstrom O, Argenius V, Ihre E, Gustafsson LE. Single-breath oxide measurements in asthmatic patients and smokers. Lancet 1994; 343:146–147.
7. Kharitonov SA, Yates D, Robbins RA, Logan-Sinclair R, Shinebourne E, Barnes PJ. Increased nitric oxide in exhaled air of asthmatic patients. Lancet 1994; 343:133–135.
8. Kharitonov SA, O'Connor BJ, Evans DJ, Barnes PJ. Allergen-induced late asthmatic reactions are associated with elevation of exhaled nitric oxide. Am J Respir Crit Care Med 1995; 151:1894–1899.
9. Massaro AF, Gaston B, Kita D, Fanta C, Stamler J, Drazen JM. Expired nitric oxide levels during treatment for acute asthma. Am J Respir Crit Care Med 1995; 152:800–803.
10. Jatakanon A, Lim S, Kharitonov SA, Chung KF, Barnes PJ. Correlation between exhaled nitric oxide, sputum eosinophils and methacholine responsiveness. Thorax 1998; 53: 91–95.
11. Dupont LJ, Rochette F, Demedts MG, Verleden GM. Exhaled nitric oxide correlates with airway hyperresponsiveness in steroid-naive patients with mild asthma. Am J Respir Crit Care Med 1998; 157:894–898.
12. Lim S, Jatakanon A, Meah S, Oates T, Chung KF, Barnes PJ. Relationship between exhaled nitric oxide and mucosal eosinophilic inflammation in mild to moderately severe asthma. Thorax 2000; 55:184–188.
13. Baraldi E, Dario C, Ongaro R, Scollo M, Azzolin NM, Panza N, Paganini N, Zacchello F. Exhaled nitric oxide concentrations during treatment of wheezing exacerbation in infants and young children. Am J Respir Crit Care Med 1999; 159:1284–1288.
14. Yates DH, Kharitonov SA, Robbins RA, Thomas PS, Barnes PJ. Effect of a nitric oxide synthase inhibitor and a glucocorticosteroid on exhaled nitric oxide. Am J Respir Crit Care Med 1995; 152:892–896.
15. Kharitonov SA, Yates DH, Barnes PJ. Regular inhaled budesonide decreases nitric oxide concentration in the exhaled air of asthmatic patients. Am J Respir Crit Care Med 1996; 153:454–457.
16. Jatakanon A, Kharitonov S, Lim S, Barnes PJ. Effect of differing doses of inhaled budesonide on markers of airway inflammation in patients with mild asthma. Thorax 1999; 54:108–114.

17. Lehtimaki L, Kankaanranta H, Saarelainen S, Turjanmaa V, Moilanen E. Inhaled flutica-
     sone decreases bronchial but not alveolar nitric oxide output in asthma. Eur Respir J
     2001; 18:635–639.
18. Donnelly LE, Barnes PJ. Expression and regulation of inducible nitric oxide synthase
     from human primary airway epithelial cells. Am J Respir Cell Mol Biol 2002; 26:
     144–151.
19. Baraldi E, Azzolin NM, Zanconato S, Dario C, Zacchello F. Corticosteroids decrease
     exhaled nitric oxide in children with acute asthma. J Pediatr 1997; 131:381–385.
20. Barnes PJ. The effect of drugs on exhaled nitric oxide. Eur Respir Rev 1999; 9:231–233.
21. Yates DH, Kharitonov SA, Barnes PJ. Effect of short- and long-acting β_2-agonists on
     exhaled nitric oxide in asthmatic patients. Eur Respir J 1997; 10:1483–1488.
22. Barnes PJ. Scientific rationale for combination inhalers with a long-acting β_2-agonists
     and corticosteroids. Eur Respir J 2002; 19:182–191.
23. Bisgaard H, Loland L, Oj JA. NO in exhaled air of asthmatic children is reduced by
     the leukotriene receptor antagonist montelukast. Am J Respir Crit Care Med 1999; 160:
     1227–1231.
24. Lim S, Tomita K, Carramori G, Jatakanon A, Oliver B, Keller A, Adcock I, Chung KF,
     Barnes PJ. Low-dose theophylline reduces eosinophilic inflammation but not exhaled
     nitric oxide in mild asthma. Am J Respir Crit Care Med 2001; 164:273–276.
25. Barnes PJ. New treatments for asthma. Eur J Int Med 2000; 11:9–20.
26. Barnes PJ. Cytokine modulators as novel therapies for asthma. Ann Rev Pharmacol
     Toxicol 2002; 42:81–98.
27. Kharitonov SA, Alving K, Barnes PJ. Exhaled and nasal nitric oxide measurement:
     recommendations. Eur Respir J 1997; 10:1683–1693.
28. Recommendations for standardized procedures for the on-line and off-line measurement
     of exhaled lower respiratory nitric oxide and nasal nitric oxide in adults and children-
     1999. Am J Respir Crit Care Med 1999; 160:2104–2117.
29. Stirling RG, Kharitonov SA, Campbell D, Robinson D, Durham SR, Chung KF, Barnes
     PJ. Increase in exhaled nitric oxide levels in patients with difficult asthma and correlation
     with symptoms and disease severity despite treatment with oral and inhaled and cortico-
     steroids. Thorax 1998; 53:1030–1034.
30. Jatakanon A, Uasaf C, Maziak W, Lim S, Chung KF, Barnes PJ. Neutrophilic inflamma-
     tion in severe persistent asthma. Am J Respir Crit Care Med 1999; 160:1532–1539.
31. Kharitonov SA, Yates DH, Chung KF, Barnes PJ. Changes in the dose of inhaled steroid
     affect exhaled nitric oxide levels in asthmatic patients. Eur J Respir Dis 1996; 9:196–201.
32. Jatakanon A, Lim S, Barnes PJ. Changes in sputum eosinophils predict loss of asthma
     control. Am J Respir Crit Care Med 2000; 161:64–72.
33. Kharitonov SA, Barnes PJ. Does exhaled nitric oxide reflect asthma control? Yes, it
     does! Am J Respir Crit Care Med 2001; 164:727–728.
34. Sippel JM, Holden We, Tilles SA, O'hollaren M, Cook J, Thukkani N, Priest J, Nelson
     B, Osborne ML. Exhaled nitric oxide levels correlate with measures of disease control
     in asthma. J Allergy Clin Immunol 2000; 106:645–650.
35. Jones SL, Kittelson J, Cowan JO, Flannery EM, Hancox RJ, McLachlan CR, Taylor
     DR. The predictive value of exhaled nitric oxide measurements in assessing changes
     in asthma control. Am J Respir Crit Care Med 2001; 164:738–743.
36. Zayasu K, Sekizawa K, Okinaga S, Yamaya M, Ohrui T, Sasaki H. Increased carbon
     monoxide in exhlaed air of asthmatic patients. Am J Respir Crit Care Med 1997; 156:
     1140–1143.

37. Horvath I, Donnelly LE, Kiss A, Paredi P, Kharitonov SA, Barnes PJ. Raised levels of exhaled carbon monoxide are associated with an increased expression of heme oxygenase-1 in airway macrophages in asthma: a new marker of oxidative stress. Thorax 1998; 53:668–672.
38. Lim S, Groneberg D, Fischer A, Oates T, Caramori G, Mattos W, Adcock I, Barnes PJ, Chung KF. Expression of heme oxygenase isoenzymes 1 and 2 in normal and asthmatic airways. Effect of inhaled corticosteroids. Am J Respir Crit Care Med 2000; 162:1912–1918.
39. Donnelly LE, Barnes PJ. Expression of heme oxygenase in human airway epithelial cells. Am J Respir Cell Mol Biol 2001; 24:295–303.
40. Yamaya M, Sekizawa K, Ishizuka S, Monma M, Sasaki H. Exhaled carbon monoxide levels during treatment of acute asthma. Eur Respir J 1999; 13:757–760.
41. Paredi P, Leckie MJ, Horvath I, Allegra L, Kharitonov SA, Barnes PJ. Changes in exhaled carbon monoxide and nitric oxide levels following allergen challenge in patients with asthma. Eur Respir J 1999; 13:48–53.
42. Uasaf C, Jatakanon A, James A, Kharitonov SA, Wilson NM, Barnes PJ. Exhaled carbon monoxide in childhood asthma. J Pediatr 1999; 135:569–574.
43. Paredi P, Shah P, Montuschi P, Sullivan P, Hodson ME, Kharitonov SA, Barnes PJ. Increased carbon monoxide in exhaled air of cystic fibrosis patients. Thorax 1999; 54: 917–920.
44. Montuschi P, Kharitonov SA, Barnes PJ. Exhaled carbon monoxide and nitric oxide in COPD. Chest 2001; 120:496–501.
45. Biernacki WA, Kharitonov SA, Barnes PJ. Exhaled carbon monoxide in patients with lower respiratory tract infection. Respir Med 2001; 95:1003–1005.
46. Paredi P, Kharitonov SA, Leak D, Shah PL, Cramer D, Hodson ME, Barnes PJ. Exhaled ethane is elevated in cystic fibrosis and correlates with carbon monoxide levels and airway obstruction. Am J Respir Crit Care Med 2000; 161:1247–1251.
47. Olopade CO, Zakkar M, Swedler WI, Rubinstein I. Exhaled pentane levels in acute asthma. Chest 1997; 111:862–865.
48. Paredi P, Kharitonov SA, Barnes PJ. Elevation of exhaled ethane concentration in asthma. Am J Respir Crit Care Med 2000; 162:1450–1454.
49. Mutlu GM, Garey KW, Robbins RA, Danziger LH, Rubinstein I. Collection and analysis of exhaled breath condensate in humans. Am J Respir Crit Care Med 2001; 164:731–737.
50. Antczak A, Nowak D, Shariati B, Krol M, Piasecka G, Kurmanowska Z. Increased hydrogen peroxide and thiobarbituric acid-reactive products in expired breath condensate of asthmatic patients. Eur Respir J 1997; 10:1235–1241.
51. Horvath I, Donnelly LE, Kiss A, Kharitonov SA, Lim S, Chung KF, Barnes PJ. Combined use of exhaled hydrogen peroxide and nitric oxide in monitoring asthma. Am J Respir Crit Care Med 1998; 158:1046–1048.
52. Dohlman AW, Black HR, Royall JA. Expired breath hydrogen peroxide is a marker of acute airway inflammation in pediatric patients with asthma. Am Rev Respir Dis 1993; 148:955–960.
53. Jobsis Q, Ratgeep HC, Hermans PWM, de Jongste JC. Hydrogen peroxide in exhaled air is increased in asthmatic children. Eur Respir J 1997; 10:519–521.
54. Emelyanov A, Fedoseev G, Abulimity A, Rudinski K, Fedoulov A, Karabanov A, Barnes PJ. Elevated concentrations of exhaled hydrogen peroxide in asthmatic patients. Chest 2001; 120:1136–1139.
55. Antczak A, Kurmanowska Z, Kasielski M, Nowak D. Inhaled glucocorticosteroids decrease hydrogen peroxide level in expired air condensate in asthmatic patients. Respir Med 2000; 94:416–421.

56. Montuschi P, Ciabattoni G, Corradi M, Nightingale JA, Collins JV, Kharitonov SA, Barnes PJ. Increased 8-isoprostane, a marker of oxidative stress, in exhaled condensates of asthmatic patients. Am J Respir Crit Care Med 1999; 160:216–220.

57. Corradi M, Montuschi P, Donnelly LE, Pesci A, Kharitonov SA, Barnes PJ. Increased nitrosothiols in exhaled breath condensate in inflammatory airway diseases. Am J Respir Crit Care Med 2001; 163:854–858.

58. Ganas K, Loukides S, Papatheodorou G, Panagou P, Kalogeropoulos N. Total nitrite/nitrate in expired breath condensate of patients with asthma. Respir Med 2001; 95: 649–654.

59. Gaston B, Sears S, Woods J, Hunt J, Ponaman M, McMahon T, Stamler JS. Bronchodilator S-nitrosothiol deficiency in asthmatic respiratory failure. Lancet 1998; 351: 1317–1319.

60. Corradi M, Montuschi P, Donnelly LE, Pesci A, Kharitonov SA, Barnes PJ. Increased nitrosothiols in exhaled breath condensate in inflammatory airway disease. Am J Respir Crit Care Med 2001; 163:854–858.

61. Hanazawa T, Kharitonov SA, Barnes PJ. Increased nitrotyrosine in exhaled breath condensate of patients with asthma. Am J Respir Crit Care Med 2000; 162:1273–1276.

62. Saleh D, Ernst P, Lim S, Barnes PJ, Giaid A. Increased formation of the potent oxidant peroxynitrite in the airways of asthmatic patients is associated with induction of nitric oxide synthase: effect of inhaled glucocorticoid. FASEB J 1998; 12:929–937.

63. Ichinose M, Sugiura H, Yamagata S, Koarai A, Shirato K. Increase in reactive nitrogen species production in chronic obstructive pulmonary disease airways. Am J Respir Crit Care Med 2000; 160:701–706.

64. Montuschi P, Kharitonov SA, Carpagnano E, Culpitt S, Russell R, Collins JV, Barnes PJ. Exhaled prostaglandin E$_2$: a new marker of airway inflammation in COPD. Am J Respir Crit Care Med 2000; 161:A821.

65. Shahid SK, Kharitonov SA, Wilson NM, Bush A, Barnes PJ. Increased interleukin-4 and decreased interferon-γ in exhaled breath condensate of asthmatic children. Am J Respir Crit Care Med 2002; 165:1290–1293.

66. Hunt JF, Fang K, Malik R, Snyder A, Malhotra N, Platts-Mills TA, Gaston B. Endogenous airway acidification. Implications for asthma pathophysiology. Am J Respir Crit Care Med 2000; 161:694–699.

67. Paredi P, Kharitonov SA, Barnes PJ. Faster rise of exhaled breath temperature in asthma. A novel marker of airway inflammation? Am J Respir Crit Care Med 2002; 165: 181–184.

68. Kumar SD, Emery MJ, Atkins ND, Danta I, Wanner A. Airway mucosal blood flow in bronchial asthma. Am J Respir Crit Care Med 1998; 158:153–156.

5

The Modulatory Effects of Carbon Monoxide on the Inflammatory Response

FRANCIS WHALEN, AUGUSTINE M. K. CHOI, and JIGME M. SETHI

University of Pittsburgh
Pittsburgh, Pennsylvania, U.S.A.

I. A Historical Perspective on Carbon Monoxide

Carbon monoxide (CO) is a molecule that has been extensively studied and much maligned since the discovery of its biological role as an asphyxiate by the French physiologist Claude Bernard in 1857. Bernard determined that CO produces asphyxia by reversibly binding to hemoglobin (1). In 1895, Haldane demonstrated that elevated partial pressures of oxygen antagonized binding of CO to hemoglobin and that experimental animals exposed to lethal CO poisoning survived when a large amount of oxygen was dissolved in their blood plasma (2). In 1944, Roughton and Darling reported that carboxyhemoglobin (COHb) shifted the oxygen-dissociation curve to the left due to the increased binding affinity of the unoccupied heme groups for oxygen (3). This of course made oxygen unloading at the tissue level more difficult. These early studies set the framework for explaining the mechanism of CO poisoning as being due to hypoxia at the tissue level. In 1949, Sjorstrand discovered that endogenously produced CO comes from the degradation of hemoglobin released during erythrocyte turnover (4). Coburn and associates reported the same findings in their work in 1967(5). In 1969, Tenhunen et al. described heme oxygenase (HO) as the enzyme responsible for the production of endogenous CO. They demonstrated that HO catalyzed the reaction that converted hemoglobin to biliverdin with CO and free iron as byproducts (6). There are three different isoforms of HO, of which HO-1 is the most studied and interesting because of its ability to be greatly induced by a wide variety of oxidative and inflammatory stressors, suggesting an important regulatory role for the enzyme.

In recent years, CO, the gaseous by-product of the reaction catalyzed by HO, has emerged as a key molecule of interest to clinical and laboratory investigators as a marker of oxidative stress, but it is increasingly apparent from in vitro and animal models of sepsis, ischemia-reperfusion, hyperoxia, and xenotransplantation that is also has a potent role in reducing oxidative and inflammatory injury (7–11). In addition, there is evidence that HO, and in particular CO, also play an important role in the physiological regulation of vascular tone (12,13). This chapter will describe how CO functions as a key molecule modulating inflammation in various disease models and outline the evidence for involvement of carbon monoxide in human airway inflammation.

II. Models of Disease and Inflammation

A. Acute Lung Injury and Sepsis

In rats exposed to lipopolysaccharide (LPS) to induce acute lung injury and sepsis, it was hypothesized that induction of HO-1 could mitigate the lethal effects of endotoxemia. Rats pretreated with hemoglobin, a potent inducer of HO-1, survived twice the lethal dose of LPS, compared to 100% mortality seen in the control group of rats exposed to a lethal dose of LPS, but pretreated with saline alone. Northern blot analysis verified that HO-1 expression was increased after hemoglobin pretreatment. In addition, pretreatment with hemoglobin resulted in significant attenuation of the neutrophilic alveolitis and lung injury and hemorrhage seen in the rats exposed to a sublethal dose of LPS alone. Importantly, tin protoporphyrin (Sn-PP), an inhibitor of HO-1, when administered along with hemoglobin prior to LPS, abrogated the hemoglobin-induced protection against endotoxic shock (14).

To elucidate the mechanism of this protection, Otterbein et al. (9) studied macrophages overexpressing HO-1 protein. These cells produced significantly less tumor necrosis factor-α (TNF-α) in response to LPS than did control macrophages that did not overexpress HO-1. Next, using wild-type RAW 264.7 macrophages, they were able to show that exposure to CO at 250 ppm significantly reduced the LPS-induced production of TNF-α from these cells, while increasing the accumulation of the anti-inflammatory cytokine IL-10. Mice given a sublethal dose of LPS in the presence of CO also produced less serum TNF-α and, interestingly, more IL-10 than mice treated with LPS alone. Since IL-10 itself can reduce TNF-α production, Otterbein et al. used IL-10–deficient mice to demonstrate that CO was still able to attenuate the TNF-α response to LPS in these mice. This indeed suggests that the anti-inflammatory effect of HO-1, at least in this model, is likely exerted through CO itself.

CO exerts these effects by a cGMP-independent pathway, and N-nitro-L-arginine methyl ester (L-NAME) was unable to attenuate the effects of CO in this model, probably by a nitric oxide (NO)–independent pathway as well. It appears that the protective effects of CO were mediated by the mitogen-activated protein kinase pathway, specifically the mitogen-actived protein kinase kinase 3 (MKK3) pathway. Thus, MKK3$^{-/-}$ knock out mice did not display the inhibitory effect of CO on TNF-α production in response to LPS, as seen in the MKK3$^{+/+}$ mice. Since CO does not affect LPS-induced TNF-α gene expression but does reduce protein expression, a posttranscriptional mechanism is likely involved (9).

B. Hyperoxia

Hyperoxia is a potent inducer of HO-1 in several cell types, and this is likely to be a protective response In vitro, human pulmonary epithelial A549 cells that are stably transfected with the rat HO-1 cDNA exhibit a marked decrease in cell growth and resistance to hyperoxia, compared with wild-type A549 cells, and both these effects can be reversed by SnPP, the HO-1 inhibitor (15). In vivo, intratracheal instillation of an adenoviral vector encoding HO-1 was used to overexpress HO-1 in the pulmonary epithelium of rats that were subsequently exposed to hyperoxia. Overexpression of HO-1 in these animals was associated with reduced pleural effusions, edema, hemorrhage, neutrophil inflammation, and apoptosis upon exposure to hyperoxia than in rats that did not overexpress HO-1(16). In another series of experiments it was shown that Sprague-Dawley rats exposed to CO at 50–500 ppm exhibited marked tolerance against hyperoxia, as compared with animals exposed to hyperoxia without prior CO exposure. Importantly, exogenous CO completely protected against hyperoxia-induced lung injury in rats in which endogenous HO-1 activity was inhibited by SnPP (10). Thus, exposure to endogenous (via increased HO-1 activity) or exogenous CO has a beneficial effect in a hyperoxic environment.

C. Lung Ischemia-Reperfusion

In a murine lung ischemia-reperfusion model, HO-1 knockout mice (*Hmox*1$^{-/-}$) demonstrated 100% mortality with ischemia-reperfusion, compared with 12% mortality of wild-type littermates. Exogenous CO (inhalation of 0.1% CO for 24 hours) protected these HO-1 knockout mice from death due to ischemia-reperfusion, and this protection was mediated by CO-driven activation of cyclic guanosine monophosphate (cGMP) and suppression of plasminogen activator inhibitor-1 (PAI-1), causing less deposition of microvascular fibrin. Thus, PAI-1 knockout mice could not be rescued from ischemic injury and fatality by exogenous CO (17).

Hypoxia is another potent inducer of the HO-1 gene. HO-1 immunostaining is increased in the bronchial epithelium and smooth muscle of guinea pigs by just 4 minutes of hypoxic breathing (100% N$_2$). This upregulation of HO-1 protein may subserve a protective bronchodilatory role, since guinea pigs exposed to exogenous CO (100%) demonstrated attenuated bronchoconstriction in response to histamine infusion (18). L-NAME could not inhibit this bronchodilatory effect of CO, thereby excluding nitric oxide (NO) as a cause of this effect.

D. Transplantation

The role of CO in modulating the immune response is exemplified by its ability to prolong graft survival in a mouse-to-rat cardiac xenotransplantation model (19). In this model rejection is prevented by brief complement inhibition by cobra venom factor (CVF) and sustained T-cell immunosuppression by cyclosporin (CsA). Mouse hearts that survive indefinitely after transplantation in rats on this regimen strongly express HO-1 in endothelial and smooth muscle cells. Hearts transplanted from HO-$1^{+/+}$ mice survived long term in this model, but hearts from HO-$1^{-/-}$ mice died soon after transplant into rats treated with CVF + CsA immunosuppression. On the other hand, inhibition of HO-1 activity with SnPP in spite of the above immunosuppression led to rapid rejection in 3–7 days, despite the use of CVF and CsA immunosuppression. This confirms that HO-1 activity is essential to graft survival by modulating the rejection process. In another elegant experiment, in which donor and recipient animals were each treated with the HO-1 inhibitor SnPP, grafts survived indefinitely in rats kept in chambers containing 250–400 ppm CO(11). Even though CO exposure ceased at 14–16 days, graft survival continued unimpeded for >50 days. Thus, exogenous CO was able to protect donor hearts from rejection in the long term, despite abrogation of endogenous HO-1 activity, and even after CO exposure had ceased—startling and exciting proof of the immunomodulatory effects of CO. Notably, grafted hearts protected against rejection by CO lacked the platelet aggregation occluding the coronary arteries that was seen in rejected grafts. A similar result was noted in an animal model of islet cell transplantation in which HO-1 upregulation protected transplanted islet cells from apoptosis mediated by pro-inflammatory cytokines and CD95 (Fas) and prolonged islet cell survival (20).

E. Vascular

Treatment of rat aortic smooth muscle cells with membrane-permeable dibutyryl cyclic adenosine monophosphate (cAMP) led to dose and time-dependent increases in HO-1 mRNA and protein and smooth muscle CO production, and this effect is not inhibited by L-glutamine, N^{G}-monomethyl-L-arginine (L-NMMA) (21). Similarly, pig arteries were transfected in vivo with adenoviral vectors encoding HO-1 leading to overexpression of HO-1 in vascular smooth muscle cells. HO-1 overexpression significantly inhibited vasoreactivity of the subsequently explanted arterial rings, an effect that was abrogated by the HO-1 inhibitor zinc protoporphyrin, but not by the ANY inhibitor L-Nω-nitro-arginine (L-NNA) (22).

   HO-1 also plays an important role in the pulmonary circulation. Rats treated with the potent HO-1 inducer nickel chloride were protected against the development of pulmonary hypertension produced by exposure to normobaric hypoxia (10% oxygen for one week) (23) ether. These experiments suggest an important modulator role of HO-1 and, presumably, CO in the maintenance of vascular tone in both the pulmonary and systemic circulations.

F. Airway Response to Aeroallergen

CO also modulates allergic inflammation. In mice sensitized to and subsequently challenged with ovalbumin, exposure to 250 ppm of CO led to marked reduction in bronchoalveolar lavage (BAL) fluid eosinophils at 24 and 48 hours, compared with similarly sensitized and challenged animals maintained in room air. Exposure to CO after sensitization and challenge also resulted in a significant decrease in BAL fluid IL-5, along with reduction in prostaglandin E_2 (PGE_2) and leukotriene B_4 (LTB_4) levels, compared to animals kept in room air (8).

III. Human Studies in Asthma

The increased burden of inflammatory cells recruited to the asthmatic airways is associated with significant local oxidative stress, reflected in part by the higher levels of hydrogen peroxide in the exhaled breath of asthmatic subjects (24). Eosinophils in asthmatics have also been shown to produce increased reactive oxidative species (25,26), contributing to greater oxidative stress and also possibly contributing to increased airway hyperresponsiveness, perpetuating the cycle (27). It follows therefore that an anti-inflammatory and antioxidant molecule like CO could potentially be of great therapeutic benefit in this disease, in part also because of its role as a bronchodilator. Thus, HO-1 expression is upregulated in the alveolar macrophages of humans with asthma as compared to controls, as are bilirubin levels in sputum (28). Human studies to date have found elevations of CO in the exhaled breath of subjects with airway inflammation, although it is unclear if this results from airway generation of CO or increased delivery of CO to the inflamed lung by the pulmonary circulation.

Exhaled CO is elevated in asthmatics, even if clinically stable, and correlates with forced expiratory volume in one second (FEV_1) and the severity of asthma (29). Treatment with inhaled corticosteroids has been shown in some studies to decrease exhaled CO to levels similar to controls. Asthmatics (nonsmokers) treated with inhaled steroids had significantly lower exhaled CO than nontreated (nonsmoking) asthmatics (30). Exhaled CO after steroid therapy was significantly less and correlated with a decrease in sputum eosinophil count as well as improvement in FEV_1 (31). Exhaled CO has been shown to be a discriminator between atopics (without active airway disease) and controls, although there was no correlation between exhaled CO and FEV_1 or concentration of methacholine required to produce 20% drop in FEV_1 (PC_{20})(31).

In a group of nonsmoking asthmatics during exacerbation, exhaled CO levels correlated inversely with peak expiratory flow rate (PEFR); treatment and resolution with steroid therapy resulted in an increase in PEFR and a decrease in exhaled CO after 7 days of therapy. Potential explanations for the decrease in exhaled CO were inhibition of the HO-1 promoter, inhibition of proinflammatory cytokines, and/or increase in NO, all via steroid therapy (32).

In another study, asthmatic subjects were given inhaled histamine or allergen to cause a reduction of FEV_1 by 20%. In the allergen challenge, there were two different groups of responders. One group had an early and late phase bronchospastic response with increases in exhaled CO preceding a reduction in FEV_1 associated with each phase. The second group consisted of subjects with the same biphasic early and late phase increases in exhaled CO, but only a late fall in the FEV_1. Thus, exhaled CO may reflect inflammatory oxidative stress not reflected in routine clinical measurements of FEV_1. Interestingly, the reduction in FEV_1 with histamine did not result in an increase in exhaled CO, showing that airway constriction did not account for the difference in exhaled CO. The combination of these findings indicate that airway caliber is not the cause for the change in exhaled CO, but that airway inflammation is likely responsible for the elevations of exhaled CO (33).

Contrary to the paradigm that increases in exhaled CO result from a protective induction of the antioxidative enzyme HO-1 in the inflamed airways of asthmatic subjects, some authors have been unable to show an increase in exhaled CO after whole lung antigen challenge (34) and have not found a correlation between the levels of exhaled isoprostanes (a marker of lipid peroxidation) and CO (35). Indeed, one study found that HO-1 was not induced in the airways of asthmatics compared to nonasthmatic controls (36). Therefore, however intriguing it may be to speculate on the protective role of HO-1 and CO in reducing inflammation in asthmatic airways, confirmatory proof is lacking.

IV. Summary

The importance of HO-1 is suggested by the fact that it is highly conserved across evolution and is ubiquitous in nature. It is not therefore surprising that a gaseous molecular end product of the reaction catalyzed by this enzyme also plays a major role as a protective anti-inflammatory and immunomodulatory agent. Since CO can modulate the activity of so many pathways involved in the inflammatory response—cytokine production, cGMP function, MAP kinase pathways, to name but a few—it is conceivable that it could one day be used clinically as an anti-inflammatory therapy. In this respect its resemblance to the other ubiquitous gaseous molecule, NO, is particularly striking. However, CO has first to overcome the baggage of its past, namely its apparent toxicity, before the beneficial effects of low doses of this remarkable gas can be harnessed in clinical medicine.

References

1. Bernard C. Lecons sur les effects de substances toxiques et medicamenteuses. Paris: Bailliere, 1857.
2. Yamaya M, Hosada M, Ishizuka S, Monma M, Matsui M, Suzuki T, Sekizawa K, Sasaki H. Relation between exhaled carbon monoxide levels and clinical severity of asthma. Clin Exp Allergy 2001, 31:417–422.
3. Roughton FJW, R. C, Darling. The effect of CO on the oxyhemoglobin dissociation curve. Am J Physiol 1944; 141:17–31.
4. Sjorstrand T. Endogenous formation of CO in man under normal and pathological conditions. Scand J Clin Lab Invest 1949; 1:201–214.
5. Coburn RF, Williams WJ, White P, Kahn SB. Production of CO from hemoglobin in vivo. J Clin Invest 1967; 46:346–356.
6. Tenhunen R, Marver HS, Schmid R. Microsomal HO—characterization of the enzyme. J Biol Chem 1969; 244:6388–6694.

7. Brouard S, Otterbein LE, Anrather J, Tobiasch E, Bach FH, Choi AM, Soares MP. Carbon monoxide generated by heme oxygenase-1 suppresses endothelial cell apoptosis. J Exp Med 2000; 192:1015–1026.

8. Chapman JT, Otterbein LE, Elias JA, Choi AM. K. Carbon monoxide attenuates aeroallergen-induced inflammation in mice. Am J Physiol 2001; 281:L209–L215.

9. Otterbein LE, Bach FH, Alam J, Soares M, Tao LuH, Wysk M, Davis RJ, Flavell RA, Choi AM. Carbon monoxide has anti-inflammatory effects involving the mitogen-activated protein kinase pathway. Nat Med 2000; 6:422–428.

10. Otterbein LE, Mantell LL, Choi AM. K. Carbon monoxide provides protection against hyperoxic lung injury. Am J Physiol 1999; 276:L688–L694.

11. Sato K, Balla J, Otterbein L, Smith RN, Brouard S, Lin Y, Csizmadia E, Sevigny J, Robson SC, Vercellotti G, Choi AM, Bach FH, Soares MP. Carbon monoxide generated by heme-oxygenase-1 suppresses the rejection of mouse-to-rat cardiac transplants. J Immunol 2001; 166:4185–4194.

12. Gaine SP, Booth G, Otterbein L, Flavahan NA, Choi AM, Wiener CM. Induction of HO-1 with hemoglobin depresses vasoreactivity in rat aorta. J Vasc Res 1999; 36: 114–119.

13. Morita T, Mitsiali, SA, Koike J, Liu Y, Kourembanas S. CO controls the proliferation of hypoxic vascular smooth muscle cells. J Biol Chem 1997; 26,2 (52):32804–32809.

14. Otterbein L, Sylvester SL, Choi AM. K. Hemoglobin provides protection against lethal endotoxemia in rats: the role of heme oxygenase-1. Am J Respir Cell Mol Biol 1995; 13:595–601.

15. Lee PJ, Alam J, Wiegand GW, Choi AM. K. Overexpression of heme oxygenase-1 in human pulmonary epithelial cells results in cell growth arrest and increased resistance to hyperoxia. Proc Natl Acad Sci USA 1996; 93:10393–10398.

16. Otterbein LE, Kolls JK, Mantell LL, Cook JL, Alam J, Choi AM. K. Exogenous administration of heme oxygenase-1 by gene transfer provides protection against hyperoxia-induced lung injury. Proc Natl Acad Sci USA 1996; 93:10393–10398.

17. Fujita T, Toda K, Karimova A, Yan S.-F., Maka Y, Yet S.-F., Pinsky DJ. Paradoxical rescue from ischemic lung injury by inhaled carbon monoxide driven by depression of fibrinolysis. Nat Med 2001; 7:598–603.

18. Cardell LO, Lou Y, Takeyama LK, Ueki FI, Lausier J, Nadel JA. Carbon monoxide, a cyclic GMP-related messenger, involved in hypoxic bronchodilation in vivo. Pulm Pharmacol Ther 1998; 11:309–315.

19. Soares MP, Lin Y, Anrather J, Csizmadia E, Takigani K, Sato K, Grey ST, Colvin RB, Choi AM, Poss KD, Bach FH. Expression of heme oxygenase-1 can determine cardiac xenograft survival. Nat Med 1998; 4:1073–1077.

20. Pilleggi A, Molano RD, Berney T, Cattan P, Vizzardelli C, Oliver R, Fraker C, Ricordi C, Pastori RL, Bach FH, Inverardi L. Heme oxygenase-1 induction in islet cells results in protection from apoptosis and improved in vivo function after transplantation. Diabetes 2001; 50(9):1983–1991.

21. Durante W, Christodoulides N, Cheng K, Peyton KJ, Sunhara RK, Schafer AI. cAMP induces heme oxygenase-1 gene expression and carbon monoxide production in vascular smooth muscle. Am J Physiol 1997; 273:H317–H323.

22. Duckers, Boehm M, True AL, Yet S.-F., San H, Park JL, Webb CR, Lee M-E., Nabel GJ, Nabel EG. Heme oxygenase-1 protects against vascular constriction and proliferation. Nat Med 2001; 7:693–698.

23. Christou H, Morita T, Hsieh C.-M., Koike H, Arkonac B, Perrella MA, Kourembanas S. Prevention of hypoxia-induced pulmonary hypertension by enhancement of endogenous heme oxygenase-1 in the rat. Circ Res 2000; 86:1224–1229.

24. Jobsis Q, Raatgeep HC, Hermans PWM, de Jongste JC. Hydrogen peroxide in exhaled air is increased in stable asthmatic children. Eur Respir J 1997; 10:519–521.
25. Sanders SP, Zweier JL, Harrison SJ, Trush MA, Rembish SJ, Liu MC. Spontaneous oxygen radical production at sites of antigen challenge in allergic subjects. Am J Respir Care Med 1995; 151:1725–1733.
26. Chanez P, Dent G, Yukawa PJ, Barnes PJ, Chung KF. Generation of oxygen free radicals from blood eosinophils from asthma patients after stimulation with PAF or phorbol ester. Eur Respir J 1990; 8:1002–1007.
27. Antczak A, Nowak D, Shariati B, Krol M, Piasecka G, Kurmanowska. Increased hydrogen peroxide and thiobarbituric acid-reactive products in expired breath condensate of asthmatic patients. Eur Respir J 1997; 10:1235–1241.
28. Horvath I, Donnelly LE, Kiss A, Paredi P, Kharitonov SA, Barnes PJ. Raised levels of exhaled carbon monoxide are associated with an increased expression of heme oxygenase-1 in airway macrophages in asthma: a new marker of oxidative stress. Thorax 1998; 53:668–672.
29. Yamaya M, Hosada M, Ishizuka S, Monma M, Matsui M, Suzuki T, Sekizawa K, Sasaki H. Relation between exhaled carbon monoxide levels and clinical severity of asthma. Clin Exp Allergy 2001; 31:417–422.
30. Zayasu K, Sekizawa K, Okinaga S, Yamaya M, Ohrui T, Hidetada S. Increased carbon monoxide in exhaled air of asthmatic patients. Am J Respir Crit Care Med 1997; 156: 1140–1143.
31. Horvath I, Barnes PJ. Exhaled monoxides in asymptomatic atopic subjects. Clin Exp Allergy 1999; 29:1276–1280.
32. Yamara M, Sekizawa K, Ishizuka S, Monma M, Sasaki H. Exhaled carbon monoxide levels during treatment of acute asthma. Eur Respir J 1999; 13:757–760.
33. Paredi P, Leckie MJ, Horvath I, Allegra L, Kharitonov SA, Barnes PJ. Changes in exhaled carbon monoxide and nitric oxide levels following allergen challenge in patients with asthma. Eur Respir J 1999; 13:48–52.
34. Khatri SB, Ozkan M, McCarthy K, Laskowski D, Hammel J, Dweik RA, Erzurum SC. Alterations in exhaled gas profile during allergen-induced asthmatic response. Am J Respir Care Med 2001; 160:1844–1848.
35. Montuschi P, Corradi M, Ciabattoni G, Nightingale J, Kharitonov SA, Barnes PJ. Increased 8-isoprostane, a marker of oxidative stress, in exhaled condensate of asthma patients. Am J Respir Care Med 1999; 160:216–220.
36. Lim S, Groneberg D, Fischer A, Oates T, Caramori G, Mattos W, Adcock I, Barnes PJ, Chung KF. Expression of heme oxygenase isoenzymes 1 and 2 in normal and asthmatic airways. Am J Respir Care Med 2000; 162:1912–1918.

6

Reactive Nitrogen Species and Tyrosine Nitration in Airway Inflammation

ALBERT van der VLIET

University of Vermont
Burlington, Vermont, U.S.A.

**JASON P. EISERICH,
BRIAN MORRISSEY,
and CARROLL E. CROSS**

University of California, Davis
Sacramento, California, U.S.A.

Although its discovery as a biological mediator only dates back about 15 years, nitric oxide (NO˙) is now widely recognized by every biologist or biochemist as a ubiquitous mediator in diverse biological processes in nearly all aspects of life. Among the classic actions of NO˙ are regulation of vascular and bronchial tone, neurotransmission, antimicrobial activity, and modulation of inflammatory-immune processes (1–3). Considerable interest has been devoted to the involvement of NO˙ in inflammation, since its production is usually dramatically increased under infectious or inflammatory conditions to provide a host defense mechanism and/or regulate the progression of inflammatory-immune processes. Many investigations have, however, insinuated that overproduction of NO˙ can also directly provoke detrimental conditions and contribute to the pathobiology of inflammatory diseases. It is generally assumed that such adverse actions of NO˙ are attributed to accelerated metabolism of NO˙ to more reactive nitrogen intermediates, due to the presence of oxidant-producing mechanisms. The multiple and often paradoxical biological effects of NO˙ form one of the major unsolved controversies in the inflammation-related diseases and have impeded efforts to implicate NO˙ as a therapeutic target in these conditions.

In an attempt to dissect the pathological actions of NO˙ (and/or its metabolites) and its normal physiological properties, much attention has been concentrated on demonstrating endogenous formation of NO˙-derived reactive nitrogen species

(RNS), usually by analysis of characteristic reaction products in biological targets. RNS can induce several covalent modifications in diverse biomolecules, including the formation of nitroso- and nitro-adducts, which presumably result in functional and/or structural changes that may somehow contribute to the pathology of disease. One such characteristic modification is nitration of the amino acid tyrosine, and detection of this modification in proteins is now often used as a diagnostic tool to identify involvement of NO$^{•}$-derived oxidants in many disease states (4–6). Moreover, there has been an increasing number of claims that protein tyrosine nitration may specifically affect certain proteins and may be causally linked to protein dysfunction or cellular injury. Here we intend to briefly overview the involvement of NO$^{•}$ and RNS in the pathophysiology of inflammatory lung diseases and to address the significance of characteristic protein modifications, with special emphasis on tyrosine nitration.

I. Nitric Oxide in Lung Inflammation: Good or Bad?

The expired breath from human subjects contains measurable amounts of NO$^{•}$, which indicates its local synthesis within the respiratory tract. Although a major fraction of expired NO$^{•}$ is thought to originate primarily from the nasal cavity and the sinuses, NO$^{•}$ is known to be generated in all areas of the respiratory tract, by both constitutive and inducible forms of NO$^{•}$ synthases (NOS). Three NOS isoforms exist, and all three are expressed in several cell types within the respiratory tract, including airway and alveolar epithelial cells, macrophages, neutrophils, mast cells, and vascular endothelial and smooth muscle cells (2). The NOS1 isoform (originally known as neuronal NOS; nNOS) is primarily found in nonadrenergic noncholinergic nerves and epithelium; NOS3 (endothelial NOS; eNOS) is observed in bronchial and large pulmonary blood vessels and in the epithelium; and NOS2 (inducible NOS; iNOS) is mostly associated with cell types that are active in inflammation, such as alveolar macrophages and also the epithelium. The expression and distribution of these NOS isoforms are species and age dependent and vary with experimental conditions. Although NOS2 is usually induced in response to inflammatory stimuli, this isoform is "constitutively" expressed in the airway epithelium, perhaps because of continuous exposure to airborne stimuli. Airway epithelial NOS2 expression is rapidly lost ex vivo, suggesting the presence of yet unknown factors in vivo that sustain continuous NOS2 expression (7). Based on studies in various NOS knockout mice, primarily NOS1 and NOS2 appear to be responsible for production exhaled NO$^{•}$ (8,9), suggesting that these are the major NO$^{•}$-producing enzymes in the lung.

During inflammatory diseases of the respiratory tract (such as acute lung injury, asthma, or bronchiectasis) or after exposure to pathogens or environmental pollutants such as ozone, local production of NO$^{•}$ in the lung is commonly enhanced, manifested by increased levels of NO$^{•}$ in expired breath. This is usually associated with induction of NOS2 in epithelial and inflammatory cells (alveolar macrophages, extravasated granulocytes) and increased respiratory tract fluid levels of the metabolic end products nitrite (NO_2^-) and/or nitrate (NO_3^-) (reviewed in Ref. 2). However, although the activation of rodent inflammatory cells (macrophages, neutrophils) generates large amounts of NO˙, the alveolar macrophage does not appear to be a major NO˙ source in the human lung (10). The increase in NOS2 expression and NO˙ production is thought to provide increased host defense against invading pathogens (3), and several studies with NOS2-deficient mice show that they are more susceptible to infections by common pathogens *Mycobacteria tuberculosis* or *Leishmania major*, although NOS2 apparently does not contribute significantly to combating infections with *Pseudomonas aeruginosa* or *Legionella pneumophilia* (11). In this regard, it is interesting to point out the dramatically reduced NOS2 expression in the respiratory epithelium of patients with cystic fibrosis, who commonly expire subnormal levels of exhaled breath NO˙ in spite of a vigorous airway inflammation (12,13). This relative lack of airway NO˙ production may be a contributing factor in the persistent infections that plague these patients (14).

In addition to antimicrobial properties, NO˙ also has several anti-inflammatory actions, and the induction of NOS2 may serve to modulate the progression of the inflammatory process by affecting leukocyte adhesion and migration into lung tissues, phagocyte oxidase activation and apoptosis, and cytokine production by, e.g., macrophages, most likely by altered gene expression due to effects on cell signaling pathways and transcription factor activation (10,15–18). The actual contribution of NO˙ to inflammatory lung diseases and the involvement of NOS2 or other NOS isozymes have been explored in several recent studies with various NOS knockout animals. However, results from such studies are unfortunately variable and sometimes inconsistent or inconclusive, primarily because of the use of different animal models that usually do not adequately mimic human disease, and also because of considerable differences between studies in endpoint measurements at variable stages. However, even though NO˙ may serve to suppress inflammation and associated tissue injury, several studies have in fact indicated that NOS2-derived NO˙ may actually contribute to injury or mortality in several models of (lung) inflammation. For instance, NOS2-deficient mice were protected from death caused by influenza virus pneumonitis (19), were less susceptible to acute lung injury by lipopolysaccharide (LPS) or after inhalation of ozone (20,21), and displayed reduced airways eosinophilia following ovalbumin immunization and challenge (22). Nevertheless, the overall role of NOS2 in these disease models is much less clear, since NOS2-deficient mice were not protected from LPS-induced mortality (23), and NOS2 deficiency did not affect airway responsiveness in ovalbumin models of asthma (24). Also, in several studies of ozone- or hyperoxia-induced lung injury, NOS2 deficiency actually resulted in dramatic increases in neutrophil influx (25,26), more consistent with the known anti-inflammatory properties of NO˙.

Overall, these findings support the concept that excessive production of NO˙ from NOS2 during inflammatory respiratory tract diseases may contribute to respiratory tract injury, although this probably depends on temporal and spacial expression patterns of NOS2 during these diseases. Importantly, recent reports also support the role for other NOS isozymes in airway diseases. Although NOS3 deficiency was found to be associated with increased airway hyperresponsiveness to, e.g., metacholine challenge (27), airway hyperreactivity in response to ovalbumin challenge in sensitized mice was actually suppressed in mice deficient in NOS1, suggesting a contribution of NOS1-derived NO$^•$ in this hyperreactivity (8,24). The recent linkage of a NOS1 gene polymorphism with human asthma (28,29), cystic fibrosis (30), and acute chest syndrome (31) further supports an important contribution of NOS1 and illustrates the complex role of NO$^•$ in these pathologies, which depends on the cellular sources and the enzymatic origin. In addition, several recent studies suggest regulation of NOS2 expression by NOS1 (9,32), further illustrating the complexities in the regulation of NO$^•$ bioactivity.

Despite the potential contribution of excessive NO$^•$ production to respiratory tract injury, protective effects of inhaled NO$^•$ against oxidant-induced cytotoxicity or lung injury have also been demonstrated in a number of investigations (e.g., Ref. 33). These protective effects are most likely conferred by the ability of NO$^•$ to inhibit leukocyte activation, adhesion and recruitment into lung parenchyma, and interference of NO$^•$ with radical-mediated oxidative processes (34,35). Administration of inhaled NO$^•$ has therefore been advocated for newborn and some adult forms of pulmonary hypertension and has also been suggested to be useful in some forms and/or stages of ARDS (36). Nevertheless, the paradox of both salutory and deleterious properties of NO$^•$ has stimulated intense research into its various biochemical properties, including its role in cellular signaling pathways, ion transport, mucus secretion, apoptosis, etc., which would be impossible to adequately cover in the context of this review. In general, the adverse effects of NO$^•$ in airway inflammation are commonly attributed to the formation of more reactive RNS, which generally result from overproduction of NO$^•$ and accelerated metabolism during inflammatory conditions, conditions often referred to as "nitrosative or nitrative stress." In the following sections, we will more specifically address the biochemical mechanisms involved in the actions of RNS, with special emphasis on tyrosine nitration.

II. A Crash Course in NO Biochemistry

Nitric oxide is an ideal signaling molecule, with high intercellular diffusibility and surprisingly selective reactivity, and carries out its biological actions mostly through interactions with heme-containing proteins and enzymes, such as guanylyl cyclase. In addition to heme centers or transition metal centers, NO$^•$ also readily reacts with other paramagnetic species, of which molecular oxygen (O_2) and superoxide anion ($O_2^{•-}$) appear to be most important from a biological perspective. Reaction with O_2 is relatively slow, is only important at high NO$^•$ levels, and in aqueous solution eventually yields nitrite (NO_2^-) via the formation of various reactive intermediates, such as dinitrogen trioxide (N_2O_3) and nitrogen dioxide ($NO_2^•$). More attention has been give to the very rapid reaction of NO$^•$ with $O_2^{•-}$ (and with other radicals) to yield peroxynitrite ($ONOO^-$) or analogous products. Peroxynitrite is unstable and very reactive to most biological molecules, and either isomerizes to nitrate (NO_3^-) or forms NO_2^- during most oxidation reactions.

In addition, NO$^•$ may also be metabolized by various iron- or heme-containing proteins, including cytochrome c oxidase (37), lipoxygenase (38), prostaglandin H synthase (39), and heme peroxidases such as myeloperoxidase (MPO) (40–42), which most likely oxidize $NO^•$ to NO_2^-. Such metabolic pathways involving phagocyte peroxidases such as MPO are expected to become more prevalent during active inflammation. Recently, an O_2-dependent $NO^•$-metabolizing flavohemoglobin has been identified in prokaryotes, fungi, and yeast, acting as a dioxygenase, and a similar activity also appears to be present in mammalian cells (43,44), catalyzing direct metabolism of $NO^•$ to NO_3^-. Collectively, the eventual biological fate of $NO^•$ is oxidation to NO_2^- and primarily NO_3^- (several heme proteins may also be active in metabolism of NO_2^- to NO_3^-), which are rapidly distributed throughout the body and excreted in the urine (45). However, the exact mechanisms involved in $NO^•$ metabolism are still rather poorly characterized and in many cases involve the intermediate formation of RNS that may target other biomolecules.

III. Nitrosative Stress: Related to Unique Protein Modifications?

Because of the rapid reaction of $NO^•$ with superoxide ($O_2^{•-}$) and its accelerated metabolism by activated heme peroxidases, the activation of oxidant-generating systems during cellular stress or inflammation can be assumed to accelerate $NO^•$ metabolism to more reactive RNS, such as $ONOO^-$, $NO_2^•$, etc. Since these RNS are capable of covalently modifying various amino acid residues, prosthetic groups in proteins, unsaturated lipids, and/or DNA bases, and thereby potentially induce structural or functional alterations, it is hypothesized that RNS may contribute significantly to the many pathophysiological processes associated with excessive $NO^•$ production (5,44,47). Among the many types of oxidative modifications induced by RNS are characteristic nitrosation and nitration reactions that are unique features of oxidative $NO^•$ biochemistry and hence are often proposed as specific features associated with nitrosative stress. Much attention has been given to reactions with various biological thiols to form *S*-nitrosothiols, which is speculated to provide a mechanism of $NO^•$ storage and transport, regulation of oxygen delivery, and regulation of various redox-sensitive signaling pathways. Similar nitrosation of amines can result in deamination of certain DNA bases, and this may be involved in mutagenic properties of $NO^•$ (47). Because *S*-nitrosation is readily reversible, it has been difficult to demonstrate *S*-nitrosation within specific cellular targets in vivo; nevertheless, there have been many convincing lines of evidence implicating *S*-nitrosation as a mechanism involved in cellular and extracellular responses to nitrosative stress (48). Another shortcoming in our current knowledge involves the exact biochemical pathways involved in such nitrosation, since it requires oxidation of $NO^•$ to N_2O_3, $ONOO^-$, or iron-$NO^•$ complexes (49). Measurements of *S*-nitrosothiols in lung lavage fluids or in exhaled breath condensates have given conflicting results, with reports of both decreased and increased levels of *S*-nitrosothiols in asthmatics, cystic fibrosis patients, etc. (50–52). Difficulties in the measurement of *S*-nitrosothiols and the comparisons of various patient populations in different disease stages undoubtedly contribute to these variable and inconsistent findings.

Other characteristic and more irreversible modifications by several RNS involve the nitration of aromatic amino acids, lipids, or DNA bases (5,34,47). In this respect, attention has mostly been focused on the amino acid tyrosine, which is a susceptible target for nitration to 3-nitrotyrosine. The formation of free or protein-associated 3-nitrotyrosine has received much recent interest, first as a biomarker for the endogenous generation of RNS in disease situations, and second as a potential novel mechanism of protein regulation, thereby implicating tyrosine nitration as a causative factor in disease development. Although such a hypothesis has received widespread popularity, definitive support for such associations is rather weak, largely because analytical methods used for nitrotyrosine analysis have been significantly hindered by artifacts during sample processing and analysis. Hence, the extent of endogenous tyrosine nitration is often overestimated and the functional significance of such protein modification in vivo is still unclear. The following paragraphs discuss more specifically the biochemical aspects of tyrosine nitration and its potential biological significance in general and in lung diseases in particular.

IV. Tyrosine Nitration: A Special Feature of Nitrosative Stress

Over the last several years, an impressive list has accumulated of respiratory tract diseases that are accompanied by increases in protein 3-nitrotyrosine levels, in either respiratory tract secretions or in lung tissues (Table 1). Importantly, all these pathologies are also associated with activated inflammatory-immune processes, conditions known to be associated with the activation of various oxidant-producing enzymes, including NAD(P)H oxidases, peroxidases, xanthine oxidase, etc. Because of generally increased generation of $O_2^{\cdot -}$ in such conditions and its diffusion-limited reaction with $NO^{\cdot}$ to form the powerful oxidizing and nitrating agent $ONOO^-$, the detection of 3-nitrotyrosine has in general been considered direct proof of endogenous formation of this oxidant. However, several recent investigations have revealed alternative biochemical pathways in the formation of nitrating RNS, which commonly involves the activation of heme proteins and peroxidases, and several studies have suggested that $ONOO^-$ generation is not the major pathway involved in the formation of nitrated tyrosine residues in biological conditions (49).

Chemical studies support the involvement of $NO_2^{\cdot}$ as the ultimate intermediate in tyrosine nitration by various RNS, which can be generated by several enzymatic and nonenzymatic mechanisms, including autoxidation of $NO^{\cdot}$, some radical-producing reactions of $ONOO^-$, or oxidation of NO_2^-. The major source of $NO_2^{\cdot}$ during conditions of active inflammation presumably involves the activation of granulocyte-derived heme peroxidases, such as myeloperoxidase and eosinophil peroxidase, to catalyze the one-electron oxidation of NO_2^-. These abundant proteins are stored in granules and secreted and activated during active inflammation as a result of the simultaneously induced respiratory burst, and are thus capable of oxidizing a host of biological substrates, among which are $NO^{\cdot}$ and/or its primary metabolite NO_2^-. The metabolite NO_2^- is normally present in all extracellular fluids at μM concentra-

Table 1 Human Respiratory Tract Diseases in Which Elevated Levels of 3-Nitrotyrosine Have Been Detected

Disease	Examined specimen	Detection method	Ref.
Adult respiratory distress syndrome	Lung tissue	Immunohistochemistry	53
	BAL fluids	ELISA	54
Acute lung injury	Lung tissue	Immunohistochemistry	55
Idiopathic pulmonary fibrosis	Lung tissue	Immunohistochemistry	56
Obliterative bronchiolitis	Lung tissue	Immunohistochemistry	57
Lung allograft inflammation	BAL fluids	ELISA, HPLC/EC	58
Asthma	Lung tissues	Immunohistochemistry	59
	Bronchial biopsies	Immunohistochemistry	60
	Exhaled breath condensate	ELISA	61
	BAL fluids	GC/MS	62
Cystic fibrosis	Expectorated sputum	HPLC/EC	63
	Sputum	ELISA	64
	Exhaled breath condensate	ELISA	65
Lung cancer	Plasma	Western blot/dot blot	66
Perennial nasal allergy	Nasal mucosa	HPLC/UV	67

tions (e.g., 0.5–3.6 μM in plasma, 10–15 μM in alveolar epithelial lining fluids, and 10–40 μM in nasal epithelial lining fluids) (49), and most likely in higher amounts as a result of enhanced NO$^{\bullet}$ production and metabolism during inflammatory conditions. Chemical studies have demonstrated that such concentrations are sufficient to allow the formation of RNS by peroxidase-catalyzed oxidation, even in the presence of more abundant alternative biological substrates (68–70). Immuno-histochemical evaluation has demonstrated that endogenous 3-nitrotyrosine is usually detected in inflammatory/infectious diseases, characterized by the infiltration and activation of leukocytes, and positive immunostaining using antinitrotyrosine antibodies is often observed in and around neutrophils, eosinophils, as well as macrophages and epithelial cells (53,55–57,59,60).

Even though protein tyrosine nitration is often found to correlate with the degree of neutrophil and/or eosinophil infiltration, unequivocal evidence of involvement of their heme peroxidases can only be presented by studies with specific inhibitors or in animal studies where their expression is silenced by targeted gene deletion. Unfortunately, no specific peroxidase inhibitors exist at present for use in in vivo studies, and although knockout animals deficient in either myeloperoxidase (MPO) or eosinophil peroxidase (EPO) are now being bred in several laboratories, no conclusive studies have yet been reported to support their critical involvement in tyrosine nitration in disease conditions. One strong piece of evidence comes from a recent study with the New Zealand white mouse, a naturally EPO-deficient mouse strain. Although this mouse responds similarly to ovalbumin sensitization challenge compared to several other generally used mouse strains with respect to the activation of eosinophilia, tyrosine nitration that occurs primarily around infiltrated eosinophils is dramatically less in EPO-deficient animals (71), and similar changes have recently been observed in EPO knockout mice (71a). Similarly, EPO-dependent pathways are also implicated in human asthma (62). More recently, nitration of liver proteins in zymosan-treated mice was found to be significantly reduced in MPO-deficient mice (42). Nevertheless, the involvement of these peroxidases, as well as the generation of nitrating RNS, in disease pathology is still open to speculation, as several studies with MPO- or EPO-deficient animals have produced unexpected or negative results (72,73). This issue needs to be further addressed, however, as common disease models do not adequately reflect the actions and fates of these peroxidases in human disease.

Collectively, formation of $NO^{\bullet}$-derived RNS during inflammatory-immune processes that are capable of inducing aromatic nitration involves multiple distinct reaction mechanisms, but most likely involves the activation of leukocyte peroxidases or related heme-proteins that can catalyze similar chemistry. Hence, it appears that MPO or other heme peroxidases may play a central role in the metabolism of $NO^{\bullet}$ and the formation of nitrating intermediates at sites of active inflammatory-immune processes (Fig. 1). With the availability of MPO- or EPO-deficient animals and further development of selective peroxidase inhibitors, the importance of MPO,

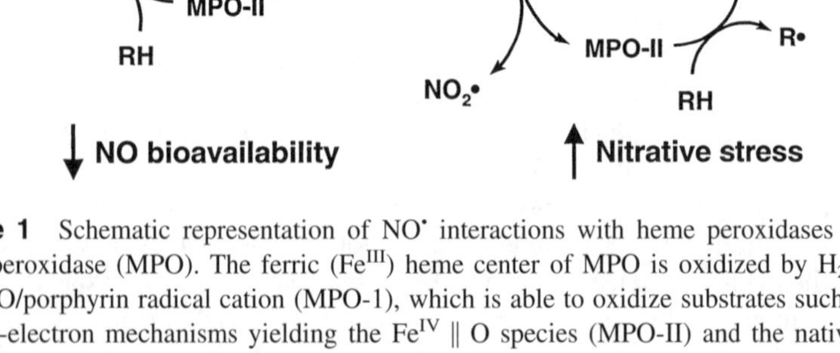

Figure 1 Schematic representation of $NO^{\bullet}$ interactions with heme peroxidases such as myeloperoxidase (MPO). The ferric (Fe^{III}) heme center of MPO is oxidized by H_2O_2 to a $Fe^{IV} \parallel$ O/porphyrin radical cation (MPO-1), which is able to oxidize substrates such as $NO^{\bullet}$ by one-electron mechanisms yielding the $Fe^{IV} \parallel$ O species (MPO-II) and the native ferric enzyme. Both MPO-I and -II can catalyze $NO^{\bullet}$ oxidation to NO_2^{-}. Additionally, formation of radical intermediates ($R^{\bullet}$) by oxidation of other substrates (RH) also accelerates removal of $NO^{\bullet}$ and suppresses its bioavailability. MPO-I is also able to oxidize NO_2^{-} to $NO_2^{\bullet}$, and can thereby contribute to (protein) tyrosine nitration during inflammatory conditions.

EPO, or related peroxidases in aromatic nitration, or their contribution to disease progression in general, will become more clear.

V. Does Tyrosine Nitration Affect Protein Structure or Function?

Although there is little doubt that 3-nitrotyrosine is generated in a number of inflammatory diseases, most likely in association with other oxidative protein modifications, it is still unclear whether protein nitration in itself has functional implications and contributes significantly to the pathobiology of respiratory tract disease. A first issue that would need to be addressed is whether tyrosine nitration occurs randomly or whether it targets certain proteins. Several recent investigations have begun to specifically address this question. First, investigations in cellular systems or in vivo have indicated that protein nitration during active inflammation primarily affects extracellular proteins (42,63), which may in part be related to slower turnover of these proteins compared to most cellular proteins. Recently, using a proteomic approach, up to 40 proteins have been identified as targets for tyrosine nitration in the lung and liver of rats following injection of lipopolysaccharide (74). The observed immunoreactive proteins were related to cell energy production, apoptosis, fatty acid metabolism, and oxidative or xenobiotic stress. Interestingly, two independent studies have indicated that mitochondrial proteins are more extensively nitrated than cytosolic proteins in liver tissues of LPS-treated rats (74,75), which may suggest mitochondria as a major cellular site of RNS formation, perhaps not surprising as they are presumably the major site of generation of intracellular oxidants.

A. Cellular Effects of Tyrosine Nitration

In several cellular studies of nitrosative stress, RNS-induced cytotoxicity or apoptosis has been associated with tyrosine nitration (76,77), but tyrosine nitration does not always parallel cell toxicity. For instance, the cytotoxicity of $ONOO^-$ is dramatically reduced in the presence of CO_2, coinciding with decreases in most oxidative modifications by $ONOO^-$, even though radical-induced modifications such as aromatic nitration are enhanced (78). Also, cytotoxic properties of heme peroxidases in the presence of H_2O_2 either are not affected by NO or NO_2^- or are in fact inhibited, despite substantial tyrosine nitration of cellular proteins (63,79). Nevertheless, although tyrosine nitration may not have acute cellular effects, such irreversible modification might have a more long-lasting impact on cellular pathways that are involved in cell proliferation or differentiation. In this respect, it is interesting to note that free 3-nitrotyrosine has been found to induce cytoskeletal changes and disrupt epithelial transport, due to microtubule disruption by selective incorporation into α-tubulin by tubulin tyrosine ligase (80,81). Nitration of protein tyrosine residues or related modifications in DNA [e.g., nitration of guanine and the formation of abasic sites (82,83)] may also be involved in disturbances of cell-signaling pathways and contribute to processes linked to mutagenesis and carcinogenesis.

B. Tyrosine Nitration and Enzyme Activity

Protein chemists have extensively used the nitrating agent tetranitromethane to investigate the location and essentiality of tyrosine residues in a large number of proteins and enzymes (5), and such studies have indicated that nitration of key tyrosine residues is often associated with a loss of either enzyme or protein function. Similarly, studies with isolated tyrosine kinase systems, in which kinase substrates were chemically nitrated or tyrosine residues were replaced with 3-nitrotyrosine, have demonstrated that tyrosine nitration results in inhibition of tyrosine phosphorylation (84,85). Efforts to demonstrate the significance of this observation in signaling pathways in cellular systems have, however, proven largely unsuccessful (86–88). Table 2 lists several recent investigations in which critical tyrosine residues have been

Table 2 Some Examples of Enzyme Systems in Which Nitration of a Critical Tyrosine Residue Has Been Implicated in Changes in Activity and/or Function

Enzyme	Nitrotyrosine analysis	Tyrosine role	Ref.
Mn-SOD	HPLC/UV, amino acid sequencing and MS/MS analysis of peptides	Catalytic acitivity?	89,90
Fe-SOD	HPLC/ESI-MS	Catalytic activity?	91
Tyrosine hydroxylase	Western blot, protein digestion, HPLC/UV analysis	Unknown	94
Glutathione-*S*-transferase	HPLC separation of tryptic fragments, MALDI/MS and HPLC/EC analysis	GSH binding and activation	95
COX-1	Protein digestion, HPLC/UV analysis and amino acid sequencing	Tyr radical in active site	96
Cytochrome P450	GC/MS and HPLC of intact protein, sequencing of tryptic fragments	Unknown, electron transfer?	97
Glutamine synthetase	HPLC and UV analysis of tryptic peptide fragments	Enzyme (in)activation	98
Cytochrome *c*	Protein digestion, HPLC/UV and MS analysis of peptides	Catalytic activity?	99
Ribonucleotide reductase	HPLC/UV analysis, protein digestion and amino acid sequencing	Catalytic activity	100
α_1-Proteinase inhibitor	Amino acid sequencing of peptide fragments	Catalytic domain	101
Surfactant protein A	Protein digestion, HPLC and MS analysis	Receptor binding, lipid aggregation	102

identified as targets for chemical nitration in vitro. The in vivo significance to these findings is, however, still unclear.

One of the early observations regarding in vivo protein targets of nitration was the finding that during human kidney allograft rejection manganese superoxide dismutase (Mn-SOD) was nitrated, and this was associated with loss of SOD activity. Interestingly, proteomic analysis of lung epithelial cell lysates or rat liver tissues after cytokine or LPS stimulation also revealed Mn-SOD as a major target for protein nitration (74). Analysis of RNS-modified recombinant Mn-SOD by proteolytic digestion, HPLC, and electrospray mass spectrometry indicated that nitration occurs primarily on Tyr[34], which is present in the active site, in addition to few other Tyr residues (89,90), suggesting that nitration of this residue may directly cause inactivation of the enzyme. Intriguingly, the Tyr[34] residue in *E. coli* Fe-SOD also appeared to be a major target for nitration by RNS; however, in this case this did not result in enzyme inactivation. Mutation studies have indicated that Tyr[34] may not be essential for catalysis, and the Y34F mutant of either Fe-SOD or Mn-SOD does not display dramatically reduced activity (91). Hence, the suggestion that nitration of Tyr[34] of SOD by RNS mediates its inactivation may be premature, even though Mn-SOD appears to be a target for nitration in vivo.

In a mouse model of Parkinson's disease using 1-methyl-4-phenyl-1,2,3,6-tetrahydropyridine (MPTP), a loss of tyrosine hydroxylase (TH) activity was observed in the striatum, in association with nitration of the enzyme (92). Studies in neuronal cells and recombinant TH further supported a causal relationship between tyrosine nitration and TH inactivation and revealed nitration primarily on Tyr[423], mutation of which resulted in ±75% reduced specific activity. Nevertheless, modification of cysteine residues by *N*-ethylmaleimide also causes enzyme inactivation, and TH cysteine oxidation by RNS may play a significant role in its inactivation (93,94).

According to proteomic analysis of liver proteins following LPS stimulation, the μ-type of glutathione-*S*-transferase (GST) appeared as a major target for tyrosine nitration (74). All GSTs contain a highly conserved essential Tyr residue within the active site (Tyr[6] in GST-μ), and biochemical studies indicated that RNS-induced inactivation of GSTs was associated with tyrosine nitration, especially in the μ-type enzyme. Further studies using trypsin digestion and MALDI-TOF and HPLC analyses revealed several Tyr residues as targets for nitration, including Tyr[6]; however, the extent of nitration was insufficient to fully account for RNS-induced enzyme inactivation, and other modifications probably contribute (95).

Based on chemical nitration mechanisms, protein tyrosyl radicals would appear to be primary targets for nitration by RNS. Indeed, the tyrosyl radical of Tyr[385] in prostaglandin H synthase appears to be such a target, and this Tyr residue is essential for cyclooxygenase activity, the tyrosyl radical being involved in hydrogen abstraction from arachidonate (96). The tyrosyl radical on Tyr[122] in the small R2 subunit of class I ribonucleotide reductase, a critical enzyme involved in DNA synthesis and repair, was also found to be a target for nitration. However, this was not the primary tyrosine target, and protein R2 inactivation could not be completely attributed to nitration, suggesting that other modifications must have contributed to inactivation (100). Moreover, no evidence exists as yet for nitration of these enzymes in vivo.

More directly relevant to the respiratory tract, $ONOO^-$ and related RNS have been found capable of nitrating tyrosine residues in several crucial proteins present in the alveolar space, including α_1-protease inhibitor and surfactant protein A (101,102). Moreover, although no direct causal links have been made, such modifications have been associated with inactivation of α_1-protease inhibitor and with a decreased ability of surfactant protein A to aggregate lipids or to bind to mannose receptors present on immune effector cells (103,104). Thus, such irreversible modifications may compromise host defense mechanisms and enable proteolytic enzymes. However, although there is some evidence for nitration of surfactant protein A in vivo in subjects with acute lung injury (105), the actual contribution of tyrosine nitration is still speculative.

Overall, there may be some compelling causal relationships between tyrosine nitration and protein structure or enzyme function in some cases, but its significance in vivo is still unclear, primarily due to a lack of reliable quantitative data. Even though there may be some convincing arguments for certain proteins as susceptible targets for nitration, there is as yet no evidence of quantitative nitration of these targets to link tyrosine nitration to overall changes in enzyme function. Many past studies that have attempted to quantitate overall tyrosine nitration may have suffered from major artifactual nitration during sample processing. The best estimates of in vivo tyrosine nitration suggest that in healthy tissues, less that 1 per 10^6 tyrosine residues is nitrated, which may increase only severalfold during intense acute inflammation (49,75). Reports of nitrotyrosine levels in extracellular proteins (e.g., serum or respiratory tract sputum) may be somewhat higher (up to 100 per 10^6 Tyr residues). Thus, is would seem difficult to envision dramatic functional implications if such a minor fraction of proteins are affected. Nevertheless, if tyrosine nitration selectively affects certain specific proteins, or proteins in specific cellular environments, the relative extent of modification of these proteins may be considerably higher. Moreover, tyrosine nitration may in fact imbue a protein with additional novel functions, e.g., akin to tyrosine phosphorylation or sulfation, in which case modification of only a small fraction of a certain protein might have significant functional consequences. The recent discovery of enzymatic denitrases in various mammalian tissues (106,107) may further attest to a potential role of tyrosine nitration as a specific signaling pathway associated with nitrosative stress.

VI. Remaining Questions and Issues

Figure 2 represents an overall scheme of the various sources and reactions of $NO^•$ in the airways and illustrates the considerable complexities in this. Despite considerable increases in our understanding of the multiple roles of $NO^•$ and RNS in airway biology and disease, there are still several unresolved questions. First, it is still not clear whether and how $NO^•$ may contribute to airway dysfunction and inflammation, as implicated from several in vivo observations. Even though good arguments can

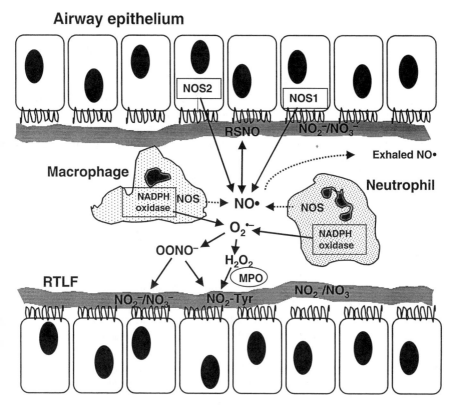

Figure 2 Schematic illustration of sources and reactions of NO$^\bullet$ within the airways. NO$^\bullet$ is produced primarily by airway epithelial cells and (at least in rodents) by inflammatory cells such as macrophages and neutrophils. Various reactions with (inflammatory) oxidants dictate the overall metabolism of NO$^\bullet$ to ONOO$^-$ or to NO$_2^-$ and NO$_3^-$ and determine the formation of *S*-nitrosothiols (RSNO) or nitrotyrosine (NO$_2$-Tyr).

be made for involvement of RNS in such cases, direct evidence for this is still weak. One technical problem is that contributions of NO$^\bullet$ to lung disease may be difficult to dissect from animal studies with unconditional NOS knockout mice. In this regard, the recent study by Steudel et al. (9) surprisingly indicated that expired NO levels are not significantly reduced in knockouts of either NOS1, NOS2, or NOS3, and was in some cases even enhanced. Another problem with, e.g., NOS2 knockout animals is that they do not adequately model the role of NOS2 in temporal situations of inflammation, where its presence may be helpful at one stage and negative in another stage. It is clear that the regulation of airway NO$^\bullet$ production is extremely complex, and may in fact involve interactions between various NOS isozymes. Consequently, measurements of expired NO$^\bullet$ in patients does not provide much useful information regarding its origin or its biological activity within the airways. In this regard, it is still unclear whether there really is a deficiency of airway NO˙ production in CF. Would augmenting NO˙ by supplementation strategies (NO˙ inhalation, arginine supplementation) improve host defense or airway inflammation, or promote even more protein nitration and injury? Similarly, this question also applies to other inflammatory lung diseases; indeed, there is some indication from animal studies that inhalation of NO˙ actually suppresses LPS-induced inflammation and protein nitration (e.g., Ref. 33).

Another important point to be made is that the generalized concept that tyrosine nitration may be involved in such adverse effects of NO˙ or RNS needs to be reconsidered. Tyrosine nitration occurs in parallel with many other oxidative modifications; dissecting a specific contribution of tyrosine nitration is extremely difficult. More generally, the biological effects of RNS most likely stretch beyond nitrosation and nitration reactions. For instance, nitrosation and oxidation of cysteine residues both result in formation of disulfides in certain proteins (e.g., phosphatases, OxyR), and the cellular responses to nitrosative and oxidative stress may largely overlap. Tyrosine nitration may really present a unique feature of nitrosative stress, but whether tyrosine nitration contributes directly to disease development still remains to be answered. At present, the presence of tyrosine nitration should only be interpreted as a marker of RNS formation during ongoing inflammatory-immune processes.

Perhaps one of the major reasons for our incomplete understanding of the roles of RNS in disease is the fact that there are still considerable technical problems with currently developed methodology to measure nitrotyrosine, nitrosothiols, etc. Such problems include lack of sensitivity, artifacts during sample preparation, and inadequate methodology to directly measure S-nitrosothiols. Continued development of improved methodology is critically needed to more accurately and conviently measure such products in vivo, ideally in association with other functional measurements, so that more adequate associations can be made between such chemical modifications and disease progression.

Acknowledgments

The authors would like to thank NIH, the American Heart Association, the University of California Tobacco-Related Disease Research Program, and the Cystic Fibrosis Foundation for research support.

References

1. Moncada S, Palmer RMJ, Higgs EA. Nitric oxide: physiology, pathophysiology, and pharmacology. Pharmacol Rev 1991; 43:109–142.
2. Gaston B, Drazen JM, Loscalzo J, Stamler JS. The biology of nitrogen oxides in the airways. Am J Respir Crit Care Med 1994; 149:538–551.
3. Fang FC. Mechanisms of nitric oxide-related antimicrobial activity. J Clin Invest 1997; 100:S43–S50.

4. Beckman JS, Koppenol WH. Nitric oxide, superoxide, and peroxynitrite: the good, the bad, and the ugly. Am J Physiol 1996; 271:C1424–C1437.

5. Beckman JS. Oxidative damage and tyrosine nitration from peroxynitrite. Chem Res Toxicol 1996; 9:836–844.

6. Ischiropoulos H. Biological tyrosine nitration: a pathophysiological function of nitric oxide and reactive oxygen species. Arch Biochem Biophys 1998; 356:1–11.

7. Pitt BR, St. Croix CM. Complex regulation of iNOS in lung. Am J Respir Cell Mol Biol 2001; 26:6–9.

8. De Sanctis GT, Mehta S, Kobzik L, Yandava C, Jiao A, Huang PL, Drazen JM. Contribution of type I NOS to expired gas NO and bronchial responsiveness in mice. Am J Physiol 1997; 273:L883–L888.

9. Steudel W, Kirmse M, Weiman J, Ullrich R, Hromi J, Zapol WM. Exhaled nitric oxide production by nitric oxide synthase-deficient mice. Am J Respir Crit Care Med 2000; 162:1262–1267.

10. Thomassen MJ, Kavuru MS. Human alveolar macrophages and monocytes as a source and target for nitric oxide. Int Immunopharmacol 2001; 1:1479–1490.

11. Nathan C. Inducible nitric oxide synthase: What difference does it make? J Clin Invest, 1997; 100:2417–2423.

12. Kelley TJ, Drumm ML. Inducible nitric oxide synthase expression is reduced in cystic fibrosis murine and human airway epithelial cells. J Clin Invest 1998; 102:1200–1207.

13. Meng QH, Springall DR, Bishop AE, Morgan K, Evans TJ, Habib S, Gruenert DC, Gyi KM, Hodson ME, Yacoub MH, Polak JM. Lack of inducible nitric oxide synthase in bronchial epithelium: a possible mechanism of susceptibility to infection in cystic fibrosis. J Pathol 1998; 184:323–331.

14. Smith AW, Green J, Eden CE, Watson ML. Nitric oxide-induced potentiation of the killing of *Burkholderia cepacia* by reactive oxygen species: implications for cystic fibrosis. J Med Microbiol 1999; 48:419–423.

15. Clancy RM, Amin AR, Abramson SB. The role of nitric oxide in inflammation and immunity. Arthritis Rheum 1998; 41:1141–1151.

16. Mannick JB, Hausladen A, Liu L, Hess DT, Zeng M, Miao QX, Kane LS, Gow AJ, Stamler JS. Fas-induced caspase denitrosylation. Science 1999; 284:651–654.

17. Raychaudhuri B, Dweik R, Connors MJ, Buhrow L, Malur A, Drazba J, Arroliga AC, Erzurum SC, Kavuru MS, Thomassen MJ. Nitric oxide blocks nuclear factor-κB activation in alveolar macrophages. Am J Respir Cell Mol Biol 1999; 21:311–316.

18. Idriss SD, Gudi T, Casteel DE, Kharitonov VG, Pilz RB, Boss GR. Nitric oxide regulation of gene transcription via soluble guanylate cyclase and type 1 cGMP-dependent protein kinase. J Biol Chem 1999; 274:9489–9493.

19. Akaike T, Noguchi Y, Ijiri S, Setoguch K, Suga M, Zheng M, Dietzschold B, Maeda B. Pathogenesis of influenza virus-induced pneumonia: involvement of both nitric oxide and oxygen radicals. Proc Natl Acad Sci USA 1996; 93:2448–2453.

20. Kristof AS, Goldberg P, Laubach V, Hussain SN. A. Role of inducible nitric oxide synthase in endotoxin-induced acute lung injury. Am J Respir Crit Care Med 1998; 158:1883–1889.

21. Kleeberger SR, Reddy SPM, Zhang L.-Y., Cho H.-Y., Jedicka AE. Toll-like receptor 4 mediates ozone-induced murine lung hyperpermeability via inducible nitric oxide synthase. Am J Physiol 2001; 280:L326–L333.

22. Xiong Y, Karupiah G, Hogan SP, Foster PS, Ramsay A. J.Inhibition of allergic airway inflammation in mice lacking nitric oxide synthase 2. J Immunol 1999; 162:445–452.

23. Laubach VE, Shesely EG, Smithies O, Sherman PA. Mice lacking inducible nitric oxide synthase are not resistant to lipopolysaccharide-induced death. Proc Natl Acad Sci USA 1995; 92:10688–10692.

24. De Sanctis GT, MacLean JA, Hamada K, Mehta S, Scott JA, Jiao A, Yandava CN, Kobzik, L, Wolyniec WW, Fabian AJ, Venugopal CS, Grasemann H, Huang PL, Drazen JM. Contribution of nitric oxide synthases 1, 2, and 3 to airway hyperresponsiveness and inflammation in a murine model of asthma. J Exp Med 1999; 189: 1621–1629.

25. Kobayashi H, Hataishi R, Mitsufuji H, Tanaka M, Jacobsen M, Tomita T, Zapol WM, Jones RC. Antiinflammatory properties of inducible nitric oxide synthase in acute hyperoxic lung injury. Am J Respir Cell Mol Biol 2001; 24:390–397.

26. Kenyon NJ, van der Vliet A, Schock BC, Okamoto T, McGrew GM, Last JA. Susceptibility to ozone-induced acute lung injury in iNOS-deficient mice. Am J Physiol 2002; 282:L540–L545.

27. Feletou M, Lonchampt M, Coge F, Galizzi J.-P., Bassoullet C, Merial C, Robineau P, Boutin JA, Huang PL, Vanhoutte PM, Canet E. Regulation of murine airway responsiveness by endothelial nitric oxide synthase. Am J Physiol 2001; 281:L258–L267.

28. Wechsler ME, Grasemann H, Deykin D, Silverman EK, Yandava CN, Israel E, Wand M, Drazen JM. Exhaled nitric oxide in patients with asthma. Association with *NOS1* genotype. Am J Respir Crit Care Med 2000; 162:2043–2047.

29. Grasemann H, Yandava CN, Storm van's Gravesande K, Deykin A, Pillari A, Ma J, Sonna LA, Lilly C, Stampfer MJ, Israel E, Silverman EK, Drazen JM. A neuronal NO synthase (NOS-1) gene polymorphism is associated with asthma. Biochem Biophys Res Commun 2000; 272:391–394.

30. Grasemann H, Knauer N, Büscher R, Hübner K, Drazen JM, Ratjen F. Airway nitric oxide levels in cystic fibrosis patients are related to a polymorphism in the neuronal nitric oxide synthase gene. Am J Respir Crit Care Med 2000; 162:2172–2176.

31. Sullivan KJ, Kissoon N, Duckworth LJ, Sandler E, Freeman B, Bayne E, Sylvester JE, Lima JJ. Low exhaled nitric oxide and a polymorphism in the NOS I gene is associated with acute chest syndrome. Am J Respir Crit Care Med 2001; 164: 2186–2190.

32. Iijima H, Duguet A, Hamid Q, Eidelman DH, Role of NNOS is eosinophilic inflammation: possible interaction with epithelial INOS expression. Am J Respir Crit Care Med 2001; 163:A195.

33. Honda K, Kobayashi H, Hataishi R, Hirano S, Fukuyama N, Nakazawa H, Tomita T. Inhaled nitric oxide reduces tyrosine nitration after lipopolysaccharide instillation into lungs of rats. Am J Respir Crit Care Med 1999; 160:678–688.

34. Rubbo H, Darley-Usmar V, Freeman BA. Nitric oxide regulation of tissue free radical injury. Chem Res Toxicol 1996; 9:809–820.

35. Kroncke K.-D., Fehsel K, Kolb-Bachofen V. Nitric oxide: cytotoxicity versus cytoprotection—how, why, when, and where? Nitric Oxide Biol Chem 1997; 1:107–120.

36. Bigetello LM, Hurford WE, Hess D. Use of inhaled nitric oxide for ARDS. Respir Care Clin North Am 1998; 3:437–458.

37. Torres J, Sharpe MA, Rosquist A, Cooper CE, Wilson MT. Cytochrome c oxidase rapidly metabolises nitric oxide to nitrite. FEBS Lett 2000; 475:263–266.

38. O'Donnell VB, Taylor KB, Parthasarathy S, Kuhn H, Koesling D, Friebe A, Bloodsworth A, Darley-Usmar VM, Freeman BA. 15-Lipoxygenase consumes nitric oxide and impairs activation of guanylate cyclase. J Biol Chem 1999; 274: 20083–20091.

39. O'Donnell VB, Coles B, Lewis MJ, Crews BC, Marnett LJ, Freeman BA. Catalytic consumption of nitric oxide by prostaglandin H synthase-1 regulates platelet function. J Biol Chem 2000; 275:38239–38244.

40. Glover RE, Koshkin V, Dunford HB, Mason RP. The rate of reaction of NO with horseradish peroxidase compounds I and II. Nitric Oxide Biol Chem 1999; 3:439–444.

41. Abu-Soud HM, Khassawneh MY, Sohn J.-T., Murray P, Haxhiu MA, Hazen SL. Peroxidases inhibit nitric oxide (NO) dependent bronchodilation: development of a model describing NO-peroxidase interactions. Biochemistry 2001; 40:11866–11875.

41a. Eiserich JP, Baldus S, Brennan ML, Ma W, Zhang C, Tousson A, Castro L, Lusis AJ, Nauseef WM, White CR, Freeman BA. Myeloperoxidase, a leukocyte-derived vascular NO oxidase. Science 2002; 296:2391–2394.

42. Baldus S, Eiserich JP, Mani A, Castro L, Figueroa M, Chumley P, Ma W, Tousson A, White CR, Bullard DC, Brennan M-L., Lusis AJ, Freeman BA. Endothelial transcytosis of myeloperoxidase confers specificity to vascular ECM proteins as targets of tyrosine nitration. J Clin Invest 2001; 108:1759–1770.

43. Gardner PR, Martin LA, Hall D, Gardner AM. Dioxygen-dependent metabolism of nitric oxide in mammalian cells. Free Rad Biol Med 2001; 31:191–204.

44. Hausladen A, Gow A, Stamler JS. Flavohemoglobin denitrosylase catalyzes the reaction of a nitroxyl equivalent with molecular oxygen. Proc Natl Acad Sci USA 2001; 98:10108–10112.

45. Parks NJ, Krohn KA, Mathis CA, Chasko JH, Geiger KR, Gregor ME, Peek NF. Nitrogen-13-labeled nitrite and nitrate: distribution and metabolism after intratracheal administration. Science 1981; 212:58–61.

46. Pryor WA, Squadrito GL. The chemistry of peroxynitrite: a product from the reaction of nitric oxide with superoxide. Am J Physiol 1995; 68:L699–L722.

47. Tamir S, Burney S, Tannenbaum SR. DNA damage by nitric oxide. Chem Res Toxicol 1996; 9:821–827.

48. Stamler JS, Lamas S, Fang FC. Nitrosylation the prototypic redox-based signaling mechanism. Cell 2001; 106:675–683.

49. Van der Vliet A, Eiserich JP, Shigenaga MK, Cross CE. Reactive nitrogen species and tyrosine nitration in the respiratory tract. Epiphenomena or a pathobiologic mechanism of disease? Am J Respir Crit Care Med 1999; 160:1–9.

50. Corradi M, Montuschi P, Donnelly LE, Pesci A, Kharitonov SA, Barnes PJ. Increased nitrosothiols in exhaled breath condensate in inflammatory airway diseases. Am J Respir Crit Care Med 2001; 163:854–858.

51. Dweik RA, Comhair SAA, Gaston B, Thunissen FB. J. M, Farver C, Thomassen MJ, Kavuru M, Hammel J, Abu-Soud HM, Erzurum SC. NO chemical events in the human airway during the immediate and late antigen-induced asthmatic response. Proc Natl Acad Sci USA 2001; 98:2622–2627.

52. Grasemann H, Gaston B, Fang K, Paul K, Ratjen F. Decreased levels of nitrosothiols in the lower airways of patients with cystic fibrosis and normal pulmonary function. J Pediatr 2001; 135:770–772.

53. Haddad IY, Pataki G, Hu P, Galliani C, Beckman JS, Matalon S. Quantitation of nitrotyrosine levels in lung sections of patients and animals with acute lung injury. J Clin Invest 1994; 94:2407–2413.

54. Sittipunt C, Steinberg KP, Ruzinski JT, Myles C, Zhu S, Goodman RB, Hudson LD, Matalon S, Martin TR. Nitric oxide and nitrotyrosine in the lungs of patients with acute respiratory distress syndrome. Am J Respir Crit Care Med 2001; 163:503–510.

55. Kooy NW, Royall JA, Ye YZ, Kelly DR, Beckman JS. Evidence for in vivo peroxyni-trite production in human acute lung injury. Am J Respir Crit Care Med 1995; 151: 1250–1254.

56. Saleh D, Barnes PJ, Giaid A. Increased production of the potent oxidant peroxynitrite in the lungs of patients with idiopathic pulmonary fibrosis. Am J Respir Crit Care Med 1997; 155:1763–1769.

57. McDermott CD, Gavita SM, Shennib H, Giaid A. Immunohistochemical localization of nitric oxide synthase and the oxidant peroxynitrite in lung transplant recipients with obliterative bronchiolitis. Transplantation 1997; 64:270–274.

58. De Andrade JA, Crow JP, Viera L, Alexander CB, Young KR, McGriffin DC, Zorn GL, Zhu S, Matalon S, and Jackson RM. Protein nitration, metabolites of reactive nitrogen species, and inflammation in lung allografts. Am J Respir Crit Care Med 2000; 161:2035–2040.

59. Kaminsky DA, Mitchell J, Carroll N, James A, Soultanakis R, Janssen Y. Nitrotyrosine formation in the airways and lung parenchyma of patients with asthma. J Allergy Clin Immunol 1999; 104:747–754.

60. Saleh D, Ernst P, Lim S, Barnes PJ, Giaid A. Increased formation of the potent oxidant peroxynitrite in the airways of asthmatic patients is associated with induction of nitric oxide synthase: effect of inhaled glucocorticoid. FASEB J 1998; 12:929–937.

61. Hanazawa T, Kharitonov SA, Barnes PJ. Increased nitrotyrosine in exhaled breath condensate of patients with asthma. Am J Respir Crit Care Med 2000; 162:1273–1276.

62. MacPherson JC, Comhair SA, Erzurum SC, Klein DF, Lipscomb MF, Kavuru MS, Samoszuk MK, Hazen SL. Eosinophils are a major source of nitric oxide-derived oxidants in severe asthma: characterization of pathways available to eosinophils for generating reactive nitrogen species. J Immunol 2001; 166:5763–5772.

63. van der Vliet A, Nguyen MN, Shigenaga MK, Eiserich JP, Marelich GP, Cross CE. Myeloperoxidase and protein oxidation in cystic fibrosis. Am J Physiol 2000; 279: L537–L546.

64. Jones KL, Hegab AH, Hillman BC, Simpson KL, Jinkins PA, Grisham MB, Owens MW, Sato E, Robbins RA. Elevation of nitrotyrosine and nitrate concentrations in cystic fibrosis sputum. Pediatr Pulmonol 2000; 30:79–85.

65. Balint B, Kharitonov SA, Hanazawa T, Donnelly LE, Shah PL, Hodson ME, Barnes PJ. Increased nitrotyrosine in exhaled breath condensate in cystic fibrosis. Eur Respir J 2001; 17:1201–1207.

66. Pignatelli B, Li CQ, Boffetta P, Chen Q, Ahrens W, Nyberg F, Mukeria A, Bruske-Hohlfeld I, Fortes C, Constantinescu V, Ischiropoulos H, Ohshima H. Nitrated and oxidized plasma proteins in smokers and lung cancer patients. Cancer Res 2001; 61: 778–784.

67. Sato M, Fukuyama N, Sakai M, Nakazawa H. Increased nitric oxide in nasal lavage fluid and nitrotyrosine formation in nasal mucosa—indices for severe perennial nasal allergy. Clin Exp Allergy 1998; 28:597–605.

68. van der Vliet A, Eiserich JP, Halliwell B, Cross CE. Formation of reactive nitrogen species during peroxidase-catalyzed oxidation of nitrite. A potential additional mecha-nism of nitric oxide-dependent toxicity. J Biol Chem 1997; 272:7617–7625.

69. Eiserich JP, Hristova M, Cross CE, Jones AD, Freeman BA, Halliwell B, van der Vliet A. Formation of nitric oxide-derived inflammatory oxidants by myeloperoxidase in neutrophils. Nature 1998; 391:393–397.

70. van Dalen CJ, Winterbourn CC, Senthilmohan R, Kettle AJ. Nitrite as a substrate and inhibitor of myeloperoxidase. Implications for nitration and hypochlorous acid production at sites of inflammation. J Biol Chem 2000; 275:11638–11644.

71. Duguet A, Iijima H, Eum S-Y., Hamid Q, Eidelman DH. Eosinophil peroxidase mediates protein nitration in allergic airway inflammation in mice. Am J Respir Crit Care Med 2001; 164:1119–1126.

71a. Brennan ML, Wu W, Fu X, Shen Z, Song W, Frost H, Vadseth C, Narine L, Lenkiewicz E, Borchers MT, Lusis AJ, Lee JJ, Lee NA, Abu-Soud HM, Ischiropoulos H, Hazen SL. A tale of two controversies: defining both the role of peroxidases in nitrotyrosine formation in vivo using eosinophil peroxidase and myeloperoxidase-deficient mice, and the nature of peroxidase-generated reactive nitrogen species. J Biol Chem 2002; 277:17415–17427.

72. Denzler KL, Borchers MT, Crosby JR, Cieslewicz G, Hines EM, Justice JP, Cormier SA, Lindenberger KA, Song W, Wu W, Hazen SL, Gleich GJ, Lee JJ, Lee NA. Extensive eosinophil degranulation and peroxidase-mediated oxidation of airway proteins do not occur in a mouse ovalbumin-challenge model of pulmonary inflammation. J Immunol 2001; 167:1672–1682.

73. Brennan M-L., Anderson MM, Shih DM, Qu X-D., Wang X, Mehta AC, Lim LL, Shi W, Hazen SL, Jacob JS, Crowley JR, Heinecke JW, Lusis AJ. Increased atherosclerosis in myeloperoxidase-deficient mice. J Clin Invest 2001; 107:419–430.

74. Aulak KS, Miyagi M, Yan L, West KA, Massillon D, Crabb JW, Stuehr DJ. Proteomic method identifies proteins nitrated in vivo during inflammatory challenge. Proc Natl Acad Sci USA 2001; 98:12056–12061.

75. Girault I, Karu AE, Schaper M, Barcellos-Hoff MH, Hagen T, Vogel DS, Ames BN, Christen S, Shigenaga MK. Immunodetection of 3-nitrotyrosine in the liver of zymosan-treated rats with a new monoclonal antibody: comparison to analysis by HPLC. Free Rad Biol Med 2001; 31:1375–1387.

76. Shin JT, Barbeito L, Mac-Millan-Crow LA, Beckman JS, Thompson JA. Acidic fibroblast growth factor enhances peroxynitrite-induced apoptosis in primary murine fibroblasts. Arch Biochem Biophys 1996; 335:32–41.

77. Estévez AG, Spear N, Manuel SM, Radi R, Henderson CE, Barbeito L, Beckman JS. Nitric oxide and superoxide contribute to motor neuron apoptosis induced by trophic factor deprivation. J Neurosci 1998; 18:923–931.

78. Lymar SV, Hurst JK. Carbon dioxide: physiological catalyst for peroxynitrite-mediated cellular damage or cellular protectant. Chem Res Toxicol 1996; 9:845–850.

79. McElhinney, Poynter ME, Kharraziha R, Hazen S, Janssen-Heininger Y. Enzymatic activity of eosinophil peroxidase causes a complex mode of death in lung epithelial cells that does not strictly depend on nitration chemistry. Free Rad Biol Med 2001; 31:S48.

80. Eiserich JP, Estévez AG, Bamberg T, Ye YZ, Beckman JS, Freeman BA. Microtubule dysfunction by post-translational nitrotyrosination of α-tubulin: a nitric oxide-dependent mechanism of cellular injury. Proc Natl Acad Sci USA 1998; 96:6365–6370.

81. Huang Y.-C., Dailey L, Zhang W.-L., Jaspers I. Nitrotyrosination of alpha-tubulin induces epithelial transport dysfunction. Free Rad Biol Med 2001; 31:S70

82. Yermilov V, Rubio J, Ohshima H. Formation of 8-nitroguanine in DNA treated with peroxynitrite in vitro and its rapid removal from DNA by depurination. FEBS Lett 1995; 376:207–210.

83. Juedes MJ, Wogan GN. Peroxynitrite-induced mutation spectra of pSP189 following replication in bacteria and in human cells. Mutat Res 1996; 349:51–61.

84. Kong S-K., Yim MB, Stadman ER, Chock PB. Peroxynitrite disables the tyrosine phosphorylation regulatory mechanism: lymphocyte-specific tyrosine kinase fails to

phosphorylate nitrated cdc2(6–20)NH$_2$ peptide. Proc Natl Acad Sci USA 1996; 93: 3377–3382.

85. Gow AJ, Duran D, Malcolm S, Ischiropoulos H. Effects of peroxynitrite-induced protein modifications on tyrosine phosphorylation and degradation. FEBS Lett 1996; 385: 63–66.

86. Li X, De Sarno P, Song L, Beckman JS, Jope RS. Peroxynitrite modulates tyrosine phosphorylation and phosphoinositide signalling in human neuroblastoma SH-SY5Y cells: attenuated effects in human 1321N1 astrocytoma cells. Biochem J 1998; 331: 599–606.

87. Mallozzi C, Di Stasi AMM, Minetti M. Peroxynitrite modulates tyrosine-dependent signal transduction pathway of human erythrocyte band 3. FASEB J 1997; 11: 1281–1290.

88. van der Vliet A, Hristova M, Cross CE, Eiserich JP, Goldkorn T. Peroxynitrite induces covalent dimerization of epidermal growth factor receptors in A431 epidermoid carcinoma cells. J Biol Chem 1998; 273:31860–31866.

89. MacMillan-Crow LA, Crow JP, Thompson JA. Peroxynitrite-mediated inactivation of manganese superoxide dismutase involves nitration and oxidation of critical tyrosine residues. Biochemistry 1998; 37:1613–1622.

90. Yakamura F, Taka H, Fujimura T, Murayama K. Inactivation of human manganese-superoxide dismutase by peroxynitrite is caused by exclusive nitration of tyrosine 34 to 3-nitrotyrosine. J Biol Chem 1998; 273:14085–14089.

91. Soulere L, Claparols C, Perie J, Hoffmann P. Peroxynitrite-induced nitration of tyrosine-34 does not inhibit *Escherichia coli* iron superoxide dismutase. Biochem J 2001; 360:563–567.

92. Ara J, Przedborski S, Naini AB, Jackson-Lewis V, Trifiletti RR, Horwitz J, Ischiropoulos H. Inactivation of tyrosine hydroxylase by nitration following exposure to peroxynitrite and 1-methyl-4-phenyl-1,2,3,6-tetrahydropyridine (MPTP). Proc Natl Acad Sci USA 1998; 95:7659–7663.

93. Kuhn DM, Aretha CW, Geddes TJ. Peroxynitrite inactivation of tyrosine hydroxylase: mediation by sulfhydryl oxidation, not tyrosine nitration. J Neurosci 1999; 19: 10289–10294.

94. Blanchard-Fillion B, Souza JM, Friel T, Jiang GCT, Vrana K, Sharov V, Barron L, Schöneich C, Quijano C, Alvarez B, Radi R, Przedborski S, Horwitz J, Ischiropoulos H. Nitration and inactivation of tyrosine hydroxylase by peroxynitrite. J Biol Chem 2001; 276:46017–46023.

95. Wong PS, Eiserich JP, Lopez CL, Jones AD, Reddy S, Cross CE, van der Vliet A. Inactivation of glutathione S-transferase by nitric oxide-derived oxidants. Exploring a role for tyrosine nitration. Arch Biochem Biophys 2001; 94:216–228.

96. Goodwin DC, Gunther MR, Hsi LC, Crews BC, Eling, TE, Mason RP, Marnett LJ. Nitric oxide trapping of tyrosyl radicals generated during prostaglandin endoperoxide synthase turnover. Detection of the radical derivative of tyrosine 385. J Biol Chem, 1998; 273:8903–8909.

97. Roberts ES, Lin H, Crowley JR, Vuletich JL, Osawa Y, Hollenberg PF. Peroxynitrite-mediated nitration of tyrosine and inactivation of the catalytic activity of cytochrome P450 2B1. Chem Res Toxicol 1998; 11:1067–1074.

98. Berlett BS, Levine RL, Stadtman ER. Carbon dioxide stimulates peroxynitrite-mediated nitration of tyrosine residues and inhibits oxidation of methionine residues of glutamine synthetase: both modifications mimic effects of adenylation. Proc Natl Acad Sci USA 1998; 95:2784–2789.

99. Cassina AM, Hodara R, Souza JM, Thomson L, Castro L, Ischiropoulos H, Freeman BA, Radi R. Cytochrome C nitration by peroxynitrite. J Biol Chem 2000; 275: 21409–21415.

100. Guittet O, Decottignies P, Serani L, Henry Y, Le Marechal P, Laprevote O, Lepoivre M. Peroxynitrite-mediated nitration of the stable free radical tyrosine residue of the ribonucleotide reductase small subunit. Biochemistry 2000; 39:4640–4648.

101. Mierzwa S, Chan SK. Chemical modification of human α1-proteinase inhibitor by tetranitromethane. Biochem J 1987; 246:37–42.

102. Greis KD, Zhu S, Matalon S. Identification of nitration sites on surfactant protein A by tandem electrospray mass spectrometry. Arch Biochem Biophys 1996; 335:396–402.

103. Zhu S, Haddad IY, Matalon S. Nitration of surfactant protein A (SP-A) tyrosine residues results in decreased mannose binding ability. Arch Biochem Biophys 1996; 333: 282–290.

104. Haddad IY, Zhou S, Ischiropoulos H, Matalon S. Nitration of surfactant protein A results in decreased ability to aggregate lipids. Am J Physiol 1996; 270:L281–L288.

105. Zhu S, Ware LB, Geiser T, Matthay MA, Matalon S. Increased levels of nitrate and surfactant protein A nitration in the pulmonary edema fluids of patients with acute lung injury. Am J Respir Crit Care Med 2001; 163:166–172.

106. Kamisaki Y, Wada K, Bian K, Balabanli B, Davis K, Martin E, Behbod F, Lee Y.-C., Murad F. An activity in rat tissues that modifies nitrotyrosine-containing proteins. Proc Natl Acad Sci USA 95:11584–11589.

107. Denitration of peroxynitrite-treated proteins by "protein nitratases" from dog prostate. Biochem Mol Biol Int 1999; 47:1061–1067.

7

S-Nitrosothiols in Lung Inflammation

HARVEY E. MARSHALL, LORETTA G. QUE, and JONATHAN S. STAMLER

Duke University Medical Center
Durham, North Carolina, U.S.A.

BENJAMIN GASTON

University of Virginia Health System
Charlottesville, Virginia, U.S.A.

I. Introduction

S-Nitrosothiols (SNOs) are complexes of nitric oxide (NO) bound to thiol groups, which are present in biological systems as proteins and low molecular weight peptides (1,2). SNOs have been regarded by some as markers of NO production [i.e., nitric oxide synthase (NOS) activity] with little inherent bioactivity. However, it has now become apparent that SNOs are critical mediators involved in several cell-signaling pathways. For example, S-nitrosylation reactions (i.e., reactions forming S-NO bonds) are involved in the regulation of p21ras (3) the ryanodine receptor (4), the N-methyl-D-aspartate (NMDA) receptor (5), caspase 3 activity (6,7), and NF-κB (p50-p65) (8). In addition, SNOs function physiologically in controlling ventilation (5) and O_2 delivery (9).

The bioactivity of SNOs in blood vessels was first recognized by Ignarro et al., who described their vasodilating properties (10). Indeed, SNO-induced vasodilation closely resembles that ascribed to endothelium-derived relaxing factor (EDRF) (11). In fact, the bioactivity of SNO is equivalent to or exceeds that of NO with regard to its effect on airway smooth muscle tone, platelet aggregation, and microbial killing (12–14). Moreover, recent studies (in vitro) have determined that S-nitrosoglutathione (GSNO) is formed in the presence of activated NOS (15). These observations—coupled with the fact that NOS activity is thiol-dependent (16)—have led some to suggest that SNOs may be a primary product of NOS activation (17).

SNOs have several advantages over NO as "NO effectors." SNOs are inherently more stable than NO at physiological pH, most having a half-life measured in hours as opposed to seconds (18). SNOs are also not as prone to the potentially deleterious interactions with O_2 and superoxide that form nitrogen dioxide (NO_2) and peroxynitrite ($OONO^-$), respectively. Moreover, SNOs can deliver NO either as nitrosonium (NO^+) or nitroxyl (NO^-) equivalents (heterolytic cleavage) or NO radical (homolytic cleavage), providing diversity in biochemical reactivity (19). Further, SNO formation can also represent a "NO reservoir," storing NO bioactivity until needed. Finally, cellular systems exist to regulate the catabolism, localization, and trafficking of SNO; comparable systems are not known for NO in eukaryotes (6,7,20).

II. SNOs in the Lung

In mammalian tissues, the concentration of SNOs varies between 10 nM and 10 μM (2,21,22). In cells with significant inducible NOS activity (NOS II) (e.g., activated macrophages), SNO levels exceed 1 μM (23). Concentrations are tightly regulated and are higher in certain cell compartments than others (6,7) and in certain tissues. For example, GSNO levels are μM in the rat medulla, but are undetectable in the thalamus, whereas levels of S-nitrosocysteinyl glycine are high in the thalamus (22,24). In no other organ system, however, is the presence and function of SNOs better delineated than in the lung.

The lung environment is highly conducive to the formation of SNOs. This is particularly true in the airways, where μM concentrations of thiol (predominantly glutathione), significant NO production in the airway epithelium (as well as resident inflammatory cells), and high oxygen tension favor synthesis of airway SNOs (2). Indeed, the endogenous formation of GSNO was first identified in the airway, where airway SNO concentrations of 100–500 nM are present at steady state but can be in excess of 1 μM in acute inflammatory conditions (Fig. 1) (2). Moreover, airway SNOs increase dramatically after exposure to inhaled NO (25,26), which is used therapeutically for such diseases as persistence of pulmonary hypertension in neonates, adult respiratory distress syndrome (ARDS), and primary pulmonary hypertension (PPH) (unpublished observations) (27–29).

While conditions that favor nitrosative chemistry and de novo SNO synthesis certainly exist in the airway lining fluid (particularly with inflammation), this does not exclude the possibility that airway SNOs are exported from resident airway cells. In fact, significant SNO concentrations are present in the respiratory epithelium and in macrophages (23,30). Moreover, immunohistochemical staining for SNO proteins in the lung reveals high concentrations of endogenous SNO proteins in airway epithelium (25,26). The fact that the airway epithelium constitutively expresses NOS II—with a marked increase in expression and activity with cytokine stimulation—further supports the notion that the epithelium is a major source of airway

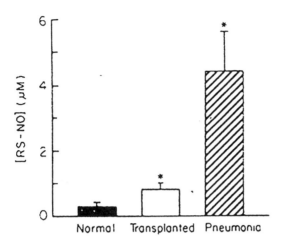

Figure 1   Distal airway S-NO levels in different patient populations. Bronchoalveolar lavage lung lining fluid S-NO concentrations in lung transplantation ($n = 9$) and pneumonia patients ($n = 3$) are greater than in normal subjects ($n = 6$) (*$p < 0.05$).

SNO (31). There is also evidence that the predominant site of SNO synthesis is the tracheal and bronchial epithelium, as the concentration of SNO is higher in fluid sampled from large airways (i.e., tracheal aspirates) than the smaller airways [i.e., bronchoalveolar lavage (BAL)] (32). Further, neurochemical stimulation of the large airways in the guinea pig causes SNO release and airway smooth muscle relaxation (33,34).

SNOs are also present in the pulmonary circulation. Proteins, rather than low-mass thiols, represent the bulk of circulating SNOs (1,21,35). The two proteins with the highest SNO concentration in the blood are hemoglobin (Hb) and albumin (9,12). NO binds to Hb not only as a nitrosothiol (on cysteine 93 of the β chain) but also as nitrosyl-heme (9). In high oxygen tension, Hb undergoes a conformational change that favors transfer of NO from the heme to the thiol, preserving NO bioactivity (9). Thus, oxygenation of Hb in the lung in essence "packages" NO for delivery to peripheral tissues. Both SNO-Hb and SNO-albumin have demonstrated bioactivity in the lung (13,36).

Several other lung cell types produce SNOs. Immunochemical studies demonstrate prominent SNO staining in the pulmonary endothelium as well as smooth muscle cells surrounding larger airways (25). Endothelial cells have also been shown to synthesize SNO in vitro (37). Interestingly, cartilage chondrocytes of large airways also show immunohistochemical evidence for the presence of SNOs. While the presence of SNOs has not been proven in pulmonary ganglia, they have been isolated from other neural cells and tissues (38) with evidence to suggest that they function in nonadrenergic, noncholinergic neurotransmission (33,34,39). Finally, SNOs are present in lymphocytes (6,7) and neutrophils (40) characteristic of various pulmonary inflammatory responses.

III. Biosynthesis of SNO

The biosynthesis of SNO commonly involves the transfer or reaction of NO^+. It is important to note that NO^+ per se is not a stable ion in solution, but exists in complexes with species that can serve as electron acceptors from NO (e.g., with Cu^+ or NO_2^-; see below). The milieu of the lung, which is rich in glutathione, O_2, and NO, provides an especially favorable environment for formation of SNOs. In the airway, for example, NO can be oxidized by O_2 to yield nitrosating and oxidizing NO_x, such as N_2O_3 and N_2O_4, that generate R-SNO species in the presence of thiols (RSH) (A). The formation of N_2O_3 and N_2O_4 also generates the end products of NO_x metabolism seen in cellular systems, NO_2^- and NO_3^- (C–F).

A. $2NO + O_2 \rightarrow 2NO_2$
B. $NO_2 + NO \rightarrow N_2O_3$
C. $2NO_2 \leftrightarrow N_2O_4$
D. $N_2O_3 \leftrightarrow NO^+ \ldots NO_2^-$
E. $N_2O_4 + H_2O \leftrightarrow HNO_2 + HNO_3$
F. $HNO_2 \leftrightarrow NO_2^- + H^+$
G. $RSH + NO^+ \rightarrow RSNO + H^+$ (R = cysteine or cysteine-containing protein or peptide)

Note that in equilibrium (D) NO_2 has served as the electron acceptor. It is important to realize, however, that while physiological conditions do support the formation of SNOs by $NO-O_2$ reactions in vivo, demonstrative proof is still lacking.

On the other hand, there is overwhelming evidence for SNO formation by NO-metal reactions in vivo. Direct S-nitrosation of thiols by metal (e.g., Fe, Cu) nitrosyl compounds in the presence of NO is well described (41–43). In particular, NO reacts with the transition metal centers (M) of proteins to form M-NO. The M-NO species supports additional nitrosative reactions with thiols (RSH/RS^-) to form RSNO. An example of in vivo SNO formation catalyzed by transition metals is ceruloplasmin, a multicopper-containing plasma protein. Expression of ceruloplasmin, which is abundant in plasma, is upregulated in the airways under inflammatory conditions, including ARDS. Type I copper, localized in one of the three copper domains of ceruloplasmin, functions as an electron acceptor in the presence of NO. The one-electron oxidation of NO from type I copper to types 2 and 3 copper in ceruloplasmin forms NO^+ coupled with a four-electron reduction of O_2 to form H_2O (44).

NO can also react directly with thiols to form SNOs in the presence of an electron acceptor such as NAD^+ via a radical intermediate, RSN·OH (45). If an electron acceptor is present, R-S-N-OH may be converted to a SNO by reduction of the acceptor.

More recently, it has been recognized that targeting of protein S-nitrosylation is exquisitely specific to consensus amino acid sequence motifs. Thus, specificity of NO binding can be conferred by acid-base and hydrophobic compartments. This cell-signaling process is similar to more thoroughly studied motifs involved in the regulation of phosphorylation. In proteins that are endogenously S-nitrosylated, acid-base and hydrophobic compartment motifs can predict regulatory cysteines modified by NO (46). Examples include NMDA receptors (47), which contain a cysteine residue within an acid-base motif, and ryanodine receptor (23), which contains a cysteine in a hydrophobic compartment motif. Of note, amino acids in the vicinity of cysteine residues that favor S-nitrosylation may be evident either in the primary sequence of the protein or in the tertiary structure (48). S-Nitrosylation of the active site cysteine, in turn, regulates protein function. Importantly, NO-protein interactions serve not only to modify protein function, but also to transport NO to sites of activity. For example, binding of O_2 to heme irons promotes binding of NO to cysteine 93 of the β chain, forming S-nitrosohemoglobin. Allosteric transition of S-nitrosohemoglobin from R to T structure during deoxygenation allows transfer of the NO group to the site of the vessels supplying the hypoxic tissue that are in need of a vasodilatory stimulus (9).

IV. SNO Bioactivities in the Lung

SNOs have many biological functions in the lung, ranging from control of ventilation/perfusion (V/Q) matching to regulation of inflammatory cell survival and activity. NOS has long been believed to play a significant role in regulating airway tone (49). SNOs formed as a result of NOS activity are potent bronchodilators. In fact, the human airway smooth muscle relaxant effects of GSNO are three times greater than NO and 100 times more powerful then theophylline (Fig. 2) (13). More significantly, endogenous airway SNOs are present in concentrations that are (1) at least 3 log orders higher than NO and (2) close to the IC_{50} for airway smooth muscle relaxation (2,50). Both protein and low-mass SNOs induce relaxation of histamine, methacholine, and LTD_4-contracted guinea pig and human airway rings (13,51). In the isolated, perfused lung, both airway and intravascular administration of SNOs induce bronchodilation, indicating that transport mechanisms from the circulation to the airways exist (52). SNO-induced bronchodilation has also been demonstrated in vivo. Aerosolized SNO decreases airway resistance in the lungs of methacholine-treated guinea pigs (53).

Importantly, SNO-induced airway smooth muscle relaxation is not dependent upon the generation of NO: hemoglobin and other NO scavengers do not significantly alter the response, particularly in the human airway (13,52). SNO-induced bronchodilation is also not dependent upon the activation of guanylate cyclase: methylene blue and other more specific guanylate cyclase inhibitors are only partially inhibitory or are noninhibitory, and the relaxant effects on the human airway are not recapitulated by 8-Br cGMP (13,54). Moreover, airways relaxed with NO return to baseline tone more rapidly then those treated with SNO, implying dissimilar mechanisms of bronchodilation (53). Of note, large, stable cell-impermeable SNOs such as S-nitrosoalbumin have IC_{50}s very close to—or greater than—smaller, cell-permeable unstable SNOs like S-nitrosocysteine (on the order of 10 μM) in relaxing human airway smooth muscle, suggesting a mechanism of action involving a cell-surface S-nitrosylation reaction (13). Interestingly, the relaxation of canine tracheal smooth muscle by GSNO is reversed upon the addition of the reducing agent 1,3-dithiothrei-

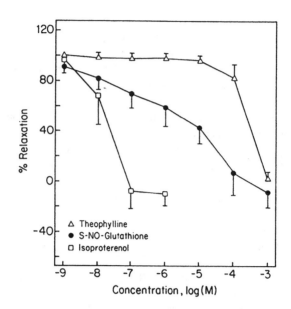

Figure 2 Comparison of relaxation effects of S-nitrosoglutathione GSNO, theophylline, and isoproterenol in human bronchi in vitro. The relaxant activity of GSNO ($n = 6$) was compared against isoproterenol ($n = 5$) and theophylline ($n = 7$) in airways contracted with 7 μm methacholine. Concentration-effect relationships reveal an order of potency: isoproterenol (squares) > GSNO (circles) > theophylline (triangles) (ANOVA; $p < 0.0005$). Results are presented as mean $\pm$ SEM.

tol (DTT), suggesting a mechanism dependent upon nitrosylation or oxidation of thiols (54). Indeed, these collective observations point to SNOs—and not NO—as the mediators of nitrogen oxide–induced bronchodilation in vivo. That is, the extent to which SNO acts to release NO radical as an "NO donor" will be the extent to which it loses its bronchodilator bioactivity.

Ventilation/perfusion (V/Q) mismatching is an important element in the pathophysiology of inflammatory diseases of the lung, and nitrogen oxides clearly play a role in regulating this process. For example, inhaled NO improves V/Q matching in acute lung injury, and endogenous NO production is required for the V/Q mismatching that occurs in sepsis (55,56). In the pulmonary circulation, SNOs are potent vasodilators with effects comparable to that of NO (57). Similar to NO, SNOs have modest effects on PVR at steady-state normoxic conditions but dramatically decrease pulmonary vascular resistance under conditions of hypoxic vasoconstriction (58). However, while both NO and SNOs dilate small pulmonary vessels equally, SNOs also have the capability to dilate larger caliber pulmonary arteries (59). Moreover, recent studies in the lung using inhaled ethyl nitrite (ENO), an NO compound with SNO-like (i.e., NO^+) properties that does not release NO radical to an appreciable extent, demonstrate more specific vasodilation of the pulmonary circulation compared to inhaled NO (60). Indeed, the pulmonary vasodilatory effect of ENO on the pulmonary vasculature is associated with a greater formation of lung SNOs, suggesting again that SNOs may be the actual effectors of pulmonary vasodilation.

SNOs affect several different functions of the airway epithelium at physiological concentrations. Both anion and cation channels on the epithelial surface are modulated by SNO (61,62). GSNO activates chloride channels in the airway epithelium, predominantly by a cGMP-dependent mechanism (62,64,65), and inhibits sodium transport in the airway through cation channels on the apical surface of the epithelium (61). Both GSNO and NO increase the ciliary beat frequency in airway epithelial cells, promoting mucus clearance from the lower airways (63).

The effect of GSNO on the cystic fibrosis (CF) epithelium is of particular importance. GSNO increases the expression and maturation of the cystic fibrosis transmembrane regulator (CFTR) chloride channel in cells homozygous for the most common mutation associated with CF (ΔF508) (66). This mutation produces a fully translated and functional CFTR protein that, because it is missing a single phenylalanine in its first ATP-binding domain, is degraded by a mechanism involving the ubiquitin/proteasome system. GSNO appears both to increase transcription of *cftr*—through increased binding of the CFTR gene promoter, SP1—and also to block the proteasomal degradation of the protein (66). Remarkably, full maturation of the protein allows expression of ΔF508 on the cell surface of CFBE4lo$^-$ (ΔF508 homozygous) airway epithelial cells, and functional Cl$^-$ transport has been documented (67) (unpublished observations). Similar results have been published using 4-phenylbutyrate, a potentially toxic agent that is now in clinical trials as a therapy for patients with the ΔF508 mutation. Unlike 4-PB, however, GSNO is an endogenous airway molecule, levels of which are low in the CF airway (68). Taken together, the ciliary prokinetic, bronchodilator, airway-hydrating, antimicrobial, and CFTR maturational effects of GSNO suggest that it may be a useful therapeutic goal to restore normal GSNO levels in the CF airway. Indeed, inhaled GSNO is well tolerated and improves oxygenation acutely in patients with CF (69).

SNOs also have important roles in regulating cellular apoptosis and proliferation that are likely to be relevant to airway remodeling, to the regeneration of lung parenchyma after acute injury, and to the inflammatory response itself (see below). For example, endogenous S-nitrosylation at the active site cysteine of caspase 3 inhibits cellular apoptosis at baseline (6,7). An appropriate cellular stimulus (e.g., Fas ligand/TNFα) induces the denitrosylation of caspase-3, resulting in the induction of apoptosis (6,70). Part of this degradation may involve regulated caspase trafficking out of the mitochondrial membrane and into the cytosol (7). On the other hand, in conditions of nitrosative stress (e.g., inflammation), higher intracellular concentrations of SNO can be pro-apoptotic, perhaps through the inhibition of NF-κB (23). Both mechanisms are likely important in the clearance of inflammatory cells from the airway and the airway remodeling that is seen in chronic asthma. Of note, GSNO promotes apoptosis of neutrophils (71), of particular interest because severe asthma (72) and CF may both be characterized by severe neutrophilic infiltration and decreased airway levels of SNO (32,68,73). Moreover, SNOs have an antiproliferative effect on airway smooth muscle cells, which may also play a role in the pathogenesis of asthma (74).

V. SNOs in Inflammation

Immune activation of many different respiratory cell types leads to the induction of NOS II and an increase in cellular NO production. Intuitively, one would expect that this increase in NOS II activity would lead (at least transiently) to a rise in intracellular SNOs. Indeed, cellular SNO levels do rise with NOS II activation in cytokine-stimulated respiratory epithelium, endothelium, and macrophages in vitro (23,30,75). SNOs produced in these immune-stimulated cells can serve several different functions. The cell might directly secrete SNOs—either into the airway lumen or into phagosomes/lysosomes—to function as antimicrobial agents (76). For example, certain microbial killing by macrophages has been shown to involve the synthesis of SNO-albumin (77), and the mechanism of NO-mediated antimicrobial activity in many cases involves a specific S-nitrosylation reaction, such as inhibitory S-nitrosylation of viral cysteine proteases (7,78).

Increasingly, however, SNOs are recognized to function more subtly as intracellular signal transducers, most notably in a number of immunomodulatory pathways. SNOs affect the transcription of inflammatory response genes in a number of different cell types. For example, nitrosylation of the prokaryotic transcription factor OxyR (79) induces transcription of proteins required for defense against the nitrosative state. In eukaryotic cells, GSNO attenuates the expression of adhesion molecules such as VCAM-1, ICAM-1, and E selectin in cytokine-stimulated endothelial cells (80). The SNO-dependent decrease in the expression of adhesion molecules may involve the same mechanism by which inhaled NO inhibits lung sequestration of neutrophils in animal models of sepsis (81). SNOs are also known to attenuate the expression of IL-1, IL-8, TNFα, and several other cytokines (82). The modulated expression of these inflammatory mediators by SNO appears to be dependent upon the inhibition of the transcription factor NF-κB. In the pulmonary system, SNOs inhibit NF-κB activation in macrophages, neutrophils, lung epithelial, smooth muscle, and endothelial cells (Fig. 3A) (8,71,83–85). Interestingly, one of the mechanisms by which SNOs (and endogenous NO) inhibit NF-κB activation is through nitrosylation of the NF-κB–activating protein dimer (p50-p65) (8,85). Nitrosylation of p50-p65 (specifically, the p50 subunit) disrupts NF-κB binding to DNA, thereby downregulating κB-dependent transcription. In addition to p50-p65, there are other proteins upstream in the NF-κB activation pathway that are targeted by SNOs, resulting in NF-κB inhibition (3,83).

Similarly, there are other transcription factors involved in lung inflammation (e.g., AP-1, HIF-1, and SP-1), the activity of which is regulated by nitrosylation (86,87). The case of HIF-1 is of particular interest because the mechanism appears to involve inhibitors of elements of the ubiquitin-proteasome system—analogous to that seen with CFTR—preventing the degradation (post-translational regulation) of its HIF-1α subunit (Fig. 3B) (87). This pathway, in turn, allows the downstream

A   B

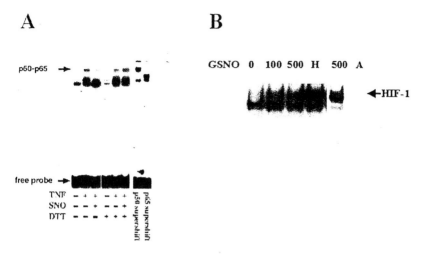

Figure 3 (A) Thiol-reversible inhibition of NF-κB by SNO in respiratory epithelial cells. A549 cells were treated with S-nitrosocysteine (1 mM) for 20 min in culture followed by stimulation with TNFα (20 ng/mL) for 30 min. Nuclear extracts were prepared with or without DTT (1 mM, in the extraction buffers. NF-κB DNA-binding activity was assessed by EMSA. Antibody supershifting of the NF-κB bands is displayed in the far right panel. Arrows denote the location of the p50–p65 heterodimer and free probe on the gel. The two bands below the p50-65 heterodimer were constitutively present and were not further characterized. (B) Nuclear proteins isolated from bovine pulmonary artery endothelial cells was treated with S-nitrosoglutathione for a period of 4 hours. HIF-1 DNA-binding activity was determined by EMSA. H, hypoxia. Further, nuclear extracts were made from bovine pulmonary artery endothelial cells treated with 100 µM GSNO in the presence (+) or absence (−) of 100 µM acivicin for 4 h.

upregulation of inflammatory enzymes such as heme oxygenase 1—and NOS II itself—in the lung.

While an important means by which SNOs affect lung inflammation appears to involve transcriptional regulation, SNOs can also target inflammatory response proteins, directly affecting their activity. Several enzymes involved in the cellular oxidative response—a crucial element of inflammation—are inhibited by nitrosylation. For example, SNOs attenuate the respiratory burst in neutrophils by inhibition of NADPH oxidase (88). S-Nitrosylation of the p47^{phox} subunit of NADPH oxidase appears to be one mechanism involved. SNOs alter cellular iron levels, a central constituent of oxidative and nitrosative chemistry, by modulating iron regulatory protein (IRP) function (89). S-Nitrosylation of IRP-2 in cytokine-stimulated macrophages prevents its interaction with the iron response element (IRE), subsequently targeting the protein for degradation in the proteasome (89). The activity of glutathione reductase is also regulated in cytokine-stimulated macrophages through nitrosylation of the enzyme, ultimately subjecting the cell to increased oxidative stress (90). On the other hand, exogenous SNO has been shown to increase cellular glutathione content in endothelial cells by augmenting the activity of γ-glutamylcysteine synthetase by a cGMP-independent mechanism (91).

Orchestration of these various potentially conflicting regulatory systems at the cell and organ system levels appears to involve precise regulation of the *composition, compartmentalization,* and *concentration* of the SNO pool. An example of *compositional* regulation is the regulation of minute ventilation at the level of the nucleus tractus solitarius, where μM GSNO levels (22) are only active as respiratory stimulants if acted upon by γ-glutamyl transpeptidase (γGT) to form S-nitrosocysteinyl glycine (92). Regulation by *compartmentalization* is illustrated by mitochondrial sequestration of S-nitrosylated (inactive) caspases, which appear to be activated by transfer to the cytosol (6,7) where they may be denitrosylated by enzymatic pathways such as glutathione-sensitive formaldehyde dehydrogenase (GS-FDH) (20). The relevance of *concentration* is illustrated by the paradoxical increase of SP1 binding with physiological (nM–low μM) airway GSNO concentrations, with paradoxical inhibition of binding by concentrators in excess of 10 μM.

A number of enzymes may regulate SNO concentrations in vitro, including xanthine/xanthine oxidase (93), thioredoxin/thioredoxin reductase (94), γGT (95), and glutathione peroxidase (96). Further, work by Liu et al. has demonstrated that catabolism of SNOs by GS-FDH may regulate intracellular SNO levels and S-nitrosylation in vivo (Fig. 4) (20). In GS-FDH knockout mice, SNO levels, including both GSNO and S-nitrosylated proteins, were increased by 60–175% compared to their wild-type littermates. Though there appears to be an equilibrium between GSNO and protein SNOs in the cytosol, GS-FDH does not metabolize high-mass SNO proteins; other "SNO-lyase" enzymes are likely to be present in cells.

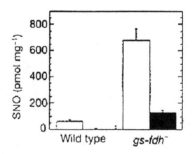

Figure 4 GSNO reductase in *S. cerevisiae* protects from nitrosative stress. Deletion of the GSNO reductase gene encoding SFA1 (GS-FDH) was accomplished in haploid Y190 cells. Increased levels of intracellular S-nitrosothiols were seen in gs-fdh mutant cells after GSNO treatment. Mid-log phase (absorbance 600 nm = 0.4–0.6) cells were cultured in the presence of 5 mM GSNO at 30°C for 2 hours. SNO signals in the whole lysate (open) and the fraction that passed through a 5K cut-off membrane (filled) were normalized against whole-cell lysate protein content. Data are the mean ± SE from three independent experiments.

VI. Asthma and Other Inflammatory Lung Diseases

The premise that high levels of airway SNOs (like exhaled NO) could serve as markers for lung inflammation would seem intuitive. After all, cellular SNO levels rise with increased expression of NOS II in cytokine-stimulated cells (23,30). Furthermore, NOS II is constitutively expressed in airway epithelium, and expression increases dramatically in some acute inflammatory conditions (97–100). It follows, then, that airway SNO levels should rise with inflammation. Indeed, in the airways of patients after lung transplantation or with acute pneumonia, airway SNOs increase 3-fold and 20-fold, respectively (2). Airway SNOs may be higher than normal in COPD (101), although these data are based on measurements in airway condensates which may not reflect true airway fluid concentrations. There is also immunohistochemical evidence for increased SNO in the airways of neonates with bronchopulmonary dysplasia (25). It is important to note that treatment with either inhaled NO or the more selective NO$^+$ donor ENO—both of which have been found to be beneficial in neonatal lung disease—increases the concentration of airway SNOs (26,60).

In asthma and cystic fibrosis, however, the situation is not as clear. In asthma, exhaled breath NO and airway fluid nitrite/nitrate are higher than in controls (13,102–105). However, airway SNO levels are actually *decreased* compared to controls in the tracheal aspirates of asthmatic children intubated for respiratory failure and in the bronchoalveolar lavage of patients with mild asthma at baseline (Fig. 5A) (32,73). Airway SNO levels seem to be lower in asthma despite the fact that airway glutathione levels are higher and airway fluid is acidified, which, coupled with the higher release of NO into the airway, favors further formation of SNOs (106–108). Following antigen challenge in mild asthmatics, BALF SNO levels rise, but only to normal (32), unlike levels of other NO_x. There are conflicting reports about whether SNOs can be measured in asthmatic exhaled breath, but, assuming they are not formed or measured as an artifact, levels may be high in some asthmatics (101) when measured indirectly—that is, when collected in the absence of airway contents. In the case of asthma, these complicated observations are best understood in the context of very rapid GSNO catabolism in the lung and airway lining fluid that has been demonstrated both in the ovalbumin-sensitized guinea pig asthma model, where particular catabolic proteins have been identified (109), and in human tracheal aspirates, where the GSNO half-life may be less than 5 min. Thus, the flux of S-nitrosothiols through the asthmatic airway surface lining fluid appears to be dramatically accelerated, with rate of catabolism in many cases outstripping synthesis. This is important, not just because SNOs have several potential salutary effects in the asthmatic airway, but also because the products of GSNO catabolism in this high-flux state—which includes ammonia, NO, hydroxylamine, and ONOO$^-$ (20,51,93,94,96)—have a broad range of bioactivities and toxicities.

SNO levels are unexpectedly low in other airway inflammatory diseases as well. In patients with CF, bronchoalveolar lavage SNO levels are virtually undetectable despite high nitrite/nitrate concentrations in the airway fluid and sputum (Fig. 5B) (68,110). These low airway SNO levels are not associated with bacterial coloni-

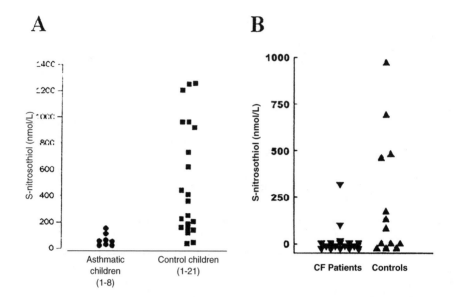

Figure 5 (A) S-Nitrosothiol concentrations in airways of children with near-fatal asthma and in control children. Tracheal S-nitrosothiol concentrations are lower in asthmatic children than in control children undergoing elective surgery. (B) SNO concentrations in BAL fluid of patients with CF and normal pulmonary function and in BAL fluid of control subjects. Each symbol represents one individual.

zation, indicating that bacterial denitrification is not involved (68). Unlike asthma, however, exhaled NO and airway NOS II expression are actually lower in CF (111,112). In fact, lower exhaled NO levels in CF seem to correlate with disease severity and exacerbations (113,114). This is particularly intriguing, as overall the biological functions of airway SNO are beneficial in CF. Both decreased synthesis and increased catabolism may be involved (66). Of note, airway SNO levels are also lower in neonates with respiratory distress syndrome who are on extracorporeal membrane oxygenation (ECMO) (2). Whether the decrease in airway SNO levels in this case was the result of the disease process or the application of ECMO is uncertain.

Clearly, there is a complex dynamic regarding the regulation of SNOs and other nitrogen oxides in lung inflammation. The idea that high airway levels of NO, nitrite/nitrate, or SNOs can represent a single surrogate marker for airways inflammation is not always valid. On the other hand, the complex metabolic relationships between SNOs and other nitrogen oxides may provide several new targets for therapeutic intervention in a broad spectrum of lung diseases.

VII. Nitrosative Defense of Colonizing Species

Bacteria are protected from SNO-mediated activation of transcription factor OxyR (79). In addition, HMP flavohemoglobin denitrosylase directly metabolizes NO and protects yeast and bacteria from the toxic effects of NO (115–117), and GS-FDH protects yeast and possibly bacteria from the antimicrobial effects of SNOs (20,115). Strategies for overcoming these defenses may provide new therapies for patients with bronchitis and pneumonia.

VIII. Summary

In summary, SNOs are endogenous species that are biologically relevant, both to normal lung physiology and to the pathophysiology of a variety of human disease states. They are more potent human airway smooth muscle relaxants than is NO itself and serve an important role in regulating airway luminal homeostasis. In addition, they have a crucial role in matching ventilation to perfusion and controlling oxygenation and oxygen delivery at several levels of the respiratory cycle. Further, tightly regulated SNO localization and catabolism appear to be relevant to many pulmonary cell-signaling processes, ranging from transcriptional regulation to protein ubiquitination. S-Nitrosylation chemistry is an important emerging concept in pulmonary biology and pathophysiology; it has already provided exciting targets for the development of new therapies.

Acknowledgments

This work was supported by the NIH and 1u19-A134607I—R01's HL 59337 and HL 69170 (BG), R01-ES-09206 (JS), K08-HL-04287 (HM), K08-HL-04171 (LQ)—and by the Henry B. Wallace Foundation (BG).

References

1. Stamler JS, et al. Nitric oxide circulates in mammalian plasma primarily as an S-nitroso adduct of serum albumin. Proc Natl Acad Sci USA 1992; 89(16):7674–7677.
2. Gaston B, et al. Endogenous nitrogen oxides and bronchodilator S-nitrosothiols in human airways. Proc Natl Acad Sci USA 1993; 90(23):10957–10961.
3. Lander HM, et al. A molecular redox switch on p21ras. Structural basis for the nitric oxide-p21ras interactions. J Biol Chem 1997; 272(7):4323–4326.
4. Xu L, et al. Activation of the cardiac calcium release channel (ryanodine receptor) by poly-S-nitrosylation. Science 1998; 279(5348):234–237.
5. Lipton SA, et al. A redox-based mechanism for the neuroprotective and neurodestructive effects of nitric oxide and related nitroso-compounds. Nature 1993; 364(6438): 626–632.
6. Mannick JB, et al. Fas-induced caspase denitrosylation. Science 1999; 284(5414): 651–654.
7. Mannick JB, et al. S-Nitrosylation of mitochondrial caspases. J Cell Biol 2001; 154(6): 1111–1116.
8. Marshall HE, Stamler JS. Inhibition of NF-kappa B by S-nitrosylation. Biochemistry 2001; 10(6):1688–1693.

9. Stamler JS, et al. Blood flow regulation by S-nitrosohemoglobin in the physiological oxygen gradient. Science 1997; 276(5321):2034–2037.

10. Ignarro LJ, et al. Mechanism of vascular smooth muscle relaxation by organic nitrates, nitrites, nitroprusside and nitric oxide: evidence for the involvement of S-nitrosothiols as active intermediates. J Pharmacol Exp Ther 1981; 218(3):739–749.

11. Creager MA, et al. N-Acetylcysteine does not influence the activity of endothelium-derived relaxing factor in vivo. Hypertension 1997; 29(2):668–672.

12. Stamler JS, et al. S-Nitrosylation of proteins with nitric oxide: synthesis and characterization of biologically active compounds. Proc Natl Acad Sci USA 1992; 89(1): 444–448.

13. Gaston B, et al. Relaxation of human bronchial smooth muscle by S-nitrosothiols in vitro. J Pharmacol Exp Ther 1994; 268(2):978–984.

14. Fang FC. Perspective series: host/pathogen interactions. Mechanisms of nitric oxide-related antimicrobial activity. J Clin Invest 1997; 99(12):2818–2825.

15. Mayer B, et al. A new pathway of nitric oxide/cyclic GMP signaling involving S-nitrosoglutathione. J Biol Chem 1998; 273(6):3264–3270.

16. Hofmann H. Schmidt HH. Thiol dependence of nitric oxide synthase. Biochemistry 1995; 34(41):13443–13452.

17. Schmidt HH, et al. No. NO from NO synthase. Proc Natl Acad Sci USA 1996; 93(25): 14492–14497.

18. Gaston B, et al. The biology of nitrogen oxides in the airways. Am J Respir Crit Care Med 1994; 149(2 Pt 1):538–551.

19. Arnelle DR, Stamler JS. NO^{+}, NO, and NO^{-} donation by S-nitrosothiols: implications for regulation of physiological functions by S-nitrosylation and acceleration of disulfide formation. Arch Biochem Biophys 1995; 318(2):279–285.

20. Liu L, et al. A metabolic enzyme for S-nitrosothiol conserved from bacteria to humans. Nature 2001; 410(6827):490–494.

21. Jia L, et al. S-Nitrosohaemoglobin: a dynamic activity of blood involved in vascular control. Nature 1996; 380(6571):221–226.

22. Kluge I, et al. S-Nitrosoglutathione in rat cerebellum: identification and quantification by liquid chromatography-mass spectrometry. J Neurochem 1997; 69(6):2599–2607.

23. Eu JP, et al. An apoptotic model for nitrosative stress. Biochemistry 2000; 39(5): 1040–1047.

24. Salt TE, et al. Novel mode of nitric oxide neurotransmission mediated via S-nitroso-cysteinyl-glycine. Eur J Neurosci 2000; 12(11):3919–3925.

25. Gow AJ, et al. Basal and stimulated protein S-nitrosylation in multiple cell types and tissues. Proc Natl Acad Sci USA 2001.

26. Lorch SA, et al. Immunohistochemical localization of protein 3-nitrotyrosine and S-nitrosocysteine in a murine model of inhaled nitric oxide therapy. Pediatr Res 2000; 47(6):798–805.

27. Hasuda T, et al. Improvement in exercise capacity with nitric oxide inhalation in patients with precapillary pulmonary hypertension. Circulation 2000; 101(17): 2066–2070.

28. Kinsella JP, et al. Inhaled nitric oxide in premature neonates with severe hypoxaemic respiratory failure: a randomised controlled trial. Lancet 1999; 354(9184):1061–1065.

29. Rossaint R, et al. Inhaled nitric oxide for the adult respiratory distress syndrome. N Engl J Med 1993; 328(6):399–405.

30. Marshall HE, Que, L, Stamler JS. Resistance of the respiratory epithelium to S-nitrososthiol-induced apoptosis. American Thoracic Society, 2001.

31. Asano K, et al. Constitutive and inducible nitric oxide synthase gene expression, regulation, and activity in human lung epithelial cells. Proc Natl Acad Sci USA 1994; 91(21): 10089–10093.

32. Dweik RA, et al. NO chemical events in the human airway during the immediate and late antigen-induced asthmatic response. Proc Natl Acad Sci USA 2001; 98(5): 2622–2627.

33. Lilly CM, et al. Modulation of vasoactive intestinal peptide pulmonary relaxation by NO in tracheally superfused guinea pig lungs. Am J Physiol 1993; 265(4 Pt 1): L410–L415.

34. Thompson DC, Altiere RJ. Differential susceptibility of tracheal contraction to nonadrenergic noncholinergic relaxation. J Pharmacol Exp Ther 1998; 284(1):19–24.

35. Tyurin VA, et al. Elevated levels of S-nitrosoalbumin in preeclampsia plasma. Circ Res 2001; 88(11):1210–1215.

36. McMahon TJ, Huang YC, Pawloski J, Stamler JS. Modulation of hypoxic pulmonary vasoconstriction by erythrocytic nitric oxide (abstr). Circulation 2001; 17:228.

37. Day BJ, et al. Transduction of nitric oxide synthase activity from endothelium to vascular smooth muscle: involvement of S-nitrosothiols. In Proceedings of the 4th International Meeting on the Biology of Nitric Oxide. Amelia Island, FL: Portland Press, 1996.

38. Jaffrey SR, et al. Protein S-nitrosylation: a physiological signal for neuronal nitric oxide. Nature Cell Biol 2001; 3(2):193–197.

39. Goemen C, et al. A possible role of S-nitrosothiols at the nitrergic relaxations in the mouse corpus cavernosum. Eur J Pharmacol 1998; 361(1):85–92.

40. Clancy RM, et al. Nitric oxide reacts with intracellular glutathione and activates the hexose monophosphate shunt in human neutrophils: evidence for S-nitrosoglutathione as a bioactive intermediary. Proc Natl Acad Sci USA 1994; 91(9):3680–3684.

41. Stamler JS, Singel, DJ, Loscalzo J. Biochemistry of nitric oxide and its redox-activated forms. Science 1992; 258(5090):1898–1902.

42. Stamler JS. Redox signaling: nitrosylation and related target interactions of nitric oxide. Cell 1994; 78(6):931–936.

43. Vanin AF, Malenkova, IV, Serezhenkov VA. Iron catalyzes both decomposition and synthesis of S-nitrosothiols: optical and electron paramagnetic resonance studies. Nitric Oxide 1997; 1(3):191–203.

44. Inoue K, et al. Nitrosothiol formation catalyzed by ceruloplasmin. Implication for cytoprotective mechanism in vivo. J Biol Chem 1999; 274(38):27069–27075.

45. Gow AJ, Buerk, DG, Ischiropoulos H. A novel reaction mechanism for the formation of S-nitrosothiol in vivo. J Biol Chem 1997; 272(5):2841–2845.

46. Hess DT, et al. S-Nitrosylation: spectrum and specificity. Nat Cell Biol 2001; 3(2): E46–49.

47. Choi YB, et al. Molecular basis of NMDA receptor-coupled ion channel modulation by S-nitrosylation. Nat Neurosci 2000; 3(1):15–21.

48. Perez-Mato I, et al. Methionine adenosyltransferase S-nitrosylation is regulated by the basic and acidic amino acids surrounding the target thiol. J Biol Chem 1999; 274(24): 17075–17079.

49. Nijkamp FP, van der Linde, HJ, Folkerts G. Nitric oxide synthesis inhibitors induce airway hyperresponsiveness in the guinea pig in vivo and in vitro. Role of the epithelium. Am Rev Respir Dis 1993; 148(3):727–734.

50. Marshall HE, Stamler JS. NO waiting to exhale in asthma. Am J Respir Crit Care Med 2000; 161(3 Pt 1):685–687.

51. Jansen A, et al. The relaxant properties in guinea pig airways of S-nitrosothiols. J Pharmacol Exp Ther 1992; 261(1):154–160.
52. Bannenberg G, et al. Characterization of bronchodilator effects and fate of S-nitrosothiols in the isolated perfused and ventilated guinea pig lung. J Pharmacol Exp Ther 1995; 272(3):1238–1245.
53. Dupuy PM, et al. Bronchodilator action of inhaled nitric oxide in guinea pigs. J Clin Invest 1992; 90(2):421–428.
54. Perkins WJ, et al. cGMP-independent mechanism of airway smooth muscle relaxation induced by S-nitrosoglutathione. Am J Physiol 1998; 275(2 Pt 1):C468–474.
55. Hermle G, et al. Ventilation-perfusion mismatch after lung ischemia-reperfusion. Protective effect of nitric oxide. Am J Respir Crit Care Med 1999; 160(4):1179–1187.
56. Ullrich R, et al. Hypoxic pulmonary blood flow redistribution and arterial oxygenation in endotoxin-challenged NOS$_2$3-deficient mice. J Clin Invest 1999; 104(10): 1421–1429.
57. McMahon TJ, Ignarro, LJ, Kadowitz PJ. Influence of Zaprinast on vascular tone and vasodilator responses in the cat pulmonary vascular bed. J Appl Physiol 1993; 74(4): 1704–1711.
58. Emery CJ. Vasodilator action of the S-nitrosothiol, SNAP, in rat isolated perfused lung. Physiol Res 1995; 44(1):19–24.
59. Guarin M, Dawson, CA, Nelin LD. The arterial site of action of nitric oxide in the neonatal pig lung determined by microfocal angiography. Lung 2001; 179(1):43–55.
60. Moya MP, et al. S-Nitrosothiol repletion by an inhaled gas regulates pulmonary function. Proc Natl Acad Sci USA 2001; 98(10):5792–5797.
61. Jain L, et al. Nitric oxide inhibits lung sodium transport through a cGMP-mediated inhibition of epithelial cation channels. Am J Physiol Lung Cell Mol Physiol 1998; 274(4):L475–484.
62. Duszyk M. Regulation of anion secretion by nitric oxide in human airway epithelial cells. Am J Physiol Lung Cell Mol Physiol 2001; 281(2):L450–457.
63. Li. D, et al. Regulation of giliary beat frequency by the nitric oxide-cyclic guanosine monophosphate signaling pathway in but airway epithelial cells. Am J Respir Cell Mol Biol 2000; 23(2):175–181.
64. Kamosinska B, et al. Role of inducible nitric-oxide synthase in regulation of whole-cell current in lung epithelial cells. J Pharmacol Exp Ther 2000; 295(2):500–505.
65. Kamosinska B et al., Nitric oxide activates chloride currents in human lung epithelial cells. Am J Physiol 1997; 272(6 Pt 1):L1098–1104.
66. Zaman K, et al. S-Nitrosoglutathione increases cystic fibrosis transmembrane regulator maturation. Biochem Biophys Res Commun 2001; 284(1):65–70.
67. Andersson C, Gaston B, Roomans GM. S-Nitrosoglutathione induces functional ΔF 508 CFTR in cultured airway epithelial cells. Biochem Biophys Res Commun 2002; 297:552–556.
68. Grasemann HMD, et al. Decreased levels of nitrosothiols in the lower airways of patients with cystic fibrosis and normal pulmonary function. J Pediatrics 1999; 135(6): 770–772.
69. Snyder A, McPherson ME, Hunt JF, Johnson M, Stamler JS, Gaston B. Acute effects of aerosolized S-Nitrosoglutathione in cystic fibrosis. Am J Respir Crit Care Med 2002; 165:922–926.
70. Li J, et al. Nitric oxide suppresses apoptosis via interrupting caspase activation and mitochondrial dysfunction in cultured hepatocytes. J Biol Chem 1999; 274(24): 17325–17333.

71. Fortenberry JD, et al. S-Nitrosoglutathione inhibits TNF-alpha-induced NFkappaB activation in neutrophils. Inflamm Res 2001; 50(2):89–95.
72. Wenzel SE, et al. Evidence that severe asthma can be divided pathologically into two inflammatory subtypes with distinct physiologic and clinical characteristics. Am J Respir Crit Care Med 1999; 160(3):1001–1008.
73. Gaston B, et al. Bronchodilator S-nitrosothiol deficiency in asthmatic respiratory failure. Lancet 1998; 351(9112):1317–1319.
74. Hamad AM, Johnson SR, Knox AJ. Antiproliferative effects of NO and ANP in cultured human airway smooth muscle. Am J Physiol Lung Cell Mol Physiol 1999; 277(5): L910–918.
75. Rubin DB, et al. Non-protein thiols flux to S-nitrosothiols in endothelial cells: an LPS redox signal. Shock 2000; 14(2):200–207.
76. De Groote MA, et al. Genetic and redox determinants of nitric oxide cytotoxicity in a *Salmonella typhimurium* model. Proc Natl Acad Sci USA 1995; 92(14):6399–6403.
77. Gobert AP, et al. Murine macrophages use oxygen- and nitric oxide-dependent mechanisms to synthesize S-nitroso-albumin and to kill extracellular trypanosomes. Infect Immun 1998; 66(9):4068–4072.
78. Saura M, et al. An antiviral mechanism of nitric oxide: inhibition of a viral protease. Immunity 1999; 10(1):21–28.
79. Hausladen A, et al. Nitrosative stress: activation of the transcription factor OxyR. Cell 1996; 86:719–729.
80. Spiecker M, et al. Differential regulation of endothelial cell adhesion molecule expression by nitric oxide donors and antioxidants. J Leukoc Biol 1998; 63(6):732–739.
81. Bloomfield GL. M. D, et al. Pretreatment with inhaled nitric oxide inhibits neutrophil migration and oxidative activity resulting in attenuated sepsis-induced acute lung injury. Crit Care Med 1997; 25(4):584–593.
82. Marshall HE, Merchant K, Stamler JS. Nitrosation and oxidation in the regulation of gene expression. FASEB J 2000; 14:1–12.
83. Peng H.-B., Libby P, Liao JK. Induction and stabilization of I-kappa B alpha by nitric oxide mediates inhibition of NF-kappa B. J Biol Chem 1995; 270(23):14214–14219.
84. Shin WS, et al. Nitric oxide attenuates vascular smooth muscle cell activation by interferon-[IMAGE]. J Biol Chem 1996; 271(19):11317–11324.
85. dela Torre A, et al. Endotoxin-mediated S-nitrosylation of p50 alters NF-kappa B-dependent gene transcription in ANA-1 murine macrophages. J Immunol 1999; 162(7): 4101–4108.
86. Nikitovic D, Holmgren A, Spyrou G. Inhibition of AP-1 DNA binding by nitric oxide involving conserved cysteine residues in Jun and Fos. Biochem Biophys Res Commun 1998; 242(1):109–112.
87. Palmer LA, Gaston B, Johns RA. Normoxic stabilization of hypoxia-inducible factor-1 expression and activity: redox-dependent effect of nitrogen oxides. Mol Pharmacol 2000; 58(6):1197–1203.
88. Park JW. Attenuation of p47phox and p67phox membrane translocation as the inhibitory mechanism of S-nitrosothiol on the respiratory burst oxidase in human neutrophils. Biochem Biophys Res Commun 1996; 220(1):31–35.
89. Kim S, Ponka P. Effects of interferon-gamma and lipopolysaccharide on macrophage iron metabolism are mediated by nitric oxide-induced degradation of iron regulatory protein 2. J Biol Chem 2000; 275(9):6220–6226.
90. Butzer U, et al. Increased oxidative stress in the RAW 264.7 macrophage cell line is partially mediated via the S-nitrosothiol-induced inhibition of glutathione reductase. FEBS Lett 1999; 445(2–3):274–278.

91. Moellering D, et al. The induction of GSH synthesis by nanomolar concentrations of NO in endothelial cells: a role for [gamma]-glutamylcysteine synthetase and [gamma]-glutamyl transpeptidase. FEBS Lett 1999; 448(2–3):292–296.

92. Lipton AJ, et al. S-Nitrosothiols signal the ventilatory response to hypoxia. Nature 2001; 413(6852):171–174.

93. Trujillo M, et al. Xanthine oxidase-mediated decomposition of S-nitrosothiols. J Biol Chem 1998; 273(14):7828–7834.

94. Nikitovic D, Holmgren A. S-Nitrosoglutathione is cleaved by the thioredoxin system with liberation of glutathione and redox regulating nitric oxide. J Biol Chem 1996; 271(32):19180–19185.

95. Hogg N, et al. S-Nitrosoglutathione as a substrate for gamma-glutamyl transpeptidase. Biochem J 1997; 23(Pt 2):477–481.

96. Hou Y, et al. Seleno compounds and glutathione peroxidase catalyzed decomposition of S-nitrosothiols. Biochem Biophys Res Commun 1996; 228(1):88–93.

97. Tracey WR, et al. Immunochemical detection of inducible NO synthase in human lung. Am J Physiol 1994; 66(6 Pt 1):L722–727.

98. Guo FH, et al. Continuous nitric oxide synthesis by inducible nitric oxide synthase in normal human airway epithelium in vivo. Proc Natl Acad Sci USA 1995; 92(17): 7809–7813.

99. Nicholson S, et al. Inducible nitric oxide synthase in pulmonary alveolar macrophages qfrom patients with tuberculosis. J Exp Med 1996; 183(5):2293–2302.

100. Redington AE, et al. Increased expression of inducible nitric oxide synthase and cyclo-oxygenase-2 in the airway epithelium of asthmatic subjects and regulation by corticosteroid treatment. Thorax 2001; 56(5):351–357.

101. Corradi M, et al. Increased nitrosothiols in exhaled breath condensate in inflammatory airway diseases. Am J Respir Crit Care Med 2001; 163(4):854–858.

102. Alving K, Weitzberg E, Lundberg JM. Increased amount of nitric oxide in exhaled air of asthmatics. Eur Respir J 1993; 6(9):1368–1370.

103. Kharitonov SA, et al. Increased nitric oxide in exhaled air of asthmatic patients. Lancet 1994; 43(8890):133–135.

104. Massaro AF, et al. Expired nitric oxide levels during treatment of acute asthma. Am J Respir Crit Care Med 1995; 152(2):800–803.

105. Hunt J, et al. Condensed expirate nitrite as a home marker for acute asthma. Lancet 1995; 346(8984):1235–1236.

106. Hunt JF, et al. Endogenous airway acidification. Implications for asthma pathophysiology. Am J Respir Crit Care Med 2000; 161(3 Pt 1):694–699.

107. Smith LJ, Houston, M, Anderson J. Increased levels of glutathione in bronchoalveolar lavage fluid from patients with asthma. Am Rev Respir Dis 1993; 147(6 Pt 1): 1461–1464.

108. Marshall HE, Stamler JS. Exhaled nitric oxide (NO), NO synthase activity, and regulation of nuclear factor (NF)-kappaB. Am J Respir Cell Mol Biol 1999; 21(3):296–297.

109. Fang K, et al. S-Nitrosoglutathione breakdown prevents airway smooth muscle relaxation in the guinea pig. Am J Physiol Lung Cell Mol Physiol 2000; 279(4):L716–721.

110. Linnane SJ, et al. Total sputum nitrate plus nitrite is raised during acute pulmonary infection in cystic fibrosis. Am J Respir Crit Care Med 1998; 158(1):207–212.

111. Kelley TJ, Drumm ML. Inducible nitric oxide synthase expression is reduced in cystic fibrosis murine and human airway epithelial cells. J Clin Invest 1998; 102(6): 1200–1207.

112. Meng QH, et al. Lack of inducible nitric oxide synthase in bronchial epithelium: a possible mechanism of susceptibility to infection in cystic fibrosis. J Pathol 1998; 184(3):323–331.

113. Grasemann H, et al. Airway nitric oxide levels in cystic fibrosis patients are related to a polymorphism in the neuronal nitric oxide synthase gene. Am J Respir Crit Care Med 2000; 162(6):2172–2176.

114. Grasemann H, et al. Decreased concentration of exhaled nitric oxide (NO) in patients with cystic fibrosis. Pediatr Pulmonol 1997; 24(3):173–177.

115. Hausladen A, Gow AJ, Stamler JS. Nitrosative stress: metabolic pathway involving the flavohemoglobin. Proc Natl Acad Sci USA 1998; 95(24):14100–14105.

116. Kim SO, et al. Anoxic function for the Escherichia coli flavohaemoglobin (Hmp): reversible binding of nitric oxide and reduction to nitrous oxide. FEBS Lett 1999; 445(2–3):389–394.

117. Gardner PR, et al. Nitric oxide dioxygenase: an enzymic function for flavohemoglobin. Proc Natl Acad Sci USA 1998; 95(18):10378–10383.

8

Contribution of Nitric Oxide Synthase Isoforms to Allergen-Induced Airway Hyperresponsiveness and Inflammation
Lessons from Murine Models

GEORGE T. De SANCTIS and EL-BDAOUI HADDAD

Aventis Pharmaceuticals
Bridgewater, New Jersey, U.S.A.

I. Introduction

A. NO in Asthma

Nitric oxide (NO), a free radical molecule, is generated from L-arginine by the actions of the enzyme NO synthase (NOS) (1). This diatomic molecule is a unique biological messenger that exists naturally in numerous cell types in the body but is not maintained at appreciable concentrations as it is rapidly converted into nitrates and nitrites as quickly as it is produced. Expired nitric oxide levels are elevated in asthmatic patients and are significantly reduced after steroid treatment (2,3). While the exact source of expired NO is unclear, it appears that the main source of NO is epithelial cells (4). This observation suggested that NO may serve as a marker for airway inflammation (3,5–7). The role of NO in asthma is controversial, with several studies reporting either beneficial effects (8–12), deleterious effects on airway function (13–16), or no effect of NO on asthmatic early and late responses (16).

Research and interest in NO as a participant in asthma has increased steadily over the past decade. In order to better understand the contribution of NO to airway function and inflammation, researchers have worked with several animal species, including the inbred mouse. In this regard, the inbred mouse has quickly established itself as the animal of choice for dissecting out the role of each of the synthase isoforms in models of asthma. In pursuit of this goal, researchers have adopted two lines of strategies. One involves the use of NOS-specific inhibitors in models of allergic asthma, and the second involves the use of targeted gene knockouts for each of the NO synthase isoforms. This chapter will provide a comprehensive review of the studies that have been undertaken in the mouse to delineate the role of each of the NOS isoforms in models of allergen-induced airway hyperresponsiveness and inflammation.

B. NO Synthase Isoforms

Several distinct isozymes of nitric oxide synthase exist. The three known nitric oxide synthase isoforms are the products of individual genes, and all catalyze the formation of NO. The current nomenclature denotes these NOSs by their historical order of cloning rather than by the cell type from which their cDNA was first cloned (17). Thus, the human genes encoding neuronal NOS (nNOS), inducible or immunological NOS (iNOS), and endothelial NOS (eNOS) are termed NOS1, NOS2, and NOS3, respectively. The tissue distribution and regulation of the three NOS isoforms are presented in Table 1. The neuronal (nNOS) and endothelial (eNOS) isoforms are also collectively known as constitutive NOS (cNOS), because they are constitutively expressed proteins and are primarily regulated by calmodulin when intracellular Ca^{2+} is elevated. NO produced by NOS1 is proposed to be a neurotransmitter in cholinergic, nonadrenergic transmission (18,19).

Type 2 NOS can be expressed by a wide variety of cell types and is inducible. Normally, resting cells do not express iNOS unless they are stimulated by an appropriate stimulus (20). The inducible (iNOS) isoform is Ca^{2+}/calmodulin independent and produces significantly higher amounts of NO than do the constitutive isoforms (eNOS and nNOS). One distinguishing feature of asthma is the upregulation of type 2 NOS, an enzyme thought to be largely responsible for the endogenous production of nitric oxide in the lung (21). Of the three enzyme isoforms identified, iNOS is currently believed to play an important role in asthma (14,20). Specifically, there is an increase in immunostaining for iNOS in the airways of asthmatics (13,21,22), and the iNOS isoform contributes most to the increase in exhaled NO concentrations observed in asthma (23). The sole role of iNOS in asthma has now been challenged

Table 1 NOS Isoforms

Isoform	Regulation	Location	Ref.
NOS1	Ca^{2+}/calmodulin	Neuronal tissue, vascular smooth muscle, skeletal muscle	125–127
NOS2	Ca^{2+} independent	Macrophages, neutrophils, T cells, epithelial cells, eosinophils, vascular smooth muscle, dendritic cells	126,128–131
NOS3	Ca^{2+}/calmodulin	Endothelial cells, B and T lymphocytes, bronchiolar epithelium	26,132

by recent data from genetic studies in asthmatics and normals. These studies have indicated a role for nNOS in the development of asthma (24,25).

Type 3 NOS or endothelial NOS (eNOS) is the isoform commonly associated with the production of endothelium-derived relaxing factor (EDRF) (26). Like nNOS, this NOS isoform is activated by raising intracellular Ca^{2+} concentrations and binding to calmodulin. In contrast to both nNOS and iNOS, this enzyme is membrane bound and not found in the soluble fraction of the cell. NOS3 has not been considered relevant to asthma until recently, when an association between a polymorphism in the endothelial NOS gene and asthma was established. While this study concluded that the eNOS gene may be associated with the development of asthma, it did not influence the severity of the disease (27).

II. Murine Models of Allergic Asthma

Murine models of allergic asthma offer distinct advantages for the study of the immune processes involved in models of allergic asthma. Unlike outbred populations which are genetically diverse, inbred strains of mice represent a homogeneous genetic population. In addition, the mouse genome has been extensively mapped and numerous transgenic and knockout mice are widely available. Therefore, these inbred strains represent a powerful genetic resource to dissect out the immune mechanisms responsible for the cellular immune responses observed in this model of allergic asthma (28–35).

There are a number of murine models of asthma, which recapitulate many of the features of asthma in humans. These features include (1) airways hyperresponsiveness, (2) elevated titers of antigen-specific IgE and IgG antibodies, (3) airway inflammation, (4) cellular infiltrates of eosinophils and lymphocytes, and (5) a Th2 cytokine secretion profile and upregulation of NOS activity. The models of allergic asthma typically involve a protocol in which mice are sensitized and challenged by varying routes of administration to a particular allergen for a defined period of time. Accordingly, these protocols represent acute and not chronic models of allergic asthma. Furthermore, while these models of allergen-induced airway hyperresponsiveness and airway inflammation replicate many of the features of asthma in humans, they do not constitute asthma per se.

It is widely believed that T cells play a central role in the regulation of immune responses in asthma. The pulmonary lymphocytes observed in these models of allergic asthma produce an array of mediators, including interleukin-3 (IL-3), IL-4, IL-5, IL-13, and granulocyte-macrophage colony-stimulating factor (GM-CSF) (28,29,36–41). The importance of these effector cells has been clearly delineated in mouse models of asthma (42–46). The two major T-cell subsets, CD4+ and CD8+ cells, respond to either exogenous, allergen-derived peptides in association with MHC class II molecules or endogenous peptides in association with MHC class 1 products, respectively (47). Furthermore, it has been shown that the CD4+ T-cell subset is largely committed to the Th2 lymphokine secretion pattern in the murine model of allergic asthma (39,44,48,49). An examination of the airway histology of mice sensitized and challenged with allergen reveals a thickening of the epithelial lining with numerous cellular infiltrates composed predominantly of eosinophils and lymphocytes (34,45,46,50–59). Figure 1 illustrates the typical histopathological features observed following antigen sensitization and challenge in wild-type mice sensitized and challenged with either PBS or ovalbumin aerosols (60). The pathological features observed in this model of allergen-induced inflammation are very similar to the histological findings observed in asthmatic airways.

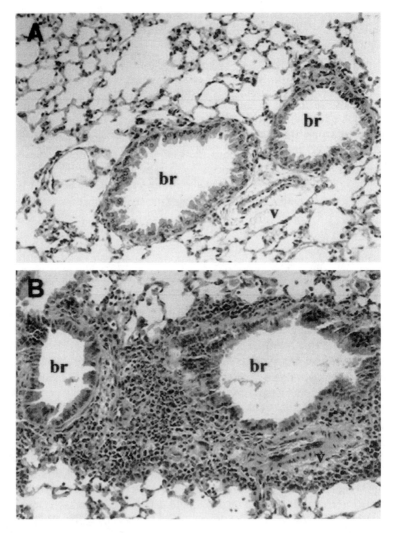

Figure 1   Typical histopathological features observed following antigen sensitization and challenge in wild-type mice sensitized and challenged with either (A) PBS or (B) ovalbumin aerosols (br = bronchiole).

Nitric oxide is upregulated in the airways of both asthmatics (13,21,22) and mice that have been immunized and challenged with ovalbumin (OVA) (35). Similarly, NO production and iNOS expression is downregulated following treatment with steroids in mice (20,61) and human asthmatics (62).

Therefore, the murine model of allergic asthma recapitulates many of the features of asthma, including airway inflammation, airway hyperresponsiveness, inflammatory infiltrates, and upregulation of NOS activity. Although this model represents an acute event induced by allergen exposure, the model is useful for understanding how the specific NOS isoforms can modify cellular immune processes germane to this model.

III. Contribution of NOS Isoforms to Allergen-Induced Airway Inflammation and Airway Hyperresponsiveness: Genetic Studies

In order to better understand the contribution of individual NOS isoforms to allergen-induced airway hyperresponsiveness (AHR) and inflammation in the mouse, investigators have sensitized and challenged various NOS single and double knockout mice along with appropriately matched wild-type controls with allergens such as ovalbumin. The use of gene knockout mice is advantageous in isolating the specific contribution of each NOS isoform and avoids the use of NOS inhibitors to dissect out the contribution of the constitutive and inducible NOS isoforms. This is important given the potential issues of inhibitor specificity and pharmacokinetic concerns. While only a few studies have been carried out to date, these have shed light on the functional role of nNOS, eNOS, and iNOS in animal models of asthma (35,63).

In the first of these two studies, Xiong and coworkers used NOS2 knockout mice to define the functional role of iNOS in a model of allergic asthma (63). Using OVA as an aeroallergen, the authors examined both airway inflammation and airway hyperresponsiveness as outcome parameters. When NOS2 knockout mice were sensitized and challenged with OVA, they reported a significant reduction in both circulatory and pulmonary eosinophil numbers when compared to wild-type controls. No differences were noted in eosinophil maturation or efflux from the bone marrow between the NOS2 knockout mice ($-/-$) and the wild-type controls (63). The significant reduction in eosinophils in the NOS2 ($-/-$) were not attributable to differences in IL-5 levels as there were no differences in cytokine levels of IL-5 from isolated lung and splenocyte CD4+ cells between the wild-type and knockout OVA-sensitized and challenged mice. There were no significant differences in either IgG1 or OVA-specific IgE between the iNOS-deficient mice and the wild-type controls. When AHR was assessed in the NOS2 $+/+$ and NOS2 $-/-$ OVA-treated animals, there were no significant differences noted between the treatment groups (Fig. 2). The results of this study reveal a clear disassociation between the allergen-induced inflammatory processes and AHR in the NOS2-deficient mice. In addition to the reduction in eosinophils described above, there were significant reductions

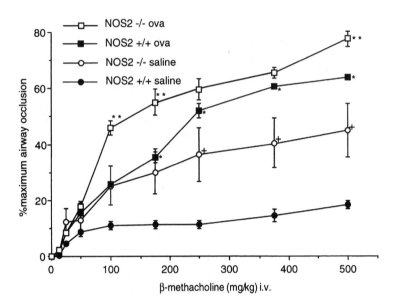

Figure 2 AHR to β-methacholine in NOS2 −/− and wild-type mice sensitized and treated with aeroallergen. Data represent the mean ± SEM for groups of five mice and are representative of two such experiments. *, $p < 0.01$ compared with saline-treated wild-type mice; **, $p < 0.05$ compared with saline-treated NOS2 −/− mice; +, $p < 0.05$ compared with saline-treated wild-type mice, each at the corresponding dose of β-methacholine. (From Ref. 63.)

in gross alterations in the structural integrity of the airway walls, microvascular leakage, mucosal edema, and mucous occlusion of the airways lumina in the NOS2-deficient mice sensitized and challenged with OVA. Analysis of macrophage and lymphocyte cell numbers in bronchoalveolar lavage fluid (BALF) from OVA-sensitized mice revealed significantly greater numbers in the NOS2-deficient mice. The cultured lymphocytes were able to secrete significantly greater amounts of IFN-γ upon restimulation in vitro. Interestingly, the enhanced production of IFN-γ in the NOS2-deficient mice was reported to be responsible for the reduction in allergen-induced airway inflammation, as in vivo depletion of this factor restored the allergen-induced inflammation to levels found in the wild-type controls (63). The findings of Xiong and coworkers (63) disagree with the conclusions of Feder and coworkers, who determined that the NO contributing to eosinophilia is not generated through the activity of iNOS (64). In their study, OVA-induced pulmonary eosinophilia was significantly reduced by L-NAME, a NOS inhibitor. The inactive isomer D-NAME had no effect. The inhibition of eosinophilia was reversed when L-NAME–treated animals were administered an excess of the NO substrate, L-arginine. Since administration of L-NIL, a selective iNOS inhibitor, had no effect, they speculated that NO derived from eNOS or NOS3 is responsible for the extravasation of eosinophils from the circulation into the lung tissue (64). The finding of no differences in methacholine-induced AHR in the iNOS $-/-$ mice is in agreement with the findings of De Sanctis and coworkers (35). In this study they reported no differences in allergen-induced AHR between the iNOS $-/-$ mice and wild-type controls treated in a similar manner. This lack of an iNOS effect on AHR was confirmed by two independent measures of bronchoconstriction (Penh and R_L) using different sensitization and challenge protocols (35).

De Sanctis and coworkers (35) carried out a comprehensive study examining the contribution of each of the three NOS isoforms. In this study mice with targeted deletions of the endothelial, neuronal, inducible, and double endothelial and neuronal NOS isoforms were studied using two models of allergen-induced airway inflammation and airway hyperresponsiveness. Since iNOS is upregulated in asthma and is believed to represent the major source of NO in the lung (65,66), De Sanctis and coworkers reasoned that NOS2 would exhibit a profound effect on airway function in a model of murine asthma. In their study iNOS was significantly upregulated in the lung tissue of the wild type, NOS1 $-/-$, NOS1 &3 $-/-$, and NOS3 $-/-$ mice sensitized and challenged with OVA (Fig. 3). The upregulation in NOS2 is similar to a finding demonstrated in the lungs of asthmatic patients (13,21). In

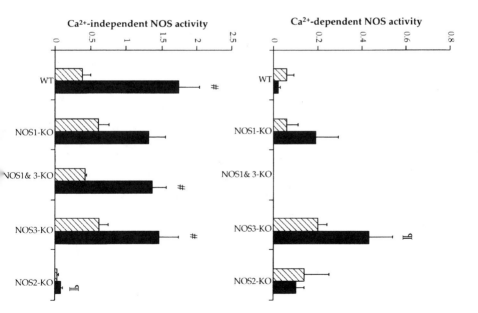

Figure 3   Assessment of calcium-dependent (cNOS, eNOS, and nNOS activity) and calcium-independent (iNOS activity) pulmonary NOS activity in OVA/PBS and OVA/OVA WT and NOS-deficient mice. Calcium-dependent (top) and calcium-independent (bottom) NOS activity was measured in whole lung preparations. Data represents means ± SEM. [#] $p <$ 0.05 compared with OVA/PBS, same genotype.[¶] $p < 0.05$ compared with WT, same treatment. Black bars, OVA/OVA; hatched bars, OVA/PBS. (From Ref. 35.)

contrast to the findings of Xiong and coworkers (63), NOS2-deficient mice exhibited no significant differences in airway inflammation or cellular recruitment into the airway space (35). The lack of an iNOS-mediated effect on allergen-induced AHR found by De Sanctis and coworkers did, however, agree with the findings of Xiong and coworkers (63). The lack of an effect of iNOS on allergen-induced AHR was confirmed in the De Sanctis study using a different immunization and challenge protocols and measurement of airway function (Fig. 4). Taken together, these two studies demonstrate that allergen-induced AHR is fully expressed in the absence of inducible NOS. To understand how basal expression of pulmonary NOS activity is expressed, De Sanctis and coworkers measured NOS activity in naïve mice that have not been treated with OVA or phosphate-buffered saline (PBS). Basally expressed levels of total NOS activity were not significantly different in NOS3-KO (eNOS knockout), NOS1-KO (nNOS knockout), NOS1 & 3-KO (nNOS and eNOS double knockout), or NOS2-KO (iNOS knockout) mice in comparison with wild-

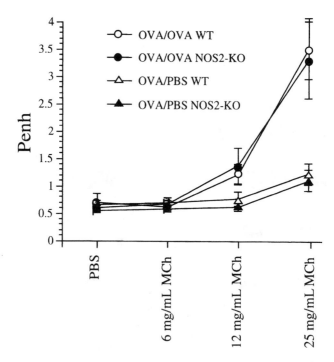

Figure 4 Airway responsiveness measured by whole-body plethysmography in awake WT (B6) and NOS2-KO mice. Penh, an index of airway obstruction, was calculated from the box pressure/time waveform after aerosolization of increasing doses of methacholine. Numerically higher values of Penh are indicative of increased airway obstruction. Dose-response curves are shown for OVA- and PBS-challenged WT and NOS2-KO mice. Data represent mean Penh values ± SEM. (From Ref. 35.)

type (WT) mice (35). The absolute level of constitutive NOS (cNOS) activity (i.e., that was attributable to eNOS and nNOS) was not affected in the single cNOS knockout strains, NOS1-KO and NOS3-KO, in comparison with the WT strain, but was significantly reduced in the double cNOS knockout (NOS1 & 3-KO) mice (35). The proportion of total NOS activity characterized as iNOS activity was not significantly different between WT, NOS1-KO, or NOS3-KO mice, but was increased in NOS1 & NOS3-KO mice, and was markedly reduced in NOS2-KO mice (35).

De Sanctis and coworkers (35) speculated that the differences in cellular recruitment between the two studies may be due to the different immunization and challenge protocols adopted in both studies. In agreement with Xiong and coworkers, there were no significant differences in the levels of OVA-specific IgE between the OVA sensitized and challenged wild-type and NOS2 $-/-$ groups.

When the airway responsiveness (AR) was ascertained in the NOS1 $-/-$, NOS3 $-/-$, and double NOS1 & 3 $-/-$ mice, the NOS1 $-/-$ and double NOS1 & 3 $-/-$ mice groups exhibited increased AR when compared to their OVA-immunized and saline-challenged controls (Fig. 5). The NOS1 $-/-$ and double NOS1 & 3 $-/-$ mice immunized and challenged with OVA (OVA/OVA) were significantly less responsive to methacholine challenge when compared to the similarly treated wild-type controls while the NOS3 $-/-$ OVA/OVA group exhibited a phenotype intermediate between the The NOS1 $-/-$ and double NOS1 & 3 $-/-$ mice and the wild-type controls. The reduction in airway hyperresponsiveness in the NOS1 $-/-$ group is supported by previous data published by De Sanctis and coworkers wherein untreated NOS1-deficient mice exhibited reduced airway responsiveness to methacholine challenge when compared to wild-type controls. Thus, the results of two studies by De Sanctis and coworkers suggest a noninflammatory link between the nNOS gene and airway responsiveness (35,50). The significant role of nNOS in this animal model of allergic asthma is intriguing given recent human data supporting a role for this particular NOS isoform in the development of asthma (24,25,67).

IV. Contribution of NOS Isoforms to Basal Airway Hyperresponsiveness: Genetic Studies

The role of each of the three NOS isoforms in basal airway responsiveness has been reported in two recent studies (50,68). While these studies do not involve an immunization and challenge protocol, differences in basal responsiveness may conceivably alter allergen-induced changes in airway responsiveness. In view of this, the results of these two studies will be presented and contrasted. The first study examining the role of NO synthases on basal airway responsiveness was carried out using mice with a targeted deletion of the nNOS gene (50). In this study De Sanctis and coworkers measured basal airway responsiveness to methacholine in nNOS $-/-$ mice and wild-type controls and reported a significant reduction in methacholine-induced airway responsiveness in the knockout group. Using chemiluminescence technology, they also reported a decrease in expired NO levels in the expirate of nNOS $-/-$ mice. They concluded that in the absence of allergenic stimulation, nNOS contributed significantly to the expired NO concentrations.

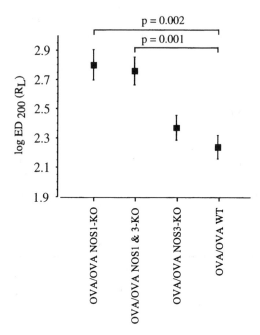

Figure 5 Airway responsiveness measured as $ED_{200}R_L$ in anesthetized OVA/OVA WT (SV129/B6) and NOS1-, NOS3-, and NOS1 & 3-deficient mice (bred on a SV129/B6 background). Airway responses were measured from the methacholine dose-response curves. The dose necessary to cause a doubling of lung resistance was calculated by log linear interpolation. The log $ED_{200}R_L$ values represent an index of airway responsiveness. There were no significant differences between the OVA/OVA WT (B6) and OVA/OVA NOS2-deficient mice. Numerically lower values are indicative of increased airway responsiveness. Data represent mean log $ED_{200}R_L$ values ± SEM. (From Ref. 35.)

    More recently, Feletou and coworkers investigated the role of NO in the regulation of murine airway responsiveness using mice with a targeted deletion of the eNOS or NOS3 gene, a nonspecific NOS inhibitor (L-NAME), and aminoguanidine, an inhibitor of iNOS (68). This study did not investigate the role of these isoforms in a murine asthma model but rather investigated the role of these isoforms on naive, non–allergen-treated mice. Using Penh as an outcome parameter, aminoguanidine did not alter basal Penh values in CD-1, C57BL/6, and eNOS −/− mice when compared to vehicle-treated animals. These results clearly demonstrated that inhibition of iNOS does not alter baseline airway responsiveness. On the other hand, when C57BL/6 and CD-1 mice were treated with L-NAME, a non-specific NOS inhibitor, airway responsiveness was significantly increased (Fig. 6) (68). The authors speculated that the increase in basal airway responsiveness was due to eNOS as inhibition of iNOS had no effect on basal airway responsiveness and previously published data by De Sanctis and coworkers reported a significant decrease in airway responsiveness

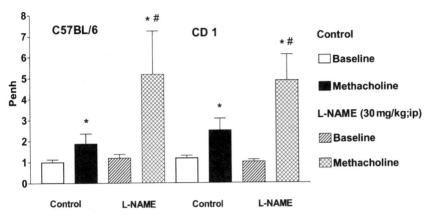

Figure 6 Inhaled methacholine (100 mM)–induced changes in airway responsiveness in unrestrained conscious C57BL/6 and CD-1 mice. Effect of *N*-nitro-L-arginine methyl ester treatment (30 mg/kg ip). Data are shown as means ± SE ($n = 5$). *Statistically significant difference with baseline ($p < 0.05$). #Statistically significant difference produced by *N*-nitro-L-arginine methyl ester treatment ($p < 0.05$). Responses in C57BL/6 mice were not significantly different from those in CD-1 mice. (From Ref. 68.)

in nNOS or NOS1-deficient mice (35). The involvement of eNOS in the study by Feletou and coworkers was further strengthened by the fact that eNOS $-/-$ mice were hyperresponsive to methacholine challenge and administration of L-NAME did not cause a further increase in airway responsiveness as noted in the CD-1 and C57BL/6 mice (68).

V. Contribution of NOS Isoforms to Allergen-Induced Airway Inflammation and Airway Hyperresponsiveness: NOS Inhibitor Studies

Several other investigators have also attempted to address the potential role of NO and NOS in airway inflammation and airway hyperreactivity by using NOS inhibitors in murine models of asthma. These studies have, however, generated controversial results (Table 2).

In agreement with the findings obtained in NOS2-KO mice (63), it has been shown that, in an allergen-driven murine lung inflammation model, administration of selective iNOS inhibitors 2-amino-5,6-dihydro-6-methyl-4*H*-1,3-thiazine (AMT) and *S*-ethylisothiourea (EIT), administered during the challenge period, significantly reduced recruitment of eosinophils and neutrophils (69). This effect was achieved through downregulation of MIP-2 and MCP-1 production (69). Also, in vitro exposure of primary cultures of murine lung fibroblasts to an NO donor, hydroxylamine, induced a dose-dependent release of MIP-2 and MCP-1 (69). NO appears, therefore,

Table 2 Summary of Effects of NOS Inhibition or NOS Knockout on Allergen-Induced Airwa
Eosinophil Recruitment and Airway Hyperresponsiveness in Mice

Strain	Inhibitor	Target	Eosinophils	AHR	Comments	R
BALB/c	L-NIL	NOS2		ND		
	AG	NOS2		ND		
	L-NAME	NS	↓	ND		
	AMT	NOS2	↓	ND	The reduced neutrophil and eosinophil accumulation was accompanied with MIP-2 and MCP-1 downregulation.	
	L-NIL	NOS2	↓	ND		
	L-NAME	NS	↓	ND		
	1400W	NOS2	=	↓	The NADPH oxidase inhibitor apocynin also reduces AHR measured using whole body plethysmography. 1400W did not impact on serum ovalbumin specific IgE	
Balb/c	1400W	NOS2	↓	↓	AHR was measured using iv methacholine as spasmogen	
CBA/J	L-NAME	NS	↑	↑	Fungal allergy model induced by Aspergillus fumigatus. The inflammatory response also comprises increased levels of CC chemokine expression	
C57BL/6	KO	NOS2	↓	=	AHR readings in OVA-challenged mice were recorded over baseline levels in control animals that were significantly greater in the NOS II mutants	
B6SV129J	KO	nNOS	ND	↓	There was also a decrease in expired NO in KO compared to WT animals	
CD-1	L-NAME	NS	ND	↑	AHR to inhaled methacholine was measured in unrestrained conscious animal using whole body plethysmography (Penh).	
CD-1	AG	NOS2	ND	=		
C57BL/6	L-NAME	NS	ND	↑		
C57BL/6	KO	NOS3	ND	↑		
C57BL/6J	KO	NOS2	↓	ND		1
SV129/C57BL/6	KO	NOS1	=	↓	AHR to iv methacholine was measured using invasive airway mechanics using Diamond box. For part of the NOS2 study, AHR was measured using whole body plethysmography	
C57BL6/J	KO	NOS 2	=	=		
SV129/C57BL/6	KO	NOS 3	=	=		
SV129/C57BL/6	KO	NOS1 + NOS3	=	↓		

AHR, airway hyperresponsiveness; =, unaltered; ↑, increase; ↓: decrease, ND: not determined, NS: nonselective, L-NAME: ?
nitro-arginine methyl ester; NMMA: NG-monomethyl-arginine; EIT: S-ethylisothiourea; AMT: 2-amino-5,6-dihydro-6-met
4H-1,3-thiazine; AG: aminoguanidine; L-NIL: L-N6-(1-iminoethyl)lysine; 1400W: N-(3-(aminomethyl)-benzyl) acetamid
See text for details.

to increase lung chemokine expression and, thereby, to facilitate influx of inflammatory cells into the airways.

Unlike the finding in NOS2-KO (35,63) Koarai and coworkers have shown that the selective iNOS inhibitor *N*-3-aminomethyl-benzyl-acetamidine-dihydrochloride (1400W) delivered via osmotic mini-pumps from 2 hours before to 24 hours after OVA challenge abrogated AHR to intavenous methacholine and to a lesser extent eosinophil accumulation into the airways when compared to vehicle-treated Balb/c mice (70). In yet another study, while treatment with the iNOS inhibitor 1400W did not significantly alter cellular influx into the airway lumen or serum ovalbumin–specific IgE in allergic mice, the inhibitor significantly inhibited ovalbumin-induced airway hyperresponsiveness in agreement with the finding by Koarai and collaborators (70). It is interesting to note that the accompanying 3-nitrotyrosine staining in eosinophils was not altered by inhibitor treatment (71). Anti-inflammatory properties have also been demonstrated with 1400W in allergic A/J mice (72). Consistent observations were reported in other species (73–75).

The role of iNOS in allergic airway inflammation has also been investigated in other studies. In allergic B6D2F1/J mice, ovalbumin challenge induced a marked eosinophilia in the BAL fluid and lung tissue 24 hours after challenge. This response was inhibited by nonselective NOS inhibitors [*N*-nitro-L-arginine methyl ester (L-NAME) and NG-monomethyl-L-arginine (NMMA)] but not by the selective iNOS inhibitor L-N6-(1-iminoethyl) lysine (L-NIL) (64). While these data suggest that NO is involved in the development of pulmonary eosinophilia in these allergic mice, it ruled out a contribution of iNOS to this process. This was further substantiated by the lack of effect of allergen challenge on iNOS protein or gene expression in the lungs or on the levels of nitrite in the BAL fluid (64). However, serum nitrite levels were increased after OVA challenge. Based on this observation, the authors speculated that after antigen challenge, the localized production of NO, possibly from pulmonary vascular endothelial cells, is involved in the extravasation of eosinophils from the circulation into the lung tissue.

Several other studies have described a beneficial effect of NO in murine asthma models. In these studies, NOS inhibitors were shown to increase or potentiate the inflammatory response, supporting a beneficial role for NO in the airways. In a fungal allergy model in CBA/J mice, L-NAME–treated mice have lower lung nitrite levels but higher airway hyperresponsiveness and inflammation after *Aspergillus fumigatus* challenge when compared to D-NAME controls (76). This inflammatory response also included increased airway and peribronchial eosinophilia and augmented levels of CC chemokine expression (76). Also, in CD-1 and C57BL/6 mice, L-NAME potentiated airway reactivity (measured as change in Penh) to methacholine (68). These findings in mice confirm previous results in other species demonstrating that administration of NOS inhibitors produce bronchial hyperresponsiveness and/or airway inflammation both in vivo and in vitro (77–80).

The discrepancies in the data generated using either NOS KO mice or NOS inhibitors may be related to several factors, including differences in sensitization and challenge protocols, or may be due to differences in genetic background of the experimental animals. The selectivity and specificity of most of the NOS inhibitors is fairly modest (81) and may account for the variable effect observed with these inhibitors. Therefore, the results generated using NOS inhibitors should be cautiously interpreted (Table 2).

VI. Contribution of NOS Isoforms to Allergen-Induced Airway Inflammation and Airway Hyperresponsiveness: Potential Cellular and Molecular Mechanisms

While the nature of the enzyme involved is still debated, most studies suggest a causal relationship between NO and airway inflammation. There are several mechanisms by which NO may recruit eosinophils into the lungs following an allergic reaction. Nitric oxide produces airway microvascular leakage (82), which may in itself augment the migration of eosinophils from the blood into the lungs. In a pleurisy model in Wistar rats, eosinophil migration induced by intrapleural injection of bradykinin, platelet-activating factor, lipopolysaccharide, and carrageenin was inhibited in animals chronically treated with L-NAME but not with the inactive enantiomer D-NAME (74). Similar results were reported in a previous study using an ex vivo eosinophil chemotaxis assay (83). Additionally, rat peritoneal eosinophils strongly express both NOS2 and NOS3 proteins, and their migratory response to both fMLP and LTB4 is inhibited by both NOS2- and NOS1/2-type inhibitors (84). As well as having local effects such as increasing vascular permeability and edema formation (82), NO also increases the production of prostaglandins through an action on cyclooxygenase enzyme (85), which may further contribute to the inflammatory process.

Inhibition of eosinophil apoptosis has also been proposed as a key mechanism for the development of blood and tissue eosinophilia in diseases such as bronchial asthma and other allergic disorders (86,87). NO has been described as a survival factor for human blood eosinophils (88) and specifically prevents Fas receptor–mediated apoptosis in freshly isolated human eosinophils (89). The underlying intracellular mechanisms involve disruption by NO of Fas receptor–mediated signaling events at the level of JNK. Therefore, NO concentrations within allergic inflammatory sites may be important in determining whether an eosinophil survives or undergoes apoptosis upon Fas ligand stimulation (89).

NO may also promote airway inflammation through mechanisms involving modulation of T-cell function (90). NO inhibits both the proliferation of Th1 cells and their production of IL-2 and IFN-γ, as demonstrated in several infectious diseases (91,92). In cloned murine T-cell lines, it has been shown that NO was an inhibitory factor of Th1-cell development, whereas it had no effect on Th2 cells (93). IFN-γ is known to inhibit Th2-cell proliferation (94). In NOS2-deficient mice (63), Xiong and colleagues have demonstrated increased IFN-γ production by cultured lymphocytes harvested from lung and spleen, suggesting that deficiency of NOS2 leads to a shift in cytokine profile. In support of this, NOS2-deficient mutant mice show enhanced Th1 responses following infection (95). NO has further been shown to promote a Th2 response in macrophages by blocking IL-12 secretion (96). Thus, production of large amounts of NO could reduce the secretion of IFN-γ, which in turn enhances the activity and stimulation of Th2 lymphocytes (6). Th2 lymphocytes are responsible for IL-4, IL-5, and IL-13 production, which are pivotal in the orchestration of asthmatic inflammation, including IgE expression and recruitment of eosinophils into the airway. While NO may play an important role in amplifying and perpetuating the Th2 cell–mediated inflammatory response in asthma (6), recent work using a murine model of airway inflammation refutes this hypothesis (69). Specifically, treatment with iNOS inhibitors either from the day of sensitization or the day of challenge induced an increased production of Th2-type cytokines (IL-4 and IL-5) with a concomitant decrease in production of Th1-type cytokine (IFN-γ). Furthermore, purified lung T cells showed the same profile of cytokine production with NOS inhibitors, namely an increase in Th2-type cytokines and a decrease in Th1-type cytokines. Similarly, in a carrageenin-induced edema murine model, it was shown that lymph node T cells from animals treated with NOS inhibitor produce less IFN-γ and more Th2-type cytokines (e.g., IL-10) (97).

There is also evidence that endogenous NO regulates the reactivity of mast cells in experimental animals (98,99). NO is produced by rat mast cells constitutively (100), and NOS inhibitors have been demonstrated not only to increase histamine release from activated mast cells in vitro (101), but also to produce all the features of mast cell–induced inflammation in vivo (102). Those data suggest that endogenous NO may protect against the effects of inhaled allergen. In addition, stem cell factor (SCF), which induces the differentiation of murine mast cells and potentiates their mediator release, has been shown to upregulate the expression of iNOS (103).

NO may also modulate lung inflammation through its interaction with the transcription factor NF-κB, which is activated by diverse inflammatory stimuli and has been causally linked to respiratory cell inflammation and pulmonary disease. NF-κB regulates many of the genes involved in the immune response, including NOS2 (104). NO or related molecules primarily inhibits NF-κB activation (105). In human alveolar macrophages, NO inhibited LPS-stimulated inflammatory cytokine production (TNF-α, IL-1β, MIP-1α) through an increase in the NF-κB inhibitory protein IκB-α (106,107). Furthermore, Raychaudhuri and colleagues have shown an inverse correlation between exhaled levels of NO and NF-κB activity in alveolar macrophages harvested from patients with asthma (106). NO has also been shown in human endothelial cells to inhibit the activation of NF-κB by inducing and stabilizing IκB-α(108,109). These observations are supportive of an anti-inflammatory and protective role for NO in asthma. In murine macrophages, however, NO has been shown to have a biphasic effect on NF-κB activity and possesses the ability to both up- and downregulate the expression of a number of proinflammatory proteins, including iNOS, COX-2, and IL-6 (110). This dual effect of NO on NF-κB may also explain in part the ability of NO to exert both pro- and anti-inflammatory influences (111,112) analyzed the function of iNOS in a murine model of hemorrhagic shock and Hierholzer and coworkers reported that the deletion of the iNOS gene in the mouse or pharmacological inhibition of iNOS by L-NIL in the rat reduced the degree of tissue injury in liver and lung. The authors further demonstrate that in the absence of iNOS the activation of NF-κB was significantly reduced in the lung and liver (113).

While NO itself is fairly nontoxic, secondary reactive nitrogen species (RNS) derived from NO are oxidants and nitrating agents. They interact with biomolecules such as proteins, carbohydrates, and lipids to modify both their structure and function, causing tissue injury and cellular dysfunction during inflammation (4,114–119). NO or RNS may lead to nitration of tyrosine residues in proteins or nitrosylation of biological constituents to form S-nitrosothiols (SNO). Peroxynitrite (ONOO$^-$) is also a potent oxidant formed by the rapid reaction of NO and superoxide (O$_2^-$). It can oxidize lipids and nitrate proteins and may therefore cause airway hyperresponsiveness and airway epithelial damage, enhances inflammatory cell recruitment, and inhibits pulmonary surfactant (13,116,117,120). ONOO$^-$ is known to inactivate human superoxide dismutase protein through exclusive nitration of tyrosine 34 (121), and reduced superoxide dismutase activity was shown in the leukocytes of asthmatic patients (122).

In comparison to healthy controls, mild well-controlled atopic asthmatics tend to have increased NO, NO$_3^-$, peroxynitrite, and nitrotyrosine, a marker of protein nitration possibly mediated by peroxynitrite (13,123). The presence of nitrotyrosine in the airway epithelium and inflammatory cells correlated inversely with methacholine PC20 and FEV$_1$, respectively (13). Administration of glucocorticoids reduced 3-nitrotyrosine staining, peroxynitite, and NOS2 expression (13). This observation, which has since been replicated (123), underscores the potential of NO to exert a toxic, oxidative effect in asthma, since tyrosine nitration may alter the function of both regulatory and structural proteins (119). Similar observations have been reported in a murine model of allergic asthma. In sensitized and OVA-challenged male A/J mice, the increased number of BALF eosinophils is accompanied by an increase in total NO$_2^-$ plus NO$_3^-$ (NO$_x$) production in BALF together with evidence for iNOS expression in airway epithelial and inflammatory cells. There was also evidence for protein nitration detected as immunostaining for 3-nitrotyrosine (3NT) in peribronchial inflammatory cells and at the epithelial surface. All these endpoints were significantly reduced by pretreatment with the specific NOS2 inhibitor 1400 W, as well as by the nonselective NOS inhibitor L-NAME (72). Furthermore, anti-IL-5 antibody, which reduced BALF eosinophilia, also decreased the number of (tyrosine nitration or nitrotyrosine formation) 3NT-positive cells in the peribronchial region and abrogated NO$_x$ in BALF (72). Recently, it was shown that both airway inflammation and AHR were dependent on the production of both NO and superoxide and may therefore involve RNS (71). Indeed, treatment of mice with the NADPH-oxidase inhibitor apocynin inhibited ovalbumin-induced airway hyperresponsiveness. Remarkably, treatment with apocynin did not alter 3-nitrotyrosine staining (71).

However, recent observations suggest that protein nitration are independent of NOS2 activity and are due rather to the action of peroxidases, including eosinophil peroxidase (EPO). In OVA-sensitized and -challenged mice, formation of 3NT in the lung was highly dependent on EPO activity rather than on expression of NOS2 or the level of production of NO metabolites. Indeed, 3NT formation was decreased in EPO-deficient New Zealand White mice after allergen challenge. In contrast, in mutant NOS2-deficient mice, 3NT formation was unaffected. These data suggest that, at least in the mouse, eosinophil peroxidase activity is a major source of protein nitration formation during allergic inflammation (124).

VII. Conclusion

The general view on the biological role of NO is that low levels of NO, as synthesized by constitutive NO synthase (NOS1 or 3), are involved in physiological events, whereas high levels of NO, as produced by NOS2, have a role in pathological processes. However, it emerges from recent studies using KO mice that NOS2 does not seem to play a major role in airway hyperreactivity, a hallmark of the asthmatic phenotype. Rather, these studies have unveiled a major role of NOS-1 in airway hyperreactivity. Although inhibitor studies argue in favor of a role of NOS2 in airway eosinophilia and inflammation in general, these data are still controversial given the selectivity issues. These controversies also highlight the complex and dichotomous role of NO in airway function. The generated controversies should not limit us but should stimulate further research into role of NO airway pathophysiology. There is no doubt that continued exploration of the role of NO in pathophysiology would yield further insights into its role in airway inflammation and airway hyperreactivity.

References

1. Sessa WC. The nitric oxide synthase family of proteins. J Vasc Res 1994; 31:131–143.
2. Kharitonov SA, Yates DH, Barnes PJ. Inhaled glucocorticoids decrease nitric oxide in exhaled air of asthmatic patients. Am J Respir Crit Care Med 1996; 153:454–457.
3. Silkoff PE, McClean PA, Slutsky AS, et al. Exhaled nitric oxide and bronchial reactivity during and after inhaled beclomethasone in mild asthma. J Asthma 1998; 35:473–479.
4. Sanders SP. Asthma, viruses, and nitric oxide. Proc Soc Exp Biol Med 1999; 220: 123–132.
5. Barnes PJ, Belvisi MG. Nitric oxide and lung disease. Thorax 1993; 48:1034–1043.
6. Barnes PJ, Liew FY. Nitric oxide and asthmatic inflammation. Immunol Today 1995; 16:128–130.
7. Lundberg JO. Airborne nitric oxide: inflammatory marker and aerocrine messenger in man. Acta Physiol Scand Suppl 1996; 633:1–27.
8. Dupuy PM, Shore SA, Drazen JM, Frostell C, Hill WA, Zapol WM. Bronchodilator action of inhaled nitric oxide in guinea pigs. J Clin Invest 1992; 90:421–428.
9. Kacmarek RM, Ripple R, Cockrill BA, Bloch KJ, Zapol WM, Johnson DC. Inhaled nitric oxide. A bronchodilator in mild asthmatics with methacholine-induced bronchospasm. Am J Respir Crit Care Med 1996; 153:128–135.
10. Gwyn DR, Lindeman KS, Hirshman CA. Inhaled nitric oxide attenuates bronchoconstriction in canine peripheral airways. Am J Respir Crit Care Med 1996; 153:604–609.
11. Hogman M, Frostell CG, Hedenstrom H, Hedenstierna G. Inhalation of nitric oxide modulates adult human bronchial tone. Am Rev Respir Dis 1993; 148:1474–1478.
12. Vaali K, Li L, Redemann B, Paakkari I, Vapaatalo H. In-vitro bronchorelaxing effects of novel nitric oxide donors GEA 3268 and GEA 5145 in guinea-pigs and rats. J Pharm Pharmacol 1996; 48:1309–1314.

13. Saleh D, Ernst P, Lim S, Barnes PJ, Giaid A. Increased formation of the potent oxidant peroxynitrite in the airways of asthmatic patients is associated with induction of nitric oxide synthase: effect of inhaled glucocorticoid. FASEB J 1998; 12:929–937.

14. Sadeghi-Hashjin G, Folkerts G, Henricks PA, et al. Peroxynitrite induces airway hyperresponsiveness in guinea pigs in vitro and in vivo. Am J Respir Crit Care Med 1996; 153:1697–1701.

15. Sugiura H, Ichinose M, Oyake T, et al. Role of peroxynitrite in airway microvascular hyperpermeability during late allergic phase in guinea pigs. Am J Respir Crit Care Med 1999; 160:663–671.

16. Taylor DA, McGrath JL, O'Connor BJ, Barnes PJ. Allergen-induced early and late asthmatic responses are not affected by inhibition of endogenous nitric oxide. Am J Respir Crit Care Med 1998; 158:99–106.

17. Moncada S, Higgs A. The L-arginine-nitric oxide pathway. N Engl J Med 1993; 329: 2002–2012.

18. Bredt DS, Snyder SH. Nitric oxide, a novel neuronal messenger. Neuron 1992; 8: 3–11.

19. Schmidt HH, Walter U. NO at work. Cell 1994; 78:919–925.

20. Robbins RA, Springall DR, Warren JB, et al. Inducible nitric oxide synthase is increased in murine lung epithelial cells by cytokine stimulation. Biochem Biophys Res Commun 1994; 198:835–843.

21. Hamid Q, Springall DR, Riveros-Moreno V, et al. Induction of nitric oxide synthase in asthma. Lancet 1993; 342:1510–1513.

22. Robbins RA, Barnes PJ, Springall DR, et al. Expression of inducible nitric oxide in human lung epithelial cells. Biochem Biophys Res Commun 1994; 203:209–218.

23. Yates DH, Kharitonov SA, Thomas PS, Barnes PJ. Endogenous nitric oxide is decreased in asthmatic patients by an inhibitor of inducible nitric oxide synthase. Am J Respir Crit Care Med 1996; 154:247–250.

24. Immervoll T, Loesgen S, Dutsch G, et al. Fine mapping and single nucleotide polymorphism association results of candidate genes for asthma and related phenotypes. Hum Mutat 2001; 18:327–336.

25. Gao PS, Kawada H, Kasamatsu T, et al. Variants of NOS1, NOS2, and NOS3 genes in asthmatics. Biochem Biophys Res Commun 2000; 267:761–763.

26. Pollock JS, Fostermann U, Mitchell JA, et al. Purification and characterization of particulate EDRF synthase from cultured and naive bovine aortic endothelial cells. Proc Natl Acad Sci USA 1991; 88:10480–10484.

27. Lee YC, Cheon KT, Lee HB, Kim W, Rhee YK, Kim DS. Gene polymorphisms of endothelial nitric oxide synthase and angiotensin-converting enzyme in patients with asthma. Allergy 2000; 55:959–963.

28. Wang J, Palmer K, Lotvall J, et al. Circulating, but not local lung, IL-5 is required for the development of antigen-induced airways eosinophilia. J Clin Invest 1998; 102: 1132–1141.

29. Kips JC, Brusselle GG, Joos GF, et al. Importance of interleukin-4 and interleukin-12 in allergen-induced airway changes in mice. Int Arch Allergy Immunol 1995; 107: 115–118.

30. Xia JQ, Rickaby DA, Kelly KJ, Choi H, Dawson CA, Kurup VP. Immune response and airway reactivity in wild and IL-4 knockout mice exposed to latex allergens. Int Arch Allergy Immunol 1999; 118:23–29.

31. Matthaei KI, Foster P, Young IG. The role of interleukin-5 (IL-5) in vivo: studies with IL-5 deficient mice. Mem Inst Oswaldo Cruz 1997; 92:63–68.

32. Wagner DD. P-selectin knockout: a mouse model for various human diseases. Ciba Found Symp 1995; 189:2–10.

33. Moqbel R. Invited editorial on "reduction of allergic airway responses in P-selectin-deficient mice" (editorial). J Appl Physiol 1997; 83:679–680.

34. Wolyniec WW, De Sanctis GT, Nabozny G, et al. Reduction of antigen-induced airway hyperreactivity and eosinophilia in ICAM-1-deficient mice. Am J Respir Cell Mol Biol 1998; 18:777–785.

35. De Sanctis GT, MacLean JA, Hamada K, et al. Contribution of nitric oxide synthases 1, 2, and 3 to airway hyperresponsiveness and inflammation in a murine model of asthma. J Exp Med 1999; 189:1621–1630.

36. Robinson DS, Hamid Q, Ying S, et al. Predominant Th2-like bronchoalveolar T-lymphocyte population in atopic asthma. N Engl J Med 1992; 326:298–304.

37. Wills-Karp M, Luyimbazi J, Xu X, et al. Interleukin-13: central mediator of allergic asthma (see comments). Science 1998; 282:2258–2261.

38. Minshall EM, Schleimer R, Cameron L, et al. Interleukin-5 expression in the bone marrow of sensitized Balb/c mice after allergen challenge. Am J Respir Crit Care Med 1998; 158:951–957.

39. Cohn L, Homer RJ, Marinov A, Rankin J, Bottomly K. Induction of airway mucus production by T helper 2 (Th2) cells: a critical role for interleukin 4 in cell recruitment but not mucus production. J Exp Med 1997; 186:1737–1747.

40. Hogan SP, Koskinen A, Foster PS. Interleukin-5 and eosinophils induce airway damage and bronchial hyperreactivity during allergic airway inflammation in BALB/c mice. Immunol Cell Biol 1997; 75:284–288.

41. Hogan SP, Foster PS, Tan X, Ramsay AJ. Mucosal IL-12 gene delivery inhibits allergic airways disease and restores local antiviral immunity. Eur J Immunol 1998; 28: 413–423.

42. Haczku A, Takeda K, Redai I, et al. Anti-CD86 (B7.2) treatment abolishes allergic airway hyperresponsiveness in mice. Am J Respir Crit Care Med 1999; 159: 1638–1643.

43. Hofstra CL, Van Ark I, Nijkamkp FP, Van Oosterhout AJ. Antigen-stimulated lung CD4+ cells produce IL-5, while lymph node CD4+ cells produce Th2 cytokines concomitant with airway eosinophilia and hyperresponsiveness. Inflamm Res 1999; 48:602–612.

44. Hogan SP, Koskinen A, Matthaei KI, Young IG, Foster PS. Interleukin-5-producing CD4+ T cells play a pivotal role in aeroallergen-induced eosinophilia, bronchial hyperreactivity, and lung damage in mice. Am J Respir Crit Care Med 1998; 157:210–218.

45. Krinzman SJ, De Sanctis GT, Cernadas M, et al. T cell activation in a murine model of asthma. Am J Physiol 1996; 271:L476–483.

46. Krinzman SJ, De Sanctis GT, Cernadas M, et al. Inhibition of T cell costimulation abrogates airway hyperresponsiveness in a murine model. J Clin Invest 1996; 98: 2693–2699.

47. Kennedy JD, Hatfield CA, Fidler SF, et al. Phenotypic characterization of T lymphocytes emigrating into lung tissue and the airway lumen after antigen inhalation in sensitized mice. Am J Respir Cell Mol Biol 1995; 12:613–623.

48. Garlisi CG, Falcone A, Hey JA, et al. Airway eosinophils, T cells, Th2-type cytokine mRNA, and hyperreactivity in response to aerosol challenge of allergic mice with previously established pulmonary inflammation. Am J Respir Cell Mol Biol 1997; 17: 642–651.

49. Keane-Myers A, Gause WC, Linsley PS, Chen SJ, Wills-Karp M. B7-CD28/CTLA-4 costimulatory pathways are required for the development of T helper cell 2-mediated allergic airway responses to inhaled antigens. J Immunol 1997; 158:2042–2049.

50. De Sanctis GT, Mehta S, Kobzik L, et al. Contribution of type I NOS to expired gas NO and bronchial responsiveness in mice. Am J Physiol 1997; 273:L883–888.

51. Zhang DH, Yang L, Cohn L, et al. Inhibition of allergic inflammation in a murine model of asthma by expression of a dominant-negative mutant of GATA-3. Immunity 1999; 11:473–482.

52. Brewer JP, Kisselgof AB, Martin TR. Genetic variability in pulmonary physiological, cellular, and antibody responses to antigen in mice. Am J Respir Crit Care Med 1999; 160:1150–1156.

53. Hamelmann E, Takeda K, Schwarze J, Vella AT, Irvin CG, Gelfand EW. Development of eosinophilic airway inflammation and airway hyperresponsiveness requires interleukin-5 but not immunoglobulin E or B lymphocytes (see comments). Am J Respir Cell Mol Biol 1999; 21:480–489.

54. Inman MD, Ellis R, Wattie J, Denburg JA, O'Byrne PM. Allergen-induced increase in airway responsiveness, airway eosinophilia, and bone-marrow eosinophil progenitors in mice (see comments). Am J Respir Cell Mol Biol 1999; 21:473–479.

55. Cieslewicz G, Tomkinson A, Adler A, et al. The late, but not early, asthmatic response is dependent on IL-5 and correlates with eosinophil infiltration. J Clin Invest 1999; 104:301–308.

56. Kaminuma O, Mori A, Ogawa K, et al. Cloned Th cells confer eosinophilic inflammation and bronchial hyperresponsiveness. Int Arch Allergy Immunol 1999; 118:136–139.

57. Temelkovski J, Hogan SP, Shepherd DP, Foster PS, Kumar RK. An improved murine model of asthma: selective airway inflammation, epithelial lesions and increased methacholine responsiveness following chronic exposure to aerosolised allergen. Thorax 1998; 53:849–856.

58. MacLean JA, Sauty A, Luster AD, Drazen JM, De Sanctis GT. Antigen-induced airway hyperresponsiveness, pulmonary eosinophilia, and chemokine expression in B cell-deficient mice. Am J Respir Cell Mol Biol 1999; 20:379–387.

59. Kung TT. Pulmonary eosinophilia and inflammation in allergic mice. Lab Anim Sci 1998; 48:61–63.

60. De Sanctis GT, MacLean JA, Qin S, et al. Interleukin-8 receptor modulates IgE production and B-cell expansion and trafficking in allergen-induced pulmonary inflammation. J Clin Invest 1999; 103:507–515.

61. Yu B, He Q, Gao Z. [The role of glucocorticosteroid and theophylline in asthmatic inflammation of murine model and the inhibition in NO production in lung]. Zhonghua Jie He He Hu Xi Za Zhi 1998; 21:664–667.

62. Guo FH, De Raeve HR, Rice TW, Stuehr DJ, Thunnissen FB, Erzurum SC. Continuous nitric oxide synthesis by inducible nitric oxide synthase in normal human airway epithelium in vivo. Proc Natl Acad Sci USA 1995; 92:7809–7813.

63. Xiong Y, Karupiah G, Hogan SP, Foster PS, Ramsay AJ. Inhibition of allergic airway inflammation in mice lacking nitric oxide synthase 2. J Immunol 1999; 162:445–452.

64. Feder LS, Stelts D, Chapman RW, et al. Role of nitric oxide on eosinophilic lung inflammation in allergic mice. Am J Respir Cell Mol Biol 1997; 17:436–442.

65. Kharitonov SA, Yates D, Springall DR, et al. Exhaled nitric oxide is increased in asthma. Chest 1995; 107:156S–157S.

66. Persson MG, Zetterstrom O, Agrenius V, Ihre E, Gustafsson LE. Single-breath nitric oxide measurements in asthmatic patients and smokers. Lancet 1994; 343:146–147.

67. Barnes KC, Neely JD, Duffy DL, et al. Linkage of asthma and total serum IgE concentration to markers on chromosome 12Q—evidence from Afro-Caribbean and Caucasian populations. Genomics 1996; 37:41–50.

68. Feletou M, Lonchampt M, Coge F, et al. Regulation of murine airway responsiveness by endothelial nitric oxide synthase. Am J Physiol Lung Cell Mol Physiol 2001; 281: L258–L267.

69. Trifilieff A, Fujitani Y, Mentz F, Dugas B, Fuentes M, Bertrand C. Inducible nitric oxide synthase inhibitors suppress airway inflammation in mice through down-regulation of chemokine expression. J Immunol 2000; 165:1526–1533.

70. Koarai A, Ichinose M, Sugiura H, Yamagata S, Hattori T, Shirato K. Allergic airway hyperresponsiveness and eosinophil infiltration is reduced by a selective iNOS inhibitor, 1400W, in mice. Pulm Pharmacol Ther 2000; 13:267–275.

71. Muijsers RB, van Ark I, Folkerts G, et al. Apocynin and 1400 W prevents airway hyperresponsiveness during allergic reactions in mice. Br J Pharmacol 2001; 134: 434–440.

72. Iijima H, Duguet A, Eum SY, Hamid Q, Eidelman DH. Nitric oxide and protein nitration are eosinophil dependent in allergen-challenged mice. Am J Respir Crit Care Med 2001; 163:1233–1240.

73. Eynott PR, Hanazawa K, Tomita K, et al. The effects of a selective inhibitor of inducible NO synthase in a brown-Norway rat model of allergic asthma. Am J Respir Crit Care Med 2000; 161:A919.

74. Ferreira HH, Bevilacqua E, Gagioti SM, et al. Nitric oxide modulates eosinophil infiltration in antigen-induced airway inflammation in rats. Eur J Pharmacol 1998; 358: 253–259.

75. Iijima H, Uchida Y, Endo T, et al. Role of endogenous nitric oxide in allergen-induced airway responses in guinea-pigs. Br J Pharmacol 1998; 124:1019–1028.

76. Blease K, Kunkel SL, Hogaboam CM. Acute inhibition of nitric oxide exacerbates airway hyperresponsiveness, eosinophilia and C-C chemokine generation in a murine model of fungal asthma. Inflamm Res 2000; 49:297–304.

77. Mehta S, Drazen JM, Lilly CM. Endogenous nitric oxide and allergic bronchial hyperresponsiveness in guinea pigs. Am J Physiol 1997; 273:L656–662.

78. Nijkamp FP, Folkerts G. Nitric oxide and bronchial hyperresponsiveness. Arch Int Pharmacodyn Ther 1995; 329:81–96.

79. Nijkamp FP, van der Linde HJ, Folkerts G. Nitric oxide synthesis inhibitors induce airway hyperresponsiveness in the guinea pig in vivo and in vitro. Role of the epithelium. Am Rev Respir Dis 1993; 148:727–734.

80. Tulic MK, Wale JL, Holt PG, Sly PD. Differential effects of nitric oxide synthase inhibitors in an in vivo allergic rat model. Eur Respir J 2000; 15:870–877.

81. Boughton Smith NK, Tinker AC. Inhibitors of nitric oxide synthase in inflammatory arthritis. Drugs 1998; 1:321–333.

82. Kuo HP, Liu S, Barnes PJ. The effect of endogenous nitric oxide on neurogenic plasma exudation in guinea-pig airways. Eur J Pharmacol 1992; 221:385–388.

83. Ferreira HH, Medeiros MV, Lima CS, et al. Inhibition of eosinophil chemotaxis by chronic blockade of nitric oxide biosynthesis. Eur J Pharmacol 1996; 310:201–207.

84. Zanardo RC, Costa E, Ferreira HH, et al. Pharmacological and immunohistochemical evidence for a functional nitric oxide synthase system in rat peritoneal eosinophils. Proc Natl Acad Sci USA 1997; 94:14111–14114.

85. Salvemini D, Misko TP, Masferrer JL, Seibert K, Currie MG, Needleman P. Nitric oxide activates cyclooxygenase enzymes. Proc Natl Acad Sci USA 1993; 90: 7240–7244.

86. Simon HU, Blaser K. Inhibition of programmed eosinophil death: a key pathogenic event for eosinophilia? Immunol Today 1995; 16:53–55.

87. Simon HU, Yousefi S, Schranz C, Schapowal A, Bachert C, Blaser K. Direct demonstration of delayed eosinophil apoptosis as a mechanism causing tissue eosinophilia. J Immunol 1997; 158:3902–3908.

88. Beauvais F, Michel L, Dubertret L. The nitric oxide donors, azide and hydroxylamine, inhibit the programmed cell death of cytokine-deprived human eosinophils. FEBS Lett 1995; 361:229–232.

89. Hebestreit H, Dibbert B, Balatti I, et al. Disruption of fas receptor signaling by nitric oxide in eosinophils. J Exp Med 1998; 187:415–425.

90. Liew FY. Regulation of lymphocyte functions by nitric oxide. Curr Opin Immunol 1995; 7:396–399.

91. Abrahamsohn IA, Coffman RL. Cytokine and nitric oxide regulation of the immunosuppression in Trypanosoma cruzi infection. J Immunol 1995; 155:3955–3963.

92. Sternberg MJ, Mabbott NA. Nitric oxide-mediated suppression of T cell responses during *Trypanosoma brucei* infection: soluble trypanosome products and interferongamma are synergistic inducers of nitric oxide synthase. Eur J Immunol 1996; 26: 539–543.

93. Taylor-Robinson AW, Liew FY, Severn A, et al. Regulation of the immune response by nitric oxide differentially produced by T helper type 1 and T helper type 2 cells. Eur J Immunol 1994; 24:980–984.

94. Gajewski TF, Goldwasser E, Fitch FW. Anti-proliferative effect of IFN-gamma in immune regulation. II. IFN-gamma inhibits the proliferation of murine bone marrow cells stimulated with IL-3, IL-4, or granulocyte-macrophage colony-stimulating factor. J Immunol 1988; 141:2635–2642.

95. Wei XQ, Charles IG, Smith A, et al. Altered immune responses in mice lacking inducible nitric oxide synthase. Nature 1995; 375:408–411.

96. Huang FP, Niedbala W, Wei XQ, et al. Nitric oxide regulates Th1 cell development through the inhibition of IL-12 synthesis by macrophages. Eur J Immunol 1998; 28: 4062–4070.

97. Ianaro A, O'Donnell CA, Di Rosa M, Liew FY. A nitric oxide synthase inhibitor reduces inflammation, down-regulates inflammatory cytokines and enhances interleukin-10 production in carrageenin-induced oedema in mice. Immunology 1994; 82: 370–375.

98. Gaboury JP, Niu XF, Kubes P. Nitric oxide inhibits numerous features of mast cell-induced inflammation. Circulation 1996; 93:318–326.

99. Salvemini D, Masini E, Pistelli P, Mannaioni PF, Vane JR. Nitric oxide: a regulatory mediator of mast cell reactivity. J Cardiovasc Pharmacol 1991; 17:S258.

100. Hogaboam CM, Befus AD, Wallace JL. Modulation of rat mast cell reactivity by IL-1 beta. Divergent effects on nitric oxide and platelet-activating factor release. J Immunol 1993; 151:3767–3774.

101. Masini E, Salvemini D, Pistelli A, Mannaioni PF, Vane JR. Rat mast cells synthesize a nitric oxide like-factor which modulates the release of histamine. Agents Actions 1991; 33:61–63.

102. Kanwar S, Wallace JL, Befus D, Kubes P. Nitric oxide synthesis inhibition increases epithelial permeability via mast cells. Am J Physiol 1994; 266:G222–229.

103. Bidri M, Ktorza S, Vouldoukis I, et al. Nitric oxide pathway is induced by Fc epsilon RI and up-regulated by stem cell factor in mouse mast cells. Eur J Immunol 1997; 27: 2907–2913.
104. Siebenlist U, Franzoso G, Brown K. Structure, regulation and function of NF-kappa B. Annu Rev Cell Biol 1994; 10:405–455.
105. Marshall HE, Stamler JS. Exhaled nitric oxide (NO), NO synthase activity, and regulation of nuclear factor (NF)-kappaB. Am J Respir Cell Mol Biol 1999; 21:296–297.
106. Raychaudhuri B, Dweik R, Connors MJ, et al. Nitric oxide blocks nuclear factor-kappaB activation in alveolar macrophages. Am J Respir Cell Mol Biol 1999; 21: 311–316.
107. Thomassen MJ, Buhrow LT, Connors MJ, Kaneko FT, Erzurum SC, Kavuru MS. Nitric oxide inhibits inflammatory cytokine production by human alveolar macrophages. Am J Respir Cell Mol Biol 1997; 17:279–283.
108. Peng HB, Libby P, Liao JK. Induction and stabilization of I kappa B alpha by nitric oxide mediates inhibition of NF-kappa B. J Biol Chem 1995; 270:14214–14219.
109. Zeiher AM, Fisslthaler B, Schray-Utz B, Busse R. Nitric oxide modulates the expression of monocyte chemoattractant protein 1 in cultured human endothelial cells. Circ Res 1995; 76:980–986.
110. Connelly L, Palacios-Callender M, Ameixa C, Moncada S, Hobbs AJ. Biphasic regulation of NF-kappa B activity underlies the pro- and anti-inflammatory actions of nitric oxide. J Immunol 2001; 166:3873–3881.
111. Hobbs AJ, Moncada S. Inducible nitric oxide synthase and inflammation. In: Willoughby DA, Tomlinson A, eds. Inducible Enzymes in the Inflammatory Response. Boston: Birkhäuser, 1999:31–54.
112. Nathan C. Inducible nitric oxide synthase: What difference does it make? J Clin Invest 1997; 100:2417–2423.
113. Hierholzer C, Harbrecht B, Menezes JM, et al. Essential role of induced nitric oxide in the initiation of the inflammatory response after hemorrhagic shock. J Exp Med 1998; 187:917–928.
114. Dweik RA, Laskowski D, Abu-Soud HM, et al. Nitric oxide synthesis in the lung. Regulation by oxygen through a kinetic mechanism. J Clin Invest 1998; 101:660–666.
115. Eiserich JP, Hristova M, Cross CE, et al. Formation of nitric oxide-derived inflammatory oxidants by myeloperoxidase in neutrophils. Nature 1998; 391:393–397.
116. Folkerts G, Kloek J, Muijsers RB, Nijkamp FP. Reactive nitrogen and oxygen species in airway inflammation. Eur J Pharmacol 2001; 429:251–262.
117. Groves JT. Peroxynitrite: reactive, invasive and enigmatic. Curr Opin Chem Biol 1999; 3:226–235.
118. Sanders SP. Nitric oxide in asthma. Pathogenic, therapeutic, or diagnostic? Am J Respir Cell Mol Biol 1999; 21:147–149.
119. van der Vliet A, Eiserich JP, Shigenaga MK, Cross CE. Reactive nitrogen species and tyrosine nitration in the respiratory tract: epiphenomena or a pathobiologic mechanism of disease? Am J Respir Crit Care Med 1999; 160:1–9.
120. Beckman JS, Koppenol WH. Nitric oxide, superoxide, and peroxynitrite: the good, the bad, and ugly. Am J Physiol 1996; 271:C1424–1437.
121. Yamakura F, Taka H, Fujimura T, Murayama K. Inactivation of human manganese-superoxide dismutase by peroxynitrite is caused by exclusive nitration of tyrosine 34 to 3-nitrotyrosine. J Biol Chem 1998; 273:14085–14089.
122. Joseph BZ, Routes JM, Borish L. Activities of superoxide dismutases and NADPH oxidase in neutrophils obtained from asthmatic and normal donors. Inflammation 1993; 17:361–370.

123. Kaminsky DA, Mitchell J, Carroll N, James A, Soultanakis R, Janssen Y. Nitrotyrosine formation in the airways and lung parenchyma of patients with asthma. J Allergy Clin Immunol 1999; 104:747–754.

124. Duguet A, Iijima H, Eum SY, Hamid Q, Eidelman DH. Eosinophil peroxidase mediates protein nitration in allergic airway inflammation in mice. Am J Respir Crit Care Med 2001; 164:1119–1126.

125. Hope BT, Michael GJ, Knigge KM. Neuronal NADPH diaphorase is a nitric oxide synthase. Proc Natl Acad Sci USA 1991; 88:2811–2814.

126. Sherman TS, Chen Z, Yuhanna IS, Lau KS, Margraf LR, Shaul PW. Nitric oxide synthase isoform expression in the developing lung epithelium. Am J Physiol 1999; 276:L383–390.

127. Silvagno F, Xia H, Bredt DS. Neuronal nitric-oxide synthase-mu, an alternatively spliced isoform expressed in differentiated skeletal muscle. J Biol Chem 1996; 271: 11204–11208.

128. Amin AR, Attur M, Vyas P, et al. Expression of nitric oxide synthase in human peripheral blood mononuclear cells and neutrophils. J Inflamm 1995; 47:190–205.

129. Asano K, Chee CB, Gaston B, et al. Constitutive and inducible nitric oxide synthase gene expression, regulation, and activity in human lung epithelial cells. Proc Natl Acad Sci USA 1994; 91:10089–10093.

130. MacPherson JC et al. Eosinophils are a major source of nitric-oxide-derived oxidants in severe asthma: characterization of pathways available to eosinophils for generating reactive nitrogen species. J Immunol 2001; 166:5763–5772.

131. Lu L et al. Induction of nitric oxide synthase in mouse dendritic cells by IFN-γ, endotoxin, and interaction with allogeneic T cells. Nitric oxide production is associated with dendritic cell apoptosis. J Immunol 1996; 157:3577–3586.

132. Reiling N et al. Nitric oxide synthase: expression of the endothelial, Ca^{2+}/calmodulin-dependent isoform in human B and T lymphocytes. Eur J Immunol 1996; 26:511–516.

9

Molecular Mechanisms of Increased Nitric Oxide in Airway Inflammation

WEILING XU and SERPIL C. ERZURUM

Lerner Research Institute
Cleveland Clinic Foundation
Cleveland, Ohio, U.S.A.

I. Nitric Oxide Synthases

Since the finding that endothelium-derived relaxing factor (EDRF) is nitric oxide (NO) (1,2), NO has been shown to be a multifunctional molecule that mediates a number of physiological processes in almost all vertebrate organ systems, including diverse functions such as smooth muscle relaxation, platelet inhibition, central and autonomic neurotransmission, tumor cell lysis, bacterial killing, and stimulation of hormonal release (3–6). NO is a diffusible gas that is produced by a group of enzymes known collectively as nitric oxide synthases (NOS, EC 1.14.13.39). These enzymes convert the amino acid L-arginine to NO and L-citrulline in the presence of oxygen and NADPH as cosubstrates, a reaction that requires several cofactors including FAD, FMN, tetrahydrobiopterin, and calmodulin (7). NO is relatively unstable and rapidly oxidized in solution to the stable metabolic end-products nitrite (NO_2^-) and nitrate (NO_3^-), which can be used as indirect markers to monitor NO formation (7). Three isoforms of NOS, which are the products of individual genes (7,8), have been identified, including two constitutive forms [neuronal (nNOS or NOS1) and endothelial (eNOS or NOS3)] and an inducible form (iNOS or NOS2) (3,5,7). In general, NOS1 and 3 are continuously expressed in endothelial and neuronal cells, respectively, and are dependent on increases in intracellular calcium to bind calmodulin, which results in enzyme activation leading to picomolar levels of

NO production (7). NOS1 is also found at relatively abundant levels in skeletal muscle (9). NOS2 is regulated at the level of transcription and mRNA stability and is expressed after exposure of cells to specific cytokines and endotoxin (4,6,7,10). NOS2 is calcium independent, avidly binding calmodulin even at low calcium concentrations intracellularly, and produces nanomolar levels of NO (7). NOS2 has been described in epithelial, endothelial, smooth muscle cells, macrophages, fibroblasts, and neutrophils. Regulation of expression of NOS2 varies in different cell types, but typically is increased by cytokines such as tumor necrosis factor alpha (TNFα), interferon gamma (IFNγ), and interleukin-1 beta (IL-1β). NOS2 expression is decreased by glucocorticoids, transforming growth factor beta (TGFβ), platelet-derived growth factor (PDGF), epidermal growth factor, insulin-like growth factor 1, and thrombin (3,5,11,12). Regulation of NOS3 at the level of transcription is less well studied, but the gene is induced by oxygen tension, shear stress, and IFNγ (3,11,13,14). Both NOS1 and 3 mRNA are increased by estrogens. NOS3, unlike 1 and 2, is membrane associated due to myristoylation of its amino-terminus end (8).

II. NO in the Lung

NO is produced in the human lung, evidenced by NO detectable in the exhaled air of humans (6–8 ppb) and NO metabolites detectable in the airway aspirate and bronchoalveolar lavage fluid (BALF) from human lungs (3,15). NO is recognized to play key roles in virtually all aspects of lung biology and has been implicated in the pathophysiology of lung diseases (16). NO in the lung is involved in pulmonary neurotransmission, host defense and bacteriostasis, airway and vascular smooth muscle relaxation, pulmonary capillary leak, inflammation, mucociliary clearance, airway mucus secretion, and cytotoxicity (3,4,8).

Cellular sources of NO in the lung include epithelial cells, endothelial cells of pulmonary arteries and veins, inhibitory nonadrenergic noncholinergic neurons, smooth muscle cells, mast cells, mesothelial cells, fibroblasts, neutrophils, lymphocytes, and macrophages (17). All three NOS isoforms are present in the human lung (3,17,18). Specifically, NOS1 is located in inhibitory nonadrenergic noncholinergic neurons in the lung, while NOS3 is found in endothelial cells and the brush border of ciliated epithelial cells (17). NOS2 is found in the epithelial cells of the airway (6,10,17,18). Although NOS2 may be induced in several types of cells in response to cytokines, endotoxin, or reactive oxygen species, NOS2 is continuously expressed in normal human airway epithelium at basal airway conditions (18). Once produced, NO is freely diffusible and enters target cells, activating soluble guanylate cyclase to produce guanosine 3',5'-cyclic monophosphate (cGMP), which mediates the majority of NO effects (7). NO also diffuses into the airway and can be measured in the gas phase (15).

Potential anatomical sources of NO in exhaled breath include the pulmonary circulation, the lower airways, and the upper airways and paranasal sinuses. NO is formed in high concentrations in the upper respiratory tract (nasopharynx and paranasal sinuses), but several studies have conclusively demonstrated that NO is also produced in the lower respiratory tract (15,18).

III. Alterations of Exhaled NO in Lung Diseases

Alterations in NO levels have been found in pulmonary diseases such as asthma, pulmonary hypertension, bronchiectasis, cystic fibrosis, and interstitial lung disease (3). Exhaled NO is increased in inflammatory airway diseases, such as asthma and upper respiratory tract infections/bronchiectasis, and reflects an increase in NOS2 activity in airway epithelial cells (3,16). Exhaled NO levels are also higher in women with lymphangioleiomyomatosis (LAM) than healthy women and are related to increased NOS3 expression in lesional smooth muscle in the lung (19). Exhaled NO levels are lower than normal in smoking individuals, and the reduction is proportionate to the number of cigarettes currently smoked. Cigarette smoke contains high levels of NO (16), which may dysregulate NOS activity and contribute to the lung injury caused by smoking (20). There is also evidence that patients with primary pulmonary hypertension (PPH) may have lower levels of expression of NOS3 in pulmonary vascular endothelial cells and lower levels of exhaled NO (21,22).

IV. Post-Translational Mechanisms Regulating NO Synthesis

NO biosynthesis is regulated at multiple levels in cells, i.e., NOS gene transcription, mRNA processing, protein expression and dimerization, and enzyme reaction kinetics (7). NO synthesis is dependent upon post-translational modifications to generate active NOS. Specifically, NOSs are synthesized as monomers and must dimerize to generate NO (7). Deletion of regions critical for NOS dimerization due to alternative splicing of the NOS2 mRNA have been identified (23). In tissue culture cells, NOS2 induction by cytokines and endotoxin results in an increase in both constitutively and alternatively spliced mRNA transcripts (23,24).

Furthermore, enzyme-catalyzed NO synthesis involves hydroxylation of arginine to generate *N*-hydroxyarginine, an enzyme-bound intermediate, which is then converted to citrulline. Intracellular concentration of arginine (several hundred mM) (25–28) has been reported to far exceed the K_m of the NO synthases (5–10 mM) (28). In this context, it would seem unlikely that arginine is ever rate limiting to the enzyme. However, arginine administration drives NO synthesis in vivo and in cell culture systems (25–28). Independent of substrate effects, arginine may regulate enzyme reaction kinetics through effects on enzyme dimerization or influences on the reduction potential of the enzyme (7). Intracellular arginine can be increased by de novo synthesis through regeneration from citrulline or transport from extracellular sources (26–28). Arginine synthetic pathways and transporter systems are induced coordinately with NOS2 induction in cell cultures. Argininosuccinate synthetase, the rate-limiting enzyme in the synthesis of arginine, is induced by endotoxin and IFNγ, suppressed by corticosteroids, and generally mirrors NOS induction in vitro

(28). Arginine is present in healthy control airway epithelial cells but is increased over threefold in asthmatic epithelial cells, suggesting coordinate induction of the arginine synthetic pathways and/or cationic amino acid transporters to support a high rate of NO synthesis in asthma (29).

V. Transcriptional Regulation of NOS2

Although translational and post-translational mechanisms are important in the regulation of NO synthesis, NOS2 is subject to predominantly transcriptional regulation (7,10,29). Healthy human airway epithelium in vivo expresses the NOS2 gene continuously at abundant mRNA levels (10,18). The human NOS2 gene is actively transcribed in airway epithelial cells in vivo using run-on transcription analyses (29). NOS2 mRNA expression in asthmatic airway epithelium is higher than controls in vivo, but not increased in asthmatics receiving inhaled corticosteroid. Several studies have shown that inhaled or intravenous corticosteroids reduce exhaled NO. In situ analysis of the asthmatic airway indicates that NOS2 expression is reduced by corticosteroids (30). In general, mechanisms by which corticosteroids regulate NOS2 gene expression in vivo are not known. In vitro, glucocorticoids inhibit NOS2 expression at multiple levels including inhibition of gene transcription, reduction of mRNA translation, and increased degradation of NOS2 protein (31–33). Increased NOS2 mRNA in asthma, which is downregulated by corticosteroid, supports an association between NOS2 expression and exhaled NO in airway inflammation.

A. Induction of the NOS2 Gene In Vitro

The molecular basis for induction of the human NOS2 gene is only partially understood (31,34,35). In contrast, regions in the murine macrophage NOS2 promotor essential for conferring inducibility of NOS2 to LPS and IFNγ have been well defined (36,37). A nuclear factor kappa B (NF-κB) element at positions -76 to -85 bp relative to the transcription start point binds members of the NF-κB/Rel family of proteins in response to LPS (38), and further upstream an IFN-stimulated response element site binds interferon regulatory factor 1 (IRF-1) upon stimulation of murine macrophage cell line (RAW 264.7 cells) with IFNγ (39). Originally identified as a transcriptional activator of IFNβ as well as IFN-inducible genes (40), IRF-1 is essential for NOS2 activation in murine macrophages (39,41). Studies suggest that IRF-1 is also important in human NOS2 gene expression (42,43). NOS2 expression parallels IRF-1 expression, with IRF-1 expression preceding NOS2 mRNA accumulation.

B. IFNγ Signaling to NOS2

IFNγ signaling to gene expression begins with a specific receptor interaction and oligomerization of receptor chains. This causes a tyrosine phosphorylation cascade, which involves activation of Janus kinases (Jak) 1 and 2, which in turn activate STAT-1. STAT-1 phosphorylation, dimerization, and translocation to the nucleus is followed by binding to regulatory DNA elements to activate transcription of interferon-stimulated genes (44). IFNγ leads to STAT-1 activation in primary human airway epithelial cells in culture (10,29,42,43), and tyrosine kinase inhibitor abolishes induction of NOS2 in airway epithelial cells (29).

C. Activation of Signal Transducers Important for NOS2 Gene Expression

Recently, STAT-1 activation has been demonstrated in the chronically inflamed asthmatic airway by nuclear localization of STAT-1 in airway epithelial cells and demonstration of phosphorylation of STAT-1 by Western analyses of epithelial cell lysates (45). The STAT-1 activation correlates with induction of IFNγ/STAT-1–stimulated genes, including IRF-1. Similarly, STAT-1 activation quantitated by electrophoretic mobility shift assays is present in healthy airways but increased in asthmatic airway epithelial cells (29). These data provide support for STAT-1 activation mediating NOS2 gene expression in human airway epithelial cells in vivo.

In general, cytokines induce NOS2 in human cell lines in vitro through transcriptional upregulation of the gene (31,34,35). Induction of NOS2 expression varies in different human cell types, but typically is increased by multiple cytokines (5,10,34,35), among which IFNγ is required for its induction. The majority of studies on the regulation of NOS2 expression in lung cells are based on the human lung adenocarcinoma cell line, A549. The effect of cytokines on human NOS2 mRNA was evaluated in A549 cells incubated with various combinations of IL-1β, TNFα, and IFNγ. The combination of IL-1β, TNFα, and IFNγ leads to maximal NOS2 induction in the A549 (10,46).

Prior work has also emphasized the importance of activator protein-1 (AP-1)–binding sites in activation of NOS2 promoter in response to cytokine combinations (34,46). Studies suggest that NF-κB activation and binding to κB DNA elements in the 5′-flanking region of the NOS2 gene play a role in the cytokine induction of NOS2 in A549 in vitro (35). Recently, inducibility of the NOS2 promoter by IFNγ or cytokines including TNFα, IFNγ, and IL-1β in A549 cells was shown to be dependent upon a 665 bp region at 4909 bp upstream of the transcription start site of the human NOS2 gene (Fig. 1). Multiple cytokine-binding sites are present in the nucleotide sequence from −5574 to −4909 bp of the NOS2 promoter (Fig. 1). Based on the consensus sequence TTN_5AA (44), this region contains two putative IFNγ activation sites termed GAS, two consensus-binding sites (TGANTCA) for AP-1 (46,47), and two consensus-binding sites (GGGRNWYYCC) for NF-κB (46,48). Exactly or partially matched sequences to γ-IRE, NF-IL6, IRF-E, and X box are also present.

Cooperative DNA binding of proteins usually involves regions in close proximity, which functionally represent a composite regulatory element (49,50). The 665 bp region of NOS2 contains several sites which may serve as composite binding elements, i.e., the 100 bp region encompassing a GAS and an AP-1 site. We have shown that NOS2 gene expression appears to require a physical interaction between c-Fos, a component of AP-1, and STAT-1 to participate in cooperative transcriptional

```
-5574   gcctccctt tctctgtctc acttcctcat tcccctcctg atgtcccctg cacttcccag

-5515   atacactact tgcccctgaa tcttgcccct tgaaccatca caccctggga ctaccccagg
                                                           NF-κB
-5455   tgccactctg tttgttgttt ctccgcctag aaggacgggc acccaggaag caaaacggga

-5395   gggcagggaa gggagggtgt tctggggagg cttgacaaga aacgaggctt ttaaaagaaa
                                                            GAS
-5335   cagcagcaaa gtgccaggcc tgcaccagcc agcttgagtc acactccagg gactcagcaa
                                            AP-1
-5275   agcttgtcca ccttcctggt ccaccctggg cctgtccatc ctggagtgac caccgggcgt
                                                                 NF-κB
-5215   ttccagtaaa aatcccttca cttcacttcc gtcatctccg agtcaggcaa ggtggtggaa
        GAS
-5155   accggggaag acctcagctt cggagctgct ggaatttgtg tgactcacgc cctccagtgg
                                                       AP-1
-5095   tcacttgaca aatgacatag ggctcacggt ctggggactt gagcttgtta gggcctcaga

-5035   accgggaggg tcccaggaat gcctcttctc aatgccttcc tttgacagct gagtggagtg

-4975   aaggccccac aggacacgtg actcgccacg ggacatgcac acacacaaat agagagtaag

-4915   agccacg
```

Figure 1   The nucleotide sequence of the 5′-flanking region of human NOS2 gene from −5574 to −4909bp (GenBank accession number AF017634). This 665bp region contains putative sequences for GAS (boxed), AP-1 (double straight underline), and NF-κB (double wavy underline).

activation of the gene. Electrophoretic mobility shift assays using extracts from A549 cells stimulated with cytokines including IFNγ, IL-1β, and TNFα demonstrate interaction of the DNA-binding proteins STAT-1 and c-Fos (Figs. 2,3).

VI. Viral Mechanisms of Airway Inflammation and Increased NO

Respiratory virus infection causes significant morbidity and mortality in human populations worldwide with a broad spectrum of clinical responses ranging from asymptomatic infection to rhinitis to viral pneumonia. Although factors dictating the severity of virus disease are complex, interaction between inherent viral properties and host cellular response ultimately determines disease outcome (51,52). The first site of viral contact with the host and main target of infection and inflammation is the airway mucosal epithelium. Epithelial cells at the airway mucosal surface have a variety of inflammatory and immune defense mechanisms to deal with virus, including expression of cytokines with chemoattractant and proinflammatory functions (53–56), e.g., NOS2 (55,57).

NO produced by NOS2 has potent antiviral activity against a number of viruses (58–62). However, NO also contributes to inflammation and injury through formation of toxic reactive nitrogen intermediates (55,57,63). In this context, development

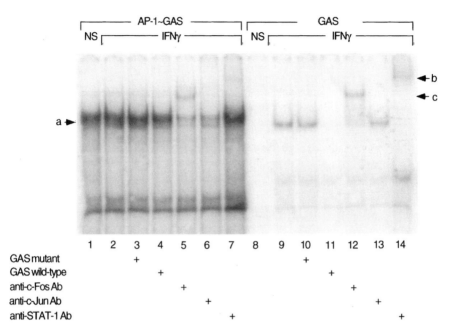

	1	2	3	4	5	6	7	8	9	10	11	12	13	14
GAS mutant			+							+				
GAS wild-type				+							+			
anti-c-Fos Ab					+							+		
anti-c-Jun Ab						+							+	
anti-STAT-1 Ab							+							+

Figure 2 Identification of the NOS2 AP-1 and GAS-binding proteins in A549 cells by electrophoretic mobility shift assays (EMSA). WCE from A549 nonstimulated (NS, lanes 1 and 8) or stimulated with IFNγ for 30 min (lanes 2–7 and 9–14) were analyzed for DNA-binding activity by EMSA using radiolabeled oligonucleotides AP-1 ~ GAS or GAS. The specificity of the binding complex (arrow a) was assessed by the addition of a 100-fold molar excess of unlabeled wild-type (lanes 4 and 11) or mutant GAS oligonucleotides (lanes 3 and 10) prior to incubation with the labeled probe. Supershift of the complex with anti-c-Fos (lanes 5, 12; arrow c) and anti-STAT-1 (lanes 7, 14; arrow b) polyclonal Ab added to binding reaction revealed that STAT-1 and c-Fos were present in the binding complexes. Supershift of the binding complex with anti-c-Jun was noted in EMSA using the AP-1 ~ GAS oligonucleotide (lane 6).

of pneumonia in a murine model of influenza infection has been linked to host NOS2 expression (57,64).

NOS2 is induced in airway epithelium by common respiratory viruses, including influenza, parainfluenza, and respiratory syncytial virus. NOS2 induction occurs in the course of viral infection in part due to IFNγ, but early in infection gene expression is induced by the viral replicative intermediate double-stranded RNA (dsRNA) through the dsRNA-activated protein kinase (PKR) (65). In support of this, NOS2 gene expression in human airway epithelial cells occurs in response to influenza A virus or synthetic dsRNA in vitro. Specifically, dsRNA leads to rapid activation of PKR, followed by activation of signaling components including NF-κB and IRF-1.

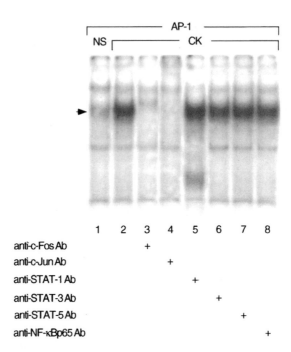

Figure 3 Identification of the NOS2 AP-1–binding proteins in A549 by EMSA. EMSA of WCE from A549 nonstimulated (lane 1) or stimulated with CK 3h (lanes 2–8) using radiolabeled AP-1 sequence. Anti-c-Fos, c-Jun, STAT-1, STAT-3, STAT-5, and NF-κBp65 polyclonal Ab were added to binding reactions to identify proteins in the binding complex (arrow). Anti-c-Fos (lane 3) and anti-c-Jun (lane 4) and perhaps anti-STAT-1 (lane 5) lead to supershift of the complex.

VII. Signal Transduction Through PKR

PKR is important for host antiviral mechanisms, as evidenced by impaired antiviral responses in mice with a homozygous targeted deletion in the PKR gene (24). First identified as a component of interferon-inducible cellular antiviral defenses, PKR exhibits two distinct kinase activities upon activation by dsRNA: autophosphorylation/activation and phosphorylation of substrates (66). One antiviral effect mediated by PKR is the phosphorylation of eukaryotic initiation factor-2a, effectively restricting viral protein translation and subsequent replication (66). In addition to effects on translation, PKR regulates transcriptional events by phosphorylation of proteins related to signal transduction pathways. For example, PKR is required for the activation of NF-κB in immortal cell lines in response to different stimuli (67). NF-κB activation by dsRNA in human airway epithelial cells is most likely due to PKR activation and phosphorylation of the inhibitor of NF-κB (IκB). Thus, PKR appears to mediate signal transduction in human airway epithelial cells in part through NF-κB. In addition, PKR may impact upon the signaling pathways through transcriptional and/or post-translational effects on IRF-1 (68). In fact, expression of IRF-1 protein in cells does not manifest functional DNA-binding activity unless a phosphorylation signal is provided (40), potentially by PKR (69,70). In support of this concept, IRF-1 protein is induced and activated by dsRNA in human airway epithelial cells.

PKR's role in signaling is essential for activation of NOS2, as assessed by experiments in murine embryo fibroblast cells (MEF) derived from mice with homozygous deletions for PKR. PKR contributes significantly to activation of signaling pathways, including NF-κB and IRF-1, which are important for proinflammatory gene expression such as NOS2 (68). Interestingly, PKR is also essential for LPS induction of NOS2 in murine cells, confirming a central role for PKR in microbial-induced signaling pathway to NOS2. On the other hand, continued NOS2 expression in PKR −/− cells exposed to a combination of IFNγ and LPS or poly IC, albeit at lower levels than in PKR +/+ cells, points out the possibility of inducible alternative signaling pathways to NOS2, which are independent of PKR (65).

VIII. Conclusion

Multiple mechanisms function coordinately to support NO synthesis in healthy airways and high-level NO synthesis in the inflamed airway. Human airway epithelium has abundant expression of NOS2 due to continuous transcriptional activation of the gene in vivo. Increased NOS2 gene expression in inflamed airways such as in asthma is associated with increased STAT-1 activation, perhaps related to increased cytokines. Viral-mediated airway NOS2 induction may occur in response to activation of PKR and downstream target signaling molecules. High levels of intracellular arginine may enhance enzyme reaction kinetics and drive NO synthesis. Importantly, multiple signal transduction pathways are specifically and coordinately activated in the airway in response to inflammation or infection, allowing cooperative transcriptional activation of the NOS2 gene. Thus, airway epithelial cells have highly efficient NO synthetic machinery, which is amplified in airway inflammation. Identification of the signaling pathways that lead to NOS expression reveal some of the underlying pathogenic mechanisms of inflammation, which may be targets for anti-inflammatory therapy in the future.

References

1. Palmer RM, Ferrige AG, Moncada S. Nitric oxide release accounts for the biological activity of endothelium-derived relaxing factor. Nature 1987; 327:524–526.
2. Ignarro LJ, Buga GM, Wood KS, Byrns RE, Chaudhuri G. Endothelium-derived relaxing factor produced and released from artery and vein is nitric oxide. Proc Natl Acad Sci USA 1987; 84:9265–9269.
3. Gaston B, Drazen JM, Loscalzo J, Stamler JS. The biology of nitrogen oxides in the airways. Am J Respir Crit Care Med 1994; 149:538–551.
4. Schmidt HH, Walter U. NO at work. Cell 1994; 78:919–925.

5. Nathan C. Nitric oxide as a secretory product of mammalian cells. FASEB J 1992; 6: 3051–3064.

6. Guo FH, Erzurum SC. Characterization of inducible nitric oxide synthase expression in human airway epithelium. Environ Health Perspect 1998; 106(suppl 5):1119–1124.

7. Stuehr DJ, Griffith OW. Mammalian nitric oxide synthases. Adv Enzymol Relat Areas Mol Biol 1992; 65:287–346.

8. Nathan C, Xie QW. Nitric oxide synthases: roles, tolls, and controls. Cell 1994; 78: 915–918.

9. Frandsen U, Lopez-Figueroa M, Hellsten Y. Localization of nitric oxide synthase in human skeletal muscle. Biochem Biophys Res Commun 1996; 227:88–93.

10. Guo FH, Uetani K, Haque SJ, et al. Interferon gamma and interleukin 4 stimulate prolonged expression of inducible nitric oxide synthase in human airway epithelium through synthesis of soluble mediators. J Clin Invest 1997; 100:829–838.

11. Nathan C, Xie QW. Regulation of biosynthesis of nitric oxide. J Biol Chem 1994; 269: 13725–13728.

12. Asano K, Chee CB, Gaston B, et al. Constitutive and inducible nitric oxide synthase gene expression, regulation, and activity in human lung epithelial cells. Proc Natl Acad Sci USA 1994; 91:10089–10093.

13. Kim N, Vardi Y, Padma-Nathan H, Daley J, Goldstein I, Saenz de Tejada I. Oxygen tension regulates the nitric oxide pathway. Physiological role in penile erection. J Clin Invest 1993; 91:437–442.

14. Shaul PW, Wells LB. Oxygen modulates nitric oxide production selectively in fetal pulmonary endothelial cells. Am J Respir Cell Mol Biol 1994; 11:432–438.

15. Dweik RA, Laskowski D, Abu-Soud HM, et al. Nitric oxide synthesis in the lung. Regulation by oxygen through a kinetic mechanism. J Clin Invest 1998; 101:660–666.

16. Barnes PJ, Belvisi MG. Nitric oxide and lung disease. Thorax 1993; 48:1034–1043.

17. Kobzik L, Bredt DS, Lowenstein CJ, et al. Nitric oxide synthase in human and rat lung: immunocytochemical and histochemical localization. Am J Respir Cell Mol Biol 1993; 9:371–377.

18. Guo FH, De Raeve HR, Rice TW, Stuehr DJ, Thunnissen FB, Erzurum SC. Continuous nitric oxide synthesis by inducible nitric oxide synthase in normal human airway epithelium in vivo. Proc Natl Acad Sci USA 1995; 92:7809–7813.

19. Dweik RA, Laskowski D, Ozkan M, Farver C, Erzurum SC. High levels of exhaled nitric oxide (NO) and NO synthase III expression in lesional smooth muscle in lymphangioleiomyomatosis. Am J Respir Cell Mol Biol 2001; 24:414–418.

20. Ischiropoulos H, Mendiguren I, Fisher D, Fisher AB, Thom SR. Role of neutrophils and nitric oxide in lung alveolar injury from smoke inhalation. Am J Respir Crit Care Med 1994; 150:337–341.

21. Giaid A, Saleh D. Reduced expression of endothelial nitric oxide synthase in the lungs of patients with pulmonary hypertension. N Engl J Med 1995; 333:214–221.

22. Kaneko FT, Arroliga AC, Dweik RA, et al. Biochemical reaction products of nitric oxide as quantitative markers of primary pulmonary hypertension. Am J Respir Crit Care Med 1998; 158:917–923.

23. Eissa NT, Yuan JW, Haggerty CM, Choo EK, Palmer CD, Moss J. Cloning and characterization of human inducible nitric oxide synthase splice variants: a domain, encoded by exons 8 and 9, is critical for dimerization. Proc Natl Acad Sci USA 1998; 95: 7625–7630.

24. Eissa NT, Strauss AJ, Haggerty CM, Choo EK, Chu SC, Moss J. Alternative splicing of human inducible nitric-oxide synthase mRNA, tissue-specific regulation and induction by cytokines. J Biol Chem 1996; 271:27184–27187.

25. Kurz S, Harrison DG. Insulin and the arginine paradox. J Clin Invest 1997; 99:369–370.
26. Hecker M, Sessa WC, Harris HJ, Anggard EE, Vane JR. The metabolism of L-arginine and its significance for the biosynthesis of endothelium-derived relaxing factor: cultured endothelial cells recycle L-citrulline to L-arginine. Proc Natl Acad Sci USA 1990; 87: 8612–8616.
27. Hammermann R, Hirschmann J, Hey C, et al. Cationic proteins inhibit L-arginine uptake in rat alveolar macrophages and tracheal epithelial cells. Implications for nitric oxide synthesis. Am J Respir Cell Mol Biol 1999; 21:155–162.
28. Baydoun AR, Emery PW, Pearson JD, Mann GE. Substrate-dependent regulation of intracellular amino acid concentrations in cultured bovine aortic endothelial cells. Biochem Biophys Res Commun 1990; 173:940–948.
29. Guo FH, Comhair SA, Zheng S, et al. Molecular mechanisms of increased nitric oxide (NO) in asthma: evidence for transcriptional and post-translational regulation of NO synthesis. J Immunol 2000; 164:5970–5980.
30. Saleh D, Ernst P, Lim S, Barnes PJ, Giaid A. Increased formation of the potent oxidant peroxynitrite in the airways of asthmatic patients is associated with induction of nitric oxide synthase: effect of inhaled glucocorticoid. FASEB J 1998; 12:929–937.
31. Geller DA, Nussler AK, Di Silvio M, et al. Cytokines, endotoxin, and glucocorticoids regulate the expression of inducible nitric oxide synthase in hepatocytes. Proc Natl Acad Sci USA 1993; 90:522–526.
32. Radomski MW, Palmer RM, Moncada S. Glucocorticoids inhibit the expression of an inducible, but not the constitutive, nitric oxide synthase in vascular endothelial cells. Proc Natl Acad Sci USA 1990; 87:10043–10047.
33. Kunz D, Walker G, Eberhardt W, Pfeilschifter J. Molecular mechanisms of dexamethasone inhibition of nitric oxide synthase expression in interleukin 1 beta-stimulated mesangial cells: evidence for the involvement of transcriptional and posttranscriptional regulation. Proc Natl Acad Sci USA 1996; 93:255–259.
34. Marks-Konczalik J, Chu SC, Moss J. Cytokine-mediated transcriptional induction of the human inducible nitric oxide synthase gene requires both activator protein 1 and nuclear factor kappaB-binding sites. J Biol Chem 1998; 273:22201–22208.
35. de Vera ME, Shapiro RA, Nussler AK, et al. Transcriptional regulation of human inducible nitric oxide synthase (NOS2) gene by cytokines: initial analysis of the human NOS2 promoter. Proc Natl Acad Sci USA 1996; 93:1054–1059.
36. Lowenstein CJ, Alley EW, Raval P, et al. Macrophage nitric oxide synthase gene: two upstream regions mediate induction by interferon gamma and lipopolysaccharide. Proc Natl Acad Sci USA 1993; 90:9730–9734.
37. Xie QW, Whisnant R, Nathan C. Promoter of the mouse gene encoding calcium-independent nitric oxide synthase confers inducibility by interferon gamma and bacterial lipopolysaccharide. J Exp Med 1993; 177:1779–1784.
38. Xie QW, Kashiwabara Y, Nathan C. Role of transcription factor NF-Kappa B/Rel in induction of nitric oxide synthase. J Biol Chem 1994; 269:4705–4708.
39. Martin E, Nathan C, Xie QW. Role of interferon regulatory factor 1 in induction of nitric oxide synthase. J Exp Med 1994; 180:977–984.
40. Harada H, Fujita T, Miyamoto M, et al. Structurally similar but functionally distinct factors, IRF-1 and IRF-2, bind to the same regulatory elements of IFN and IFN-inducible genes. Cell 1989; 58:729–739.
41. Kamijo R, Harada H, Matsuyama T, et al. Requirement for transcription factor IRF-1 in NO synthase induction in macrophages. Science 1994; 263:1612–1615.

42. Uetani K, Arroliga ME, Erzurum SC. Double-stranded rna dependence of nitric oxide synthase 2 expression in human bronchial epithelial cell lines BET-1A and BEAS-2B. Am J Respir Cell Mol Biol 2001; 24:720–726.

43. Uetani K, Thomassen MJ, Erzurum SC. Nitric oxide synthase 2 through an autocrine loop via respiratory epithelial cell-derived mediator. Am J Physiol Lung Cell Mol Physiol 2001; 280:L1179–1188.

44. Haque SJ, Williams BR. Signal transduction in the interferon system. Semin Oncol 1998; 25:14–22.

45. Sampath D, Castro M, Look DC, Holtzman MJ. Constitutive activation of an epithelial signal transducer and activator of transcription (STAT) pathway in asthma. J Clin Invest 1999; 103:1353–1361.

46. Chu SC, Marks-Konczalik J, Wu HP, Banks TC, Moss J. Analysis of the cytokine-stimulated human inducible nitric oxide synthase (iNOS) gene: characterization of differences between human and mouse iNOS promoters. Biochem Biophys Res Commun 1998; 248:871–878.

47. Shaulian E, Karin M. AP-1 in cell proliferation and survival. Oncogene 2001; 20: 2390–2400.

48. Taylor BS, de Vera ME, Ganster RW, et al. Multiple NF-kappaB enhancer elements regulate cytokine induction of the human inducible nitric oxide synthase gene. J Biol Chem 1998; 273:15148–15156.

49. Chinenov Y, Kerppola TK. Close encounters of many kinds: Fos-Jun interactions that mediate transcription regulatory specificity. Oncogene 2001; 20:2438–2452.

50. Zhang X, Wrzeszczynska MH, Horvath CM, Darnell JE, Jr. Interacting regions in Stat3 and c-Jun that participate in cooperative transcriptional activation. Mol Cell Biol 1999; 19:7138–7146.

51. Garcia-Sastre A, Durbin RK, Zheng H, et al. The role of interferon in influenza virus tissue tropism. J Virol 1998; 72:8550–8558.

52. Kagnoff MF, Eckmann L. Epithelial cells as sensors for microbial infection. J Clin Invest 1997; 100:6–10.

53. Matsukura S, Kokubu F, Noda H, Tokunaga H, Adachi M. Expression of IL-6, IL-8, and RANTES on human bronchial epithelial cells, NCI-H292, induced by influenza virus A. J Allergy Clin Immunol 1996; 98:1080–1087.

54. Zhu Z, Tang W, Ray A, et al. Rhinovirus stimulation of interleukin-6 in vivo and in vitro. Evidence for nuclear factor kappa B-dependent transcriptional activation. J Clin Invest 1996; 97:421–430.

55. Tanaka K, Nakazawa H, Okada K, Umezawa K, Fukuyama N, Koga Y. Nitric oxide mediates murine cytomegalovirus-associated pneumonitis in lungs that are free of the virus. J Clin Invest 1997; 100:1822–1830.

56. Hayden FG, Fritz R, Lobo MC, Alvord W, Strober W, Straus SE. Local and systemic cytokine responses during experimental human influenza A virus infection. Relation to symptom formation and host defense. J Clin Invest 1998; 101:643–649.

57. Akaike T, Noguchi Y, Ijiri S, et al. Pathogenesis of influenza virus-induced pneumonia: involvement of both nitric oxide and oxygen radicals. Proc Natl Acad Sci USA 1996; 93:2448–2453.

58. Karupiah G, Xie QW, Buller RM, Nathan C, Duarte C, MacMicking JD. Inhibition of viral replication by interferon-gamma-induced nitric oxide synthase. Science 1993; 261: 1445–1448.

59. Croen KD. Evidence for antiviral effect of nitric oxide. Inhibition of herpes simplex virus type 1 replication. J Clin Invest 1993; 91:2446–2452.

60. Mannick JB, Asano K, Izumi K, Kieff E, Stamler JS. Nitric oxide produced by human B lymphocytes inhibits apoptosis and Epstein-Barr virus reactivation. Cell 1994; 79: 1137–1146.

61. Fang FC. Perspectives series: host/pathogen interactions. Mechanisms of nitric oxide-related antimicrobial activity. J Clin Invest 1997; 99:2818–2825.

62. Zaragoza C, Ocampo CJ, Saura M, McMillan A, Lowenstein CJ. Nitric oxide inhibition of coxsackievirus replication in vitro. J Clin Invest 1997; 100:1760–1767.

63. Adler H, Beland JL, Del-Pan NC, et al. Suppression of herpes simplex virus type 1 (HSV-1)-induced pneumonia in mice by inhibition of inducible nitric oxide synthase (iNOS, NOS2). J Exp Med 1997; 185:1533–1540.

64. Karupiah G, Chen JH, Mahalingam S, Nathan CF, MacMicking JD. Rapid interferon gamma-dependent clearance of influenza A virus and protection from consolidating pneumonitis in nitric oxide synthase 2-deficient mice. J Exp Med 1998; 188:1541–1546.

65. Uetani K, Der SD, Zamanian-Daryoush M, et al. Central role of double-stranded RNA-activated protein kinase in microbial induction of nitric oxide synthase. J Immunol 2000; 165:988–996.

66. Meurs E, Chong K, Galabru J, et al. Molecular cloning and characterization of the human double-stranded RNA-activated protein kinase induced by interferon. Cell 1990; 62:379–390.

67. Kumar A, Haque J, Lacoste J, Hiscott J, Williams BR. Double-stranded RNA-dependent protein kinase activates transcription factor NF-kappa B by phosphorylating I kappa B. Proc Natl Acad Sci USA 1994; 91:6288–6292.

68. Kumar A, Yang YL, Flati V, et al. Deficient cytokine signaling in mouse embryo fibroblasts with a targeted deletion in the PKR gene: role of IRF-1 and NF-kappaB. Embo J 1997; 16:406–416.

69. Watanabe N, Sakakibara J, Hovanessian AG, Taniguchi T, Fujita T. Activation of IFN-beta element by IRF-1 requires a posttranslational event in addition to IRF-1 synthesis. Nucleic Acids Res 1991; 19:4421–4428.

70. Kirchhoff S, Koromilas AE, Schaper F, Grashoff M, Sonenberg N, Hauser H. IRF-1 induced cell growth inhibition and interferon induction requires the activity of the protein kinase PKR. Oncogene 1995; 11:439–445.

10

Regulation of Nitric Oxide Synthesis by Inducible Nitric Oxide Synthase

PAWEL KOLODZIEJSKI and N. TONY EISSA

Baylor College of Medicine
Houston, Texas, U.S.A.

Nitric oxide (NO), a noxious unstable gas, a byproduct of automobile exhaust, electric power stations, and lighting, has been discovered in the human body to be a crucial participant in a multitude of functions ranging from signal transduction, neurotransmission, vasodilatation, protein modification, and host defense to inflammation (1,2). Since that discovery in 1987, there has been almost unprecedented intense interest in studying NO roles and regulation. That interest has resulted in thousands of scientific articles and a Nobel prize award for the discovery. Rather than attempting an exhaustive review of the literature, this chapter provides a brief overview of how inducible nitric oxide synthase (iNOS) is regulated, with special emphasis on opportunities for therapeutic strategies targeting iNOS.

I. Nitric Oxide: The Mouse That Roars

The best known mechanism of action of NO is through its binding to the heme moiety of guanelyl cyclase leading to an increase in cGMP levels that is responsible for NO vasodilator effect. However, this mechanism does not account for many effector functions for NO that have become known as cGMP-independent mechanisms (3). How does such a small short-lived molecule exert so many functions? Several explanations are proposed to explain this phenomenon. They include the production by NO at different sites inside the cell, by different cell types, and by different nitric oxide synthase (NOS) isoforms. But the most compelling argument for the diversity of NO functions stems from its ability to link to proteins, a process known as nitrosylation. Nitrosylation of proteins modifies their functions and allows NO "function" to be transferred well beyond its point of synthesis (4,5).

II. Nitric Oxide Synthases

Nitric oxide is synthesized from L-arginine by NOS isoforms (Fig. 1). The reaction catalyzed by NOS utilizes L-arginine as a substrate and requires molecular oxygen and reducing equivalents in the form of NADPH. The products of the reaction are NO and citrulline (6). As a signaling molecule, NO is produced by two constitutive calcium (Ca^{2+})-dependent isoforms, neuronal NOS (nNOS or NOS1) and endothelial NOS (eNOS or NOS3) (Table 1). Ca^{2+}-activated calmodulin (CaM) binds to and transiently activates constitutive NOS dimers. Due to the transient nature of elevated Ca^{2+} levels, the activity of NO produced is short-lived. As an agent of inflammation and cell-mediated immunity, NO is produced by a Ca^{2+}-independent cytokine-inducible NOS (iNOS or NOS2) (6–8). Calmodulin is tightly bound to iNOS even at basal Ca^{2+} levels (9), and therefore iNOS is notably distinguished from the constitutive isoforms by its prolonged production of a relatively large amount of NO. The high output production of NO is suited for iNOS function as a host-defense agent. However, it has become clear that the high output production of NO is also responsible for its cytotoxicity (10).

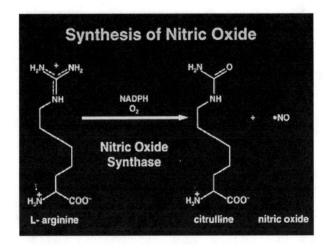

Figure 1   The reaction catalyzed by NOS. L-Arginine is converted to cirtulline and NO. The nitrogen atom in NO is derived from L-arginine. The reaction requires molecular oxygen and reducing equivalents in the form of NADPH. (From Ref. 15.)

Table 1   Human NOS Isoforms

Enzyme type	Expression	Gene locus	Molecular mass	Ca^{2+}
NOS1	Constitutive	12	150	Yes
NOS2	Inducible	17	131	No
NOS3	Constitutive	7	135	Yes

III. Nitric Oxide Synthesis by iNOS

The human iNOS gene, containing 26 exons, encodes a protein of 131 kDa (Fig. 2) (11,12). Like other NOSs, iNOS protein has three domains: (1) an amino-terminal oxygenase domain (residues 1–504) that binds heme, tetrahydrobiopterin (H_4B), and L-arginine and forms the active site where NO synthesis takes place; (2) a carboxy-terminal reductase domain (residues 537–1153) that binds FMN, FAD, and NADPH; and (3) an intervening CaM-binding domain (residues 505–536) that regulates electron transfer between the oxygenase and reductase domains (6,8). During NO synthesis the reductase flavins acquire electrons from NADPH and transfer them to the heme iron, which permits them to bind and activate O_2 and catalyze NO synthesis.

For the synthesis of NO, similar to other NOS isoforms, iNOS is active only as a homodimer in which the subunits align in a head-to-head manner, with the oxygenase domains forming a dimer and the reductase domains existing as independent monomeric extensions (13). The presence of the substrate L-arginine and the cofactors heme and H_4B promotes dimer formation by iNOS, but whether or not any of these agents is absolutely required for iNOS dimerization in vivo is not yet clear (13,14). Residues involved in binding of heme (Cys^{200}) (15), L-arginine (Glu^{377}) (16), and H_4B (Gly^{456}, Ala^{459}) (17) have been determined. However, the mechanism of dimer formation/dissociation, the exact requirements of dimerization, and the roles of cofactors and critical residues involved remain to be elucidated.

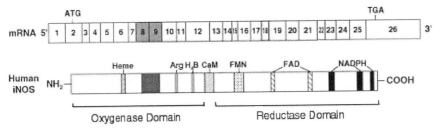

Figure 2   A diagram of iNOS and the exon-structure of the mRNA with the putative cofactor binding sites for heme, L-arginine, H_4B, CaM, FMN, FAD, and NADPH. The domain encoded by exons 8–9 is highlighted.

IV. Nitric Oxide in the Lung

The lungs contain many cell types that express one or more NOS isforms. Of particular interest is the "constitutive" expression of iNOS in airway epithelial cells (18,19).
When airway epithelial cells are removed and cultured in vitro iNOS expression is
rapidly lost (19). The cause for this loss has been partially explained by the presence
of in vivo factors that are required to maintain the expression (20,21). Additionally,
it could be related to loss of the differentiation state of epithelial cells. It has been
shown that iNOS expression is related to the cell state of differentiation. In airway
epithelial cells cultured in vitro on air–liquid interface, differentiation into mucus
phenotype was associated with spontaneous expression of iNOS (22). In all cases,
when airway epithelial cells are stimulated by cytokines, they produce much higher
levels of iNOS than their baseline (20–22).

The cytokine most critical in human iNOS induction in airways is interferon
(IFN)-γ. Synergism is provided with tumor necrosis factor (TNF)-α and interleukin
(IL)-1β. This synergism is believed to be due to a physical interaction between the
transcription factors IRF-1 and NFκB (23). In addition, STAT-1 activation by IFN-
γ is needed for maximal induction of iNOS (24). Other transcription factors involved
in iNOS induction include AP-1 and nuclear factor interleukin-6 (25,26). Depending
on the stimulus of iNOS induction, different upstream signaling pathways are involved. Janus kinases, Raf-protein kinase, mitogen-activated protein kinase, and
protein kinase C increase iNOS transcription, whereas phosphoinositide-3-kinase
and protein tyrosine phosphatase inhibit iNOS transcription (25–27). Although iNOS
is markedly upregulated in asthma, cytokines that favor the asthma Th2 response
do not seem responsible for iNOS induction. To the contrary, iNOS induction is
inhibited by IL-10 and IL-13 (28–30). Nevertheless, levels of IFN-γ are elevated
in asthmatic subjects compared to normals, and in both cases they increases in
response to segmental allergen challenge (31).

While iNOS is readily induced in murine macrophages, its expression in human
macrophages is controversial. Although iNOS has been found in human macrophages
during infection or inflammation, it has been difficult to demonstrate any functional
activity for iNOS in human macrophages either in vitro on in vivo (26,32). Some
of the difference has been suggested to be that, unlike mouse and rat macrophages,
human macrophages do not synthesize the iNOS cofactor H_4B. The differences
among species are not limited to human and mouse macrophages. Caprine, lapine,
and porcine macrophages do not seem to generate NO, whereas bovine macrophages
do (32,33).

The endothelial NOS isoform is present predominantly in endothelial cells.
Since endothelial cells provide a large surface area of the lung, it is reasonable to
assume that endothelial NOS contribute to exhaled NO. Due to its large production
of NO, the inducible form, however, is accredited with the large contribution to
exhaled NO, particularly in conditions where iNOS is upregulated, such as in asthma
(31,34,35). The endothelial NOS is also present in epithelial cells and human macrophages (36–38). Its role in these cells is not yet established. The neuronal form has

been implicated in the pathogenesis of airway hyperreactivity in mouse experimental asthma (39).

V. Nitric Oxide and Airway Inflammation of Asthma

As elsewhere in the body, NO in the airways is implicated in nonspecific host defense against inhaled microbes. In addition, NO has been shown to affect ciliary beat frequency, mucus secretion, and plasma exudation (40). It has been recognized, however, that overproduction of NO by iNOS could cause tissue damage that outweighs its potential benefit for host defense (10,41). One such example is the surprising observation that genetic deficiency of iNOS substantially protects mice from death caused by influenza A virus. In this infection, the inflammatory response appears to be a more important cause of mortality than the cytopathic effects of the virus, and iNOS appears to contribute substantially to the inflammation (42).

Overproduction of NO by iNOS has been implicated in the pathogenesis of airway inflammation of asthma (31,43,44). It has been clearly shown that both exhaled NO and airway epithelial iNOS are increased in asthma (31,43). Further, their levels return towards normal after treatment with corticosteroids (31,43). In addition, the increase in iNOS in the airways of asthmatic patients was found to be associated with increased formation of peroxynitrite (44). Peroxynitrite, formed by the rapid reaction of NO with superoxide, is a strong oxidant that has been implicated in the nitrosylation of tyrosine residues on proteins, cytotoxic tissue injury, and DNA damage. It causes airway hyperresponsiveness and airway epithelial damage, enhances inflammatory cell recruitment, and inhibit pulmonary surfactant. Peroxynitrite may contribute to airway obstruction and hyperresponsiveness and epithelial damage in asthma and thus be responsible for the "collateral damage" caused by overproduction of NO by iNOS. Peroxynitrite in asthmatic airways was reduced following inhibition of iNOS with corticosteroid treatment (44). Therefore, reduction of NO and peroxynitrite production in asthma can be achieved by targeting iNOS.

In addition to airway inflammation, overproduction of NO by iNOS has been implicated in the pathogenesis of other inflammatory syndromes, e.g., transplant rejection, inflammatory bowel disease, rheumatoid arthritis, and septic shock (10,41). Although iNOS upregulation may not be a primary event in all these diseases, the proinflammatory effects of iNOS contribute to their pathophysiology. Therefore, attenuation of iNOS, particularly in those disease where inflammation is not the consequence of infection such as in asthma, is potentially beneficial (10,41). Understanding the regulation of NO synthesis by iNOS is a prerequisite for strategies of modulating NO.

VI. Structural Diversity and Alternative Splicing of iNOS mRNA

Understanding how cells control the level of NO production is fundamental to efforts aimed at its regulation. In this context, in vivo regulation of NOSs, both transcriptional and post-translational, has been the subject of intensive investigation. The molecular diversity of iNOS mRNA generated by alternative splicing may represent one such regulation. We studied the transcription initiation sites and the structure of the 5′-untranslated region in the human iNOS gene. Despite the presence of a TATA box in the promoter region, multiple transcription initiation sites were observed upstream from the main TATA-directed initiation site. The TATA-independent iNOS mRNA transcripts were upregulated by cytokines. The 5′-untranslated region contains eight partially overlapping open reading frames upstream of the putative iNOS ATG, which may be involved in translational regulation of human iNOS mRNA (46).

We have also demonstrated that the human iNOS gene has the capacity to produce different isoforms by alternative splicing of its mRNA. Four sites of alternative splicing were identified; these included deletion of (1) exon 5, (2) exons 8 and 9, (3) exons 9, 10, and 11, and (4) exons 15 and 16. The deduced amino acid sequences of the iNOS splice variants cDNAs predict one truncated protein (resulting from exon 5 deletion) and three iNOS proteins with in-frame deletions. Analyses of mRNA from various human tissues were consistent with tissue-specific regulation of iNOS alternative splicing. In cultured cells, iNOS induction by cytokines was associated with an increase in alternatively spliced mRNA transcripts (47).

Since the four sites of alternative splicing result in deletion of conserved sequences, it is unlikely that any of these splice variants by themselves would be capable of generating NO. It seems more likely that alternative splicing may be involved in modifying the kinetics of NO synthesis or conferring new functions to NOS. Modulation of NO synthesis by alternatively spliced variants could be achieved through the formation of heterodimers. Lee et al. (48) demonstrated, by co-expression, that truncated mutants of endothelial NOS formed heterodimers with wild-type endothelial NOS and exerted a dominant negative effect on its activity. Since the cytochrome *c* reductase activity of the carboxyl terminus of iNOS is equivalent to that of full-length iNOS (13), the function of some of these variants could be similar to other cytochrome P-450 reductase proteins. A similar pattern of alternative splicing of mRNA with an in-frame deletion of 105 amino acids in the oxygenase domain has been reported for mouse and human neuronal NOS (49,50) as well as for NOS cloned from *Drosphila* (51). The presence of a conserved pattern of alternative splicing in vertebrates and flies among various NOSs suggests a common function for the resulting isoforms.

VII. Human iNOS Subdomain Encoded by Exons 8 and 9

Post-translational subunit dimerization of iNOS represents a potential critical locus for therapeutic interventions aimed at controlling its activity. Such a strategy would require understanding the specific requirements for iNOS dimerization. We have demonstrated that the subdomain encoded by exons 8 and 9 is critical for dimer formation and NO production (Fig. 2) (52). To identify the critical residues in the exon 8 and 9 subdomain for iNOS dimerization and NO synthesis, we performed alanine-scanning mutagenesis. Based on the crystal structures, 16 conserved amino acids, judged to be involved in catalytic activity and/or dimer formation, were selected for the analysis. Alanine was chosen because it eliminates the side chain without altering the main-chain conformation and it does not impose electrostatic or steric effects (53). The resulting iNOS mutants were characterized following their expression in the human embryonic kidney (HEK) 293 epithelial cell line, a line that does not express any NOS genes (15,52). The mutagenesis study identified four amino acids in the exon 8 and 9 subdomain to be critical for iNOS activity, three of which also influence dimerization. These residues are strictly conserved among all NOS isoforms and across species (54).

iNOS activity, measured by the enzyme ability to produce NO, reflects the presence of functional reductase and oxygenase domains. We hypothesized that the inability of the iNOS-Ala mutants to produce NO may reflect a defect in the oxygenase domain activity. Using an *E. coli* expression system, we produced, purified, and characterized wild-type iNOS and iNOS-Ala mutants. The functional integrity of the oxygenase domain was selectively tested by measuring the H_2O_2-supported oxidation of L-N^{ω}-hydroxy-L-Arg (55,56). We demonstrated that the iNOS mutants' inabilities to synthesize NO were due to selective defects in the oxygenase domain activity (57). Interestingly, deletion of exons 8 and 9 in human iNOS does not include substrate/cofactor binding, but it does include structural elements important for the global iNOS oxygenase fold. Deletions or point mutations within this subdomain can modulate the dimerization and heme function from a distal site.

VIII. Critical Role of Asp280 of Human iNOS in Substrate Binding and Subunit Interactions

Detailed characterization of the Asp280-Ala (iNOSD280A) mutant revealed that it retains a functional reductase domain, as measured by its ability to reduce cytochrome *c*. Gel permeation chromatography confirmed that the Asp280-Ala mutant exists as a dimer, but in contrast to wild-type iNOS, urea-generated monomers of the mutant fail to reassociate into dimers when incubated with L-Arg and H_4B, suggesting inadequate subunit interaction. In contrast to wild-type iNOS, which seems to exist in an equilibrium mixture of monomers and dimers, iNOSD280A is in a "locked" dimer position. These data suggest that replacing Asp280 with Ala brings a unique incorrigible defect in subunit interaction that results in an inactive dimmer (57).

Spectral analysis revealed that Asp280-Ala mutant does not bind L-Arg. This indicates that, in addition to dimerization, proper subunit interaction is required for substrate binding. Asp280 forms a hydrogen-bonding network with Arg 388 and residues Asp382 and Glu 377, which participate in substrate binding and the dimer interface (58,59). Thus, mutation of human Asp280 removes important buttressing hydrogen bonds for conserved residues that stabilize substrate binding. This mechanism of "remote control" destabilization results in impairment of substrate binding.

Moreover, Asp280 mutation to Ala adversely affects oxygenase subunit association The latter, by causing improper subunit interaction, lead to the assembly of a "defec-tive" dimer. Future studies will evaluate the utility of iNOSD280A as a potentia dominant negative iNOS mutant that may inactivate wild-type iNOS by forming locked and inactive heterodimers (57).

IX. iNOS Subcellular Localization

NO is a labile molecule that carries out important biological roles both within the cell in which it is synthesized as well as in interactions with nearby cells and mole-cules (60–62). Since NO may be either stabilized or degraded through its interactions with diverse intracellular or extracellular moieties, the localization of iNOS within the cell can influence the biological role and fate of the NO produced. Detailed studies of the subcellular localization of eNOS and nNOS provided much insight into the biological functions of these isoforms. eNOS is targeted, primarily by acyla-tion, to plasmalemmal caveolae (63). *N*-Myristoylation and cysteine palmitoylation influence eNOS membrane targeting as well (64,65). Mislocation of eNOS caused by mutation of the *N*-myristoylation or cysteine palmitoylation sites reduces enzyme activity, suggesting that intracellular targeting of eNOS is critical for NO production (66). Plasmalemmal caveolae serve as sites for the sequestration of signaling mole-cules, e.g. receptors, G proteins, and protein kinases. Targeting of eNOS to the caveolae may facilitate the activation of eNOS by establishing local environment in which NOS-coupled signaling molecules are in propinquity. Although nNOS was first characterized from neuronal tissues as a soluble (cytosolic) protein, it is now clear that it is localized in specialized postsynaptic densities (67). The membrane localization is due to the amino-terminal PDZ/GLGF motif that mediates protein-protein interactions with the postsynaptic density proteins PSD-95 and PSD-93. In skeletal muscles sarcolemma, nNOS undergoes an important association with the cytoskeletal dystrophin complex, and there is selective loss of sarcolemmal nNOS in Duchenne muscular dystrophy transgenic mice lacking the endogenous dystrophin gene (68).

In contrast to other NOS isoforms, most studies on iNOS have dealt with the biochemical characterization of purified soluble iNOS (8). A significant portion of iNOS, however, seems to reside in the subcellular particulate (membrane) fraction. Whereas iNOS isolated from rat neutrophils (69) or transformed macrophages (70) is primarily cytosolic, approximately 25% of the iNOS in the murine macrophage cell line RAW264.7 (71) and 40% of iNOS isolated from primary mouse peritoneal macrophages are membrane associated (72). In the latter cells, iNOS is present in intracellular vehicles, possibly reflecting a locale for NO-dependent killing of opsonized intracellular microorganisms. Alternatively, localization of iNOS may compartmentalize enzyme near critical substrates or cofactors. It remains to be estab-lished if iNOS is similarly targeted in other cells, e.g., epithelial cells. Generally, there seems to be a greater membrane association for human iNOS. In human neutro-phils, >90% of iNOS is tightly membrane-associated and exists in perinuclear distribution (73). Our studies suggest that human iNOS is present in both soluble and particulate fraction of human embryonic kidney (HEK) 293 epithelial cells expressing exogenous human iNOS (52; unpublished observations).

X. iNOS Inhibitors

The use of selective inhibitors of iNOS has been advocated as a novel therapeutic approach for several inflammatory diseases, including asthma (41,74). Inhibition of the activity of an enzyme can be accomplished by inhibition of its synthesis, inhibition of its catalytic activity, or acceleration of its degradation. Inhibition of iNOS synthesis can be done using corticosteroids (6,10). However, corticosteroid effects are not specific to iNOS, and their long-term use is associated with various side effects. The catalytic activity of iNOS can be inhibited using L-arginine analog (41,75). A prototype of a commonly used such inhibitor is N^w-nitro-L-arginine methyl ester (L-NAME). However, a major difficulty in the use of these compounds is their lack of specificity for the iNOS isoform. Because of the undesirable side effects associated with inhibition of the other NOS isoforms, much effort has been expended in the search for selective inhibitors of iNOS. Amidine-containing substrate analog form a "second generation" of iNOS inhibitors, and they include S-ethylisothiourea ($K_i = 14.7$ nM) and 2-amino-5,6-dihydro-6-methyl-4H-1,3-thiazine ($K_i = 4.2$ nM) (76). Although they are more potent than first generation inhibitors, they are only slightly selective for iNOS. A "third generation" of iNOS inhibitors are represented by heme ligands. The presence of heme in the NOS active site and its critical function in NOS catalysis led to the discovery of heme-binding imidazole-containing compounds as NOS inhibitors. Screening of an encoded combinatorial chemical library, designed based on a structurally related series of compounds of a pyrimidineimidazole core, resulted in the discovery of a class of allosteric potent and selective inhibitors of iNOS. The prototype compound of this class acts by binding to iNOS monomer's heme, where it occupies the active site in such a way that it grossly perturbs key structural elements and allosterically disrupts protein-protein interactions at the dimer interface (77). These compounds have no effect against already formed iNOS dimers, since they cannot gain access to the heme site in the dimer (77,78). Since dimerization is required for iNOS activity, these newly discovered allosteric inhibitors may make iNOS more vulnerable to degradation by altering its tertiary structure and thus preventing its dimerization.

XI. iNOS Degradation

It has been increasingly recognized that, in addition to mRNA transcription, cells titrate their gene expression using a sophisticated system of protein proteolysis (79,80). This degradation process thus has to be highly selective and tightly regulated. In recent years, major advances in our understanding of protein degradation led to several important drug developments, such as tissue plasminogen activator and protease inhibitors that selectively inhibit the HIV protease or angiotensin-converting enzyme. The degradation pathway and rate of protein turnover for any of the NOS isoforms are not well studied. Potentially, acceleration of iNOS degradation may prove to be an efficient approach for NO modulation, since the process of targeting cellular proteins for degradation is highly selective (79,81).

To determine the degradation pathway of iNOS, HEK293 cells with stable expression of human iNOS were incubated in the presence of various degradation pathway inhibitors. The 26S proteasome, a large multisubunit protease, is responsible for the selective degradation of a number of short-lived regulatory proteins whose activity must be tightly regulated, such as NF-κB, STAT-1, fos/jun, and cyclins. Treatment with the specific proteasomal inhibitor lactacystin resulted in accumulation of iNOS, indicating that these inhibitors blocked its degradation. Moreover, proteasomal inhibition blocked iNOS degradation when NO synthesis was inhibited by L-NAME. Furthermore, proteasonal inhibition blocked degradation of an iNOS splice variant that lacked capacity to dimerize and of an iNOS mutant that lacks L-arginine–binding ability, suggesting that iNOS is targeted by proteasomes, notwithstanding its capacity to produce NO, dimerize, or bind the substrate. Although our data suggest that the ability of iNOS to synthesize NO or to form dimers is not required for its targeting for degradation, they do not indicate whether or not inactive iNOS or iNOS monomer is preferentially targeted for degradation (82). In contrast to proteasomal inhibitors, the calpain inhibitor calpastain and lysosomal inhibitors E64, leupeptin, pepstatin A, chloroquine, and NH_4Cl did not lead to significant accumulation of iNOS. Thus, the proteasome is the primary degradation pathway for iNOS (82).

XII. Dichotomous Effect of Proteasomal Inhibition on Cytokine-Induced Human iNOS

NF-κB is a major transcription factor involved in the inducible expression of iNOS (25,83). Proinflammatory stimuli activate NF-κB through a tightly regulated cascade of phosphorylation, ubiquitination, and proteasomal proteolysis of a physically associated class of inhibitor molecules, the best characterized of which is IκBα. Therefore, proteasomal inhibitors block the degradation of already phosphorylated and ubiquitinated IκBα, thus aborting NF-κB activation (84,85). We hypothesized that the proteasome regulates iNOS on two distinct levels: at the transcriptional level, by degrading IκBα and thus activating NF-κB, and at the posttranslational level, by degrading iNOS protein. To test this hypothesis we used a cytokine mixture of IL-1β, TNF-α, and IL-6 to induce iNOS expression in RT4 cells, a human urinary bladder transitional cell papilloma cell line (47,86). Addition of proteasomal inhibitors 1 hour prior to cytokine stimulation prevented iNOS induction. The inhibitory effect on iNOS induction was due to inhibition of IκBα degradation (87). In contrast, proteasomal inhibitors added to RT4 cells 48 hours following cytokine induction of iNOS led to a dose-dependent accumulation of iNOS. Thus, there is a dichotomous effect of proteasomal inhibition on cytokine-induced human iNOS. Similar results were obtained using murine macrophage cell line RAW 264.7 stimulated by LPS to induce iNOS expression (7,47). These studies indicate that targeting iNOS to the proteasome occurs in both human and murine cells and it occurs independently of the mechanism of iNOS induction, e.g., by transfection (HEK293), cytokines (RT4), or LPS (RAW 264.7).

XIII. Role of Ubiquitination in iNOS Degradation

Ubiquitination is a well-established signal that targets proteins for degradation through either the proteosome pathway or the lysosomes (79,88). Degradation of a protein via the ubiquitin pathway involves two distinct steps: tagging the protein by covalent attachment of multiple ubiquitin molecules and degradation of the targeted protein with the release of free and to-be-reutilized ubiquitin. Initially, the C-terminal Gly of ubiquitin is activated to a high-energy thiol ester intermediate in a reaction catalyzed by the ubiquitin-activating enzyme, E1. Following activation, the E2 (ubiquitin-conjugating enzyme) transfers ubiquitin from E1 to the substrate that is bound to an ubiquitin-protein ligase, E3. An isopeptide bond is formed between the activated C-terminal Gly of ubiquitin and a Lys residue of the substrate. Release of ubiquitin (deubiquitination) is carried out by ubiquitin C-terminal hydrolases (isopeptidases) (79,81). Traditionally, it has been thought that all substrates of the proteasome pathway must be ubiquitinated as a prelude to their destruction. Detection of ubiquitinated proteins and their accumulation following proteosome inhibition have been the traditional criteria used to determine if a specific protein is degraded by the ubiquitin-proteasome system. However, recent studies revealed that some proteins, e.g., p21[Cip1], that are known to be ubiquitinated do not require ubiquitination prior to undergoing proteasomal degradation (89). These studies suggest that ubiquitination in these proteins may serve other functions rather than signaling proteolysis (90). These studies further illustrate that ubiquitination of a protein is insufficient to conclude that the protein degradation must proceed through a ubiquitinated intermediate. It is not known if the accumulated iNOS following proteasomal inhibition is ubiquitinated and whether or not ubiquitination of iNOS is required for its degradation. A role for ubiquitination in iNOS degradation is yet to be elucidated. In this context, future studies on iNOS degradation will need to address two key questions: (1) Is human iNOS ubiquitinated? and (2) Is iNOS ubiquitination required for its degradation? If the answer for both questions, turns out to be affirmative, the specific ubiquitin ligase (E3) that is responsible for iNOS ubquitination will need to be identified and characterized. Since the specificity of the ubiquitination process is dependent on the interaction between the ubiquitin ligase and the substrate, the E3 ubiquitin ligase specific for iNOS will be a major target for any efforts directed at modulation of iNOS degradation.

It has become clear that cells control the level of their gene expression, in part, through their control over protein degradation. Understanding the regulation of iNOS degradation will reveal how cells control the level of NO synthesis during inflammation and host defense. For instance, it has been already shown that in activated mouse peritoneal macrophages, enhancement of iNOS degradation partially contributes to the mechanisms of suppression of NO release by transforming growth factor-β (91). Recently, Fell-Bosco et al. reported that, in human colon carcinoma cells, caveolin-1 downregulates iNOS via the proteasome pathway (92). Potentially, acceleration of iNOS degradation may prove to be an efficient approach for NO modulation since the process of targeting cellular proteins for degradation is highly selective (79,80,93).

Acknowledgments

Supported by The American Lung Association, The Methodist Foundation, a T. T. Chao Scholar Award, and an award from the National Institutes of Health (5T32HL07747-08).

References

1. Lowenstein CJ, Dinerman JL, Snyder SH. Nitric oxide: A physiologic messenger. Ann Intern Med 1994; 120:227–237.

2. Palmer RM, Ferrige AG, Moncada S. Nitric oxide release accounts for the biological activity of endothelium-derived relaxing factor. Nature 1987; 327:524–526.

3. McDonald LJ, Murad F. Nitric oxide and cyclic GMP signaling. Proc Soc Exp Biol Med 1996; 211:1–6.

4. Stamler JS, Jaraki O, Osborne J, Simon DI, Keaney J, Vita J, Singel D, Valeri CR, Loscalzo J. Nitric oxide circulates in mammalian plasma primarily as an S-nitroso adduct of serum albumin. Proc Natl Acad Sci USA 1992; 89:7674–7677.

5. Gaston B, Reilly J, Drazen JM, Fackler J, Ramdev P, Arnelle D, Mullins ME, Sugarbaker DJ, Chee C, Singel DJ, Loscalzo J, Stamler JS. Endogenous nitrogen oxides and broncho-dilator S-nitrosothiols in human airways. Proc Natl Acad Sci USA 1993; 90: 10957–10961.

6. Marletta MA. Nitric oxide synthase: aspects concerning structure and catalysis. Cell 1994; 78:927–930.

7. Xie Q-W, Cho HJ, Calaycay J, Mumford RA, Swiderek KM, Lee TD, Ding A, Troso T, Nathan C. Cloning and characterization of inducible nitric oxide synthase from mouse macrophages. Science 1992; 256:225–228.

8. Stuehr DJ. Mammalian nitric oxide synthases. Biochim Biophys Acta 1999; 1411: 217–230.

9. Cho HJ, Xie QW, Calaycay J, Mumford RA, Swiderek KM, Lee TD, Nathan C. Calmodulin is a subunit of nitric oxide synthase from macrophages. J Exp Med 1992; 176: 599–604.

10. Nathan C. Inducible nitric oxide synthase: what difference does it make? J Clin Invest 1997; 100:2417–2423.

11. Geller DA, Lowenstein CJ, Shapiro RA, Nussler AK, Di Silvio M, Wang SC, Nakayama DK, Simmons RL, Snyder SH, Billiar TR. Molecular cloning and expression of inducible nitric oxide synthase from human hepatocytes. Proc Natl Acad Sci USA 1993; 90: 3491–3495.

12. Chartrain NA, Geller DA, Koty PP, Sitrin NF, Nussler AK, Hoffman EP, Billiar TR, Hutchinson NI, Mudgett JS. Molecular cloning, structure, and chromosomal localization of the human inducible nitric oxide synthase gene. J Biol Chem 1994; 269:6765–6772.

13. Ghosh DK, Stuehr DJ. Macrophage NO. synthase: characterization of isolated oxygenase and reductase domains reveals a head-to-head subunit interaction. Biochemistry 1995; 34:801–807.

14. Baek JK, Thiel BA, Lucas S, Stuehr DJ. Macrophage nitric oxide synthase subunits: purification, characterization, and role of prosthetic groups and substrate in regulating their association into a dimeric enzyme. J Biol Chem 1993; 268:21120–21129.

15. Xie Q-W, Leung M, Fuortes M, Sassa S, Nathan C. Complementation analysis of mutants of nitric oxide synthase reveals that the active site requires two hemes. Proc Natl Acad Sci USA 1996; 93:4891–4896.

16. Gachhui R, Gosh DK, Wu C, Parkinson J, Crane BR, Stuehr DJ. Mutagenesis of acidic residues in the oxygenase domain of inducible nitric-oxide synthase identifies a glutamate involved in arginine binding. Biochemistry 1997; 36:5097–5103.

17. Cho HJ, Martin E, Xie Q-W, Sassa S, Nathan C. Inducible nitric oxide synthase: identification of amino acid residues essential for dimerization and binding of tetrahydrobiopterin. Proc Natl Acad Sci USA 1995; 92:11514–11518.

18. Kobzik L, Bredt DS, Lowenstein CJ, Drazen J, Gaston B, Sugarbaker D, Stamler JS. Nitric oxide synthase in human and rat lung: immunocytochemical and histochemical localization. Am J Respir Cell Mol Biol 1993; 9:371–377.

19. Guo FH, De Raeve HR, Rice TW, Stuehr DJ, Thunissen FB. J. M, Erzurum SC. Continuous nitric oxide synthesis by inducible nitric oxide synthase in normal human airway epithelium in vivo. Proc Natl Acad Sci USA 1995; 92:7809–7813.

20. Guo FH, Uetani K, Haque SJ, Williams BR, Dweik RA, Thunnissen FB, Calhoun W, Erzurum SC. Interferon gamma and interleukin 4 stimulate prolonged expression of inducible nitric oxide synthase in human airway epithelium through synthesis of soluble mediators. J Clin Invest 1997; 100:829–838.

21. Uetani K, Thomassen MJ, Erzurum SC. Nitric oxide synthase 2 through an autocrine loop via respiratory epithelial cell-derived mediator. Am J Physiol Lung Cell Mol Physiol 2001; 280:L1179–1188.

22. Norford D, Koo JS, Gray T, Alder K, Nettesheim P. Expression of nitric oxide synthase isoforms in normal human tracheobronchial epithelial cells in vitro: dependence on retinoic acid and the state of differentiation. Exp Lung Res 1998; 24:355–366.

23. Saura M, Zaragoza C, Bao C, McMillan A, Lowenstein CJ. Interaction of interferon regulatory factor-1 and nuclear factor κB during activation of inducible nitric oxide synthase transcription. J Mol Biol 1999; 289:459–471.

24. Gao J, Morrison DC, Parmely TJ, Russell SW, Murphy WJ. An interferon-gamma-activated site (GAS) is necessary for full expression of the mouse iNOS gene in response to interferon-gamma and lipopolysaccharide. J Biol Chem 1997; 272:1226–1230.

25. Marks-Konczalik J, Chu SC, Moss J. Cytokine-mediated transcriptional induction of the human inducible nitric oxide synthase gene requires both activator protein 1 and nuclear factor k-B-binding sites. J Biol Chem 1998; 273:22201–22208.

26. Bogdan C. Nitric oxide and the immune response. Nat Immunol 2001; 2:907–916.

27. Kristof AS, Marks-Konczalik J, Moss J. Mitogen-activated protein kinases mediate activator protein-1-dependent human inducible nitric-oxide synthase promoter activation. J Biol Chem 2001; 276:8445–8452.

28. Berkman N, Robichaud A, Robbins RA, Roesems G, Haddad EB, Barnes PJ, Chung KF. Inhibition of inducible nitric oxide synthase expression by interleukin-4 and interleukin-13 in human lung epithelial cells. Immunology 1996; 89:363–367.

29. Wright K, Ward SG, Kolios G, Westwick J. Activation of phosphatidylinositol 3-kinase by interleukin-13. An inhibitory signal for inducible nitric-oxide synthase expression in epithelial cell line HT-29. J Biol Chem 1997; 272:12626–12633.

30. Berkman N, Robichaud A, Robbins RA, Roesems G, Haddad EB, Barnes PJ, Chung KF. Inhibition of inducible nitric oxide synthase expression by interleukin-4 and interleukin-13 in human lung epithelial cells. Immunology 1996; 89:363–367.

31. Guo FH, Comhair SAA, Zheng S, Dweik RA, Eissa NT, Thomassen MJ, Calhoun W, Erzurum SC. Molecular mechanisms of increased nitric oxide (NO) in asthma: evidence for transcriptional and post-translational regulation of NO synthesis. J Immunol 2000; 164:5970–5980.

32. Schneemann M, Schoedon G. Species differences in macrophage NO production are important; Bogdan C. Response. Nat Immunol 2002; 3:102.

33. Jungi TW, Adler H, Adler B, Thony M, Krampe M, Peterhans E. Inducible nitric oxide synthase of macrophages. Present knowledge and evidence for species-specific regulation. Vet Immunol Immunopathol 1996; 54:323–330.

34. Dweik RA, Laskowski D, Abu-Soud HM, Kaneko F, Hutte R, Stuehr DJ, Erzurum SC. Nitric oxide synthesis in the lung. Regulation by oxygen through a kinetic mechanism. J Clin Invest 1998; 101:660–666.

35. Steudel W, Kirmse M, Weimann J, Ullrich R, Hromi J, Zapol WM. Exhaled nitric oxide production by nitric oxide synthase-deficient mice. Am J Respir Crit Care Med 2000; 162:1262–1267.

36. Shaul PW, North AJ, Wu LC, Wells LB, Brannon TS, Lau KS, Michel T, Margraf LR, Star RA. Endothelial nitric oxide synthase is expressed in cultured human bronchiolar epithelium. J Clin Invest 1994; 94:2231–2236.

37. German Z, Chambliss KL, Pace MC, Arnet UA, Lowenstein CJ, Shaul PW. Molecular basis of cell-specific endothelial nitric-oxide synthase expression in airway epithelium. J Biol Chem 2000; 275:8183–8189.

38. Macrophages in lung tissue from patients with pulmonary emphysema express both inducible and endothelial nitric oxide synthase. Mod Pathol 1998; 11:648–655.

39. De Sanctis GT, MacLean JA, Hamada K, et al. Contribution of nitric oxide synthases 1, 2, and 3 to airway hyperresponsiveness and inflammation in a murine model of asthma. J Exp Med 1999; 189:1621–1630.

40. Gaston, Drazen JM, Loscalzo J, Stamler JS. The biology of nitrogen oxides in the airways. Am J Respir Crit Care Med 1994; 149:538–551.

41. Hobbs AJ, Higgs A, Moncada S. Inhibition of nitric oxide synthase as a potential therapeutic target. Annu Rev Pharamacol Toxicol 1999; 39:191–220.

42. Karupiah G, Chen J.-H., Mahalingam S, Nathan CF, MacMicking JD. Rapid Interferon-γ-dependent clearance of influenza A virus and protection from consolidating pneumonitis in nitric oxide synthase 2-deficient mice. J Exp Med 1998; 188:1541–1546.

43. Massaro AF, Mehta S, Lilly CM, Kobzik L, Reilly JJ, Drazen JM. Elevated nitric oxide concentrations in isolated lower airway gas of asthmatic subjects. Am J Respir Crit Care Med 1996; 153:1510–1514.

44. Saleh D, Ernst P, Lim S, Barnes PJ, Giaid A. Increased formation of the potent oxidant peroxynitrite in the airways of asthmatic patients is associated with induction of nitric oxide synthase: effect of inhaled glucocorticoid. FASEB J 1998; 12:929–937.

45. Baraldi E, Azzolin NM, Zanconato S, Dario C, Zaccheloo F. Corticosteroids decrease exhaled nitric oxide in children with acute asthma. J Pediatr 1997; 131:381–385.

46. Chu SC, Wu H.-P., Banks TC, Eissa NT, Moss J. Structural diversity in the 5'-untranslated region of cytokine-stimulated human inducible nitric oxide synthase mRNA. J Biol Chem 1995; 270:10625–10630.

47. Eissa NT, Strauss AJ, Haggerty CM, Choo EK, Chu SC, Moss J. Alternative splicing of human inducible nitric-oxide synthase mRNA: tissue-specific regulation and induction by cytokines. J Biol Chem 1996; 271:27184–27187.

48. Lee CM, Robinson LJ, Michel T. Oligomerization of endothelial nitric oxide synthase: evidence for a dominant negative effect of truncation mutants. J Biol Chem 1995; 270: 27403–27406.

49. Hall AV, Antoniou H, Wang Y, Cheung AH, Arbus AM, Olson SL, Lu WC, Kau C.-L., Marsden PA. Structural organization of the human neuronal nitric oxide synthase gene (NOS1). J Biol Chem 1994; 269:33082–33090.

50. Iwasaki T, Hori H, Hayashi Y, Nishino T, Tamura K, Oue S, Iizuka T, Ogura T, Esumi H. Characterization of mouse nNOS2, a natural variant of neuronal nitric-oxide synthase produced in the central nervous system by selective alternative splicing. J Biol Chem 1999; 274:17559–17566.

51. Regulski M, Tully T. Molecular and biochemical characterization of dNOS: a *Drosophila* Ca^{2+}/calmodulin-dependent nitric oxide synthase. Proc Natl Acad Sci USA 1995; 92:9072–9076.

52. Eissa NT, Yuan J, Haggerty CM, Choo EK, Moss J. Cloning and characterization of human inducible nitric oxide synthase splice variants: a domain, encoded by exons 8 and 9, is critical for dimerization. Proc Natl Acad Sci USA 1998; 95:7625–7630.

53. Cunningham BC, Wells JA. High-resolution epitope mapping of hGH-receptor interactions by alanine-scanning mutagenesis. Science 1989; 244:1081–1085.

54. Eissa NT, Haggerty CM, Palmer CD, Patton W, Moss J. Identification of residues critical for enzymatic activity in the domain encoded by exons 8 and 9 of the human inducible nitric oxide synthase. Am J Respir Cell Mol Biol 2001; 24:616–620.

55. Ghosh DK, Wu C, Pitters E, Moloney M, Werner ER, Mayer B, Stuehr DJ. Characterization of the inducible nitric oxide synthase oxygenase domain identifies a 49 amino acid segment required for subunit dimerization and tetrahydrobiopterin interaction. Biochemistry 1997; 36:10609–10619.

56. Pufahl RA, Wishnok JS, Marletta MA. Hydrogen peroxide-supported oxidation of NG-hydroxy-L-arginine by nitric oxide synthase. Biochemistry 1995; 34:1930–1941.

57. Ghosh DK, Rashid MB, Crane B, Taskar V, Mast M, Misukonis M, Weinberg JB, Eissa NT. Characterization of key residues, in the subdomain encoded by exons 8–9 of human inducible nitric oxide synthase: a critical role for Asp 280 in substrate binding and subunit interactions. Proc Natl Acad Sci USA 2001; 98:10392–10397.

58. Chen P.-F., Tsai A.-L., Berka V, Wu KK. Mutation of Glu-361 in human endothelial nitric-oxide synthase selectively abolishes L-arginine binding without perturbing the behavior of heme and other redox centers. J Biol Chem 1997; 272:6114–6118.

59. Crane BR, Arvai AS, Ghosh DK, Wu C, Getzoff ED, Stuehr DJ, Tainer JA. Structure of Nitric Oxide Synthase Oxygenase Dimer with Pterin and Substrate. Science 1998; 279:2121–2126.

60. Michel T, Feron O. Nitric oxide synthases: which, where, how, and why? J Clin Invest 1997; 100:2146–2152.

61. Barouch LA, Harrison RW, Skaf MW, Rosas GO, Cappola TP, Kobeissi ZA, Hobai IA, Lemmon CA, Burnett AL, O'Rourke B, Rodriguez ER, Huang PL, Lima JA, Berkowitz DE, Hare JM. Nitric oxide regulates the heart by spatial confinement of nitric oxide synthase isoforms. Nature 2002; 416:337–339.

62. Kanai AJ, Pearce LL, Clemens PR, Birder LA, VanBibber MM, Choi SY, de Groat WC, Peterson J. Identification of a neuronal nitric oxide synthase in isolated cardiac mitochondria using electrochemical detection. Proc Natl Acad Sci USA 2001; 98: 14126–14131.

63. Shaul PW, Smart EJ, Robinson LJ, German Z, Yuhanna IS, Ying Y, Anderson RGW, Michel T. Acylation targets endothelial nitric-oxide synthase to plasmalemmal caveolae. J Biol Chem 1996; 271:6518–6522.

64. Liu J, Sessa WC. Identification of covalently bound aminoterminal myristic acid in endothelial nitric oxide synthase. J Biol Chem 1994; 269:11691–11694.

65. García-Cardeña G, Oh P, Liu J, Schnitzer JE, Sessa WC. Targeting of nitric oxide synthase to endothelial cell caveolae via palmitoylation: implications for nitric oxide signaling. Proc Natl Acad Sci USA 1996; 93:6448–6453.

66. Sessa WC, García-Cardeña G, Liu J, Keh A, Pollock JS, Bradley J, Thiru S, Braverman IM, Desai KM. The Golgi association of endothelial nitric oxide synthase is necessary for the efficient synthesis of nitric oxide. J Biol Chem 1995; 270:17641–17644.

67. Brenman JE, Chao DS, Gee SH, McGee AW, Craven SE, Santillano DR, Wu Z, Huang F, Xia H, Peters MF, Froehner SC, Bredt DS. Interaction of nitric oxide synthase with the postsynaptic density protein PSD-95 and α1-syntrophin mediated by PDZ domains. Cell 1996; 84:757–767.

68. Brenman JE, Chao DS, Xia H, Aldape K, Bredt DS. Nitric oxide synthase complexed with dystrophin and absent from skeletal muscle sarcolemma in Duchenne muscular dystrophy. Cell 1995; 82:743–752.

69. Yui Y, Hattori R, Kosuga K, Eizawa H, Hiki S, Ohkawa S, Ohnishi K, Terao S, Kawai C. Calmodulin-independent nitric oxide synthase from rat polymorphonuclear neutrophils. J Biol Chem 1991; 266:3369–3371.

70. Stuehr DJ, Cho HJ, Kwon NS, Weise MF, Nathan CF. Purification and characterization of the cytokine-induced macrophage nitric oxide synthase: an FAD- and FMN-containing flavoprotein. Proc Natl Acad Sci USA 1991; 88:7773–7777.

71. Vodovotz Y, Russell D, Xie Q.-w., Bogdan C, Nathan C. Vesicle membrane association of nitric oxide synthase in primary mouse macrophages. J Immunol 1995; 154: 2914–2925.

72. Schmidt HH. H. W, Warner TD, Nakane M, Förstermann U, Murad F. Regulation and subcellular location of nitrogen oxide synthase in RAW264.7 macrophages. Mol Pharmacol 1992; 41:615–624.

73. Wheeler MA, Smith SD, García-Cardeña G, Nathan CF, Weiss RM, Sessa WC. Bacterial infection induces nitric oxide synthase in human neutrophils. J Clin Invest 1997; 99: 110–116.

74. Barnes PJ, Liew FY. Nitric oxide and asthmatic inflammation. Immunol Today 1995; 16:128–130.

75. Stuehr DJ, Griffith OW. Mammalian nitric oxide synthases. Adv Enzymol Relat Areas Mol Biol 1992; 65:287–346.

76. Nakane M, Klinghofer V, Kuk JE, Donnelly JL, Budzik GP, Pollock JS, Basha F, Carter GW. Novel potent and selective inhibitors of inducible nitric oxide synthase. Mol Pharmacol 1995; 47:831–834.

77. McMillan K, Adler M, Auld DS, Baldwin JJ, Blasko E, Browne LJ, Chelsky D, Davey D, Dolle RE, Eagen KA, Erickson S, Feldman RI, Glaser CB, Mallari C, Morrissey MM, Ohlmeyer MH, Pan G, Parkinson JF, Phillips GB, Polokoff MA, Sigal NH, Vergona R, Whitlow M, Young TA, Devlin JJ. Allosteric inhibitors of inducible nitric oxide synthase dimerization discovered via combinatorial chemistry. Proc Natl Acad Sci USA 2000; 97:1506–1511.

78. Blasko E, Glaser CB, Devlin JJ, Xia W, Feldman RI, Polokoff MA, Phillips GB, Whitlow M, Auld DS, McMillan K, Ghosh S, Stuehr DJ, Parkinson JF. Mechanistic studies with potent and selective inducible nitric-oxide synthase dimerization inhibitors. J Biol Chem 2002; 277:295–302.

79. Ciechanover A, Schwartz AL. The ubiquitin-proteasome pathway: the complexity and myriad functions of proteins death. Proc Natl Acad Sci USA 1998; 95:2727–2730.

80. Lee DH, Goldberg AL. Proteasome inhibitors: valuable new tools for cell biologists. Trends Cell Biol 1998; 8:397–403.

81. Hershko A, Ciechanover A. The ubiquitin system. Annu Rev Biochem 1998; 67: 425–479.

82. Musial A, Eissa NT. Inducible nitric oxide synthase is regulated by the proteasome degradation pathway. J Biol Chem 2001; 276:24268–24273.

83. Xie Q.-w., Kashiwabara Y, Nathan C. Role of transcription factor NF-kappa B/Rel in induction of nitric oxide synthase. J Biol Chem 1994; 269:4705–4708.

84. Gosh S, May M, Kopp E, NF-kB and Rel proteins: evolutionarily conserved mediators of immune responses. Annu Rev Immunol 1998; 16:225–260.

85. Karin M, Ben-Neriah Y. Phosphorylation meets ubiqitination: The control of NF-kB activity. Annu Rev Immunol 2000; 18:621–663.

86. Knour A, Krause SW, Rehli M, Kreutz M, Andreesen R. Human monocytes induce a carcinoma cell line to secrete high amounts of nitric oxide. J Immunol 1996; 157: 2109–2115.

87. Neish AS, Gewirtz AT, Zeng H, Young AN, Hobert ME, Karmali V, Rao AS, Madra JL. Prokaryotic regulation of epithelial responses by inhibition of I-κB-α ubiquitination. Science 2000; 289:1560–1563.

88. Hicke L. Getting' down with ubiquitin: turning off cell-surface receptors, transporters and channels. Trends Cell Biol 1999; 9:107–112.

89. Sheaff RJ, Singer JD, Swanger J, Smitherman M, Roberts JM, Clurman BE. Proteasomal turnover of p21^{Cip1} does not require p21^{Cip1} ubiquitination. Mol Cell 2000; 5:403–410.

90. Verma R, Deshaies RJ. A proteasome howdunit: the case of the missing signal. Cell 2000; 101:341–344.

91. Vodovotz Y, Bogdan C, Paik J, Xie Q.-w., Nathan C. Mechanisms of suppression of macrophage nitric oxide release by transforming growth factor beta. J Exp Med 1993; 178: 605–613.

92. Felley-Bosco E, Bender FC, Courjault-Gautier F, Bron C, Quest AFG. Caveolin-1 down-regulates inducible nitric oxide synthase via the proteasome pathway in human colon carcinoma cells. Proc Natl Acad Sci USA 2000; 97:14334–14339.

93. Wickner S, Maurizi MR, Gottesman S. Posttranslational quality control: folding, refolding, and degrading proteins. Science 1999; 286:1888–1893.

11

Novel Strategies for Selective Inhibition of Inducible Nitric Oxide Synthase

JOHN F. PARKINSON

Berlex Biosciences
Richmond, California, U.S.A.

I. Introduction

The presence of a high-output, cytokine-inducible nitric oxide synthase (iNOS) (Fig. 1) in cells of the immune system was defined during the late 1980s by Hibbs, Tannenbaum, Marletta, Stuehr, Nathan, and their colleagues (1–4). Since these pioneering efforts, the role of iNOS in the physiology and pathophysiology of the immune and other organ systems has been explored extensively using iNOS inhibitors of varying pharmacological specificity and also transgenic knockout (iNOS$^{-/-}$) mice. What has emerged from over a decade of intense academic and industrial research on iNOS is a large body of evidence that iNOS plays a pivotal role in the physiological responses of the immune system and in the pathogenesis of diverse acute and chronic immune disorders (5,6).

For many of these disorders, including septic and hemorrhagic shock, acute respiratory distress syndrome (ARDS), rheumatoid arthritis (RA), osteoarthritis (OA), inflammatory bowel disease (IBD), transplant allograft rejection, and asthma, there are high unmet clinical needs for new treatment modalities. These needs are manifold. There is a lack of efficacious and safe agents available to the clinician, e.g., for the treatment of septic shock and ARDS. Some diseases are resistant to available therapeutics such as nonsteroidal anti-inflammatory drugs (NSAID), e.g., OA and IBD. There are also concerns about short- and long-term drug side effects,

199

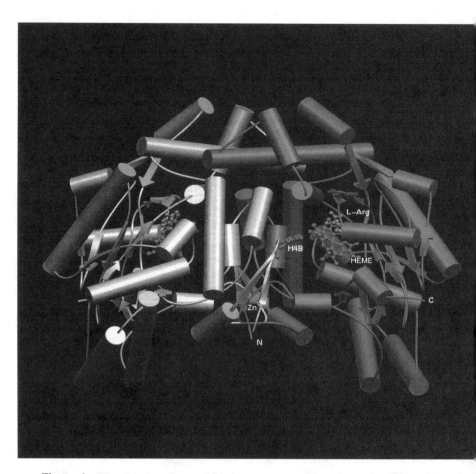

Figure 1 The crystal structure of human iNOS oxygenase domain. The figure shows the Cα trace of the oxygenase domain of human inducible nitric oxide synthase solved at 2.55 Å resolution (34). The monomer subunits of the oxygenase dimer are shown with α-helices presented as cylinders and β-strands as arrows. The heme prosthetic unit (HEME), cofactor tetrahydrobiopterin (H4B), and substrate L-arginine (L-Arg) are indicated. A zinc tetrathiolate center (ZnS_4) that promotes dimer stability is also shown at bottom center (Zn). The dimer interface comprises ~ 2800 $Å^2$.

particularly in children (e.g., asthma), but also in multidrug treatment regimens with complex drug-drug interactions (e.g., transplant rejection). A large investment has been made by the pharmaceutical industry to identify highly potent and selective iNOS inhibitors as novel therapeutics for the treatment of these diseases. This investment has been rewarded in recent years with substantial progress towards achieving this goal. Very specific pharmacological agents for inhibiting iNOS in vitro and in vivo are now available. These can be used to rigorously test "established" and new therapeutic concepts for iNOS inhibitors and also to explore the physiological functions of iNOS and hence the potential side effects for this novel class of drugs. The reader is referred to several reviews that cover first-generation and relatively nonselective iNOS inhibitors (7–10). The purpose of the current review is to assess the state of the art, with an emphasis on the most recent developments. Where possible, cross-reference will be made to in vivo studies on airway inflammation and lung physiology/pathophysiology that have been made with highly selective iNOS inhibitors. Where this is not possible, references will be provided to studies in other systems that are directly relevant, on a mechanistic basis, to the airway biologist.

II. Criteria for Establishing iNOS Selectivity

A. The Mythology of Selectivity

As reviewed extensively by Knowles and colleagues (10), there has been longstanding confusion regarding the "selectivity" of various classes of NOS inhibitors. This relates to both their NOS isoform selectivity and general pharmacological selectivity against other enzyme and receptor targets. For example, reference has been made to aminoguanidine as a "selective" iNOS inhibitor and to 7-nitroindazole as a "selective" neuronal NOS (nNOS) inhibitor. These compounds, however, have only minimal NOS isoform selectivity and cross-react with other pathways in vivo (10). The interpretation of results obtained with these and other less specific NOS inhibitors is thus highly problematic, and the perpetuation of this "selectivity" terminology needs better clarification.

B. Mechanism of Action: Slow-Binding and Rapidly Reversible Effects

Further confusion arises from the fact that different NOS inhibitor classes have different modes of action against the NOS isoforms that impact their selectivity ratio quite dramatically. In the case of several highly potent and selective iNOS inhibitors, it has become clear that optimization toward iNOS inhibition has yielded slow-binding, mechanism-based, irreversible or pseudo-irreversible iNOS inhibitors (10). The confusion arises due to the fact that these potent inhibitors are also rapidly reversible inhibitors of endothelial NOS (eNOS) and nNOS at higher concentrations. High-bolus doses of such compounds in vivo will likely lead to rapid eNOS and nNOS inhibition, with more selective inhibition of iNOS over time. The potential for profound local and possibly systemic eNOS and nNOS inhibition thus exists even when using a well-defined selective iNOS inhibitor, i.e., a selective iNOS inhibitor can have nonselective effects if used inappropriately. The investigator needs to be aware of these considerations in designing both in vitro and in vivo experiments with any given iNOS inhibitor such that the assignment of an observed function to iNOS and not to eNOS or nNOS can be made with confidence.

C. Cellular Permeability and Functional Selectivity

Another level of complexity arises from cellular permeability. Substrate-based L-arginine analog inhibitors of iNOS must enter cells in order to exert their effects. Many L-arginine analogs are polar molecules that are not expected to be readily cell-permeable. It is thus necessary to show that a potent and selective iNOS inhibitor identified at the enzyme assay level is also potent and selective against iNOS at the cellular level. The relationship between K_i for iNOS, eNOS, and nNOS inhibition in enzyme assays versus IC_{50} for NOS isoform inhibition in cells is an important criterion of selectivity.

NOS isoform inhibition can be measured in cells using measurements of NO release (e.g., NO metabolites in cell culture medium) or in cell lysates using the $[^{14}C]$-L-arginine to $[^{14}C]$-L-citrulline NOS activity assays. For the direct approaches, some convincing selectivity data have been generated in cell-based assays using recombinant NOS isoforms expressed in heterologous cells. This type of cellular selectivity data, however, is not reported for all iNOS inhibitor classes. For the functional approach, well-defined pharmacological assays, particularly in rodent systems, are available for each NOS isoform, but functional selectivity criteria are also lacking in some cases.

These are important parameters to consider under circumstances where multiple NOS isoforms are expressed in the same cell type or tissue. From a functional perspective, the problems to be confronted and the value of appropriate test systems can be illustrated by example. Let us consider aortic ring organ cultures treated in vitro with pro-inflammatory cytokines such as lipopolysaccharide (LPS), tumor necrosis factor alpha (TNFα), or interleukin-1β (IL-1β). In this setting it is well established that the endothelium is expressing both eNOS and iNOS and that the vascular smooth muscle is expressing iNOS. This is the basis for iNOS-dependent vascular dysfunction observed as hyporeactivity to contractile mediators such as phenylephrine (PE) (11–13) and is an in vitro correlate for iNOS-dependent severe hypotension in endotoxemia and sepsis (14,15). Thus a comparison of the vascular responses of normal to cytokine-treated vessels can be used rigorously to test the hypothesis that a given class of iNOS inhibitors truly has functional selectivity for iNOS versus eNOS. For a truly selective iNOS inhibitor the following functional selectivity criteria can be envisioned. In normal vessels, the IC_{50} for inhibition of basal and ACh-stimulated NO responses (eNOS) should be $>>IC_{50}$ for iNOS inhibition in a defined cell-based iNOS assay (selectivity ratio 1). In cytokine-treated vessels, the IC_{50} for inhibition of cytokine-induced PE hyporeactivity (iNOS) should be $\sim IC_{50}$ observed in the iNOS cell-based assay. Moreover, a selective iNOS inhibitor should normalize the vascular response to ACh (eNOS) and IC_{50} for nonselective inhibition of this response should be $>>IC_{50}$ for PE hyporeactivity (selectivity ratio 2). Ideally, selectivity ratio 1 = selectivity ratio 2.

The purpose of this exercise is to illustrate to the investigator that there are means by which the selectivity of iNOS inhibitors can be established using appropriate pharmacological assays for iNOS, eNOS, and nNOS function in vitro. This review will seek to highlight the inhibitor classes for which functional iNOS selectivity criteria have been established and are pharmacologically useful.

D. Evidence for In Vivo and Ex Vivo iNOS Selectivity

The next criterion to establish is iNOS selectivity in vivo or ex vivo. The simplest method for testing iNOS inhibition in vivo is the use of LPS-induced endotoxemia models in rodents (16,17). Bolus injection of LPS results in rapid induction of iNOS enzyme activity in multiple tissues (lung, liver, heart, kidney, small and large intestines, etc.) within approximately 3 hours (18). Expression of iNOS lasts up to 24 hours and is associated with large increases (10 to 20-fold) in circulating plasma/serum nitrite plus nitrate (NOx) levels from 6 to 18 hours. Plasma NOx levels are readily measured using modifications of the Griess reagent assay, and post-LPS measurement of this parameter at 6 hours is routinely used for assessing iNOS inhibition in vivo (16,17). The ED_{50} or IC_{50} in this assay for a given dose and route of administration (i.v., s.c., i.p., or p.o.) provides a measure of iNOS potency in vivo (mg/kg). The validity of this approach is that the percent inhibition of plasma NOx levels can be correlated directly to the percent inhibition of iNOS enzyme activity in organ homogenates ex vivo (18). For rapidly reversible iNOS inhibitors the ex vivo measurements are complicated by inhibitor washout during sample preparation, but the assay is more robust for the new generation of highly potent and selective iNOS inhibitors, which are slow binding and have high affinity for iNOS.

Establishing in vivo selectivity for iNOS versus eNOS and nNOS inhibition is more problematic (10). For nonselective eNOS inhibition, increase in mean arterial pressure has been used but is a less sensitive physiological readout for eNOS inhibition than other in vivo endpoints, such as systemic vascular resistance (10). More direct measurements of eNOS-dependent vascular reactivity can be made in vivo both in large and small vessel preparations but have rarely been used to establish in vivo iNOS selectivity criteria versus eNOS. Likewise, the effect of iNOS inhibitors on vascular reactivity in vessel preparations ex vivo is rarely reported.

For nNOS inhibition in vivo the situation is even less satisfactory. Gastric transit or emptying time has been used as an indicator of nNOS inhibition (19), but like blood pressure measurements for eNOS, this method suffers from lack of sensitivity and specificity. There are in vitro and in vivo preparations of specific and sensitive nNOS-mediated responses that can be used to establish iNOS versus nNOS selectivity, such as electrical field stimulation of the gastric fundus (20). However, the ED_{50} of selective iNOS inhibitors in such assays are not generally reported. An alternative to these functional assays is to measure the effect of selective iNOS inhibitors on nNOS enzyme activity in tissues ex vivo. This NOS isoform is distributed in selected tissues, and activity can be measured ex vivo in gastrocnemius muscle and specific brain areas such as cerebellum (21). Such assays have been used to establish that nonselective NOS inhibitors such as N^G-nitro-L-arginine methyl can lead to prolonged nNOS inhibition in vivo (22). This type of information could yield valuable information on the central nervous system (CNS) permeability of iNOS inhibitor classes and the potential for CNS side effects due to nNOS inhibition.

E. Evidence for General Pharmacological Selectivity

It is important to clarify what information is known about the nonspecific effects of selective iNOS inhibitor classes on other enzymatic and receptor pathways in vitro and their general tolerance and pharmacological specificity in vivo. This review will highlight where such information is available for the state-of-the-art iNOS inhibitors and can be used by the investigator to assess the suitability of each class for use in acute and chronic experiments.

F. Pharmacokinetic and Pharmacodynamic Considerations

There are many acute and chronic animal models with which to study the physiological and pathophysiological functions of iNOS in vivo. The investigator should thus have at hand relevant pharmacokinetic information on the plasma half-life, absorption, and oral availability, biodistribution, and clearance of selective iNOS inhibitors. The in vivo assays for iNOS in LPS-treated animals (plasma NOx) also provide a means to assess the onset and duration of action of these compounds, i.e., pharmacodynamic responses. For many nonselective NOS inhibitors that are frequently used, this type of information is generally completely lacking and has had to be established empirically in the laboratory. For the state-of-the-art selective iNOS inhibitors, due to the proprietary nature of this information a complete picture is not yet available but will be provided in this chapter wherever possible. The investigator should obtain this type of information from his or her industrial collaborator, as it is essential in the design of successful and convincing in vivo experiments.

G. Summary of iNOS Selectivity Criteria

This review will focus on iNOS inhibitors with proven in vitro selectivity for iNOS versus eNOS or nNOS with a selectivity ratio ~50 or higher (IC_{50} or K_i in enzyme assays). Frequently used nonselective iNOS inhibitors that do not meet this criterion include L-NAME, L-NMMA, aminoguanidine, and isothioureas. The profiles of these and many other first-generation iNOS inhibitors have been reviewed (7–9). These selectivity criteria also exclude a recently described highly potent cyclic amidine–based iNOS inhibitor ONO-1714 (23), which has shown some efficacy in bacterial sepsis–induced lung injury in mice (24) and hemodynamic endpoints in LPS-treated dogs (25). ONO-1714 has only 10-fold selectivity for iNOS versus eNOS in enzyme assays (23) and appears to have a narrow therapeutic range in vivo (24). In addition, no enzymatic or functional selectivity for iNOS versus nNOS has been reported.

In addition, the chapter will also focus on compounds that are useful for selective iNOS inhibition both in vitro *and* in vivo and which have met some or all of the following criteria:

iNOS versus eNOS and nNOS inhibition in enzyme assays: selectivity ratio > 50

iNOS versus eNOS and nNOS inhibition in cell-based assays: selectivity ratio > 10

Functional pharmacological iNOS selectivity in vitro: selectivity ratio > 10

Potency versus iNOS established in vivo

Selectivity versus eNOS and nNOS established in vivo or ex vivo

General pharmacological selectivity and in vivo tolerance defined
Pharmacokinetic and pharmacodynamic information available

III. Inhibitor Classes

This section will first cover well-known and recently described L-arginine substrate–based analogs that directly inhibit the enzyme activity of dimeric human iNOS (10). The remainder of this section will review recently described pyrimidylimidazole-based compounds. These are a novel class of potent and selective iNOS inhibitors that function by an unprecedented mechanism of action: potent inhibition of the assembly of inactive iNOS monomers into iNOS dimers (26,27).

A. L-Arginine Analogs

Substrate-based L-arginine analogs (Fig. 2 and Table 1) directly inhibit the enzymatic activity of dimeric iNOS (10).

New iNOS Inhibitors with Undefined In Vivo Profiles

A series of thienopyridines (28) and dihydro-1-isoquinolinamines (29) were recently described by Astra-Zeneca Pharmaceuticals. The thienopyridines provided a reasonably potent compound (IC_{50} = 89 nM), but with only ~10-fold selectivity versus eNOS and little to no selectivity versus nNOS in enzyme assays. Potency in a cell-based assay for iNOS was 2.2 μM, illustrating the point that competitive L-arginine analogs lose potency in cells due to cell permeability issues and the presence of competing L-arginine (1 mM in the culture medium). Data for the thienopyridine

Table 1 Potency and Selectivity of iNOS Inhibitor Classes

Inhibitor	IC_{50} or Ki (μM)			Selectivity ratio	
	iNOS	eNOS	nNOS	e/i	n/i
L-NIL	1.6	49	37	49	23
3,4-Dihydro-1-isoquinolinamine	0.16	>100	16	~1000	100
Heterocyclic amidine	2.4	1363	26	>500	11
1400W[a]	0.007	50	2	>5000	>250
GW273629[b]	8	1000	630	>125	78
GW274150[b]	1.4	466	145	333	104

[a] Ki for 1400W in iNOS is determined from slow-binding experiments (43).

[b] GW273629 and GW274150 are also slow-binding iNOS inhibitors; the IC_{50} values for these compounds determined under reversible conditions likely underestimate iNOS potency and thus e/i and n/i selectivity ratios (10).

L-NIL

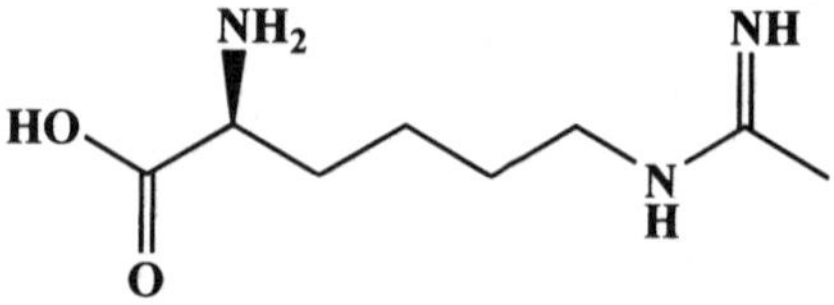

1400W

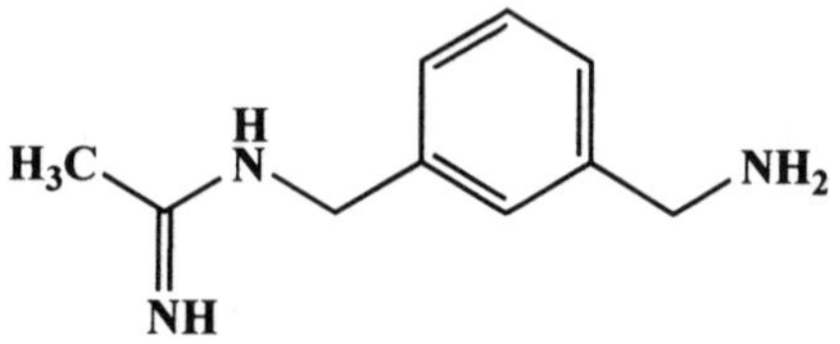

3,4-Dihydro-1-isoquinolinamine
Astra-Zeneca

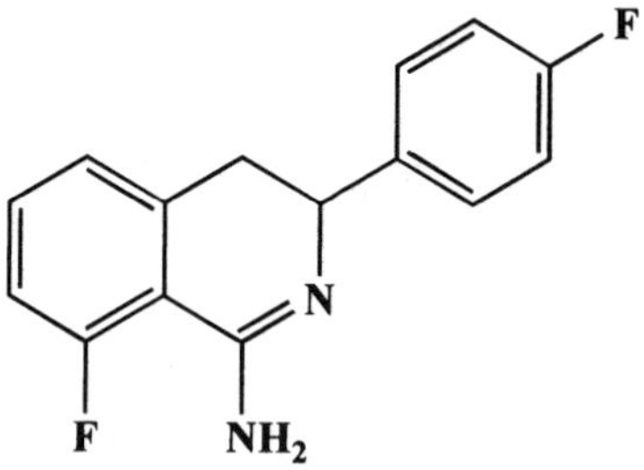

Heterocyclic amidine
Pharmacia

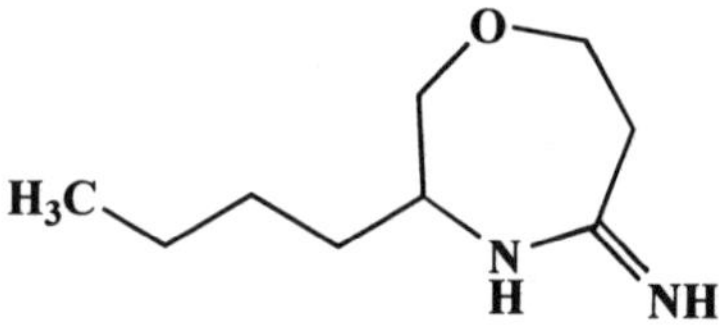

GW273629
GlaxoSmithKline

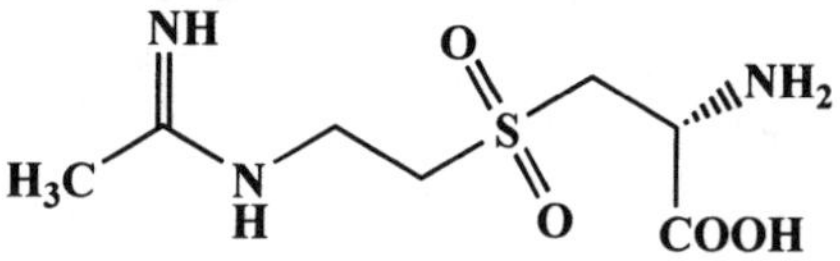

GW274150
GlaxoSmithKline

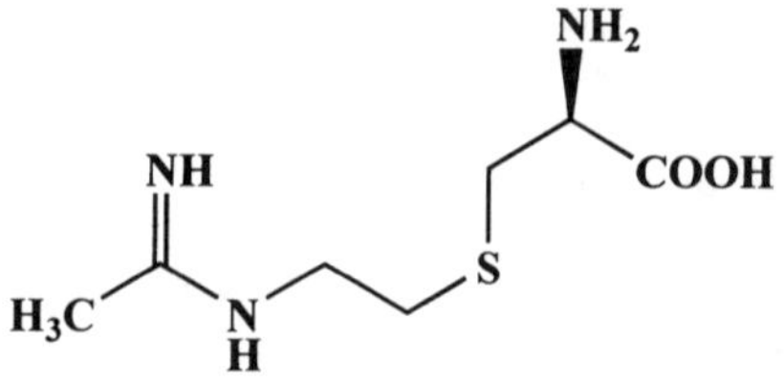

Figure 2 Selective iNOS inhibitors. The figure shows the chemical structures of compounds that target iNOS via direct inhibition of the enzyme active site and are classical substrate-based analogs. The potency and selectivity of these compounds are summarized in Table 1.

series also confirmed that the in vitro iNOS selectivity did not translate to in vivo effects: ED_{50} for LPS-induced plasma NOx (iNOS) and mean arterial pressure (eNOS) were similar. These results highlight the difficulties in identifying potent and selective iNOS inhibitors suitable for in vivo use. A more promising dihydro-1-isoquinolinamine was identified (Fig. 2): $IC_{50} = 160$ nM for human iNOS, with 100- and 1000-fold versus nNOS and eNOS, respectively. Potency in cell-based assays was considerably weaker ($IC_{50} = 83$ uM), and no in vivo data have yet been reported.

Scientists at Pharmacia Corporation have also explored heterocyclic amidine inhibitors of iNOS related in structure to ONO-1714 (30). While generally much weaker ($IC_{50} = 0.15$ to >10 μM) than ONO-1714, a compound with 500-fold iNOS versus eNOS selectivity was identified (Fig. 2). Selectivity versus nNOS, however, was lacking (12-fold at best), and no cellular or in vivo parameters have been published.

These novel chemical strategies towards iNOS inhibition illustrate a common hurdle that has been encountered in the field: optimizing inhibitor potency and selectivity toward iNOS versus eNOS has met with much greater success than selectivity for iNOS versus nNOS. Interestingly this has been observed both for the L-arginine analogs *and* the novel iNOS dimerization inhibitors described below. The results strongly suggest that iNOS and nNOS are more structurally related to each other than to eNOS. The advent of rational drug design using the published crystal structures for iNOS and eNOS (31–34) may help to solve these problems in the longer run. It should be noted, however, that a crystal structure for nNOS is still lacking and that pharmaceutical companies are already using crystal structure and molecular modeling information in the elaboration of selective iNOS inhibitor structure-activity relationships. It thus remains to be proven that structural biology information can be used to rationally design de novo a highly potent iNOS inhibitor ($IC_{50} < 10$ nM) that is truly selective versus both eNOS and nNOS (selectivity ratio > 1000 against both isoforms).

N^6-Iminoethyl-L-Lysine (L-NIL)

Under reversible conditions, L-NIL (Fig. 2) is a relatively weak inhibitor of iNOS ($IC_{50} = 1.6$ μM) with 49- and 23-fold selectivity versus eNOS and nNOS enzyme activity in vitro, respectively (10). Inhibition by L-NIL progresses to irreversibility over time and results in heme loss from iNOS (35). L-NIL inhibits iNOS in cytokine-stimulated astrocytes with $IC_{50} \sim 25$ μM (36). The functional iNOS versus eNOS selectivity of L-NIL was confirmed by comparison of its effects to L-NAME and dexamethasone on vasodilator and vasoconstrictor reactivities with and without LPS treatment (37). Functional nNOS selectivity was measured in the electrical field stimulated pig gastric fundus (20). L-NIL was the least potent nNOS inhibitor of a series tested ($EC_{50} = 840$ μM). Thus, L-NIL has a functional selectivity ratio of ~33 for iNOS versus nNOS. Since selectivity for iNOS versus eNOS and nNOS has thus been established, L-NIL can be considered a weak and selective iNOS inhibitor suitable for in vivo experimentation.

Several investigators have used L-NIL to study airway and lung biology in vivo. Feder et al. (38) studied allergic pulmonary eosinophilia in mice sensitized and challenged with ovalbumin (OVA). Eosinophilia post-OVA challenge was significantly reduced by L-NAME, partially reduced by aminoguanidine and L-NMMA, but not affected by L-NIL. Since no iNOS was induced in the lungs by OVA challenge, the authors concluded that lung-derived NO from eNOS or nNOS, rather than iNOS, contributed to eosinophilia in this model. Turnage et al. (39) reported that L-NIL reduced intestinal ischemia/reperfusion-induced secondary lung microvascular permeability in rats, whereas L-NAME exacerbated this response. The authors reported iNOS expression in the lungs in this model.

L-NIL has been used to examine vasoconstriction, vasodilation, and blood flow responses in the lung. Despite increased iNOS expression in the lungs, constrictor responses to U-46619 and pulmonary hemodynamics were not altered by L-NIL, but were affected by L-NAME in rats with pulmonary hypertension due to chronic hypoxia (40). In LPS-treated rats, L-NIL inhibited enhanced exhaled NO by 83%, whereas L-NAME had no effect (37). In addition, L-NIL but not L-NAME inhibited transient increases in acetylcholine- or bradykinin-induced pulmonary artery pressure of isolated lungs. In control lungs L-NAME, but not L-NIL, attenuated acetylcholine- or bradykinin-induced vasodilation. The authors concluded that selective iNOS inhibition attenuated LPS-induced vasoconstrictor responses while preserving endothelium (eNOS)–dependent functions. Zapol and colleagues recently developed a model of hypoxic pulmonary vasoconstriction (HPV) via left mainstem bronchus occlusion (LMBO) in mice (41). LMBO-induced HPV was impaired in LPS-treated mice, and this impairment was absent in iNOS$^{-/-}$ mice. The impaired HPV response due to LPS could be prevented by L-NIL.

Taken together, these studies in the normal, allergic, and acutely injured lung show that L-NIL can be used to explore the role of iNOS in the airways with moderate success. These are remarkable results for a compound with moderate potency and relatively low pharmacological selectivity. However, the doses of L-NIL used in these studies were not shown to specifically inhibit iNOS enzyme activity in the target tissue without comprising eNOS or nNOS enzyme activity. In some studies functional selectivity versus eNOS inhibition was shown, but functional selectivity versus nNOS functions in the lung was not established. With this caveat in mind, the investigator should put the results with L-NIL into context with the more potent and selective inhibitors described below.

1400W (N-[3-Aminomethyl)benzyl]acetamidine)

1400W (Table 1 and Fig. 2) is a mechanism-based, slow-binding, and slowly reversible inhibitor of human iNOS with a steady state $K_i < 7$ nM and selectivity versus eNOS and nNOS of 5000 and 250-fold, respectively (42). Weak enzyme inhibition of eNOS and nNOS is rapidly reversibly. 1400W has $IC_{50} \sim 0.8$ μM against LPS-stimulated rat smooth muscle iNOS versus $IC_{50} \sim 300$ μM against rat aortic ring endothelial NOS, establishing high (~ 500-fold) iNOS versus eNOS functional selectivity (42). Definitive data on functional nNOS selectivity have not been reported for 1400W but can be inferred from the in vivo results summarized below.

Despite acute CNS toxicity at high bolus doses (>50 mg/kg i.v.), 1400W has a significant therapeutic ratio in vivo. In LPS-treated rodents, 1400W selectively inhibits iNOS-dependent delayed vascular leak in multiple organs (ED_{50} ~0.2–0.6 mg/kg). No effects on early vascular leak or hemodynamics were reported and are in contrast to effects observed with L-NAME (42,43). An in vivo iNOS versus eNOS selectivity ratio of at least 50–70 can thus be estimated. 1400W was thus the first highly selective iNOS inhibitor described for which enzymatic, functional, and in vivo selectivity criteria were clearly established.

There are now more than 60 publications describing the pharmacology of 1400W in vitro and in vivo. Several have reported on the affects of 1400W on pulmonary pathophysiology. *Helicobacter pylori* LPS-induced pulmonary vascular leak is inhibited by 1400W (44). Mice sensitized and challenged with OVA were treated with 1400W in osmotic minipumps (45). OVA challenge increased iNOS expression in airway epithelium and infiltrating inflammatory cells. 1400W blocked tracheal eosinophilia by 50% and completely prevented airway hyperreactivity (AHR). Similar salutary effects of 1400W in allergic airway inflammation have been observed (46).

GW273629 and GW274150

GlaxoSmithKline recently described two highly selective acetamidine-based iNOS inhibitors (10,47): a sulfide GW273629 and a sulfone GW274150 (Table 1 and Fig. 2). Under reversible conditions, IC_{50} for iNOS inhibition are 8 and 1.2 μM, respectively, with high selectivity versus eNOS (125- and 333-fold, respectively) and nNOS (78- and 104-fold, respectively). These are also reported to be NADPH-dependent, slow-binding iNOS inhibitors. Steady-state conditions are required to fully delineate the true potency and selectivity of these compounds.

Preliminary in vivo data for these compounds were reported at the First International Meeting of the Nitric Oxide Society (48). GW273629 is orally available in rats (%F = 60) with a short plasma half-life (1.2 h), whereas GW274150 has higher oral availability (% F = 100) with a longer plasma half-life (4.3 h). Both compounds are eliminated via renal excretion. ED_{50} in the LPS-induced plasma NOx assay in mice was 10 mg/kg for GW273629 (measured at 4–6 h) versus 3 mg/kg for GW274150 (measured at 18 h). Both compounds prevented delayed vascular leak in LPS-treated rodents without exacerbating acute vascular leak, confirming in vivo iNOS versus eNOS selectivity. Efficacy was shown in various inflammation models where iNOS has been reported to play a pathogenic role. These included prevention of hypotension and increased survival in endotoxemic rodents, prevention of postoperative ileus and inhibition of inflammatory as well as neuropathic pain. Published in vivo findings include prevention of NSAID-induced intestinal injury and jejunal microvascular leakage in rats by GW273629 (49). To date there are no published in vivo data with GW274150.

In summary, both GW273629 and GW274150 are potent and highly selective iNOS inhibitors that appear well tolerated, efficacious, and selective for iNOS inhibition in vivo. The profile of GW273629 suggests potential utility as an i.v. or short-acting oral drug in acute or subchronic indications, whereas GW274150 may offer an opportunity for oral use in chronic indications. Further information on the clinical development profiles of these compounds is eagerly awaited.

B. iNOS Dimerization Inhibitors

A completely novel approach to potent and highly selective iNOS inhibition has been achieved via the discovery of iNOS dimerization inhibitors (26,27). These compounds were discovered by high-capacity screening of pyrimidylimidazole-based combinatorial chemistry libraries in a cell-based human iNOS assay using cytokine-stimulated A-172 astrocytoma cells (26). Examples of six compounds are shown in Figure 3. To date these are the most potent inhibitors of iNOS reported in cell-based assays (IC_{50} in the pM to nM range; Table 2). It must be recognized that the potential for imidazole-based compounds to function as iNOS dimerization

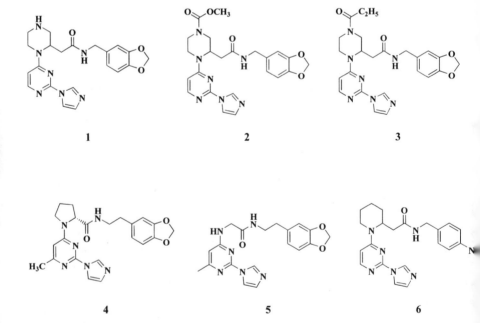

Figure 3 Potent and selective iNOS dimerization inhibitors. The figure shows the structures of six pyrimidylimidazole-based compounds that were recently discovered using A-172 astrocytoma cell–based assays of human iNOS (26,27). The potency and dimerization selectivity of these compounds is summarized in Tables 2 and 3. The compounds prevent assembly of iNOS monomers into active iNOS dimers (see Fig. 4–6).

Table 2 Potency of iNOS Dimerization Inhibitors

iNOS dimerization inhibitor	A-172 cell-based assay, IC_{50} (nM)	Radioligand binding assay, apparent K_d (nM)
1	0.50	0.73
2	0.74	2.2
3	0.38	1.8
4	0.49	0.09
5	1.20	0.33
6	270	27

The structures of the iNOS dimerization inhibitors are shown in Figure 2. Inhibitors were tested for iNOS potency (IC_{50}) in human A-172 astrocytoma cells stimulated with IL-1β, TNFα, and IFNγ. Nitrite accumulation in cell culture medium was measured after 24 hours. Inhibitor affinity (K_d) to purified human iNOS monomers was determined using [^{3}H]-Compound 3 in competitive binding experiments using a rapid filtration radioligand-binding assay. The correlation between cellular potency and monomer binding affinity demonstrates excellent cellular permeability.
Source: Data derived from Ref. 27.

inhibitors was also discovered completely independently by Stuehr and colleagues (50). The antifungal imidazoles described by this group are >1000-fold less potent than the current pyrimidylimidazole-based inhibitors and do not have the pharmacological potency or selectivity expected for therapeutic application as iNOS inhibitors.

There are several salient mechanistic features of these novel iNOS dimerization inhibitors:

1. iNOS inhibition occurs via ligation of the heme in nascent iNOS monomers and the formation of a "dead-end" iNOS monomer-inhibitor complex (Fig. 4).
2. Exposure of cytokine-stimulated cells to the dimerization inhibitors leads to accumulation of iNOS monomers within cells that retain flavoprotein reductase activity, but no heme-dependent NO or L-citrulline formation from the substrate L-arginine (Fig. 5).
3. The potency (IC_{50}) of dimerization inhibitors in cells is not affected by L-arginine and only minimally by biopterin supplementation in tissue culture medium. The inhibitors thus do not appear to compete directly with L-arginine and H4B-binding sites.
4. Crystallographic studies show that the inhibitors coordinate the heme in the iNOS monomer, disrupt helices 7a and 8, and furthermore displace the critical L-arginine–binding Glu-371 residue from the active site (Fig. 6).

These findings confirm that the inhibitors function by allosteric regulation of protein-protein and protein-substrate molecular recognition in the iNOS monomer.

These key findings were corroborated in mechanistic studies where dimerization inhibitor interactions were studied directly via radioligand binding and in vitro

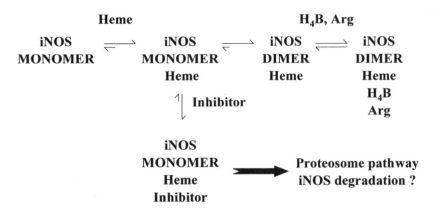

Figure 4 Mechanism of action of iNOS dimerization inhibitors. The figure shows a schematic of iNOS monomer-dimer equilibria and the effects of iNOS dimerization inhibitors. Insertion of heme into iNOS monomers initiates rapid formation of a heme-containing iNOS dimer. Substrate and H4B binding further stabilize the iNOS dimer. The dimerization inhibitors ligate the heme in the iNOS monomer and form a high-affinity, ternary monomer-heme-inhibitor complex that has no enzymatic NOS activity. This "dead-end" inhibitor complex may be targeted for degradation by the proteasome pathway.

dimerization assays with purified human or murine iNOS monomer (27). These studies confirmed a strong correlation between monomer binding affinity and inhibitor potency in the cell-based iNOS assay (Table 2). In distinct contrast to the competitive inhibitors of L-arginine (reviewed above), which have been frequently shown to have much lower potency in cells than in enzyme assays (often several log orders), the iNOS dimerization inhibitors exhibit exceptional cellular permeability. In contrast to the direct iNOS enzyme inhibitors, however, the iNOS dimerization inhibitors do not inhibit preformed enzymatically active iNOS, eNOS, or nNOS dimers, even after prolonged incubation ($IC_{50} >> 100$ μM). Thus, only newly formed iNOS monomers can be targeted with this approach, at least in an acute setting. This finding is confirmed by the loss of potency of the dimerization inhibitors versus iNOS when added to cell cultures several hours after cytokine stimulation.

The discovery of the iNOS dimerization inhibitors lead to the need to develop assay systems to explore the selectivity versus inhibiting eNOS and nNOS dimerization. This was achieved by *de novo* transient expression of human iNOS, eNOS, and nNOS in BSC-1 cells using vaccinia virus expression vectors (26). These studies revealed that the dimerization inhibitors are generally highly selective for iNOS versus eNOS dimerization (ratio > 1000). In contrast, a range of selectivities was observed for inhibition of nNOS dimerization. Examples of two compounds are summarized in Table 3. These results confirm that highly potent iNOS dimerization inhibitors that have high selectivity for iNOS versus eNOS and nNOS dimerization and that also have no appreciable inhibitory effect on preformed eNOS or nNOS dimers have been identified and optimized.

A

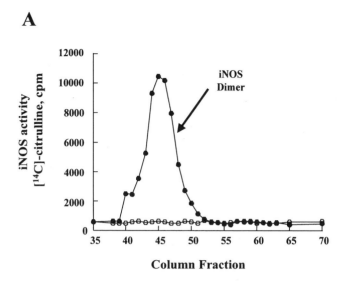

B

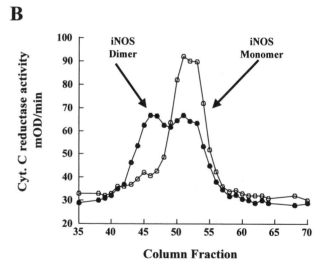

Figure 5 Dimerization inhibitors lead to iNOS monomer accumulation. The figure shows size exclusion chromatograms of cellular extracts prepared from RAW 264.7 cells treated with LPS and IFNγ and grown overnight in the presence (open symbols) or absence (filled symbols) of the iNOS dimerization inhibitor Compound 2 (10 uM). Column fractions were assayed for NOS activity ($[^{14}C]$-citrulline, cpm), which is present only in iNOS dimers (A) and cytochrome C reductase activity (mOD/min), which is present in both iNOS dimers and monomers (B). Dimeric iNOS activity is seen in cytokine-treated extracts but is absent when cells are treated with Compound 2. Cytokine-treated cells contain a mixture of iNOS monomers and dimers with reductase activity that collapses to a single monomer peak in the presence of Compound 2. The monomers have reductase activity but no NOS activity. (From Ref. 26.)

A   B

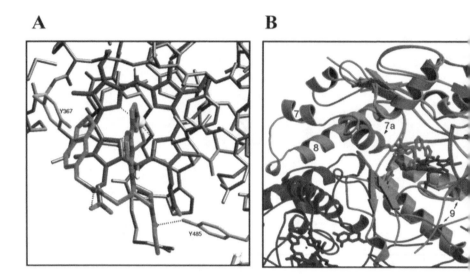

Figure 6   Crystal structure of iNOS monomer-inhibitor complex. The figure shows the co-crystal of Compound 2 in complex with the murine iNOS monomer (N-terminal 114 mutant) (A) Compound 2 ligates the heme iron (yellow) via the imidazole moiety (green and blue and adopts a U-shaped conformation, projecting the benzodioxolane moiety (green and red back into the heme pocket. This moiety displaces from the heme pocket the Glu371 side chain in helix 7a that is critical for L-arginine binding. (B) Monomer structural change: induced by Compound 2 are shown. The murine iNOS dimer interface is shown (light and dark blue monomers) with the monomer-inhibitor complex overlaid (yellow). Helices 8, 7 (light blue), and 7a (red, with Glu371 side chain shown), normally seen in the iNOS monomer and dimer structures, are disordered in the monomer-inhibitor complex. Helix 9 is ordered but displaced. The data support direct effects of the inhibitor on iNOS monomer structure via interruption of protein-heme, protein-substrate, and protein-protein interactions essentia for dimerization. This represents an unprecedented mechanism and approach for selective iNOS inhibition. (from Ref. 26.)

Table 3   NOS Dimerization Selectivity

Assay	Compound 2, IC_{50} (nM)	Compound 4, IC_{50} (nM)
A-172 cells	0.7	0.5
iNOS dimerization[a]	18	20
nNOS dimerization[a]	108	12400
	Selectivity = 6	Selectivity = 620
eNOS dimerization[a]	19800	>30000
	Selectivity = 1100	Selectivity ≥1500

[a] The selectivity of iNOS dimerization inhibitors was evaluated in cell-based assays of de novo human iNOS, nNOS, and eNOS transient expressed in BSC-1 cells using vaccinia virus vectors as described in Ref. 26.

Functional and cellular selectivity for the iNOS dimerization inhibitors has been established via several approaches. Compound 2 (Fig. 2) did not appreciably inhibit recombinant human nNOS activity expressed in HEK-239 cells when tested at 10 μM for ~7 days (K. McMillan, unpublished observations). The nNOS selectivity of Compound 2 in cell-based systems is thus >1000. For eNOS selectivity, functional effects for Compound 2 were tested in rat aortic ring cultures treated overnight with or without IL-1β to induce iNOS. Compound 2 dose-dependently prevented iNOS-dependent hyporeactivity to PE (ED_{50} < 100 nM) with no effects on acetylcholine-induced, eNOS-dependent relaxation (K. Kauser, unpublished observations). In control rings, Compound 2 had no effect on basal NO release at concentrations up to 100 μM (J. Post, unpublished observations). The functional iNOS/eNOS selectivity in these assays was ~1000.

Compound 4 was also evaluated for general selectivity against a panel of >60 pharmacologically relevant receptor and enzyme activities at concentrations of 10–100 μM. No significant inhibition of any target (>50%) was observed, confirming the high general pharmacological selectivity of this inhibitor (G. B. Phillips and J. F. Parkinson, unpublished observations). Imidazole-based compounds are known cytochrome P450 inhibitors. The iNOS dimerization inhibitors do not exhibit broad P450 cross-reactivity, but have been found to inhibit CYP-3A4 (27). The IC_{50} of Compound 4 for CYP-3A4 is ~150 nM in a microsomal benzyloxyresorufin assay and ~1 μM in a cell-based testosterone hydroxylase assay (27). Compound 4 is thus ~300- to 2000-fold selective for inhibiting iNOS dimerization in cells than CYP-3A4. Since CYP-3A4 is the most abundant drug metabolizing P450 in humans, the iNOS dimerization inhibitors have the potential to cause drug-drug interactions in vivo. Further optimization of this parameter in newer compounds from this class is in progress.

Figure 7 shows that Compound 2 dose-dependently inhibits LPS-induced elevations in plasma NOx in both mice and rats. The ED_{50} for Compound 2 was ~1 mg/kg. Compound 4 has similar potency in vivo. To establish in vivo selectivity for the iNOS dimerization inhibitors, Compound 4 has been dosed chronically at 30 mg/kg b.i.d. in rats. No inhibition of eNOS functional responses in aortic rings or nNOS activity in tissue extracts of gastrocnemius muscles was observed ex vivo (J. Post, R. Fitch, and G. Burton, unpublished observations). The in vivo selectivity ratio of Compound 4 is thus >>30 versus both eNOS and nNOS.

Depending on species, Compounds 2 and 4 have variable oral availability (%F = 20–90%) with moderate plasma half-life (1–3 h). A hepatobiliary elimination route has been observed, with evidence for accelerated clearance after chronic dosing for some compounds in the series in rodent species, but not in higher-order animals (B. Subramanyam, unpublished observations).

Preliminary data on the in vivo efficacy of iNOS dimerization inhibitors were reported at the First International Meeting of the Nitric Oxide Society (52,53). Compound 4 significantly attenuated soft tissue inflammation in adjuvant-induced arthritis in Lewis rats as assessed by soft tissue swelling and x-ray analysis of joint disease (52). Oral efficacy for Compound 4 was established in an endocrinological assay (53). It has been established that iNOS is expressed at uterus implantation sites of

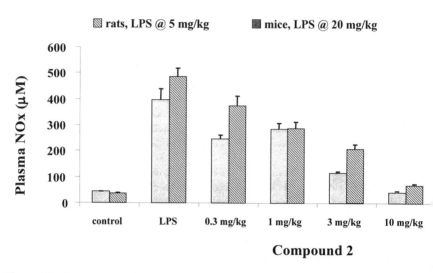

Compound 2

Figure 7   Compound 2 inhibits iNOS in endotoxemic rodents. The figure shows the plasma NOx assay for iNOS inhibition in endotoxin (LPS)–treated rats and mice. The large increase in iNOS-dependent plasma NOx levels seen 6 hrs post-LPS is inhibited dose-dependently by Compound 2 (dosed 1 hour post-LPS) with ED_{50} ~ 1 mg/kg in both species. (Adapted from Ref. 26.)

fertilized ova in rodents, where iNOS may function to promote inflammation-driven angiogenesis and tissue remodeling (54). Aminoguanidine and L-NAME inhibit implantation in rodents when dosed during the peri-implantation period in combination with antiprogestins (55). As in this previous study, the iNOS dimerization inhibitors were found not to block implantation when dosed alone. However, a dose-dependent synergistic effect with the antiprogestin (30- to 100-fold shift in antiprogestin dose-response) was observed (53). The synergistic effects were obtained at doses of Compound 4 ~100-fold lower than for aminoguanidine (55). These results serve to remind us of the important functions for iNOS in normal physiological processes. They also establish a novel concept for postcoital contraception.

In summary, the results for the selective iNOS dimerization inhibitors establish that they are a novel strategy for potent and highly selective iNOS inhibition both in vitro and in vivo. Systemic and oral efficacy has been established. The compounds are well tolerated for acute and chronic dosing in animal models of inflammation at bolus doses at least as high as 30–50 mg/kg. The iNOS dimerization inhibitors are currently being evaluated in animal models of endotoxemia, acute cardiopulmonary and renal dysfunction in the setting of severe ARDS, and cardiac allograft transplantation. Salutary effects have been observed on numerous clinically relevant efficacy endpoints in these models and will be the subject of future publications.

IV. Overall Summary and Future Perspectives

A retrospective analysis has shown that L-NIL and 1400W, which are widely commercially available and relatively inexpensive, remain the most accessible reagents of choice for selective iNOS inhibition in vitro and in vivo. However, several new classes of iNOS inhibitors have recently emerged through the perseverance of the pharmaceutical industry. These can be broadly divided into two classes:

1. Compounds with high iNOS versus eNOS selectivity, but relatively low iNOS versus nNOS selectivity: These include ONO-1714, the dihydro-1-isoquinolinamines described by Astra-Zeneca, and heterocyclic amidines described by Pharmacia. For the latter two series, clear evidence of efficacy and in vivo selectivity versus eNOS and nNOS has yet to be published.

2. Compounds with potency versus iNOS and high selectivity toward *both* eNOS and nNOS established in vivo. To date, these include GW273629, GW274150, and the pyrimidylimidazole-based iNOS dimerization inhibitors (e.g., Compounds 2 and 4).

For these series, published data have confirmed their in vivo selectivity and therapeutic potential.

These are exciting times for the selective iNOS inhibitor field as we can expect progress on several fronts. The most advanced compounds that have been publicly disclosed appear to all intents and purposes like drugs, and we can anticipate progress in phase I/II clinical studies for these in the relatively near future. The transition from preclinical to clinical research marks a major step forward for the field. These studies will begin to reveal compound-specific liabilities but, more importantly, the short- and long-term mechanism-related side effect profiles of selective iNOS inhibitors and how they may impact therapeutic applications. There are competing approaches with new inhibitor series that can exploit the solved crystal structures of the NOS isoforms in rational design of second generation drugs. Despite the high sequence and structural homology of the NOS isoforms within the catalytic domain, selectivity has been achieved by the perseverance of those that have stayed the course in the case of the substrate-based inhibitors and by serendipity, combined with hard work, in the case of the dimerization inhibitors. It is anticipated that better things are yet to come on this front. The availability of potent and highly selective iNOS inhibitors opens the door for new, more efficient and definitive research into the known and as-yet-unknown physiological and pathophysiological functions of iNOS in cell biology and in vivo. As we have seen in this review, airway biologists have helped tremendously to define the iNOS past and will certainly have a major impact on the iNOS future with the new tools available to them.

Acknowledgments

I wish to thank the many contributions of colleagues at Berlex Biosciences, Richmond, CA, and Pharmacopeia Inc., Princeton, NJ, for their scientific excellence and inspiration on the iNOS project team. I am indebted to Dr. Richard Knowles (GlaxoSmithKline, Stevenage, UK), Dr. Pamela Manning (Pharmacia Corp., St. Louis, MO), and their many colleagues for provocative discussions about new "selective" iNOS inhibitors. Many thanks are also due to the NOS crystallographers: Dr. Tom Poulos (University of California, Irvine, CA) and Dr. Jon Tainer (Scripps Research Institute, La Jolla, CA).

References

1. Hibbs JB. Jr, Vavrin Z, Taintor RR. L-Arginine is required for expression of the activated macrophage effector mechanism causing selective metabolic inhibition in target cells. J Immunol 1987; 138:550–565.
2. Miwa M, Stuehr DJ, Marletta MA, Wishnok JS, Tannenbaum SR. Nitrosation of amines by stimulated macrophages. Carcinogenesis 1987; 8:955–958.
3. Stuehr DJ, Marletta MA. Mammalian nitrate biosynthesis: mouse macrophages produce nitrite and nitrate in response to *Escherichia coli* lipopolysaccharide. Proc Natl Acad Sci USA 1985; 82:7738–7742.
4. Ding AH, Nathan CF, Stuehr DJ. Release of reactive nitrogen intermediates and reactive oxygen intermediates from mouse peritoneal macrophages. Comparison of activating cytokines and evidence for independent production. J Immunol 1988; 141:2407–2412.
5. Nathan C. Inducible nitric oxide synthase: what difference does it make? J Clin Invest 1997; 100:2417–2423.
6. Bogdan C. Nitric oxide and the immune response. Nat Immunol 2001; 2:907–916.
7. Babu BR, Griffith OW. Design of isoform-selective inhibitors of nitric oxide synthase. Curr Opin Chem Biol 1998; 2:491–500.
8. Parkinson JF, Devlin JJ, Phillips GB. Nitric oxide synthase inhibitors. In: Rubanyi G, ed. The Pathophysiology and Clinical Applications of Nitric Oxide. Harwood: Academic, 1998:505–521.
9. Parkinson JF, NOS inhibitors I—substrate analogs and heme ligands. In: Mayer B, ed. Handbook of Experimental Pharmacology—Nitric Oxide. Vol. 143. Heidelberg: Springer-Verlag, 1999:111–135.
10. Alderton WK, Cooper CE, Knowles RG. Nitric oxide synthases: structure, function and inhibition. Biochem J 2001; 357:593–615.
11. Joly GA, Ayres M, Chelly F, Kilbourn RG. Effects of NG-methyl-L-arginine, NG-nitro-L-arginine, and aminoguanidine on constitutive and inducible nitric oxide synthase in rat aorta. Biochem Biophys Res Commun 1994; 199:147–154.
12. Joly GA, Ayres M, Kilbourn RG. Potent inhibition of inducible nitric oxide synthase by geldanamycin, a tyrosine kinase inhibitor, in endothelial, smooth muscle cells, and in rat aorta. FEBS Lett 1997; 403:40–44.
13. O'Brien AJ, Wilson AJ, Sibbald R, Singer M, Clapp LH. Temporal variation in endotoxin-induced vascular hyporeactivity in a rat mesenteric artery organ culture model. Br J Pharmacol 2001; 133:351–360.
14. Hom GJ, Grant SK, Wolfe G, Bach TJ, MacIntyre DE, Hutchinson NI. Lipopolysaccharide-induced hypotension and vascular hyporeactivity in the rat: tissue analysis of nitric oxide synthase mRNA and protein expression in the presence and absence of dexamethasone, NG-monomethyl-L-arginine or indomethacin. J Pharmacol Exp Ther 1995; 272:452–459.

15. MacMicking JD, Nathan C, Hom G, Chartrain N, Fletcher DS, Trumbauer M, Stevens K, Xie QW, Sokol K, Hutchinson N, et al. Altered responses to bacterial infection and endotoxic shock in mice lacking inducible nitric oxide synthase. Cell 1995; 81:641–650.

16. Szabo C, Southan GJ, Thiemermann C. Beneficial effects and improved survival in rodent models of septic shock with S-methylisothiourea sulfate, a potent and selective inhibitor of inducible nitric oxide synthase. Proc Natl Acad Sci USA 1994; 91: 12472–12476.

17. Tracey WR, Tse J, Carter G. Lipopolysaccharide-induced changes in plasma nitrite and nitrate concentrations in rats and mice: pharmacological evaluation of nitric oxide synthase inhibitors. J Pharmacol Exp Ther 1995; 272:1011–1015.

18. Thiemermann C, Szabo C, Mitchell JA, Vane JR. Vascular hyporeactivity to vasoconstrictor agents and hemodynamic decompensation in hemorrhagic shock is mediated by nitric oxide. Proc Natl Acad Sci USA 1993; 90:267–271.

19. Mashimo H, Kjellin A, Goyal RK. Gastric stasis in neuronal nitric oxide synthase-deficient knockout mice. Gastroenterology 2000; 119:766–773.

20. Dick JM, Lefebvre RA. Influence of different classes of NO synthase inhibitors in the pig gastric fundus. Naunyn Schmiedebergs Arch Pharmacol 1997; 356:488–494.

21. Forstermann U, Gath I, Schwarz P, Closs EI, Kleinert H. Isoforms of nitric oxide synthase. Properties, cellular distribution and expressional control. Biochem Pharmacol 1995; 50:1321–1332.

22. Dwyer MA, Bredt DS, Snyder SH. Nitric oxide synthase: irreversible inhibition by L-NG-nitroarginine in brain in vitro and in vivo. Biochem Biophys Res Commun 1991; 176:1136–1141.

23. Naka M, Nanbu T, Kobayashi K, Kamanaka Y, Komeno M, Yanase R, Fukutomi T, Fujimura S, Seo HG, Fujiwara N, Ohuchida S, Suzuki K, Kondo K, Taniguchi NA. potent inhibitor of inducible nitric oxide synthase, ONO-1714, a cyclic amidine derivative. Biochem Biophys Res Commun 2000; 270:663–667.

24. Okamoto I, Abe M, Shibata K, Shimizu N, Sakata N, Katsuragi T, Tanaka K. Evaluating the role of inducible nitric oxide synthase using a novel and selective inducible nitric oxide synthase inhibitor in septic lung injury produced by cecal ligation and puncture. Am J Respir Crit Care Med 2000; 162:716–722.

25. Mitaka C, Hirata Y, Yokoyama K, Makita K, Imai T. A selective inhibitor for inducible nitric oxide synthase improves hypotension and lactic acidosis in canine endotoxic shock. Crit Care Med 2001; 29:2156–2161.

26. McMillan K, Adler M, Auld DS, Baldwin JJ, Blasko E, Browne LJ, Chelsky D, Davey D, Dolle RE, Eagan KA, Erickson S, Feldman R, Glaser CB, Mallari C, Morrissey MM, Ohlmeyer MHJ, Pan G, Parkinson JF, Phillips GB, Polokoff MA, Sigal NH, Young TA, Vergona R, Whitlow M, Devlin JJ. Allosteric inhibitors of inducible nitric oxide synthase dimerization discovered via combinatorial chemistry. Proc Natl Acad Sci USA 2000; 97:1506–1511.

27. Blasko E, Glaser CB, Devlin JJ, Xia W, Feldman RI, Polokoff MA, Phillips GB, Whitlow M, Auld DS, McMillan K, Ghosh S, Stuehr DJ, Parkinson JF. Mechanistic studies with potent and selective inducible nitric-oxide synthase dimerization inhibitors. J Biol Chem 2002; 277:295–302.

28. Beaton H, Boughton-Smith N, Hamley P, Ghelani A, Nicholls DJ, Tinker AC, Wallace AV. Thienopyridines: nitric oxide synthase inhibitors with potent in vivo activity. Bioorg Med Chem Lett 2001; 11:1027–1030.

29. Beaton H, Hamley P, Nicholls DJ, Tinker AC, Wallace AV. 3,4-Dihydro-1-isoquinolinamines: a novel class of nitric oxide synthase inhibitors with a range of isoform selectivity and potency. Bioorg Med Chem Lett 2001; 11:1023–1026.

30. Moormann AE, Metz S, Toth MV, Moore WM, Jerome G, Kornmeier C, Manning P Hansen DW. Jr., Pitzele BS, Webber RK. Selective heterocyclic amidine inhibitors o human inducible nitric oxide synthase. Bioorg Med Chem Lett 2001; 11:2651–2653.

31. Crane BR, Arvai AS, Gachhui R, Wu C, Ghosh DK, Getzoff ED, Stuehr DJ, Taine JA. The structure of nitric oxide synthase oxygenase domain and inhibitor complexes Science 1997; 278:425–431.

32. Crane BR, Arvai AS, Ghosh DK, Wu C, Getzoff ED, Stuehr DJ, Tainer JA. Structure of nitric oxide synthase oxygenase dimer with pterin and substrate. Science 1998; 279 2121–2126.

33. Raman CS, Li H, Martasek P, Kral V, Masters BS, Poulos TL. Crystal structure o constitutive endothelial nitric oxide synthase: a paradigm for pterin function involving a novel metal center. Cell 1998; 95:939–950.

34. Li H, Raman CS, Glaser CB, Blasko E, Young TA, Parkinson JF, Whitlow M, Poulos TL. Crystal structures of zinc-free and -bound heme domain of human inducible nitric oxide synthase. Implications for dimer stability and comparison with endothelial nitric oxide synthase. J Biol Chem 1999; 274:21276–21284.

35. Wolff DJ, Lubeskie A, Gauld DS, Neulander MJ. Inactivation of nitric oxide synthase and cellular nitric oxide formation by N6-iminoethyl-L-lysine and N5-iminoethyl-L ornithine. Eur J Pharmacol 1998; 350:325–334.

36. Li W, Xia J, Sun GY. Cytokine induction of iNOS and sPLA2 in immortalized astrocytes (DITNC): response to genistein and pyrrolidine dithiocarbamate. J Interferon Cytokine Res 1999; 19:121–127.

37. Fischer LG, Horstman DJ, Hahnenkamp K, Kechner NE, Rich GF. Selective iNOS inhibition attenuates acetylcholine- and bradykinin-induced vasoconstriction in lipopoly saccharide-exposed rat lungs. Anesthesiology 1999; 91:1724–1732.

38. Feder LS, Stelts D, Chapman RW, Manfra D, Crawley Y, Jones H, Minnicozzi M Fernandez X, Paster T, Egan RW, Kreutner W, Kung TT. Role of nitric oxide on eosinophilic lung inflammation in allergic mice. Am J Respir Cell Mol Biol 1997; 17 436–442.

39. Turnage RH, Wright JK, Iglesias J, LaNoue JL, Nguyen H, Kim L, Myers S. Intestina reperfusion-induced pulmonary edema is related to increased pulmonary inducible nitric oxide synthase activity. Surgery 1998; 124:457–462.

40. Resta TC, O'Donaughy TL, Earley S, Chicoine LG, Walker BR. Unaltered vasoconstric tor responsiveness after iNOS inhibition in lungs from chronically hypoxic rats. Am J Physiol 1999; 276:L122–130.

41. Ullrich R, Bloch KD, Ichinose F, Steudel W, Zapol WM. Hypoxic pulmonary bloo flow redistribution and arterial oxygenation in endotoxin-challenged NOS2-deficien mice. J Clin Invest 1999; 104:1421–1429.

42. Garvey EP, Oplinger JA, Furfine ES, Kiff RJ, Laszlo F, Whittle BJ, Knowles RG 1400W is a slow, tight binding, and highly selective inhibitor of inducible nitric-oxide synthase in vitro and in vivo. J Biol Chem 1997; 272:4959–4963.

43. Laszlo F, Whittle BJ. Actions of isoform-selective and non-selective nitric oxide syn thase inhibitors on endotoxin-induced vascular leakage in rat colon. Eur J Pharmacol 1997; 334:99–102.

44. Whittle BJ, Morschl E, Pozsar J, Moran AP, Laszlo F. Helicobacter pylori lipopolysac charide provokes iNOS-mediated acute systemic microvascular inflammatory responses in rat cardiac, hepatic, renal and pulmonary tissues. J Physiol Paris 2001; 95:257–259

45. Koarai A, Ichinose M, Sugiura H, Yamagata S, Hattori T, Shirato K. Allergic airway hyperresponsiveness and eosinophil infiltration is reduced by a selective iNOS inhibitor 1400W, in mice. Pulm Pharmacol Ther 2000; 13:267–275.

46. Iijima H, Duguet A, Eum SY, Hamid Q, Eidelman DH. Nitric oxide and protein nitration are eosinophil dependent in allergen-challenged mice. Am J Respir Crit Care Med 2001; 163:1233–1240.

47. Young RJ, Beams RM, Carter K, Clark HA, Coe DM, Chambers CL, Davies PI, Dawson J, Drysdale MJ, Franzman KW, French C, Hodgson ST, Hodson HF, Kleanthous S, Rider P, Sanders D, Sawyer DA, Scott KJ, Shearer BG, Stocker R, Smith S, Tackley MC, Knowles RG. Inhibition of inducible nitric oxide synthase by acetamidine derivatives of hetero-substituted lysine and homolysine. Bioorg Med Chem Lett 2000; 10:597–600.

48. Knowles RG, Clayton NM, Dawson J. Selective inhibition of iNOS as a potential therapeutic strategy for inflammatory disease (abstr). Nitric Oxide 2000; 4:200.

49. Evans SM, Whittle BJ. Interactive roles of superoxide and inducible nitric oxide synthase in rat intestinal injury provoked by non-steroidal anti-inflammatory drugs. Eur J Pharmacol 2001; 429:287–296.

50. Sennequier N, Wolan D, Stuehr DJ. Antifungal imidazoles block assembly of inducible NO synthase into an active dimer. J Biol Chem 1999; 274:930–938.

51. Fitch R, Vergona R, Wang J, Post J, Kauser K, Burton G, Kenrick M, Mallari C, Devlin J, Phillips G, Perez H, Parkinson J. Pharmacological selectivity and therapeutic potential of iNOS dimerization inhibitors (abstr). Nitric Oxide 2000; 4:201.

52. Hess-Stumpp H, Garfield RE, Parkinson J, Chwalisz K. Synergistic effect of an antiprogestin and a selective dimerization inhibitor of inducible nitric oxide synthase in blocking implantation (abstr). Nitric Oxide 2000; 4:199.

53. Purcell TL, Given R, Chwalisz K, Garfield RE. Nitric oxide synthase distribution during implantation in the mouse. Mol Hum Reprod 1999; 5:467–475.

54. Chwalisz K, Winterhager E, Thienel T, Garfield RE. Synergistic role of nitric oxide and progesterone during the establishment of pregnancy in the rat. Hum Reprod 1999; 14:542–552.

12

Leukocyte Recruitment in Allergic Pulmonary Inflammation

BRUCE S. BOCHNER

The Johns Hopkins University School of Medicine
Baltimore, Maryland, U.S.A.

I. Introduction

Accumulation in tissues of subsets of leukocytes, especially eosinophils, basophils, and Th2 lymphocytes, is a hallmark of asthma and other forms of chronic allergic inflammation (1,2). The notion that these cells play central roles in allergic diseases is supported by the identification of their mediators at sites of allergic inflammatory responses and the reduction of these cells and their mediators during the resolution of allergic reactions (reviewed in Ref. 3). Selective migration of these cells also occurs following the instillation of allergen into the airways during human experimental late phase responses (LPRs). For example, eosinophils can account for 60% or more of the cells entering the lumen of the lower airways after introduction of allergen by segmental challenge (4). Basophil numbers in the lower airway also increase during the LPR, often by more than 100-fold, and can account for as many as 3% of the total infiltrating cells (5). The vast majority of infiltrating T cells in the lung are CD4 + memory cells displaying a cytokine pattern typical for Th2 cells, including production of IL-4 and IL-5 (1).

Because eosinophils, basophils, and Th2 lymphocytes are preferentially attracted to allergic airway inflammatory sites, where they contribute to disease pathophysiology, mechanisms must exist that favor their recruitment into the affected tissues. The current paradigm of leukocyte recruitment contends that adhesion molecules, chemokines, and possibly other chemotactic factors work in concert with cytokines to direct selective leukocyte migration. Indeed, each tissue in the body, including the lung, may have its own unique pathway for facilitating inflammatory responses (6–8). This chapter will review our current understanding of how soluble and cell surface inflammatory molecules work in concert to mediate events critical to cellular recruitment to the lung during allergic inflammatory responses, with a particular emphasis on human studies. The reader is also referred to other recent reviews focusing on similar topics but with a greater emphasis on animal models (9–11).

II. General Molecular Mechanisms Involved in Inflammatory Responses

Regardless of the cell type or tissue involved, the process of leukocyte recruitment into tissues during an inflammatory response is believed to involve a series of steps. The earliest events begin when circulating cells undergo margination, resisting the shear forces associated with blood flow (Fig. 1) (7,12). Adhesion molecules are

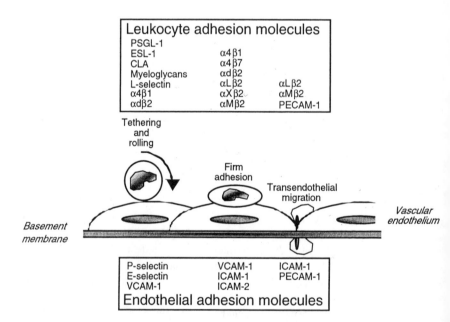

Figure 1 Adhesion molecules on leukocytes and endothelium and their role during cell recruitment. PSGL-1: P-selectin glycoprotein-1; ESL-1: E-selectin ligand-1; CLA: cutaneous lymphocyte antigen; PECAM: platelet endothelial cell adhesion molecule; VCAM: vascular cell adhesion molecule; ICAM: intercellular adhesion molecule. Integrins are designated using common names for their α and β subunits. (From Ref. 156.)

necessary for these interactions to occur, and it is now believed that selectins (L-selectin, P-selectin, and E-selectin) and their carbohydrate-containing counterligands (including those expressing sialyl-Lewis X) mediate the initial margination steps involving tethering and rolling. Subsequent to selectin and selectin ligand interactions, the processes of firm leukocyte adhesion and transendothelial migration are initiated. These events involve different subsets of adhesion molecules termed integrins and immunoglobulin gene superfamily members (7,13). Examples of the former include the β1 and β2 integrins, while examples of the latter include VCAM-1 (vascular cell adhesion molecule-1) and ICAM-1 (intercellular adhesion molecule-1). There can be exceptions to this rule. For example, integrins such as α4β1 and αdβ2 can contribute to cell rolling (14,15).

Among the β2 integrins, LFA-1 and Mac-1 are particularly important during the process of firm adhesion, transendothelial, and transepithelial migration of leukocytes, regardless of cell type. It is felt that the activation state of these integrins may be more important than their relative levels of cell surface expression in determining adhesive function (16). This is an event in which chemokines (see below), via specific seven transmembrane, G-protein–coupled receptors, are felt to play an important role in shaping the cellular makeup of an inflammatory infiltrate. For example, it has been proposed that exposure to chemokines at or near the endothelial luminal surface rapidly increases affinity of the LFA-1/ICAM-1 interaction and that this activation is critical for leukocyte capture on the endothelial cell (7,16). This mechanism may be similar for the α4 integrins, because activation of T cells or eosinophils through seven transmembrane receptors has been reported to alter their adhesion to VCAM-1, ICAM-1, or MAdCAM-1 (17–19). Ultimately, cells must detach from endothelium prior to directional migration; other events, such as chemokine-induced regulation of function and redistribution of integrins on the cell surface, are thought to mediate these processes (20).

III. Specific Molecular Mechanisms Involved in Allergic Inflammatory Responses

The allergic inflammatory response is a complex tissue reaction involving a variety of cells, chemical mediators, and cytokines (21,22). Ultimately, the nature of the allergen, the route of exposure, and the organ affected determines not only the symptoms of the particular type of allergic reaction but also the mechanisms involved in the inflammatory process. Allergic reactions in the lungs involve IgE antibody and are regulated by antigen-specific Th2 cells that accumulate and expand in number. Acute responses primarily involve effects of the release of preformed mediators from mast cells, along with rapidly but newly generated substances such as prostaglandins and leukotrienes (e.g., histamine, PGD2, and LTC4, respectively). In addition, allergen exposure causes release of other substances that facilitate the recruitment of eosinophils, basophils, and Th2 lymphocytes to the site, and this is subsequently influenced by cytokines derived from recruited antigen-specific Th2 lymphocytes (1,23). However, it is the combined contributions of soluble factors released from tissue-resident cells, such as mast cells, dendritic cells, endothelial cells, and epithelial cells, that ultimately shapes the response to allergen exposure (6).

In allergic respiratory diseases, recruitment of allergic inflammatory cells to a tissue site exposed to allergen is regulated by a particular network of cytokines (1,6,13). These include cytokines that activate vascular endothelial cells to express adhesion molecules, those that prolong survival and potentiate (or "prime") circulating leukocyte functions, and those that stimulate cells, such as the respiratory epithelium, to release chemoattractants (e.g., chemokines) that influence migration.

A. Endothelial Activating Cytokines

The potential role of endothelial adhesion molecules in allergic diseases has been reviewed (12,13). Indeed, there are numerous examples of animal studies implicating adhesion molecules in allergic airway inflammation. By employing genetically manipulated mice, blocking monoclonal antibodies, or specific pharmacological antagonists, studies suggest roles for VCAM-1/VLA-4 (24–34), ICAM-1/β2 integrins (26,32,35–38), ICAM-2 (39), E-selectin (40), and P-selectin (32,37,41), with little or no contribution by PECAM-1 (42) or selectin ligands (43). The role of L-selectin varies from major effect to no effect depending on the model (31,32,36,44). Overall, the roles of VCAM-1, ICAM-1, and P-selectin in these models appear to be most prominent.

The cytokines first discovered to influence endothelial cell adhesiveness were TNFα and IL-1. These cytokines are unique in that they are capable, albeit with differing kinetics, to induce a wide range of endothelial adhesion molecules. Some, such as E-selectin, appear de novo within a few hours, while others, such as VCAM-1, take 24–48 hours to become maximally expressed. Other constitutively expressed adhesion molecules, such as ICAM-1, are upregulated. In contrast, examples of selective adhesion molecule induction on endothelium include enhancement of expression of ICAM-1 by IFNγ and induction of VCAM-1 by IL-4 and IL-13 (45,46). Furthermore, these latter two cytokines synergize with IL-1 or TNFα in promoting expression of VCAM-1 (47).

In animals, eosinophil influx has been observed following injection of IL-1 into the skin of rats (48) and after IL-4 injection into the skin or peritoneum of mice (49). Production of IL-4 and IL-13 in the lungs of mice is associated with inflammatory changes that are reminiscent of asthma (50–53). Other murine studies demonstrated a potential role of TNFα in allergic disease pathophysiology, based initially on finding antigen-induced release of TNFα from mast cells (54). Subsequent studies in animal models of inflammation, including those induced by allergen, provided further support for this notion (55–62). Thus, IgE-dependent production of cytokines, such as TNFα, perhaps acting synergistically with IL-4 or IL-13, can lead to a unique pattern of infiltrating cells, especially eosinophils, basophils, and Th2 cells (6).

B. Leukocyte Survival–Promoting and Priming Cytokines

Certain cytokines, such as IL-3, IL-5, and GM-CSF, dramatically and selectively prolong eosinophil and basophil survival (63,64). For mast cells, the equivalent cytokine is stem cell factor (65). The ability of these cells to release mediators and to adhere to various tissue substrates in the presence of these cytokines is also altered (66–69). So, too, are their chemotactic and transendothelial migration responses (67,70–72). Furthermore, these cytokines alter expression and function of adhesion molecules on eosinophils and basophils (23). The sources of most of these cytokines include activated Th2 cells, epithelial cells, eosinophils themselves, and other cells (1,21,22). These cytokines are detected in the airways and at other sites following antigen challenge, and their neutralization in animal models can have profound inhibitory effects on eosinophil numbers and airways inflammation (73).

C. Chemokines and Other Chemoattractants

Differences in chemokine receptor expression among leukocyte subtypes are certain to play a major role in selective cell recruitment (Fig. 2) (1,6). For example, expression of CCR4 and CCR8, as well as perhaps CCR3, has been associated with the Th2 phenotype (74–76), although this remains somewhat controversial (77–79) (see also below). In contrast, expression of CCR5 and CXCR3 has been associated with Th1 cells (74,76,80). Thus, the state of activation, differentiation, or priming can influence which chemokine receptors are expressed and, based upon the type of chemokine encountered within a given tissue site, can determine which subsets of leukocytes are recruited into a particular tissue.

Besides possible expression on lymphocytes, expression of CCR3 is relatively limited and includes eosinophils, basophils, and mast cells (23). These are the primary cells that respond to eotaxin and related chemokines. Based on studies with antagonists and in knockout animals, CCR3 and eotaxin seem to play particularly important roles in homing of eosinophils to the gut (81–83). CCR3-dependent pathways for airway recruitment of eosinophils in these models have also been demon-

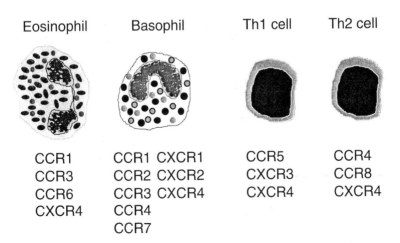

Figure 2 Chemokine receptor expression on human eosinophils, basophils, and T cells.

strated (84,85), but to date, most impressive have been studies of CCR8-deficient mice, where the greatest inhibition of allergic inflammation has been observed (86). This is in contrast to data with CCR4 knockout mice, where no effect was seen (87), and CCR3-deficient mice, where airway eosinophils were reduced but an unexpected increase in baseline airway hyperreactivity and mast cell numbers was observed (88). However, human eosinophils also express CCR1, CCR6, CXCR4, and an as-yet-unidentified, non-CCR4 receptor for the chemokine MDC (89–92), while basophils express CCR1, CCR2, CCR4, CXCR1, CXCR2, CXCR4, and probably others (Fig. 2) (69,93,94). Therefore, additional chemokine-dependent pathways may exist that contribute to their accumulation in vivo (89–92). Other chemoattractants have been implicated, including C3a (95), leukotriene C4 (LTC4) (96), and prostaglandin D2 (PGD2) (97), the latter acting via a recently identified receptor termed CRTH2 expressed by eosinophils, basophils, and Th2 cells (98). What are sorely needed are studies in asthmatic patients with selective antagonists; these should be forthcoming.

Besides the cellular specificity, the pattern of chemokine production within tissues can be tissue-specific. One example is the lymph node–selective production of the chemokine SLC. For naive T cells, interactions with high endothelial venules are stimulated by SLC via activation of its receptor, CCR7. Subsequently, their positional localization within the lymph node may then be controlled by production of another chemokine, MIP-3β (also via CCR7), within the T-cell zone (99,100). Another example is in the gastrointestinal tract, where homing of lymphocytes to sites in Peyer's patches and lamina propria involves initial interactions via the gut-specific adhesion molecule MAdCAM-1 and its leukocyte ligand α4β7 integrin (101). These interactions can be stimulated by the chemokine TECK (via CCR9), produced by the small intestine and also by intestinal epithelial cells, but not in skin or lymph nodes (102,103).

In contrast to lymph node and gut homing, recruitment of memory T cells to the skin during allergic cutaneous inflammation appears to involve initial endothelial interactions via E-selectin and its glycosylated ligand CLA, perhaps stimulated by the chemokine TARC (via CCR4) (79,104). Subsequent localization within tissues may then be controlled by local production of other chemokines such as CTACK (via CCR10) (105,106) or LARC (via CCR6) (107) and interactions between β1 integrins and tissue matrix proteins such as collagen (108).

Of particular relevance to allergic airway inflammation is the observation that airway epithelium is a major, if not the predominant, source of chemokine production (109). This initial observation was made in nasal polyps (110), and subsequent studies using primary respiratory epithelial cells and epithelial cell lines have clearly demonstrated production of key chemokines such as eotaxin, RANTES, MCP-4, and TARC (111–114). Notable in the in vitro cell culture systems was the profound ability of cytokines, such as TNFα, IL-4, IL-13, and IFNγ, either alone or in combination, to stimulate synthesis of a wide variety of chemokines (111,112,115–117). Equally remarkable was the ability of glucocorticoids, a major therapeutic agent in asthma, to inhibit epithelial chemokine production (111,118).

IV. Mechanisms of Cellular Recruitment to the Lungs in Allergic Asthma: In Vivo Human Studies

Evidence that asthma is an inflammatory disease has been gained from four major approaches (1,2). The first approach, histological examination of airway tissue from autopsy and biopsy, has revealed epithelial shedding, airway wall thickening with deposition of excess amounts of matrix proteins (e.g., collagen) in the subbasement membrane region, and hypertrophy and hyperplasia of smooth muscle and mucus glands. The disease is also characterized by copious quantities of mucus, dead and dying eosinophils and basophils, and eosinophil proteins at areas of epithelial destruction and in the lumen of the airways.

A second approach to the study of asthma utilizes physiological measurements of lung function and airways reactivity (119). Such studies have demonstrated that asthma is characterized by the presence of variable airway obstruction and bronchial hyperreactivity, the latter being correlated with asthma severity. Bronchial hyperreactivity, the hallmark of asthma, is a state of enhanced sensitivity of the airways of asthmatic subjects to the bronchoconstricting effects of inhaled stimuli such as histamine or methacholine, which for normal individuals has little or no effect, even at higher concentrations. The etiology of bronchial hyperreactivity is unknown, but may result from abnormalities in smooth muscle, in lung elastic recoil, in neuronal control of the airway muscle, in epithelial structure or function, edema of the airways, or a combination of these factors.

A third approach to the study of asthma utilizes bronchoalveolar lavage (BAL). Results using this technique have confirmed autopsy and biopsy studies that suggested that asthma was a disease of inflammation. BAL studies have demonstrated a correlation of the severity of the disease with elevations in mast cell numbers, eosinophil numbers, and eosinophil proteins. A variety of inflammatory mediators are elevated in lavage fluids taken from asthmatics, including histamine, prostanoids, leukotrienes, mast cell tryptase, cytokines (e.g., IL-5, GM-CSF), and chemokines (120–122). The precise roles and relative importance of each of these mediators remain to be determined.

A fourth approach to the study of asthma has been the use of experimental allergen challenge tests (123). In these tests, administration of allergen to the lungs (inhalational or whole lung challenge) or to a section of the lung via a bronchoscope (segmental challenge) induces physiological responses associated with the appearance of inflammatory mediators and cells. To generalize, the allergen-induced physiological response caused by whole lung challenge is characterized by acute constriction of the airways occurring within minutes, and resolving within 2 hours (the acute phase response), followed, in a proportion of subjects, by a late phase airflow obstruction occurring many hours later (the LPR). While the physiological responses to whole lung challenge are more dramatic than with segmental challenge, the latter provides a greater localized cellular and mediator response (124,125). Indeed, BAL following the acute response reveals markedly elevated concentrations of mast cell–derived mediators. The late inflammatory response following allergen challenge is characterized by the influx of large numbers of eosinophils and some basophils (4,120,123,124). Both early and late responses are accompanied by increases in vascular permeability and worsening bronchial reactivity (126), but the changes in vascular permeability do not, by themselves, explain the changes in airways hyperreactivity (125).

Despite clear evidence that asthma is an inflammatory disease, the exact role of adhesion molecules, cytokines, chemokines, and other molecules in cell recruitment to the lungs is less clear compared to skin, gut, and lymph node homing. Part of the difficulty is that human lungs do not normally contain secondary lymphoid organs, so-called BALT (bronchus-associated lymphoid tissue), that are present in other mammals (127–129). Therefore, it may be misleading to extrapolate to humans results from studies examining leukocyte trafficking to lungs in animals, such as rabbits, rats, and mice, that do contain BALT (127). Regardless, the last decade has seen tremendous progress in efforts to document the local adhesion molecule, cytokine, and chemokine milieu in a variety of diseases, including asthma. While by necessity these are mostly correlative studies, they provide absolutely critical support in humans for paradigms derived from in vitro and animal data. Based on this and other information, momentum is building for the development and testing of novel antagonists of each of these types of molecules. It is these kinds of studies that ultimately will formally test the hypothesis that specific adhesion molecules, cytokines, and chemokines play key roles in allergic inflammatory events in the lungs.

A. Role of Adhesion Molecules in Human Asthma

Expression of endothelial adhesion molecules has been examined using immunohistochemistry following experimental allergen challenge and bronchoscopic biopsy. Endobronchial allergen challenge resulted in increased endothelial VCAM-1 staining and epithelial ICAM-1 staining, with a significant correlation between these parameters and eosinophil influx (130). In nonhuman primates, allergen inhalation resulted in E-selectin expression on the airway vascular endothelium within 6 hours (40). There is additional indirect evidence that endothelial activation also occurs within the human airway following intrabronchial allergen challenge. Increased levels of soluble forms of E-selectin, ICAM-1, and VCAM-1 are observed in BAL fluids (131–134). In one of these studies there was a correlation with eosinophil influx and levels of both IL-4 and IL-5 (133), while in another, prednisone reduced levels of soluble E-selectin in BAL fluids (134).

In asthma, studies are somewhat contradictory, perhaps because of differences in patient severity or treatment. One study examining bronchial mucosal biopsies from normal subjects and mild allergic asthmatics found similar levels of endothelial ICAM-1 and E-selectin, despite an increased number of eosinophils in the mucosa of the asthmatics (135). Another study compared endothelial adhesion molecule expression in airway biopsies from subjects with mild allergic and nonallergic asthma as well as normal controls (130). Constitutive expression of ICAM-1, VCAM-1, and E-selectin was observed in all groups. Endothelial staining for ICAM-1 and E-selectin, not VCAM-1, was significantly increased in the nonallergic asthmatic group only, while epithelial staining for ICAM-1 was increased in both groups of asthmatic subjects. A third study comparing eosinophil numbers and VCAM-1 staining in asthmatics before and after 8 weeks treatment with inhaled budesonide or formoterol revealed that both treatments reduced eosinophil numbers, but only in the budesonide-treated subjects was this accompanied by a reduction in VCAM-1 (136). Analysis of the nonallergic asthmatics was complicated by the inclusion of subjects with more severe disease and higher medication requirements. Correlations were seen between eosinophil infiltration and endothelial ICAM-1 and E-selectin, while the correlation with endothelial VCAM-1 did not quite reach statistical significance. Subsequent studies of patients with more active disease, including moderately symptomatic asthmatics, showed strong endothelial staining for VCAM-1 and ICAM-1 (136–138). Staining correlated with levels of IL-4 in the airway, suggesting that cytokines appropriate for such endothelial activation were produced locally. While there is relatively little information on the adhesive function of circulating cells in asthma, there is one report of enhanced eosinophil adhesiveness for VCAM-1 and ICAM-1 in asthmatics (139). Increased serum levels of soluble ICAM-1 and E-selectin, but not VCAM-1, have been measured among patients admitted for exacerbations of asthma (140), while in another study, increased levels of soluble VCAM-1 were reported in asthmatics (141).

With respect to the adhesion phenotype of "lung-homing" lymphocytes, it has been shown that the majority of T cells in normal airways are CD4 + and CD45RO +. Some (but relatively few) express $\alpha 4 \beta 7$ integrin, VLA-1, and the intraepithelial lymphocyte marker $\alpha E \beta 7$ integrin, although the latter is found more commonly on lung CD8 + cells (142–144). Lung lymphocytes do not express either the skin-homing structure CLA or $\alpha 4 \beta 7$ integrin (144,145). Intraepithelial lymphocytes are observed in normal and inflamed airways, and based on studies of explanted human bronchial tissue into SCID mice, these cells appear to be long-lived (146,147). However, the importance of $\alpha E \beta 7$ integrin in lung homing has been questioned by the finding that mice deficient in αE integrins have normal numbers of lung T cells, although their numbers at other mucosal sites, such as gut, were diminished (147,148). Finally, altered expression and function of adhesion molecules occurs on eosinophils and basophils during their allergen-induced movement from the circulation into tissues. For example, analysis of adhesion molecules on eosinophils recovered from either sputum or BAL after antigen challenge revealed increased expression of CD11b, CD11c, CD69, and ICAM-1, diminished L-selectin and VLA-4, and little or no change in CD11a or CD32 (131,149–152).

Adhesion molecules in the lung have also been studied in the context of potential changes induced during successful pharmacotherapy. For example, treatment of asthmatics with inhaled corticosteroids reduced the tissue eosinophilia without changing ICAM-1 or E-selectin expression (135), while in another study both eosinophils and VCAM-1 were reduced (153). In the allergen challenge model, treatment with glucocorticoids not only suppressed the allergen-induced inflammation, but also inhibited endothelial activation (130,134). However, direct proof of adhesion molecule involvement in allergic diseases will, by necessity, require the use of specific adhesion molecule antagonists (154–156). Although no published data exist for allergic diseases in humans, antibodies to adhesion molecules, such as ICAM-1 and VLA-4, have been administered in clinical trials (157–159). These efforts have been motivated in large part by success seen in animal studies. Blocking monoclonal antibodies have been used successfully in a variety of animal models of allergic inflammatory conditions of the airways and skin (28,154–156, 160). Sometimes infusion of adhesion molecule antibodies failed to inhibit cell influx, yet still resulted in "clinical" benefit, or local application was more effective than systemic administration, perhaps because of effects on cell function (24,33,161). In addition to antibodies, a wide variety of pharmaceutical agents are being tested for their ability to prevent cell recruitment by blocking adhesion molecules (28,162–165). Ultimately, however, information on the role of adhesion molecules in allergic diseases in vivo must await results of planned or ongoing studies with antagonists in humans.

B. Role of Cytokines in Human Asthma

There is ample evidence for the presence of each of the previously mentioned cytokines in allergic pulmonary inflammation in vivo (166). Methods including immuno-histochemistry, in situ hybridization, and ELISA have clearly documented the presence of TNFα, IL-4, IL-5, IL-13, and GM-CSF in asthmatic lung and following allergen challenge (1,167–175). Eosinophils obtained from peripheral blood or by BAL after antigen challenge display a primed phenotype and a pronounced potentiation of transendothelial migration quite reminiscent of that induced by in vitro culture with cytokines (131,176,177). Treatment with glucocorticoids reduces the levels of these cytokines (178–180). Furthermore, inhalation of IL-4 or IL-5 by volunteers worsens the asthmatic phenotype, including eosinophilia and bronchial reactivity (181,182). Early studies with an inhaled, soluble form of the IL-4 receptors were promising (183,184), but subsequent phase 3 clinical trials have been disappointing. Additional antagonists of both IL-4 and IL-13 are under development. Systemic administration of GM-CSF or IL-5 enhances numbers of eosinophils and enhances their expression of CCR3 (185–187). Treatment of allergic asthmatics with a humanized anti-IL-5 antibody reduced numbers of circulating eosinophils and allergen-induced sputum eosinophils, although the efficacy of this agent in asthma remains uncertain (188,189). Finally, trials of anti-TNFα drugs in asthma, such as etanercept, are underway, but data from such studies are not yet published.

C. Role of Chemokines in Human Asthma

Eosinophil and basophil accumulation during allergic diseases of the airways, including asthma, appears to be mediated by the same array of chemokines that function in other tissues. This makes CCR3 an attractive target for therapeutic intervention in allergic inflammation (190, 191). Methods used to come to this conclusion include analysis of sputum, bronchoalveolar lavage and biopsies for CCR3-active chemokines including the eotaxins, RANTES, mucosae-associated epithelial chemokine (MEC), MCP-3, and MCP-4 (109,122,192–194). Given the pronounced ability of respiratory epithelium to produce these chemokines following exposure to Th2 cytokines, especially in conjunction with TNFα (111,112,117,118), their role in selective recruitment of eosinophils is strongly suggested. Indeed, local challenge of human subjects with RANTES or eotaxin, both CCR3-active chemokines, stimulated local eosinophil (and to a lesser degree basophil) influx (195–197). Other lung-resident cells capable of producing these same chemokines include fibroblasts and smooth muscle (122,198). In addition to CCR3-active chemokines, other chemokines implicated in animal models of asthma include SDF-1 (199), a potentially important ligand for eosinophils, basophils, and T cells, which functions via its receptor CXCR4 (92,93).

With respect to the chemokine receptor phenotype of "lung-homing" lymphocytes, recent efforts have focused on those receptors expressed by Th2 cells (8). Initially, it was proposed that CCR3 may be important for recruitment of Th2 cells (200), but most subsequent studies of allergic inflammation in human airways have failed to support this notion (144,201). Another proposed pathway for T-cell recruitment to the lung involves the epithelial-derived cytokine IL-16, acting via its receptor CD4, but its potency as a chemoattractant is relatively modest (202,203). Most recently, it has been reported that the chemokine receptors CCR4 and CCR8 are highly expressed on Th2 cells (75,104,204). Ligands for CCR4, such as the chemokine TARC, are produced in asthmatic airways (114,205). TARC is produced by both endothelial cells and epithelial cells (104,114). One study found increased CCR4 expression compared to blood on lung T cells from asthmatics (205), while another did not (144). The role of another CCR4-active chemokine, MDC, has also been implicated in eosinophil migration (91), but its role in the asthmatic airway is less clear (114). Perhaps most impressive was expression of CCR8 by airway T cells in bronchial biopsies of asthmatics (205). Whether its ligand, I-309, is overexpressed in asthma has not been reported.

V. Conclusions

The human immune system has evolved clever mechanisms for regulating tissue-specific leukocyte accumulation during inflammatory responses. Many tissues have been designed with unique patterns of adhesion molecules, along with specific arrays of chemokines, to direct subsets of leukocytes via selective interactions mediated by adhesion ligands and chemokine receptors. This new knowledge gives additional importance to the role played by tissue resident cells, such as endothelium, epithelium, and dendritic cells, in orchestrating the cellular makeup of inflammatory infiltrates in tissues such as the lung (Fig. 3). The fact that allergic reactions involve numerous cytokines, adhesion molecules, and chemokines and are highly orchestrated processes makes it difficult to sort out the relative importance of each protein. One of the challenges we now face is to determine the relative importance, in allergic disease, of each of these molecules. The impending availability of specific pharmacological antagonists should soon shed light on this issue.

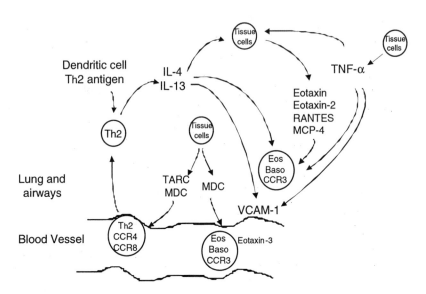

Figure 3 Possible roles of adhesion molecules, cytokines, and chemokines in recruitment of eosinophils, basophils, and Th2 cells to the airway during allergic inflammation. Tissue cells can include mast cells, basophils, eosinophils, T cells, and epithelium.

References

1. Busse WW, Lemanske RF, Jr. Asthma. N Engl J Med 2001; 344:350–362.
2. Kepley CL, McFeeley PJ, Oliver JM, Lipscomb MF. Immunohistochemical detection of human basophils in postmortem cases of fatal asthma. Am J Respir Crit Care Med 2001; 164:1053–1058.
3. Bochner BS, Undem BJ, Lichtenstein LM. Immunological aspects of allergic asthma. Annu Rev Immunol 1994; 12:295–335.
4. Liu MC, Hubbard WC, Proud D, Stealey B, Galli S, Kagey-Sobotka A, Bleecker ER, Lichtenstein LM. Immediate and late inflammatory responses to ragweed antigen challenge of the peripheral airways in asthmatics: cellular, mediator, and permeability changes. Am Rev Respir Dis 1991; 144:51–58.
5. Guo CB, Liu MC, Galli SJ, Bochner BS, Kagey-Sobotka A, Lichtenstein LM. Identification of IgE-bearing cells in the late-phase response to antigen in the lung as basophils. Am J Respir Cell Mol Biol 1994; 10:384–390.
6. Bochner BS. Road signs guiding leukocytes along the inflammation superhighway. J Allergy Clin Immunol 2000; 106:817–828.
7. von Andrian UH, Mackay CR. T-cell function and migration. N Engl J Med 2000; 343:1020–1034.
8. D'Ambrosio D, Mariani M, Panina-Bordignon P, Sinigaglia F. Chemokines and their receptors guiding T lymphocyte recruitment in lung inflammation. Am J Respir Crit Care Med 2001; 164:1266–1275.
9. Doerschuk C. Leukocyte trafficking in alveoli and airway passages. Respir Res 2000; 1:136–140.

10. Broide D, Sriramarao P. Eosinophil trafficking to sites of allergic inflammation. Immunol Rev 2001; 179:163–172.

11. Lloyd CM, Gonzalo JA, Coyle AJ, Gutierrez-Ramos JC. Mouse models of allergic airway disease. Adv Immunol 2001; 77:263–295.

12. Davenpeck K, Bochner BS. Leukocyte-blood vessel interactions. In: Zweiman B, Schwartz LB, eds. Inflammatory Mechanisms in Allergic Disease. New York: Marcel Dekker, Inc., 2002:125–141.

13. Bochner BS. Cellular adhesion in inflammation. In: Middleton E, C. Reed, E. Ellis, Adkinson NF, Yunginger J, Busse W, eds. Allergy Principles and Practice. 5th ed. St. Louis: Mosby, 1998:94–107.

14. Sriramarao P, von Andrian UH, Butcher EC, Bourdon MA, Broide DH. L-selectin and very late antigen-4 integrin promote eosinophil rolling at physiological shear rates in vivo. J Immunol 1994; 153:4238–4246.

15. Kikuchi M, Tachimoto M, Hudson SA, Bochner BS, Phorbol myristate acetate (PMA) alters human eosinophil expression of α4β1 and αdβ2 integrins and adhesion to VCAM-1 under static and flow conditions (abstr). J Allergy Clin Immunol 2000; 105: S258.

16. Dustin ML. Adhesion molecules. In: Austen KF, Frank MM, Atkinson JP, Cantor H, eds. Samter's Immunological Diseases. 10th ed. Philadelphia: Lippincott Williams & Wilkins, 2001:155–166.

17. Butcher EC, Williams M, Youngman K, Rott L, Briskin M. Lymphocyte trafficking and regional immunity. Adv Immunol 1999; 72:209–253.

18. Kitayama J, Mackay CR, Ponath PD, Springer TA. The C-C chemokine receptor CCR3 participates in stimulation of eosinophil arrest on inflammatory endothelium in shear flow J Clin Invest 1998; 101:2017–2024.

19. Tachimoto H, Burdick M, Hudson SA, Kikuchi M, Konstantopoulous K, Bochner BS. CCR3-active chemokines promote rapid detachment of eosinophils from VCAM-1 in vitro. J Immunol 2000; 165:2748–2754.

20. Sanchez-Madrid F, del Pozo M. Leukocyte polarization in cell migration and immune interactions. EMBO J 1999; 18:501–511.

21. Kay AB, Allergy and allergic diseases. Part 2. N Engl J Med 2001; 344:109–113.

22. Kay AB, Allergy and allergic diseases. Part 2. N Engl J Med 2001; 344:30–37.

23. Bochner BS, Schleimer RP. Mast cells, basophils, and eosinophils: distinct but overlapping pathways for recruitment. Immunol Reviews 2001; 179:5–15.

24. Abraham WM, Sielczak MW, Ahmed A, Cortes A, Lauredo IT, Kim J, Pepinsky B, Benjamin CD, Leone DR, Lobb RR, Weller PF. α4-Integrins mediate antigen-induced late bronchial responses and prolonged airway hyperresponsiveness in sheep. J Clin Invest 1994; 93:776–787.

25. Abraham WM, Gill A, Ahmed A, Sielczak MW, Lauredo IT, Botinnikova Y, Lin KC, Pepinsky B, Leone DR, Lobb RR, Adams SP. A small-molecule, tight-binding inhibitor of the integrin α4β1 blocks antigen-induced airway responses and inflammation in experimental asthma in sheep. Am J Respir Crit Care Med 2000; 162:603–611.

26. Das AM, Williams TJ, Lobb R, Nourshargh S. Lung eosinophilia is dependent on IL-5 and the adhesion molecules CD18 and VLA-4, in a guinea-pig model. Immunology 1995; 84:41–46.

27. Chin J, Hatfield C, Winterrowd G, Brashler J, Vonderfecht S, Fidler S, Griffin R, Kolbasa K, Krzesicki R, Sly L, Staite N, Richards I. Airway recruitment of leukocytes in mice is dependent on α4-integrins and vascular cell adhesion molecule-1. Am J Physiol 1997; 272:L219–29.

28. Bochner BS. Targeting VLA-4 integrin function: potential therapeutic implications. In: Mousa SA, ed. Cell Adhesion Molecules Matrix Proteins in Health and Disease. Georgetown, TX: Springer-Verlag and Landes Bioscience, 1998:113–131.

29. Rabb HA, Olivenstein R, Issekutz TB, Renzi PM, Martin JG. The role of the leukocyte adhesion molecules VLA-4, LFA-1, and Mac-1 in allergic airway responses in the rat. Am J Respir Crit Care Med 1994; 149:1186–1191.

30. Pretolani M, Ruffie C, Silva JRLE, Joseph D, Lobb RR, Vargaftig BB. Antibody to very late activation antigen 4 prevents antigen-induced bronchial hyperreactivity and cellular infiltration in the guinea pig airways. J Exp Med 1994; 180:795–805.

31. Fryer AD, Costello RW, Yost BL, Lobb RR, Tedder TF, Steeber DA, Bochner BS. Antibody to VLA-4, but not to L-selectin, protects neuronal M2 muscarinic receptors in antigen-challenged guinea pig airways. J Clin Invest 1997; 99:2036–2044.

32. Gonzalo JA, Lloyd CM, Kremer L, Finger E, Martinez C, Siegelman MH, Cybulsky M, Gutierrez-Ramos JC. Eosinophil recruitment to the lung in a murine model of allergic inflammation—the role of T cells, chemokines, and adhesion receptors. J Clin Invest 1996; 98:2332–2345.

33. Henderson WR, Chi EY, Albert RK, Chu SJ, Lamm WJE, Rochon Y, Jonas M, Christie PE, Harlan JM. Blockade of CD49d (α4 integrin) on intrapulmonary but not circulating leukocytes inhibits airway inflammation and hyperresponsiveness in a mouse model of asthma. J Clin Invest 1997; 100:3083–3092.

34. Kanehiro A, Takeda K, Joetham A, Tomkinson A, Ikemura T, Irvin CG, Gelfand EW. Timing of administration of anti-VLA-4 differentiates airway hyperresponsiveness in the central and peripheral airways in mice. Am J Respir Crit Care Med 2000; 162: 1132–1139.

35. Gundel RH, Wegner CD, Torcellini CA, Letts LG. The role of intercellular adhesion molecule-1 in chronic airway inflammation. Clin Exp Allergy 1992; 22:569–575.

36. Keramidaris E, Merson TD, Steeber DA, Tedder TF, Tang ML. L-selectin and intercellular adhesion molecule 1 mediate lymphocyte migration to the inflamed airway/lung during an allergic inflammatory response in an animal model of asthma. J Allergy Clin Immunol 2001; 107:734–738.

37. Broide DH, Sullivan S, Gifford T, Sriramarao P. Inhibition of pulmonary eosinophilia in P-selectin- and ICAM-1-deficient mice. Am J Respir Cell Mol Biol 1998; 18:218–225.

38. Wolyniec WW, De Sanctis GT, Nabozny G, Torcellini C, Haynes N, Joetham A, Gelfand EW, Drazen JM, Noonan TC. Reduction of antigen-induced airway hyperreactivity and eosinophilia in ICAM-1-deficient mice. Am J Respir Cell Mol Biol 1998; 18:777–785.

39. Gerwin N, Gonzalo JA, Lloyd C, Coyle AJ, Reiss Y, Banu N, Wang BP, Xu H, Avraham H, Engelhardt B, Springer TA, Gutierrez-Ramos JC. Prolonged eosinophil accumulation in allergic lung interstitium of ICAM-2-deficient mice results in extended hyperresponsiveness. Immunity 1999; 10:9–19.

40. Gundel RH, Wegner CD, Torcellini CA, Clarke CC, Haynes N, Rothlein R, Smith CW, Letts LG. Endothelial leukocyte adhesion molecule-1 mediates antigen-induced acute airway inflammation and late-phase airway obstruction in monkeys. J Clin Invest 1991; 88:1407–1411.

41. De Sanctis GT, Wolyniec WW, Green FH, Qin S, Jiao A, Finn PW, Noonan T, Joetham AA, Gelfand E, Doerschuk CM, Drazen JM. Reduction of allergic airway responses in P-selectin-deficient mice. J Appl Physiol 1997; 83:681–687.

42. Miller M, Sung KL, Muller WA, Cho JY, Roman M, Castaneda D, Nayar J, Condon T, Kim J, Sriramarao P, Broide DH. Eosinophil tissue recruitment to sites of allergic

inflammation in the lung is platelet endothelial cell adhesion molecule independent. J Immunol 2001; 167:2292–2297.

43. Broide DH, Miller M, Castaneda D, Nayar J, Cho JY, Roman M, Ellies LG, Sriramarao P. Core 2 oligosaccharides mediate eosinophil and neutrophil peritoneal but not lung recruitment. Am J Physiol Lung Cell Mol Physiol 2002; 282:L259–L266.

44. Fiscus LC, Van Herpen J, Steeber DA, Tedder TF, Tang ML. L-selectin is required for the development of airway hyperresponsiveness but not airway inflammation in a murine model of asthma. J Allergy Clin Immunol 2001; 107:1019–1024.

45. Schleimer RP, Sterbinsky SA, Kaiser J, Bickel CA, Klunk DA, Tomioka K, Newman W, Luscinskas FW, Gimbrone MA, Jr, McIntyre BW, Bochner BS. Interleukin-4 induces adherence of human eosinophils and basophils but not neutrophils to endothelium: association with expression of VCAM-1. J Immunol 1992; 148:1086–1092.

46. Bochner BS, Klunk DA, Sterbinsky SA, Coffman RL, Schleimer RP. Interleukin-13 selectively induces vascular cell adhesion molecule-1 (VCAM-1) expression in human endothelial cells. J Immunol 1995; 154:799–803.

47. Thornhill MH, Haskard DO. IL-4 regulates endothelial cell activation by IL-1, tumor necrosis factor, or IFN-γ. J Immunol 1990; 145:865–872.

48. Sanz MJ, Weg VB, Bolanowski MA, Nourshargh S. IL-1 is a potent inducer of eosinophil accumulation in rat skin—inhibition of response by a platelet-activating factor antagonist and an anti-human IL-8 antibody. J Immunol 1995; 154:1364–1373.

49. Moser R, Groscurth P, Carballido JM, Bruijnzeel PLB, Blaser K, Heusser CH, Fehr J. Interleukin-4 induces tissue eosinophilia in mice: Correlation with its in vitro capacity to stimulate the endothelial cell-dependent selective transmigration of human eosinophils. J Lab Clin Med 1993; 122:567–575.

50. Lukacs NW, Strieter RM, Chensue SW, Kunkel SL. Interleukin-4-dependent pulmonary eosinophil infiltration in a murine model of asthma. Am J Respir Cell Mol Biol 1994; 10:526–532.

51. Rankin JA, Picarella DE, Geba GP, Temann UA, Prasad B, Dicosmo B, Tarallo A, Stripp B, Whitsett J, Flavell RA. Phenotypic and physiologic characterization of transgenic mice expressing interleukin 4 in the lung: lymphocytic and eosinophilic inflammation without airway hyperreactivity. Proc Natl Acad Sci USA 1996; 93: 7821–7825.

52. Wills-Karp M, Luyimbazi J, Xu XY, Schofield B, Neben TY, Karp CL, Donaldson DD. Interleukin-13: central mediator of allergic asthma. Science 1998; 282:2258–2261.

53. Zhu Z, Homer RJ, Wang Z, Chen Q, Geba GP, Wang J, Zhang Y, Elias JA. Pulmonary expression of interleukin-13 causes inflammation, mucus hypersecretion, subepithelial fibrosis, physiologic abnormalities, and eotaxin production. J Clin Invest 1999; 103: 779–788.

54. Gordon JR, Galli SJ. Mast cells as a source of both preformed and immunologically inducible TNF-α/cachectin. Nature 1990; 346:274–276.

55. Wershil BK, Wang ZS, Gordon JR, Galli SJ. Recruitment of neutrophils during IgE-dependent cutaneous late phase reactions in the mouse is mast cell-dependent—partial inhibition of the reaction with antiserum against tumor necrosis factor-α. J Clin Invest 1991; 87:446–453.

56. Nagai H, Sakurai T, Abe T, Matsuo A, Musoh K, Tsunematsu M, Inagaki N. TNFα participates in an IgE-mediated cutaneous reaction in mast cell deficient, WBB6F1-W/Wv mice. Inflamm Res 1996; 45:136–40.

57. Sanz MJ, Hartnell A, Chisholm P, Williams C, Davies D, Weg VB, Feldmann M, Bolanowski MA, Lobb RR, Nourshargh S. Tumor necrosis factor α-induced eosinophil

accumulation in rat skin is dependent on α4 integrin/vascular cell adhesion molecule-1 adhesion pathways. Blood 1997; 90:4144–4152.

58. Sanz MJ, Marinova-Mutafchieva L, Green P, Lobb RR, Feldmann M, Nourshargh S. IL-4-induced eosinophil accumulation in rat skin is dependent on endogenous TNF-α and α4 integrin/VCAM-1 adhesion pathways. J Immunol 1998; 160:5637–5645.

59. Sakurai T, Inagaki N, Nagai H. The effect of anti-tumor necrosis factor (TNF)-alpha monoclonal antibody on allergic cutaneous late phase reaction in mice. Life Sci 1994; 54:L291–L295.

60. Renzetti LM, Paciorek PM, Tannu SA, Rinaldi NC, Tocker JE, Wasserman MA, Gater PR. Pharmacological evidence for tumor necrosis factor as a mediator of allergic inflammation in the airways. J Pharmacol Exp Ther 1996; 278:847–853.

61. Gater PR, Renzetti LM. Ro 45–2081, a TNF receptor fusion protein, prevents inflammatory responses in the airways. Agents Actions Suppl 1998; 49:67–71.

62. Broide DH, Stachnick G, Castaneda D, Nayar J, Sriramarao P. Inhibition of eosinophilic inflammation in allergen-challenged TNF receptor p55/p75- and TNF receptor p55-deficient mice. Am J Respir Cell Mol Biol 2001; 24:304–311.

63. Schleimer RP, Benenati SV, Friedman B, Bochner BS. Do cytokines play a role in leukocyte recruitment and activation in the lungs? Am Rev Respir Dis 1991; 143: 1169–1174.

64. Rothenberg ME. Mechanisms of disease: eosinophilia. N Engl J Med 1998; 338: 1592–1600.

65. Galli SJ. New concepts about the mast cell. N Engl J Med 1993; 328:257–265.

66. Yuan Q, Austen KF, Friend DS, Heidtman M, Boyce JA. Human peripheral blood eosinophils express a functional c-kit receptor for stem cell factor that stimulates very late antigen 4 (VLA-4)-mediated cell adhesion to fibronectin and vascular cell adhesion molecule 1 (VCAM-1). J Exp Med 1997; 186:313–323.

67. Vliagoftis H, Metcalfe DD. Cell adhesion molecules in mast cell adhesion and migration. In: Bochner BS, ed. Adhesion Molecules in Allergic Diseases. New York: Marcel Dekker, Inc., 1997:151–172.

68. Kita H, Adolphson CR, Gleich GJ. Biology of eosinophils. In: E. Middleton J, Reed CE, Ellis EF, N. F. Adkinson J, Yunginger JW, Busse W, eds. Allergy Principles and Practice. 5th ed. St. Louis: Mosby, 1998:242–260.

69. Bochner BS, Schroeder J. Basophils. In: Austen KF, Frank MM, Atkinson JP, Cantor H, eds. Samter's Immunological Diseases. 6th ed. Philadelphia: Lippincott Williams & Wilkins, 2001:244–253.

70. Ebisawa M, Bochner BS, Schleimer RP. Eosinophil-endothelial interactions and trans-endothelial migration. In: Bochner BS, eds. Adhesion Molecules in Allergic Diseases. New York: Marcel Dekker, Inc., 1997:173–186.

71. Shahabuddin S, Ponath P, Schleimer RP. Migration of eosinophils across endothelial cell monolayers: interactions among IL-5, endothelial-activating cytokines, and C-C chemokines. J Immunol 2000; 164:3847–3854.

72. Yamamoto H, Sedgwick JB, Vrtis RF, Busse WW. The effect of transendothelial migration on eosinophil function. Am J Respir Cell Mol Biol 2000; 23:379–388.

73. Lukacs NW, Kunkel SL, Strieter RM, Evanoff HL, Kunkel RG, Key ML, Taub DD. The role of stem cell factor (c-kit ligand) and inflammatory cytokines in pulmonary mast cell activation. Blood 1996; 87:2262–2268.

74. Zingoni A, Soto H, Hedrick JA, Stoppacciaro A, Storlazzi CT, Sinigaglia F, D'Ambrosio D, O'Garra A, Robinson D, Rocchi M, Santoni A, Zlotnik A, Napolitano M.

The chemokine receptor CCR8 is preferentially expressed in Th2 but not Th1 cells. J Immunol 1998; 161:547–551.

75. D'Ambrosio D, Iellem A, Bonecchi R, Mazzeo D, Sozzani S, Mantovani A, Sinigaglia F. Selective up-regulation of chemokine receptors CCR4 and CCR8 upon activation of polarized human type 2 Th cells. J Immunol 1998; 161:5111–5115.

76. Yamamoto J, Adachi Y, Onoue Y, Adachi YS, Okabe Y, Itazawa T, Toyoda M, Seki T, Morohashi M, Matsushima K, Miyawaki T. Differential expression of the chemokine receptors by the Th1- and Th2-type effector populations within circulating CD4 + T cells. J Leukoc Biol 2000; 68:568–574.

77. Annunziato F, Cosmi L, Galli G, Beltrame C, Romagnani P, Manetti R, Romagnani S, Maggi E. Assessment of chemokine receptor expression by human Th1 and Th2 cells in vitro and in vivo. J Leukoc Biol 1999; 65:691–699.

78. Ying S, Meng Q, Zeibecoglou K, Robinson DS, Macfarlane A, Humbert M, Kay AB. Eosinophil chemotactic chemokines (eotaxin, eotaxin-2, RANTES, monocyte chemoattractant protein-3 (MCP-3), and MCP-4), and C-C chemokine receptor 3 expression in bronchial biopsies from atopic and nonatopic (intrinsic) asthmatics. J Immunol 1999; 163:6321–6329.

79. Andrew DP, Ruffing N, Kim CH, Miao W, Heath H, Li Y, Murphy K, Campbell JJ, Butcher EC, Wu L. C-C Chemokine Receptor 4 expression defines a major subset of circulating nonintestinal memory T cells of both Th1 and Th2 potential. J Immunol 2001; 166:103–111.

80. Qin S, Rottman JB, Myers P, Kassam N, Weinblatt M, Loetscher M, Koch AE, Moser B, Mackay CR. The chemokine receptors CXCR3 and CCR5 mark subsets of T cells associated with certain inflammatory reactions. J Clin Invest 1998; 101:746–754.

81. Matthews AN, Friend DS, Zimmerrmann N, Sarafi MN, Luster AD, Pearlman E, Wert SE, Rothenberg ME. Eotaxin is required for the baseline level of tissue eosinophils. Proc Natl Acad Sci USA 1998; 95:6273–6278.

82. Mishra A, Hogan SP, Lee JJ, Foster PS, Rothenberg ME. Fundamental signals that regulate eosinophil homing to the gastrointestinal tract. J Clin Invest 1999; 103: 1719–1727.

83. Mishra A, Hogan SP, Brandt EB, Rothenberg ME. Peyer's patch eosinophils: identification, characterization, and regulation by mucosal allergen exposure, interleukin-5, and eotaxin. Blood 2000; 96:1538–1544.

84. Rothenberg ME, MacLean JA, Pearlman E, Luster AD, Leder P. Targeted disruption of the chemokine eotaxin partially reduces antigen-induced tissue eosinophilia. J Exp Med 1997; 185:785–790.

85. Dabbagh K, Xiao Y, Smith C, Stepick-Biek P, Kim SG, Lamm WJ, Liggitt DH, Lewis DB. Local blockade of allergic airway hyperreactivity and inflammation by the poxvirus-derived pan-CC-chemokine inhibitor vCCI. J Immunol 2000; 165: 3418–3422.

86. Chensue SW, Lukacs NW, Yang TY, Shang X, Frait KA, Kunkel SL, Kung T, Wiekowski MT, Hedrick JA, Cook DN, Zingoni A, Narula SK, Zlotnik A, Barrat FJ, O'Garra A, Napolitano M, Lira SA. Aberrant in vivo T helper type 2 cell response and impaired eosinophil recruitment in CC chemokine receptor 8 knockout mice. J Exp Med 2001; 193:573–584.

87. Chvatchko Y, Hoogewerf AJ, Meyer A, Alouani S, Juillard P, Buser R, Conquet F, Proudfoot AE, Wells TN, Power CA. A key role for CC chemokine receptor 4 in lipopolysaccharide-induced endotoxic shock. J Exp Med 2000; 191:1755–1764.

88. Gerard C, Rollins BJ. Chemokines and disease. Nature Immunol 2001; 2:108–115.

89. Heath H, Qin SX, Rao P, Wu LJ, LaRosa G, Kassam N, Ponath PD, Mackay CR. Chemokine receptor usage by human eosinophils—the importance of CCR3 demonstrated using an antagonistic monoclonal antibody. J Clin Invest 1997; 99:178–184.

90. Sullivan SK, McGrath DA, Liao F, Boehme SA, Farber JM, Bacon KB. MIP-3α induces human eosinophil migration and activation of the mitogen-activated protein kinases (p42/p44 MAPK) J Leukoc Biol 1999; 66:674–682.

91. Bochner BS, Bickel CA, Taylor ML, MacGlashan DW, Jr, Gray PW, Raport CJ, Godiska R. Macrophage derived chemokine (MDC) induces human eosinophil chemotaxis in a CCR3- and CCR4-independent manner. J Allergy Clin Immunol 1999; 103: 527–532.

92. Nagase H, Miyamasu M, Yamaguchi M, Fujisawa T, Ohta K, Yamamoto K, Morita Y, Hirai K. Expression of CXCR4 in eosinophils: functional analyses and cytokine-mediated regulation. J Immunol 2000; 164:5935–5943.

93. Jinquan T, Jacobi HH, Jing C, Reimert CM, Quan S, Dissing S, Poulsen LK, Skov PS. Chemokine stromal cell-derived factor 1α activates basophils by means of CXCR4. J Allergy Clin Immunol 2000; 106:313–320.

94. Schleimer R, Bickel C, White J, Lim L, Bochner B, MacGlashan D, Jr. Chemokine responses in purified human basophils (abstr). J Allergy Clin Immunol 2002; 109;574.

95. Humbles AA, Lu B, Nilsson CA, Lilly C, Israel E, Fujiwara Y, Gerard NP, Gerard C. A role for the C3a anaphylatoxin receptor in the effector phase of asthma. Nature 2000; 406:998–1001.

96. Holgate ST, Bradding P, Sampson AP. Leukotriene antagonists and synthesis inhibitors: new directions in asthma therapy. J Allergy Clin Immunol 1996; 98:1–13.

97. Matsuoka T, Hirata M, Tanaka H, Takahashi Y, Murata T, Kabashima K, Sugimoto Y, Kobayashi T, Ushikubi F, Aze Y, Eguchi N, Urade Y, Yoshida N, Kimura K, Mizoguchi A, Honda Y, Nagai H, Narumiya S. Prostaglandin D2 as a mediator of allergic asthma. Science 2000; 287:2013–2017.

98. Hirai H, Tanaka K, Yoshie O, Ogawa K, Kenmotsu K, Takamori Y, Ichimasa M, Sugamura K, Nakamura M, Takano S, Nagata K. Prostaglandin D2 selectively induces chemotaxis in T helper type 2 cells, eosinophils, and basophils via seven-transmembrane receptor CRTH2. J Exp Med 2001; 193:255–261.

99. Campbell JJ, Butcher EC. Chemokines in tissue-specific and microenvironment-specific lymphocyte homing. Curr Opin Immunol 2000; 12:336–341.

100. Cyster JG. Chemokines and cell migration in secondary lymphoid organs. Science 1999; 286:2098–2102.

101. Briskin M. Pathways of cell recruitment to mucosal surfaces. In: Bochner BS, eds. Adhesion Molecules in Allergic Diseases. New York: Marcel Dekker, 1997: 105–128.

102. Wurbel MA, Philippe JM, Nguyen C, Victorero G, Freeman T, Wooding P, Miazek A, Mattei MG, Malissen M, Jordan BR, Malissen B, Carrier A, Naquet P. The chemokine TECK is expressed by thymic and intestinal epithelial cells and attracts double- and single-positive thymocytes expressing the TECK receptor CCR9. Eur J Immunol 2000; 30:262–271.

103. Kunkel EJ, Campbell JJ, Haraldsen G, Pan J, Boisvert J, Roberts AI, Ebert EC, Vierra MA, Goodman SB, Genovese MC, Wardlaw AJ, Greenberg HB, Parker CM, Butcher EC, Andrew DP, Agace WW. Lymphocyte CC. chemokine receptor 9 and epithelial thymus-expressed chemokine (TECK) expression distinguish the small intestinal immune compartment: epithelial expression of tissue-specific chemokines as an organizing principle in regional immunity. J Exp Med 2000; 192:761–768.

104. Campbell JJ, Haraldsen G, Pan J, Rottman J, Qin S, Ponath P, Andrew DP, Warnke R, Ruffing N, Kassam N, Wu L, Butcher EC. The chemokine receptor CCR4 in vascular recognition by cutaneous but not intestinal memory T cells. Nature 1999; 400:776–780.

105. Morales J, Homey B, Vicari AP, Hudak S, Oldham E, Hedrick J, Orozco R, Copeland NG, Jenkins NA, McEvoy LM, Zlotnik A, CTACK, a skin-associated chemokine that preferentially attracts skin-homing memory T cells. Proc Natl Acad Sci USA 1999; 96:14470–14475.

106. Homey B, Wang W, Soto H, Buchanan ME, Wiesenborn A, Catron D, Muller A, McClanahan TK, Dieu-Nosjean MC, Orozco R, Ruzicka T, Lehmann P, Oldham E, Zlotnik A. Cutting edge: the orphan chemokine receptor G protein-coupled receptor-2 (GPR-2, CCR10) binds the skin-associated chemokine CCL27 (CTACK/ALP/ILC). J Immunol 2000; 164:3465–3470.

107. Fitzhugh DJ, Naik S, Caughman SW, Hwang ST. Cutting edge: C-C chemokine receptor 6 is essential for arrest of a subset of memory T cells on activated dermal microvascular endothelial cells under physiologic flow conditions In vitro. J Immunol 2000; 165:6677–6681.

108. de Fougerolles AR, Sprague AG, Nickerson-Nutter CL, Chi-Rosso G, Rennert PD, Gardner H, Gotwals PJ, Lobb RR, Koteliansky VE. Regulation of inflammation by collagen-binding integrins $\alpha 1\beta 1$ and $\alpha 2\beta 1$ in models of hypersensitivity and arthritis. J Clin Invest 2000; 105:721–729.

109. Ying S, Kay A. Chemokines in allergic asthma. In: Rothenberg ME, ed. Chemokines in Allergic Disease. New York: Marcel Dekker, 2000:383–402.

110. Beck LA, Stellato C, Beall LD, Schall TJ, Leopold D, Bickel CA, Baroody F, Bochner BS, Schleimer RP. Detection of the chemokine RANTES and endothelial adhesion molecules in nasal polyps. J Allergy Clin Immunol 1996; 98:766–780.

111. Stellato C, Beck LA, Gorgone GA, Proud D, Schall TJ, Ono SJ, Lichtenstein LM, Schleimer RP. Expression of the chemokine RANTES by a human bronchial epithelial cell line: modulation by cytokines and glucocorticoids. J Immunol 1995; 155:410–418.

112. Stellato C, Collins P, Li H, White J, Ponath PD, Newman W, Soler D, Bickel C, Liu M, Bochner BS, Williams T, Schleimer RP. Production of the novel C-C-chemokine MCP-4 by airway cells and comparison of its biological activity to other C-C chemokines. J Clin Invest 1997; 99:926–936.

113. Lilly CM, Nakamura H, Kesselman H, NaglerAnderson C, Asano K, Garcia-Zepeda EA, Rothenberg ME, Drazen JM, Luster AD. Expression of eotaxin by human lung epithelial cells—induction by cytokines and inhibition by glucocorticoids. J Clin Invest 1997; 99:1767–1773.

114. Sekiya T, Miyamasu M, Imanishi M, Yamada H, Nakajima T, Yamaguchi M, Fujisawa T, Pawankar R, Sano Y, Ohta K, Ishii A, Morita Y, Yamamoto K, Matsushima K, Yoshie O, Hirai K. Inducible expression of a Th2-type CC chemokine thymus- and activation-regulated chemokine by human bronchial epithelial cells. J Immunol 2000; 165:2205–2213.

115. Sauty A, Dziejman M, Taha RA, Iarossi AS, Neote K, Garcia-Zepeda EA, Hamid Q, Luster AD. The T cell-specific CXC chemokines IP-10, Mig, and I-TAC are expressed by activated human bronchial epithelial cells. J Immunol 1999; 162:3549–3558.

116. Matsukura S, Stellato C, Georas SN, Casolaro V, Plitt JR, Miura K, Kurosawa S, Schindler U, Schleimer RP. Interleukin-13 upregulates eotaxin expression in airway epithelial cells by a STAT6-dependent mechanism. Am J Respir Cell Mol Biol 2001; 24:755–761.

117. Matsukura S, Stellato C, Plitt JR, Bickel C, Miura K, Georas SN, Casolaro V, Schleimer RP. Activation of eotaxin gene transcription by NF-kappa B and STAT6 in human airway epithelial cells. J Immunol 1999; 163:6876–6883.

118. Stellato C, Matsukura S, Fal A, White J, Beck LA, Proud D, Schleimer RP. Differential regulation of epithelial-derived C-C chemokine expression by IL-4 and the glucocorticoid budesonide. J Immunol 1999; 163:5624–5632.

119. Cockcroft DW, Hargreave FE. Airway hyperresponsiveness Am Rev Respir Dis 1990; 142:497–500.

120. Liu MC, Bleecker ER, Lichtenstein LM, Kagey-Sobotka A, Niv Y, McLemore TL, Permutt S, Proud D, Hubbard WC. Evidence for elevated levels of histamine, prostaglandin D_2, and other bronchoconstricting substances in the airways of mild asthmatic subjects Am Rev Respir Dis 1990; 142:126–132.

121. Broide DH, Lotz M, Cuomo AJ, Coburn DA, Federman EC, Wasserman SI. Cytokines in symptomatic asthma airways. J Allergy Clin Immunol 1992; 89:958–967.

122. Ghaffar O, Christodoulopoulos P, Hamid Q. Cellular sources of chemokines in allergic diseases. In: Rothenberg ME, eds. Chemokines in Allergic Disease. New York: Marcel Dekker, 2000:403–424.

123. Peters SP, Zangrilli JG, Fish JE. Late phase allergic reactions. In: Middleton E, C. Reed, F. Ellis, Adkinson NF, J. Yunginger, W. Busse, eds. Allergy Principles and Practice. 5th ed. St. Louis: Mosby, 1998:342–355.

124. Calhoun WJ, Jarjour NN, Gleich GJ, Stevens CA, Busse WW. Increased airway inflammation with segmental versus aerosol antigen challenge. Am Rev Respir Dis 1993; 147:1465–1471.

125. Peebles RS, Jr, Wagner EM, Liu MC, Proud D, Hamilton RG, Togias A. Allergen-induced changes in airway responsiveness are not related to indices of airway edema. J Allergy Clin Immunol 2001; 107:805–811.

126. Cockcroft DW. Airway responses to inhaled allergens. Can Respir J 1998; 5(suppl A): 7A–14A.

127. Pabst R, Gehrke I. Is the bronchus-associated lymphoid tissue (BALT) an integral structure of the lung in normal mammals, including humans? Am J Respir Cell Mol Biol 1990; 3:131–135.

128. Berman J. Lymphocytes in the lung: should we continue to exalt only BALT? Am J Respir Cell Mol Biol 1990; 3:101–102.

129. Richmond I, Pritchard GE, Ashcroft T, Avery A, Corris PA, Walters EH. Bronchus associated lymphoid tissue (BALT) in human lung: its distribution in smokers and non-smokers. Thorax 1993; 48:1130–1134.

130. Bentley AM, Durham SR, Robinson DS, Menz G, Storz C, Cromwell O, Kay AB, Wardlaw AJ. Expression of endothelial and leukocyte adhesion molecules intercellular adhesion molecule-1, E-selectin, and vascular cell adhesion molecule-1 in the bronchial mucosa in steady-state and allergen-induced asthma. J Allergy Clin Immunol 1993; 92:857–868.

131. Georas SN, Liu MC, Newman W, Beall WD, Stealey BA, Bochner BS. Altered adhesion molecule expression and endothelial activation accompany the recruitment of human granulocytes to the lung following segmental antigen challenge. Am J Respir Cell Mol Biol 1992; 7:261–269.

132. Takahashi N, Liu MC, Proud D, Yu XY, Hasegawa S, Spannhake EW. Soluble intracellular adhesion molecule 1 in bronchoalveolar lavage fluid of allergic subjects following segmental antigen challenge. Am J Respir Crit Care Med 1994; 150:704–709.

133. Zangrilli JG, Shaver JR, Cirelli RA, Cho SK, Garlis CG, Falcone A, Cuss FM, Fish JE, Peters SP. sVCAM-1 levels after segmental challenge correlate with eosinophil influx, IL-4 and IL-5 production, and the late phase response. Am J Respir Crit Care Med 1995; 151:1346–1353.

134. Liu MC, Proud D, Lichtenstein LM, Hubbard WC, Bochner BS, Stealey BA, Breslin L, Xiao H, Freidhoff LR, Schroeder JT, Schleimer RP. Effects of prednisone on the cellular responses and release of cytokines and mediators after segmental allergen challenge of asthmatic subjects. J Allergy Clin Immunol 2001; 108:29–38.

135. Montefort S, Roche WR, Howarth PH, Djukanovic R, Gratziou C, Carroll M, Smith L, Britten KM, Haskard D, Lee TH, Holgate ST. Intercellular adhesion molecule-1 (ICAM-1) and endothelial leukocyte adhesion molecule-1 (ELAM-1) expression in the bronchial mucosa of normal and asthmatic subjects. Eur Respir J 1992; 5:815–823.

136. Gossct P, Tillie-Leblond I, Janin A, Marquette CH, Copin MC, Wallaert B, Tonnel AB. Increased expression of ELAM-1, ICAM-1, and VCAM-1 on bronchial biopsies from allergic asthmatic patients. Ann NY Acad Sci 1994; 725:163–172.

137. Ohkawara Y, Yamauchi K, Maruyama N, Hoshi H, Ohno I, Honma M, Tanno Y, Tamura G, Shirato K, Ohtani H. In situ expression of the cell adhesion molecules in bronchial tissues from asthmatics with air flow limitation: in vivo evidence of VCAM-1/VLA-4 interaction in selective eosinophil infiltration. Am J Respir Cell Mol Biol 1995; 12:4–12.

138. Fukuda T, Fukushima Y, Numao T, Ando N, Arima M, Nakajima H, Sagara H, Adachi T, Motojima S, Makino S. Role of interleukin-4 and vascular cell adhesion molecule-1 in selective eosinophil migration into the airways in allergic asthma. Am J Respir Cell Mol Biol 1996; 14:84–94.

139. Hakansson L, Bjornsson E, Janson C, Schmekel B. Increased adhesion to vascular cell adhesion molecule-1 and intercellular adhesion molecule-1 of eosinophils from patients with asthma. J Allergy Clin Immunol 1995; 96:941–950.

140. Montefort S, Holgate ST. Expression of cell adhesion molecules in asthma. In: Bochner BS, eds. Adhesion Molecules in Allergic Diseases. New York: Marcel Dekker, Inc., 1997:315–338.

141. Koizumi A, Hashimoto S, Kobayashi T, Imai K, Yachi A, Horie T. Elevation of serum soluble vascular cell adhesion molecule-1 (sVCAM-1) levels in bronchial asthma. Clin Exp Immunol 1995; 101:468–473.

142. Erle DJ, Brown T, Christian D, Aris R. Lung epithelial lining fluid T cell subsets defined by distinct patterns of $\beta7$ and $\beta1$ integrin expression. Am J Respir Cell Mol Biol 1994; 10:237–244.

143. Erle DJ, Pabst R. Intraepithelial lymphocytes in the lung: a neglected lymphocyte population. Am J Respir Cell Mol Biol 2000; 22:398–400.

144. Campbell JJ, Brightling CE, Symon FA, Qin S, Murphy KE, Hodge M, Andrew DP, Wu L, Butcher EC, Wardlaw AJ. Expression of chemokine receptors by lung T cells from normal and asthmatic subjects. J Immunol 2001; 166:2842–2848.

145. Leung DYM, Picker LJ. Adhesion pathways controlling recruitment responses of lymphocytes during allergic inflammatory reactions in vivo. In: Bochner BS, eds. Adhesion Molecules in Allergic Diseases. New York: Marcel Dekker, 1997:297–314.

146. Fournier M, Lebargy F, Le Roy Ladurie F, Lenormand E, Pariente R. Intraepithelial T-lymphocyte subsets in the airways of normal subjects and of patients with chronic bronchitis. Am Rev Respir Dis 1989; 140:737–742.

147. Goto E, Kohrogi H, Hirata N, Tsumori K, Hirosako S, Hamamoto J, Fujii K, Kawano O, Ando M. Human bronchial intraepithelial T lymphocytes as a distinct T-cell subset:

their long-term survival in SCID-Hu chimeras. Am J Respir Cell Mol Biol 2000; 22: 405–411.

148. Schon MP, Arya A, Murphy EA, Adams CM, Strauch UG, Agace WW, Marsal J, Donohue JP, Her H, Beier DR, Olson S, Lefrancois L, Brenner MB, Grusby MJ, Parker CM. Mucosal T lymphocyte numbers are selectively reduced in integrin alpha E (CD103)-deficient mice. J Immunol 1999; 162:6641–6649.

149. Hansel TT, Walker C. The migration of eosinophils into the sputum of asthmatics: the role of adhesion molecules. Clin Exp Allergy 1992; 22:345–356.

150. Kroegel C, Liu MC, Hubbard WM, Lichtenstein LM, Bochner BS. Blood and bronchoalveolar eosinophils in allergic subjects following segmental antigen challenge: surface phenotype, density heterogeneity, and prostanoid production. J Allergy Clin Immunol 1994; 93:725–734.

151. Matsumoto K, Appiah-Pippim J, Schleimer RP, Bickel CA, Beck LA, Bochner BS. CD44 and CD69 represent different types of cell surface activation markers for human eosinophils. Am J Respir Cell Mol Biol 1998; 18:860–866.

152. Bochner BS. Systemic activation of basophils and eosinophils: markers and consequences. J Allergy Clin Immunol 2000; 106:S292–S302.

153. Wilson SJ, Wallin A, Della-Cioppa G, Sandstrom T, Holgate ST. Effects of budesonide and formoterol on NFκB, adhesion molecules, and cytokines in asthma. Am J Respir Crit Care Med 2001; 164:1047–1052.

154. Bochner BS. Cellular adhesion and its antagonism. J Allergy Clin Immunol 1997; 100: 581–585.

155. Schleimer RP, Bochner BS. The role of adhesion molecules in allergic inflammation and their suitability as targets of antiallergic therapy. Clin Exp Allergy 1998; 28:15–23.

156. Bochner BS. Adhesion molecule antagonism: an overview. In: Hansel TT, Barnes P, eds. New Drugs for Asthma, Allergy and COPD. Progress in Respiratory Research. Basel: Karger, 2001:298–301.

157. Kavanaugh A. Overview of cell adhesion molecules and their antagonism. In: Bochner BS, ed. Cell Adhesion Molecules in Allergic Disease. New York: Marcel Dekker, 1997:1–24.

158. Tubridy N, Behan PO, Capildeo R, Chaudhuri A, Forbes R, Hawkins CP, Hughes RA, Palace J, Sharrack B, Swingler R, Young C, Moseley IF, MacManus DG, Donoghue S, Miller DH. The effect of anti-α4 integrin antibody on brain lesion activity in MS. Neurology 1999; 53:466–472.

159. Miller D, Khan O, Sheremata W, Blumhardt L, Rice G, O'Connor P. Results of a double-blind, randomized, placebo-controlled, phase II trial of Antegren (natalizumab) in subjects with relapsing multiple sclerosis. Multiple Sclerosis 2001; 7:s16.

160. Lobb RR. Adhesion molecule antagonists in animal models of asthma. In: Bochner BS, ed. Adhesion Molecules in Allergic Diseases. New York: Marcel Dekker, Inc. 1997:396–406.

161. Wegner CD, Gundel RH, Letts LG. Expression and probable roles of cell adhesion molecules in lung inflammation. Chest 1992; 101:34S–39S.

162. Berens KL, Vanderslice P, Dupre B, Dixon RA. F. Selectin antagonists. In: Hansel TT, Barnes P, eds. New Drugs for Asthma, Allergy and COPD. Progress in Respiratory Research. Basel: Karger, 2001:306–309.

163. Adams SP, Lobb RR. Small-molecule VLA-4 antagonists. In: Hansel TT, Barnes P, eds. New Drugs for Asthma, Allergy and COPD. Progress in Respiratory Research. Basel: Karger, 2001:302–305.

164. Richards IM, Khare Slatter V. ICAM-1 and VCAM-1 antagonists. In: Hansel TT, Barnes P, eds. New Drugs for Asthma, Allergy and COPD. Progress in Respiratory Research. Basel: Karger, 2001:310–313.

165. Peebles RS, Bochner BS, Schleimer RP. Pharmacologic regulation of adhesion molecule function and expression. In: Ruffolo J, Hollinger MA, eds. Inflammation: Mediators and Pathways. Boca Raton, FL.: CRC Press, 1995:29–97.

166. Hamid QA, Minshall EM. Molecular pathology of allergic disease: I: Lower airway disease. J Allergy Clin Immunol 2000; 105:20–36.

167. Walker C, Bode E, Boer L, Hansel TT, Blaser K, Virchow JC, Jr. Allergic and nonallergic asthmatics have distinct patterns of T-cell activation and cytokine production in peripheral blood and bronchoalveolar lavage. Am Rev Respir Dis 1992; 146:109–115.

168. Robinson DS, Hamid Q, Ying S, Tsicopoulos A, Barkans J, Bentley AM, Corrigan C, Durham SR, Kay AB. Predominant Th2-like bronchoalveolar T-lymphocyte population in atopic asthma. N Engl J Med 1992; 326:298–304.

169. Ying S, Robinson DS, Varney V, Meng Q, Tsicopoulos A, Moqbel R, Durham SR, Kay AB, Hamid Q. TNFα mRNA expression in allergic inflammation. Clin Exp Allergy 1991; 21:745–750.

170. Bradding P, Mediwake R, Feather IH, Madden J, Church MK, Holgate ST, Howarth PH. TNFα is localized to nasal mucosal mast cells and is released in acute allergic rhinitis Clin Exp Allergy 1995; 25:406–415.

171. Hamilos DL, Leung DYM, Wood R, Bean DK, Song YL, Schotman E, Hamid Q. Eosinophil infiltration in nonallergic chronic hyperplastic sinusitis with nasal polyposis is associated with endothelial VCAM-1 upregulation and expression of TNF-α. Am J Respir Cell Mol Biol 1996; 15:443–450.

172. Weinberger MS, Davidson TM, Broide DH. Differential expression of vascular cell adhesion molecule mRNA and protein in nasal mucosa in response to IL-1 or tumor necrosis factor. J Allergy Clin Immunol 1996; 97:662–671.

173. Broide DH, Firestein GS. Endobronchial allergen challenge in asthma. Demonstration of cellular source of granulocyte macrophage colony-stimulating factor by in situ hybridization. J Clin Invest 1991; 88:1048–1053.

174. Massey W, Friedman B, Kato M, Cooper P, Kagey-Sobotka A, Lichtentein LM, Schleimer RP. Appearance of IL-3 and GM-CSF activity at allergen-challenged cutaneous late-phase reaction sites. J Immunol 1993; 150:1084–1092.

175. Ohnishi T, Kita H, Weiler D, Sur S, Sedgwick JB, Calhoun WJ, Busse WW, Abrams JS, Gleich GJ. IL-5 is the predominant eosinophil-active cytokine in the antigen-induced pulmonary late-phase reaction. Am Rev Respir Dis 1993; 147:901–907.

176. Ebisawa M, Liu MC, Yamada T, Kato M, Lichtenstein LM, Bochner BS, Schleimer RP. Eosinophil transendothelial migration induced by cytokines II. The potentiation of eosinophil transendothelial migration by eosinophil-active cytokines. J Immunol 1994; 152:4590–4597.

177. Gauvreau GM, O'Byrne PM, Moqbel R, Velazquez J, Watson RM, Howie KJ, Denburg JA. Enhanced expression of GM-CSF in differentiating eosinophils of atopic and atopic asthmatic subjects. Am J Respir Cell Molec Biol 1998; 19:55–62.

178. Robinson D, Hamid Q, Ying S, Bentley A, Assoufi B, Durham S, Kay AB. Prednisolone treatment in asthma is associated with modulation of bronchoalveolar lavage cell interleukin-4, interleukin-5, and interferon-γ cytokine gene expression. Am Rev Respir Dis 1993; 148:401–406.

179. Sousa AR, Poston RN, Lane SJ, Nakhosteen JA, Lee TH. Detection of GM-CSF in asthmatic bronchial epithelium and decrease by inhaled corticosteroids. Am Rev Respir Dis 1993; 147:1557–1561.

180. Davies RJ, Wang JH, Trigg CJ, Devalia JL. Expression of GM-CSF, IL-8 and RANTES bronchial epithelium of mild asthmatics is down regulated by inhaled beclomethasone dipropionate. Int Arch Allergy Immunol 1994; 107:428–429.

181. Shi HZ, Deng JM, Xu H, Nong ZX, Xiao CQ, Liu ZM, Qin SM, Jiang HX, Liu GN, Chen YQ. Effect of inhaled interleukin-4 on airway hyperreactivity in asthmatics. Am J Respir Crit Care Med 1998; 157:1818–1821.

182. Shi HZ, Xiao CQ, Zhong D, Qin SM, Liu Y, Liang GR, Xu H, Chen YQ, Long XM, Xie ZF. Effect of inhaled interleukin-5 on airway hyperreactivity and eosinophilia in asthmatics. Am J Respir Crit Care Med 1998; 157:204–209.

183. Borish LC, Nelson HS, Lanz MJ, Claussen L, Whitmore JB, Agosti JM, Garrison L. Interleukin-4 receptor in moderate atopic asthma—a phase I/II randomized, placebo-controlled trial. Am J Respir Crit Care Med 1999; 160:1816–1823.

184. Borish LC, Nelson HS, Corren J, Bensch G, Busse WW, Whitmore JB, Agosti JM. Efficacy of soluble IL-4 receptor for the treatment of adults with asthma. J Allergy Clin Immunol 2001; 107:963–970.

185. Groopman JE, Mitsuyasu RT, DeLeo MJ, Oette DH, Golde DW. Effect of recombinant human granulocyte-macrophage colony-stimulating factor on myelopoiesis in the acquired immunodeficiency syndrome. N Engl J Med 1987; 317:593–598.

186. Stirling RG, van Rensen EL, Barnes PJ, Chung KF. Interleukin-5 induces CD34(+) eosinophil progenitor mobilization and eosinophil CCR3 expression in asthma. Am J Respir Crit Care Med 2001; 164:1403–1409.

187. van Rensen EL, Stirling RG, Scheerens J, Staples K, Sterk PJ, Barnes PJ, Chung KF. Evidence for systemic rather than pulmonary effects of interleukin-5 administration in asthma. Thorax 2001; 56:935–940.

188. Leckie MJ, Brinke A, Khan J, Diamant Z, O'Connor BJ, Walls CM, Mathur AK, Cowley HC, Chung KF, Djukanovic R, Hansel TT, Holgate ST, Sterk PJ, Barnes PJ. Effects of an interleukin-5 blocking monoclonal antibody on eosinophils, airway hyper-responsiveness, and the late asthmatic response. Lancet 2000; 356:2144–2148.

189. O'Byrne PM, Inman MD, Parameswaran K. The trials and tribulations of IL-5, eosinophils, and allergic asthma J Allergy Clin Immunol 2001; 108:503–508.

190. Barnes PJ. Therapeutic strategies for allergic diseases. Nature 1999; 402:B31–38.

191. Barnes P. New directions in allergic diseases: mechanism-based anti-inflammatory therapies. J Allergy Clin Immunol 2000; 106:5–16.

192. Nickel R, Beck LA, Stellato C, Schleimer RP. Chemokines and allergic disease. J Allergy Clin Immunol 1999; 104:723–742.

193. Berkman N, Ohnona S, Chung FK, Breuer R. Eotaxin-3 but not eotaxin gene expression is upregulated in asthmatics 24 hours after allergen challenge. Am J Respir Cell Mol Biol 2001; 24:682–687.

194. Pan J, Kunkel EJ, Gosslar U, Lazarus N, Langdon P, Broadwell K, Vierra MA, Genovese MC, Butcher EC, Soler D. A novel chemokine ligand for CCR10 and CCR3 expressed by epithelial cells in mucosal tissues. J Immunol 2000; 165:2943–2949.

195. Kuna P, Alam R, Ruta U, Gorski P. RANTES induces nasal mucosal inflammation rich in eosinophils, basophils, and lymphocytes in vivo Am J Respir Crit Care Med 1998; 157:873–879.

196. Hanazawa T, Antuni JD, Kharitonov SA, Barnes PJ. Intranasal administration of eotaxin increases nasal eosinophils and nitric oxide in patients with allergic rhinitis. J Allergy Clin Immunol 2000; 105:58–64.

197. Beck LA, Dalke S, Leiferman KM, Bickel CA, Hamilton R, Rosen H, Bochner BS, Schleimer RP. Cutaneous injection of RANTES causes eosinophil recruitment: comparison of nonallergic and allergic human subjects. J Immunol 1997; 159:2962–2972.

198. Teran LM. CCL chemokines and asthma. Immunol Today 2000; 21:235–242.
199. Gonzalo J, Lloyd C, Peled A, Delaney T, Coyle A, Gutierrez-Ramos J. Critical involvement of the chemotactic axis CXCR4/stromal cell-derived factor-1α in the inflammatory component of allergic airway disease. J Immunol 2000; 165:499–508.
200. Sallusto F, Mackay CR, Lanzavecchia A. Selective expression of the eotaxin receptor CCR3 by human T helper 2 cells. Science 1997; 277:2005–2007.
201. Ying S, Robinson DS, Meng Q, Rottman J, Kennedy R, Ringler DJ, Mackay CR, Daugherty BL, Springer MS, Durham SR, Williams TJ, Kay AB. Enhanced expression of eotaxin and CCR3 mRNA and protein in atopic asthma. Eur J Immunol 1997; 27: 3507–3516.
202. Arima M, Plitt J, Stellato C, Bickel C, Motojima S, Makino S, Fukuda T, Schleimer RP. Expression of interleukin-16 by human epithelial cells. Am J Respir Cell Mol Biol 1999; 21:684–692.
203. Krug N, Cruikshank WW, Tschernig T, Erpenbeck VJ, Balke K, Hohlfeld JM, Center DM, Fabel H. Interleukin 16 and T-cell chemoattractant activity in bronchoalveolar lavage 24 hours after allergen challenge in asthma. Am J Respir Crit Care Med 2000; 162:105–111.
204. Sallusto F, Lanzavecchia A, Mackay CR. Chemokines and chemokine receptors in T-cell priming and Th1/Th2- mediated responses. Immunol Today 1998; 19:568–574.
205. Panina-Bordignon P, Papi A, Mariani M, Di Lucia P, Casoni G, Bellettato C, Buonsanti C, Miotto D, Mapp C, Villa A, Arrigoni G, Fabbri LM, Sinigaglia F. The C-C chemokine receptors CCR4 and CCR8 identify airway T cells of allergen-challenged atopic asthmatics. J Clin Invest 2001; 107:1357–1364.

13

Neutrophil Emigration in the Lungs

CLAIRE M. DOERSCHUK

Case Western Reserve University
Cleveland, Ohio, U.S.A.

I. Introduction

The lungs serve two major functions: gas exchange and host defense. The very large surface area in contact with the external environment makes host defense a critical function. Many aspects of the anatomy and physiology of the lungs are well suited for host defense. The structure of the airways results in the deposition of inhaled microorganisms and particulate matter on the mucous lining of the airways, and airway epithelial cells are equipped with cilia that move the inhaled pathogens back up the airway into the pharynx, where they are swallowed. The epithelial cells are capable of responding to inhaled matter by generating regulatory cytokines, chemokines, and other mediators that can initiate an inflammatory response. Any pathogens or particulates that reach the alveolar spaces encounter the alveolar macrophages, which phagocytose and kill many pathogens without initiating recruitment of other leukocytes. The capillary blood contains a high concentration of neutrophils, often termed the marginated pool, which is readily recruitable if needed.

When the lung parenchymal cells are unable to destroy the inhaled stimulus, an inflammatory response is initiated. In the large proximal airways, this response is driven by the epithelial cells and the immune cells that reside in the airway wall. Alveolar macrophages that are crawling up the airway tree may also contribute. In the distal airways and the airspaces, host defense is regulated primarily by alveolar macrophages and dendritic cells. Contributions by alveolar type II cells and the recruited neutrophils also play an important role in initiating, amplifying, and modulating the inflammatory response. In addition to differences in cell types within the large and small airways of the lungs, these two regions of the lungs are served by separate circulations that deliver neutrophils and plasma-derived mediators to the tissue. The large airways are supplied by the bronchial circulation, while the pulmonary circulation serves the distal lung parenchyma. Important differences in anatomy and expression of modulatory molecules by these circulations are described later in this chapter. The diseases that affect these two regions are also different. Asthma, bronchiectasis, chronic bronchitis, and infectious bronchitis are diseases of the large airways, while pneumonia, radiation pneumonitis, interstitial fibrosis, emphysema, and acute respiratory distress syndrome demonstrate pathology focused on the small airways and airspaces.

The response of neutrophils to inflammatory stimuli within the lungs involves a series of sequential processes that include recognition of stimulus, sequestration, adhesion, diapedesis, and migration into the lung parenchyma (Fig. 1). These pro-

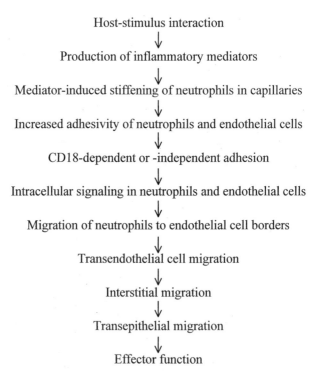

Figure 1 Postulated response of neutrophils to inflammatory stimuli in the lungs. This sequence describes the events that occur for each neutrophil when it arrives at a site of inflammation.

cesses occur during virtually all inflammatory diseases, including pneumonia, acute and chronic bronchitis, acute respiratory distress syndrome (ARDS), asthma, emphysema, and interstitial lung diseases. Similar to other immune cells, neutrophils are a double-edged sword; they are beneficial to the host in their extraordinary abilities to destroy microorganisms and repair lung damage, but these abilities are detrimental to the host when directed toward parenchymal cells or when control mechanisms are lost. This beneficial/detrimental behavior can be considered as a delicate balance—for example, an altered balance due to the leakage of mediators such as reactive oxygen species (ROS) or elastase into the environment during intracellular killing. Alternatively, the damaging effects may represent a dysregulated response, resulting in premature or excessive production and release of injurious mediators. While both these perspectives are likely important, they suggest different therapeutic targets.

As we learn more about innate immunity and the acute inflammatory response, several concepts are becoming clear. First, while many aspects of the inflammatory response are common to any stimulus that recruits neutrophils, there are important differences between the mechanisms and pathways through which neutrophils are recruited in response to a particular stimulus. For example, some stimuli induce neutrophil emigration through adhesion pathways that require the CD11/CD18 adhesion complex expressed on leukocytes, while other stimuli elicit emigration through other pathways. These differences in mechanisms may allow important opportunities to modulate the inflammatory response more selectively, leaving at least some aspects of host defense intact. Second, understanding host defense in the lungs requires a synthesis of reductionistic and integrative approaches, both of which clearly have their limitations and can be misleading in isolation, as well as consideration of cardiovascular function and regulation of release of neutrophils from the bone marrow, since both modulate the inflammatory response within the lungs and offer opportunities for therapeutic intervention. This chapter will consider each step in the recruitment of neutrophils from their sequestration within the microvasculature through their adhesion and migration into the lung tissue, focusing on the inflammatory response in the distal lung parenchyma where our knowledge is more complete. Differences between the response to individual stimuli will be acknowledged. Questions that remain unclear will be highlighted, as well as opportunities for new therapeutic interventions. To clarify often confusing nomenclature, the term "margination" will be used to describe the increased concentration of neutrophils in capillaries of noninflamed lungs, and "sequestration" will be used to describe the process through which neutrophils accumulate within the microvasculature of inflamed lungs in preparation for migration or for endothelial cell injury.

II. Recognition of a Stimulus and Initiation of Inflammation

Alveolar macrophages interact with organisms through a large number of receptors that recognize molecules expressed by microorganisms. These include Fc receptors,

complement receptors, pattern recognition receptors including mannose and scavenger receptors, surfactant protein A receptors, toll-like receptors, CD14, and others
(1–19). Few of these are specific to any particular organism, and the innate immune
response likely depends on the balance of receptors utilized by any particular organism. Within the large airways, epithelial cells also express receptors that mediate
adhesion of pathogens.

These receptors induce intracellular signaling pathways that result in production of mediators. For example, alveolar macrophages and other cells express members of the toll-like receptor (TLR) family (9–15). These molecules initiate signaling
that leads to activation and nuclear translocation of the transcription factor, NF-κB
NF-κB is present in the cytosol of many cells including epithelial cells, alveolar
macrophages, and endothelial cells complexed to a family of inhibitors, I-κB
(9,21–25). Upon activation of TLR4 and other TLR family members, a number of
intracellular events occur that include association of the activated TLR with the
adaptor protein MyD88, which associates with IRAK to phosphorylate TRAF6
which activates both the MAPK kinases and the IKK complex. The IKK complex
initiates phosphorylation of I-κB, which leads to ubiquitination of I-κB and proteolysis by proteasomes. NF-κB is thus separated from its inhibitor, and the activated
complex is translocated to the nucleus. This transcription factor regulates many
aspects of the inflammatory response through increasing the gene transcripts of
molecules such as TNF-α, IL-1, IL-8 and other chemokines, and ICAM-1 and other
adhesion molecules.

NF-κB signaling is a major regulator of acute inflammatory responses induced
by many stimuli in the lungs and other organs, including *Escherichia coli* LPS, *E
coli*, *Pseudomonas aeruginosa*, and IgG immune complexes, induce nuclear translocation of NF-κB (21,26–31). This transcription factor appears to regulate both acute
and chronic inflammation in the large and small airways, and it is present in virtually
all cells, including bronchial epithelial cells, alveolar macrophages, and endothelial
cells. Pharmacological inhibition, while not always entirely specific, has demonstrated this important regulatory role in many inflammatory responses. How this
transcription factor is regulated and how it functions to induce production of transcripts has received much attention and is not yet certain.

The NF-κB complex is a heterodimer composed of two subunits. The RelA
(p65) and the p50 subunits appear to be most commonly translocated during the
acute inflammatory response (4,26–38). The roles of these individual subunits in
gene transcription and how each interacts with other regulatory proteins in the nucleus are topical questions. Mice deficient in RelA die early in utero from hepatic
necrosis, but mice deficient in both TNF-α receptor 1 (TNFR1) and RelA survive
for 2–4 weeks (32). In response to lipopolysaccharide (LPS) instilled into the airways
at age 3–5 days, the RelA/TNFR1-deficient mice have defects in the production of
gene transcripts for at least two chemokines (KC and MIP-2) and the adhesion
molecule ICAM-1 (32). Furthermore, they have a major defect in neutrophil emigration into the airspaces of the lungs that is not present in wild-type mice or mice
deficient in only TNFR1 (32). However, curiously, when these mice die at 2–4
weeks of age, the airspaces contain numerous neutrophils, and the inciting pathogen

appears to be *Pasteurella pneumotropia* (32), suggesting that neutrophil emigration does not necessarily require Re1A and that the inciting pathogen determines which signaling pathway will be utilized. Other acute inflammatory reactions may also not require NF-κB, at least for their induction.

The role of the p50 subunit is even more complex and appears to depend upon the particular inflammatory response and the organ. It can have both pro- and anti-inflammatory effects. For example, the survival of p50-deficient mice following inhalation of *Mycobacterium tuberculosis* was less than that of wild-type mice, and the expression of iNOS, IL-2, interferon-γ (IFN-γ), and TNF-α mRNA were less (33). Survival following intraperitoneal instillation of *Streptococcus pneumoniae* was also less (34). The translocation of NF-κB to nuclei and the production of TNF-α, IL-1α and IL-1β, and IL-6 was less following ionizing radiation in p50-deficient compared with wild-type mice (35). Alternatively, p50 may downregulate inflammation in other circumstances. For example, the development of tolerance to LPS requires p50 (36). Transient transfection of p50 in macrophages decreases TNF-α production (36,37). A polymorphism in the promoter region of the TNF-α gene that prevents binding of p50 homodimers decreases TNF-α production (38). Few data are available evaluating its function in innate immunity within the lungs.

NF-κB regulates the expression of TNF-α and IL-1. These molecules appear to have considerable redundancy in the pathways they recruit in the lungs. For example, mice deficient in either TNFR1 or IL-1 receptor 1 (IL-1R1) have no defect in neutrophil emigration in response to *E. coli*. Mice deficient in both TNF receptors R1 and R2 demonstrated increased neutrophil emigration and a defect in clearance of this organism (30). In contrast, deficiency of both TNFR1 and IL-1R1 resulted in a defect in neutrophil emigration (31). Moreover, the role of these molecules was dependent on the organism. Neutrophil emigration induced by *S. pneumoniae* was actually enhanced without an observable decrease in bacterial clearance in mice deficient in TNFR1 and IL-1R1 (39). Taken together, these studies suggest that IL-1 and TNF-α are important in *E. coli*–induced emigration, that each may compensate for absence of the other, and that TNF-α may be involved in the clearance of *E. coli*.

In addition to being regulated by NF-κB, TNF-α and IL-1 also regulate this complex by signaling through their respective receptors to enhance nuclear translocation of NF-κB. However, while NF-κB translocation to nuclei within liver homogenates of mice with *E. coli* pneumonia was prevented by deficiency of both TNFR1 and IL-1R1, there was no defect in NF-κB translocation in lung tissue of these same mice (31). Furthermore, superoxide generated by NADPH oxidase in neutrophils and monocytes/macrophages and other *N*-acetylcysteine–inhibitable oxidants are required for full activation of NF-κB within the lungs in response to intraperitoneal instillation of *E. coli* LPS (40,41), but when the LPS is aerosolized into the lungs, NADPH oxidase–generated superoxide is not required (41). Clearly, our understanding of NF-κB activation and activity is incomplete, and the potential of this molecule and its subunits in therapeutic modulation of host defense and inflammation is not yet realized. In addition, the role of other transcription factors in regulating the inflammatory response in the lungs, including AP-1 and the Jak/STAT pathways, are similarly exciting and unresolved (42–50).

III. Neutrophil Sequestration Within the Capillaries

With the exception of the hepatic sinusoids, neutrophils emigrate primarily through the postcapillary venules within the systemic circulation. Sequestration in these vessels occurs through rolling and is mediated by the selectins (51–54). In the lungs, however, much of the neutrophil sequestration and emigration occurs through the pulmonary capillaries, which are too narrow to allow rolling (55–68). The role of recognized adhesion molecules has been examined by evaluating the role of adhesion molecules in neutrophil sequestration induced by inflammatory mediators including complement protein 5 fragments, IL-8, and fMLP (69–75). Intravascular injection of these mediators induces virtually complete neutropenia within 1 minute, and the site of neutrophil sequestration is the pulmonary capillary bed (70). Studies investigating the role of L-selectin and CD11/CD18 showed that neither was required for sequestration within the pulmonary capillaries (69,72,76). Moreover, if both these molecules were simultaneously blocked, neutrophil sequestration was still not inhibited (72). However, once the neutrophils were sequestered, both L-selectin and CD11/CD18 were critical to keep these neutrophils within the capillary bed for more than 4–7 minutes (69,72). Even when CD11/CD18, P-selectin, E-selectin, and the integrins α4 and α5 are simultaneously blocked using a combination of antibodies, neutrophil sequestration in response to the tripeptide fMLP was prevented by only 50–60% (72).

These studies suggested that mechanisms other than neutrophil-endothelial adhesion appear to mediate the initial events in neutrophil sequestration. Inflammatory mediators initiate a number of changes in neutrophils that alter their mechanical properties. Binding of mediators to receptors on neutrophil membranes induces changes that include a transient decrease in the neutrophil's ability to deform, increases in cell volume, and changes in shape, prolonging or preventing neutrophil transit through the lung capillaries (77–86). Changes in deformability are most likely to result in the observed sequestration because they occur most rapidly. Thus, understanding the mechanical properties of neutrophils and their role in neutrophil trafficking became important.

In healthy lungs, the mechanical properties of neutrophils are critical in their trafficking through the capillary bed (60,61). The pulmonary capillaries contain a concentration of neutrophils 40–65 times that found in the large vessels (55,60,63). Differences in the capillary transit times of neutrophils and red blood cells (RBC) appear to explain the increase in concentration of neutrophils. If two cell types enter and leave a network in the same respective concentrations but one cell type requires longer than the second to pass through this network, then the concentration of the first cell type will be increased within the network relative to the second. Studies comparing the transit of neutrophils and RBC showed that 78 ± 3% of rabbit neutrophils and 87 ± 2% of dog neutrophils had longer pulmonary transit times than RBC (55,56,87). Using videomicroscopy, Lien and colleagues demonstrated that the transit of neutrophils through the pulmonary capillary bed of alveoli just beneath the pleura required a median time of 26 seconds and a mean time of 6.1 seconds (63). This transit time contrasted with that of plasma or RBC, which have capillary transit times ranging from 1.4 to 4.2 seconds (62,88). Videomicroscopy also showed that neutrophils do not simply move slowly, but rather in hops (63). The prolonged transit time was primarily due to the time they spent stopped.

The diameter of spherical neutrophils measures 6–8 μm, while the diameter of pulmonary capillary segments measure 2–15 μm, and at least 40–60% of the segments require neutrophils to change their shape to pass through (56,62,89). Because one capillary pathway contains about 40–100 segments, most neutrophils must change their shape during passage from an arteriole to a venule. In fact, measurements of neutrophil shape demonstrated that neutrophils in arterioles were nearly round (shape factors of 1.1 ± 0.1) while neutrophils within the pulmonary capillaries were elongated [shape factors of 1.5 ± 0.2 (56,58)]. The hops observed by videomicroscopy suggest that neutrophils stop when they reach a narrow segment and require time to change their shape. The slower deformation of neutrophils compared to RBC, which simply fold to enter a narrow capillary, likely account for the increased transit time. These deformations are likely maintained until the neutrophils appear in the venules, since the relaxation times of deformed neutrophils are much longer than the time needed to pass through the junctions of segments or through wide segments (90–93). Computational modeling studies demonstrated that only 1% of the capillary segments must be narrower than spherical neutrophils to stop 50% of these cells (94). Simulations of blood flow through a single septum showed that preferential patterns of flow occur due to anatomical variability in capillary segment dimensions, suggesting that neutrophils may not be delivered to the smaller segments (95,96). In addition, computational estimates of the distribution of pressure drops along segments showed that when a segment is blocked (as occurs when neutrophils stop), the pressure gradient increases within that segment and in surrounding segments, but falls to nearly unperturbed levels within a distance of three segments (95). Since the pressure gradient along a capillary segment is likely to be the driving force for changes in neutrophil shape, these studies suggest that margination of one neutrophil may decrease margination within adjacent segments. Furthermore, studies to determine if capillary segment diameters are an important criteria in neutrophil margination examined the effect of narrowing capillary diameter on neutrophil transit using forced expiratory maneuvers in humans or application of positive end-expiratory pressure in rabbits. Both studies showed that a transient venous-arterial gradient in circulating neutrophil counts occurred following either intervention, suggesting that narrowing capillaries lengthened neutrophil transit times through this bed (97,98). Moreover, a patient with pulmonary telangiectasia whose vessels were sufficiently wide to allow passage of 30 μm microspheres had shortened neutrophil transit times (99). Taken together, these data suggest that the increased concentration of neutrophils present within the pulmonary capillary bed appears due to the structural characteristics of the capillary bed and the mechanical properties of neutrophils that cause them to deform more slowly the RBC, lengthening their pulmonary capillary transit time. We and others postulate that this prolonged transit time of neutrophils is helpful in host defense, as it allows these cells time to sense the presence of an inflammatory process.

Thus, the mechanical properties of neutrophils are critical in normal trafficking within the pulmonary circulation, and a reduction in deformability induced by inflammatory mediators will lengthen the capillary transit times and/or stop neutrophils, resulting in sequestration of neutrophils at inflammatory sites. The long transit times of neutrophils gives these cells time to sample the pulmonary environment. The mechanical properties of leukocytes have been studied in vitro using several techniques, including measurements of the pressure required to aspirate a leukocyte into a micropipette, the force needed to indent the leukocyte's cytoplasm, the pressure or flow needed to pass leukocytes through a polycarbonate filter with 5 μm pores, and most recently magnetic twisting cytometry (100,101). Many inflammatory mediators including complement fragments and fMLP induce stiffening of neutrophils in less than 0.5 minutes. This stiffening is inhibited by cytochalasin B but not colchicine, suggesting that actin rearrangements but not microtubular reassembly are required for stiffening (81,101–106). This stiffening appears to occur due to cytoskeletal rearrangements that include the polymerization of monomeric globular (G) actin to filamentous (F) actin into a subcortical shell beneath the plasma membrane.

Many in vivo observations have provided support for the hypothesis that changes in mechanical properties of neutrophils are induced by inflammatory mediators and result in sequestration, although definitive causal evidence for the role of deformability in sequestration has not yet been obtained. For example, neutrophils that sequester in the pulmonary capillaries of rabbits within 1.5 minutes following infusion of complement fragments are more spherical than neutrophils normally marginated within these vessels, supporting the hypothesis that mediators decrease the deformability of neutrophils and result in sequestration (107). Furthermore, pretreatment of neutrophils with cytochalasin D prevents fMLP-induced sequestration in vivo within the lungs of rabbits (106). Definitive studies addressing the causal relationship between deformability and sequestration await the development of agents that prevent the deformability changes but not other neutrophil responses.

Thus, these stimulus-induced changes in the mechanical properties of neutrophils appear critical in lengthening the transit times of neutrophils and resulting in sequestration. The intracellular signaling pathways initiated by inflammatory mediators, most of which bind to members of the seven transmembrane spanning, G-protein linked serpentine family of receptors, that cause this very rapid remodeling of the cytoskeleton remain an important question. While our knowledge of signaling pathways for many neutrophil functions such as superoxide production, degranulation, and motility has progressed rapidly of late, tyrosine kinases and phosphatases, MAP kinases, cyclic nucleotides, and other molecules appear less clear in the events that lead to the rapid remodeling (108–114). Calcium fluxes are clearly required, as is the small GTPase rac2 (115), while pertussis toxin-inhibitable G-linked proteins, NADPH oxidase-generated superoxide, and iNOS-generated nitric oxide are not (unpublished observations), but the roles of other molecules remain controversial and may likely depend on the stimulus and the circumstances.

The changes in the mechanical properties induced by inflammatory mediators thus results in lengthening of capillary transit times, likely allowing subsequent events in the activation cascade of neutrophils that result in firm adhesion. This reduction in the deformability of neutrophils is reversible by 5–20 minutes, even if the stimulus is still present (80,83,84,85). Then, the shape changes needed for adhesion and migration, including flattening and formation of pseudopods, follow and may be facilitated by these initial cytoskeletal rearrangements.

Whether these observations are pertinent to neutrophil sequestration within the bronchial microvasculature is unclear and unlikely. The bronchial circulation has many of the attributes of other systemic vessels, but its drainage system is unusual in that more than 85% of the systemic blood flow to the bronchial circulation returns to the left ventricle. Anastomoses between the bronchial and pulmonary circulations have been identified at the precapillary, capillary, and postcapillary levels. The diameters of the bronchial microvasculature have not been definitively measured under physiological conditions, but they appear to be larger than the pulmonary capillaries. The bronchial vessels appear to have a small marginated pool, and about 50% of the neutrophils take longer to pass through these vessels than RBC (116), but this may be an overestimate due to anastomoses at the precapillary level of the pulmonary circulation. To my knowledge, no studies have examined the mechanisms of neutrophil sequestration in the bronchial microvasculature.

IV. Adhesion of Neutrophils to Endothelial Cells and Migration Toward Endothelial Borders

A. Overview

Although adhesion molecules do not appear to mediate the initial events in the sequestration of neutrophils, they are needed for neutrophils to remain sequestered in the pulmonary capillaries for more than a few minutes. Blockade of either L-selectin or CD11/CD18 results in release of neutrophils from the lungs following fMLP or complement fragment-induced sequestration (69,71,72,73,76). Platelets also accumulate in the lungs (117–119), and platelet-neutrophil interactions likely contribute to the behavior of neutrophils. Adhesion and migration are mediated through at least two different adhesion pathways, one requiring the CD11/CD18 complex and another that does not (120). These pathways are discussed in detail below, and understanding these pathways is critical for understanding the inflammatory process and targeting therapies. Adhesion induces intracellular signaling within both neutrophils and endothelial cells. Subsequent events include migration of neutrophils to the borders of endothelial cells and transendothelial migration, which in some inflammatory processes requires the adhesion molecule, PECAM-1 (121).

B. CD11/CD18-Dependent and -Independent Adhesion Pathways

In the systemic microvasculature, most acute neutrophil emigration requires the CD11/CD18 complex for adhesion and migration in postcapillary venules. In the pulmonary capillaries, however, neutrophil emigration into the distal airspaces can occur through at least two adhesion pathways, one that requires the CD11/CD18 adhesion complex and one that does not (Table 1) (120,122–130). Which adhesion pathway is selected depends upon the stimulus. Neutrophil emigration requires CD11/CD18 when elicited by *E. coli, P. aeruginosa, E. coli* endotoxin, IgG immune complexes, IL-1, and PMA, while emigration in response to *S. pneumoniae*, Group B *Streptococcus, S. aureus*, hydrochloric acid, hyperoxia, KC, and complement protein C5a occurs through CD11/CD18-independent pathways. Even in neutrophil emigration requiring CD11/CD18, only 70–80% of migration is blocked when the function of CD11/CD18 is inhibited. In the systemic circulation, virtually all stimuli tested including *S. pneumoniae, S. aureus*, hydrochloric acid, and C5a induce CD11/CD18-dependent emigration, with complete block of emigration in the absence of functional CD11/CD18 (120,122,126,128,131). The major exception is neutrophil sequestration within the liver, where CD11/CD18 and ICAM-1 are often not required (132,133).

Many of these studies utilized reagents that blocked only one site on the CD11/CD18 heterodimer, leaving open the possibility that another site on this complex mediated the observed CD11/CD18-independent neutrophil emigration. Mice with a complete deficiency of the CD18 molecule have extraordinarily high neutrophil counts measuring 5–40 or more times greater than wild-type mice (134,135), similar to the patients with this genetic deficiency. Neutrophil emigration into either *E. coli* LPS or *S. pneumoniae* pneumonia was actually increased in CD18 null compared to wild-type mice (135). However, the increase was not as great as the increase in circulating count. Since the relationship between circulating and emigrating neutrophils is complex and not linear, these data were impossible to interpret. Mice were

Table 1   Adhesion Pathways Elicited by In Vivo Stimuli Within the Distal Airways

---

Stimuli eliciting primarily CD11/CD18-dependent adhesion and migration
    E. coli (128)
    P. aeruginosa (124,127)
    E. coli endotoxin (120)
    IgG immune complexes (126)
    IL-1 (122)
    PMA (120)
Stimuli eliciting CD11/CD18-independent adhesion and migration
    S. pneumoniae (120)
    Group B *Streptococcus* (129)
    S. aureus (128)
    Hydrochloric acid (120,125)
    Hyperoxia (123)
    KC (130)
    Complement protein C5a (122)

---

therefore generated that had both CD18 null and wild-type neutrophils circulating by lethally irradiating wild-type mice and reconstituting their bone marrows with a mixture of CD18 null and wild-type stem cells obtained from 14-day fetal livers. In these mice, the CD18 null neutrophils showed the predicted defect in emigration into the airspaces in response to *E. coli* LPS when compared to wild-type neutrophils in the same mouse (136). However, CD18 null neutrophils showed no defect when emigration was induced by *S. pneumoniae* (136). These studies indicated that the CD11/CD18-independent emigration observed using blocking antibodies did not require any part of the CD11/CD18 adhesion complex.

CD18-independent mechanisms of neutrophil emigration have been identified in three different in vitro systems. First, neutrophil chemotaxis along glass toward lysed RBC did not require CD11/CD18 when the space between the glass surface and the coverslip was less than 14 μm, but CD11/CD18 was required when the coverslip was more than 17 μm above the surface (137). These data suggest that neutrophil adhesion and crawling induced by the same stimulus may be regulated differently when neutrophils are in a confined space where mechanical contacts parallel to the surface may facilitate crawling. Second, neutrophil emigration through human umbilical cord endothelial cells in response to fMLP required CD11/CD18, but this complex was not required when IL-8 or sputum sol was the stimulus (138). Third, neutrophil emigration through pulmonary arterial endothelial cells was CD11/CD18-independent when induced by IL-8 and LTB4, but again, CD11/CD18 was required in response to fMLP (139). These studies suggest that the mediators (or the balance of mediators) produced by a stimulus may determine which adhesion pathway is elicited. Although whether these systems mimic the CD18-independent emigration of neutrophils that occurs in the pulmonary microvasculature remains to be determined, they will hopefully provide an approach to determine the molecules important in CD18-independent emigration and the mechanisms through which this adhesion pathway(s) is regulated.

As mentioned above, the selectin of an adhesion pathway appears to be determined by the stimulus. In addition, interactions between a stimulus and the lung appear important, since the same stimulus induces CD11/CD18-dependent adhesion in the peritoneum or the skin but CD11/CD18-independent adhesion in the lungs. ICAM-1 is the major endothelial cell ligand for the CD11/CD18 adhesion complex, leading to the hypothesis that increased ICAM-1 expression results in CD11/CD18-dependent emigration. In fact, stimuli that elicit CD11/CD18-dependent neutrophil emigration such as *E. coli* LPS and *Pseudomonas aeruginosa* do induce expression of ICAM-1mRNA, while stimuli such as *S. pneumoniae* that elicit CD11/CD18-independent emigration do not. Moreover, studies using ultrastructural immunohistochemistry and colloidal gold labeling showed that the expression of ICAM-1 on pulmonary capillary endothelium was increased in response to *E. coli* LPS and not during CD11/CD18-independent emigration induced by *S. pneumoniae* (140). In contrast, upregulation of ICAM-1 on the alveolar type II cells was increased during emigration elicited by either stimulus (140). These data suggested that whether a particular stimulus increases the expression of ICAM-1 on capillary endothelium may determine which adhesion pathway is utilized and that perhaps that these pathways might more accurately be called ICAM-1 dependent and independent.

These studies led to the hypothesis that the signaling pathways and the expression of cytokines and chemokines induced by a particular stimulus determines which adhesion pathway is selected. The ICAM-1 gene is regulated by pro-inflammatory cytokines, including TNF-α and IL-1. As mentioned in Sec. II, mice deficient in both TNFR1 and IL-1R1 demonstrate a defect in neutrophil emigration in response to *E. coli* but not *S. pneumoniae* (31,39). Many genes critical in the inflammatory process, including TNF-α and ICAM-1, have NF-κB–binding sites and are regulated by this transcription factor. Observations made by many investigators have shown that IgG immune complexes, *E. coli*, *E. coli* LPS, and *P. aeruginosa* induce nuclear translocation of NF-κB (21,26–31). In contrast, NF-κB translocation in response to *S. pneumoniae* occurs later. Furthermore, as mentioned in Sec. II, neutrophil emigration induced by *E. coli* LPS in mice deficient in the RelA subunit of NF-κB is less than in mice of the same genotype that express this molecule (32).

The in vitro observations demonstrating that IL-8 and LTB4 induce CD11/CD18-independent adhesion and fMLP elicits CD11/CD18-dependent emigration suggest that the particular array of chemoattractants produced in response to a pathogen may also influence the mechanisms that lead to an inflammatory response. There are few data to address this hypothesis as yet, although the chemoattractants do vary depending on the organism. It is curious to note, however, that IL-8 gene transcription does require NF-κB. The role of chemokines and their receptors in innate immunity have been reviewed by several authors (4,141–146). Chemokines play at least two roles in the response of neutrophils during pulmonary inflammation. First, chemokines expressed on endothelial cells or in the capillary blood may contribute to the initial sequestration of neutrophils by binding to serpentine receptors on marginating neutrophils, reducing their ability to deform and pass through narrow capillaries, as discussed in detail in Sec. II. Second, extravascular chemokines may induce chemotaxis toward the stimulus. Elegant studies by Butcher and colleagues (147–150) have described how the generation of chemotactic and haptotactic gradients and interactions between the many receptors for these mediators on neutrophils results in directed neutrophil migration in vitro. The application of these ideas to directed migration in the lungs will be exciting. Furthermore, the observations in vitro that the balance of chemokines and other chemotactic mediators such as LTB4 may regulate the selection of adhesion pathways (138,139) makes understanding the interactions between the vast number of chemokines, their regulation, their receptors, and their overlapping and distinct functions exciting.

Taken together, these data suggest that the wide variety of receptor-mediated interactions between the microorganism or other inflammatory stimulus and the host underlie the differences in the host's response to stimuli through differences in signaling, transcription factors, and mediators that are produced (1–19). Understanding how the host interacts with particular pathogens and the subsequent downstream signaling remains an important question. The hope is that this focus will lead to the targeting of immunosuppressive or immuno-enhancing therapies toward specific pathogens or classes of pathogens and preservation of other host defense pathways.

The complexities and the gaps in our understanding of adhesion pathways and the regulation of acute inflammation are enormous. There are in all likelihood more than one CD11/CD18-independent pathway of neutrophil emigration. Moreover, the pathways recruited by different stimuli may reflect the lung cell types with which they first interact and the compartment where the signal is perceived. For example, unilateral intrabronchial instillation of hydrochloric acid in rat lungs induces CD11/CD18-independent neutrophil sequestration and emigration in the area of pneumonia but induces CD11/CD18-dependent sequestration in the contralateral lung of the same rat (125). Intravenous infusion of complement fragments induces neutrophil sequestration that requires CD11/CD18 after neutrophils are initially trapped in the lungs (69), and intravenous activation of complement proteins by cobra venom factor induces neutrophil sequestration that requires CD11/CD18 (151), but instillation of C5 fragments induces CD11/CD18-independent neutrophil emigration into the alveolar spaces (122). In contrast, injection of LPS induces CD11/CD18-independent neutrophil sequestration in the pulmonary microvasculature (105), while intrabronchial LPS induced CD11/CD18-dependent neutrophil emigration (120).

While the receptors, transcription factors, cytokines, and chemokines that regulate CD11/CD18-dependent emigration are becoming clear, current understanding of CD11/CD18-independent emigration pathways is very hazy, and there is likely more than one pathway. Several candidates for the adhesion molecules have been suggested. For example, Ridger and colleagues demonstrated that α2 (CD49b) and α4 (CD49d, VLA-4) mediated CD11/CD18-independent emigration included by KC (130). Burns and coworkers suggested that α4β1 and α5β1 mediate the CD11/CD18-independent portion of LPS-induced emigration (152). In contrast, α4β1 plays only a very small role in mediating CD11/CD18-independent emigration induced by *S. pneumoniae*. It is also important to note that VCAM-1 does not appear to be expressed on capillary endothelium during inflammation, so the ligand for α4β1 is not yet clear. No information is yet available about the regulation of CD11/CD18-independent pathways.

Finally, the applicability of these adhesion pathways in neutrophil emigration in the bronchial circulation should be considered. Bronchial endothelial cells constitutively express ICAM-1 and P-selectin, and these molecules as well as E-selectin and VCAM-1 are inducible during inflammation. In contrast, the pulmonary capillaries express only ICAM-1, either constitutively or during the inflammatory process. While far fewer studies have examined the function of adhesion molecules in emigration through the bronchial vessels and the airways, to my knowledge, CD11/CD18 is crucial and no CD18-independent pathways have been described.

C. Intracellular Signaling Induced by CD11/CD18 Adhesion

When neutrophils adhere to endothelial cells through either L-selectin or CD11/CD18-ICAM-1 interactions, a series of signaling events are initiated (153–159). Neutrophils become flattened and begin to migrate toward the junctions of the endothelial cells. The biomechanical events that occur within these cells are very complex and vary regionally within the cells as they begin to crawl. The mechanisms also may be different. For example, microtubular reassembly is not needed for sequestration of neutrophils but is required during migration of neutrophils into an inflamed focus (160). Schmid-Schoenbein and colleagues showed that the leading edge of both pseudopodia and lamelopodia are filled with actin filaments and devoid of granules, and pseudopods are stiffer than the body, as shown using micropipette aspiration (161). Yanai and colleagues demonstrated, using laser tweezers to grab individual granules, that the granules in the lamelopodia are easier to oscillate in response to a given force than granules in the body or the tail of adherent neutrophils (162). These studies suggest that the mechanical properties of crawling leukocytes are very dynamic and rigorously controlled (163). Ligation of adhesion molecules induces signals that also influence cytoskeletal structure and many neutrophil functions, including phagocytosis, assembly and function of the NADPH oxidase complex, and degranulation. The regulation of cytoskeletal rearrangement and the interaction between the cytoskeleton and adhesion molecules recognizing ligands on endothelial cells or matrix molecules is a critical focus of interest, particularly when considered in light of the therapeutic opportunities to enhance adhesion and crawling but prevent premature activation of the more destructive functions of neutrophils.

Neutrophil-endothelial cell adhesion also results in activation of intracellular signaling pathways within the pulmonary microvascular endothelial cells. For example, binding of ICAM-1 by neutrophils initiates intracellular signaling pathways that result in cytoskeletal rearrangements within endothelial cells by 2 minutes of adhesion (100,164,165) (Fig. 2). This remodeling is mimicked by crosslinking ICAM-1 and results in increased stiffness of the endothelial cells (164). These changes do not occur on pulmonary arterial endothelial cells but only on microvascular cells, which are the site of neutrophil emigration. This remodeling required ICAM-1–initiated signaling, and ICAM-1 rapidly forms large aggregates. Through signaling pathways that are not yet clearly defined, xanthine dehydrogenase is proteolytically cleaved to the active xanthine oxidase form, and superoxide and downstream ROS are formed. These ROS lead to phosphorylation of p38 MAP kinase, which phosphorylates heat shock protein 27, an actin-binding protein. Nitric oxide and myosin light chain kinase-mediated actin-myosin contraction appear not to play a role (100,164). Most importantly, these cytoskeletal rearrangements appear required for neutrophils migrate to the borders of the endothelial cells, since inhibitors of p38 activity and of F-actin modulation prevent this process (100,164,165). Many steps in the signaling remain to be clarified, as well as the role of heat shock protein 27. Why this cytoskeletal rearrangement is needed and how it facilitates neutrophil migration along the endothelial surface also are not clear.

V. Neutrophil Migration Across the Parenchyma and into the Airways and Airspaces

The geometry of the pulmonary capillary endothelial cells appears complex. Calculations estimating the numbers of capillary segments and capillary endothelial cells in human lungs have suggested that one endothelial cell covers three capillary seg-

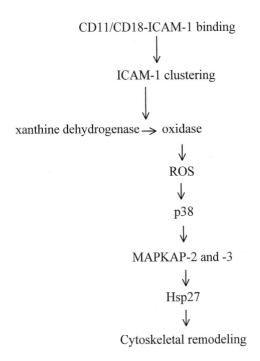

CD11/CD18-ICAM-1 binding

↓

ICAM-1 clustering

↓

xanthine dehydrogenase → oxidase

↓

ROS

↓

p38

↓

MAPKAP-2 and -3

↓

Hsp27

↓

Cytoskeletal remodeling

Figure 2 Postulated endothelial cell signaling pathway induced by neutrophil adhesion to pulmonary microvascular endothelial cells (as described in Refs. 100, 164, and 165).

ments (60), providing a very unusual three-dimensional structure. In venules and in confluent human umbilical vein endothelial cell cultures, neutrophil emigration preferentially occurs at the tri-cellular junctions where three endothelial cells come together (166–168). However, how the borders of the capillary endothelial cells come together is not clear.

The borders of endothelial cells are thought to be the site of neutrophil egress. The pathway of neutrophil emigration out of the pulmonary capillaries and into the alveolar spaces has been elegantly described by Walker and colleagues using serial reconstructions of electron microscopic sections (67,68). Cross-sectioned pulmonary capillaries have a thin and a thick region of their wall. On the thin-walled side, the endothelial and alveolar type I epithelial basal laminae are fused and the capillary segment often bulges into the alveolar space. On the thick-walled side, the basal laminae are separated by a small amount of connective tissue containing collagen, elastin, reticulin, proteoglycans, and scattered mesenchymal cells. About 80% of the borders of endothelial cells are located at the intersections of the thick and thin wall of the capillaries where the two basal laminae separate, while 15% of the borders are located on the thick wall (67). The endothelial basal lamina contains slit-like defects beneath the junctions, and fibroblast extensions reach these holes. Fibroblasts cross the interstitium from the endothelium to the epithelium, and fibroblast extensions interact with alveolar type II cell processes that protrude through defects in the epithelial basal lamina. Furthermore, these studies showed that in response to *S. pneumoniae*, neutrophils migrate out of capillaries between two endothelial cells and through the slit-like defects in the endothelial basal lamina, disrupting the fibroblast-endothelial cell contact (67). They then migrate along or near the disrupted fibroblast and the extracellular matrix of the thick wall until they reach the hole in the epithelial basal lamina where the type II cell is in contact with fibroblast. Neutrophils disrupt this fibroblast/type II cell contact, pass through the epithelial basal lamina into the intercellular space, and emerge between a type I and type II epithelial cell into the alveolar space (67,68). No neutrophils were observed to migrate between two type I cells. These studies suggest that neutrophil migration through the narrow interstitium of the alveolo-capillary wall is a very organized and regulated process involving neutrophil-fibroblast and neutrophil-matrix interactions. Critical questions that remain to be examined is the role of matrix and fibroblast adhesion and the signaling pathways that regulate this complex and extraordinary process.

The specific contributions of leukocyte adhesion molecules such as CD11/CD18 that bind to both endothelial cell ligands and connective tissue matrix to neutrophil migration through the matrix of the alveolo-capillary wall are difficult to evaluate in vivo, since blockade of endothelial cell adhesion will mask any role for the complex in matrix migration. Neutrophil migration through fibroblast monolayers in vitro requires both CD11/CD18 and β1 integrin (169). However, CD11/CD18 is not required for neutrophil migration through endothelial cell basement membranes and subjacent interstitial matrix (170). Interestingly, however, CD11/CD18 ligation induces surface expression of β1 integrin (171), and ligation of β1 integrin modules CD11/CD18-mediated adhesion to fibronectin (172). Ridger and colleagues showed that β1 integrins were required for neutrophil migration into alveolar spaces through either LPS-induced CD11/CD18-dependent or KC-induced CD11/CD18-independent pathways, and that this integrin was mediating neutrophil-matrix interactions (130). The roles of the α subunits of β1 integrins, other integrins, and matrix molecule receptors to migration through connective tissue remain to be determined.

Another interesting and unresolved question concerns the role of neutrophil elastase and other proteases in neutrophil emigration across the endothelium and through the interstitium. Some studies provide evidence indicating that membrane-bound or released neutrophil elastase is required for neutrophil transmigration across endothelium (179), while others indicate that it is not (174). Studies of either elastase deficient or gelatinase B–deficient mice showed no defect in neutrophil emigration, suggesting no absolute requirement for these molecules in emigration (175,176), although other roles for these enzymes during inflammation and repair have been demonstrated.

VI. Recruitment of Neutrophils from Bone Marrow

The bone marrow is the home of myeloid stem cells and the site of neutrophil production. The release of mature and immature neutrophils from the bone marrow during the inflammatory response has unique importance to the pulmonary microvasculature because it is the first capillary bed that these newly released neutrophils will encounter. Mediators produced in the lungs are potent inducers of bone marrow release, as instilling saline or carbon particles into the lungs initiates neutrophil release from the bone marrow (177,178). In the absence of inflammation, the circulating half-life of neutrophils is only 4–8 hours (179), and release from the bone marrow is continuously occurring to maintain a constant concentration of neutrophils in the blood. The regulation of normal maintenance levels of neutrophils has not been determined. During most inflammatory processes, large numbers of neutrophils are recruited from the bone marrow. As discussed below, many properties of these neutrophils are different from those of neutrophils that have been circulating. Understanding the processes mediating release of neutrophils from the bone marrow and their behavior in the pulmonary microvasculature will provide insights into new approaches to modulate host defense and the inflammatory response.

Neutrophils develop within the parenchyma of the bone marrow, and the process of maturation requires about 3 days. As they mature, they move toward the venous sinusoids (180–189). The wall of the sinusoids consists of three layers, an adventitial lining layer, the endothelial cell basement membrane, and the endothelial cells, which contain diaphragmed fenestrae through which the neutrophils exit the bone marrow into the vascular lumen (183,186,187). The venous sinusoids normally contain increased numbers of neutrophils compared to the concentration of neutrophils in circulating blood, suggesting that the sinusoids contain a marginated pool of neutrophils (190).

While the process of hematopoiesis has been extensively studied and much has been learned about the mediators and pathways of proliferation and differentiation, the process through which mature neutrophils are released from the bone marrow, either normally or in response to inflammatory mediators, is far less clear. Inflammatory mediators induce the release of both morphologically mature neutrophils and immature ones with poorly segmented nuclei, and most are also potent activators of many neutrophil functions (74,180). When inflammatory mediators are infused intravascularly, release of neutrophils peaks at 1.0–1.5 hours after injection of LTB4, C5a, and IL-8 and at 3–4 hours after fMLP, PAF, and TNF-α, suggesting that mediator-induced neutrophilia happens too quickly to result from increased hematopoiesis (180–182,191).

The role of adhesion molecules in the adherence of neutrophils to the bone marrow stroma or other cellular constituents of the bone marrow or to the sinusoidal wall and their role in release are not clear. CD11/CD18-mediated adhesion plays a role in poorly defined aspects of maturation (192,193). L-selectin expression is higher on neutrophils in the bone marrow than on those in the sinusoids, suggesting that cleavage of L-selectin may be a prerequisite for release of neutrophils into the circulation (190). However, pretreatment of rabbits with antibodies against either L-selectin or CD18 did not prevent or enhance neutrophil release in response to fMLP, C5a, or TNF-α (181), and neither L-selectin–nor CD11/CD18-deficient mice appear to have defects in neutrophil release (73,135), suggesting that these molecules are not required for emigration of neutrophils out of the marrow. During maturation, α2,6-sialyltransferase mRNA increases, and specific proteins become sialylated, and this change is associated with a decrease in binding to fibronectin and cultured bone marrow stroma (194). The role this sialylation may play in bone marrow release is intriguing. Proteases may also play a role in this process. However, while antibodies against gelatinase B (MMP-9) prevented release of hematopoietic progenitor cells from the bone marrow (195), mice deficient in either gelatinase B or neutrophil elastase do not appear to have defects in neutrophil release, suggesting that these proteases are not required (175,176).

Recent observations have suggested that the effect of inflammatory mediators on bone marrow release may occur much more rapidly than previously described and that mediator-induced neutropenia may be masking release (69,70,119). For example, the total number of neutrophils that accumulated in the pulmonary capillaries during a 15-minute infusion of complement fragments was more than twice as large as the sum of the total circulating pool and the pool normally marginated within the pulmonary capillaries (69,70). This discrepancy was due to release of neutrophils from the bone marrow, which was measured by comparing the circulating neutrophil counts in blood from the distal inferior vena cava with those in samples obtained from the aorta (119). These studies showed that complement fragments or fMLP (but not endotoxin) induced released of neutrophils from the bone marrow into the venous circulation within 7 minutes, that the released neutrophils immediately sequestered in the lungs during infusion of complement fragments and were not present in the arterial blood, and that the number of neutrophils released from the bone marrow could completely account for the observed discrepancy in sequestered neutrophil numbers (119). This rapid release was not inhibited by colchicine, suggesting the microtubular rearrangements in either neutrophils or endothelial cells were not required (101).

The neutrophils that are released from the bone marrow appear phenotypically different from those that have been circulating. As mentioned above, L-selectin expression is highest on neutrophils in the bone marrow, and levels decrease as neutrophils age in the circulation (119,196,190). Newly released neutrophils expressed more L-selectin than ones that had been circulating. In fact, neutrophils that expressed low or no L-selectin were more often apoptotic compared to ones with high levels (196). Morphologically mature neutrophils or bands in the bone marrow are stiffer and less deformable (101,197), and they have decreased NADPH oxidase activity, decreased superoxide production in response to fMLP and PMA, decreased alkaline phosphatase activity, decreased ingestion of Oil Red O–coated particles, and less degranulation (198,199). The maturation time of neutrophils in the bone marrow is shortened during pneumonia (200). While this rapid maturation may account for phenotypic functional differences in studies of patients with pneumonia, it cannot account for differences seen following rapid mobilization following infusion of mediators or very acute pneumonia (201,202). Newly released neutrophils preferentially sequester in the capillary bed during endotoxemia and at sites of *S. pneumoniae* pneumonia due to either poor deformability or increased adhesivity, but they are slower to migrate into the pulmonary parenchyma (203–205). This defect in migration is particularly evident if bacteremia as well as pneumonia is ongoing (204). Taken together, these data suggest that neutrophils in the bone marrow have not yet developed all functional capacities, that the inflammatory response accelerates the release of morphologically mature but functionally immature neutrophils, and that these neutrophils preferentially sequester in the pulmonary capillaries but are poor to migrate and participate in host defense. Understanding the mechanisms of bone marrow release and using this knowledge to modulate the numbers of responding neutrophils may impact on many disease processes.

VII. Summary of Mechanisms, Questions for the Future, and Opportunities for Therapeutic Interventions

The response of neutrophils to inflammatory stimuli within the lungs involves a series of sequential processes that include recognition of the inflamed site, sequestration, adhesion, diapedesis, and migration into the lung parenchyma. These processes occur during virtually all inflammatory diseases, including pneumonia, bronchitis, acute respiratory distress syndrome, chronic obstructive pulmonary disease, asthma, and interstitial lung diseases. There is a delicate balance between the highly beneficial effects of host defense and the ability of the inflammatory response to induce injury. The mechanisms underlying the initial recognition and stopping of neutrophils in the pulmonary capillaries and the subsequent emigration and/or injury are complex and involve a sequential series of events for each neutrophil, all ongoing simultaneously during the acute inflammatory response (Fig. 1). This sequential process involves complex events regulating interactions between mechanical and adhesive properties of both neutrophils and endothelial cells. Initial changes in the cytoskeleton may stiffen the neutrophils and prevent them from deforming, while subsequent dynamic cytoskeletal remodeling of neutrophils and endothelial cells results in crawling and transendothelial migration. Emigration of neutrophils can occur through at least two adhesion pathways: one that requires the CD11/CD18 adhesion complex and one that does not. Which pathway is selected is determined by the stimulus and the signaling pathways that are initiated. Migration through the interstitium and into the airways is also highly regulated. Neutrophils released from the bone marrow traffic first through the pulmonary microvasculature, and the phenotype of these newly released neutrophils impacts on pulmonary host defense. The many recent studies underline the complexity of neutrophil responses and host defense and the uncertainties of our knowledge.

The opportunities for modulation of this process are numerous and will expand as our knowledge of the inflammatory process grows. A few possibilities are summarized in Table 2. For example, how does the initial interaction of the stimulus with the host determine the cascade of cytokines and other mediators that dictate the adhesion pathways to be utilized? Understanding the signaling pathways and their differences and commonalities could permit modulation of specific pathways without alterations in others to prevent lung injury or to enhance particular arms of innate immunity. One could even imagine an individualized drug therapy for a patient's particular organism based on rapid analysis of the organism's receptor, toxin, and

Table 2 Potential Opportunities for Therapeutic Interventions to Modulate the Inflammatory Response

Process	Effect of intervention
Host-stimulus interaction	Modulation of signaling pathway to influence the inflammatory pathway
Bone marrow release of neutrophils	Modulation of the number of neutrophils released
Signaling pathways that lead to neutrophil cytoskeletal rearrangements	Modulation of neutrophil sequestration
Signaling initiated by neutrophil-endothelial cell adhesion	Modulation of neutrophil-induced endothelial cell injury
Balance of cytokine production	Selection of CD18-dependent or –independent pathways
Molecules mediating CD11/CD18-independent adhesion	Modulation of one adhesion pathway without altering others
Mechanical and adhesive properties of crawling neutrophils	Modulation of efficiency and damage
Chemoattractant-directed migration	Maximizing effectiveness of migration and minimizing injury
Neutrophil–connective tissue cell and matrix adhesion	Modulation of edema and injury induced by migration

mediator expression arrays. Individualized anti-inflammatory therapy based on the balance of pro- and anti-inflammatory mediators and functional polymorphisms might also be a goal of the future. How does release of neutrophils from the bone marrow occur, and can the number of neutrophils that reach an inflamed site be modulated up or down, depending on the patient's needs? What are the intracellular signaling pathways that regulate the rapid remodeling of the neutrophil's cytoskeleton and result in sequestration? The signaling that leads to cytoskeletal remodeling and stiffening appear novel to neutrophils, and targeting specific signaling molecules may be beneficial. What are the signaling pathways that are initiated by neutrophil-endothelial cell adhesion, as well as in neutrophil adhesion to fibroblasts and epithelial cells, and what is their function? The potential to enhance migration of neutrophils along cells and decrease neutrophil-mediated injury is tantalizing. What adhesion molecules, if any, mediate CD11/CD18-independent adhesion? How are these adhesion molecules regulated, is their potential for injuring cells more or less than CD11/CD18, and could they serve as a drug target? How do chemoattractants induce directed migration of neutrophils? How is migration through the matrix regulated, and are there opportunities for modulating accumulation of edema and parenchymal injury? How is inflammation limited or resolved? Even the basic mechanisms through which an inflammatory reaction occurs are not yet clear. Comparison of gene transcripts in infected and healthy hosts are providing abundant information and demonstrating differences between organs (206), and similar studies are underway comparing responses to individual organism. Much remains to understand host defense and innate immunity, to modulate it, and to effectively and innovatively treat infections and other inflammatory disease.

Acknowledgments

Supported by HL 48106, HL 33009, HL 52466, and a Clinical Scientist Award in Translational Research from the Burroughs Wellcome Fund.
I would like to thank James C. Hogg, Joseph P. Mizgerd, Qin Wang, and my many colleagues and coworkers for years of exciting and wonderful interactions. I also thank Lynnette Wettstein for help in the preparation of this manuscript. I apologize to the many scientists who have made invaluable contributions to our understanding of neutrophil emigration in the lungs but were not mentioned in this review due simply to space limitations.

References

1. Kimbrell DA, Beutler B. The evolution and genetics of innate immunity. Nat Rev Genet 2001; 2:256–267.
2. Pulendran B, Palucka K, Banchereau J. Sensing pathogens and tuning immune responses. Science 2001; 293:253–256.
3. Beutler B, Poltorak A. Sepsis and evolution of the innate immune response. Crit Care Med 2001; 29:S2–S7.
4. Lentsch AB, Ward PA. Regulation of experimental lung inflammation. Resp Physiol 2001; 128:17–22.
5. Linehan SA, Martinez-Pomares L, Gordon S. Macrophage lectins in host defense. Microb Infect 2000; 2:279–288.
6. Platt N, Gordon S. Is the class A macrophage scavenger receptor (SR-A) multifunctional?—The mouse's tale. J Clin Invest 2001; 108:649–654.
7. Linehan SA, Martinez-Pomares L, Gordon S. Mannose receptor and scavenger receptor: two macrophage pattern recognition receptors with diverse functions in tissue homeostasis and host defense. Adv Exp Med Biol 2000; 479:1–14.
8. Wright JR, Borron P, Brinker KG, Folz RJ. Surfactant protein A regulation of innate and adaptive immune responses in lung inflammation. Am J Respir Cell Mol Biol 2001; 24:513–517.
9. Akira S. Toll-like receptors and innate immunity. Adv Immunol 2001; 78:1–56.
10. Akira S, Takeda K, Kaisho T. Toll-like receptors: critical proteins linking innate and acquired immunity. Nat Immunol 2001; 2:675–680.
11. Medzhitov R, Janeway C Jr. The toll receptor family and microbial recognition. Trends Microbiol 2000; 8:452–456.
12. Zhang G, Ghosh S. Molecular mechanisms of NF-kappaB activation induced by bacterial lipopolysaccharide through toll-like receptors. J Endotoxin Res 2000; 6:453–457.
13. Martin TR. Recognition of bacterial endotoxin in the lungs. Am J Respir Cell Mol Biol 2000; 23:128–132.
14. Guha M, Mackman N. LPS induction of gene expression in human monocytes. Cell Signal 2001; 13:85–94.

15. Bradley JR, Pober JS. Tumor necrosis factor receptor-associated factors (TRAFs). Oncogene 2001; 20:6482–6491.
16. Aderem A. Role of toll-like receptors in inflammatory response in macrophages. Crit Care Med 2001; 29:S16–S18.
17. Ulevitch RJ. New therapeutic targets revealed through investigations of innate immunity. Crit Care Med 2001; 29:S8–S12.
18. Landmann R, Muller B, Zimmerli W. CD14, new aspects of ligand and signal diversity. Microb Infect 2000; 2:295–304.
19. Frevert CW, Matute-Bello G, Skerrett SJ, Goodman RB, Kajikawa O, Sittipunt C, Martin TR. Effect of CD14 blockade in rabbits with escherichia coli pneumonia and sepsis. J Immunol 2000; 164:5439–5445.
20. Abraham E. NF-kappaB activation. Crit Care Med 2000; 28:N100–N104.
21. Christman JW, Sadikot RT, Blackwell TS. The role of nuclear factor-kappa B in pulmonary diseases. Chest 2000; 117:1482–1487.
22. Hatada EN, Krappmann D, Scheidereit C. NF-kappaB and the innate immune response. Curr Opin Immunol 2000; 12:52–58.
23. Israel A. The IKK complex: an integrator of all signals that activate NF-kappaB? Trends Cell Biol 2000; 10:129–133.
24. Janssen-Heininger YM, Poynter ME, Baeuerle PA. Recent advances towards understanding redox mechanisms in the activation of nuclear factor kappaB. Free Radic Biol Med 2000; 28:1317–1327.
25. Karin M, Delhase M. The I kappa B kinase (IKK) and NF-kappa B: key elements of proinflammatory signalling. Semin Immunol 2000; 12:85–98.
26. Blackwell TS, Lancaster LH, Blackwell TR, Venkatakrishnan A, Christman JW. Differential NF-kappaB activation after intratracheal endotoxin. Am J Physiol 1999; 277: L823–L830.
27. Lentsch AB, Czermak BJ, Bless NM, Van Rooijen N, Ward PA. Essential role of alveolar macrophages in intrapulmonary activation of NF-kappaB. Am J Respir Cell Mol Biol 1999; 20:692–698.
28. Lentsch AB, Czermak BJ, Bless NM, Ward PA. NF-kappaB activation during IgG immune complex-induced lung injury: requirements for TNF-alpha and IL-1beta but not complement. Am J Pathol 1998; 152:1327–1336.
29. Lentsch AB, Jordan JA, Czermak BJ, Diehl KM, Younkin EM, Sarma V, Ward PA. Inhibition of NF-kappaB activation and augmentation of IkappaBbeta by secretory leukocyte protease inhibitor during lung inflammation. Am J Pathol 1999; 154: 239–247.
30. Mizgerd JP, Peschon JJ, Doerschuk CM. Roles of tumor necrosis factor receptor signaling during murine *E. coli* pneumonia. Am J Respir Mol Cell Biol 2000; 22:85–91.
31. Mizgerd JP, Spieker MR, Doerschuk CM. Early response cytokines and innate immunity: essential roles for TNF receptor 1 and type I IL-1 receptor during *Escherichia coli* pneumonia in mice. J Immunol 2001; 166:4042–4048.
32. Alcamo E, Mizgerd JP, Horwitz BH, Bronson R, Beg AA, Scott M, Doerschuk CM, Hynes RO, Baltimore D. Targeted mutation of TNF receptor I rescues the RelA-deficient mouse and reveals a critical role for NF-κB in leukocyte recruitment. J Immunol 2001; 167:1592–1600.
33. Yamada H, Mizuno S, Reza-Gholizadeh M, Sugawara I. Relative importance of NF-κB p50 in mycobacterial infection. Infect Immun 2001; 69:7100–7105.
34. Sha WC, Liou C, Tuomanen EI, Baltimore D. Targeted disruption of the p50 subunit of NF-κB leads to multifocal defects in immune responses. Cell 1995; 80:321–330.

35. Zhou D, Yu T, Chen G, Brown SA, Yu Z, Mattson MP, Thompson JS. Effects of NF-κB1 (p50) targeted gene disruption on ionizing radiation-induced NF-κB activation and TNFα, IL-1α, IL-1β, and IL-6 mRNA expression in vivo. Int J Radiat Biol 2001; 77:763–772.

36. Bohuslav J, Kravchenko VV, Parry GCN, Erlich JH, Gerondakis S, Mackman N, Ulevitch RJ. Regulation of an essential innate immune response by the p50 subunit of NF-κB. J Clin Invest 1998; 102:1645–1652.

37. Baer M, Dillner A, Schwartz RC, Sedon C, Nedospasov S, Johnson PF. Tumor necrosis factor alpha transcription in macrophages is attenuated by an autocrine factor that preferentially induced NF-kappaB p50. Mol Cell Biol 1998; 18:5678–5689.

38. Udalova IA, Richardson A, Denys A, Smith C, Ackerman H, Foxwell B, Kwiatkowski D. Functional consequences of a polymorphism affecting NF-kappaB p50-p50 binding to the TNF promoter region. Mol Cell Biol 2000; 20:9113–9119.

39. Hashimoto I, Doerschuk CM. TNF and IL-1 are not required for the acute inflammatory response to *S. pneumoniae* in mice (abstr). Am J Respir Crit Care Med 2001; 163: A427.

40. Blackwell TS, Blackwell TR, Holden EP, Christman BW, Christman JW. In vivo antioxidant treatment suppresses nuclear factor-κB activation and neutrophilic lung inflammation. J Immunol 1996; 157:1630–1637.

41. Koay MA, Christman JW, Segal BH, Venkatakrishnan A, Blackwell TR, Holland SM, Blackwell TS. Impaired pulmonary NF-κB activation in response to lipopolysaccharide in NADPH oxidase-deficient mice. Infect Immun 2001; 69:5991–5996.

42. Kyriakis JM. Activation of the AP-1 transcription factor by inflammatory cytokines of the TNF family. Gene Exp 1999; 7:217–231.

43. Wisdom R. AP-1: one switch for many signals. Exp Cell Res 1999; 253:180–185.

44. Macian F, Lopez-Rodriguez C, Rao A. Partners in transcription: NFAT and AP-1. Oncogene 2001; 20:2476–2489.

45. Bromberg J, Chen X. STAT proteins: signal tranducers and activators of transcription. Methods Enzymol 2001; 333:138–151.

46. Leonard WJ. Role of Jak kinases and STATs in cytokine signal transduction. Int J Hematol 2001; 73:271–277.

47. Ivashkiv LB. Jak-STAT signaling pathways in cells of the immune system. Rev Immunogenet 2000; 2:220–230.

48. Ihle JN. The STAT family in cytokine signaling. Curr Opin Cell Biol 2001; 13: 211–217.

49. Sehgal PB. STAT-signalling through the cytoplasmic compartment—consideration of a new paradigm. Cell Signal 2000; 12:525–535.

50. Greenhalgh CJ, Hilton DJ. Negative regulation of cytokine signaling. J Leukoc Biol 2001; 70:348–356.

51. Ley K, Gaehtgens P, Fennie C, Singer MS, Lasky LA, Rosen SD. Lectin-like cell adhesion molecule 1 mediates leukocyte rolling in mesenteric venules in vivo. Blood 1991; 77:2553–2555.

52. von Andrian UH, Chambers JD, McEvoy LM, Bargatze RF, Arfors KE, Butcher EC. Two-step model of leukocyte-endothelial cell interaction in inflammation: distinct roles for LECAM-1 and the leukocyte beta 2 integrins in vivo. Proc Natl Acad Sci USA 1991; 88:7538–7542.

53. Tozeren A, Ley K. How do selectins mediate leukocyte rolling in venules? Biophys J 1992; 63:700–709.

54. Bevilacqua MP, Nelson RM. Selectins. J Clin Invest 1993; 91:379–387.

55. Doerschuk CM, Allard MF, Martin BA, MacKenzie A, Hogg JC. Marginated pool of neutrophils in lungs of rabbits. J Appl Physiol 1987; 63:1806–1815.
56. Doerschuk CM, Beyers N, Coxson HO, Wiggs B, Hogg JC. Comparison of neutrophil and capillary diameters and their relation to neutrophil sequestration in the lung. Appl Physiol 1993; 74:3040–3045.
57. Downey GP, Worthen GS, Henson PM, Hyde DM. Neutrophil sequestration and migration in localized pulmonary inflammation: capillary localization and migration across the interalveolar septum. Am Rev Respir Dis 1993; 147:168–176.
58. Gebb SA, Graham JA, Hanger CC, Godbey PS, Capen RL, Doerschuk CM, Wagner Jr WW. Sites of leukocyte sequestration in the pulmonary microcirculation. J Appl Physiol 1995; 79:493–497.
59. Henson PM, McCarthy BS, Larsen GL, Webster RO, Giclas PC, Dreisin RB, King TE, Shaw JO. Complement fragments, alveolar macrophages, and alveolitis. Am J Pathol 1979; 97:93–110.
60. Hogg JC. Neutrophil kinetics and lung injury. Physiol Rev 1987; 67:1249–1295.
61. Hogg JC. Neutrophil kinetics in the pulmonary circulation. In: The Pulmonary Circulation and Acute Lung Injury. Mount Kisco: Futura, 1991: 253–269.
62. Hogg JC, McLean T, Martin BA, Wiggs B. Erythrocyte transit and neutrophil concentration in the dog lung. J Appl Physiol 1988; 65:1217–1225.
63. Lien DC, Wagner WW Jr, Capen RL, Haslett C, Hanson WL, Hofmeister SE, Henson PM, Worthen GS. Physiologic neutrophil sequestration in the canine pulmonary circulation. J Appl Physiol 1987; 62:1236–1243.
64. Lien DC, Henson RL, Hyde DM. Neutrophil kinetics in the pulmonary microcirculation during acute inflammation. Am Rev Respir Dis 1993; 147:168–176.
65. Loosli CG, Baker RF. Acute experimental pneumonococcal (type I) pneumonia in the mouse: The migration of leukocytes from the pulmonary capillaries into the alveolar spaces as revealed by the electron microscope. Trans Am Clin Climatol Assoc 1962; 74:15–28.
66. Shaw JO. Leukocytes in chemotactic fragment-induced lung inflammation. Am J Pathol 1980; 101:283–302.
67. Walker DC, Behzad AR, Chu F. Neutrophil migration through preexisting holes in the basal laminae of alveolar capillaries and epithelium during streptococcal pneumonia. Microvasc Res 1995; 50:397–416.
68. Behzad AR, Chu F, Walker DC. Fibroblasts are in a position to provide directional information to migrating neutrophils during pneumonia in rabbit lungs. Microvasc Res 1996; 51:303–316.
69. Doerschuk CM. The role of CD18-mediated adhesion in neutrophil sequestration induced by infusion of activated plasma in rabbits. Am J Respir Cell Mol Biol 1992; 7: 140–148.
70. Doerschuk CM, Allard MF, Hogg JC. Neutrophil kinetics in rabbits during infusion of zymosan-activated plasma. J Appl Physiol 1989; 67:88–95.
71. Doerschuk CM, Mizgerd JP, Kubo H, Qin L, Kumasaka T. Adhesion molecules and cellular biomechanical changes in acute lung injury: Giles F. Filley Lecture. Chest 1999; 116:37S–43S.
72. Kubo H, Doyle NA, Graham L, Bhagwan SD, Quinlan WM, Doerschuk CM. L- and P-selectin and CD11/CD18 in intracapillary neutrophil sequestration in rabbit lungs. Am J Respir Crit Care Med 1999; 159:267–274.
73. Lundberg C, Wright SD. Relation of the CD11/CD18 family of leukocyte antigens to the transient neutropenia caused by chemoattractants. Blood 1990; 76:1240–1245.

74. Terashima T, English D, Hogg JC, Van Eeden SF. Release of polymorphonuclear leukocytes from the bone marrow by interleukin-8. Blood 1998; 92:1062–1069.
75. Burns JA, Issekutz TB, Yagita H, Issekutz AC. The β2, α4, α5 integrins and selectins mediate chemotactic factor and endotoxin-enhanced neutrophil sequestration in the lung. Am J Pathol 2001; 158:1809–1819.
76. Doyle NA, Bhagwan SD, Meek BB, Kutkoski GJ, Steeber DA, Tedder TF, Doerschuk CM. Neutrophil margination, sequestration and emigration in L-selectin mutant mice. J Clin Invest 1997; 99:526–533.
77. Downey GP, Grinstein S, Sue-A-Quan A, Czaban B, Chan CK. Volume regulation in leukocytes: requirement for an intact cytoskeleton. J Cell Physiol 1995; 163:96–104.
78. Grinstein S, Foskett JK. Ionic mechanisms of cell volume regulation in leukocytes. Annu Rev Physiol 1990; 52:399–414.
79. Grinstein S, Furuya W, Cragoe EJ. Volume changes in activated human neutrophils: the role of Na^+/H^+ exchange. J Cell Physiol 1986; 128:33–40.
80. Howard TH, Oresajo CO. The kinetics of chemotactic peptide-induced change in F-actin content, F-actin distribution, and the shape of neutrophils. J Cell Biol 1985; 101:1078–1085.
81. Inano H, English D, Doerschuk CM. Effect of zymosan-activated plasma on the deformability of rabbit polymorphonuclear leukocytes and the role of the cytoskeleton. J Appl Physiol 1992; 73:1370–1376.
82. Nash GB, Jones JG, Mikita J, Christopher B, Dormandy JA. Effects of preparative procedures and of cell activation on flow of white cells through micropore filters. Br J Haematol 1988; 70:171–176.
83. Packman CH, Lichtman MA. Activation of neutrophils: measurement of actin conformational changes by flow cytometry. Blood Cells 1990; 16:193–207.
84. Pecsvarady Z, Fisher TC, Fabok A, Coates TD, Meiselman HJ. Kinetics of granulocyte deformability following exposure to chemotactic stimuli. Blood Cells 1992; 18:333–352.
85. Wallace PJ, Westo RP, Packman CH, Lichtman MA. Chemotactic peptide-induced changes in neutrophil actin conformation. J Cell Biol 1984; 99:1060–1065.
86. Worthen GS, Henson PM, Rosengren S, Downey GP, Hyde DM. Neutrophils increase volume during migration in vivo and in vitro. Am J Respir Cell Mol Biol 1994; 10:1–7.
87. Martin BA, Wright JL, Thommasen H, Hogg JC. Effect of pulmonary blood flow on the exchange between the circulating and marginating pool of polymorphonuclear leukocytes in dog lungs. J Clin Invest 1982:1277–1285.
88. Presson RGJ, Graham JA, Hanger CC, Godbey PS, Gebb SA, Sidner RA, Glenny RW, Wagner WW Jr. Distribution of pulmonary capillary red blood cell transit times. J Appl Physiol 1995; 79:382–388.
89. Wiggs BR, English D, Quinlan WM, Doyle NA, Hogg JC, Doerschuk CM. The contributions of capillary pathway size and neutrophil deformability to neutrophil transit through rabbit lungs. J Appl Physiol 1994; 77:463–470.
90. Evans E. Structural model for passive granulocyte behavior based on mechanical deformation and recovery after deformation tests. In: White Cell Mechanics: Basic Science and Clinical Aspects. Proceedings of a symposium held at the Kroc Foundation, Santa Ynez Valley, California, May 2–6, 1983. New York: Liss, 1984: 53–71.
91. Schmid-Schonbein GW, Usami S, Skalak R, Chien S. Interaction of leukocytes and erythrocytes in capillary and post-capillary vessels. Microvasc Res 1980; 19:45–70.

274   *Doerschuk*

92. Sung KLP, Dong C, Schmid-Schobein GW, Chien S, Skalak R. Leukocyte relaxation properties. Biophys J 1988; 54:331–336.
93. Tran-Son-Tay R, Needham D, Yeung A, Hochmuth RM. Time-dependent recovery of passive neutrophils after large deformation. Biophys J 1991; 60:856–866.
94. Hanger CC, Wagner WW, Jr, Janke SJ, Lloyd TC, Jr, Capen RL. Computer simulation of neutrophil transit through the pulmonary capillary bed. J Appl Physiol 1993; 74: 1647–1652.
95. Dhadwal A, Wiggs B, Doerschuk CM, Kamm RD. Effects of anatomic variability on blood flow and pressure gradients in the pulmonary capillaries. J Appl Physiol 1997; 83:1711–1720.
96. Huang Y, Doerschuk CM, Kamm RD. Computational modeling of RBC and neutrophil transit through the pulmonary capillaries. J Appl Physiol 2001; 90:545–564.
97. Markos J, Doerschuk CM, English D, Wiggs BR, Hogg JC. Effect of positive end-expiratory pressure on leukocyte transit in rabbit lungs. J Appl Physiol 1993; 74: 2627–2633.
98. Markos J, Hooper RO, Kavanagh-Gray D, Wiggs BR, Hogg JC. Effect of raised alveolar pressure on leukocyte retention in the human lung. J Appl Physiol 1990; 69: 214–221.
99. Selby C, Drost E, Wraith PK, MacNee W. In vivo neutrophil sequestration within lungs of humans is determined by in vitro "filterability." J Appl Physiol 1991; 71: 1996–2003.
100. Wang Q, Doerschuk CM. Neutrophil-induced changes in the biomechanical properties of endothelial cells: the roles of ICAM-1 and reactive oxygen species. J Immunol 2000; 164:6487–6494.
101. Saito H, Lai J, Rogers R, Doerschuk CM. The mechanical properties of rat bone marrow and circulating neutrophils and their responses to inflammatory mediators. Blood. In press.
102. Buttrum SM, Drost EM, MacNee W, Goffin E, Lockwood CM, Hatton R, Nash GB. Rheological response of neutrophils to different types of stimulation. J Appl Physiol 194; 77:1801–1810.
103. Downey GP, Doherty DE, Schwab B, III, Elson EL, Henson PM, Worthen GS. Retention of leukocytes in capillaries: role of cell size and deformability. J Appl Physiol 1990; 69:1767–1778.
104. Downey GP, Worthen GS. Neutrophil retention in model capillaries: deformability, geometry, and hydrodynamic forces. J Appl Physiol 1988; 65:1861–1871.
105. Erzurum SC, Downey GP, Doherty DE, Schwab B, III, Elson EL, Worthen GS. Mechanisms of lipopolysaccharide-induced neutrophil retention. Relative contributions of adhesive and cellular mechanical properties. J Immunol 1992; 149:154–162.
106. Worthen GS, Schwab BI, Elson EL, Downey GP. Mechanics of stimulated neutrophils: cell stiffening induces retention in capillaries. Science 1989; 245:183–186.
107. Motosugi H, Graham L, Noblitt TW, Doyle NA, Quinlan WM, Li Y, Doerschuk CM. Changes in neutrophil actin and shape during sequestration induced by complement fragments in rabbits. Am J Pathol 1996; 149:963–973.
108. Brumell JH, Chan CK, Butler J, Borregaard N, Siminovitch KA, Grinstein S, Downey GP. Regulation of Src homology 2-containing tyrosine phosphatase 1 during activation of human neutrophils. Role of protein kinase C. J Biol Chem 1997; 272:875–882.
109. Downey GP, Butler JR, Brumell J, Borregaard N, Kjeldsen L, Sue-A-Quan AK, Grinstein S. Chemotactic peptide-induced activation of MEK-2, the predominant iso-

form in human neutrophils. Inhibition by wortmannin. J Biol Chem 1996; 271: 21005–21011.

110. Downey GP, Butler JR, Tapper H, Fialkow L, Saltiel AR, Rubin BB, Grinstein S. Importance of MEK in neutrophil microbicidal responsiveness. J Immunol 1998; 160: 434–443.

111. Knall C, Worthen GS, Johnson GL. Interleukin 8-stimulated phosphatidylinositol-3-kinase activity regulates the migration of human neutrophils independent of extracellular signal-regulated kinase and p38 mitogen-activated protein kinases. Proc Natl Acad Sci USA 1997; 94:3052–3057.

112. Knall C, Young S, Nick JA, Buhl AM, Worthen GS. Johnson GL. Interleukin-8 regulation of the Ras/Raf/mitogen-activated protein kinase pathway in human neutrophils. J Biol Chem 1996; 271:2832–2838.

113. Nick JA, Avdi NJ, Young SK, Knall C, Gerwins P, Johnson GL, Worthen GS. Common and distinct intracellular signaling pathways in human neutrophils utilized by platelet activating factor and FMLP. J Clin Invest 1997; 99:975–986.

114. Nick JA, Avdi NJ, Young SK, Lehman LA, McDonald PP, Frasch SC, Billstrom MA, Henson PM, Johnson GL, Worthen GS. Selective activation and functional significance of p38alpha mitogen-activated protein kinase in lipopolysaccharide-stimulated neutrophils. J Clin Invest 1999; 103:851–858.

115. Roberts AW, Kim C, Zhen L, Lowe JB, Kapur R, Petryniak B, Spaetti A, Pollock JD, Borneo JB, Bradford GB, Atkinson SJ, Dinauer MC, Williams DA. Deficiency of the hematopoietic cell-specific Rho family GTPase Rac2 is characterized by abnormalities in neutrophil function and host defense. Immunity 1999; 10:183–196.

116. Baile EM, Pare PD, Ernest D, Dodek PM. Distribution of blood flow and neutrophil kinetics in bronchial vasculature of sheep. J Appl Physiol 1997; 82:1466–1471.

117. Issekutz AC, Ripley M. The effect of intravascular neutrophil chemotactic factors on blood neutrophil and platelet kinetics. Am J Hematol 1986; 21:157–171.

118. Issekutz AC, Ripley M, Jackson JR. Role of neutrophils in the deposition of platelets during acute inflammation. Lab Invest 1983; 49:716–724.

119. Kubo H, Graham L, Doyle NA, Quinlan WM, Hogg JC, Doerschuk CM. Complement fragment-induced release of neutrophils from bone marrow and sequestration within pulmonary capillaries in rabbits. Blood 1998; 92:283–290.

120. Doerschuk CM, Winn RK, Coxson HO, Harlan JM. CD18-dependent and -independent mechanisms of neutrophil emigration in the pulmonary and systemic microcirculation of rabbits. J Immunol 1990; 144:2327–2333.

121. Vaporciyan AA, DeLisser HM, Yan HC, Mendiguren II, Thom SR, Jones ML, Ward PA, Albelda SM. Involvement of platelet-endothelial cell adhesion molecule-1 in neutrophil recruitment in vivo. Science 1993; 262(5139):1580–1582.

122. Hellewell PG, Young SK, Henson PM, Worthen GS. Disparate role of the β_2-integrin CD18 in the local accumulation of neutrophils in pulmonary and cutaneous inflammation in the rabbit. Am J Respir Cell Mol Biol 1994; 10:391–398.

123. Keeney SE, Mathews MJ, Haque AK, Rudloff HE, Schmalstieg FC. Oxygen-induced lung injury in the guinea pig proceeds through CD18-independent mechanisms. Am J Respir Crit Care Med 1994; 149:311–319.

124. Kumasaka T, Doyle NA, Quinlan WM, Graham L, Doerschuk CM. The role of CD11/CD18 in neutrophil emigration during acute and recurrent *Pseudomonas aeruginosa*-induced pneumonia in rabbits. Am J Pathol 1996; 148:1287–1305.

125. Motosugi H, Quinlan WM, Bree M, Doerschuk CM. Role of CD11b in focal acid-induced pneumonia and contralateral lung injury in rats. Am J Respir Crit Care Med 1998; 157:192–198.

126. Mulligan MS, Wilson GP, Todd RF, Smith CW, Anderson DC, Varani J, Issekutz TB, Miyasaka M, Tamatani T, Rusche JR, Vaporciyan AA, Ward PA. Role of β_1, β_2 integrins and ICAM-1 in lung injury following deposition of IgG and IgA immune complexes. J Immunol 1993; 150:2407–2417.

127. Qin L, Quinlan WM, Doyle NA, Graham L, Sligh JE, Takei F, Beaudet AL, Doerschuk CM. The roles of CD11/CD18 and ICAM-1 in acute *Pseudomonas aeruginosa*-induced pneumonia in mice. J Immunol 1996; 157:5016–5021.

128. Ramamoorthy C, Sasaki SS, Su DL, Sharar SR, Harlan JM, Winn RK. CD18 adhesion blockade decreases bacterial clearance and neutrophil recruitment after intrapulmonary *E. coli*, but not after *S. aureus*. J Leuk Biol 1997; 61:167–172.

129. Sherman MP, Johnson JT, Rothlein R, Hughes BJ, Smith CW, Anderson DC. Role of pulmonary phagocytes in host defense against Group B streptococci in preterm versus term rabbit lung. J Infect Dis 1992; 166:818–826.

130. Ridger VC, Wagner BE, Wallace WAH, Hellewell PG. Differential effects of CD18, CD29, and CD49 integrin subunit inhibition on neutrophil migration in pulmonary inflammation. J Immunol 2001; 166:3484–3490.

131. Arfors KE, Lundberg C, Lindbom L, Lundberg K, Beatty PG, Harlan JM. A monoclonal antibody to the membrane glycoprotein complex CDw18 (LFA) inhibits PMN accumulation and plasma leakage in vivo. Blood 1987; 69:338–343.

132. Jaeschke H, Smith CW. Mechanisms of neutrophil-induced parenchymal cell injury. J Leuk Biol 1997; 61:647–653.

133. Wong J, Johnston B, Lee SS, Bullard DC, Smith CW, Beaudet AL, Kubes P. A minimal role for selectins in the recruitment of leukocytes into the inflamed liver microvasculature. J Clin Invest 1997; 99:2782–2790.

134. Scharfetter-Kochanek J, Lu H, Norman K, van Nood N, Munoz F, Grabbe S, McArthur M, Lorenzo I, Kaplan S, Ley K, Smith CW, Montgomery CA, Rich S, Beaudet AL. Spontaneous skin ulceration and defective T cell function in CD18 null mice. J Exp Med 1998; 188:119–126.

135. Mizgerd JP, Kubo H, Kutkoski GJ, Bhagwan SD, Scharffetter-Kochanek K, Beaudet AL, Doerschuk CM. Neutrophil emigration in the skin, lungs, and peritoneum: different requirements for CD11/CD18 revealed by CD18-deficient mice. J Exp Med 1997; 186: 1357–1364.

136. Mizgerd JP, Horwitz BH, Quillen HC, Scott ML, Doerschuk CM. Effects of CD18 deficiency on the emigration of murine neutrophils during pneumonia. J Immunol 1999; 163:995–999.

137. Malawista SE, de Buisfleury CA. Random locomotion and chemotaxis of human blood polymorphonuclear leukocytes (PMN) in the presence of EDTA: PMN in close quarters require neither leukocyte integrins nor external divalent cations. Proc Natl Acad Sc USA 1997; 94:11577–11582.

138. Morland CM, Morland BJ, Darbyshire PJ, Stockley RA. Migration of CD18-deficient neutrophils in vitro: evidence for a CD18-independent pathway induced by IL-8. Biochim Biophys Acta 2000; 1500:70–76.

139. Mackarel AJ, Russell KJ, Brady CS, FitzGerald MX, O'Connor CM. Interleukin-8 and leukotriene-B$_4$, but not formylmethionyl leucylphenylalanine, stimulate CD18 independent migration of neutrophils across human pulmonary endothelial cells in vitro. Am J Respir Cell Mol Biol 2000; 23:154–161.

140. Burns AB, Takei F, Doerschuk CM. Quantitation of ICAM-1 expression in mouse lung during pneumonia. J Immunol 1994; 153:3189–3198.

141. Bless NM, Huber-Lang M, Guo RF, Warner RL, Schmal H, Czermak BJ, Shanley TP, Crouch LD, Lentsch AB, Sarma V, Mulligan MS, Friedl HP, Ward PA. Role of CC chemokines (macrophage inflammatory protein-1 beta, monocyte chemoattractant protein-1, RANTES), in acute lung injury in rats. J Immunol 2000; 164:2650–2659.

142. Martin TR. Lung cytokines and ARDS: Roger S. Mitchell Lecture. Chest 1999; 116: 2S–8S.

143. Moore TA, Standiford TJ. The role of cytokines in bacterial pneumonia: an inflammatory balancing act. Proc Assoc Am Physicians 1998; 110:297–305.

144. Strieter RM, Kunkel SL, Keane MP, Standiford TJ. Chemokines in lung injury: Thomas A. Neff Lecture. Chest 1999; 116:103S–110S.

145. Czermak BJ, Friedl HP, Ward PA. Role and regulation of chemokines in rodent models of lung inflammation. ILAR J 1999; 40:1–5.

146. Zhang P, Summer WR, Bagby GJ, Nelson S. Innate immunity and pulmonary host defense. Immunol Rev 2000; 173:39–51.

147. Campbell JJ, Butcher EC. Chemokines in tissue-specific and microenvironment-specific lymphocyte homing. Curr Opin Immunol 2000; 12:336–341.

148. Foxman EF, Kunkel EJ, Butcher EC. Integrating conflicting chemotactic signals-the role of memory in leukocyte navigation. J Cell Biol 1999; 147:577–588.

149. Campbell JJ, Faxman EF, Butcher EC. Chemoattractant receptor cross talk as a regulatory mechanism in leukocyte adhesion and migration. Eur J Immunol 1997; 27: 2571–2578.

150. Foxman EF, Campbell JJ, Butcher EC. Multistep navigation and the combinatorial control of leukocyte chemotaxis. J Cell Biol 1997; 139:1349–1360.

151. Mulligan MS, Varani J, Warren JS, Till GO, Smith CW, Anderson DC, Todd RF, III, Ward PA. Roles of beta 2 integrins of rat neutrophils in complement- and oxygen radical-mediated acute inflammatory injury. J Immunol 1992; 148:1847–1857.

152. Burns JA, Issekutz TB, Yagita H, Issekutz AC. The $\alpha_4\beta_1$ (very late antigen (VLA)-4, CD49d/CD29) and $\alpha_5\beta_1$ (VLA-5, CD49e/CD29) integrins mediate β_2 (CD11/CD18) integrin-independent neutrophil recruitment to endotoxin-induced lung inflammation. J Immunol 2001; 166:4644–4649.

153. Axelsson L, Hellberg C, Melander F, Smith D, Smith D, Zheng L, Andersson T. Clustering of beta(2)-integrins on human neutrophils activates dual signaling pathways to PtdIns 3-kinase. Exp Cell Res 2000; 256:257–263.

154. Simon SI, Cherapanov V, Nadra I, Waddell TK, Seo SM, Wang Q, Doerschuk CM, Downey GP. Signaling functions of L-selectin: alterations in the cytoskeleton and co-localization with CD18. J Immunol 1999; 163:2891–2901.

155. Smolen JE, Petersen TK, Koch C, O'Keefe SJ, Hanlon WA, Seo S, Pearson D, Fossett MC, Simon SI. L-selectin signaling of neutrophil adhesion and degranulation involves p38 mitogen-activated protein kinase. J Biol Chem 2000; 275:15876–15884.

156. Waddell TK, Fialkow L, Chan CK, Kishimoto TK, Downey GP. Signaling functions of L-selectin. Enhancement of tyrosine phosphorylation and activation of MAP kinase. J Biol Chem 1995; 270:15403–15411.

157. Walzog B, Seifert R, Zakrzewicz A, Gaehtgens P, Ley K. Cross-linking of CD18 in human neutrophils induces an increase of intracellular free Ca2+, exocytosis of azurophilic granules, quantitative up-regulation of CD18, shedding of L-selectin, and actin polymerization. J Leukoc Biol 1994; 56:625–635.

158. Willeke T, Behrens S, Scharffetter-Kochanek K, Gaehtgens P, Walzog B. Beta2 integrin (CD11/CD18)-mediated signaling involves tyrosine phosphorylation of c-Cb1 in human neutrophils. J Leukoc Biol 2000; 68:284–292.

159. Yan SR, Beron G. Antibody-induced engagement of beta2 integrins in human neutrophils causes a rapid redistribution of cytoskeletal proteins, Src-family tyrosine kinases, and p72syk that precedes de novo actin polymerization. J Leukoc Biol 1998; 64: 401–408.

160. Mueller GM, Quinlan WM, Doyle NA, Doerschuk CM. The role of cytoskeletal proteins in neutrophil emigration induced by *Streptococcus pneumoniae* in rabbit lungs. Am J Respir Crit Care Med 1994; 150:455–461.

161. Schmid-Schönbein GW, Skalak R, Sung KLP, Chien S. Human leukocytes in the active state. In: Bagge U, Born GVR, Gaehtgens P, eds. White Blood Cells. Morphology and Rheology as Related to Function The Hague: Martinus Nijhoff, 1982:21–31.

162. Yanai M, Butler JP, Suzuki T, Kanda A, Kurachi M, Tashiro H, Sasaki H. Intracellular elasticity and viscosity in the body, leading, and trailing regions of locomoting neutrophils. Am J Physiol 1999; 277:C432–C440.

163. Stossel TP, Hartwig JH, Janmey PA, Kwiatkowski DJ. Cell crawling two decades after Abercrombie. Biochem Soc Symp 1999; 65:267–280.

164. Wang Q, Chiang ET, Lim M, Lai J, Rodgers R, Jamney PA, Shepro D, Doerschuk CM. Changes in the biomechanical properties of neutrophils and endothelial cells during adhesion. Blood 2001; 97:660–668.

165. Wang Q, Doerschuk CM. The p38 mitogen-activated protein kinase mediates cytoskeletal remodeling in pulmonary microvascular endothelial cells upon intercellular adhesion molecule-1 ligation. J Immunol 2001; 166:6877–6884.

166. Walker DC, MacKenzie A, Hosford S. The structure of the tricellular region of endothelial tight junctions of pulmonary capillaries analyzed by freeze-fracture. Microvasc Res 1994; 48:259–281.

167. Burns AR, Bowden RA, MacDonell SD, Walker DC, Odebunmi TO, Donnachie EM, Simon SI, Entman ML, Smith CW. Analysis of tight junctions during neutrophil transendothelial migration. J Cell Sci 2000; 113:45–57.

168. Burns AR, Walker DC, Brown ES, Thurmon LT, Bowden RA, Keese CR, Simon SI, Entman ML, Smith CW. Neutrophil transendothelial migration is independent of tight junctions and occurs preferentially at tricellular corners. J Immunol 1997; 159: 2893–2903.

169. Shang XZ, Issekutz AC, Beta 2 (CD18) and beta 1 (CD29) integrin mechanisms in migration of human polymorphonuclear leucocytes and monocytes through lung fibroblast barriers: shared and distinct mechanisms. Immunology 1997; 92:527–535.

170. Sixt M, Hallmann R, Wendler O, Scharffetter-Kochanek K, Sorokin LM. Cell adhesion and migration properties of beta 2-integrin negative polymorphonuclear granulocytes on defined extracellular matrix molecules-relevance for leukocyte extravasation. J Biol Chem 2001; 276:18878–18887.

171. Werr J, Eriksson EE, Hedqvist P, Lindbom L. Engagement of beta2 integrins induces surface expression of beta 1 integrin receptors in human neutrophils. J Leukoc Biol 2000; 68:553–560.

172. van den Berg JM, Mul FP, Schippers E, Weening JJ, Roos D, Kuijpers TW. Beta1 integrin activation on human neutrophils promotes beta2 integrin-mediated adhesion to fibronectin. Eur J Immunol 2001; 31:276–284.

173. Delclaux C, Delacourt C, d'Ortho M-P, Boyer V, Lafuma C, Harf A. Role of gelatinase B and elastase in human polymorphonuclear neutrophil migration across basement membrane. Am J Respir Cell Mol Biol 1996; 14:288–295.

174. Mackarel AJ, Cottell DC, Russell KJ, FitzGerald MX, O'Connor CM. Migration of neutrophils across human pulmonary endothelial cells is not blocked by matrix metallo-

proteinase or serine protease inhibitors. Am J Respir Cell Mol Biol 1999; 20: 1209–1219.

175. Belaaouaj A, McCarthy R, Baumann M, Gao Z, Ley TJ, Abraham SN, Shapiro SD. Mice lacking neutrophil elastase reveal impaired host defense against gram negative bacterial sepsis. Nat Med 1998; 4:615–618.

176. Betsuyaku T, Shipley JM, Liu Z, Senior RM. Neutrophil emigration in the lungs, peritoneum, and skin does not require gelatinase B. Am J Respir Cell Mol Biol 1999; 20:1303–1309.

177. Cohen AB, Batra GK. Bronchoscopy and lung lavage induced bilateral pulmonary neutrophil influx and blood leukocytosis in dogs and monkeys. Am Rev Respir Dis 1980; 122:239–247.

178. Terashima T, Wiggs B, English D, Hogg JC, Van Eeden SF. Phagocytosis of small carbon particles (PM10) by alveolar macrophages stimulates the release of polymorphonuclear leukocytes from bone marrow. Am J Respir Crit Care Med 1997; 155: 1441–1447.

179. Bicknell S, Van Eeden S, Hayashi S, Hards J, English D, Hogg JC. A non-radioisotopic method for tracing neutrophils in vivo using 5′-bromo-2′-deoxyuridine. Am J Respir Cell Mol Biol 1994; 10:16–23.

180. Jagels MA, Hugli TE. Neutrophil chemotactic factors promote leukocytosis. A common mechanism for cellular recruitment from bone marrow. J Immunol 1992; 148: 1119–1128.

181. Jagels MA, Hugli TE. Mechanisms and mediators of neutrophilic leukocytosis. Immunopharmacology 1994; 28:1–18.

182. Petrides PE, Dittmann KH. How do normal and leukemic white blood cells egress from the bone marrow? Morphological facts and biochemical riddles. Blut 1990; 61: 3–13.

183. Campbell FB. Ultrastructural studies of transmural migration of blood cells in the bone marrow of rats, mice and guinea pigs. Am J Anat 1972; 135:521–536.

184. DeBruyn PPH, Breen PC, Thomas TB. The microcirculation of the bone marrow. Anat Rec 1970; 168:55–68.

185. DeSaint-Georges L, Miller SC. The microcirculation of bone and marrow in the diaphysis of the rat hemopoietic long bones. Anat Rec 1992; 233:169–177.

186. Tavassoli M, Shaklai M. Absence of tight junctions in endothelium of marrow sinuses: possible significance for marrow cell egress. Br J Haematol 1979; 41:303–307.

187. Weiss L. Transmural cellular passage in vascular sinuses of rat bone marrow. Blood 1970; 36:189–208.

188. Wickramasinghe SN. Observations on the ultrastructure of sinusoids and reticular cells in human bone marrow. Clin Lab Haemat 1991; 13:263–278.

189. Wilkins BS. Histology of normal haemopoiesis: bone marrow histology. Intl J Pathol 1992; 45:645–649.

190. Van Eeden SF, Miyagashima R, Haley L, Hogg JC. A possible role for L-selectin in the release of polymorphonuclear leukocytes from bone marrow. Am J Physiol 1997; 272:H1717–H1724.

191. Jagels MA, Chambers JD, Arfors KE, Hugli TE. C5a- and tumor necrosis factor-α-induced leukocytosis occurs independently of β_2 integrins and L-selectin: differential effects on neutrophil adhesion molecule expression in vivo. Blood 1995; 85: 2900–2909.

192. Horwitz BH, Mizgerd JP, Scott ML, Doerschuk CM. Mechanisms of granulocytosis in the absense of CD18. Blood 2001; 97:1578–1583.

193. Papayannopoulou T, Priestley GV, Nakamoto B, Zafiropoulos V, Scott LM, Harlan JM. Synergistic mobilization of hemopoietic progenitor cells using concurrent β1 and β2 integrin blockage or β2-deficient mice. Blood 2001; 97:1282–1288.

194. Le Marer N, Skacel PO. Up-regulation of α2,6 sialylation during myeloid maturation: a potential role in myeloid cell release from the bone marrow. J Cell Physiol 1999; 179:315–324.

195. Pruijt JFM, Fibbe WE, Laterveer L, Pieters RA, Lindley IJD, Paemen L, Masure S, Willemze R, Opdenakker G. Prevention of interleukin-8-induced mobilization of hematopoietic progenitor cells in rhesus monkeys by inhibitory antibodies against the metalloproteinase gelatinase B (MMP-9). Proc Natl Acad Sci USA 1999; 96: 10863–10868.

196. Matsuba KT, Van Eeden SF, Bicknell SG, Walker BAM, Hayashi S, Hogg JC. Apoptosis in circulating PMN: increased susceptibility in L-selectin-deficient PMN. Am J Physiol 1997; 272:H2852–H2858.

197. Lichtman MA. Cellular deformability during maturation of the myeloblast: Possible role in marrow egress. N Engl J Med 1970; 283:943–948.

198. Berkow RL, Dodson RW. Purification and functional evaluation of mature neutrophils from human bone marrow. Blood 1986:853–860.

199. Rosalia DL, McKenna PJ, Gee MH, Albertine KH. Infusion of zymosan-activated plasma affects neutrophils in peripheral blood and bone marrow in sheep. J Leukoc Biol 1992; 52:501–515.

200. Terashima T, Wiggs B, English D, Hogg JC, Van Eeden SF. Polymorphonuclear leukocyte transit times in bone marrow during streptococcal pneumonia. Am J Physiol 1996; 271:L587–L592.

201. McKenna PJ, Rosalia DL, Ishihara Y, Albertine KH, Staub NC, Gee MH. Downregulation of blood and bone marrow neutrophils decreases expression of acute lung injury in sheep. Am J Physiol 1992; 263:H1492–H1498.

202. Zimmermann B, Dalhoff K, Braun J. Impaired neutrophil exocytosis in patients with severe pneumonia. Intensive Care Med 1999; 25:44–51.

203. Lawrence E, Van Eeden S, English D, Hogg JC. Polymorphonuclear leukocyte (PMN) migration in streptococcal pneumonia: comparison of older PMN with those recently released from the marrow. Am J Respir Cell Mol Biol 1996; 14:217–224.

204. Sato Y, Van Eeden SF, English D, Hogg JC. Bacteremic pneumococcal pneumonia: bone marrow release and pulmonary sequestration of neutrophils. Crit Care Med 1998; 26:501–509.

205. Van Eeden SF, Kitagawa Y, Klut ME, Lawrence E, Hogg JC. Polymorphonuclear leukocytes released from the bone marrow preferentially sequester in lung microvessels. Microcirculation 1997; 4:369–380.

206. Chinnaiyan AM, Huber-Lang, M, Kumar-Sinha C, Barrette TR, Shankar-Sinha S, Sarma VJ, Padgaonkar VA, Ward PA. Molecular signatures of sepsis: multiorgan gene expression profiles of systemic inflammation. Am J Pathol 2001; 159:1199–1209.

14

Dendritic Cells

A. KAROLINA PALUCKA and JACQUES BANCHEREAU

Baylor Institute for Immunology Research
Dallas, Texas, U.S.A.

I. Introduction

Dendritic cells (DCs) are antigen-presenting cells (APCs), unique in their ability to control immune responses. DC progenitors in the bone marrow give rise to circulating precursors that home to the tissue where they reside as immature cells with high phagocytic capacity. Recent studies suggest that immature DCs are important in the establishment/maintenance of peripheral tolerance. Upon microbial invasion, immature DCs capture the microbe, become activated either by microbial components or the proinflammatory molecules released by the damaged tissue, and then migrate to the draining lymphoid organs. Meanwhile, DCs undergo maturation, that is, they express a novel set of surface molecules, particularly costimulatory molecules, and digest/process the microbes to present their derivatives (peptides, oligosaccharides, and lipids) on MHC class I and II as well as CD1 molecules. These complexes allow selection and activation of rare Ag-specific T cells, thereby initiating immune responses. DCs present Ag to CD4 + –T cells, which further activate the DC and also stimulate other immune effectors including Ag-specific CD8 + T cells and B cells as well as non–Ag-specific macrophages, eosinophils, and natural killer (NK) cells. Just as lymphocytes are composed of different subsets with specific effector functions (B, NK, and T cells), DCs are composed of distinct subsets with specific regulatory functions. Given this central role in controlling immunity, DCs represent logical targets for many clinical situations, including resistance to tumors and infectious agents.

II. Features of Dendritic Cells

A. Discovery and Function

It took hundreds of millions of years of evolution to endow the upper vertebrates with a system that efficiently copes with the myriad of microbes that invade them every day. Such protection is ensured by the action of the immune system that is composed of two limbs—innate and adaptive (1)—and is controlled by a special set of cells: the dendritic cells (DCs). The innate immune system, the most ancient one, includes proteins such as complement factors, interferons, and several cell types such as natural killer (NK) cells and phagocytic cells. These cells recognize microbes and their products through receptors, i.e., proteins expressed on the cell surface, which are encoded by single genes. The evolutionary younger adaptive immune system is based on B and T lymphocytes, which through genetic rearrangement express specific receptors. These clones carry immunological memory, i.e., a memory of the antigen (e.g., a microbe-specific molecule) encounter that permits them to swiftly mount a response upon reexposure. Upon microbe invasion, B and T cells eventually become antibody-producing cells and cytotoxic T cells (CTLs), respectively. B cells can directly recognize native antigens. In contrast, T cells recognize fragments of the antigens bound to MHC class I and II molecules expressed on antigen presenting cells (APCs), which present peptides to CD8 + and CD4 + T cells, respectively. The CD1 molecules can also present microbial nonprotein antigens to T cells as well as natural killer cells. Thus, different microbial components can be presented to different immune effectors, thereby explaining how vertebrates can survive thousands of threatening microbes.

DCs, first identified in the epidermis in 1868 by Langerhans, were rediscovered in spleen a century later by Steinman (2). Knowledge of DC physiology started to progress at a high pace following the discovery, in the early 1990s, of culture systems that permitted in vitro generation of large numbers of mouse (3) and human DCs (4–6). Currently, human DCs are generated in vitro from (1) bone marrow progenitors cultured in GM-CSF and TNF and (2) blood monocytes cultured with GM-CSF and IL-4/IL-13 (reviewed in Ref. 7).

Besides their rarity, the complexity of DCs lies in their different maturation stages, their different subsets, and their plasticity. Currently, two major DC subsets can be found in human blood: (1) the myeloid DCs, which can differentiate into either Langerhans cells, uniquely expressed in stratified epithelia such as skin and mucosa or interstitial DCs, expressed in all other tissues; (2) the plasmacytoid DCs (pDCs), which upon viral encounter promptly secrete large amounts of type I interferon (Fig. 1). Therefore, circulating DCs, each representing ~0.5% of white mononuclear cells, initially act as members of the innate immunity constituting the first barrier to the expansion of intruding microbes. Importantly these cells subsequently differentiate into DCs able to induce immune responses, thus acting as members of adaptive immunity.

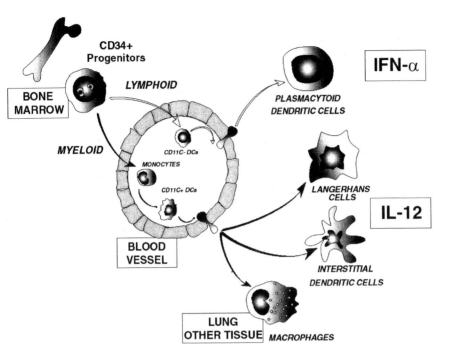

Figure 1 DC progenitors give rise to myeloid (monocytes and CD11c + DCs) and lymphoid (CD11c − plasmacytoid DCs) precursors. Upon interaction with inflamed endothelium monocytes differentiate into CD11c + blood DCs which give rise to Langerhans cells, interstitial DCs, and macrophages. Differentiation of plasmacytoid DCs from CD34 + progenitors (45) can be blocked by Id2 and Id3 overexpression suggesting their lymphoid origin (46). Thus, circulating blood precursors give rise to all tissular DC subsets. Plasmacytoid DCs secrete large amounts of type I interferon, while myeloid DCs secrete IL-12. Thus, DCs are an inherent component of the innate immunity.

While much of the knowledge about DCs came from either Langerhans cells or in vitro generated DCs, this review will highlight their role in lung pathophysiology, for which the readers are referred to earlier reviews (8,9). The epithelial surfaces of lungs and airways face, as the gastrointestinal tract, the decision of mounting or not mounting an immune response to the mixture of antigens, mostly ubiquitous nonpathogenic antigens from plant (pollen) and animal origin interspersed with some pathogenic microbes (viruses and bacteria). In the conductive airways, the majority of antigens are removed by the overlying mucociliary escalator, and a small proportion is then handled by the epithelial APCs, mostly composed of DCs. The antigenic particles that reach alveolar surfaces of the deep lung are mostly processed by the macrophage populations that sit on the alveolar surface, with a few being processed by the DCs below the epithelium. Recent studies point to the importance of DCs in the maintenance of immunological homeostasis within the lungs (8,9).

B. Different Maturation Stages

Immature DCs

DCs are present throughout the respiratory tract, most particularly in the epithelium of the airways and the lung parenchyma. Studies in rats have shown that DCs in airway epithelium and lung walls show half-lives of 2 and 7–10 days, respectively, while those for skin DCs are >21 days. Only gut DCs show a half-life comparable to those from lungs, likely reflecting the close contact with microbes and their products. This rapid turnover is actually further accelerated during acute inflammation as an influx of DCs can be measured within 2 hours of a challenge, while it takes more than 4 hours to get neutrophil infiltration. The recruitment time appears comparable whether it is in response to a productive viral challenge or in response to a soluble antigen to which the individual has been primed (10–14).

One of the most important functions of the tissular immature DCs is to capture microbes and their products, collectively referred to as antigens (Ags), to present them to the effectors, the lymphocytes (Fig. 2). The capture of Ags is accomplished through several mechanisms, including (1) macropinocytosis; (2) receptor-mediated endocytosis via C-type lectins or Fcγ receptors; (3) phagocytosis of particulate live and nonlive antigens (reviewed in Refs. 7,15); and (4) internalization of heat shock proteins (16). Captured antigens are targeted to endosomal compartments for MHC class II loading and subsequent presentation to CD4 T cells (17,18). DCs are able to load their MHC class I molecules with peptides derived from endogenous proteins. However, DCs exhibit a property unique among APCs, that is, the ability to load class I molecules with peptides derived from exogenous antigens. This mechanism, called cross-presentation or cross-priming, permits presentation of antigens from immune complexesr dying/opsonized cells (19–22). Once DCs have captured Ags, they start a complex maturation program that occurs as they migrate into the draining secondary lymphoid organ and makes them APCs. Airway epithelial surfaces, as well as gastrointestinal surfaces, present the challenge of not yielding uncontrolled DC activation, which could be provided by the numerous saprophyte, nonpathogenic microbes that are in contact with epithelia. This necessitates the existence of dampening mechanisms to keep DC activation within defined limits. Local macrophages may initiate these inhibitory properties, possibly through the secretion of NO as well as cytokines such as IL-10 and TGF-β.

Mature DCs

DCs have evolved to promptly mature in response to pathogenic microbes and their products. Conversely, these pathogens have designed a variety of strategies to avoid the maturation of DCs that will elicit immune responses, eventually resulting in the elimination of the pathogen, a defeat with regards to the pathogen vantage point. Numerous factors induce and/or regulate DC maturation, including products of the microbes themselves or products of the tissular microenvironment. Pathogen-related molecules include lipopolysaccharides (LPS) (which bind to TollR4), peptidoglycan, lipoteichoic acid (which binds to TollR2/TollR6), flagellin (which binds to Toll-5),

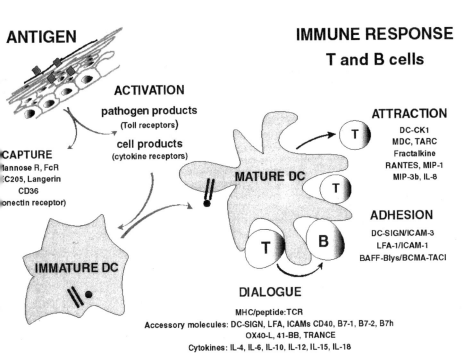

Figure 2 The main function of immature tissue-residing DCs, the differentiation of which is a subject to microenvironmental regulation, is antigen capture. Following antigen capture and activation either by signals from surrounding cells and/or pathogen products, DCs migrate to lymphoid organs. Mature antigen-presenting DCs display peptide-MHC complexes and co-stimulatory molecules, allowing selection, expansion, and differentiation of antigen-specific lymphocytes. DCs display an array of molecules at different stages of differentiation and/or maturation. Given the enormous progress in genomics and proteomics approaches, we are likely to uncover the molecular pathways regulating DC functions and explaining their crucial role in the induction, regulation, and maintenance of immune responses.

CpG nucleotides from demethylated bacterial DNA (which bind to TollR9), as well as double-stranded RNA from viruses (which binds to TollR3) (23–27). The micro-environment contributes through the release of cytokines such as TNF, IL-1, IL-6, and IL-10 (reviewed in Refs. 7,28), as well as mediators including eicosanoids such as PGE2 and leukotrienes, which affect the migration and polarization of DCs. All mediators of DC maturation trigger their migration to secondary lymphoid organs, where the DC can present peptide-MHC complexes to naïve T cells. The migration of maturing DCs involves a coordinated action of several chemokines. After antigen uptake, inflammatory stimuli turn off the expression on immature DCs of CCR6 (the receptor to MIP-3α that attract immature DCs) (reviewed in Ref. 7) and upregulate CCR7 (receptor to MIP-3β and 6Ckine). Consequently, maturing DCs will leave the inflamed tissues and enter the lymph stream, potentially directed by 6Ckine, which is expressed on lymphatic vessels. Mature DCs entering the draining lymph nodes will be directed into the paracortical area in response to MIP-3β and/or 6Ckine by cells spread over the T-cell zone. The newly arriving DCs produce chemokines that attract T cells, B cells, and possibly more DCs (29) (Fig. 2). The initial contact between DCs and resting T cells seems to be mediated by a transient, high-affinity interaction between DC-SIGN on DCs and the adhesion molecule ICAM-3 on T cells (30) and is followed by involvement of other adhesion molecules and their corresponding ligands (ICAM-1/LFA-1, LFA-3/CD2). Following TCR engagement, an intimate contact, often referred to as "the immunological synapse," evolves where multiple interactions between co-stimulatory molecules on DCs and their ligands on T cells result in final DC maturation and T-cell activation (31). T-cell signals such as CD40-L and RANK contribute to the full maturation of the DCs (reviewed in Ref. 7). The induced antigen-specific CD4 T cells then orchestrate other effectors of the immune system, including CD8 T cells, B cells, and NK cells. However, DCs can directly present antigens to CD8 T cells as well as B cells and NK cells (see below). Thus, DCs induce a diverse immune response involving multiple effectors of both cellular and humoral immunity.

III. Dendritic Cell Subsets

A. Humans

The existence of distinct DC subsets was found in different studies on (1) skin DCs (32), (2) DCs generated in vitro by culture of CD34 + hematopoietic progenitors (HPC) (33), and (3) blood DC precursors (34). Human skin contains two subsets with distinct localization: LCs within the epidermis, characterized by the expression of CD1a and Birbeck granules, and interstitial (dermal) DCs (intDCs), lacking Birbeck granules but expressing coagulation factor XIIIa. These two subsets also emerge in cultures of CD34 + HPC driven by GM-CSF and TNF (33), and most interestingly these subsets have common as well as unique functions (35), For example, intDCs, but not LCs, are able to induce the differentiation of naive B cells into immunoglobulin-secreting plasma cells. IntDCs demonstrate a high efficiency of Ag capture—about 10-fold higher than that of LCs. They also express high levels of nonspecific esterases, markers of the lysosomal compartment, while LCs do not. While no unique function has yet been formally attributed to LCs, there are hints that they may be particularly efficient activators of cytotoxic CD8 T cells.

Two subsets of DC precursors circulate in the blood: (1) lineage negative CD11c + myeloid DCs (mDCs), which derive from monocytes, and (2) CD11c − IL-3Rα + plasmacytoid DCs (pDCs) (7,36). Both monocytes and mDCs can give rise to interstitial DC (under the influence of GM-CSF and IL-4 or TNF), Langerhans cells (in the presence of TGF-β), and macrophages (in the presence of M-CSF or GM-CSF) (35,37,38). Distinct factors regulate the survival and differentiation of pDCs (25,39–43). These cells die rapidly after isolation and are critically dependent on IL-3 for survival and CD40-L for maturation. pDCs can be further distinguished from mDCs by differential expression of immunoglobulin-like transcripts (ILTs), with pDCs being ILT1 − /ILT3 + and CD11c + DCs being ILT1 + /ILT3 + . They have unique properties such as the expression of lymphoid antigens (39), the ability to produce large amounts of type I interferon (43), and the ability to polarize T cells differently than mDCs with a proportion induced toward the production of IL-4 and IL-5 (type 2 cells) (42). Because pDCs and mDCs carry a different set of toll-like receptors, they are likely to respond to different microbes or to turn on different immune responses to a given microbe. In particular, pDCs but not mDCs express Toll9R (receptor for microbial demethylated DNA) and Toll7R (of yet unknown specificity). Conversely, mDCs, but not pDCs, express Toll2R, Toll4R, and Toll6R, receptors to peptidoglycan, LPS, and flagellin, respectively (44). Thus, the different DC subsets initiate the response to a large variety of microbes and generate different immune responses to a single microbe, thus increasing the chances of successfully controlling the microbial invasion (Fig. 3).

Studies on pDCs are confronting the challenge of their difficult isolation, but recent studies demonstrate the possibility to generate them in vitro from CD34 + hematopoietic progenitors in response to FLT3-L (45). Interestingly, their differentiation can be blocked by overexpression of Id2 and Id3 proteins, which also inhibit the development of lymphoid cells but not myeloid ones (46). Therefore, the phenotypic analysis and the blockade of pDC ontogeny with transcription factors that specifically inhibit the lymphoid lineage suggest that pDCs may indeed be members of the lymphoid system. Systemic administration to humans over several days of Flt3-L increases both mDCs and pDCs in blood, while that of G-CSF increases only

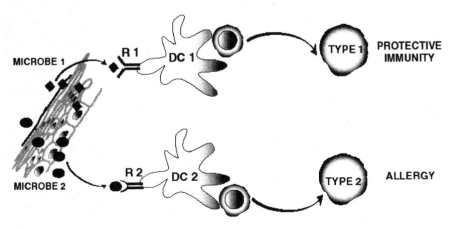

Figure 3 Different DC subsets are targeted by different pathogens via unique set of receptors expressed by DCs. This results in different types of immune responses, and consequently the interaction of a given pathogen with a given subset of DC determines the outcome, which is protective or deleterious immunity.

pDC (36,47,48). pDCs are not restricted to blood, as they can be found in lymphoid organs such as thymus and lymph nodes, in central nervous system (CNS) fluid and are increased in inflamed tissues such as tonsils, skin from lupus patients, and allergen-challenged nasal mucosa (49).

B. Mice

Early studies have distinguished mouse DCs into two major subsets: the myeloid CD8-subset and the lymphoid CD8+ subset. CD8α+ and CD8α− DCs differ in phenotype, localization, and function. Both subsets express high levels of CD11c class II MHC, and the costimulatory molecules CD86 and CD40. CD8α+ DCs are localized in the T-cell–rich areas of the periarteriolar lymphatic sheaths (PALS) in the spleen and lymph nodes (50–52). In contrast, CD8α− DCs are in the marginal zone (51,53). The CD8α+ DCs make higher levels of IL-12 and are more phagocytic than CD8α− DCs (50,54,55). While in vitro, the CD8α+ DCs were reported to prime allogeneic CD4 and CD8 T cells less efficiently than CD8α− DCs (56,57) in vivo, both subsets appear to prime antigen-specific CD4+ T cells efficiently (54,58). These splenic subsets perform different functions. Myeloid DCs, which secrete IL-12, induce type 1 responses while lymphoid DCs, unable to produce IL-12, induce type 2 responses.

Recent years have produced a change in the way we look at mouse DC subsets. Indeed, CD8 was found to also represent an activation marker of Langerhans cells. Furthermore, both committed hematopoietic lymphoid and myeloid progenitors were found to yield both CD8+ and CD8− DCs, therefore ruling out the concept that CD8 was distinguishing myeloid from lymphoid DCs (59–64). Most recently, a common precursor population yielding CD8+ and CD8− murine DCs but devoid of myeloid or lymphoid differentiation potential has been characterized (65). Finally, a novel mouse DC subset, the equivalent to human pDCs, has been identified based on its ability to produce type 1 IFN (66–68). Thus, despite critical differences in their approaches, mouse and human DC biologists are getting closer to a consensus. A pathway of plasmacytoid DCs, possibly of lymphoid origin, coexists with a myeloid pathway that includes human Langerhans cells and interstitial DCs and mouse CD8+ and CD4+ DCs. It is not yet clear how these different human and mouse myeloid DCs correspond because these subsets are studied in different cell sources in different assays.

IV. Functional Heterogeneity of DC Subsets

A. Type 1 and Type 2 T Cells

Type 1 and type 2 cells have been considered as the two extremes of T-cell polarization (69). While initially proposed for CD4+ T-helper cells, this paradigm has now been extended to CD8+ T cells as well as NK and NKT cells (70–72). There is now evidence that either polarized DCs or distinct DC subsets may provide T cells with the different cytokines/molecules microenvironments that determine the classes of immune response, e.g., type 1 versus type 2. In mice, splenic CD8α+ DCs prime naïve CD4 T cells to make Th1 cytokines in a process involving IL-12, while splenic CD8α − DCs prime naïve CD4 T cells to make Th2 cytokines (54,58). In humans, the picture is less clear. CD40-ligand (CD40-L)–activated monocyte-derived DCs prime Th1 responses via IL-12–dependent mechanism, while IL-3 + CD40-L–activated pDCs have been shown to secrete negligible amounts of IL-12 and prime Th2 responses (42). However, the polarizing effects of DC subsets may be susceptible to microenvironmental signals, which could instruct a given DC subset to elicit different Th responses. Indeed, monocyte-derived DCs can induce T cells to make IL-4, rather than IFN-γ, when (1) the DCs are used in low numbers (73) (2) the DCs are exposed to factors such as prostaglandin E2 (PGE2), corticosteroids, or IL-10, or (3) upon prolonged activation in vitro (74–77). Furthermore, pDCs, when stimulated by virus, secrete IFN-α, which drives Th1 responses in humans (78), and mature into DCs that can induce T cells to produce IFN-γ and IL-10 (79). Thus, both the type of DC subset as well as microenvironmental signals are important for Th polarization. Pulmonary DCs permanently sample and present antigens in the lung, leading to the preferential induction of Th2 responses (reviewed in Refs. 8,9). Freshly isolated antigen-pulsed lung DCs appear to prime selectively for Th2-dependent antibody responses, mirroring the normal "Th2 default" that is observed when animals encounter aerosolized Ag for the first time. Repeated challenge further enhances Th2-dependent antibody production without stimulating the production of Th1-dependent antibodies. Upon maturation with GM-CSF, DCs, now able to secrete IL-12 rather than IL-10, can stimulate type 1 immune responses (80).

B. Tolerance, Regulatory T Cells, and Tolerizing DCs

The immune system must discriminate between and appropriately respond to both pathogenic and innocuous antigens. While the thymus permits the deletion of autoreactive T cells, the peripheral immune system has evolved several mechanisms to maintain a state of tolerance to innocuous antigens, which indeed include components of self. In particular, clonal deletion is complemented by anergy and active suppression by regulatory T cells. Regulatory (Tr) lymphocytes display inhibitory activity on other immune cells, which are believed to be central to the prevention of autoimmune diseases, allergies, transplant rejection, and immune-deficiency disorders (reviewed in Refs. 81–83). Different subsets of CD4 + and CD8 + T cells show regulatory activities that are mediated either by immunosuppressive cytokines or by contact-dependent mechanisms. In both humans and rodents, CD4 + CD25 + lymphocytes represent the best-characterized Tr cell population. After TCR-triggering, CD4 + CD25 + Tr cells are anergic and express CTLA-4, a co-stimulatory receptor that delivers a negative signal to T cells. A distinct subset of CD4 + Tr cells, isolated by expanding human T cells primed with alloantigens in the presence of IL-10, was termed type 1 Tr cells. These cells inhibit both naïve and memory T cells in an antigen-specific manner via a mechanism that is partially dependent on the production of the immunoregulatory cytokines IL-10 and TGF-β. Similarly, within the human CD8 + subset, there exist antigen-specific Tr cells that suppress CD4 + T-helper cell activity by producing IL-10. There is a population of human

Tr cells that are characterized by their CD8 + CD28 − phenotype and are referred to as T-suppressor (Ts) cells (84).

There is now information about the role of DCs in the generation of these Tr cells, all indicating a critical role for IL-10 in the establishment of these Tr cells. Repetitive in vitro stimulation with Ag-loaded APCs, immature DCs in particular (85), can lead to the emergence of regulatory T cells, producing large amounts of IL-4 and IL-10, whose supernatant can block the activation of fresh T cells. IL-10 may also convert DC function to the induction of antigen-specific anergy, thus leading to the state of tolerance against tumor tissue (86,87). The generation of immature tolerizing DCs is best obtained by blocking transduction of NF-κB either using pharmacological agents such as N-acetyl-cysteine (88,89) or triggering the ILT3 and ILT4 surface molecules that deliver negative intracellular signals to myeloid cells through the expression of ITIM motifs (90). Lung DCs appear to play a key role in the development of allergen CD4 + T-cell unresponsiveness that protects against the development of Th2 responses and allergen-induced airway hyperreactivity, a cardinal feature of asthma (91,92). Then, IL-10 producing phenotypically mature DCs is generated, which induces the development of Tn cells (92).

C. Regulation of B Lymphocytes

Beside activating naive T cells, DC can directly enhance the proliferation of naive and memory B cells and their differentiation into antibody-secreting plasma cells. DC enhance differentiation of CD40-activated memory B cells towards IgG-secreting cells through secretion of the soluble IL6Rα gp80, which complexes to IL-6 (93). Interstitial DCs, but not Langerhans cells, also permit the switching of naive B cells into IgA-producing cells. Most strikingly, the switching of naive B cells into cells producing IgA2, the mucosal Ig, could only be obtained by addition of DCs to the cultures of naïve B cells (94). Thus, DC subsets have the capacity to directly regulate B-cell responses. In order to generate a humoral immune response, antigen-specific CD4 + T-helper and antigen-specific B cells must interact. Within paracortical areas of the secondary lymphoid organs, interdigitating DCs select the rare antigen-specific T and B cells. As recently demonstrated in vivo in the rat, DCs can also capture and retain unprocessed antigen, then transfer it to naive B cells to initiate a specific Th2-associated antibody response (95). This could be the role of the GCDC population localized within germinal centers and originally described as an "antigen-transporting cell" (96,97), which could display the antigen to both T and B cells.

D. Effectors of Innate Immunity

DCs at different stages of differentiation can regulate effectors of innate immunity such as NK cells and NK T cells. Both direct cell-cell interactions and indirect cytokine-mediated interactions have been implicated (98–100). Precursors of pDC may activate NK cells through the release of IFN-α, thereby leading to enhanced antiviral and antitumor activity of NK cells (25,43). DCs at later stages of differentiation may regulate the activity of NK/NK T cells (101) through the release of IL-12, IL-15, and IL-18 (102,103). However, NK cells can reciprocally regulate DCs, and the interaction between activated human NK cells and DCs may provide a "control switch" for the immune system (99). Indeed, NK cells can enhance DC maturation, possibly through TNF-α (98). However, NK cells are also capable of lysis of immature DCs via NKp30 receptor (100), thus bringing about a novel regulatory pathway in immune responses.

V. DCs in Diseases

The importance of DCs in the control of immunity may explain why no human syndrome has been yet reported to exist with a total deficit of DCs, while deficits of T and B cells are now well characterized. The central role of DCs may also explain several pathologies as it can be easily imagined that too much or too little or too skewed function of DCs can contribute to disease pathogenesis. For instance, our recent studies have demonstrated that systemic lupus erythematosus (SLE) may be due to hyperactivation of DCs (104). There, unabated production of type I interferon, possibly by pDCs, results in the activation of monocytes into cells with functions of DCs. These circulating DCs are able to capture the circulating nucleosomes, the origin of which remain an enigma, and present them to autoreactive lymphocytes, which are usually delected either in the thymus or the bone marrow or kept under control through peripheral tolerance mechanisms, which are currently thought to be essentially dependent on immature DCs.

Increased numbers of DCs in the lung have been found in smokers as well as lung transplant patients undergoing chronic rejection. Allergic respiratory diseases including allergic rhinitis and atopic asthma are associated with increased numbers of DCs in the nasal and bronchial mucosa, respectively. The chronic airway inflammation, in both atopic and nonatopic asthma, is associated with CD4+ T cells expressing Th2 cytokines. A skewed DC function could easily facilitate local activation of allergen-specific Th2 cells. Such Th2 skewing by lung-associated DCs goes beyond local regulation as myeloid DCs injected into respiratory system travel to draining lymph nodes and prime T cells making IL-4 and IL-5 (105). The molecular mechanisms of such Th2-skewed priming remain to be unraveled, but a few candidates can be considered. Thus, increased expression of GM-CSF by epithelial cells may modulate DC to skew T-cell response toward type 2 (101–108). Other critical cytokines may include recently identified IL-25, the injection of which into mice results in IL-4, IL-5, and IL-13 gene expression as well as Th2-like responses (109). One of the hallmarks of IL-25–induced clinical symptoms are eosinophilic infiltrates in the lung (109). Another important issue to be resolved is which subset of DC is critical for development of Th2 immunity in the lung as well as how long the DC can retain antigen to support Th2 T cells locally. A recent study, based on the use of a Leishmania antigen (LACK) as an inducer of allergic airway inflammation, provided evidence for the presence of long-lived antigen-retaining DCs in the lung (91). In this model, aerosol administration of LACK to LACK-sensitized mice results in the persistence of LACK-specific Th2 T cells. Surprisingly, bronchoalveolar lavage fluid contained a long-lived DC subset loaded with LACK. This subset shows a unique phenotype that suggests them to be pDCs. Therefore, the sensitization of animals with a low dose of antigen skews the ensuing immune response as a consequence of alteration in DC recruitment and mobilization.

The mobilization of different DC subsets may eventually lead to understanding of the development of atopic diseases. Holt proposed that the key etiological factor in atopic disease may not be the initial acquisition of allergen-specific Th2-skewed immunity, but a failure of immune deviation mechanisms, which in nonatopic individuals redirect the early Th2 immune response towards Th1 ones (9). Such immune deviation mechanisms would develop as a consequence of child exposure to bacterial and viral stimuli, which mostly skew immunity toward type 1. In this model, certain infectious agents that fail to stimulate type 1 immunity, such as rhinosyncytial virus, enhance the development of atopy (Fig. 3).

VI. Conclusions

The ultimate challenge of exploiting DC for therapeutic strategies, either as vaccines to increase immunity or as targets for instance in asthma, is to modulate them in vivo. Before this can be accomplished, several issues need to be resolved, including the identification of unique molecules expressed on DC subsets, and the molecular pathways determining the type of immunity induced by a given DC subset. These milestones will enable one to design vectors that would target a given DC subset and deliver a desired modulatory signal, for instance, to correct immune deviation mechanisms and skew early type 2 immunity to type 1, thus preventing development of asthma.

References

1. Fearon DT, Locksley RM. The instructive role of innate immunity in the acquired immune response. Science 1996; 272(5258):50–53.
2. Steinman RM, Cohn ZA, Identification of a novel cell type in peripheral lymphoid organs of mice. I Morphology, quantitation, tissue distribution. J Exp Med 1973; 137(5):1142–1142.
3. Inaba K, et al. Generation of large numbers of dendritic cells from mouse bone marrow cultures supplemented with granulocyte/macrophage colony-stimulating factor. J Exp Med 1992; 176(6):1693–1702.
4. Caux C, et al. GM-CSF and TNF-alpha cooperate in the generation of dendritic Langerhans cells. Nature 1992; 360(6401):258–261.
5. Sallusto F, Lanzavecchia A. Efficient presentation of soluble antigen by cultured human dendritic cells is maintained by granulocyte/macrophage colony-stimulating factor plus interleukin 4 and downregulated by tumor necrosis factor alpha. J Exp Med 1994; 179(4):1109–1118.
6. Romani N, et al. Proliferating dendritic cell progenitors in human blood. J Exp Med 1994; 180(1):83–93.
7. Banchereau J, et al. Immunobiology of dendritic cells. Ann Rev Immunol 2000; 18: 767–812.

8. Lambrecht BN. The dendritic cell in allergic airway diseases: a new player to the game. Clin Exp Allergy 2001; 31(2):206–218.

9. Holt PG. Antigen presentation in the lung. Am J Respir Crit Care Med 2000; 162(4 Pt 2):S151–S156.

10. Holt PG, et al. Origin and steady-state turnover of class II MHC-bearing dendritic cells in the epithelium of the conducting airways. J Immunol 1994; 153(1):256–261.

11. McWilliam AS, et al. Rapid dendritic cell recruitment is a hallmark of the acute inflammatory response at mucosal surfaces. J Exp Med 1994; 179(4):1331–1336.

12. McWilliam AS, et al. Dendritic cells are recruited into the airway epithelium during the inflammatory response to a broad spectrum of stimuli. J Exp Med 1996; 184(6): 2429–2432.

13. McWilliam AS, Marsh AM, Holt PG. Inflammatory infiltration of the upper airway epithelium during Sendai virus infection: involvement of epithelial dendritic cells. J Virol 1997; 71(1):226–236.

14. Xia W, Pinto CE, Kradin RL. The antigen-presenting activities of Ia+ dendritic cells shift dynamically from lung to lymph node after an airway challenge with soluble antigen. J Exp Med 1995; 181(4):1275–1283.

15. Banchereau J, Steinman RM. Dendritic cells and the control of immunity. Nature 1998; 392(6673):245–252.

16. Srivastava PK, et al. Heat shock proteins come of age: primitive functions acquire new roles in an adaptive world. Immunity 1998; 8(6):657–665.

17. Cella M, et al. Inflammatory stimuli induce accumulation of MHC class II complexes on dendritic cells [see comments]. Nature 1997; 388(6644):782–787.

18. Inaba K, et al. Efficient presentation of phagocytosed cellular fragments on the major histocompatibility complex class II products of dendritic cells. J Exp Med 1998; 188(11):2163–2173.

19. Albert ML, Sauter B, Bhardwaj N. Dendritic cells acquire antigen from apoptotic cells and induce class I-restricted CTLs. Nature 1998; 392(6671):86–89.

20. Rodriguez A, et al. Selective transport of internalized antigens to the cytosol for MHC class I presentation in dendritic cells. Nat Cell Biol 1999; 1(6):362–368.

21. Berard F, et al. Cross-priming of naive CD8 T cells against melanoma antigens using dendritic cells loaded with killed allogeneic melanoma cells. J Exp Med 2000; 192(11): 1535–1544.

22. Dhodapkar KM, et al. Antitumor monoclonal antibodies enhance cross-presentation of cellular antigens and the generation of myeloma-specific killer T cells by dendritic cells. J Exp Med 2002; 195(1):125–133.

23. Sparwasser T, et al. Bacterial DNA and immunostimulatory CpG oligonucleotides trigger maturation and activation of murine dendritic cells. Eur J Immunol 1998; 28(6): 2045–2054.

24. Hartmann G, Weiner GJ, Krieg AM. CpG DNA: a potent signal for growth, activation, and maturation of human dendritic cells. Proc Natl Acad Sci USA 1999; 96(16): 9305–9310.

25. Cella M, et al. Plasmacytoid monocytes migrate to inflamed lymph nodes and produce large amounts of type I interferon. Nat Med 1999; 5(8):919–923.

26. Rescigno M, Borrow P. The host-pathogen interaction: new themes from dendritic cell biology. Cell 2001; 106(3):267–270.

27. Underhill DM, Ozinsky A. Toll-like receptors: key mediators of microbe detection. Curr Opin Immunol 2002; 14(1):103–110.

28. Kalinski P, et al. T-cell priming by type-1 and type-2 polarized dendritic cells: the concept of a third signal. Immunol Today 1999; 20(12):561–567.

29. Sallusto F, Lanzavecchia A, Mackay CR. Chemokines and chemokine receptors in T-cell priming and Th1/Th2-mediated responses. Immunol Today 1998; 19(12):568–574.

30. Geijtenbeek TB, et al. Identification of DC-SIGN, a novel dendritic cell-specific ICAM-3 receptor that supports primary immune responses. Cell 2000; 100(5):575–585.

31. Krummel MF, Davis MM. Dynamics of the immunological synapse: finding, establishing and solidifying a connection. Curr Opin Immunol 2002; 14:66–74.

32. Cerio R, et al. Characterization of factor XIIIa positive dermal dendritic cells in normal and inflamed skin. Br J Dermatol 1989; 121(4):421–431.

33. Caux C, et al. CD34 + hematopoietic progenitors from human cord blood differentiate along two independent dendritic cell pathways in response to GM-CSF + TNF alpha. J Exp Med 1996; 184(2):695–706.

34. O'Doherty U, et al. Human blood contains two subsets of dendritic cells, one immunologically mature and the other immature. Immunology 1994; 82(3):487–493.

35. Caux C, et al. CD34 + hematopoietic progenitors from human cord blood differentiate along two independent dendritic cell pathways in response to granulocyte-macrophage colony-stimulating factor plus tumor necrosis factor alpha: II. Functional analysis. Blood 1997; 90(4):1458–1470.

36. Pulendran B, et al. Flt3-ligand and granulocyte colony-stimulating factor mobilize distinct human dendritic cell subsets in vivo. J Immunol 2000; 165(1):566–572.

37. Palucka KA, et al. Dendritic cells as the terminal stage of monocyte differentiation. J Immunol 1998; 160(9):4587.

38. Ito T, et al. A CD1a+/CD11c+ subset of human blood dendritic cells is a direct precursor of Langerhans cells. J Immunol 1999; 163(3):1409–1419.

39. Grouard G, et al. The enigmatic plasmacytoid T cells develop into dendritic cells with interleukin (IL)-3 and CD40-ligand. J Exp Med 1997; 185(6):1101–1111.

40. Olweus J, et al. Dendritic cell ontogeny: a human dendritic cell lineage of myeloid origin. Proc Natl Acad Sci USA 1997; 94(23):12551–12556.

41. Palucka K, Banchereau J. Dendritic cells: a link between innate and adaptive immunity. J Clin Immunol 1999; 19(1):12–25.

42. Rissoan MC, et al. Reciprocal control of T helper cell and dendritic cell differentiation. Science 1999; 283:1183–1186.

43. Siegal FP, et al. The nature of the principal type 1 interferon-producing cells in human blood. Science 1999; 284(5421):1835–1837.

44. Kadowaki N, et al. Subsets of human dendritic cell precursors express different toll-like receptors and respond to different microbial antigens. J Exp Med 2001; 194(6):863–869.

45. Blom B, et al. Generation of interferon alpha-producing predendritic cell (pre-DC)2 from human CD34(+) hematopoietic stem cells. J Exp Med 2000; 192(12):1785–1796.

46. Spits H, et al. Id2 and Id3 inhibit development of CD34+ stem cells into pre-DC2 but not into pre-DC1: evidence for a lymphoid origin of pre-DC2. J Exp Med 2000; 192.

47. Arpinati M, et al. Granulocyte-colony stimulating factor mobilizes T helper 2-inducing dendritic cells [see comments]. Blood 2000; 95(8):2484–2490.

48. Maraskovsky E, et al. In vivo generation of human dendritic cell subsets by Flt3 ligand. Blood 2000; 96(3):878–884.

49. Jahnsen FL, et al. Experimentally induced recruitment of plasmacytoid (CD123high) dendritic cells in human nasal allergy. J Immunol 2000; 165(7):4062–4068.

50. Pulendran B, et al. Developmental pathways of dendritic cells in vivo: distinct function, phenotype, and localization of dendritic cell subsets in FLT3 ligand-treated mice. J Immunol 1997; 159(5):2222–2231.

51. De Smedt T, et al. Regulation of dendritic cell numbers and maturation by lipopolysaccharide in vivo. J Exp Med 1996; 184(4):1413–1424.

52. Steinman RM, Pack M, Inaba K. Dendritic cells in the T-cell areas of lymphoid organs. Immunol Rev 1997; 156:25–37.

53. Reis e Sousa C, et al. In vivo microbial stimulation induces rapid CD40 ligand-independent production of interleukin 12 by dendritic cells and their redistribution to T cell areas [see comments]. J Exp Med 1997; 186(11):1819–1829.

54. Maldonado-Lopez R, et al. CD8alpha+ and CD8alpha− subclasses of dendritic cells direct the development of distinct T helper cells in vivo. J Exp Med 1999; 189(3): 587–592.

55. Ohteki T, et al. Interleukin 12-dependent interferon gamma production by CD8alpha+ lymphoid dendritic cells. J Exp Med 1999; 189(12):1981–1986.

56. Suss G, Shortman K. A subclass of dendritic cells kills CD4 T cells via Fas/Fas-ligand-induced apoptosis. J Exp Med 1996; 183(4):1789–1796.

57. Kronin V, et al. A subclass of dendritic cells regulates the response of naive CD8 T cells by limiting their IL-2 production. J Immunol 1996; 157(9):3819–3827.

58. Pulendran B, et al. Distinct dendritic cell subsets differentially regulate the class of immune response in vivo. Proc Natl Acad Sci USA 1999; 96(3):1036–1041.

59. Merad M, et al. Differentiation of myeloid dendritic cells into CD8alpha-positive dendritic cells in vivo. Blood 2000; 96(5):1865–1872.

60. Martin P, et al. Concept of lymphoid versus myeloid dendritic cell lineages revisited: both CD8alpha(−) and CD8alpha(+) dendritic cells are generated from CD4(low) lymphoid-committed precursors. Blood 2000; 96(7):2511–2519.

61. Anjuere F, et al. Langerhans cells develop from a lymphoid-committed precursor. Blood 2000; 96(5):1633–1637.

62. Anjuere F, et al. Langerhans cells acquire a CD8+ dendritic cell phenotype on maturation by CD40 ligation. J Leukoc Biol 2000; 67(2):206–209.

63. Martinez del Hoyo G, et al. CD8alpha+ dendritic cells originate from the CD8alpha− dendritic cell subset by a maturation process involving CD8alpha, DEC-205, and CD24 up-regulation. Blood 2002; 99(3):999–1004.

64. Traver D, et al. Development of CD8alpha-positive dendritic cells from a common myeloid progenitor. Science 2000; 290(5499):2152–2154.

65. del Hoyo GM, et al. Characterization of a common precursor population for dendritic cells. Nature 2002; 415(6875):1043–1047.

66. Nakano H, Yanagita M, Gunn MD. CD11c(+)B220(+)Gr-1(+) cells in mouse lymph nodes and spleen display characteristics of plasmacytoid dendritic cells. J Exp Med 2001; 194(8):1171–1178.

67. Bjorck P. Isolation and characterization of plasmacytoid dendritic cells from Flt3 ligand and granulocyte-macrophage colony-stimulating factor-treated mice. Blood 2001; 98(13):3520–3526.

68. Asselin-Paturel C, et al. Mouse type I IFN-producing cells are immature APCs with plasmacytoid morphology. Nat Immunol 2001; 2(12):1144–1150.

69. Mosmann TR, Coffman RL. TH1 and TH2 cells: different patterns of lymphokine secretion lead to different functional properties. Annu Rev Immunol 1989; 7:145–173.

70. Benlagha K, Bendelac A. CD1d-restricted mouse V alpha 14 and human V alpha 24 T cells: lymphocytes of innate immunity. Semin Immunol 2000; 12(6):537–542.

71. Lee PT, et al. Distinct functional lineages of human valpha24 natural killer T cells. J Exp Med 2002; 195(5):637–641.

72. Terabe M, et al. NKT cell-mediated repression of tumor immunosurveillance by IL-13 and the IL-4R-STAT6 pathway. Nat Immunol 2000; 1(6):515–520.

73. Tanaka H, et al. Human monocyte-derived dendritic cells induce naive T cell differentiation into T helper cell type 2 (Th2) or Th1/Th2 effectors. Role of stimulator/responder ratio. J Exp Med 2000; 192(3):405–412.

74. Kalinski P, et al. Final maturation of dendritic cells is associated with impaired responsiveness to IFN-gamma and to bacterial IL-12 inducers: decreased ability of mature dendritic cells to produce IL-12 during the interaction with Th cells. J Immunol 1999; 162(6):3231–3236.

75. Vieira PL, et al. Development of Th1-inducing capacity in myeloid dendritic cells requires environmental instruction. J Immunol 2000; 164(9):4507–4512.

76. Langenkamp A, et al. Kinetics of dendritic cell activation: impact on priming of TH1, TH2 and nonpolarized T cells. Nat Immunol 2000; 1:311–316.

77. Lanzavecchia A, Sallusto F. Dynamics of T lymphocyte responses: intermediates, effectors, and memory cells. Science 2000; 290(5489):92–97.

78. Parronchi P, et al. Effects of interferon-alpha on cytokine profile, T cell receptor repertoire and peptide reactivity of human allergen-specific T cells. Eur J Immunol 1996; 26(3):697–703.

79. Kadowaki N, et al. Natural interferon alpha/beta-producing cells link innate and adaptive immunity. J Exp Med 2000; 192(2):219–226.

80. Stumbles PA, et al. Resting respiratory tract dendritic cells preferentially stimulate T helper cell type 2 (Th2) responses and require obligatory cytokine signals for induction of Th1 immunity. J Exp Med 1998; 188(11):2019–2031.

81. Roncarolo MG, et al. Type 1 T regulatory cells. Immunol Rev 2001; 182:68–79.

82. Sakaguchi S, et al. Immunologic tolerance maintained by CD25 + CD4 + regulatory T cells: their common role in controlling autoimmunity, tumor immunity, and transplantation tolerance. Immunol Rev 2001; 182:18–32.

83. Shevach EM, et al. Control of autoimmunity by regulatory T cells. Adv Exp Med Biol 2001; 490:21–32.

84. Cortesini R, et al. CD8 + CD28 − T suppressor cells and the induction of antigen-specific, antigen-presenting cell-mediated suppression of Th reactivity. Immunol Rev 2001; 182:201–206.

85. Jonuleit H, et al. Induction of interleukin 10-producing, nonproliferating CD4(+) T cells with regulatory properties by repetitive stimulation with allogeneic immature human dendritic cells. J Exp Med 2000; 192(9):1213–1222.

86. Enk AH, et al. Dendritic cells as mediators of tumor-induced tolerance in metastatic melanoma. Int J Cancer 1997; 73(3):309–316.

87. Steinbrink K, et al. Interleukin-10-treated human dendritic cells induce a melanoma-antigen-specific anergy in CD8(+) T cells resulting in a failure to lyse tumor cells. Blood 1999; 93(5):1634–1642.

88. Yoshimura S, et al. Role of NFkappaB in antigen presentation and development of regulatory T cells elucidated by treatment of dendritic cells with the proteasome inhibitor PSI. Eur J Immunol 2001; 31(6):1883–1893.

89. Verhasselt V, et al. N-Acetyl-L-cysteine inhibits primary human T cell responses at the dendritic cell level: association with NF-kappaB inhibition. J Immunol 1999; 162(5): 2569–2574.

90. Chang CC, et al. Tolerization of dendritic cells by T(S) cells: the crucial role of inhibitory receptors ILT3 and ILT4. Nat Immunol 2002; 3(3):237–243.

91. Julia V, et al. A restricted subset of dendritic cells captures airborne antigens and remains able to activate specific T cells long after antigen exposure. Immunity 2002; 16(2):271–283.

92. Akbari O, DeKruyff RH, Umetsu DT. Pulmonary dendritic cells producing IL-10 mediate tolerance induced by respiratory exposure to antigen. Nat Immunol 2001; 2(8): 725–731.

93. Dubois B, et al. Dendritic cells enhance growth and differentiation of CD40-activated B lymphocytes [see comments]. J Exp Med 1997; 185(5):941–951.

94. Fayette J, et al. Human dendritic cells skew isotype switching of CD40-activated naive B cells towards IgA1 and IgA2. J Exp Med 1997; 185(11):1909–1918.

95. Wykes M, et al. Dendritic cells interact directly with naive B lymphocytes to transfer antigen and initiate class switching in a primary T-dependent response. J Immunol 1998; 161(3):1313–1319.

96. Grouard G, et al. Dendritic cells capable of stimulating T cells in germinal centres. Nature 1996; 384(6607):364–367.

97. Szakal AK, Kosco MH, Tew JG. Microanatomy of lymphoid tissue during humoral immune responses: structure function relationships. Annu Rev Immunol 1989; 7: 91–109.

98. Gerosa F, et al. Reciprocal activating interaction between natural killer cells and dendritic cells. J Exp Med 2002; 195(3):327–333.

99. Piccioli D, et al. Contact-dependent stimulation and inhibition of dendritic cells by natural killer cells. J Exp Med 2002; 195(3):335–341.

100. Ferlazzo G, et al. Human dendritic cells activate resting natural killer (NK) cells and are recognized via the NKp30 receptor by activated NK cells. J Exp Med 2002; 195(3): 343–351.

101. Fernandez NC, et al. Dendritic cells directly trigger NK cell functions: cross-talk relevant in innate anti-tumor immune responses in vivo. Nat Med 1999; 5(4):405–411.

102. Shah PD. Dendritic cells but not macrophages are targets for immune regulation by natural killer cells. Cell Immunol 1987; 104(2):440–445.

103. Geldhof AB, et al. Interleukin-12-activated natural killer cells recognize B7 costimulatory molecules on tumor cells and autologous dendritic cells. Blood 1998; 91(1): 196–206.

104. Blanco P, et al. Induction of dendritic cell differentiation by IFN-alpha in systemic lupus erythematosus. Science 2001; 294(5546):1540–1543.

105. Lambrecht BN, et al. Myeloid dendritic cells induce Th2 responses to inhaled antigen, leading to eosinophilic airway inflammation. J Clin Invest 2000; 106(4):551–559.

106. Stampfli MR, et al. GM-CSF transgene expression in the airway allows aerosolized ovalbumin to induce allergic sensitization in mice. J Clin Invest 1998; 102(9): 1704–1714.

107. Christensen PJ, et al. Regulation of rat pulmonary dendritic cell immunostimulatory activity by alveolar epithelial cell-derived granulocyte macrophage colony-stimulating factor. Am J Respir Cell Mol Biol 1995; 13(4):426–433.

108. Wang J, et al. Transgenic expression of granulocyte-macrophage colony-stimulating factor induces the differentiation and activation of a novel dendritic cell population in the lung. Blood 2000; 95(7):2337–2345.

109. Fort MM, et al. IL-25 induces IL-4, IL-5, and IL-13 and Th2-associated pathologies in vivo. Immunity 2001; 15(6):985–995.

15

Roles of Mast Cells in Airway Hyperreactivity, Inflammation and Remodeling, and Immunoregulation in Asthma

JOHN L. FAUL and STEPHEN J. GALLI

Stanford University School of Medicine
Stanford, California, U.S.A.

I. Introduction

While it is generally accepted that mast cell activation is critical for the expression of the acute bronchoconstriction provoked by allergen challenge in subjects with atopic asthma, there is much less agreement about the roles of mast cells in the late phase reactions or chronic allergic inflammation associated with this disorder (reviewed in Refs. 1–6). In this chapter we shall discuss the characteristics of the mast cell that enable it to act as both an important effector cell and as a potential immunoregulatory cell in asthma and other allergic diseases. Although many potential mechanisms may contribute to mast cell activation in subjects with asthma, including those involving complement (7,8), neurotrophins, or neuropeptides (9–11), the c-*kit* ligand stem cell factor (12–14), T-cell–derived products (15), and products of bacteria or viruses (16–18) (see other chapters in this volume), we shall focus on the role of IgE in eliciting mast cell function in this setting. We shall present evidence, much of it derived from in vivo studies in mice, indicating that mast cells can indeed contribute importantly to the expression of IgE-dependent late phase reactions, IgE-dependent enhancement of airway hyperreactivity and certain features of chronic allergic inflammation in the airways. As a subtheme, we shall consider two important issues that contribute to the "controversy" about the relevance of the findings obtained in murine asthma "models" to our understanding of asthma in humans: the redundancy and complexity of effector and immunoregulatory mechanisms in IgE-associated immune responses and certain differences in these processes in mice and humans.

II. Mast Cell Biology: Natural History, Changes in Atopic Asthma, and Heterogeneity

A. Natural History

Mast cells are derived from hematopoietic progenitor cells and, except for the small numbers of mast cells that reside in the bone marrow, maturation typically occurs in the peripheral tissues (19–23). Interactions between the tyrosine kinase receptor c-kit, which is expressed on the surface of mast cells and their precursors, and the c-kit ligand stem cell factor (SCF), are essential for mast cell development and survival in both mice and rats and, probably, also in humans (19,21,23–25). In certain circumstances, SCF can also directly induce mast cell mediator release and enhance mast cell mediator release in response to other signals, including those mediated by IgE-dependent mechanisms (21,25–28). However, in vitro studies indicate that many other cytokines/growth factors besides SCF may also influence mast cell populations through effects on the cells' survival, proliferation, phenotype, or function (1–3,5,22,23).

Mast cells are well positioned anatomically to participate in allergic reactions in the airways and other surfaces exposed to the environment. Unlike mature basophils, mature mast cells do not normally circulate in the blood but are widely distributed throughout normal connective tissues, where they often lie adjacent to blood and lymphatic vessels, near or within nerves and beneath epithelial surfaces, such as those of the respiratory and gastrointestinal systems and skin (1–3,5,19–22,29). Mast cell numbers in normal tissues exhibit considerable variation according to anatomical site, and these "baseline" numbers of mast cells can change, sometimes strikingly, in association with certain inflammatory or immunological reactions (1–3,5,19–22,29). For example, a greater than 10-fold expansion of mast cell populations can occur in mice at sites of infection with some intestinal parasites that induce a strong Th2 response, and this process is dependent on both the c-kit ligand, SCF, and IL-3 (30).

B. Changes in Mast Cells in Atopic Asthma

Increased numbers of mast cells have been reported in tissues affected by chronic allergic inflammation in humans (31–33). However, while some studies found that certain subjects with asthma have increased numbers of mast cells in the mucosa of the airways (32,34,35), others did not (36,37). In some cases of fatal asthma, numbers of morphologically identifiable mast cells in the airways can be decreased compared to values obtained from normal controls, a finding that has been attributed to the loss of the cells' cytoplasmic granule staining as a result of the extensive activation and degranulation of the cells in this setting (32,38). However, other studies demonstrated marked increases in mast cells (34) and/or basophils (34,39) in the airways of subjects with fatal asthma. In another study, no differences were detected in the numbers of epithelial or airway wall mast cells in patients with mild-moderate as opposed to fatal asthma (40).

A study of surgically resected lung tissue from patients with lung cancer demonstrated that numbers of mast cells were increased in the airway muscularis of specimens that exhibited evidence of prior sensitization to common aeroallergens as opposed to those that did not (40). Moreover, cases of fatal asthma can exhibit marked increases in mast cells in many regions in the airways, including within smooth muscle bundles in the bronchioles (34). The extent to which these findings may be reflective of a correlation of mast cell numbers in the airway muscularis with asthma per se, or with the severity of asthma, and the pathophysiological importance of any such association remain to be determined. However, these findings raise the possibility that some of the changes in mast cell numbers of potential importance in asthma may occur in anatomical locations that ordinarily are poorly sampled in endobronchial biopsy specimens.

C. Mast Cell Heterogeneity

In addition to being able to undergo changes in their anatomical distribution or numbers, studies in both humans and experimental animals show that mast cell populations can vary in many aspects of their phenotype, including morphology, histochemistry, mediator content, and response to stimuli of activation (1–3,5,19–21,23,29). This aspect of mast cell biology has been called "mast cell heterogeneity." The practical implication of these findings is the recognition that, to understand the relevance of "mast cells" to a particular biological response, one ideally should study those mast cells that actually participate in that response in vivo. This is not as simple as it may seem, since mast cells in a specific anatomical location can undergo alterations in phenotype during the course of immunological or inflammatory responses, and some of these changes may be reversible (1–3,5,19–21,23,29). The analysis of airway mast cells in humans presents special challenges: the amount of airway tissue available for study from subjects with asthma generally is very small and is typically derived primarily from superficial layers of the airway; pulmonary mast cells isolated from surgical specimens may undergo alterations in phenotype and function as a result of the isolation procedure itself; and the maintenance of mast cells (from any source) in vitro may also induce potentially significant changes in their properties.

III. Model for Analyzing Mast Cell Development and Function and Potential Therapeutic Targets In Vivo: Mast Cell Knock-In Mice

IgE-associated immune responses in asthma and other settings typically involve the coordinated and potentially redundant activities of several cell types; under these circumstances, characterizing the specific contributions of a single cell can be difficult. To investigate the roles of mast cells in such settings, this problem can be addressed by using genetically mast cell–deficient Kit^W/Kit^{W-v} mice (19,21,42–47). Kit^W/Kit^{W-v} mice are anemic and virtually lack tissue mast cells, germ cells, melano-cytes, and interstitial cells of Cajal (19,21,42–47). These defects reflect conse-quences of the animals' mutations affecting both copies of c-*kit*, which result in a marked reduction in the c-kit–dependent signaling in the affected lineages; thus, such cells respond poorly, or not at all, to stimulation with the kit ligand, SCF (21,24). However, mast cell activity can be selectively reconstituted in Kit^W/Kit^{W-v} mice to compare the expression of biological responses in tissues that differ solely in containing, or virtually lacking, mast cells (21,42–47). Selective repair of the mast cell deficiency of Kit^W/Kit^{W-v} mice (i.e., correction of the animals' profound mast cell deficiency without alteration of other defects related to the effects of animals' c-*kit* mutations) may be achieved by the adoptive transfer of bone mar-row–derived cultured mast cells (BMCMCs) of wild-type origin (42). Alternatively, one may substitute other mast cell populations that express genetically determined abnormalities in products that potentially affect the cells' development, survival, phenotype, or function (21,42,46–48).

For example, it is now possible to generate mouse mast cells in vitro in large numbers from mouse embryonic stem (ES) cells including ES cells that express certain "embryonic lethal" genotypes (46,47,49). Such ES cell–derived mast cells (ESMCs) not only can be analyzed in vitro, but also can survive and express mast cell function in vivo after adoptive transfer into the skin or peritoneal cavity of Kit^W/Kit^{W-v} mice (46,47). This approach permits the production of Kit^W/Kit^{W-v} mice that selectively contain mast cells of defined genotype, for comparison to Kit^W/Kit^{W-v} mice that selectively contain adoptively transferred populations of (+/+) mast cells. This general approach may be used for studies of mast cell survival, development, and function, as well as for analyzing the roles of specific mast cell–associated molecules (e.g., surface receptors, elements of signaling pathways, transcription factors, or secreted products) in mouse models of allergic diseases or other adaptive or pathological biological responses. An additional use of this approach is the evalua-tion, in adult mice in vivo, of the results of the genetic manipulation of potential "therapeutic targets" in asthma and other disorders (46,49).

When Kit^W/Kit^{W-v} mice are injected i.d., i.p., or i.v. with phenotypically "imma-ture" mast cells (BMCMCs) of cogenic +/+ origin, the recipient "mast cell knock-in mice" develop tissue mast cell populations of donor origin whose ultrastructural and histochemical characteristics are similar to those of the corresponding mast cell populations in the tissues of normal mice (42). However, depending on such factors as the route of BMCMC administration and the interval after BMCMC transfer at which the properties of the adaptively transferred mast cell population are assessed, the numbers, anatomical distribution, and mediator content of mast cells in "mast cell knock-in mice," may not be identical to those in the corresponding wild-type (+/+) mice (42). For example, Kit^W/Kit^{W-v} mice injected i.v. with +/+ BMCMCs develop, in comparison to the congenic +/+ mice of the same age, fewer mast cells in the trachea but more mast cells in the periphery of the lungs (50,51). Such mice also appear to develop few or no mast cells in the heart (52) or the central nervous system (53).

These and other potentially important "nuances" of this system should be kept in mind when one is interpreting the results of work conducted using this approach. For example, depending on the anatomical site, relatively low levels of activation of mast cell degranulation and mediator release in normal mice can result in near maximal expression of some of the pathological consequences associated with the mast cell–dependent biological response elicited at this site (such as the swelling of the skin induced by SCF/c-kit–dependent mast cell activation) (27). By contrast, other features of the same locally induced reaction (such as the amount of SCF- and mast cell–dependent fibrin deposition in the skin at sites of SCF injection) can exhibit a more direct positive relationship to the extent of mast cell degranulation induced in that setting (27).

IV. Mast Cell Mediators

A. Introduction

Mast cells contain, or elaborate on appropriate stimulation, a diverse array of potent biologically active products, which can have many different potential effects in inflammation, tissue remodeling, and organ function at sites of mast cell activation. (Fig. 1) (1–5,29,54). The recent introduction of various approaches to perform massively parallel, genome-wide analyses of mast cell transcriptional responses has resulted in the identification of many more products (and therefore many potential mast cell–associated "therapeutic targets") that can contribute to the mast cell's ability to influence the pathophysiology of asthma and other disorders (55,56). Some of these products are stored preformed in the cells' cytoplasmic granules, while others are synthesized upon appropriate cell activation. Cytokines and chemokines are the most recently identified group of mast cell products; it appears that some of these, e.g., TNF-α (57–59) and vascular permeability factor/vascular endothelial cell growth factor (VPF/VEGF) (60,61), can be released by activated mast cells from both preformed and newly synthesized pools.

B. Preformed Mediators

Mediators stored preformed in the cytoplasmic granules of mouse or human mast cells include histamine (mouse and rat, but not human, mast cells also contain serotonin), proteoglycans, serine proteases, carboxypeptidase A, small amounts of sulfatases and exoglycosidases, and major basic protein (long thought to represent an "eosinophil-specific" product) (1–5,29,54,55). Studies in genetically mast cell–deficient and cogenic normal mice indicate that mast cells account for nearly all of the histamine stored in normal tissues, with the exception of the glandular stomach and the central nervous system (62).

Mouse and human mast cell populations contain variable mixtures of heparin and chondroitin sulfate proteoglycans (1–3). Mast cell proteoglycans probably have several biological functions both within and outside of the cells (1–3,29,63). By ionic interactions, they bind histamine, neutral proteases, and carboxypeptidase, and they contribute to the packaging and storage of these molecules within the secretory

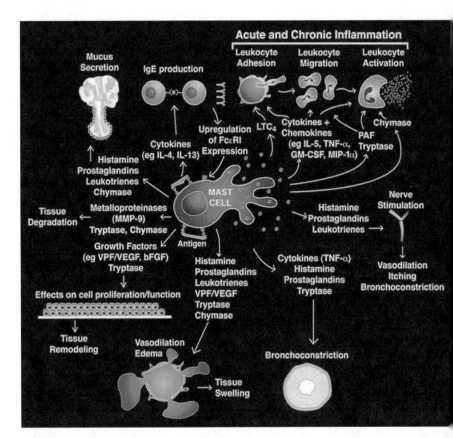

Figure 1 Diagrammatic representation of some of the major mediators, cytokines, and growth factors that are produced upon IgE- and antigen-dependent activation of mast cells and the potential contributions of these products to various features of the acute, late phase and chronic inflammation that is associated with asthma and other allergic diseases. It must be kept in mind that (1) different individual mast cells may vary in their ability to express certain products, especially individual proteases (tryptases, chymases), cytokines, chemokines and growth factors; (2) the fact that a particular mediator can exert a particular effect (in vitro or after administration in vivo) does not prove that such an effect is critical to the expression of allergic inflammation during actual disease processes in vivo; (3) other effector cell types that participate in allergic inflammation can produce some of the same mediators as mast cells; (4) basophils, which express high levels of FcεRI and can produce a spectrum of mediators that is similar but not identical to that of mast cells, once recruited to these responses may have functions that partially overlap with those of the mast cells. (From Ref 54.)

granules (64,65). When the granule matrices are exposed to physiological conditions of pH and ionic strength during degranulation, the various mediators associated with the proteoglycans dissociate at different rates—histamine very rapidly but tryptase and chymase much more slowly (1). In addition to regulating the kinetics of release of mediators from the granule matrices, proteoglycans can also regulate the activity of some of the associated mediators.

Neutral proteases are the major protein component of mast cell secretory granules. By weight, tryptase is the major enzyme stored in the cytoplasmic granules of human mast cells, and this neutral protease occurs in most, if not all, human mast cell populations (1,66). Human mast cell tryptase is a serine endopeptidase that exists in the granule in active form as a tetramer of 134 kDa containing subunits of 31–35 kDa, each of which contains an active site. Tryptase has also been identified in human basophils and may be increased in the basophils of subjects with allergic disorders (66,67). Recent evidence indicates that there may be multiple forms of human tryptase, derived from distinct transcripts and genes; the biological significance of these findings is not yet clear (68,69). Mast cell chymase is also a serine protease that is stored in the active form (as a monomer with a molecular weight of 30 kDa) in the granules of some, but not all, human mast cells (1). Many human lung mast cells lack chymase, as determined by immunohistochemical analysis (1,66). A discussion of the diverse potential biological functions of the many mouse and rat mast cell proteases that have been identified, or of the human mast cell proteases, is beyond the scope of this review (other chapters in this volume deal with this topic). However, in the case of the mouse system, transgenic mice that lack expression of specific proteases will be very valuable resources for defining the specific roles of these mediators in vivo (29,70).

C. Newly Synthesized Lipid Mediators

The most important mast cell–derived lipid mediators are the cyclooxygenase and lipoxygenase metabolites of arachidonic acid, which have potent inflammatory activities and which may also play a role in modulating the release process itself (71,72). The major cyclooxygenase product of mast cells is prostaglandin D_2 (PGD_2), and the major lipoxygenase products derived from mast cells are the sulfidodopeptide leukotrienes (LTs): LTC_4 and its peptidolytic derivatives, LTD_4 and LTE_4. Human mast cells can produce LTB_4, although in much smaller quantities than PGD_2 or LTC_4 (71,72), and some mast cell populations represent a potential source of PAF (73).

D. Cytokines and Chemokines

Several lines of evidence indicate that certain mature, "resting" (nonactivated) mouse (57–59) or human (74–76) mast cells contain preformed stores of TNF-α available for immediate release upon appropriate stimulation of the cells. Certain mast cell populations may also have preformed stores of VPF/VEGF (60,61). Many other cytokines have been identified in various mast cell populations by immunohisto-chemical or immunocytochemical methods; these may represent additional cytokines that can be released in part from "stored" pools (75). Thus, in IgE-dependent reactions, mast cells are likely to represent an important initial source of TNF-α, VPF/VEGF, and perhaps several other cytokines.

Mast cells represent a potential source of many cytokines and chemokines and growth factors that might influence IgE-associated allergic inflammation, and the synthesis and release of many of these products can be induced via IgE-dependent mechanisms. For example, certain mouse mast cells activated via the FcεRI contain increased levels of mRNA for many cytokines, including IL-1α, IL-3, IL-4, IL-5, IL-6, IL-13, GM-CSF, TGF-β, TNF-α, VPF/VEGF, IFN-γ, and the chemokines MIP-1α, MIP-1β, MCAF (MCP-1), MARC, and I-309, and/or secrete substances with the corresponding bioactivities, including IL-1, IL-3, IL-4, IL-6, IL-9, IL-13, GM-CSF, and TNF-α (54,74). The list of cytokines/chemokines/growth factors associated with various populations of purified or in vitro–derived human mast cells (or detected in human mast cells in situ) includes IL-3, -4, -5, -6, -8, -10, -11, -13, -16, TNF-α, VPF/VEGF, GM-CSF, SCF, bFGF, and MIP-1α (54,56,77–93), and enhanced gene expression for many more cytokines and chemokines has been identified using cDNA microarray analysis in populations of in vitro–derived mast cells that have been activated via the FcεRI (56).

V. The High-Affinity Receptor for IgE (FcεRI)

A. Introduction

Because another chapter in this volume deals primarily with this topic, we shall mention only a few points of direct relevance to the role of mast cells in asthma. In humans, mast cells are thought to express immunologically specific effector function in allergic disorders primarily as a result of their ability to bind IgE antibodies to FcεRI, the high-affinity receptor for IgE; aggregation of the FcεRI upon binding of allergen to multiple cell-bound IgE antibodies activates mast cells to release all classes of mediators (94,95). The expression of FcεRI on the surface of mouse mast cells appears to occur early in their differentiation and/or maturation (22,96–98), and mature mouse mast cells can express FcεRI in excess of 10^5 per cell (99). In normal mice, FcεRI are detectable only on mast cells and basophils (95). Human mast cells and basophils also express large numbers of FcεRI on their cell surface; however, at least under some circumstances, many other potential effector cells in humans, including Langerhans cells, blood monocytes and macrophages, circulating dendritic cells, and eosinophils also may express at least small numbers of this receptor (95). Thus, many cells in addition to mast cells and basophils may contribute to the expression of IgE-associated immune reactions in humans.

On the other hand, mouse mast cells express FcγRIII (which utilizes the same β and γ chains as FcεRI), as do mouse monocytes and macrophages, neutrophils, and natural killer cells (95). FcγRIII can bind IgG$_1$ antibodies, which typically are produced along with IgE antibodies during Th2 responses in mice (5,95,100). The widespread distribution of FcγRIII on various mouse effector cells permits these cells, in addition to mast cells and basophils, to participate in the expression of IgE- (and IgG$_1$) associated immune responses in mice.

B. Regulation of FcεRI Surface Expression by IgE—Implications for Asthma

Levels of FcεRI surface expression on mouse or human mast cells and basophils can be regulated by levels of IgE (92,83,101–104), at least in part via IgE-dependent stabilization of the expression of FcεRI on the cell surface (reviewed in Refs. 5,102–105). Such IgE-dependent upregulation of FcεRI expression permits mouse or human mast cells to exhibit IgE-dependent mediator release upon challenge with lower concentrations of specific antigen or anti-IgE and/or to secrete increased amounts of preformed and lipid mediators at a given level of challenge, as well as to produce strikingly higher levels of certain cytokines and growth factors (60,83,92,102).

This work thus identifies a potentially important mechanism for enhancing the expression of effector cell function in IgE-dependent allergic reactions or immunological responses to parasites. Because this process also can increase the ability of various mast cell populations to produce IL-4 (102), IL-13 (84,92), and MIP-1α (83), all of which can promote IgE production (reviewed in Refs. 83,84,92,102), IgE-dependent upregulation of FcεRI expression may also be part of a positive feedback mechanism for inducing further production of IgE and thereby promoting a persistent "Th2 bias" of the immune system in subjects with parasite infections or allergic diseases associated with high levels of IgE.

VI. Mast Cell Functions in IgE-Associated Immune Responses

A. Introduction

The effector phases of IgE-associated immune responses can be conceptualized as occurring in three temporal patterns: (1) acute reactions, which develop within seconds or minutes of allergen exposure; (2) late-phase reactions, which develop within hours of allergen exposure, often after at least some of the effects of the acute reaction have partially diminished; and (3) chronic allergic inflammation, which can persist for days to years (5).

B. Acute Allergic Reactions

Passive cutaneous anaphylaxis (PCA) represents one of the simplest experimental models of an acute allergic reaction. In this model, IgE (and/or, in mice, IgG$_1$) antibodies of defined allergenic specificity are injected into the skin, and, at a suitable interval thereafter (for IgE-dependent PCA reactions typically 24–48 hours), the specific allergen is administered intravenously, inducing mast cell activation and augmented vascular permeability (reviewed in Refs. 5,106). Mast cell–deficient Kit^W/Kit^{W-v} mice are not able to express detectable PCA reactions (106–108). By contrast, IgE-dependent PCA reactions can be readily expressed in Kit^W/Kit^{W-v} mice at cutaneous sites that have been selectively repaired of their mast cell deficiency, by prior injection of either BMCMCs (106–108) or ESMCs (46). Similar approaches have been used to show that essentially all of the assessed acute consequences of IgE-dependent reactions elicited in the mouse respiratory tract upon systemic challenge with anti-IgE, including reductions in both pulmonary dynamic compliance and conductance (109,110), as well as the enhancement of airway reactivity to methacholine that is detected minutes after anti-IgE challenge (50), are also mast cell–dependent.

Based on this evidence, it appears very likely that mast cells are essential for the expression of at least the major features of IgE-dependent acute allergic reactions in mice, including the consequences of these reactions in the respiratory system. In one setting, the anaphylaxis associated observed in mice sensitized to penicillin V (111), an apparently IgE-dependent acute immunological response, can be elicited in the essential absence of mast cells in Kit^W/Kit^{W-v} mice. While pharmacological evidence suggests that PAF is a key mediator of this response, its source remains to be determined (111). As the only other cell in the mouse known to express FcεRI, the basophil represents a prime suspect.

C. Mast Cell–Leukocyte Cytokine Cascades: A Mechanism by Which Mast Cells Can Contribute to Late Phase Reactions and Chronic Allergic Inflammation

Several groups have shown that various features of late phase reactions or chronic allergic inflammation can be expressed in the airways of mice that lack IgE, B cells, or mast cells (112–120). In part because of such work, interest has focused increasingly on eosinophils and Th2 lymphocytes as key effector cells of these phases of allergic inflammation (121–126). While this remains an important area of research, we feel that the key question is not whether IgE and mast cells, as opposed to basophils, eosinophils, or T cells, are mainly responsible for the pathology associated with chronic allergic diseases (because in different settings it is likely that each type of effector cell may be important), but to identify the extent to which particular clinically significant characteristics of these disorders reflect the specific contributions of distinct potential effector cell types.

Our group has formulated the hypothesis that a "mast cell–leukocyte cytokine cascade" can critically contribute to the initiation, amplification, and perpetuation of IgE-associated allergic inflammation in the airways and other sites (5,45,77,127). Specifically, we propose that the activation of mast cells through the FcεRI can initiate both the acute and late phase components of the response, the latter orchestrated in part through the release of TNF-α and other cytokines and chemokines that can influence the recruitment and function of additional effector cells, including eosinophils, basophils, neutrophils, and T cells. These recruited cells then promote the further progression of the inflammatory response by providing additional sources of certain cytokines that may also be produced by mast cells stimulated by ongoing exposure to allergen, as well as new sources of cytokines and other mediators that may not be produced by mast cells.

Certain mast cell cytokines, such as TNF-α, VPF/VEGF, and TGF-β, may also contribute to chronic allergic inflammation through effects on fibroblasts, vascular endothelial cells, and other cells resident at the sites of these reactions (60,128,129).

Finally, mast cell activation may directly or indirectly promote the release of cytokines from certain other cells resident in the tissues (e.g., in the respiratory tract, such cells would include alveolar macrophages, eosinophils, bronchial epithelial cells, vascular endothelial cells, fibroblasts, epithelial cells, and nerves); together, the diverse cytokines that are released in these responses then contribute to the vascular and epithelial changes and to the tissue remodeling, angiogenesis, and fibrosis that can be so prominent in IgE-associated chronic allergic inflammation and many other disorders associated with mast cell activation and leukocyte infiltration. Moreover, at certain points in the natural history of these complex processes, cytokines and other mediators derived from mast cells, or from eosinophils or other recruited cells, may also contribute to the downregulation of the response.

D. The Potential Role of Mast Cell–Derived TNF-α in Asthma

While mast cells can produce a very large number of cytokines and chemokines, the potential role of one of these, TNF-α, in the pathophysiology of IgE-dependent inflammation has been studied in some detail. Studies in "mast cell knock-in mice" showed that mast cells were required for essentially all of the leukocyte infiltration observed in the skin after challenge with IgE and specific antigen and that ~50% of such IgE- and mast cell–dependent leukocyte infiltration was inhibitable with a neutralizing antibody to recombinant mouse TNF-α (107). Other mast cell–derived mediators, including histamine, serotonin, and leukotienes, probably also contribute to mast cell–associated leukocyte infiltration in this setting. Granulocyte recruitment in this system was affected minimally, if at all, in mice that lacked either P-selection or E-selectin, but was essentially eliminated in mice that lacked both of these selectins (130); such IgE- and mast cell–dependent granulocyte recruitment could be suppressed by treatment with cyclosporin A (CsA) or dexamethasone (131). The latter findings (131) are consistent with the hypothesis that at least some of the therapeutic benefit of drugs such as corticosteroids and CsA, both in asthma and in other IgE-associated inflammatory disorders (132), may reflect the ability of these agents to interfere with multiple steps in the pathogenesis of mast cell–leukocyte cytokine cascades, including the mast cell–dependent production of TNF-α and other cytokines.

However, the actual importance of TNF-α in asthma, whether derived from mast cells or other sources, is not yet clear. TNF-α can induce bronchial hyperresponsiveness in rats (133) or humans (134). TNF-α can also induce hyperresponsiveness (135,136) and proliferation (137) of human airway smooth muscle cells in vitro. Moreover, Bradding et al. (75) reported that TNF-α expression is upregulated in the airway mucosa of subjects with allergic asthma and that this expression of TNF-α occurs predominantly in mast cells and monocytes/macrophages; no TNF-α immunoreactivity was localized in either T cells or eosinophils. Ohkawara et al. (138) found that three resident cell populations in human lung fragments—mast cells, tissue and alveolar macrophages, and bronchial epithelial cells,—expressed TNF-α by immunohistochemistry 4 hours after anti-IgE challenge in vitro whereas no cells exhibited TNF-α immunoreactivity in specimens incubated with medium alone. Taken together, this work suggests that "normal" human lung mast cells might exhibit low levels of TNF-α, but that expression of the cytokine can be upregulated in mast cells challenged via the FcɛRI.

Notably, studies of OVA-induced immune responses in mice deficient in TNF-α receptors 1 and 2 indicate that a lack of these receptors can moderately reduce (139) or increase (140) antigen-dependent airway eosinophil recruitment and has either no detectable effect (139) or can enhance (140) antigen-induced airway hyperreactivity (AHR) (139,140). OVA-induced eosinophil recruitment to BAL fluid was moderately reduced in mice treated with an anti-TNF-α antibody (141) or in TNF-α $-/-$ mice (142), but TNF-α $-/-$ mice did not exhibit reduced numbers of tissue eosinophils (142). Moreover, OVA-induced AHR in OVA-sensitized mice was significantly greater in TNF-α $-/-$ mice than in wild-type controls (142). The reason(s) for the divergent results in the various studies are not clear. However, all of these studies tested mice that were sensitized with OVA using alum as an adjuvant, a method that appears to favor the development of mast cell–independent airway AHR and eosinophil recruitment (51).

VII. Mast Cells and the Airway Hyperreactivity and Eosinophil-Rich Inflammation Associated with Asthma

Are mast cells important in orchestrating either airway hyperreactivity or eosinophil infiltration into the airways, two major hallmarks of human asthma? Initial studies of "asthma models" in mice suggested that the answer to this question is no. For example, at least four studies using mast cell–deficient Kit^W/Kit^{W-v} mice reported that mast cells were not essential for the development either of antigen-induced infiltration of the airways with eosinophils (112–114,117) or AHR to cholinergic stimulation (117). However, in each of these studies the investigators used strong procedures of antigen sensitization and challenge, such as immunizing the mice with an antigen admixed with alum as an adjuvant—approaches that favor the production of strong immunological responses.

These studies prove that, under the conditions of antigen sensitization and challenge tested, mast cells are not essential for antigen-induced eosinophil infiltration, or AHR. However, human subjects with asthma often express dramatic pathophysiological responses after sensitization and challenge with very low doses of specific antigen (143,144). In settings such as this (i.e., in "naturally" sensitized subjects exposed to low doses of antigen), mast cells may serve as critical "amplifiers" of IgE-associated inflammation and its potential consequences, including eosinophil infiltration (4). In accord with this hypothesis, Kung et al. (145), using a protocol in which aerosol challenge with OVA was performed only twice on a single day, found that eosinophil infiltration of the airways in Kit^W/Kit^{W-v} mice was ≤50% of that in the $+/+$ mice. Subsequently, using "mast cell knock-in mice," Williams and Galli (51) showed that mast cells can importantly contribute to the recruitment of eosinophils to the airways in a model of asthma that does not employ alum as an adjuvant during sensitization with antigen. While some antigen-dependent eosinophil recruitment was detected in mast cell–deficient mice even in this "asthma model," levels of tissue eosinophils were ~70% lower than those in identically sensitized and challenged wild-type or mast cell–reconstituted Kit^W/Kit^{W-v} mice (51). Based on these findings, we hypothesize that mast cells can indeed be critical in regulating eosinophil infiltration during allergic inflammation in mice, but that this role may be undetectable or dispensable in models that induce strong immune responses, such as when alum or other adjuvants are used for sensitization or when challenge is performed with large doses of antigen.

The specific mechanisms by which mast cells might regulate eosinophil recruitment and/or activation in mouse models remain to be determined, but it seems reasonable to suggest that chemokines, and particularly eotaxin, may be involved. Mast cells can contribute to eotaxin-induced eosinophil accumulation in vivo (146); mast cell–deficient Kit^W/Kit^{W-v} mice exhibit a delayed peak of eosinophil influx, as well as reduced numbers of peritoneal eosinophils, after i.p. injection of eotaxin (147); and mast cell fibroblast co-culture promotes enhanced production of eotaxin by the mast cells, a process that can be enhanced further by TNF-α (148). Moreover, human lung mast cells represent potential sources of IL-5 and GM-CSF (75,79,80,85,87), and these cytokines also can enhance eosinophil recruitment and/or activation.

While airway eosinophil infiltration and AHR to cholinergic stimulation often are observed together in mouse "models" of asthma, there is as yet no proof that the former is required for the latter. Nevertheless, our studies of mice sensitized to OVA in the absence of alum showed that normal (+ / +) mice exhibited significantly enhanced OVA-induced AHR to aerosol methacholine challenge compared to mast cell–deficient Kit^W/Kit^{W-v} mice, as assessed by whole body plethysmography in nonanesthetized mice, and that values for AHR in OVA-sensitized, OVA-challenged mast cell knock-in Kit^W/Kit^{W-v} mice were statistically indistinguishable from those in the + / + mice (51). Notably, OVA-sensitized, saline-challenged + / + mice exhibited more AHR to methacholine than did mast cell–deficient Kit^W/Kit^{W-v} mice, whereas the mast cell-knock-in Kit^W/Kit^{W-v} mice exhibited an intermediate level of AHR response that differed significantly from that of either the + / + or Kit^W/Kit^{W-v} groups (51). This result has at least two possible explanations: (1) the observed differences are partly dependent on mast cells and partly on non–mast cell–related consequences of the c-*kit* mutations in Kit^W/Kit^{W-v} mice; (2) the differences are entirely mast cell–dependent, but the magnitude of the effect reflects differences in the numbers, anatomical distribution, phenotype, or function of mast cells in + / + vs. mast cell knock-in Kit^W/Kit^{W-v} mice (51).

In a study in which airway responses to *intravenous* acetylcholine chloride was measured in anesthetized, artificially ventilated mice, Kobayashi et al. (149) detected a significant mast cell–dependent component of OVA-induced AHR in mice that were sensitized and challenged with OVA using a relatively "weak" protocol, but which included immunization with OVA in alum. Using a stronger protocol of OVA challenge, no significant difference in AHR was observed between + / + and Kit^W/Kit^{W-v} mice (149).

Taken together, the work of Williams and Galli (51) and Kobayashi et al. (149) are in accord in showing that relatively "weak" protocols of antigen sensitization and challenge can reveal important contributions of mast cells to antigen-induced AHR and cholinergic stimulation that may be masked under other conditions.

VIII.   Mast Cells and Tissue Remodeling

Persistent chronic allergic inflammation can result in remodeling of the affected tissues, and these structural changes can be associated with functional alterations. For instance, some patients with asthma develop irreversible changes in lung function, despite apparently appropriate and aggressive anti-inflammatory therapy (150), and many subjects with asthma exhibit a decline in lung function over time (151,152). Moreover, airway tissues from patients with asthma can exhibit structural abnormalities such as smooth muscle hypertrophy, mucus gland hyperplasia, blood vessel proliferation, and collagen deposition beneath the epithelial basement membrane (153–156).

We feel that it is too soon to conclude whether, let alone to what extent, mast cells contribute to the tissue remodeling associated with chronic allergic inflammation. However, several lines of evidence strongly suggest that mast cells may indeed have important roles in this process. As summarized in Figure 1, mast cell–derived proteases, cytokines, growth factors, and other mediators have been shown to have a number of in vitro or in vivo effects that are consistent with the hypothesis that mast cells can promote tissue remodeling. For example, it was recently shown that human skin, lung, and synovial mast cells are strongly positive for matrix metalloproteinase 9 (MMP9) by immunhistochemistry (157). Because they can promote the degradation of extracellular matrix, matrix metalloproteinases are believed to play a role in the pathogenesis of certain disorders associated with tissue remodeling (158). Various populations of mast cells also have been identified as sources of several growth-promoting peptide mediators, including TNF-α, VPF/VEGF, FGF-2 (also known as basic fibroblast growth factor or bFGF), PDGF, TGF-β, and NGF (57–61,74–76,90,128,159); in aggregate, these products might contribute to the neovascularization, connective tissue remodeling and/or reepithelialization associated with chronic tissue remodeling, in the context of asthma and in other settings.

However, there are very few studies that assess the actual importance of mast cells as sources of such growth factors, or as effectors of tissue remodeling, in vivo. In "mast cell knock-in mice," the increased expression of Type I collagen mRNA observed at sites of IgE-dependent PCA reactions in vivo was entirely mast cell–dependent (128); parallel in vitro studies suggested that mast cell–dependent enhancement of skin fibroblast collagen mRNA expression was mediated largely by TGF-β1 and TNF-α (128,129). TFG-β1 can also markedly upregulate the ability of mouse bone marrow–derived mast cells to produce and store the mucosal mast cell beta chymase, mouse mast cell protease-1 (160). On the other hand, expression of gelatinase B (MMP9) by dog mast cells can be induced by SCF but is downregulated by TGF-β (161). Finally, it appears that human mast cells can themselves represent a potential source of SCF (89,162,163), which can be cleaved by human mast cell–derived chymase to release soluble biologically active SCF from the cell membrane associated form of the molecule (162,164). Taken together with evidence that SCF itself can induce mast cell activation and release of VPF/VEGF and other mediators (27,29,60), these findings suggest that mast cells can participate in intricate paracrine and autocrine networks that may both contribute to tissue remodeling and influence mast cell numbers and function.

Because many studies have indicated that the airway epithelium in subjects with asthma can exhibit injury and repair, including enhanced proliferation of epithelial cells (165–167), Williams and Galli (51) used the thymidine analogue bromodeoxyuridine (BrdU) to quantify proliferating cells in the tracheal and bronchiolar epithelium of mice that were challenged with OVA after sensitization by injecting OVA i.p. either with or without alum. Although statistically significant, albeit modest, antigen-induced increases in proliferating cells were observed in mast cell–deficient Kit^W/Kit^{W-v} mice, significantly higher numbers of BrdU + cells were observed in the airway epithelial layers of antigen-challenged + / + mice; notably, this was true whether the mice had been sensitized with OVA with or without alum (51). While the mechanisms by which mast cells contribute to epithelial proliferation in this setting remain to be determined (both direct and indirect effects may be involved), the findings support the hypothesis that mast cells can importantly influence certain aspects of "airway remodeling," at least in mouse "models" of asthma.

IX. Conclusions

Studies in mast cell–deficient and "mast cell-knock in" mice support the notion that mast cells not only represent the key effector cells of acute IgE-dependent reactions in the airway and other sites, but also can contribute significantly to certain features of IgE-associated late phase reactions and to chronic allergic inflammation in "asthma models." However, even in the mouse, the mechanisms that regulate allergic inflammation are complex and can exhibit significant redundancy, and this may be especially true of the late phase and chronic aspects of allergic inflammatory responses in the airways. Thus, given the experimental conditions that are often used to produce robust "asthma models" in mice (often involving antigen sensitization with adjuvants, and both sensitization and challenge with high doses of antigen), certain important features of allergic inflammation, such as eosinophil infiltration or airway hyperreactivity to cholinergic stimulation, clearly can be elicited in mice by mechanisms that are entirely mast cell–independent (4,51,112–114,117).

The effector mechanisms of allergic inflammation in humans are unlikely to be any less complex or redundant than those in mouse. And, in humans, one does not generally have the opportunity to analyze the expression of these reactions in subjects with defined mutations that affect various potential components of immunological or inflammatory responses. Nevertheless, we believe that the available data from humans, when taken together with the findings from murine systems, support two unifying hypotheses (both of which can much more readily be tested in mice than in humans).

1. As effector cells, mast cells function to amplify many of the acute, late phase, and chronic features of asthma, and this role can be enhanced when levels of IgE are high. It is now clear that the FcεRI β chain functions as a molecular "amplifier" of signaling through this receptor, an effect that can markedly upregulate the magnitude of the mediator release induced in response to FcεRI aggregation (168,169). Moreover, certain mutations that result in amino acid substitutions in the human β chain have been linked to atopic disease (see reviews in Refs. 95,168,169). In addition, IgE-dependent upregulation of FcεRI expression both permits the cell to exhibit mediator release at lower concentrations of specific antigen or anti-IgE (92,83,102,103,170) and primes such cells to produce strikingly higher levels of certain mediators, including IL-4 and other cytokines (60,92,83,103), under optimal conditions of antigen challenge. This mechanism can promote enhanced IgE-dependent mast cell (and basophil) effector function, not only in the setting of acute reactions to allergen exposure of the airways, but also in late phase reactions and chronic allergic inflammation. Indeed, the mast cell seems to be superbly equipped functionally, as well as strategically positioned anatomically, to represent a critical initiator and amplifier of IgE-dependent immune responses, in asthma and other settings.

2. Mast cells represent potential "immunoregulatory" cells in asthma. In addition to their function as effector cells in allergic inflammation, there are at least three mechanisms by which mast cells might contribute to the development or persistence of Th2 responses; antigen processing/presentation (171–173), antigen transport through epithelial barriers (174,175), and the production of immunoregulatory cytokines (as discussed above). Although the extent to which each of these three potential functions is important in the development of Th2 responses in vivo remains to be determined (even in mice and rats), the notion that mast cells may have immunoregulatory function in IgE-associated responses is intriguing. Both mouse and human mast cells can produce IL-4 and IL-13, and perhaps other cytokines (e.g., MIP-1α), which can enhance IgE production. This fact, taken together with the findings demonstrating IgE-dependent upregulation of FcεRI surface expression, suggest a potential positive feedback mechanism (↑ IgE→ ↑ FcεRI → ↑ antigen-, IgE-, and FcεRI-dependent release of IL-4 (102), IL-13 (84), and/or other cytokines, e.g., MIP-1α (83) → ↑ IgE) by which mast cells (and possibly basophils) may enhance the further evolution, and persistence, of Th2-biased, IgE-associated immune responses. Mast cells and basophils also may enhance IgE production via expression of the CD40 ligand (84,176). Finally, in vitro studies in mice indicate that the binding of IgE to FcεRI, even in the absence of specific antigen, can have effects that promote mast cell survival under conditions when concentrations of mast cell survival/growth factors otherwise would be limiting (177,178). And, in some circumstances, the binding of certain monoclonal IgE antibodies to mouse mast cells appears to be able to induce the cells to secrete cytokines, at least in vitro (178)!

The clinical significance of many of these new findings largely remains to be established. However, this work clearly supports a complex, but more unified, view of the pathogenesis of allergic diseases, which proposes that both T cells and mast cells (and other FcεRI+ cells, such as basophils) can have both effector cell and

mmunoregulatory roles in these disorders. This hypothesis has a number of interest-
ng implications with respect to existing, and proposed, therapeutic approaches for
sthma and other allergic disease.

References

1. Schwartz LB, Huff TF. Biology of mast cells. In: Middleton EJ, Reed CE, Ellis EF, Yunginger JW, Adkinson NF Jr, Busse WW, eds. Allergy: Principles and Practice. Vol. 1. St. Louis, MO: Mosby-Year Book, 1998:261.
2. Metcalfe DD, Baram D, Mekori YA. Mast cells. Physiol Rev 1997; 77:1033–1079.
3. Wedemeyer J, Galli SJ. Mast cells and basophils. In: Rich RR, Fleisher TA, Shearer WT, Kotzin BL, Schroeder AW Jr, eds. Clinical Immunology: Principles and Practice. 2nd ed. London: Mosby, 2001; 23:1–23.13.
4. Galli SJ. Complexity and redundancy in the pathogenesis of asthma: reassessing the roles of mast cells and T cells. J Exp Med 1997; 186:343–347.
5. Galli SJ, Lantz CS. Allergy. In: Paul WE, ed. Fundamental Immunology. 4th ed. Philadelphia: Lippincott-Raven Press, 1999:1137–1184.
6. Busse WW, Lemanske RF Jr. Asthma. N Engl J Med 2001; 344:350–362.
7. Humbles AA, Lu B, Nilsson CA, Lilly C, Israel E, Fujiwara Y, Gerard NP, Gerard C. A role for the C3a anaphylatoxin receptor in the effector phase of asthma. Nature 2000; 406:998–1001.
8. Karp CL, Grupe A, Schadt E, Ewart SL, Keane-Moore M, Cuomo PJ, Kohl J, Wahl L, Kuperman D, Germer S, Aud D, Peltz G, Wills-Karp M. Identification of complement factor 5 as a susceptibility locus for experimental allergic asthma. Nat Immunol 2000; 1:221–226.
9. Kraneveld AD, Nijkamp FP. Tachykinins and neuro-immune interactions in asthma. Int Immunopharmacol 2001; 1:1629–1650.
10. Carr MJ, Hunter DD, Undem BJ. Neurotrophins and asthma. Curr Opin Pulm Med 2001; 7:1–7.
11. Braun A, Quarcoo D, Schulte-Herbrüggen O, Lommatzsch, Hoyle G, Renz H. Nerve growth factor induces airway hyperresponsiveness in mice. Int Arch Allergy Immunol 2001; 124:205–207.
12. Undem BJ, Lichtenstein LM, Hubbard WC, Meeker S, Ellis JL. Recombinant stem cell factor-induced mast cell activation and smooth muscle contraction in human bronchi. Am J Respir Cell Mol Biol 1994; 11:646–650.
13. Campbell E, Hogaboam C, Lincoln P, Lukacs NW. Stem cell factor-induced airway hyperreactivity in allergic and normal mice. Am J Pathol 1999; 154:1259–1265.
14. Finotto S, Buerke M, Lingnau K, Schmitt E, Galle PR, Neurath MF. Local administration of antisense phosphorothioate oligonucleotides to the c-kit ligand, stem cell factor, suppresses airway inflammation and IL-4 production in a murine model of asthma. J Allergy Clin Immunol 2001; 107:279–286.
15. van Houwelingen A, van der Avoort LA, Heuven-Nolsen D, Kraneveld AD, Nijkamp FP. Repeated challenge with dinitrobenzene suphonic acid in dinitrofluorobenzene-sensitized mice results in vascular hyperpermeability in the trachea: a role for tachykinins. Br J Pharmacol 1999; 127:1583–1588.
16. Folkerts G, Busse WW, Nijkamp FP, Sorkness R, Gern JE. Virus-induced airway hyperresponsiveness and asthma. Am J Respir Crit Care Med 1998; 157:1708–1720.

17. Martin RJ, Kraft M, Chu, HW, Berns EA, Cassell GH. A link between chronic asthma and chronic infection. J Allergy Clin Immunol; 2001: 595–601.
18. Galli SJ, Maurer, Lantz CS. Mast cells as sentinels of innate immunity. Curr Opin Immunol 1999; 11:53–59.
19. Kitamura Y. Heterogeneity of mast cells and phenotypic changes between subpopulations. Annu Rev Immunol 1989; 127:191–198.
20. Galli SJ. Biology of disease. New insights into "the riddle of the mast cells": Microenvironmental regulation of mast cell development and phenotype heterogeneity. Lab Invest 1990; 62:5–33.
21. Galli SJ, Zsebo KM, Geissler EN. The kit ligand, stem cell factor. Adv Immunol 1994; 55:1–96.
22. Rodewald H-R, Dessing M, Dvorak AM, Galli SJ. Identification of a committed precursor for the mast cell lineage. Science 1996; 271:818–822.
23. Galli SJ. Mast cells and basophils. Curr Opin Hematol 2000; 7:32–39.
24. Broudy VC. Stem cell factor and hematopoiesis. Blood 1997; 90:1345–1364.
25. Costa JJ, Demetri GD, Harrist TJ, Dvorak AM, Hayes DF, Merica EA, Menchaca DM, Gringeri AJ, Schwartz LB, Galli SJ. Recombinant human stem cell factor (kit ligand) promotes human mast cell and melanocyte hyperplasia and functional activation in vivo. J Exp Med 1996; 183:2681–2686.
26. Bischoff SC, Dahinden CA, c-kit ligand: a unique potentiator of mediator release by human lung mast cells. J Exp Med 1992; 175:237–244.
27. Wershil BK, Tsai M, Geissler EN, Zsebo KM, Galli SJ. The rat c-*kit* ligand, stem cell factor, induces c-*kit* receptor-dependent mouse mast cell activation in vivo. Evidence that signaling through the c-*kit* receptor can induce expression of cellular function. J Exp Med 1992; 175:245–255.
28. Gagari E, Tsai M, Lantz CS, Fox LG, Galli SJ. Differential release of mast cell interleukin-6 via c-*kit*. Blood 1997; 89:2654–2663.
29. Huang C, Sali A, Stevens RL. Regulation and function of mast cell proteases in inflammation. J Clin Immunol 1998; 18:169–183.
30. Lantz CS, Boesiger J, Song C-H, Mach N, Kobayashi T, Mulligan RC, Nawa Y, Dranoff G, Galli SJ. Role for interleukin-3 in mast cell and basophil development and in immunity to parasites. Nature 1998; 392:90–93.
31. Church MK, Okayama Y, Bradding P. The role of the mast cell in acute and chronic allergic inflammation. Ann NY Acad Sci 1994; 725:13–21.
32. Jeffery PK. Comparative morphology of the airways in asthma and chronic obstructive pulmonary disease. Am J Respir Crit Care Med 1994; 150:S6–S13.
33. Miyachi Y, Kurosawa M. Mast cells in clinical dermatology. Australas J Dermatol 1998; 39:14–18.
34. Koshino T, Teshima S, Fukushima N, Takaishi T, Hirai K, Miyamoto Y, Arai Y, Sano Y, Ito K, Morita Y. Identification of basophils by immunohistochemistry in the airways of post-mortem cases of fatal asthma. Clin Exp Allergy 1993; 23:919–25.
35. Karjalainen EM, Laitinen A, Sue-Chu M, Altraja A, Bjermer L, Laitinen LA. Evidence of airway inflammation and remodeling in ski athletes with and without bronchial hyperresponsiveness to methacholine. Am J Respir Crit Care Med 2000; 161: 2086–2091.
36. Djukanovic R, Wilson JW, Britten KM, Wilson SJ, Walls AF, Roche WR, Howarth PH, Holgate ST. Quantitation of mast cells and eosinophils in the bronchial mucosa of symptomatic atopic asthmatics and healthy control subjects using immunohistochemistry. Am Rev Respir Dis 1990; 142:863–871.

37. Bradley BL, Azzawi M, Jacobson M, Assoufi B, Collins JV, Irani AMA, Schwartz LB, Durham SR, Jeffery PK, Kay AB. Eosinophils, T-lymphocytes, mast cells, neutrophils, and macrophages in bronchial biopsy specimens from atopic subjects with asthma: comparison with biopsy specimens from atopic subjects without asthma and normal control subjects and relationship to bronchial hyperresponsiveness. J Allergy Clin Immunol 1991; 88:661–673.

38. Kay AB. Pathology of mild, severe, and fatal asthma. Am J Respir Crit Care Med 1996; 154(2 Pt 2):S66–69.

39. Kepley CL, McFeeley PJ, Oliver JM, Lipscomb MF. Immunohistochemical detection of human basophils in postmortem cases of fatal asthma. Am J Respir Crit Care Med 2001; 164:1053–1058.

40. Synek M, Beasley R, Frew AJ, Goulding D, Holloway L, Lampe FC, Roche WR, Holgate ST. Cellular infiltration of the airways in asthma of varying severity. Am J Respir Crit Care Med 1996; 154:224–230.

41. Ammit AJ, Bekir SS, Johnson PR, Hughes JM, Armour CL, Black JL. Mast cell numbers are increased in the smooth muscle of human sensitized isolated bronchi. Am J Respir Crit Care Med 1997; 155:1123–1129.

42. Nakano T, Sonoda T, Hayashi C, Yamatodani A, Kanayama Y, Yamamura T, Asai H, Yonezawa T, Kitamura Y, Galli SJ. Fate of bone marrow-derived cultured mast cells after intracutaneous, intraperitoneal and intravenous transfer into genetically mast cell-deficient W/Wᵛ mice. Evidence that cultured mast cells can give rise to both connective tissue type and mucosal mast cells. J Exp Med 1985; 162:1025–1043.

43. Galli SJ, Kitamura Y. Animal model of human disease. Genetically mast cell-deficient W/Wᵛ and Sl/Slᵈ mice: their value for the analysis of the roles of mast cells in biological responses in vivo. Am J Pathol 1987; 127:191–198.

44. Nakano T, Kanakura Y, Nakahata T, Matsuda H, Kitamura Y. Genetically mast cell-deficient W/Wᵛ mice as a tool of differentiation and function of mast cells. Fed Proc 1987; 46:1920–1923.

45. Galli SJ. New concepts about the mast cell. N Engl J Med 1993; 328:257–265.

46. Tsai M, Wedemeyer J, Ganiatsas S, Tam S-Y, Zon LI, Galli SJ. In vivo immunological function of mast cells derived from embryonic stem cells: an approach for the rapid analysis of even embryonic lethal mutations in adult mice in vivo. Proc Natl Acad Sci USA 2000; 97:9186–9190.

47. Tsai M, Tam S-Y, Wedemeyer J, Galli SJ. Mast cells derived from embryonic stem cells: a model system for studying effects of genetic manipulations on mast cell development, phenotype, and function in vitro and in vivo. Int J Hematol 2002; 75:345–349.

48. Sylvestre DL, Ravetch JV. A dominant role for mast cell Fc receptors in the arthus reaction. Immunity 1996; 5:387–390.

49. Garrington TP, Ishizuka T, Papst PJ, Chayama K, Webb S, Yujiri T, Sun W, Sather S, Russell DM, Gibson SB, Keller G, Gelfand EW, Johnson GL. MEKK2 gene disruption causes loss of cytokine production in response to IgE and c-Kit ligand stimulation of ES cell-derived mast cells. EMBO J 2000; 19:5387–5395.

50. Martin TR, Takeishi T, Katz HR, Austen KF, Drazen JM, Galli SJ. Mast cell activation enhances airway responsiveness to methacholine in the mouse. J Clin Invest 1993; 91:1176–1182.

51. Williams CM, Galli SJ. Mast cells can amplify airway reactivity and features of chronic inflammation in an asthma model in mice. J Exp Med 2000; 192:455–462.

52. Hara M, Ono K, Hwang M-W, Iwasaki A, Okada M, Nakatani K, Sasayama S, Matsumori A. Evidence for a role of mast cells in the evolution to congestive heart failure. J Exp Med 2002; 195:375–381.

53. Secor VH, Secor WE, Gutekunst CA, Brown MA. Mast cells are essential for early onset and severe disease in a murine model of multiple sclerosis. J Exp Med 2000 191:813–822.

54. Williams CM, Galli SJ. The diverse potential effector and immunoregulatory roles of mast cells in allergic disease. J Allergy Clin Immunol. 2000; 105:847–859.

55. Nakajima T, Matsumoto K, Suto H, Tanaka K, Ebisawa M, Tomita H, Yuki K, Katsunuma T, Akasawa A, Hashida R, Sugita Y, Ogawa H, Ra C, Saito H. Gene expression screening of human mast cells and eosinophils using high-density oligonucleotide probe arrays: abundant expression of major basic protein in mast cells. Blood 2001; 98 1127–1134.

56. Sayama K, Diehn M, Matsuda K, Lunderius, Tsai M, Tam S-Y, Botstein D, Brown PO, Galli SJ. Transcriptional response of human mast cells stimulated via the FcεRI and identification of mast cells as a source of IL-11. BMC Immunol 2002; 3:5.

57. Young JD-E, Liu C-C, Butler G, Cohn ZA, Galli SJ. Identification, purification, and characterization of a mast cell-associated cytolytic factor related to tumor necrosis factor. Proc Natl Acad Sci USA 1987; 84:9175–9179.

58. Gordon JR, Galli SJ. Mast cells as a source of both preformed and immunologically inducible TNF-alpha/cachectin. Nature 1990; 346:274–276.

59. Gordon JR, Galli SJ. Release of both preformed and newly synthesized tumor necrosis factor-α (TNF-α)/cachectin by mouse mast cells stimulated by the FcεRI. A mechanism for the sustained action of mast cell-derived TNF-α during IgE-dependent biological responses. J Exp Med 1991; 174:103–107.

60. Boesiger J, Tsai M, Maurer M, Yamaguchi M, Brown LF, Claffey KP, Dvorak HF Galli SJ. Mast cells can secrete VPF/VEGF and exhibit enhanced release after IgE dependent upregulation of FcεRI expression. J Exp Med 1998; 188:1135–1145.

61. Grutzkau A, Kruger-Krasagakes S, Baumeister H, Schwartz C, Kogel H, Welker P Lippert U, Henz BM, Moller A. Synthesis, storage and release of vascular endothelia growth factor/vascular permeability factor (VEGF/VPF) by human mast cells: implications for the biological significance of VEGF206. Mol Biol Cell 1998; 9:875–884.

62. Yamatodani A, Maeyama K, Watanabe T, Wada H, Kitamura Y. Tissue distribution of histamine in a mutant mouse deficient in mast cells: clear evidence for the presence of non-mast-cell histamine. Biochem Pharmacol 1982; 31:305–309.

63. Page C. The role of proteoglycans in the regulation of airways inflammation and airways remodeling. J Allergy Clin Immunol 2000; 105:S518–S521.

64. Humphries DE, Wong GW, Friend DS, Gurish MF, Qiu WT, Huang C, Sharpe AH, Stevens RL. Heparin is essential for the storage of specific granule proteases in mast cells. Nature 1999; 400:769–772.

65. Forsberg E, Pejler G, Ringvall M, Lunderius C, Tomasini-Johansson B, Eriksson I Ledin J, Hellman L, Kjellen L. Abnormal mast cells in mice deficient in a heparin-synthesizing enzyme. Nature 1999; 400:773–776.

66. Schwartz LB. Tryptase: a clinical indicator of mast cell-dependent events. Allergy Proc 1994; 15:119–123.

67. Li L, Li Y, Reddel SW, Cherrian M, Friend DS, Stevens RL, Krilis SA. Identification of basophilic cells that express mast cell granule proteases in the peripheral blood of asthma allergy and drug-reactive patients. J Immunol 1998; 161:5079–5086.

68. Caughey GH. Of mites and men: trypsin-like proteases in the lungs. Am J Respir Cell Mol Biol 1997; 16:621–628.

69. Pallaoro M, Fejzo MS, Shayesteh L, Blount JL, Caughey GH. Characterization of genes encoding known and novel human mast cell tryptases on chromosome 16p13.3 J Biol Chem 1999; 274:3355–3362.

70. Wastling JM, Knight P, Ure J, Wright S, Thornton EM, Scudamore CL, Mason J, Smith A, Miller HR. Histochemical and ultrastructural modification of mucosal mast cell granules in parasitized mice lacking the β-chymase, mouse mast cell protease-1. Am J Pathol 1998; 153:491–504.

71. Silverman ES, Drazen JM. Genetic variations in the 5-lipoxygenase core promoter. Description and functional implications. Am J Respir Crit Care Med 2000; 161: S77–80.

72. Salvi SS, Krishna MT, Sampson AP, Holgate ST. The anti-inflammatory effects of leukotriene-modifying drugs and their use in asthma. Chest 2001; 119:1533–1546.

73. Mencia-Huerta JM, Lewis RA, Razin E, Austen KF. Antigen-initiated release of platelet-activating factor (PAF-acether) from mouse bone marrow-derived mast cells sensitized with monoclonal IgE. J Immunol 1983; 131:2958–2964.

74. Walsh LJ, Trinchieri G, Waldorf HA, Whitaker D, Murphy GF. Human dermal mast cells contain and release tumor necrosis factor α which induces endothelial leukocyte adhesion molecule 1. Proc Natl Acad Sci USA 1991; 88:4220–4224.

75. Bradding P, Roberts JA, Britten KM, Montefort S, Djukanovic R, Mueller R, Heusser CH, Howarth PH, Holgate ST. Interleukin-4, -5, -6 and tumour necrosis factor-α in normal and asthmatic airways: evidence for the human mast cell as a source of these cytokines. Am J Respir Cell Mol Biol 1994; 10:471–480.

76. Okayama Y, Ono Y, Nakazawa T, Church MK, Mori M. Human skin mast cells produce TNF-α by substance P. Int Arch Allergy Immunol 1998; 117(suppl):48–51.

77. Gordon JR, Burd PR, Galli SJ. Mast cells as a source of multifunctional cytokines. Immunol Today 1990; 11:458–464.

78. Bradding P, Feather IH, Howarth PH, Mueller R, Roberts JA, Britten K, Bews JP, Hunt TC, Okayama Y, Heusser CH. Interleukin 4 is localized to and released by human mast cells. J Exp Med 1992; 176:1381–1386.

79. Jaffe JS, Glaum MC, Raible DG, Post TJ, Dimitry E, Govindarao D, Wang Y, Schulman ES. Human lung mast cell IL-5 gene and protein expression: temporal analysis of upregulation following IgE-mediated activation. Am J Respir Cell Mol Biol 1995; 13: 665–675.

80. Okayama Y, Petit-Frère C, Kassel O, Semper A, Quint D, Tunon-de-Lara MJ, Bradding P, Holgate ST, Church MK. IgE-dependent expression of mRNA for IL-4 and IL-5 in human lung mast cells. J Immunol 1995; 155:1796–1808.

81. Jaffe JS, Raible DG, Post TJ, Wang Y, Glaum MC, Butterfield JH, Schulman ES. Human lung mast cell activation leads to IL-13 mRNA expression and protein release. Am J Respir Cell Mol Biol 1996; 15:473–481.

82. Bradding P. Human mast cell cytokines. Clin Exp Allergy 1996; 26:13–19.

83. Yano K, Yamaguchi M, de Mora F, Lantz CS, Butterfield JH, Costa JJ, Galli SJ. Production of macrophage inflammatory protein-1α by human mast cells: increased anti-IgE-dependent secretion after IgE-dependent enhancement of mast cell IgE binding ability. Lab Invest 1997; 77:185–193.

84. Pawankar R, Okuda M, Yssel H, Okumura K, Ra C. Nasal mast cells in perenial allergic rhinitics exhibit increased expression of the FcεRI, CD40L, IL-4, and IL-13, and can induce IgE synthesis in B cells. J Clin Invest 1997; 99:1492–1499.

85. Bressler RB, Lesko J, Jones ML, Wasserman M, Dickason RR, Huston MM, Cook SW, Huston DP. Production of IL-5 and granulocyte-macrophage colony-stimulating factor by naive human mast cells activated by high-affinity IgE receptor ligation. J Allergy Clin Immunol 1997; 99:508–554.

86. Rumsaeng V, Cruikshank WW, Foster B, Prussin C, Kirshenbaum AS, Davis TA, Kornfeld H, Center DM, Metcalfe DD. Human mast cells produce the CD4+ T lymphocyte chemoattractant factor, IL-16. J Immunol 1997; 159:2904–2410.

87. Okayama Y, Kobayashi H, Ashman LK, Dobashi K, Nakazawa T, Holgate ST, Church MK, Mori M. Human lung mast cells are enriched in the capacity to produce granulocyte-macrophage colony stimulating factor in response to IgE-dependent stimulation. Eur J Immunol 1998; 28:708–715.

88. Kobayashi H, Okayama Y, Ishizuka T, Pawankar R, Ra C, Mori M. Production of IL-13 by human lung mast cells in response to Fcε receptor cross-linkage. Clin Exp Allergy 1998; 28:1219–1227.

89. Zhang S, Anderson DF, Bradding P, Coward WR, Baddeley SM, MacLeod JD, McGill JI, Church MK, Holgate ST, Roche WR. Human mast cells express stem cell factor. J Pathol 1998; 186:59–66.

90. Qu Z, Kayton RJ, Ahmadi P, Liebler JM, Powers MR, Planck SR, Rosenbaum JT. Ultrastructural immunolocalization of basic fibroblast growth factor in mast cell secretory granules. Morphological evidence for bFGF release through degranulation. J Histochem Cytochem 1998; 46:1119–1128.

91. Ishizuka T, Okayama Y, Kobayashi H, Mori M. Interleukin-10 is localized to and released by human lung mast cells. Clin Exp Allergy 1999; 10:1424–1432.

92. Yamaguchi M, Sayama K, Yano K, Lantz CS, Noben-Trauth N, Ra C, Costa JJ, Galli SJ. IgE enchances Fcε receptor I expression and IgE-dependent release of histamine and lipid mediators from human umbilical cord blood-derived mast cells: synergistic effect of IL-4 and IgE on human mast cell Fcε receptor I expression and mediator release. J Immunol 1999; 162:5455–5465.

93. Ishizuka T, Okayama Y, Kobayashi H, Mori M. Interleukin-3 production by mast cells from human lung. Inflammation 1999; 23:25–35.

94. Metzger H. The receptor with high affinity for IgE. Immunol Rev 1992; 125:37–48.

95. Turner H, Kinet J-P. Signalling through the high-affinity IgE receptor FcεRI. Nature 1999; 402(suppl):B24–B30.

96. Rottem M, Barbieri S, Kinet J-P, Metcalfe DD. Kinetics of the appearance of FcεRI-bearing cells in interleukin-3-dependent mouse bone marrow cultures: correlation with histamine content and mast cell maturation. Blood 1992; 79:972–980.

97. Lantz CS, Huff TF. Murine KIT+ lineage bone marrow progenitors express FcγRI but do not express FcεRI until mast cell granule formation. J Immunol 1995; 154:355–362.

98. Kinzer CA, Keegan AD, Paul WE. Identification of FcεRIneg mast cells in mouse bone marrow cultures. Use of a monoclonal anti-p161 antibody. J Exp Med 1995; 182:575–579.

99. Sterk AR, Ishizaka T. Binding properties of IgE receptors on normal mouse mast cells. J Immunol 1982; 128:838–843.

100. Miyajima I, Dombrowicz D, Martin TR, Ravetch JV, Kinet J-P, Galli SJ. Systemic anaphylaxis in the mouse can be mediated largely through IgG1 and FcγRIII. Assessment of the cardiopulmonary changes, mast cell degranulation, and death associated with active or IgE- or IgG$_1$-dependent passive anaphylaxis. J Clin Invest 1997; 99:901–914.

101. Lantz CS, Yamaguchi M, Oettgen HC, Katona IM, Miyajima I, Kinet J-P, Galli SJ. IgE regulates mouse basophil FcεRI expression in vivo. J Immunol 1997; 158:2517–2521.

102. Yamaguchi M, Lantz CS, Oettgen HC, Katona IM, Fleming T, Miyajima I, Kinet JP, Galli SJ. IgE enhances mouse mast cell FcεRI expression in vitro and in vivo. Evidence

for a novel amplification mechanism In IgE-dependent reactions. J Exp Med 1997; 158:11438–11445.

103. MacGlashan DW Jr, Bochner BS, Adelman DC, Jardieu PM, Togias A, McKenzie-White J, Sterbinsky SA, Hamilton RG, Lichtenstein LM. Down-regulation of FcεRI expression on human basophils during in vivo treatment of atopic patients with anti-IgE antibody. J Immunol 1997; 158:1438–1445.

104. Shaikh N, Rivera J, Hewlett BR, Steak RH, Zhu F-G, Marshall JS. Mast cell FcεRI expression in the rat intestinal mucosa and tongue is enhanced during *Nippostrongylus brasiliensis* infection and can be up-regulated by in vivo administration of IgE. J Immunol 1997; 158:3805–3812.

105. MacGlashan Jr. D, Lichtenstein LM, MacKenzie-White J, Chichester K, Henry AJ, Sutton BJ, Gould HJ. Upregulation of FcεRI on human basophils by IgE antibody is mediated by the interaction of IgE with FcεRI. J Allergy Clin Immunol 1999; 104: 1841–1849.

106. Wershil BK, Mekori YA, Murakami T, Galli SJ. ^{125}I-Fibrin deposition in IgE-dependent immediate hypersensitivity reactions in mouse skin. Demonstration of the role of mast cells using genetically mast cell-deficient mice locally reconstituted with cultured mast cells. J Immunol 1987; 139:2605–2614.

107. Wershil BK, Wang Z-S, Gordon JR, Galli SJ. Recruitment of neutrophils during IgE-dependent cutaneous late phase responses in the mouse is mast cell dependent: partial inhibition of the reaction with antiserum against tumor necrosis factor-α. J Clin Invest 1991; 87:446–453.

108. Mekori YA, Galli SJ. [125I]fibrin deposition occurs at both early and late intervals of IgE-dependent or contact sensitivity reactions elicited in mouse skin. Mast cell-dependent augmentation of fibrin deposition at early intervals in combined IgE-dependent and contact sensitivity reactions. J Immunol 1990; 145:3719–3727.

109. Martin TR, Galli SJ, Katona IM, Drazen JM. Role of mast cells in anaphylaxis. Evidence for the importance of mast cells in the pulmonary alterations and death induced by anti-IgE in mice. J Clin Invest 1989; 83:1375–1383.

110. Takeishi T, Martin TR, Katona IM, Finkelman FD, Galli SJ. Differences in the expression of the cardiopulmonary alterations associated with anti-immunoglobulin E-induced or active anaphylaxis in mast cell-deficient and normal mice. Mast cells are not required for the cardiopulmonary changes associated with certain fatal anaphylactic responses. J Clin Invest 1991; 88:598–608.

111. Choi IH, Shin YM, Park JS, Lee MS, Han EH, Chai OH, Im SY, Ha TY, Lee HK. Immunoglobulin E-dependent active fatal anaphylaxis in mast cell-deficient mice. J Exp Med 1998; 188: 1587–1592.

112. Nogami M, Suko M, Okudaira H, Miyamonto T, Shiga J, Ito M, Kasuya S. Experimental pulmonary eosinophilia in mice by *Ascaris suum* extract. Am Rev Respir Dis 1990; 414:1289–1295.

113. Brusselle GG, Kips JC, Tavernier JH, van der Heyden JG, Cuvelier CA, Pauwels RA, Bluethmann H. Attenuation of allergic airway inflammation in IL-4 deficient mice. Clin Exp Allergy 1994; 24:73–80.

114. Nagai H, Yamaguchi S, Tanaka H. The role of interleukin-5 (IL-5) in allergic airway hyperresponsiveness in mice. Ann NY Acad Sci 1996; 796:91–96.

115. Korsgren M, Erjefalt JS, Korsgren O, Sundler F, Persson CG. Allergic eosinophilrich inflammation develops in lungs and airways of B cell-deficient mice. J Exp Med 1997; 185:885–892.

116. Mehlhop PD, van de Rijn M, Goldberg AB, Brewer JP, Kurup VP. Martin TR, Oettgen HC. Allergen-induced bronchial hyperreactivity and eosinophilic inflammation occur in the absence of IgE in a mouse model of asthma. Proc Natl Acad Sci USA 1997; 94:1344–1349.

117. Takeda K, Hamelmann E, Joetham A, Shultz LD, Larsen GL, Irvin CG, Gelfand EW. Development of eosinophilic airway inflammation and airway hyperresponsiveness in mast cell-deficient mice. J Exp Med 1997; 186:449–454.

118. Corry DB, Grunig G, Hadeiba H, Kurup VP, Warnock ML, Sheppard D, Rennick DM, Locksley RM. Requirements for allergen-induced airway hyperreactivity in T and B cell-deficient mice. Mol Med 1998; 4:344–355.

119. Hamelmann E, Cieslewicz G, Schwarze J, Ishizuka T, Joetham A, Heusser C, Gelfand EW. Anti-interleukin 5 but not anti-IgE prevents airway inflammation and airway hyperresponsiveness. Am J Respir Crit Care Med 1999; 160:934–941.

120. MacLean JA, Sauty A, Luster AD, Drazen JM, De Sanctis GT. Antigen-induced airway hyperresponsiveness, pulmonary eosinophilia, and chemokine expression in B cell-deficient mice. Am J Respir Cell Mol Biol 1999; 20:379–387.

121. Galli SJ, Gordon JR, Wershil BK, Costa JJ, Elovic A, Wong DT. et al. Mast cells and eosinophil cytokines in allergy and inflammation. In: Gleich GJ, Kay AB, eds. Eosinophils: Immunological and Clinical Aspects. New York: Marcel Dekker, 1994: 255–280.

122. Kay AB, Barata L, Meng Q, Durham SR, Ying S. Eosinophils and eosinophil-associated cytokines in allergic inflammation. Int Arch Allergy Immunol 1997; 113:196–199.

123. Kay AB. T cells as orchestrators of the asthmatic response. Ciba Found Symp 1997; 206:56–70.

124. Capron M, Desreumaux P. Immunobiology of eosinophils in allergy and inflammation. Res Immunol 1997; 148:29–33.

125. Gleich GJ. Mechanisms of eosinophil-associated inflammation. J Allergy Clin Immunol 2000; 105:651–663.

126. Romagnani S. The role of lymphocytes in allergic disease. J Allergy Clin Immunol 2000; 105:399–408.

127. Galli SJ, Costa JJ. Mast cell-leukocyte cytokine cascades in allergic inflammation. Allergy 1995; 50:851–862.

128. Gordon JR, Galli SJ. Promotion of mouse fibroblast collagen gene expression by mast cells stimulated via the FcεRI. Role for mast cell-derived transforming growth factor β and tumor necrosis factor α. J Exp Med 1994; 180:2027–2037.

129. Kendall JC, Li XH, Galli SJ, Gordon JR. Promotion of mouse fibroblast proliferation by IgE-dependent activation of mouse mast cells: role for mast cell tumor necrosis factor α and transforming growth factor β. J Allergy Clin Immunol 1997; 99:113–123

130. de Mora F, Williams CMM, Frenette PS, Wagner DD, Hynes RO, Galli SJ. P- and E-selectins are required for the leukocyte recruitment, but not the tissue swelling associated with IgE, and mast cell-dependent inflammation in mouse skin. Lab Invest 1998; 78:497–505.

131. Wershil BK, Furuta GT, Lavigne JA, Roy Choudhury A, Wang Z-S, Galli SJ. Dexamethasone or cyclosporin A suppresses mast cell-leukocyte cytokine cascades. Multiple mechanisms of inhibition of IgE- and mast cell-dependent cutaneous inflammation in the mouse. J Immunol 1995; 154:1391–1398.

132. Barnes PJ. Therapeutic strategies for allergic diseases. Nature 1999; 402(suppl): B31–B8.

133. Kips JC, Tavernier J, Pauwels A. Tumor necrosis factor causes bronchial hyperresponsiveness in rats. Am Rev Respir Dis 1992; 145:332–336.
134. Thomas PS, Yates DH, Barnes PJ. Tumor necrosis factor-α increases airway responsiveness and sputum neutrophilia in normal human subjects. Am J Respir Crit Care Med 1995; 52:76–80.
135. Amrani Y, Chen H, Panettieri RA Jr. Activation of tumor necrosis factor receptor 1 in airway smooth muscle: a potential pathway that modulates bronchial hyper-responsiveness in asthma? Respir Res 2000; 1:49–53.
136. Page S, Ammit AJ, Black JL, Armour CL. Human mast cell and airway smooth muscle cell interactions: implications for asthma. Am J Physiol Lung Cell Mol Physiol 2001; 281:L1313–L1323.
137. Amrani Y, Panettieri RA, Jr, Frossard N, Bronner C. Activation of the TNF-α-p55 receptor induces myocyte proliferation and modulates agonist-evoked calcium transients in cultured human tracheal smooth muscle cells. Am J Respir Cell Mol Biol 1996; 15:55–63.
138. Ohkawara Y, Yamauchi K, Tanno Y, Tamura G, Ohtani H, Nagura H, Ohkuda K, Takishima T. Human lung mast cells and pulmonary macrophages produce tumour necrosis factor-α in sensitized lung tissue after IgE receptor triggering. Am J Respir Cell Mol Biol 1992; 7:385–392.
139. Broide D, Stachnick G, Castaneda D, Nayar J. and Sriramarao P. Inhibition of eosinophilic inflammation in allergen-challenged TNF receptor p55/p75- and TNF receptor p55-deficient mice. Am J Respir Cell Mol Biol 2001; 24:304–311.
140. Rudmann DG, Moore MW, Tepper JS, Aldrich MC, Pfeiffer JW, Hogenesch H, Tumas DB. Modulation of allergic inflammation in mice deficient in TNF receptors. Am J Physiol Lung Cell Mol Physiol 2000; 279:L1047–L1057.
141. Randolph DA, Stephens R, Carruthers CJL, Chaplin DD. Cooperation between Th1 and Th2 cells in a murine model of eosinophilic airway inflammation. J Clin Invest 1999; 104:1021–1029.
142. Kanehiro A, Lahn M, Makela MJ, Dakhama A, Fujita M, Joetham A, Mason RJ, Born W, Gelfand EW. Tumor necrosis factor-α negatively regulates airway hypperresponsiveness through γδ T cells. Am J Respir Crit Care Med 2001; 164:2229–2238.
143. MacIntyre D, Boyd G. Factors influencing the occurrence of a late reaction to allergen challenge in atopic asthmatics. Clin Allergy 1984; 14:311–317.
144. Sulakelidze I, Inman MD, Rerecich T, O'Bryne PM. Increases in airway eosinophils and interleukin-5 with minimal bronchoconstriction during repeated low-dose allergen challenge in atopic asthmatics. Eur Respir J 1998; 11:821–827.
145. Kung TT, Stelts D, Zurcher JA, Jones H, Umland SP, Kreutner W, Egan RW, Chapman RW. Mast cells modulate allergic pulmonary eosinophilia in mice. Am J Respir Cell Mol Biol 1995; 12:404–409.
146. Das AM, Flower RJ, Perretti M. Resident mast cells are important for eotaxin-induced eosinophil accumulation in vivo. J Leukoc Biol 1998; 64:156–162.
147. Harris RR, Komater VA, Marett RA, Wilcox DM, Bell RL. Effect of mast cell deficiency and leukotriene inhibition on the influx of eosinophils induced by eotaxin. J Leukoc Biol 1997; 62:688–691.
148. Hogaboam C, Kunkel SL, Strieter RM, Taub DD, Lincoln P, Standiford TJ, Lukacs NW. Novel role of transmembrane SCF for mast cell activation and eotaxin production in mast cell-fibroblast interactions. J Immunol 1998; 160:6166–6171.
149. Kobayashi T, Miura T, Haba T, Sato M, Serizawa I, Nagai H, Ishizaka K. An essential role of mast cells in the development of airway hyperresponsiveness in a murine asthma model. J Immunol 2000; 164:3855–3861.

150. Jeffery PK, Godfrey RW, Adelroth E, Nelson F, Rogers A, Johansson SA. Effects of treatment on airway inflammation and thickening of basement membrane reticular collagen in asthma. A quantitative light and electron microscopic study. Am Rev Respir Dis 1992; 145:890–899.

151. Peat JK, Woolcock AJ, Cullen K. Rate of decline of lung function in subjects with asthma. Eur J Respir Dis 1987; 20:171–179.

152. Brown PJ, Greville HW, Finucane KE. Asthma and irreversible airflow obstruction. Thorax 1984; 39:131–136.

153. Wilson JW. What causes airway remodeling in asthma? Clin Exp Allergy 1998; 28: 534–536.

154. Li X, Wilson JW. Increased vascularity of the bronchial mucosa in mild asthma. Am J Respir Crit Care Med 1997; 156:229–233.

155. Roche WR. Fibroblasts and asthma. Clin Exp Allergy 1991; 21:545–548.

156. Brewster LEP, Howarth PH, Djukanovic R, Wilson J, Holgate ST, Roche WR. Myofibroblasts and subepithelial fibrosis in bronchial asthma. Am J Respir Cell Mol Biol 1990; 3:507–511.

157. Kanbe N, Tanaka A, Kanbe M, Itakura A, Kurosawa M, Matsuda H. Human mast cells produce matrix metalloproteinase 9. Eur J Immunol 1999; 29:2645–2649.

158. Shapiro SD, Senior RM. Matrix metalloproteinases. Matrix degradation and more. Am J Respir Cell Mol Biol 1999; 20:1100–1102.

159. Leon A, Buriani A, Dal Toso R, Fabris M, Romanello S, Aloe L, Levi-Montalcini R. Mast cells synthesize, store, and release nerve growth factor. Proc Natl Acad Sci USA 1994; 26:3739–3743.

160. Miller HR, Wright SH, Knight PA, Thornton EM. A novel function for transforming growth factor-β1: upregulation of the expression and the IgE-independent extracellular release of a mucosal mast cell granule-specific β-chymase, mouse mast cell protease-1. Blood 1999; 93:3473–3486.

161. Fang KC, Wolters PJ, Steinhoff M, Bidgel A, Blount JL, Caughey GH. Mast cell expression of gelatinase A and B is regulated by kit ligand and TGF-β. J Immunol 1999; 162:5528–5535.

162. de Paulis A, Minopoli G, Dal Piaz F, Pucci P, Russo T, Marone G. Novel autocrine and paracrine loops of the stem cell factor/chymase network. Int Arch Allergy Immunol 1999; 118:422–425.

163. Welker P, Grabbe J, Gibbs B, Zuberbier T, Henz BM. Human mast cells produce and differentially express both soluble and membrane-bound stem cell factor. Scand J Immunol 1999; 49:495–500.

164. Longley BJ, Tyrrell L, Ma Y, Williams DA, Halaban R, Langley K, Lu HS, Schechter NM. Chymase cleavage of stem cell factor yields a bioactive, soluble product. Proc Natl Acad Sci USA 1997; 94:9017–9021.

165. Busse W, Elias J, Sheppard D, Banks-Schlegal S. Airway remodeling and repair. Am J Respir Crit Care Med 1999; 160:1035–1042.

166. Holgate ST, Lackie PM, Davies DE, Roche WR, Walls AF. The bronchial epithelium as a key regulator of airway inflammation and remodeling in asthma. Clin Exp Allergy 1999; 29(suppl 2):90–95.

167. Holgate ST. The inflammation-repair cycle in asthma: the pivotal role of the airway epithelium. Clin Exp Allergy 1998; 28(suppl 5):97–103.

168. Lin S, Cicala C, Scharenberg AM, Kinet J-P. The FcϵRIβ subunit functions as an amplifier of FcϵRIγ-mediated cell activation signals. Cell 1996; 85:985–995.

169. Dombrowicz D, Lin S, Flamand V, Brini AT, Koller BH, Kinet JP. Allergy-associated FcRβ is a molecular amplifier of IgE- and IgG-mediated in vivo responses. Immunity 1998; 8:517–529.

170. Hsu C, MacGlashan D Jr. IgE antibody up-regulates high affinity IgE binding on murine bone marrow-derived mast cells. Immunol Lett 1996; 52:129–134.

171. Banovac K, Neylan D, Leone J, Ghandur-Mnaymneh L, Rabinovitch A. Are the mast cells antigen presenting cells? Immunol Invest 1989; 18:901–906.

172. Tkaczyk C, Villa I, Peronet R, David B, Mecheri S. FcεRI-mediated antigen endocytosis turns IFN-γ-treated mouse mast cells from inefficient into potent antigen-presenting cells. Immunology 1999; 97:333–430.

173. Frandji P, Tkaczyk C, Oskeritzian C, Lapeyre J, Peronet R, David B, Guillet JG, Mecheri S. Presentation of soluble antigens by mast cells: upregulation by interleukin-4 and granulocyte/macrophage colony-stimulating factor and downregulation by interferon-γ. Cell Immunol 1995; 163:37–46.

174. Yang PC, Berin MC, Perdue MH. Enhanced antigen transport across rat tracheal epithelium induced by sensitization and mast cell activation. J Immunol 1999; 163: 2769–2776.

175. Berin MC, Kiliaan AJ, Yang PC, Groot JA, Kitamura Y, Perdue MH. The influence of mast cells on pathways of transepithelial antigen transport in rat intestine. J Immunol 1998; 161:2561–2566.

176. Gauchat JF, Henchoz S, Mazzei G, Aubry JP, Brunner T, Blassey H, Life P, Talabot D, Flores-Romo L, Thompson J, et al. Induction of human IgE synthesis in B cells by mast cells and basophils. Nature 1993; 365:340–343.

177. Asai K, Kitaura J, Kawakami Y, Yamagata N, Tsai M, Cargbone DP, Liu F-T, Galli SJ, Kawakami T. Regulation of mast cell survival by IgE. Immunity 2001; 14:791–800.

178. Kalesnikoff J, Huber M, Lam V, Damen JE, Zhang J, Siraganian RP, Krystal G. Monomeric IgE stimulates signaling pathways in mast cells that lead to cytokine production and cell survival. Immunity 2001; 14:801–811.

16

Mast Cell Exocytosis in Airway Inflammation

ROBERTO ADACHI

Baylor College of Medicine
Houston VA Medical Center
Houston, Texas, U.S.A.

RUPESH NIGAM

Baylor College of Medicine
Houston, Texas, U.S.A.

BURTON F. DICKEY

M.D. Anderson Cancer Center
Baylor College of Medicine
Houston VA Medical Center
Houston, Texas, U.S.A.

I. Introduction

The central role of mast cell activation in acute allergic reactions, including asthma, is well known (1,2). Increasingly, the participation of mast cells in perpetuating the chronic phase of allergic inflammation is being recognized (3,4). For these reasons, suppression of mast cell function is an important part of the treatment of allergic inflammation. However, protective roles of mast cells in initiating host defense against bacterial pathogens have recently been identified (5). Thus, therapeutic suppression of mast cell function should be selective so that maladaptive and troublesome allergic activation is eliminated without impairing essential defense functions. Mast cells are activated both through a specific IgE-mediated immune mechanism as well as through innate mechanisms mediated by complement (6), lectins (7), and other pathways (8). Since it appears that there is no important protective role of IgE-dependent immunity of the airways in contemporary Western societies (9), whereas the protective roles of mast cells appear to all be mediated by innate immune mechanisms (10), therapeutic targeting of IgE-dependent mast cell activation is an attractive strategy being pursued by several pharmaceutical companies (see Chap. 43). However, this strategy is only partially effective (11), possibly because mast cells are also activated by non–IgE-dependent mediators in allergic inflammation, such as adenosine (see Chap. 31). An alternative strategy would be to target signal transduction pathways downstream of the IgE receptor and other allergic-responsive receptors, while leaving those downstream of critical innate immune receptors intact. A third possibility would be to selectively target distinct mast cell effector mechanisms.

In both innate and specific immunity, mast cells function principally by releasing inflammatory mediators that either activate target cells (e.g., histamine-induced smooth muscle contraction and increase in endothelial permeability) or initiate biochemical changes in the extracellular milieu (e.g., heparin-dependent modulation of fibrin formation) (1). While mast cells have been shown to be capable of additional immune functions, such as phagocytosis (12,13) and antigen presentation (14,15), other cell types carry out these other functions more effectively. Several of the inflammatory mediators released by mast cells have already been targeted therapeutically, including histamine and cysteinyl-leukotrienes (see Chap. 29), and others are targets of current drug development, including individual mast cell proteases (see Chap. 17), cytokines, and chemokines. In view of the large number of inflammatory mediators released by activated mast cells (1), targeting individual mediators may be impractical if several are shown to be important. Since many of these mediators are released by common effector mechanisms, targeting the release of mediators could be an effective therapeutic strategy if the protective and pathological functions of mast cells can be separated at this level.

II. Mast Cell Effector Responses

Once stimulated, mast cells have three principal effector responses: exocytic release of preformed inflammatory mediators stored in their granules (degranulation) (16,17), de novo synthesis and release of eicosanoids (18,19), and de novo generation and release of cytokines and chemokines (20) (Fig. 1). The process of mast cell degranulation will be the focus of this chapter, and the other two responses that do not depend on regulated exocytosis will be described here only briefly.

As in other cells, eicosanoids in mast cells are synthesized in the cytoplasm and exported by transmembrane transporters to the extracellular space (21–23). Among eicosanoids, the most abundant prostaglandin produced by stimulated mast cells is PGD_2 (24,25), and the most abundant cysteinyl-leukotriene is LTC_4 (26–28). When released extracellularly, these two eicosanoids exert potent bronchoconstrictive, vasodilatory, and chemoattractive effects (1). The metabolism and role in inflammation of these mast cell products are discussed in detail in Chapter 29.

Immunohistochemical analysis of bronchial biopsies from asthmatic patients (29,30) and of nasal biopsies from patients with allergic rhinitis (31) has revealed that mast cells are an important source of cytokines and chemokines. In one study, mast cells accounted for 90% of the IL-4 and IL-6 immunoreactive cells seen in mucosal biopsies (30). Mast cells are known to release the cytokines IL-3 (32), IL-4 (33,34), IL-5 (35,36), IL-6 (37,38), IL-9 (39), IL-13 (40,41), IL-16 (42), TNFα (43,44), GM-CSF (35,38) IFNγ (43,45), and TGFβ (46,47), and many chemokines such as IL-8 (48,49) and others (50). The roles of these products in airway inflamma-

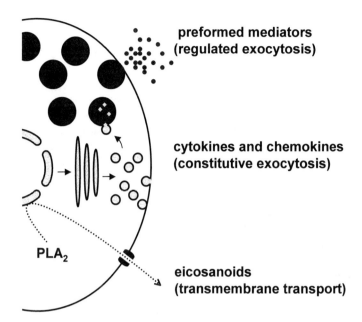

Figure 1 Schematic depiction of mast cell effector responses. Upon activation, mast cells secrete preformed mediators stored in their granules (large dark gray vesicles) by regulated exocytosis. The mediators released into the extracellular space (small dark gray circles) include biogenic amines, glycosaminoglycans, and proteases. Stimulation also induces the transcription of cytokines and chemokines (light gray diamonds), which are newly synthesized and transported through the perinuclear endoplasmic reticulum and Golgi apparatus (light gray compartments), then released from small post-Golgi vesicles (small light gray vesicles) by constitutive exocytosis. Some of these small post-Golgi vesicles fuse laterally (small arrows) with the secretory granules, resulting in a small amount of cytokines stored and secreted through this compartment (see text). Eicosanoids are also newly synthesized; phospholipase A_2 (PLA_2) releases arachidonic acid, mainly from the nuclear membrane, to be used as a substrate for the synthesis of prostanoids and leukotrienes. These products (dotted line) are then secreted by specific transporter proteins present at the plasma membrane.

tion are discussed in detail elsewhere in this volume. In most cells, cytokines and chemokines are released by constitutive exocytosis of small post-Golgi vesicles (51,52), and regulation of their synthesis and release is primarily at the level of transcription (53). The same is true for mast cells (54–57), but after stimulation a small amount of some cytokines such as TNFα and IL-4, but not IL-5, are found in mast cell granules (58–60), suggesting a convergence of regulated and constitutive secretory pathways. It is possible that, after stimulation, some cytokine-containing post-Golgi vesicles are redirected to the endosomal or lysosomal compartments where regulated secretory granules originate (61). Cytokines packed in the granules, although present in small amounts, will render a stimulated mast cell "primed" for future activation events so that it can release some cytokines immediately without waiting for their transcription and translation (Fig. 1).

Although it was long thought that mast cells have monotonic effector responses to all stimuli, there is evidence suggestive of the contrary. Cross-linking of surface FcεRI is the most effective physiological stimulus known, powerfully eliciting all three mast cell effector responses: degranulation, release of eicosanoids, and secretion of cytokines and chemokines (62). However, different stimuli may induce different responses. For example, incubation of mouse bone marrow-derived mast cells with stem cell factor leads to activation of mast cells via c-kit, resulting in release of IL-6 but not of leukotriene C_4 or preformed granule mediators (36). Also, rat peritoneal mast cells that release histamine and IL-6 when stimulated by FcεRI cross-linking secrete only histamine when exposed to a calcium ionophore and release only IL-6 when exposed to lipopolysaccharide (LPS) (63). These experiments prove not only that mast cells can selectively respond to different stimuli, but also that one effector response does not necessarily depend on the activation of the others, offering the possibility of artificially modulating one of the mast cell responses without affecting the others.

III. Protective Roles of Mast Cells

Mast cells have been mostly known for their roles in allergic reactions (64) and IgE-mediated specific immunity against parasitic infestation (65,66). More recently their involvement in defense against bacterial infections has been described, and mast cells are now recognized as an important component of the innate immune system (67). Their essential role in host defense against acute bacterial infections was proven in vivo by studying the responses of the mast cell–deficient mouse strain WBB6F$_1$-W/W^v (W/W^v) in bacterial peritonitis and pneumonia models, compared with the responses of normal congenic mice and of mast cell–reconstituted W/W^v mice. In these experiments, all infected W/W^v mice died, while 70% of congenic controls were able to control and clear the infection (68,69). Furthermore, reconstitution of W/W^v mice with mast cells derived from bone marrow from congenic controls rendered them resistant to the infection (68,69). These and other experiments also proved that the protective effects of mast cells depend on the early recruitment of neutrophils to the site of infection (6,68,69), which is mediated, at least in part, by mast cell activation through complement receptors and toll-like 4 receptor (6,70,71) and by the release from mast cells of TNFα (68,69) and LTB$_4$ (72). Also, increasing the total number of mast cells present in mice by administration of stem cell factor improved survival of infected mice (73). Together, these experiments suggest that mast cells play important roles in innate immunity via the production of eicosanoids and cytokines. Because the secretion of these products does not depend on regulated exocytosis, it is possible that an agent that can specifically block regulated exocytosis in mast cells will prevent the release of the preformed inflammatory mediators stored in their granules and attenuate allergic reactivity without impairing the protective roles of mast cells.

IV. Mast Cell Granule Contents

The most striking morphological characteristic of mast cells is the numerous granules present in their cytoplasm. These granules are large exocytic vesicles that contain a variety of proteases, biogenic amines, and sometimes a small amount of cytokines, all of them tightly packed around a core of heavily sulfated anionic proteoglycans (74).

A. Proteases

Mast cell tryptases and chymases constitute the main protein components of the mast cell granule and play multiple roles in airway inflammation. Together, these enzymes activate receptors and metalloproteinases, inactivate fibrinogen and neuropeptides, induce the expression of adhesion proteins by endothelium and of chemokines and mucus by epithelium, and are fibrogenic and angiogenic (1). These proteases are described in detail in Chapter 17.

B. Cytokines

While some mast cells contain TNFα (58,59) and IL-4 (60) in their secretory granules, the amount of cytokines present in the granules is so small when compared with levels produced by transcriptional activation (20) that they may not have a major physiological effect.

C. Amines

Only mast cells and basophils produce histamine, the first mediator implicated in the pathophysiology of asthma. Compared to control subjects, asthmatic patients manifest bronchial hyperreactivity to nebulized histamine (75), and histamine is present in the bronchoalveolar lavage fluid of patients with allergic asthma (76,77). Four histamine receptors (HR) have been cloned (78,79), and H1R is mainly responsible for the effects of histamine on the airways (80). Histamine causes contraction of bronchial smooth muscle (81), a response that can be modulated by prostaglandins (82), leukotrienes (83), and mast cell proteases (84), and it also induces proliferation of cultured airway smooth muscle cells (85). Histamine causes vasodilation in the airways and plasma extravasation at the level of postcapillary venules (86), though its precise role in causing airway edema in human asthma has not been fully defined (87). Histamine induces the production of multiple inflammatory cytokines by endothelial (88,89) and epithelial cells (90) and is also a potent mucus secretagogue (91). Mucus secretion is perhaps the only effect of histamine in the lung known to depend on H2R (92). Based on animal models, it has always been assumed that at least part of the bronchoconstrictor effect of histamine is mediated via cholinergic reflexes (93–95), but studies in humans are controversial (96). In different combinations, the four HR have been described in inflammatory cells. Histamine was one of the first selective eosinophil chemoattractants and activators to be described (97,98), and it also stimulates alveolar macrophages (99), but has an inhibitory effect on mast cells (100). Histamine has many effects on lymphocytes, including stimulation of the production by CD8+ T cells of IL-16, one of the most potent chemotactic factors for CD4+ T lymphocytes (101). Dendritic cells (important antigen-presenting cells that initiate the polarization of Th cells) that mature in the presence of histamine fail to produce IL-12 despite the presence of IFNγ, but instead increase their production of IL-10, and polarize naïve CD4+ T cells toward a Th2 phenotype (102,103). When exposed to histamine, splenocytes decrease their production of IFNγ and increase their production of IL-5 and IL-10 (104), mature Th1 cells decrease their production of IFNγ (105), and differentiated Th2 cells show a dose-dependent increase of IL-13 production (106). In summary, histamine is not only an important mediator during the early phase of the asthmatic response (e.g., smooth muscle contraction, tissue edema, and mucus hypersecretion), but it also affects the chronic phase by attracting and activating inflammatory cells and biasing the immune system toward a type 2 response. Serotonin, in contrast, is not found in human mast cell granules (though it is the major amine stored in rodent mast cells), and it does not have a bronchoconstrictive effect on human airways (107).

D. Proteoglycans

The sulfated proteoglycans in the core of a mast cell granule consist of a serine- and glycine-enriched protein backbone (serglycin) with multiple side chains of glycosaminoglycans (108). In some mast cells, the most abundant side chains are the heavily sulfated pentasaccharide units of heparin glycosaminoglycans, while in others it is the less negatively charged chondroitin sulfate (109). This differential content of heavily anionic heparin chains explains the distinctive histological staining and metachromasia of some mast cell granules (110,111) that was used in initial attempts to classify mast cells into different phenotypes (112). The density of anionic charge given by heparin to granules also explains their higher content of histamine (113). The presence of heparin is necessary for the expression and storage of some proteases, such as mouse mast cell protease-4 (mMCP-4), mMCP-5, and mMC-carboxypeptidase A (mMC-CPA) (114,115). In vitro and in vivo studies have proven that the differential expression of glycosaminoglycans and proteases in mast cell granules is determined by the microenvironment in which they develop and the stimuli to which they are exposed and that the phenotypes are reversible (109,116,117). Even though the amount of heparin released by mast cells is too small to have a systemic effect or to exert the anti-inflammatory and bronchoprotective effects seen when pharmacological doses are given systemically or applied topically by inhalation (118), the secreted matrix proteoglycans can exert a local effect. They may act as chemotactic agents (116), activate inflammatory cells, and modulate local coagulation and fibrinolytic processes (116), either directly (119), or indirectly through modulation of protease activity (120,121). Heparin allows the association of mast cell proteases into homotetramers (122) or heterotetramers (123) needed for their enzymatic activation (124), and it also protects these proteases from natural inhibitors (125).

By targeted disruption of the glucosaminyl *N*-deacetylase/*N*-sulfotransferase-2 (NDST-2) gene, two groups generated mice that were unable to sulfate heparin glycosaminoglycans, and therefore lack true heparin (114,115). Peritoneal mast cells from these mutant mice have only a few, small, weakly staining granules (115). They also contain less than 10% of the histamine found in peritoneal mast cells from control animals (115). Granules from these mast cells lack protease activity and have no measurable levels of mMCP-4, mMCP5, and mMC-CPA, despite the fact that mRNA levels for these enzymes are normal. Nevertheless, when acute inflammation was induced by intraperitoneal injection of IgE and anti-IgE antibody, the deletant mice exhibited a neutrophilic influx to the site of inflammation comparable to that of the controls (115), probably secondary to intact synthesis and secretion of cytokines and leukotrienes. This supports the idea that blocking the release of preformed granule mediators by inhibition of regulated exocytosis may not interfere with the important role of mast cells in innate immunity.

V. Overview of Regulated Exocytosis

Recent evidence from a variety of biochemical and genetic approaches has revealed a conserved mechanism of exocytosis from yeast to humans (126–128). The central components are SNARE proteins that are localized on transport vesicles (v-SNAREs, such as VAMP), and on the target (i.e., plasma) membrane (t-SNAREs, such as Syntaxin and SNAP-25). These bind tightly to each other, forming a parallel four-helix bundle known as the core complex (129). Coiling of the four helices brings together the opposing membranes, resulting in complete fusion. Additional proteins regulate these processes, as shown in Figure 2.

A SNARE domain near the C-terminus (transmembrane region) of Syntaxin is necessary for binding other SNAREs, as well as the calcium sensor Synaptotagmin (130). The N-terminus of Syntaxin contains three internal coils that fold back onto the SNARE domain in the basal state (closed conformation), preventing unregulated SNARE-SNARE interactions (131). Munc18 binds the closed conformation of Syntaxin along its entire cytoplasmic length, forming a stable complex that is an essential intermediate in opening Syntaxin's conformation (131,132). Munc13, a peripheral plasma membrane protein, binds to the N-terminus of Syntaxin at the same site as Munc18, displacing Munc18 from Syntaxin. This interaction leads to the transition of Syntaxin to an open conformation that forms a binary complex with SNAP-25 (t-SNARE complex) (133–135).

Rab3 proteins anchored on the granule membrane are exocytic isoforms of a large family of Ras-related GTPases that facilitate this process, perhaps through indirect activation of Munc13 (136,137). The cytoplasmic C2 domains of Synaptotagmin, an integral vesicle membrane protein thought to be the principal calcium sensor of the exocytic machinery (138), can penetrate the lipid bilayer of the plasma membrane in a calcium-dependent manner (139). This may anchor the secretory vesicles to the plasma membrane, allowing VAMP (the v-SNARE) and the binary t-SNARE (Syntaxin and SNAP-25) complex to form a tertiary complex (core complex)

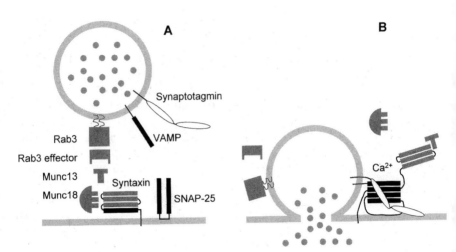

Figure 2 Schematic depiction of regulated exocytosis. (A) Resting: The v-SNARE (VAMP) and the t-SNAREs (Syntaxin and SNAP-25) are located on the secretory granule membrane and the plasma membrane, respectively. Syntaxin, in a closed conformation (see text), is bound to Munc18. Rab GTPases on the granules activate Munc13 through Rab effectors, such as RIM. (B) Fusion: Dissociation of the Munc18-Syntaxin complex by Munc13 opens the Syntaxin conformation. The Synaptotagmin C2B domain binds to the plasma membrane, allowing the SNARE motifs of VAMP, Syntaxin, and SNAP-25 to form a four-helix bundle, with two helices contributed by SNAP-25 and one helix each by Syntaxin and VAMP. In the presence of calcium-bound Synaptotagmin, further coiling of the helical core complex results in close apposition and penetration of the lipid bilayer structure of granule and plasma membranes. This results in membrane fusion and exocytic release of granule contents.

(140). Synaptotagmin may then regulate the process of tight coiling (zippering) of the core complex that leads to fusion (138).

The relative importance and precise roles of each of these proteins have been investigated through selective deletion of the corresponding genes in neurons of mice, flies, and worms, followed by analysis of synaptic vesicle exocytosis. In such models, deletion of the SNAREs (i.e., Syntaxin, SNAP-25, VAMP) (141–144) or of molecules that directly regulate Syntaxin conformation (i.e., Munc18, Munc13) (145,146) results in severe defects in exocytosis, while milder defects are seen with more distal regulators such as Rab GTPases (147).

VI. Regulated Exocytosis in Mast Cells

Many paralogs of the components of the neuronal exocytic machinery have been described in mast cells. Two nonneuronal isoforms of SNAP-25 are known, SNAP-23 (149) and SNAP-29 (150); in mast cells, SNAP-23 has been found to be part of the SNARE complex that mediates exocytosis (151,152). Similar to SNAP-25, SNAP-23 has two SNARE motifs and forms complexes with Syntaxin isoforms to yield a t-SNARE complex, and then with VAMP isoforms to form the full core complex (153,154). Studies using anti-SNAP-23 antibodies in streptolysin permeabilized rat peritoneal mast cells revealed that SNAP-23 was necessary for calcium– and GTPγS-dependent exocytosis. They also showed that in resting mast cells SNAP-23 is located on the plasma membrane, and that upon cell stimulation it translocated to the membrane of the secretory granules, an event that preceded actual exocytosis (152). It has been postulated that this translocation, unique so far to mast cells, is necessary for compound exocytosis, a phenomenon that involves fusion of secretory granules among themselves before their final fusion to the plasma membrane. Homotypic fusion among secretory granules would also require a t- and v-SNARE interaction, and SNAP-23 would form part of the t-SNARE complex (152). In another study, overexpression of wild-type SNAP-23 in RBL-2H3 mast cells increased stimulated exocytosis, an effect proven to be due to a specific interaction of SNAP-23 with VAMP because overexpression of a mutant SNAP-23 able to form complexes with Syntaxin but unable to bind VAMP in vitro and in vivo had no effect on exocytosis (155). SNAP-23 seems to be one of the few SNARE proteins that stimulates exocytosis when overexpressed, and it could be that in mast cells the expression of this protein is a limiting factor in regulated exocytosis.

Syntaxins-2, -3, and -4 have been identified in mast cells, but only Syntaxin-4 seems to be able to form a SNARE complex with SNAP-23 and a VAMP (152). Also, overexpression of Syntaxin-4 but not of Syntaxins-2 and -3 caused inhibition of degranulation in RBL-2H3 mast cells (152). A similar phenomenon is seen with Syntaxin-1 in neurons, where the excess or defect of this protein causes a dose-dependent inhibition of regulated exocytosis (142).

Very little is known about VAMPs in mast cells. VAMP-2,-3,-7, and -8 have been identified in mast cells, and the only evidence of the involvement in exocytosis of one of them, VAMP-8, is its co-localization with serotonin-containing granules in RBL-2H3 mast cells and its ability to form core complexes with SNAP-23 and Syntaxin-4 (152).

Synaptotagmins-2, -3, and -5 haven been identified in mast cells (156). By immunofluorescent microscopy and cell fractionation studies using a nonspecific anti-Synaptotagmin antibody, anti-Synaptotagmin immunoreactivity was identified at the level of the secretory granules (157). Overexpression in RBL-2H3 mast cells of Synaptotagmin-1, which is not a mast cell isoform, resulted in its targeting to secretory granules and potentiation of calcium-induced mast cell degranulation (157). On the other hand, Synaptotagmin-2 co-fractionated in RBL-2H3 mast cells with lysosomes that are part of the secretory compartment in mast cells and had a negative effect on calcium-induced exocytosis (156). No studies about the localization and function of Synaptotagmins-3 and 5 in mast cells have been published. Although in neurons Synaptotagmin-3 seems to be a plasma membrane protein (158,159), in pancreatic β-cells and insulin-secreting cell lines, Synaptotagmin-3 colocalized with insulin-containing vesicles by fractionation studies (160,161) and by confocal microscopy (162), and overexpression of this protein conferred greater calcium sensitivity for exocytosis (162). The 13 mammalian Synaptotagmins (163) can be classified based on the calcium affinities of their C2A domains in complex with phospholipids (164), a property that may be functionally important given that there is a precise correlation between the different calcium affinities and the inhibitory effects of Synaptotagmin C2A domains on calcium-triggered exocytosis in PC12 cells (159). While the Synaptotagmin-2 C2A domain has a relatively low calcium affinity, the calcium affinity of Synaptotagmin-3 and Synaptotagmin-5 C2A domains is high (159,165) and within the range of intracellular calcium transients observed during mast cell activation (166,167), suggesting that if a Synaptotagmin has a facilitatory role in mast cell exocytosis, it would be Synaptotagmin-3 or -5 and not Synaptotagmin-2.

All three isoforms of Munc18 are transcriptionally expressed in mast cells (unpublished observations). Quantitatively, Munc18-2 mRNA is the most abundant, followed by Munc18-3 and Munc18-1, but Munc18-3 is the functional isoform of our unpublished observations.

The introduction of a poorly hydrolyzable form of GTP, GTPγS, into mast cells causes complete degranulation (16), indicating the participation of GTPases in secretion. Based on the involvement of Rab3A in neuronal exocytosis (168), it was postulated that a Rab3 isoform could be one of the GTPases mediating this phenomenon in mast cells. By RT-PCR, ribonuclease protection assays, and immunoblotting from the rat mast cell line RBL-2H3, it was found that the predominant Rab3 expressed in mast cells was Rab3D (169,170), an isoform expressed in many nonneuronal tissues (171,172). By immunofluorescence microscopy, Rab3D localized on rat peritoneal mast cell granules and translocated to the plasma membrane upon stimulated exocytosis (169).

Overexpression of wild-type and mutant Rab3D in RBL-2H3 mast cells decreased stimulated exocytosis (170). In the same studies, Rab3A was also found, but it was present in the cytosolic fraction, and overexpression of wild-type or mutant proteins had minimal effects on exocytosis (169,170). Although these studies prove that Rab3D is part of the mast cell exocytic machinery and that it plays a role in regulating mast cell degranulation, there is no definite proof that it is the only GTPase involved in exocytosis. Other Rabs, like Rab37, have also been found associated with mast cell secretory granules, but their functional roles have not been elucidated (173). Also, there is evidence that activation of members of the Rho family of monomeric GTPases (Rho, Rac, Cdc42) play important roles in mast cell secretion (174).

SCAMPs (secretory carrier membrane proteins) are a family of ubiquitous membrane proteins associated with transporter vesicles. Of the three isoforms, SCAMP-1 is the most abundant in mast cells and is found associated with secretory granules. Patch-clamping of mast cells from the SCAMP-1 KO mouse revealed that the initial rise in membrane capacitance triggered by GTPγS was normal, but the final capacitance was reduced, in association with an increase in the proportion of reversible events. Therefore, SCAMP-1 is not essential, but promotes the full execution of exocytosis in mast cells (175).

Although the signaling cascades triggered by FcεRI crosslinking have been characterized (62), the transduction pathway connecting IgE receptors to the exocytic machinery remains incompletely defined. Activation of the Lyn/Syk protein tyrosine kinases induces translocation and phosphorylation of phospholipase-C (PLC) isoforms and phosphoinositide 3-kinase (PI3K). Subsequent PLCγ-mediated formation of inositol 3,4,5-phosphate and diacylglycerol leads to calcium release from internal stores and activation of protein kinase C (PKC), respectively, while PI3K mediates calcium influx through phosphatidylinositol (3,4,5)-trisphosphate–sensitive calcium channels (176,177). The transient elevation of intracellular calcium concentration is necessary for mast cell degranulation (166,167), and the effects of calcium in mast cell exocytosis are mediated at least in part through its binding to Synaptotagmin (156,157). PKC phosphorylates multiple components of the exocytic machinery including Munc18, SNAP-25, Synaptotagmin, and Syntaxin (178).

Phosphorylation of Munc18 reduces its affinity for Syntaxin and may promote secretion (179). Also, β phorbol esters/diacylglycerol bind and activate Munc13, stimulating exocytosis (180), and calcium/calmodulin-dependent protein kinase II phosphorylates Synaptotagmin (181). Rak3D (Rab3D-associated kinase) is a Rab3D interacting protein isolated from mast cells that phosphorylates Syntaxin-4 but not Syntaxins-2 or -3. The phosphorylation of Syntaxin-4 by Rak3D decreases its affinity for SNAP-23, and the kinase activity of Rak3D decreases after FcεRI-induced calcium-dependent mast cell activation, suggesting a possible mechanism by which stimulation modulates the competence of the mast cell exocytic machinery (182).

VII. Conclusions

Mast cells play important roles in allergic reactions and in the innate immune response to infections. They have three fundamental effector responses: degranulation, release of eicosanoids, and release of cytokines. During degranulation, mast cells release many preformed inflammatory mediators by regulated exocytosis. Inflammatory mediators stored in mast cell granules appear to be mainly involved in the generation of allergic reactions and parasite defense, but do not appear to be necessary for the beneficial role of mast cells in defense against bacteria. Because the process of regulated exocytosis in mast cells uses the same basic molecular machinery as other cells, it might be possible to selectively inhibit mast cell degranulation by applying what we have learned from other cellular systems.

References

1. Hart PH. Regulation of the inflammatory response in asthma by mast cell products. Immunol Cell Biol 2001; 79:149–153.
2. Busse WW, Lemanske RF, Jr. Asthma. N Engl J Med 2001; 344:350–362.
3. Page S, Ammit AJ, Black JL, Armour CL. Human mast cell and airway smooth muscle cell interactions: implications for asthma. Am J Physiol Lung Cell Mol Physiol 2001; 281:L1313–L1323.
4. Bingham CO, Austen KF. Mast-cell responses in the development of asthma. J Allergy Clin Immunol 2000; 105:S527–S534.

5. Malaviya R, Abraham SN. Mast cell modulation of immune responses to bacteria. Immunol Rev 2001; 179:16–24.
6. Prodeus AP, Zhou X, Maurer M, Galli SJ, Carroll MC. Impaired mast cell-dependent natural immunity in complement C3-deficient mice. Nature 1997; 390:172–175.
7. Malaviya R, Ross E, Jakschik BA, Abraham SN. Mast cell degranulation induced by type 1 fimbriated *Escherichia coli* in mice. J Clin Invest 1994; 93:1645–1653.
8. Abraham SN, Malaviya R. Mast cell modulation of the innate immune response to enterobacterial infection. Adv Exp Med Biol 2000; 479:91–105.
9. Sutton BJ, Gould HJ. The human IgE network. Nature 1993; 366:421–428.
10. Abraham SN, Malaviya R. Mast cells in infection and immunity. Infect Immun 1997; 65:3501–3508.
11. Milgrom H, Fick RB, Jr, Su JQ, Reimann JD, Bush RK, Watrous ML, Metzger WJ. Treatment of allergic asthma with monoclonal anti-IgE antibody. N Engl J Med 1999; 341:1966–1973.
12. Malaviya R, Ross EA, MacGregor JI, Ikeda T, Little JR, Jakschik BA, Abraham SN. Mast cell phagocytosis of FimH-expressing enterobacteria. J Immunol 1994; 152: 1907–1914.
13. Arock M, Ross E, Lai-Kuen R, Averlant G, Gao Z, Abraham SN. Phagocytic and tumor necrosis factor alpha response of human mast cells following exposure to gram-negative and gram-positive bacteria. Infect Immun 1998; 66:6030–6034.
14. Poncet P, Arock M, David B. MHC class II-dependent activation of CD4 + T cell hybridomas by human mast cells through superantigen presentation. J Leukoc Biol 1999; 66:105–112.
15. Frandji P, Oskeritzian C, Cacaraci F, Lapeyre J, Peronet R, David B, Guillet JG, Mecheri S. Antigen-dependent stimulation by bone marrow-derived mast cells of MHC class II-restricted T cell hybridoma. J Immunol 1993; 151:6318–6328.
16. Fernandez JM, Neher E, Gomperts BD. Capacitance measurement reveals stepwise fusion events in degranulating mast cells. Nature 1984; 312:453–455.
17. Lawson D, Raff MC, Gomperts B, Fewtrell C, Gilula NB. Molecular events during membrane fusion. A study of exocytosis in rat peritoneal mast cells. J Cell Biol 1977; 72:242–259.
18. Peters SP, MacGlashan DW, Jr, Schulman ES, Schleimer RP, Hayes EC, Rokach J, Adkinson NF, Jr, Lichtenstein LM. Arachidonic acid metabolism in purified human lung mast cells. J Immunol 1984; 132:1972–1979.
19. Schleimer RP, Davidson DA, Lichtenstein LM, Adkinson NF, Jr. Selective inhibition of arachidonic acid metabolite release from human lung tissue by antiinflammatory steroids. J Immunol 1986; 136:3006–3011.
20. Kobayashi H, Ishizuka T, Okayama Y. Human mast cells and basophils as sources of cytokines. Clin Exp Allergy 2000; 30:1205–1212.
21. Lam BK, Xu K, Atkins MB, Austen KF. Leukotriene C4 uses a probenecid-sensitive export carrier that does not recognize leukotriene B4. Proc Natl Acad Sci USA 1992; 89:11598–11602.
22. Bartosz G, Konig J, Keppler D, Hagmann W. Human mast cells secreting leukotriene C4 express the MRP1 gene-encoded conjugate export pump. Biol Chem 1998; 379: 1121–1126.
23. Leier I, Jedlitschky G, Buchholz U, Keppler D. Characterization of the ATP-dependent leukotriene C4 export carrier in mastocytoma cells. Eur J Biochem 1994; 220:599–606.
24. Lewis RA, Soter NA, Diamond PT, Austen KF, Oates JA, Roberts LJ. Prostaglandin D2 generation after activation of rat and human mast cells with anti-IgE. J Immunol 1982; 129:1627–1631.

25. Lewis RA, Holgate ST, Roberts LJ, Oates JA, Austen KF. Preferential generation of prostaglandin D2 by rat and human mast cells. Kroc Found Ser 1981; 14:239–254.
26. Razin E, Mencia-Huerta JM, Stevens RL, Lewis RA, Liu FT, Corey E, Austen KF. IgE-mediated release of leukotriene C4, chondroitin sulfate E proteoglycan, beta-hexosaminidase, and histamine from cultured bone marrow-derived mouse mast cells. J Exp Med 1983; 157:189–201.
27. Razin E, Mencia-Huerta JM, Lewis RA, Corey EJ, Austen KF. Generation of leukotriene C4 from a subclass of mast cells differentiated in vitro from mouse bone marrow. Proc Natl Acad Sci USA 1982; 79:4665–4667.
28. Heavey DJ, Ernst PB, Stevens RL, Befus AD, Bienenstock J, Austen KF. Generation of leukotriene C4, leukotriene B4, and prostaglandin D2 by immunologically activated rat intestinal mucosa mast cells. J Immunol 1988; 140:1953–1957.
29. Ghaffar O, Laberge S, Jacobson MR, Lowhagen O, Rak S, Durham SR, Hamid Q. IL-13 mRNA and immunoreactivity in allergen-induced rhinitis: comparison with IL-4 expression and modulation by topical glucocorticoid therapy. Am J Respir Cell Mol Biol 1997; 17:17–24.
30. Bradding P, Roberts JA, Britten KM, Montefort S, Djukanovic R, Mueller R, Heusser CH, Howarth PH, Holgate ST. Interleukin-4, -5, and -6 and tumor necrosis factor-α in normal and asthmatic airways: evidence for the human mast cell as a source of these cytokines. Am J Respir Cell Mol Biol 1994; 10:471–480.
31. Bradding P, Feather IH, Wilson S, Bardin PG, Heusser CH, Holgate ST, Howarth PH. Immunolocalization of cytokines in the nasal mucosa of normal and perennial rhinitic subjects. The mast cell as a source of IL-4, IL-5, and IL-6 in human allergic mucosal inflammation. J Immunol 1993; 151:3853–3865.
32. Razin E, Leslie KB, Schrader JW. Connective tissue mast cells in contact with fibroblasts express IL-3 mRNA. Analysis of single cells by polymerase chain reaction. J Immunol 1991; 146:981–987.
33. Okayama Y, Petit-Frére C, Kassel O, Semper A, Quint D, Tunon-de-Lara MJ, Bradding P, Holgate ST, Church MK. IgE-dependent expression of mRNA for IL-4 and IL-5 in human lung mast cells. J Immunol 1995; 155:1796–1808.
34. Pawankar R, Okuda M, Yssel H, Okumura K, Ra C. Nasal mast cells in perennial allergic rhinitics exhibit increased expression of the Fc epsilonRI, CD40L, IL-4, and IL-13, and can induce IgE synthesis in B cells. J Clin Invest 1997; 99:1492–1499.
35. Bressler RB, Lesko J, Jones ML, Wasserman M, Dickason RR, Huston MM, Cook SW, Huston DP. Production of IL-5 and granulocyte-macrophage colony-stimulating factor by naive human mast cells activated by high-affinity IgE receptor ligation. J Allergy Clin Immunol 1997; 99:508–514.
36. Gagari E, Tsai M, Lantz CS, Fox LG, Galli SJ. Differential release of mast cell interleukin-6 via c-kit. Blood 1997; 89:2654–2663.
37. Hultner L, Szots H, Welle M, Van Snick J, Moeller J, Dormer P. Mouse bone marrow-derived IL-3-dependent mast cells and autonomous sublines produce IL-6. Immunology 1989; 67:408–413.
38. Gomi K, Zhu FG, Marshall JS. Prostaglandin E2 selectively enhances the IgE-mediated production of IL-6 and granulocyte-macrophage colony-stimulating factor by mast cells through an EP1/EP3-dependent mechanism. J Immunol 2000; 165:6545–6552.
39. Stassen M, Arnold M, Hultner L, Muller C, Neudorfl C, Reineke T, Schmitt E. Murine bone marrow-derived mast cells as potent producers of IL-9: costimulatory function of IL-10 and kit ligand in the presence of IL-1. J Immunol 2000; 164:5549–5555.

40. Toru H, Pawankar R, Ra C, Yata J, Nakahata T. Human mast cells produce IL-13 by high-affinity IgE receptor cross-linking: enhanced IL-13 production by IL-4-primed human mast cells. J Allergy Clin Immunol 1998; 102:491–502.

41. Kobayashi H, Okayama Y, Ishizuka T, Pawankar R, Ra C, Mori M. Production of IL-13 by human lung mast cells in response to Fcepsilon receptor cross-linkage. Clin Exp Allergy 1998; 28:1219–1227.

42. Rumsaeng V, Cruikshank WW, Foster B, Prussin C, Kirshenbaum AS, Davis TA, Kornfeld H, Center DM, Metcalfe DD. Human mast cells produce the CD4$^+$ T lymphocyte chemoattractant factor, IL-16. J Immunol 1997; 159:2904–2910.

43. Williams CM, Coleman JW. Induced expression of mRNA for IL-5, IL-6, TNF-alpha, MIP-2 and IFN-gamma in immunologically activated rat peritoneal mast cells: inhibition by dexamethasone and cyclosporin A. Immunology 1995; 86:244–249.

44. Csonga R, Prieschl EE, Jaksche D, Novotny V, Baumruker T. Common and distinct signaling pathways mediate the induction of TNF-alpha and IL-5 in IgE plus antigen-stimulated mast cells. J Immunol 1998; 160:273–283.

45. Gupta AA, Leal-Berumen I, Croitoru K, Marshall JS. Rat peritoneal mast cells produce IFN-gamma following IL-12 treatment but not in response to IgE-mediated activation. J Immunol 1996; 157:2123–2128.

46. Moller A, Henz BM, Grutzkau A, Lippert U, Aragane Y, Schwarz T, Kruger-Krasagakes S. Comparative cytokine gene expression: regulation and release by human mast cells. Immunology 1998; 93:289–295.

47. Gordon JR, Galli SJ. Promotion of mouse fibroblast collagen gene expression by mast cells stimulated via the Fc epsilon RI. Role for mast cell-derived transforming growth factor beta and tumor necrosis factor alpha. J Exp Med 1994; 180:2027–2037.

48. Lin TJ, Issekutz TB, Marshall JS. Human mast cells transmigrate through human umbilical vein endothelial monolayers and selectively produce IL-8 in response to stromal cell-derived factor-1alpha. J Immunol 2000; 165:211–220.

49. Moller A, Lippert U, Lessmann D, Kolde G, Hamann K, Welker P, Schadendorf D, Rosenbach T, Luger T, Czarnetzki BM. Human mast cells produce IL-8. J Immunol 1993; 151:3261–3266.

50. Wakahara S, Fujii Y, Nakao T, Tsuritani K, Hara T, Saito H, Ra C. Gene expression profiles for FcepsilonRI, cytokines and chemokines upon FcepsilonRI activation in human cultured mast cells derived from peripheral blood. Cytokine 2001; 16:143–152.

51. Zhu FG, Gomi K, Marshall JS. Short-term and long-term cytokine release by mouse bone marrow mast cells and the differentiated KU-812 cell line are inhibited by brefeldin A. J Immunol 1998; 161:2541–2551.

52. Marquardt DL, Alongi JL, Walker LL. The phosphatidylinositol 3-kinase inhibitor wortmannin blocks mast cell exocytosis but not IL-6 production. J Immunol 1996; 156:1942–1945.

53. Henkel G, Brown MA. PU.1 and GATA: components of a mast cell-specific interleukin 4 intronic enhancer. Proc Natl Acad Sci USA 1994; 91:7737–7741.

54. Baumgartner RA, Yamada K, Deramo VA, Beaven MA. Secretion of TNF from a rat mast cell line is a Brefeldin A-sensitive and a calcium/protein kinase C-regulated process. J Immunol 1994; 153:2609–2614.

55. Hural JA, Kwan M, Henkel G, Hock MB, Brown MA. An intron transcriptional enhancer element regulates IL-4 gene locus accessibility in mast cells. J Immunol 2000; 165:3239–3249.

56. Sherman MA, Secor VH, Lee SK, Lopez RD, Brown MA. STAT6-independent production of IL-4 by mast cells. Eur J Immunol 1999; 29:1235–1242.

57. Sherman MA, Nachman TY, Brown MA. Cutting edge: IL-4 production by mast cells does not require c-maf. J Immunol 1999; 163:1733–1736.

58. Beil WJ, Login GR, Galli SJ, Dvorak AM. Ultrastructural immunogold localization of tumor necrosis factor-a to the cytoplasmic granules of rat peritoneal mast cells with rapid microwave fixation. J Allergy Clin Immunol 1994; 94:531–536.

59. Bacci S, Rucci L, Riccardi-Arbi R, Borghi-Cirri MB. Colocalization of tumor necrosis factor-alpha and nitric oxide-synthase immunoreactivity in mast cell granules of nasal mucosa. Histol Histopathol 1998; 13:1011–1014.

60. Wilson SJ, Shute JK, Holgate ST, Howarth PH, Bradding P. Localization of interleukin (IL)-4 but not IL-5 to human mast cell secretory granules by immunoelectron microscopy. Clin Exp Allergy 2000; 30:493–500.

61. Dragonetti A, Baldassarre M, Castino R, Demoz M, Luini A, Buccione R, Isidoro C. The lysosomal protease cathepsin D is efficiently sorted to and secreted from regulated secretory compartments in the rat basophilic/mast cell line RBL. J Cell Sci 2000; 113(Pt 18):3289–3298.

62. Turner H, Kinet JP. Signalling through the high-affinity IgE receptor Fc epsilonRI. Nature 1999; 402:B24–B30.

63. Leal-Berumen I, Conlon P, Marshall JS. IL-6 production by rat peritoneal mast cells is not necessarily preceded by histamine release and can be induced by bacterial lipopolysaccharide. J Immunol 1994; 152:5468–5476.

64. Wedemeyer J, Tsai M, Galli SJ. Roles of mast cells and basophils in innate and acquired immunity. Curr Opin Immunol 2000; 12:624–631.

65. Oku Y, Itayama H, Kamiya M. Expulsion of Trichinella spiralis from the intestine of W/Wv mice reconstituted with haematopoietic and lymphopoietic cells and origin of mucosal mast cells. Immunology 1984; 53:337–344.

66. Knight PA, Wright SH, Lawrence CE, Paterson YY, Miller HR. Delayed expulsion of the nematode Trichinella spiralis in mice lacking the mucosal mast cell-specific granule chymase, mouse mast cell protease-1. J Exp Med 2000; 192:1849–1856.

67. Galli SJ, Wershil BK. The two faces of the mast cell. Nature 1996; 381:21–22.

68. Echtenacher B, Mannel DN, Hultner L. Critical protective role of mast cells in a model of acute septic peritonitis. Nature 1996; 381:75–77.

69. Malaviya R, Ikeda T, Ross E, Abraham SN. Mast cell modulation of neutrophil influx and bacterial clearance at sites of infection through TNF-alpha. Nature 1996; 381: 77–80.

70. Gommerman JL, Oh DY, Zhou X, Tedder TF, Maurer M, Galli SJ, Carroll MC. A role for CD21/CD35 and CD19 in responses to acute septic peritonitis: a potential mechanism for mast cell activation. J Immunol 2000; 165:6915–6921.

71. Supajatura V, Ushio H, Nakao A, Okumura K, Ra C, Ogawa H. Protective roles of mast cells against enterobacterial infection are mediated by Toll-like receptor 4. J Immunol 2001; 167:2250–2256.

72. Malaviya R, Abraham SN. Role of mast cell leukotrienes in neutrophil recruitment and bacterial clearance in infectious peritonitis. J Leukoc Biol 2000; 67:841–846.

73. Maurer M, Echtenacher B, Hultner L, Kollias G, Mannel DN, Langley KE, Galli SJ. The c-kit ligand, stem cell factor, can enhance innate immunity through effects on mast cells. J Exp Med 1998; 188:2343–2348.

74. Galli SJ. New concepts about the mast cell. N Engl J Med 1993; 328:257–265.

75. Curry JJ. The action of histamine on the respiratory tract in normal and asthmatic subjects. J Clin Invest 1946; 25:785–791.

76. Casale TB, Wood D, Richerson HB, Trapp S, Metzger WJ, Zavala D, Hunning hake GW. Elevated bronchoalveolar lavage fluid histamine levels in allergic asthmatic are associated with methacholine bronchial hyperresponsiveness. J Clin Invest 1987 79:1197–1203.

77. Rankin JA, Kaliner M, Reynolds HY. Histamine levels in bronchoalveolar lavage from patients with asthma, sarcoidosis, and idiopathic pulmonary fibrosis. J Allergy Clin Immunol 1987; 79:371–377.

78. Nakamura T, Itadani H, Hidaka Y, Ohta M, Tanaka K. Molecular cloning and characterization of a new human histamine receptor, HH4R. Biochem Biophys Res Commun 2000; 279:615–620.

79. Oda T, Morikawa N, Saito Y, Masuho Y, Matsumoto S. Molecular cloning and characterization of a novel type of histamine receptor preferentially expressed in leukocytes J Biol Chem 2000; 275:36781–36786.

80. Arrang JM, Drutel G, Garbarg M, Ruat M, Traiffort E, Schwartz JC. Molecular and functional diversity of histamine receptor subtypes. Ann NY Acad Sci 1995; 757 314–323.

81. Marthan R, Crevel H, Guenard H, Savineau JP. Responsiveness to histamine in human sensitized airway smooth muscle. Respir Physiol 1992; 90:239–250.

82. Knight DA, Stewart GA, Thompson PJ. Prostaglandin E2, but not prostacyclin inhibit histamine-induced contraction of human bronchial smooth muscle. Eur J Pharmacol 1995; 272:13–19.

83. Ellis JL, Undem BJ. Role of cysteinyl-leukotrienes and histamine in mediating intrinsic tone in isolated human bronchi. Am J Respir Crit Care Med 1994; 149:118–122.

84. Johnson PR, Ammit AJ, Carlin SM, Armour CL, Caughey GH, Black JL. Mast cell tryptase potentiates histamine-induced contraction in human sensitized bronchus. Eur Respir J 1997; 10:38–43.

85. Panettieri RA, Yadvish PA, Kelly AM, Rubinstein NA, Kotlikoff MI. Histamine stimulates proliferation of airway smooth muscle and induces c-fos expression. Am J Physiol 1990; 259:L365–L371.

86. Webber SE, Salonen RO, Widdicombe JG. H1- and H2-receptor characterization in the tracheal circulation of sheep. Br J Pharmacol 1988; 95:551–561.

87. Evans TW, Rogers DF, Aursudkij B, Chung KF, Barnes PJ. Regional and time-dependent effects of inflammatory mediators on airway microvascular permeability in the guinea pig. Clin Sci (Lond) 1989; 76:479–485.

88. Delneste Y, Lassalle P, Jeannin P, Joseph M, Tonnel AB, Gosset P. Histamine induces IL-6 production by human endothelial cells. Clin Exp Immunol 1994; 98:344–349.

89. Jeannin P, Delneste Y, Gosset P, Molet S, Lassalle P, Hamid Q, Tsicopoulos A, Tonnel AB. Histamine induces interleukin-8 secretion by endothelial cells. Blood 1994; 84 2229–2233.

90. Noah TL, Paradiso AM, Madden MC, McKinnon KP, Devlin RB. The response of human bronchial epithelial cell line to histamine: intracellular calcium changes and extracellular release of inflammatory mediators. Am J Respir Cell Mol Biol 1991; 5 484–492.

91. Irokawa T, Nagaki M, Shimura S, Sasaki T, Yamaya M, Yamauchi K, Shirato K HMT regulates histamine-induced glycoconjugate secretion from human airways in vitro. Respir Physiol 1997; 108:233–240.

92. Tamaoki J, Nakata J, Takeyama K, Chiyotani A, Konno K. Histamine H2 receptor mediated airway goblet cell secretion and its modulation by histamine-degrading enzymes. J Allergy Clin Immunol 1997; 99:233–238.

93. Benson MK, Graf PD. Bronchial reactivity: interaction between vagal stimulation and inhaled histamine. J Appl Physiol 1977; 43:643–647.
94. Kikuchi Y, Okayama H, Okayama M, Sasaki H, Takishima T. Interaction between histamine and vagal stimulation on tracheal smooth muscle in dogs. J Appl Physiol 1984; 56:590–595.
95. Benson MK, Graf PD. Bronchial reactivity: interaction between vagal stimulation and inhaled histamine. J Appl Physiol 1977; 43:643–647.
96. Casterline CL, Evans R, Ward GW, Jr. The effect of atropine and albuterol aerosols on the human bronchial response to histamine. J Allergy Clin Immunol 1976; 58: 607–613.
97. Clark RA, Gallin JI, Kaplan AP. The selective eosinophil chemotactic activity of histamine. J Exp Med 1975; 142:1462–1476.
98. Clark RA, Sandler JA, Gallin JI, Kaplan AP. Histamine modulation of eosinophil migration. J Immunol 1977; 118:137–145.
99. Cluzel M, Liu MC, Goldman DW, Undem BJ, Lichtenstein LM. Histamine acting on a histamine type 1 (H1) receptor increases beta-glucuronidase release from human lung macrophages. Am J Respir Cell Mol Biol 1990; 3:603–609.
100. Bissonnette EY. Histamine inhibits tumor necrosis factor alpha release by mast cells through H2 and H3 receptors. Am J Respir Cell Mol Biol 1996; 14:620–626.
101. Mashikian MV, Tarpy RE, Saukkonen JJ, Lim KG, Fine GD, Cruikshank WW, Center DM. Identification of IL-16 as the lymphocyte chemotactic activity in the bronchoalveolar lavage fluid of histamine-challenged asthmatic patients. J Allergy Clin Immunol 1998; 101:786–792.
102. Mazzoni A, Young HA, Spitzer JH, Visintin A, Segal DM. Histamine regulates cytokine production in maturing dendritic cells, resulting in altered T cell polarization. J Clin Invest 2001; 108:1865–1873.
103. Caron G, Delneste Y, Roelandts E, Duez C, Bonnefoy JY, Pestel J, Jeannin P. Histamine polarizes human dendritic cells into Th2 cell-promoting effector dendritic cells. J Immunol 2001; 167:3682–3686.
104. Osna N, Elliott K, Chaika O, Patterson E, Lewis RE, Khan MM. Histamine utilizes JAK-STAT pathway in regulating cytokine production. Int Immunopharmacol 2001; 1:759–762.
105. Osna N, Elliott K, Khan MM. The effects of histamine on interferon gamma production are dependent on the stimulatory signals. Int Immunopharmacol 2001; 1:135–145.
106. Elliott KA, Osna NA, Scofield MA, Khan MM. Regulation of IL-13 production by histamine in cloned murine T helper type 2 cells. Int Immunopharmacol 2001; 1: 1923–1937.
107. Barnes PJ. Histamine and serotonin. Pulm Pharmacol Ther 2001; 14:329–339.
108. Stevens RL, Austen KF. Proteoglycans of the mast cell. Kroc Found Ser 1981; 14: 69–88.
109. Galli SJ. New insights into "the riddle of the mast cells": microenvironmental regulation of mast cell development and phenotypic heterogeneity. Lab Invest 1990; 62:5–33.
110. Enerback L. Mast cells in rat gastrointestinal mucosa. I. Effects of fixation. Acta Pathol Microbiol Scand 1966; 66:289–302.
111. Enerback L. Mast cells in rat gastrointestinal mucosa. 2. Dye-binding and metachromatic properties. Acta Pathol Microbiol Scand 1966; 66:303–312.
112. Beil WJ, Schulz M, Wefelmeyer U. Mast cell granule composition and tissue location—a close correlation. Histol Histopathol 2000; 15:937–946.

113. Uvnas B. Recent observations on mechanisms of storage and release of mast cell histamine. Applicability to other biogenic amines. Agents Actions Suppl 1992; 36 23–33.

114. Humphries DE, Wong GW, Friend DS, Gurish MF, Qiu WT, Huang C, Sharpe AH Stevens RL. Heparin is essential for the storage of specific granule proteases in mast cells. Nature 1999; 400:769–772.

115. Forsberg E, Pejler G, Ringvall M, Lunderius C, Tomasini-Johansson B, Kusche-Gullberg M, Eriksson I, Ledin J, Hellman L, Kjellen L. Abnormal mast cells in mice deficient in a heparin-synthesizing enzyme. Nature 1999; 400:773–776.

116. Friend DS, Ghildyal N, Austen KF, Gurish MF, Matsumoto R, Stevens RL. Mast cell that reside at different locations in the jejunum of mice infected with *Trichinella spiralis* exhibit sequential changes in their granule ultrastructure and chymase phenotype. Cell Biol 1996; 135:279–290.

117. Friend DS, Ghildyal N, Gurish MF, Hunt J, Hu X, Austen KF, Stevens RL. Reversible expression of tryptases and chymases in the jejunal mast cells of mice infected with *Trichinella spiralis*. J Immunol 1998; 160:5537–5545.

118. Lever R, Page C. Glycosaminoglycans, airways inflammation and bronchial hyperresponsiveness. Pulm Pharmacol Ther 2001; 14:249–254.

119. Lassila R, Lindstedt K, Kovanen PT. Native macromolecular heparin proteoglycan exocytosed from stimulated rat serosal mast cells strongly inhibit platelet-collagen interactions. Arterioscler Thromb Vasc Biol 1997; 17:3578–3587.

120. Tchougounova E, Pejler G. Regulation of extravascular coagulation and fibrinolysis by heparin-dependent mast cell chymase. FASEB J 2001; 15:2763–2765.

121. Tchougounova E, Forsberg E, Angelborg G, Kjellen L, Pejler G. Altered processing of fibronectin in mice lacking heparin a role for heparin-dependent mast cell chymase in fibronectin degradation. J Biol Chem 2001; 276:3772–3777.

122. Hallgren J, Karlson U, Poorafshar M, Hellman L, Pejler G. Mechanism for activation of mouse mast cell tryptase: dependence on heparin and acidic pH for formation of active tetramers of mouse mast cell protease 6. Biochemistry 2000; 39:13068–13077.

123. Huang C, Morales G, Vagi A, Chanasyk K, Ferrazzi M, Burklow C, Qiu WT, Feyfan E, Sali A, Stevens RL. Formation of enzymatically active, homotypic, and heterotypic tetramers of mouse mast cell tryptases. Dependence on a conserved Trp-rich domain on the surface. J Biol Chem 2000; 275:351–358.

124. Pereira PJ, Bergner A, Macedo-Ribeiro S, Huber R, Matschiner G, Fritz H, Sommerhof CP, Bode W. Human beta-tryptase is a ring-like tetramer with active sites facing a central pore. Nature 1998; 392:306–311.

125. Lindstedt L, Lee M, Kovanen PT. Chymase bound to heparin is resistant to its natural inhibitors and capable of proteolyzing high density lipoproteins in aortic intimal fluid Atherosclerosis 2001; 155:87–97.

126. Bock JB, Scheller RH. SNARE proteins mediate lipid bilayer fusion. Proc Natl Acad Sci USA 1999; 96:12227–12229.

127. Gonzalez LJ, Scheller RH. Regulation of membrane trafficking: structural insights from a Rab/effector complex. Cell 1999; 96:755–758.

128. Carr CM, Novick PJ. Membrane fusion. Changing partners. Nature 2000; 404:347–349

129. Sutton RB, Fasshauer D, Jahn R, Brunger AT. Crystal structure of a SNARE complex involved in synaptic exocytosis at 2.4 A resolution. Nature 1998; 395:347–353.

130. Wu MN, Fergestad T, Lloyd TE, He Y, Broadie K, Bellen HJ. Syntaxin 1A interacts with multiple exocytic proteins to regulate neurotransmitter release in vivo. Neuron 1999; 23:593–605.

131. Dulubova I, Sugita S, Hill S, Hosaka M, Fernandez I, Sudhof TC, Rizo J. A conformational switch in syntaxin during exocytosis: role of munc18. EMBO J 1999; 18: 4372–4382.

132. Jahn R. Sec1/Munc18 proteins: mediators of membrane fusion moving to center stage. Neuron 2000; 27:201–204.

133. Sassa T, Harada S, Ogawa H, Rand JB, Maruyama IN, Hosono R. Regulation of the UNC-18-caenorhabditis elegans syntaxin complex by UNC-13. J Neurosci 1999; 19: 4772–4777.

134. Betz A, Okamoto M, Benseler F, Brose N. Direct interaction of the rat unc-13 homologue Munc13-1 with the N terminus of syntaxin. J Biol Chem 1997; 272:2520–2526.

135. Nicholson KL, Munson M, Miller RB, Filip TJ, Fairman R, Hughson FM. Regulation of SNARE complex assembly by an N-terminal domain of the t-SNARE Sso1p. Nat Struct Biol 1998; 5:793–802.

136. Knight DA, Lim S, Scaffidi AK, Roche N, Chung KF, Stewart GA, Thompson PJ. Protease-activated receptors in human airways: upregulation of PAR-2 in respiratory epithelium from patients with asthma. J Allergy Clin Immunol 2001; 108:797–803.

137. Schimmoller F, Simon I, Pfeffer SR. Rab GTPases, directors of vesicle docking. J Biol Chem 1998; 273:22161–22164.

138. Augustine GJ. How does calcium trigger neurotransmitter release? Curr Opin Neurobiol 2001; 11:320–326.

139. Bai J, Wang P, Chapman ER. C2A activates a cryptic Ca(2+)-triggered membrane penetration activity within the C2B domain of synaptotagmin I. Proc Natl Acad Sci USA 2002; 99:1665–1670.

140. Hu K, Carroll J, Fedorovich S, Rickman C, Sukhodub A, Davletov B. Vesicular restriction of synaptobrevin suggests a role for calcium in membrane fusion. Nature 2002; 415:646–650.

141. Schulze KL, Broadie K, Perin MS, Bellen HJ. Genetic and electrophysiological studies of *Drosophila* syntaxin-1A demonstrate its role in nonneuronal secretion and neurotransmission. Cell 1995; 80:311–320.

142. Wu MN, Littleton JT, Bhat MA, Prokop A, Bellen HJ. ROP, the *Drosophila* Sec1 homolog, interacts with syntaxin and regulates neruotransmitter release in a dosage-dependent manner. EMBO J 1997; 17:127–139.

143. Washbourne P, Thompson PM, Carta M, Costa ET, Mathews JR, Lopez-Bendito G, Molnar Z, Becher MW, Valenzuela CF, Partridge LD, Wilson MC. Genetic ablation of the t-SNARE SNAP-25 distinguishes mechanisms of neuroexocytosis. Nat Neurosci 2002; 5:19–26.

144. Schoch S, Deak F, Konigstorfer A, Mozhayeva M, Sara Y, Sudhof TC, Kavalali ET. SNARE function analyzed in synaptobrevin/VAMP knockout mice. Science 2001; 294:1117–1122.

145. Verhage M, Mala AS, Plomp JJ, Brussaard AB, Heeroma JH, Vermeer H, Toonen RF, Hammer RE, van den Berg TK, Missler M, Geuze HJ, Sudhof TC. Synaptic assembly of the brain in the absence of neurotransmitter secretion. Science 2000; 287: 864–869.

146. Augustin I, Rosenmund C, Sudhof TC, Brose N. Munc13-1 is essential for fusion competence of glutamatergic synaptic vesicles. Nature 1999; 400:457–461.

147. Leenders AG, Lopes da Silva FH, Ghijsen WE, Verhage M. Rab3a is involved in transport of synaptic vesicles to the active zone in mouse brain nerve terminals. Mol Biol Cell 2001; 12:3095–3102.

148. Voets T, Moser T, Lund PE, Chow RH, Geppert M, Sudhof TC, Neher E. Intracellular calcium dependence of large dense-core vesicle exocytosis in the absence of synaptotagmin I. Proc Natl Acad Sci USA 2001; 98:11680–11685.

149. Ravichandran V, Chawla A, Roche PA. Identification of a novel syntaxin- and synaptobrevin/VAMP-binding protein, SNAP-23, expressed in non-neuronal tissues. J Biol Chem 1996; 271:13300–13303.

150. Steegmaier M, Yang B, Yoo JS, Huang B, Shen M, Yu S, Luo Y, Scheller RH. Three novel proteins of the syntaxin/SNAP-25 family. J Biol Chem 1998; 273:34171–34179.

151. Guo Z, Turner C, Castle D. Relocation of the t-SNARE SNAP-23 from lamellipodia-like cell surface projections regulates compound exocytosis in mast cells. Cell 1998; 94:537–548.

152. Paumet F, Le Mao J, Martin S, Galli T, David B, Blank U, Roa M. Soluble NSF attachment protein receptors (SNAREs) in RBL-2H3 mast cells: functional role of syntaxin 4 in exocytosis and identification of a vesicle-associated membrane protein 8-containing secretory compartment. J Immunol 2000; 164:5850–5857.

153. St Denis JF, Cabaniols JP, Cushman SW, Roche PA. SNAP-23 participates in SNARE complex assembly in rat adipose cells. Biochem J 1999; 338 (Pt 3):709–715.

154. Flaumenhaft R, Croce K, Chen E, Furie B, Furie BC. Proteins of the exocytotic core complex mediate platelet alpha-granule secretion. Roles of vesicle-associated membrane protein, snap-23, and syntaxin 4. J Biol Chem 1999; 274:2492–2501.

155. Vaidyanathan VV, Puri N, Roche PA. The last exon of SNAP-23 regulates granule exocytosis from mast cells. J Biol Chem 2001; 276:25101–25106.

156. Baram D, Adachi R, Medalia O, Tuvim M, Dickey BF, Mekori YA, Sagi-Eisenberg R. Synaptotagmin II negatively regulates Ca^{2+}-triggered exocytosis of lysosomes in mast cells. J Exp Med 1999; 189:1649–1658.

157. Baram D, Linial M, Mekori YA, Sagi-Eisenberg R. Ca^{2+}-dependent exocytosis in mast cells is stimulated by the Ca^{2+} sensor, synaptotagmin I. J Immunol 1998; 161: 5120–5123.

158. Butz S, Fernandez-Chacon R, Schmitz F, Jahn R, Sudhof TC. The subcellular localizations of atypical synaptotagmins III and VI. J Biol Chem 1999; 274:18290–18296.

159. Sugita S, Shin OH, Han W, Lao Y, Sudhof TC. Synaptotagmins form a hierarchy of exocytotic Ca(2+) sensors with distinct Ca(2+) affinities. EMBO J 2002; 21: 270–280.

160. Mizuta M, Kurose T, Miki T, Shoji-Kasai Y, Takahashi M, Seino S, Matsukura S. Localization and functional role of synaptotagmin III in insulin secretory vesicles in pancreatic beta-cells. Diabetes 1997; 46:2002–2006.

161. Brown H, Meister B, Deeney J, Corkey BE, Yang SN, Larsson O, Rhodes CJ, Seino S, Berggren PO, Fried G. Synaptotagmin III isoform is compartmentalized in pancreatic beta-cells and has a functional role in exocytosis. Diabetes 2000; 49:383–391.

162. Gao Z, Reavey-Cantwell J, Young RA, Jegier P, Wolf BA. Synaptotagmin III/VII isoforms mediate Ca^{2+}-induced insulin secretion in pancreatic islet beta-cells. J Biol Chem 2000; 275:36079–36085.

163. Von Poser C, Sudhof TC. Synaptotagmin 13: structure and expression of a novel synaptotagmin. Eur J Cell Biol 2001; 80:41–47.

164. Sudhof TC, Rizo J. Synaptotagmins: C_2-domain proteins that regulate membrane traffic. Neuron 1996; 17:379–388.

165. Sutton RB, Ernst JA, Brunger AT. Crystal structure of the cytosolic C2A-C2B domains of synaptotagmin III. Implications for Ca(+2)-independent snare complex interaction. J Cell Biol 1999; 147:589–598.

166. Kim TD, Eddlestone GT, Mahmoud SF, Kuchtey J, Fewtrell C. Correlating Ca^{2+} responses and secretion in individual RBL-2H3 mucosal mast cells. J Biol Chem 1997; 272:31225–31229.

167. Kuchtey J, Fewtrell C. Protein kinase C activator PMA reduces the $Ca(2+)$ response to antigen stimulation of adherent RBL-2H3 mucosal mast cells by inhibiting depletion of intracellular $Ca(2+)$ stores. J Cell Physiol 1999; 181:113–123.

168. Fischer von Mollard G, Sudhof TC, Jahn R. A small GTP-binding protein dissociates from synaptic vesicles during exocytosis. Nature 1991; 349:79–81.

169. Tuvim MJ, Adachi R, Chocano JF, Moore RH, Lampert RM, Zera E, Romero E, Knoll BJ, Dickey BF. Rab3D, a small GTPase, is localized on mast cell secretory granules and translocates to the plasma membrane upon exocytosis. Am J Respir Cell Mol Biol 1999; 20:79–89.

170. Roa M, Paumet F, Le Mao J, David B, Blank U. Involvement of the ras-like GTPase rab3d in RBL-2H3 mast cell exocytosis following stimulation via high affinity IgE receptors. J Immunol 1997; 159:2815–2823.

171. Baldini G, Scherer PE, Lodish HF. Nonneuronal expression of rab3A: induction during adipogenesis and association with different intracellular membranes than rab3D. Proc Natl Acad Sci USA 1995; 92:4284–4288.

172. Adachi R, Nigam R, Tuvim MJ, DeMayo F, Dickey BF. Genomic organization, chromosomal localization, and expression of the murine RAB3D gene. Biochem Biophys Res Commun 2000; 273:877–883.

173. Masuda ES, Luo Y, Young C, Shen M, Rossi AB, Huang BC, Yu S, Bennett MK, Payan DG, Scheller RH. Rab37 is a novel mast cell specific GTPase localized to secretory granules. FEBS Lett 2000; 470:61–64.

174. Pinxteren JA, O'Sullivan AJ, Larbi KY, Tatham PE, Gomperts BD. Thirty years of stimulus-secretion coupling: from $Ca(2+)$ to GTP in the regulation of exocytosis. Biochimie 2000; 82:385–393.

175. Fernandez-Chacon R, De Toledo GA, Hammer RE, dhof TC. Analysis of SCAMP1 function in secretory vesicle exocytosis by means of gene targeting in mice. J Biol Chem 1999; 274:32551–32554.

176. Kinet JP. The high-affinity IgE receptor (Fc epsilon RI): from physiology to pathology. Annu Rev Immunol 1999; 17:931–972.

177. Marom Z, Shelhamer J, Berger M, Frank M, Kaliner M. Anaphylatoxin C3a enhances mucous glycoprotein release from human airways in vitro. J Exp Med 1985; 161:657–668.

178. Hilfiker S, Augustine GJ. Regulation of synaptic vesicle fusion by protein kinase C. J Physiol (Lond) 1999; 515:1.

179. De Vries KJ, Geijtenbeek A, Brian EC, de Graan PN, Ghijsen WE, Verhage M. Dynamics of munc18-1 phosphorylation/dephosphorylation in rat brain nerve terminals. Eur J Neurosci 2000; 12:385–390.

180. Rhee JS, Betz A, Pyott S, Relm K, Varoqueaux F, Augustin I, Hesse D, Sudhof TC, Takahashi M, Rosenmund C, Brose N. Beta phorbol ester- and diacylglycerol-induced augmentation of transmitter release is mediated by Munc13s and not by PKCs. Cell 2002; 108:121–133.

181. Hilfiker S, Pieribone VA, Nordstedt C, Greengard P, Czernik AJ. Regulation of synaptotagmin I phosphorylation by multiple protein kinases. J Neurochem 1999; 73:921–932.

182. Pombo I, Martin-Verdeaux S, Iannascoll B, Le Mao J, Deriano L, Rivera J, Blank U. IgE receptor type I-dependent regulation of a Rab3D-associated kinase: a possible link in the calcium-dependent assembly of SNARE complexes. J Biol Chem 2001; 276:42893–42900.

17

Mast Cell Proteases

KENNETH C. FANG and GEORGE H. CAUGHEY

University of California at San Francisco
San Francisco, California, U.S.A.

I. Introduction

Mast cell proteases attract the attention of scientists and clinicians alike because they are the major proteins stored and secreted by mast cells and are useful markers of mast cell activation (1,2). For many years they have provided a basis for distinguishing mast cell subpopulations and, more recently, have emerged as targets for development of drugs to treat allergic diseases. These enzymes have been comprehensively reviewed in the past (1–3). This chapter provides an updated overview of major proteases expressed by mast cells, emphasizing enzymes that are secreted and are known or suspected to contribute to asthma and other varieties of allergic inflammation (see Table 1).

II. Serine Proteases

A. Tryptases

Intracellular Tryptic Enzymes in Mast Cells

Serine-class proteases use the side chain of the amino acid serine to attack and hydrolyze links between amino acids in target peptides and proteins. In most human mast cells, the dominant serine proteases are termed "tryptases" because, like trypsin,

Table 1 Mast Cell Proteases

Protease	Suspected actions in asthma
Serine class	
Tryptases	
α	Uncertain; may be catalytically inactive
βI, II, & III	Destroy bronchodilating peptides
	Promote subepithelial fibrosis and smooth muscle hyperplasia
	Activate stromelysin and degrade matrix
	Recruit inflammatory cells
	Enhance bronchoconstriction
	Activate PAR-2
γ	Unclear; probably membrane anchored
Chymase	Degrades and remodels matrix
	Stimulates gland cell secretion
	Regulates of vessel caliber and growth via angiotensin II
Cathepsin G	Actions resemble those of chymase
	Inflicts epithelial damage
Tissue plasminogen activator	Influences tissue remodeling and response to injury
Metallo class	
Gelatinases A & B	Promote epithelial remodeling and angiogenesis
	Promote inflammatory cell infiltration
Collagenase	Promotes airway epithelial and vascular remodeling
Stromelysin	Promotes epithelial remodeling
Carboxypeptidase A	Destroys vasoactive peptides
Thiol class	
DPPI/Cathepsin C	Activation of chymase, cathepsin G, and tryptases

they cleave peptides after lysine or arginine (4). When first sighted over four decades ago (5), mast cell tryptic enzymes were noted to be active intracellularly, an unusual feature not true of pancreatic trypsinogen, which is secreted as an inactive zymogen and activated extracellularly. Tryptase activity was detected in several mammals but was especially prominent in humans, where it was unusually resistant to circulating inhibitors of most other trypsin-like proteases and provoked inflammation when injected into skin (6,7). Tryptases were characterized in highly purified form in the early 1980s (8–10) and the first cDNAs and genes were cloned by the end of the decade (11–13), revealing distinct structural and enzymatic differences between tryptases and other members of the fecund family of trypsin-like serine proteases.

α-Tryptases

We now know a great deal more about tryptases. They are expressed mainly in mast cells and to a limited extent in basophils (14–16). Human mast cells express up to three major isoforms: α, β, and γ. α-Tryptase behaves idiosyncratically (12,17). Unlike β, α is secreted constitutively rather than being stored with histamine and heparin in secretory granules. Due to a mutation in its propeptide, α may be incapable of conversion to an enzymatically competent form (18) and has never been isolated from human tissues as an active protease. However, when provisioned with an artificial propeptide that is removed in vitro, recombinant α is weakly active but with activity towards peptidic substrates sharply reduced compared with human β and other mammalian tryptases (19). α-Tryptase is the major tryptase circulating in the bloodstream at baseline in most individuals and can reach high levels in systemic mastocytosis (20), perhaps in its inactive, proenzyme form (21). High baseline serum levels may also be a risk factor for severe allergic reactions to *Hymenoptera* venom (22). Because α is secreted constitutively, blood levels are thought to reflect total mast cell burden. However, genetic deficiency of α-tryptase is fairly common (23) with an individual inheriting zero, one, or two α genes. Indeed, it appears that α alleles compete with βl alleles at one tryptase locus, with a second locus being occupied exclusively by βII and βIII alleles (24). Thus, individuals inherit as few as two or as many as four β alleles. It remains to be determined whether differences in inheritance of α- and β-tryptase genes affect susceptibility to allergic diseases or responses to treatment.

β-Tryptases

β-Isoforms are the major tryptases stored in secretory granules and are released in parallel with histamine (25). Their appearance in blood after systemic mast cell degranulation helps to diagnose pre- and postmortem anaphylaxis. They are also the isoforms purified from extracts of tissues or mast cell preparations. Three types of β have been identified, I, II, and III, which are 98–99% identical in amino acid sequence. There is no evidence of functional differences between the β isoforms (17). Indeed, βI and II have been expressed recombinantly and compared directly, with no difference in substrate preferences (26). Tryptases purified from human tissues are likely to represent a mixture of β-isoforms. β-Tryptases are stored and secreted as self-compartmentalized, noncovalent assemblages of four catalytically competent subunits, as demonstrated by the structure derived from crystals of βII (27). This tetramer is donut-shaped, with each active site facing a central cavity (Fig. 1). Substrates and inhibitors gain access to tryptase catalytic sites by entering the cavity. This toroidal configuration is the basis for the exceptional resistance of β-tryptases to circulating protease inhibitors, most of which are too large to enter the cavity. Following exocytosis from the secretory granule, human β-tryptase remains associated with heparin proteoglycan, which stabilizes the tetramer against dissociation into inactive monomers.

Natural Substrates of β-Tryptases

Not surprisingly, given the small size of the central cavity, β-tryptases are not general proteases like trypsins but do avidly hydrolyze a variety of small peptide-based substrates. Identified natural targets include the neuropeptides vasoactive intestinal

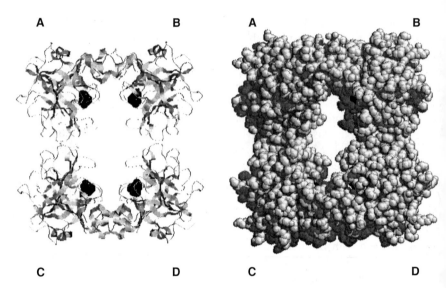

Figure 1 Structure of the human mast cell β-tryptase tetramer. These images were created in RasMol using the crystallographic coordinates of protein database file 1AOL (see Ref. 27). The left panel shows the four subunits (A–D) of the tryptase tetramer in ribbon format, with a small inhibitor (black space-filling model) occupying each of the four active sites, which face a central pore. The right panel shows a space-filling model of the entire tetramer (gray), plus inhibitor (black), revealing the restricted nature of the active sites. This structure reveals the basis of tryptase's resistance to circulating antiproteases, which are too big to gain access to the active sites in the central pore. The outside edges of the catalytic domains of tryptase released from mast cells are bridged by heparin, which stabilizes the tetrameric configuration.

peptide and calcitonin gene–related peptide (28,29) Tryptase-mediated inactivation of these peptides may limit the activity of these peptides in bronchorelaxation and cutaneous flare responses in the context of neurogenic inflammation. β-Tryptases also generate bradykinins by activating prekallikrein (30) or by acting on fragments of kininogen that first are hydrolyzed by a general protease, such as neutrophil elastase (31). In some instances, tryptases hydrolyze protein targets that would seem too large to enter the tetramer's central cavity. These targets include fibrinogen (32) and the proenzyme forms of stromelysin (33) and urokinase (34). Presumably these and other large substrates possess dangling ends or projecting loops that can reach the interior of the cavity. Some targets of tryptase may be proteins anchored to the cell surface. Among these are proteinase-activated receptor-2 (PAR-2) (35,36), which may provide a molecular link between tryptase release and stimulation of nerves, airway epithelium, and mitogenic responses (37). Tryptase hydrolyzes synthetic peptides based on PAR-2 activation sequence with efficiency similar to that of pancreatic trypsin (36,38). However, tryptase is weaker than trypsin in activating intact PAR-2 on the cell surface (38) and PAR-2's sensitivity to activation by tryptase depends on its degree of posttranslational modification by glycosylation, as well as on the amount of heparin with which it is associated (39). These observations suggest that access of PAR-2's activation sequence to tryptase catalytic sites is easily blocked.

Roles of β-Tryptases in Airway Responsiveness and Fibrosis

Several studies suggest a connection between tryptase release and airway hyperresponsiveness (40–43). The mechanisms are not yet clear but may relate to hydrolysis of bronchodilating peptides (29) and cell surface proteins regulating calcium flux (40) or to spread of mast cell degranulation signals (44). In vitro, β-tryptases are mitogenic for several types of cells, including fibroblasts (45), airway smooth muscle cells (46), and epithelial cells (47). Some of these effects may be mediated by PAR-2, but others not. Additionally, when exposed to human fibroblasts, β-tryptases stimulate chemotaxis (48) and collagen synthesis (49). These effects on fibroblasts support the possibility that tryptase promotes subendothelial fibrosis and collagen deposition in chronic asthma.

Roles of β-Tryptases in Anticoagulation, Fibrinolysis, and Angiogenesis

In the vicinity of the degranulating mast cell, β-tryptases may help to create a "fibrin-free zone" by destroying fibrin's precursor, fibrinogen (32,50), and by activating urokinase (34), which then activates plasmin to degrade polymerized fibrin. In this respect, tryptases act concertedly with heparin, a component of the secretory granule to which β-tryptase remains attached after exocytosis. These anticoagulant and profibrinolytic effects of the secreted tryptase-heparin complex may facilitate egress of extravasated host defense proteins and inflammatory cells to sites of tissue invasion or injury signaled by mast cell degranulation, β-Tryptases also stimulate release of IL-8 from epithelial and endothelial cells (47,51) and degranulation of nearby mast cells. These actions may explain why β-tryptase injected into skin (7,52) or lung promotes neutrophil accumulation (53). When placed in the airways of mast cell–deficient mice, human β-tryptase partially protects the animals from *Klebsiella pneumoniae* infection (53), presumably by recruiting neutrophils. Tryptases also induce endothelial cells to form tube-like structures (54,55) and thus may play a role in endothelial differentiation and angiogenesis.

Development of β-Tryptase Inhibitors

Because of the suspected importance of tryptases in human disease, several laboratories have developed tryptase inhibitors for research and clinical applications. This is challenging because of the resistance of β-tryptases to inactivation by natural inhibitor proteins. The first high-potency, reversible inhibitors of human β-tryptases identified were dibasic aromatic compounds, such as BABIM (bis-5-amidino-2-benzimidazolyl methane) (56). BABIM supported the importance of tryptases in

asthma by inhibiting airway inflammation, bronchoconstriction, and hyperresponsiveness in a sheep model of allergic airway inflammation (41). However, BABIM
and closely similar compounds are not selective for β-tryptase, especially in comparison with trypsin (56–58). The recognition that BABIM and its relatives inactivate
tryptase and trypsin by forming a ternary complex involving enzyme, inhibitor, and
Zn^{2+} (59) led to the development of potent inhibitors with higher selectivity (60).
The first tryptase inhibitor to be tested in humans was the peptidic compound APC-
366, which was efficacious in sheep (41) but was comparatively weak, slow-acting,
and nonselective as a human β-tryptase inhibitor. This compound showed a small
but statistically significant reduction in late asthmatic responses in a phase Ia trial
(61). Subsequent pharmaceutical development has focused on nonpeptidic compounds of higher potency, selectivity, and bioavailability. This includes the dibasic
aromatic inhibitor APC-2059, which has advanced to human testing in trials of
psoriasis, ulcerative colitis, and asthma (62). Two of the more innovative attempts
to boost selectivity involve creating divalent inhibitors bridging active sites across
β-tryptase's most unique feature, its central cavity (63,64). Several other dibasic,
aromatic tryptase inhibitors are active in animal models of allergic inflammation
(65,66). Although later-generation dibasic inhibitors are potent and selective, they
tend to have low oral absorption. Some success with developing more absorbable
inhibitors has been achieved (67). A natural inhibitor protein derived from the medicinal leech has also been identified (68). Unlike most natural inhibitors, it is small
enough to fit within β-tryptase's central cavity (69) β-Tryptase inactivation by two
larger proteins, lactoferrin and myeloperoxidase, is slow in onset. These proteins,
which are not classical protease inhibitors, appear to destabilize the active tetramer
by competing for tryptase-bound heparin (70,71), which may be an endogenous
mechanism by which the heparin-bound β-tryptase tetramer is inactivated following
secretion.

γ-Tryptases

The most recently described member of the human mast cell tryptase family is γ,
which differs from α and β most notably in containing a predicted membrane anchor
(24,72). It is the product of a separate gene locus, which is the telomeric neighbor
of βII/βIII. Its enzymatic behavior and function are not known. However, it is likely
to differ from α and β in mode of activation and tendency to oligomerize; moreover,
its expression appears to be more tissue-restricted and less robust than that of β-
tryptases. Because it is predicted to be membrane-anchored and is not known to be
released in a soluble form, it may act at the cell surface, perhaps in the context of
cell-cell contact.

B. Chymase and Cathepsin G

Human chymase and cathepsin G are structurally related serine proteases stored in
(and secreted from) granules of MC_C and MC_{TC} mast cells (14,73–76). Both enzymes are highly charged and bind strongly to polyanionic proteoglycans, such as
heparin. The genes encoding these enzymes are next-door neighbors on chromosome

14q11.1–.2 (77). Despite similarities in protein structure (Fig. 2) and chromosomal location, the enzymes differ in expression and behavior. Whereas chymase expression is limited primarily to mast cells, cathepsin G is expressed in neutrophils as well as mast cells (73,78). Chymase is decidedly chymotryptic in its substrate preferences, avidly hydrolyzing targets containing aromatic amino acids, whereas cathepsin G is weaker and much less specific, hydrolyzing after either basic or aromatic amino acids. Chymase-expressing mast cells are a much higher percentage of the mast cell population in human airway tissues (79) than in the pulmonary parenchyma. Human chymase's most outstanding attribute is its ability to convert angiotensin I to vasoactive angiotensin II. Chymase is even more efficient than angiotensin-converting enzyme in this regard and appears to be the major extravascular generator of angiotensin II in humans. Chymase-mediated angiotensin II generation may be responsible for acute vasomotor effects, such as endotoxin-mediated vasoconstriction (80) as well as slower-to-develop effects such as vascular stenosis after angioplasty (81). The importance of chymase-generated angiotensin II in airway disease is unclear, although it could play a role in vascular remodeling. Chymase also cleaves procolla-

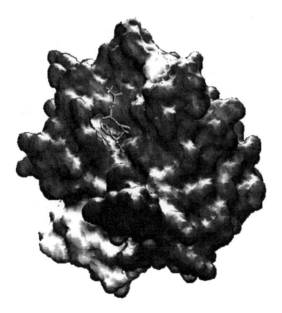

Figure 2 Structure of the human α-chymase monomer. This image was created in Swiss-PdbViewer based on the coordinates of protein database file 1 pjp (see Ref. 76). In this view, the substrate-binding site faces frontward in the center of the chymase catalytic domain, which is surface-contoured to reveal the topography of the active site. The upper section of the active site is occupied by a succinyl-Ala-Ala-Pro-Phe-based peptide depicted by the stick model. Prominent features of the substrate-binding site include a deep hydrophobic cleft accommodating the substrate phenyalanine's aromatic side chain, as shown, and a wide shelf at the base of active site.

gen I to initiate fibril formation, degrades gelatin and collagen VI (55,82), and influences matrix turnover indirectly by activating metalloproteinases (see below). By solubilizing latent transforming growth factor β1 from extracellular matrix, chymase may also stimulate fibroblast growth and matrix protein deposition (83). Therefore, chymase may help to remodel airway tissues in the setting of chronic allergic inflammation. Chymase also may regulate airway hyperresponsiveness by cleaving big endothelin to generate novel trachea-constricting endothelins (84). Chymase induction of mucus secretion from airway submucosal serious cells (85) and cleavage of degranulated chondroitin sulfate (86) suggest that its proteolytic activity may also influence airway gland secretions and patency. Based on this and other evidence of roles for chymase in cardiac, vascular, and pulmonary disease, several groups of investigators have developed potent and selective inhibitors of chymase, so that we may soon have a test of its importance in humans (87–89).

C. Tissue-Type Plasminogen Activator

Human lung mast cells express and secrete tissue-type plasminogen activator (tPA) (90). The importance of mast cell production of this enzyme is not yet established. Presumably, like heparin, tryptase and tryptase-activated urokinase, mast cell tPA helps to maintain the aforementioned fibrin-free zone in the vicinity of activated mast cells. Unlike many other tPA-secreting cells, mast cells release tPA without co-secreting plasminogen activator inhibitors, thereby increasing the likelihood of generating fibrinolytic plasmin near mast cells.

III. Matrix Metalloproteinases

A. Matrix Metalloproteinases in Inflammation

Hydrolysis of matrix proteins by a family of zinc-dependent matrix metalloproteinases (MMPs) regulates tissue invasion by inflammatory cells and deposition of extracellular proteins (91). MMPs may regulate critical aspects of airway inflammation and remodeling, which contribute to the development of irreversible airflow obstruction in chronic disease. Activity of MMPs in a given milieu depends upon secretion by a variety of inflammatory, epithelial, and mesenchymal cells, conversion of secreted proenzymes into active forms (Fig. 3), and control of activity by tissue inhibitors of metalloproteinases (TIMPs) (91). Mast cells secrete gelatinase-, collagenase-, and stromelysin-class MMPs and also secrete some of the four characterized TIMPs (92–100). Mast cells also use tryptase and chymase to regulate local MMP activity (33,96–99,101–103).

B. Mast Cell Gelatinases

Proteolysis of gelatin is a defining characteristic of the gelatinase class of MMPs, which include gelatinases A (MMP-2) and B (MMP-9). Gelatinase B is the principal MMP implicated in allergic airway remodeling (91). Progelatinase B, like other pro-MMPs, is inactive due to coordination of the active site zinc cation by a sulfhydryl

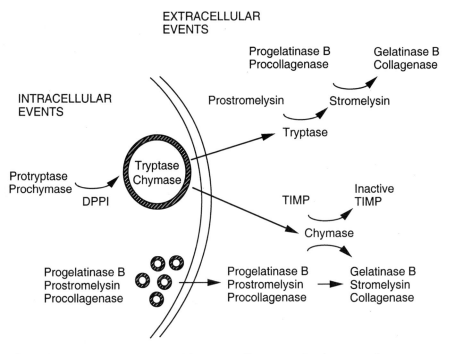

Figure 3 Activation cascades involving mast cell proteases. Prochymase and protryptases are activated intracellularly by removal of propeptide by dipeptidyl peptidase I, with or without assistance from other activating enzymes. Preactivated chymase and tryptases are stored in secretory granules along with histamine and heparin and are released in a regulated fashion in response to stimuli such as antigen-bound IgE crosslinking surface-expressed FcεRI. By contrast, mast cell pro-MMPs, such as progelatinase B, prostromelysin, and procollagenase, are released from separate granule compartments through largely constitutive pathways as inactive proenzymes, which can also be complexed with inhibitor. Secreted chymase activates the proenzyme forms of these MMPs by cleaving the proenzymes and, in the case of inhibitor-bound progelatinase B, by destroying enzyme-bound TIMP-1. Tryptases are not able to activate procollagenase and progelatinases directly, but do so indirectly by activating prostromelysin, which then activates other MMPs. Thus, MMP activation is coupled to exocytotic release of mast cell serine proteases.

group of the cysteine residue in the propeptide. Disruption of this so-called cysteine switch activates the zymogen, which undergoes autoproteolysis to additional active and inactive forms (104). Proteolytic activation of progelatinase B occurs via removal of the prodomain by serine proteases such as mast cell chymase (96,97), and by other MMPs such as collagenase, stromelysin (105), matrilysin, and gelatinase A (106). Zymography detects gelatinases via degradation of gelatin imbedded in polyacrylamide gels (107), revealing 92 kDa progelatinase B and other isoforms, including a ~200 kDa homodimer, and active forms of 68, 84, and 88 kDa generated by autoproteolysis (96). It should be stressed that inactive zymogens and TIMP-bound gelatinases cleave gelatin after electrophoresis due to electrophoretic dissociation of the TIMP-gelatinase complex and detergent-induced disruption of the cysteine switch. For this reason, demonstration of activity by zymography does not necessarily predict activity in solution and in the native state. Nonetheless, zymography is a highly sensitive method of assessing relative abundance of proenzyme and cleaved forms of gelatinases.

Mast cells in human and canine lung tissues, established mast cell lines, and mast cells derived from peripheral or cord blood secrete gelatinase B, whose expression can be induced by phorbol ester, lipopolysaccharide, or by co-culture with T cells activated by tumor necrosis factor (94,96–98,108,109). Mast cells and neutrophils both store gelatinase B in granules, which may serve as a reservoir for controlled exocytosis (108,110). c-Kit ligand upregulates gelatinase B expression in canine mast cells via intracellular signaling pathways involving phospholipase C, protein kinase C, and calcium. This upregulation is attenuated by transforming growth factor-α (98). By contrast, ligation of kit receptor on mouse bone marrow–derived or IC-2 mast cells downregulates gelatinase B production (93).

C. Activation of Mast Cell Gelatinases

Hydrolysis of MMP prodomains by tryptase and chymase involves activation cascades unique to mast cells. Tryptase and chymase activate progelatinase B via indirect and direct pathways, respectively. As already noted, tryptase activates prostromelysin (33), which in turn activates progelatinase B (105). Chymase, however, cleaves progelatinase B directly to remove the prodomain, an event accelerated by heparin. Chymase-activated gelatinase B is less active than the enzyme activated by trypsin, which cleaves a different site. The lower activity of chymase-generated gelatinase B may be due to the absence of an NH_2-terminal phenylalanine, resulting in a disordered NH_2-terminal hexapeptide affecting substrate interactions (96,97). Since mast cells store tryptases and chymase in granules separate from those containing gelatinase B, progelatinase activation by these proteases depends on mast cell activation and degranulation. At present, mast cells are the sole example of cells that activate an MMP by co-secreting an activating enzyme (96). Chymase also regulates progelatinase B activity by cleaving TIMP-1, destroying its inhibitory capacity. Chymase hydrolyzes TIMP-1 in both its free and gelatinase-complexed forms. Chymase-mediated destruction of gelatinase-bound TIMP-1 increases gelatinolytic activity, suggesting that chymase can reverse the effect of TIMP inhibition (99).

D. Gelatinases in Asthma

Inhibition of gelatinase B by TIMP-1 predicts that the ratio of TIMP-1 to gelatinase B in airway lumen and extracellular interstitium affects development of subepithelial fibrosis and inflammatory cell recruitment. Clinical studies identify gelatinase B and TIMP-1 as the major MMP and TIMP in bronchial biopsies (111), sputum, and bronchoalveolar lavage fluid (BAL) in asthmatics (112). Compared to levels in healthy patients, an excess of TIMP-1 over gelatinase B prevails in sputum (113) and BAL (112) from untreated, stable asthmatics. Thus, TIMP-1 is overexpressed relative to gelatinase B in stable asthma. Furthermore, activated forms of gelatinase B are absent (112). By contrast, an excess of gelatinase B and free gelatinolytic activity exists in the BAL from patients with uncontrolled asthma or those with a severe exacerbation (114).

Since several cell types involved in asthmatic inflammation secrete gelatinase B and TIMP-1, their main cellular source in asthmatic airways is unclear. In addition to mast cells, sources of gelatinase B may include epithelial cells (115), airway smooth muscle cells (116), eosinophils (117), macrophages (112), and neutrophils (110). Dexamethasone attenuates synthesis of gelatinase B and TIMP-1 by alveolar macrophages from healthy subjects (118) and patients with asthma, regardless of inhaled steroid use (119). In addition, low TIMP-1:gelatinase B ratios are found in subjects with little or no improvement in FEV_1 with steroid use, suggesting that poorly reversible bronchial fibrosis may predominate over inflammation in these patients (120). Inhaled corticosteroids reduce the size of the reticular basement membrane and decrease gelatinase B immunoreactivity, while that of TIMP-1 increases (121). Investigations of mechanical stress on human bronchial epithelial cells (in an in vitro system without inflammatory cells) demonstrate stress-induced increases in gelatinase B and decreases in TIMP-1 expression, lowering the TIMP-1:gelatinase B ratio (122). A mouse model of allergen-induced airway inflammation demonstrates that gelatinase A and B levels increase in BAL fluid following ovalbumin inhalation in sensitized animals, with infiltration of inflammatory cells. Airway administration of TIMP or a synthetic MMP inhibitor reduced antigen-induced inflammatory cell infiltration, while TIMP decreased antigen-induced airway hyperresponsiveness (123). These data implicate gelatinases in inflammatory cell recruitment and the development of airway hyperresponsiveness.

E. Gelatinases in Angiogenesis

Increased vascularity of the bronchial mucosa in asthma suggests that angiogenesis occurs during airway remodeling and may contribute to the development of irreversible airflow obstruction. Bronchial biopsies from patients with mild asthma demonstrate an increase in the number and size of blood vessels (124), which correlates with airflow hyperresponsiveness and changes in FEV_1 (125). Gelatinase B regulates signaling of endothelial cells in remodeling tissues by releasing sequestered angiogenic activators, as shown by delayed angiogenesis in bone growth plates in gelatinase B-null mice (126). By releasing chymase, which activates progelatinase B, mast cells switch tissues to an angiogenic phenotype. During activation of angiogenesis in a murine model of squamous epithelial carcinogenesis, mast cells infiltrate premalignant tissues and accumulate around capillaries and epithelial basement membranes where they degranulate and release stored tryptase and chymase. Attenuation of early neoplasia in mast cell–deficient mice suggests the possible importance of secreted mast cell serine proteases in initiating tissue angiogenesis (55).

F. Nongelatinase Mast Cell MMPs

Mast cells also secrete other subclasses of MMPs implicated in tissue remodeling. Hydrolysis of collagens I–III, VII, and X is a distinguishing characteristic of the collagenase class of MMPs, which includes interstitial (MMP-1) or neutrophil (MMP-8) collagenase and collagenase-3 (MMP-13) (127). Both cultured HMC-1 mast cells and tryptase- and chymase-positive human tissue mast cells express collagenases (100), which are implicated in airway and vascular remodeling (92,128–130). Mast cell serine proteases activate procollagenase in a manner analogous to their activation of progelatinase B. Tryptase cannot cleave the proenzyme, but rather participates indirectly by first activating prostromelysin, which then activates procollagenase (33). By contrast, human, canine, and rat chymases directly cleave and activate procollagenase (101–103). Co-localization of collagenase to mast cells and evidence of mast cell degranulation in remodeling pulmonary arteries support a role for tryptase and chymase in procollagenase activation in vivo (92,128). Immunohistochemical techniques detect increased collagenase in asthmatic airway smooth muscle, while tissue extracts reveal marked increases in collagenase compared to healthy controls. Since collagenase cleavage of insulin-like growth factor (IGF)–binding protein modulates IGF activity in airway smooth muscle cells, collagenase may induce asthmatic smooth muscle hyperplasia and airway obstruction (129). Immunolocalization of collagenase to mast cells during hypoxia-induced pulmonary artery remodeling suggests that recruitment of collagenase-expressing mast cells to the adventitia and media of hypertensive vessels may play a role in the restoration of normal vascular architecture (92,128). Additionally, co-expression of tryptase and collagenase by cells in atherosclerotic lesions suggests that mast cells and degranulation of procollagenase-activating serine proteases may destabilize arterial plaques (130).

Mast cells also express members of the stromelysin subclass of MMPs, which overlap with gelatinases in substrate specificity, but also cleave additional proteins (127). In bone marrow–derived murine mast cells, stromelysin localizes to granules (95). Endobronchial biopsies of asthmatic airways reveal stromelysin immunoreactivity in mast cells, eosinophils, and neutrophils, and also in epithelium and extracellular matrix (131). As noted elsewhere in this chapter, human tryptase and chymase directly activate stromelysin. Although activated stromelysins are present in the epithelial lining fluid in asthmatics, the extent of their contribution to asthmatic airway remodeling is unclear (114).

G. Pharmacological Inhibition of MMPs in Airway Inflammation

Targeting individual MMPs as an approach to the management of asthma is a challenging objective due to broad overlap in substrate specificity among MMPs. There is also a wide overlap in MMP selectivity among endogenous TIMPs. Not surprisingly, perhaps, it has been difficult to design inhibitors to target specific MMPs. Synthetic inhibitors of MMPs include collagen peptidomimetics, nonpeptidic inhibitors of the active site, tetracycline derivatives, and bisphosphonates. Batimastat and marimastat are broad-spectrum, pseudopeptide hydroxamate derivatives, which mimic the structure of collagen and bind reversibly to the active site and chelate the catalytic zinc. Marimastat is an orally bioavailable form under investigation as an antineoplastic agent. Nonpeptidic inhibitors include agents synthesized based on crystallographic analysis of MMP active sites, a strategy potentially enabling targeting of specific subclasses. These orally bioavailable inhibitors demonstrate antitumor activity in preclinical models and are current under study in phase I and II trials (127). Derivatives of tetracycline not only inhibit MMP activity, but also regulate production of MMPs, thus supporting investigation of these agents in diseases in which MMP activity is amplified. In addition to classic tetracycline antibiotics, newer tetracycline analogues lacking antimicrobial activity interfere with collagenase and gelatinase activities. Chemically modified tetracyclines, such as Col-3 (metastat), which demonstrate several pharmacological advantages and antitumor effects are also being investigated. Bisphosphonate agents inhibit MMP activity and attenuate expression of MMPs, although their mechanism of action remains unclear (127).

Investigations of synthetic MMP inhibitors in animal models of lung disease suggest that pharmacological modulation of MMP activity may benefit those with asthma and acute lung injury. Synthetic MMP inhibitors inhibit inflammatory cell infiltration to the airway lumen in a murine ovalbumin model of asthma (123) and attenuate recruitment of inflammatory cells, airway epithelial thickening, mucus accumulation, MMP-9 activity, and airway hyperresponsiveness in a murine model of toluene diisocyanate–induced asthma (132). Batimastat inhibits the development of pulmonary fibrosis in a murine bleomycin model of acute lung injury, attenuates recruitment of macrophages and lymphocytes, and reduces activity of gelatinases A and B (133). Similarly, prinomastat blocks lung injury induced by high volume mechanical ventilation (134). A chemically modified nonantibiotic tetracycline, CMT-3, prevented histopathological changes of acute lung injury induced by cardiopulmonary bypass (135). Since lung diseases such as asthma involve many processes including inflammatory cell recruitment, airway hyperresponsiveness, angiogenesis, and extracellular cell matrix remodeling, beneficial effects of MMP inhibitors on one pathway may be deleterious effects on another. Expression and activation of MMPs also may be temporally regulated in response to injury. Thus, the timing and duration of administration of MMP inhibitors may be important. The current lack of selectivity for a given MMP among available inhibitors increases the likelihood that undesired inhibition of other MMPs in a subclass will yield unexpected side effects.

IV. Exopeptidases

A. Dipeptidylpeptidase I

Mast cells are also generously endowed with exopeptidases, which remove one or two amino acids from an end of susceptible peptide and protein targets. One of these enzymes is the cysteine protease dipeptidyl peptidase I (DPPI) otherwise known as cathepsin C, which removes dipeptides from polypeptide amino termini. DPPI is expressed in many cells, but is particularly abundant in granulated cells containing serine proteases, such as tryptase and chymase, in the case of mast cells. Although DPPI is largely an intracellular enzyme of lysosomes, degranulating mast cells secrete DPPI, which can degrade extracellular peptides and proteins such as angiotensin and fibronectin (136,137). However, this capacity appears to be limited compared with that of mast cell serine proteases and MMPs. In the mast cell, DPPI's most important role may be to activate chymase and tryptase intracellularly from proenzyme forms. This relationship is clearer for prochymases, which are activated be removal of an acidic dipeptide from the amino terminus of the zymogen. In vitro, inhibitors of DPPI reduce production of active chymase (138); furthermore, purified mast cell DPPI activates recombinant prochymase (136). In vivo proof of DPPI's importance in this regard has been obtained from DPPI-null mice, which lack active chymase (39). Data generated in vitro suggest a role for DPPI in activating human pro-β-tryptase in the second phase of a two-step process (18). The importance of DPPI in the activation of tryptases is partially supported by the finding of reduced levels of mouse tryptase mMCP-6 in DPPI-null mice (139). Some active tryptase remains, however, suggesting the presence of an alternative but less efficient pathway for tryptase activation.

B. Mast Cell Carboxypeptidase A

The chymase-containing MC_{TC} subset of human mast cells produce a Zn^{2+}-dependent metallocarboxypeptidase that differs from the more extensively studied pancreatic carboxypeptidases. The mast cell carboxypeptidase is the product of a separate gene and preferentially removes aromatic amino acids from target carboxy termini. Because of this specificity, it may be specialized to act sequentially with chymase, which hydolyzes internal sites in its targets leaving a carboxy-terminal residue at the site of cleavage, which is then removed by carboxypeptidase. A relationship between carboxypeptidase and chymase is further suggested by colocalization of the two enzymes in secretory granules and in macromolecular complexes with proteoglycan following exocytosis (140). Targets hydrolyzed by mast cell carboxypeptidase A include proteins, such as apolipoprotein B, and vasoactive peptides (141). However, the importance of this ex、peptidase in allergic disease remains to be established.

Acknowledgments

This work is supported by NIH grant HL-24136 and by the University of California Tobacco-Related Disease Research Program.

References

1. Schwartz LB. Neutral proteases of mast cells. In: Hanson LA, Shakib F, eds. Monographs in Allergy. Vol. 27. Basel: Karger, 1990:165.

2. Caughey GH, ed. Mast Cell Proteases in Immunology and Biology. New York: Marcel Dekker, 1995:354.

3. Caughey GH. Of mites and men: trypsin-like proteases in the lungs. Am J Respir Cell Mol Biol 1997; 16:621–628.

4. Lagunoff D, Benditt EP. Proteolytic enzymes of mast cells. Ann NY Acad Sci 1963; 103:185–198.

5. Glenner GG, Cohen LA. Histochemical demonstration of a species-specific trypsin-like enzyme in mast cells. Nature 1960; 185:846–847.

6. Fraki JE, Hopsu-Havu VK. Human skin proteases: separation and characterization of two alkaline proteases, one splitting trypsin and the other chymotrypsin substrates. Arch Dermatol Res 1975; 253:261–276.

7. Fraki JE. Human skin proteases: effect of separated proteases on vascular permeability and leukocyte emigration in skin. Acta Dermatovener 1977; 57:393–398.

8. Schwartz LB, Lewis RA, Austen KF. Tryptase from human pulmonary mast cells. Purification and characterization. J Biol Chem 1981; 256:11939–11943.

9. Tanaka T, McRae BJ, Cho K, et al. Mammalian tissue trypsin-like enzymes. Comparative reactivities of human skin tryptase, human lung tryptase, and bovine trypsin with peptide 4-nitroanilide and thioester substrates. J Biol Chem 1983; 258:13552–13557.

10. Smith TJ, Hougland MW, Johnson DA. Human lung tryptase. Purification and characterization. J Biol Chem 1984; 259:11046–11051.

11. Vanderslice P, Craik CS, Nadel JA, Caughey GH. Molecular cloning of dog mast cell tryptase and a related protease: structural evidence of a unique mode of serine protease activation. Biochemistry 1989; 28:4148–4155.

12. Miller JS, Westin EH, Schwartz LB. Cloning and characterization of complementary DNA for human tryptase. J Clin Invest 1989; 84:1188–1195.

13. Vanderslice P, Ballinger SM, Tam EK, Goldstein SM, Craik CS, Caughey GH. Human mast cell tryptase: multiple cDNAs and genes reveal a multigene serine protease family. Proc Natl Acad Sci USA 1990; 87:3811–3815.

14. Irani AA, Schechter NM, Craig SS, DeBlois G, Schwartz LB. Two types of human mast cells that have distinct neutral protease compositions. Proc Natl Acad Sci USA 1986; 83:4464–4468.

15. Xia H-Z, Kepley CL, Sakai K, Chelliah J, Irani A-M. A, Schwartz LB. Quantitation of tryptase, chymase, FcεRIa, and FcεRIγ mRNAs in human mast cells and basophils by competitive reverse transcription-polymerase chain reaction. J Immunol 1995; 154: 5472–5480.

16. Li L, Li Y, Reddel SW, et al. Identification of basophilic cells that express mast cell granule proteases in the peripheral blood of asthma, allergy, and drug-reactive patients. J Immunol 1998; 161:5079–86.

17. Pallaoro M, Fejzo MS, Shayesteh L, Blount JL, Caughey GH. Characterization of genes encoding known and novel human mast cell tryptases on chromosome 16p 13.3. J Biol Chem 1999; 274:3355–3362.

18. Sakai K, Ren S, Schwartz LB. A novel heparin-dependent processing pathway for human tryptase: autocatalysis followed by activation with dipeptidyl peptidase I. J Clin Invest 1996; 97:988–995.

19. Huang C, Li L, Krilis SA, et al. Human tryptases α and β/II are functionally distinct due, in part, to a single amino acid difference in one of the surface loops that forms the substrate-binding cleft. J Biol Chem 1999; 274:19670–19676.

20. Schwartz LB, Sakai K, Bradford TR, et al. The alpha form of human tryptase is the predominant type present in blood at baseline in normal subjects and is elevated in those with systemic mastocytosis. J Clin Invest 1995; 96:2702–2710.

21. Kanthawatana S, Carias K, Arnaout R, Hu J, Irani AM, Schwartz LB. The potential clinical utility of serum α-protryptase levels. J Allergy Clin Immunol 1999; 103: 1092–1099.

22. Ludolph-Hauser D, Rueff F, Fries C, Schopf P, Przybilla B. Constitutively raised serum concentrations of mast-cell tryptase and severe anaphylactic reactions to Hymenoptera stings. Lancet 2001; 357:361–362.

23. Guida M, Riedy M, Lee D, Hall J. Characterization of two highly polymorphic human tryptase loci and comparison with a newly discovered monkey tryptase ortholog. Pharmacogenetics 2000; 10:389–396.

24. Caughey GH, Raymond WW, Blount JL, et al. Characterization of human γ-tryptases, novel members of the chromosome 16p mast cell tryptase and prostasin gene families. J Immunol 2000; 164:6566–6575.

25. Schwartz LB, Lewis RA, Seldin D, Austen KF. Acid hydrolases and tryptase from secretory granules of dispersed human lung mast cells. J Immunol 1981; 126: 1290–1294.

26. Harris JL, Niles A, Burdick K, et al. Definition of the extended substrate specificity determinants for β-tryptases I and II. J Biol Chem 2001; 276:34941–34947.

27. Pereira PJB, Bergner A, Macedo-Ribeiro S, et al. Human β-tryptase is a ring-like tetramer with active sites facing a central pore. Nature 1998; 392:306–311.

28. Caughey GH, Leidig F, Viro NF, Nadel JA. Substance P and vasoactive intestinal peptide degradation by mast cell tryptase and chymase. J Pharmacol Exp Ther 1988; 244:133–137.

29. Tam EK, Caughey GH. Degradation of airway neuropeptides by human lung tryptase. Am J Respir Cell Mol Biol 1990; 3:27–32.

30. Imamura T, Dubin A, Moore W, Tanaka R, Travis J. Induction of vascular permeability enhancement by human tryptase: dependence on activation of prekallikrein and direct release of bradykinin from kininogens. Lab Invest 1996; 74:861–870.

31. Kozik A, Moore RB, Potempa J, Imamura T, Rapala-Kozik M, Travis J. A novel mechanism for bradykinin production at inflammatory sites. Diverse effects of a mixture of neutrophil elastase and mast cell tryptase versus tissue and plasma kallikreins on native and oxidized kininogens. J Biol Chem 1998; 273:33224–33229.

32. Schwartz LB, Bradford TR, Littman BH, Wintroub BU. The fibrinolytic activity of purified tryptase from human lung mast cells. J Immunol 1985; 135:2762–2767.

33. Gruber BL, Marchese MJ, Suzuki K, et al. Synovial procollagenase activation by human mast cell tryptase. Dependence upon matrix metalloproteinase 3 activation. J Clin Invest 1989; 84:1657–1662.

34. Stack MS, Johnson DA. Human mast cell tryptase activates single-chain urinary-type plasminogen activator (pro-urokinase). J Biol Chem 1994; 269:9416–9419.

35. Corvera CU, Dery O, McConalogue K, et al. Mast cell tryptase regulates rat colonic myocytes through proteinase-activated receptor 2. J Clin Invest 1997; 100:1383–1393.

36. Molino M, Barnathan ES, Numerof R, et al. Interactions of mast cell tryptase with thrombin receptors and PAR-2. J Biol Chem 1997; 272:4043–4049.

37. Steinhoff M, Vergnolle N, Young SH, et al. Agonists of proteinase-activated receptor 2 induce inflammation by a neurogenic mechanism. Nat Med 2000; 6:151–158.

38. Schmidlin F, Amadesi S, Vidil R, et al. Expression and function of proteinase-activated receptor 2 in human bronchial smooth muscle. Am J Respir Crit Care Med 2001; 164: 1276–1281.

39. Compton SJ, Renaux B, Wijesuriya SJ, Hollenberg MD. Glycosylation and the activation of proteinase-activated receptor 2 (PAR(2)) by human mast cell tryptase. Br J Pharmacol 2001; 134:705–718.

40. Sekizawa K, Caughey GH, Lazarus SC, Gold WM, Nadel JA. Mast cell tryptase causes airway smooth muscle hyperresponsiveness in dogs. J Clin Invest 1989; 83:175–179.

41. Clark JM, Abraham WM, Fishman CE, et al. Tryptase inhibitors block allergen-induced airway and inflammatory responses in allergic sheep. Am J Respir Crit Care Med 1995; 152:2076–2083.

42. Johnson PRA, Ammit AJ, Carlin SM, Armour CL, Caughey GH, Black JL. Mast cell tryptase potentiates histamine-induced contraction in human sensitized bronchus. Eur Resp J 1997; 10:38–43.

43. Berger P, Compton SJ, Molimard M, et al. Mast cell tryptase as a mediator of hyperresponsiveness in human isolated bronchi. Clin Exp Allergy 1999; 29:804–812.

44. Molinari JF, Scuri M, Moore WR, Clark J, Tanaka R, Abraham WM. Inhaled tryptase causes bronchoconstriction in sheep via histamine release. Am J Respir Crit Care Med 1996; 154:649–653.

45. Ruoss SJ, Hartmann T, Caughey GH. Mast cell tryptase is a mitogen for cultured fibroblasts. J Clin Invest 1991; 88:493–499.

46. Brown JK, Tyler CL, Jones CA, Ruoss SJ, Hartmann T, Caughey GH. Tryptase, the dominant secretory granular protein in humans mast cells, is a potent mitogen for cultured dog tracheal smooth muscle cells. Am J Respir Cell Mol Biol 1995; 13: 227–236.

47. Cairns JA, Walls AF. Mast cell tryptase is a mitogen for epithelial cells—stimulation of IL-8 production and intercellular adhesion molecule-1 expression. J Immunol 1996; 156:275–283.

48. Gruber BL, Kew RR, Jelaska A, et al. Human mast cells activate fibroblasts: tryptase is a fibrogenic factor stimulating collagen messenger ribonucleic acid synthesis and fibroblast chemotaxis. J Immunol 1997; 158:2310–2317.

49. Cairns JA, Walls AF. Mast cell tryptase stimulates synthesis of type I collagen in human lung fibroblasts. J Clin Invest 1997; 99:1313–1321.

50. Thomas VA, Wheeless CJ, Stack MS, Johnson DA. Human mast cell tryptase fibrinogenolysis: kinetics, anticoagulation mechanism, and cell adhesion disruption. Biochemistry 1998; 37:2291–2298.

51. Compton SJ, Cairns JA, Holgate ST, Walls AF. The role of mast cell tryptase in regulating endothelial cell proliferation, cytokine release, and adhesion molecule expression: tryptase induces expression of mRNA for IL-1 βand IL-8 and stimulates the selective release of IL-8 from human umbilical vein endothelial cells. J Immunol 1998; 161:1939–1946.

52. He SH, Walls AF. Human mast cell tryptase: a stimulus of microvascular leakage and mast cell activation. Eur J Pharmacol 1997; 328:89–97.

53. Huang C, De Sanctis GT, O'Brien PJ, et al. Evaluation of the substrate specificity of human mast cell tryptase β1 and demonstration of its importance in bacterial infections of the lung. J Biol Chem 2001; 276:26276–26284.

54. Blair RJ, Meng H, Marchese MJ, et al. Human mast cells stimulate vascular tube formation. Tryptase is a novel, potent angiogenic factor. J Clin Invest 1997; 99: 2691–2700.

55. Coussens LM, Raymond WW, Bergers G, et al. Inflammatory mast cells upregulate angiogenesis during squamous epithelial carcinogenesis. Genes Dev 1999; 13: 1382–1397.

56. Caughey GH, Raymond WW, Bacci E, Lombardy RJ, Tidwell RR. Bis(5-amidino-2-benzimidazolyl)methane and related amidines are potent, reversible inhibitors of mast cell tryptases. J Pharmacol Exp Ther 1993; 264:676–682.

57. Sturzebecher J, Prasa D, Sommerhoff CP. Inhibition of human mast cell tryptase by benzamidine derivatives. Biol Chem Hoppe Seyler 1992; 373:1025–1030.

58. Kam CM, Hernandez MA, Patil GS, et al. Mammalian tissue trypsin-like enzymes: substrate specificity and inhibitory potency of substituted isocoumarin mechanism-based inhibitors, benzamidine derivatives, and arginine fluoroalkyl ketone transition-state inhibitors. Arch Biochem Biophys 1995; 316:808–814.

59. Katz BA, Clark JM, Finer-Moore JS, et al. Design of potent selective zinc-mediated serine protease inhibitors. Nature 1998; 391:608–612.

60. Janc JW, Clark JM, Warne RL, Elrod KC, Katz BA, Moore WR. A novel approach to serine protease inhibition: kinetic characterization of inhibitors whose potencies and selectivities are dramatically enhanced by zinc(II). Biochemistry 2000; 39:4792–4800.

61. Krishna MT, Chauhan AJ, Little L, et al. Effect of inhaled APC 366 on allergen-induced bronchoconstriction and airway hyperresponsiveness to histamine in atopic subjects. Am J Respir Crit Care Med. 1998; 157:A456.

62. Rice KD, Wang VR, Gangloff AR, et al. Dibasic inhibitors of human mast cell tryptase. Part 2: Structure-activity relationships and requirements for potent activity. Bioorg Med Chem Lett 2000; 10:2361–2366.

63. Burgess LE, Newhouse BJ, Ibrahim P, et al. Potent selective nonpeptidic inhibitors of human lung tryptase. Proc Natl Acad Sci USA 1999; 96:8348–8352.

64. Schaschke N, Matschiner G, Zettl F, et al. Bivalent inhibition of human β-tryptase. Chem Biol 2001; 8:313–327.

65. Ono S, Kuwahara S, Takeuchi M, Sakashita H, Naito Y, Kondo T. Syntheses and evaluation of amidinobenzofuran derivatives as tryptase inhibitors. Bioorg Med Chem Lett 1999; 9:3285–3290.

66. Wright CD, Havill AM, Middleton SC, et al. Inhibition of allergen-induced pulmonary responses by the selective tryptase inhibitor 1,5-bis-[4-[(3-carbamimidoyl-benzenesulfonylamino)-methyl] -phenoxy]-pentane (AMG-126737). Biochem Pharmacol 1999; 58:1989–1996.

67. Combrink KD, HB GI, Meanwell NA, et al. 1,2-Benzisothiazol-3-one 1,1-dioxide inhibitors of human mast cell tryptase. J Med Chem 1998; 41:4854–4860.

68. Sommerhoff CP, Sollner C, Mentele R, Piechottka GP, Auerswald EA, Fritz H. A Kazal-type inhibitor of human mast cell tryptase: isolation from the medicinal leech Hirudo medicinalis, characterization, and sequence analysis. Biol Chem Hoppe-Seyler 1994; 375:685–694.

69. Stubbs MT, Morenweiser R, Sturzebecher J, et al. The three-dimensional structure of recombinant leech-derived tryptase inhibitor in complex with trypsin. Implications for the structure of human mast cell tryptase and its inhibition. J Biol Chem 1997; 272: 19931–19937.

70. Elrod KC, Moore WR, Abraham WM, Tanaka RD. Lactoferrin, a potent tryptase inhibitor, abolishes late-phase airway responses in allergic sheep. Am J Respir Crit Care Med 1997; 156:375–381.

71. Cregar L, Elrod KC, Putnam D, Moore WR. Neutrophil myeloperoxidase is a potent and selective inhibitor of mast cell tryptase. Arch Biochem Biophys 1999; 366:125–130.

72. Wong GW, Tang Y, Feyfant E, et al. Identification of a new member of the tryptase family of mouse and human mast cell proteases which possesses a novel COOH-terminal hydrophobic extension. J Biol Chem 1999; 274:30784–30793.

73. Salvesen G, Farley D, Shuman J, Przybyla A, Reilly C, Travis J. Molecular cloning of human cathepsin G: structural similarity to mast cell and cytotoxic T lymphocyte proteinases. Biochemistry 1987; 26:2289–2293.

74. Caughey GH, Zerweck EH, Vanderslice P. Structure, chromosomal assignment, and deduced amino acid sequence of a human gene for mast cell chymase. J Biol Chem 1991; 266:12956–12963.

75. Hof P, Mayr I, Huber R, et al. The 1.8 A crystal structure of human cathepsin G in complex with Suc-Val-Pro-PheP-(OPh)2: a Janus-faced proteinase with two opposite specificities. EMBO J 1996; 15:5481–5491.

76. Pereira PJB, Wang ZM, Rubin H, et al. The 2.2 Å crystal structure of human chymase in complex with succinyl-Ala-Ala-Pro-Phe-chloromethylketone: structural explanation for its dipeptidyl carboxypeptidase specificity. J Mol Biol 1999; 286:163–173.

77. Caughey GH, Schaumberg TH, Zerweck EH, et al. The human mast cell chymase gene (CMA1): mapping to the cathepsin G/granzyme gene cluster and lineage-restricted expression. Genomics 1993; 15:614–620.

78. Schechter NM, Irani AM, Sprows JL, Abernethy J, Wintroub B, Schwartz LB. Identification of a cathepsin G-like proteinase in the MCTC type of human mast cell. J Immunol 1990; 145:2652–2661.

79. Matin R, Tam EK, Nadel JA, Caughey GH. Distribution of chymase-containing mast cells in human bronchi. J Histochem Cytochem 1992; 40:781–786.

80. Suzuki H, Caughey GH, Gao X-P, Rubinstein I. Mast cell chymase-like protease(s) modulates Escherichia coli lipopolysaccharide-induced vasomotor dysfunction in skeletal muscle in vivo. J Pharmacol Exp Therap 1998; 284:1156–1164.

81. Shiota N, Okunishi H, Takai S, et al. Tranilast suppresses vascular chymase expression and neointima formation in balloon-injured dog carotid artery. Circulation 1999; 99:1084–1090.

82. Kielty CM, Lees M, Shuttleworth CA, Woolley D. Catabolism of intact type VI collagen microfibrils: susceptibility to degradation by serine proteinases. Biochem Biophys Res Commun 1993; 191:1230–1236.

83. Taipale J, Lohi J, Saarinen J, Kovanen PT, Keski-Oja J. Human mast cell chymase and leukocyte elastase release latent transforming growth factor-β1 from the extracellular matrix of cultured human epithelial and endothelial cells. J Biol Chem 1995; 270:4689–4696.

84. Nakano A, Kishi F, Minami K, Wakabayashi H, Nakaya Y, Kido H. Selective conversion of big endothelins to tracheal smooth muscle-constricting 31-amino acid-length endothelins by chymase from human mast cells. J Immunol 1997; 159:1987–1992.

85. Sommerhoff CP, Caughey GH, Finkbeiner WE, Lazarus SC, Basbaum CB, Nadel JA. Mast cell chymase. A potent secretagogue for airway gland serous cells. J Immunol 1989; 142:2450–2456.

86. Sommerhoff CP, Ruoss SJ, Caughey GH. Mast cell proteoglycans modulate the secretagogue, proteoglycanase, and amidolytic activities of dog mast cell chymase. J Immunol 1992; 148:2859–2866.

87. Aoyama Y, Uenaka M, Kii M, et al. Design, synthesis and pharmacological evaluation of 3-benzylazetidine-2-one-based human chymase inhibitors. Bioorg Med Chem 2001; 9:3065–3075.

88. Akahoshi F, Ashimori A, Sakashita H, et al. Synthesis, structure-activity relationships, and pharmacokinetic profiles of nonpeptidic difluoromethylene ketones as novel inhibitors of human chymase. J Med Chem 2001; 44:1297–1304.

89. Groutas WC, Schechter NM, He S, Yu H, Huang P, Tu J. Human chymase inhibitors based on the 1,2,5-thiadiazolidin-3-one-1, 1-dioxide scaffold. Bioorg Med Chem Lett 1999; 9:2199–2204.

90. Sillaber C, Baghestanian M, Bevec D, et al. The mast cell as site of tissue-type plasminogen activator expression and fibrinolysis. J Immunol 1999; 162:1032–1041.

91. Woessner JF, Jr. Matrix metalloproteinases and their inhibitors in connective tissue remodeling. FASEB J 1991; 5:2145–2154.

92. Tozzi CA, Thakker-Varia S, Yu SY, et al. Mast cell collagenase correlates with regression of pulmonary vascular remodeling in the rat. Am J Respir Cell Mol Biol 1998; 18:497–510.

93. Tanaka A, Arai K, Kitamura Y, Matsuda H. Matrix metalloproteinase-9 production, a newly identified function of mast cell progenitors, is downregulated by c-kit receptor activation. Blood 1999; 94:2390–2395.

94. Kanbe N, Tanaka A, Kanbe M, Itakura A, Kurosawa M, Matsuda H. Human mast cells produce matrix metalloproteinase 9. Eur J Immunol 1999; 29:2645–2649.

95. Brownell E, Fiorentino L, Jolly G, et al. Immunolocalization of stromelysin-related protein in murine mast cell granules. Int Arch Allergy Immunol 1995; 107:333–335.

96. Fang KC, Raymond WW, Lazarus SC, Caughey GH. Dog mastocytoma cells secrete a 92-kD gelatinase activated extracellularly by mast cell chymase. J Clin Invest 1996; 97:1589–1596.

97. Fang KC, Raymond WW, Blount JL, Caughey GH. Dog mast cell α-chymase activates progelatinase B by cleaving the Phe[88]-Gln[89] and Phe[91]-Glu[92] bonds of the catalytic domain. J Biol Chem 1997; 272:25628–25635.

98. Fang KC, Wolters PJ, Steinhoff M, Bidgol A, Blount JL, Caughey GH. Mast cell expression of gelatinases A and B is regulated by kit ligand and TGF-β. J Immunol 1999; 162:5528–5535.

99. Frank BT, Rossall JC, Caughey GH, Fang KC. Mast cell tissue inhibitor of metalloproteinase-1 is cleaved and inactivated extracellularly by α-chymase. J Immunol 2001; 166:2783–2792.

100. Di Girolamo N, Wakefield D. In vitro and in vivo expression of interstitial collagenase/ MMP-1 by human mast cells. Dev Immunol 2000; 7:131–142.

101. Saarinen J, Kalkkinen N, Welgus HG, Kovanen PT. Activation of human interstitial procollagenase through direct cleavage of the Leu[83]-Thr[84] bond by mast cell chymase. J Biol Chem 1994; 269:18134–18140.

102. Suzuki K, Lees M, Newlands GF, Nagase H, Woolley DE. Activation of precursors for matrix metalloproteinases 1 (interstitial collagenase) and 3 (stromelysin) by rat mast-cell proteinases I and II. Biochem J 1995; 305:301–306.

103. Lees M, Taylor DJ, Woolley DE. Mast cell proteinases activate precursor forms of collagenase and stromelysin, but not of gelatinases A and B. Eur J Biochem 1994; 223:171–177.

104. Van Wart HE, Birkedal-Hansen H. The cysteine switch: a principle of regulation of metalloproteinase activity with potential applicability to the entire matrix metalloproteinase gene family. Proc Natl Acad Sci USA 1990; 87:5578–5582.

105. Ogata Y, Enghild JJ, Nagase H. Matrix metalloproteinase 3 (stromelysin) activates the precursor for the human matrix metalloproteinase 9. J Biol Chem 1992; 267: 3581–3584.

106. Fridman R, Toth M, Pena D, Mobashery S. Activation of progelatinase B (MMP-9) by gelatinase A (MMP-2). Cancer Res 1995; 55:2548–2555.
107. Hibbs MS, Hasty KA, Seyer JM, Kang AH, Mainardi CL. Biochemical and immunological characterization of the secreted forms of human neutrophil gelatinase. J Biol Chem 1985; 260:2493–2500.
108. Baram D, Vaday GG, Salamon P, Drucker I, Hershkoviz R, Mekori YA. Human mast cells release metalloproteinase-9 on contact with activated t cells: juxtacrine regulation by TNF-alpha. J Immunol 2001; 167:4008–4016.
109. Tanaka A, Yamane Y, Matsuda H. Mast cell MMP-9 production enhanced by bacterial lipopolysaccharide. J Vet Med Sci 2001; 63:811–813.
110. Kjeldsen L, Bainton DF, Sengelov H, Borregaard N. Structural and functional heterogeneity among peroxidase-negative granules in human neutrophils: identification of a distinct gelatinase-containing granule subset by combined immunocytochemistry and subcellular fractionation. Blood 1993; 82:3183–3191.
111. Hoshino M, Nakamura Y, Sim J, Shimojo J, Isogai S. Bronchial subepithelial fibrosis and expression of matrix metalloproteinase-9 in asthmatic airway inflammation. J Allergy Clin Immunol 1998; 102:783–788.
112. Mautino G, Henriquet C, Jaffuel D, Bousquet J, Capony F. Tissue inhibitor of metalloproteinase-1 levels in bronchoalveolar lavage fluid from asthmatic subjects. Am J Respir Crit Care Med 1999; 160:324–330.
113. Vignola AM, Riccobono L, Mirabella A, et al. Sputum metalloproteinase-9/tissue inhibitor of metalloproteinase-1 ratio correlates with airflow obstruction in asthma and chronic bronchitis. Am J Respir Crit Care Med 1998; 158:1945–1950.
114. Lemjabbar H, Gosset P, Lamblin C, et al. Contribution of 92 kDa gelatinase/type IV collagenase in bronchial inflammation during status asthmaticus. Am J Respir Crit Care Med 1999; 159:1298–1307.
115. Vliagoftis H, Schwingshackl A, Milne CD, et al. Proteinase-activated receptor-2-mediated matrix metalloproteinase-9 release from airway epithelial cells. J Allergy Clin Immunol 2000; 106:537–545.
116. Foda HD, George S, Rollo E, et al. Regulation of gelatinases in human airway smooth muscle cells: mechanism of progelatinase A activation. Am J Physiol 1999; 277: L174–182.
117. Ohno I, Ohtani H, Nitta Y, et al. Eosinophils as a source of matrix metalloproteinase-9 in asthmatic airway inflammation. Am J Respir Cell Mol Biol 1997; 16:212–219.
118. Shapiro SD, Campbell EJ, Kobayashi DK, Welgus HG. Dexamethasone selectively modulates basal and lipoplysaccharide-induced metalloproteinase and tissue inhibitor of metalloproteinase production by human alveolar macrophages. J Immunol 1991; 146:2724–2729.
119. Mautino G, Oliver N, Chanez P, Bousquet J, Capony F. Increased release of matrix metalloproteinase-9 in bronchoalveolar lavage fluid and by alveolar macrophages of asthmatics. Am J Respir Cell Mol Biol 1997; 17:583–591.
120. Bosse M, Chakir J, Rouabhia M, Boulet LP, Audette M, Laviolette M. Serum matrix metalloproteinase-9; tissue inhibitor of metalloproteinase-1 ratio correlates with steroid responsiveness in moderate to severe asthma. Am J Respir Crit Care Med 1999; 159: 596–602.
121. Hoshino M, Takahashi M, Takai Y, Sim J. Inhaled corticosteroids decrease subepithelial collagen deposition by modulation of the balance between matrix metalloproteinase-9 and tissue inhibitor of metalloproteinase-1 expression in asthma. J Allergy Clin Immunol 1999; 104:356–363.

122. Swartz MA, Tschumperlin DJ, Kamm RD, Drazen JM. Mechanical stress is communicated between different cell types to elicit matrix remodeling. Proc Natl Acad Sci USA 2001; 98:6180–6185.

123. Kumagai K, Ohno I, Okada S, et al. Inhibition of matrix metalloproteinases prevents allergen-induced airway inflammation in a murine model of asthma. J Immunol 1999; 162:4212–4219.

124. Li X, Wilson JW. Increased vascularity of the bronchial mucosa in mild asthma. Am J Respir Crit Care Med 1997; 156:229–233.

125. Orsida BE, Li X, Hickey B, Thien F, Wilson JW, Walters EH. Vascularity in asthmatic airways: relation to inhaled steroid dose. Thorax 1999; 54:289–295.

126. Vu TH, Shipley JM, Bergers G, et al. MMP-9/gelatinase B is a key regulator of growth plate angiogenesis and apoptosis of hypertrophic chondrocytes. Cell 1998; 93:411–422.

127. Hidalgo M, Eckhardt SG. Development of matrix metalloproteinase inhibitors in cancer therapy. J Natl Cancer Inst 2001; 93:178–193.

128. Riley DJ, Thakker-Varia S, Wilson FJ, Polani GJ, Tozzi CA. Role of proteolysis and apoptosis in regression of pulmonary vascular remodeling. Physiol Res 2000; 49: 577–585.

129. Rajah R, Nachajon RV, Collins MH, Hakonarson H, Grunstein MM, Cohen P. Elevated levels of the IGF-binding protein protease MMP-1 in asthmatic airway smooth muscle. Am J Respir Cell Mol Biol 1999; 20:199–208.

130. Johnson JL, Jackson CL, Angelini GD, George SJ. Activation of matrix-degrading metalloproteinases by mast cell proteases in atherosclerotic plaques. Arterioscler Thromb Vasc Biol 1998; 18:1707–1715.

131. Dahlen B, Shute J, Howarth P. Immunohistochemical localisation of the matrix metalloproteinases MMP-3 and MMP-9 within the airways in asthma. Thorax 1999; 54: 590–596.

132. Lee YC, Song CH, Lee HB, et al. A murine model of toluene diisocyanate-induced asthma can be treated with matrix metalloproteinase inhibitor. J Allergy Clin Immunol 2001; 108:1021–1026.

133. Corbel M, Caulet-Maugendre S, Germain N, Molet S, Lagente V, Boichot E. Inhibition of bleomycin-induced pulmonary fibrosis in mice by the matrix metalloproteinase inhibitor batimastat. J Pathol 2001; 193:538–545.

134. Foda HD, Rollo EE, Drews M, et al. Ventilator-Induced Lung Injury Upregulates and Activates Gelatinases and EMMPRIN. Attenuation by the synthetic matrix metalloproteinase inhibitor, prinomastat (AG3340). Am J Respir Cell Mol Biol 2001; 25:717–724.

135. Carney DE, Lutz CJ, Picone AL, et al. Matrix metalloproteinase inhibitor prevents acute lung injury after cardiopulmonary bypass. Circulation 1999; 100:400–406.

136. Caughey GH, Raymond WW, Wolters PJ. Angiotensin II generation by mast cell α- and β-chymases. Biochim Biophys Acta 2000; 1480:245–257.

137. Wolters PJ, Laig-Webster M, Caughey GH. Dipeptidyl peptidase I cleaves matrix-associated proteins and is expressed mainly by mast cells in normal dog airways. Am J Respir Cell Mol Biol 2000; 22:183–190.

138. McGuire MJ, Lipsky PE, Thiele DL. Generation of active myeloid and lymphoid granule serine proteases requires processing by the granule thiol protease dipeptidyl peptidase I. J Biol Chem 1993; 268:2458–2467.

139. Wolters PJ, Pham CT, Muilenburg DJ, Ley TJ, Caughey GH. Dipeptidyl peptidase I is essential for activation of mast cell chymases, but not tryptases, in mice. J Biol Chem 2001; 276:18551–18556.

40. Goldstein SM, Leong J, Schwartz LB, Cooke D. Protease composition of exocytosed human skin mast cell protease-proteoglycan complexes: tryptase resides in a complex distinct from chymase and carboxypeptidase. J Immunol 1992; 148:2475–2482.
41. Goldstein SM. Mast cell carboxypeptidase: structure and regulation of gene expression. In: Caughey GH. ed. Mast Cell Proteases in Immunology and Biology. New York: Marcel Dekker, 1995:109–126.

18

Peroxidases and Asthma

MICHAEL E. GREENBERG and STANLEY L. HAZEN

Cleveland Clinic Foundation
Cleveland, Ohio, U.S.A.

I. Introduction

This chapter is based upon the following ideas, which are discussed subsequently in greater detail: (1) asthma is an inflammatory disorder; (2) a prominent feature of the inflammatory response is cellular injury and oxidative tissue damage; and (3) inflammatory cells such as eosinophils and neutrophils participate in tissue injury through the release of heme peroxidases and formation of reactive oxidant species. The most abundant proteins in eosinophils and neutrophils are their respective heme peroxidase, eosinophil peroxidase (EPO), and myeloperoxidase (MPO). Their normal function is to inflict oxidative damage upon invading parasites and pathogens as part of innate host defenses. However, the reactive species formed by peroxidases can also injure host/normal tissues. We have exploited formation of specific brominated and chlorinated targets as tools for monitoring molecular signatures for EPO- and MPO-dependent oxidative injury. Using this approach, we recently demonstrated that eosinophils and neutrophils use EPO- and MPO-generated oxidants to promote oxidative damage of lung and airways proteins in severe asthma as well as following allergen challenge in subjects with mild asthma. However, even in the presence of plasma levels of halides, both EPO and MPO can use numerous alternative cosubstrates, generating an array of free radicals and reactive oxidant species. Thus,

373

leukocytes have potential for inflicting oxidative modifications on proteins and lipids in asthmatic airways via numerous pathways.

A key task then becomes defining the nature of the oxidation reactions that are mediated by leukocyte peroxidases and the extent to which they occur during asthma. In this chapter we will review the evidence demonstrating that peroxidases through the use of an ever-growing milieu of physiological substrates, generate powerful oxidizing species capable of modifying biological targets, thereby contributing to the development of asthma. We will detail the chemical reactions catalyzed by leukocyte peroxidases and their products, initially identified in vitro, and discuss those for which there is now data confirming their presence in vivo. Based on data accrued from recent in vitro, organ chamber, animal model, and human clinical studies, we will evaluate the peroxidase-mediated reactions that may be most relevant in contributing to acute and chronic complications of asthma. Finally, we will discuss future research directions, peroxidases and their reactive products as potential therapeutic targets, and the potential role of peroxidase oxidation products as novel diagnostic markers to predict or monitor disease progression, severity, and response to therapy.

II. Leukocytes and Asthma

Eosinophil recruitment to the lung and airways is one of the earliest cellular hall marks of asthma (1–4). Their role as participants in the pathogenesis of the disease however, has not yet been established. Upon stimulation, eosinophils release cyto toxic granule proteins including EPO, major basic protein, eosinophilic cation pro tein, and eosinophil-derived neurotoxin (1–5). Eosinophils and their granule constit uents are enriched in blood, sputum, bronchoalveolar lavage (BAL), and bronchia tissues of asthmatic subjects. They have also been used as markers of asthma, a an index of disease severity, and as an indirect indicator of inflammation and the response of the disease to therapies (6–10). A role for eosinophils in the pathogenesi of asthma is suggested by the observations that numerous eosinophil-derived prod ucts promote many of the pathophysiological features of asthma. These include but are not limited to, denudation of airway epithelium, destruction of epithelia morphology, increased microvascular permeability and edema, and hyperreactivit (11–20). Eosinophils in culture release proinflammatory lipid-derived second mes sengers such as platelet-activating factor and eicoisanoid oxidation products that can serve as chemotactic factors, bronchoconstrictors, and mucostimulatory agent (7,21–24). Collectively, these observations have suggested that eosinophils are majo effector cells in asthma and play a critical role in the pathogenesis of the disease.

Recent studies, however, have questioned the link between eosinophils and the development of specific features of asthma, such as induction of airway hyperre activity. Interleukin 5 (IL-5) derived from Th2 cells is the primary cytokine responsi ble for eosinophil differentiation and survival (25). In a recent clinical trial with humanized anti-IL-5 monoclonal antibody, no reduction in airway hyperresponsive ness to histamine 1 and 4 weeks following treatment was observed (26). In this study a single dose of antibody was shown to decrease sputum and blood eosinophilia for up to 4 weeks and 16 weeks, respectively. Whether levels of EPO were diminished within asthmatic airway tissues following anti-IL-5 treatment was not assessed. This is particularly relevant since EPO is known to be a long-lived protein that may remain in tissues at sites of eosinophil activation. For example, in numerous cancers EPO is detected by immunostaining despite the absence of eosinophils, suggesting that once released it may persist for long periods of time (27,28).

A potential role for neutrophils in asthma and its chronic complications, such as development of airways remodeling, is receiving increased attention. Neutrophils are typically observed in sputum, bronchial biopsies, and BAL of asthmatics, but in relatively low numbers (29–31). Significant increases in neutrophils are observed in the late-phase reaction after allergen challenge (32,33), in many cases of fatal asthma (34,35), nocturnal asthma (36), in long-standing asthma even during periods of remission (37), and in patients with steroid responsive intractable asthma (38). Suggested mechanisms potentially linking neutrophils and asthma and remodeling include leukocyte-dependent expression of transforming growth factor β, matrix metalloprotease activity, matrix deposition, production of mucostimulatory eicosanoids, activation of elastase, and inactivation of α 1-antitrypsin (21,39–43). A role of MPO-generated oxidants in activation of protease cascades, including those of matrix metalloproteases, elastase, and plasminogen, has been suggested at sites of inflammation (44–49). A role for EPO- or MPO-generated oxidants in asthma and airways remodeling has not been examined.

III. Oxidative Reactions Mediated by Eosinophils and Neutrophils

As essential constituents of the innate immune system, the granulocytic white blood cells eosinophils and neutrophils generate an arsenal of chemical weapons with which to combat invading microbes. The reactive species they form, however, also have the potential to harm host tissue and contribute to inflammatory injury. EPO and MPO play roles in host defense against parasites and pathogens, while lactoperoxidase (LPO) participates in barrier functions on mucosal surfaces such as tracheal lining fluid and within exocrine gland secretions including saliva, tears, and milk (50–53). All share a high degree of structural and sequence similarity and rely upon peroxide as the major source of oxidizing equivalents for catalysis (54,55).

A. The Respiratory Burst

During leukocyte (eosinophil, neutrophil, and monocyte) activation, NADPH oxidase is activated and reduced oxygen species such as $O_2^{\cdot-}$ (superoxide anion) and its dismutation product, H_2O_2 (hydrogen peroxide), are rapidly formed (56–58).

Formation of $O_2^{\bullet-}$ during the respiratory burst is a characteristic feature of activated leukocytes (59–61). The significance of this reaction in leukocyte-mediated host defenses is underscored by the profound increase in susceptibility to suppurative infections in individuals with a functional defect in the NADPH oxidase complex, a condition known as chronic granulomatous disease (62). Formation of $O_2^{\bullet-}$ by the plasma membrane complex of eosinophils is a primary source of reduced oxygen species by the leukocytes, and production of $O_2^{\bullet-}$ in this disorder is ablated (59,61,63). Thus, the components of the NADPH complex of eosinophils share many features with their brethren leukocyte, neutrophils. The respiratory burst of eosinophils is remarkable in comparison with that of other leukocytes for a prodigious capacity to generate $O_2^{\bullet-}$. Activated eosinophils generate 3 to 10 times as much $O_2^{\bullet-}$ as a corresponding number of neutrophils (63–65).

B. The Peroxidase Cycle

Leukocytes have enzymes that amplify the oxidative properties of H_2O_2, the peroxidases EPO and MPO. These abundant heme proteins are stored in granules and secreted during leukocyte activation (54,66–69). EPO and MPO are members of the mammalian peroxidase superfamily, which also includes LPO, thyroid peroxidase, and prostaglandin H synthase. Like the others, EPO contains a heme group in the form of an iron (Fe) protoporphyrin IX ring (70). EPO is comprised of a 55 kDa heavy chain and a $\sim$ 15 kDa light chain processed from a 70 kDa polyprotein precursor (70). MPO, a distinct gene product from EPO, is the most abundant protein stored in neutrophil and monocyte granules and is secreted during neutrophil and monocyte activation (54).

The overall reactions of EPO are similar to those of the other members of the mammalian peroxidase family [see Eqs. (1)–(3)]. The ground state (ferric or Fe^{III}) of the enzyme uses H_2O_2 as initial substrate to generate Compound I, a ferryl (Fe^{IV} = O) π cation radical intermediate [Eq. (1)]. This two-electron ($2e^-$) equivalent oxidized form of EPO can undergo two sequential one-electron reduction steps generating Compound II, followed by the ground state ferric form, while concomitantly catalyzing two one-electron oxidation reactions of a reducing substrate [Eqs. (2) and (3)]. Examples of one-electron reducing substrates for EPO and MPO include tyrosine, nitrite (NO_2^-), and nitric oxide (NO, nitrogen monoxide), yielding tyrosyl radical, nitrogen dioxide ($^{\bullet}NO_2$), and nitrosonium cation (NO^+), respectively (71–79).

$$E\ (Fe^{III},\ R)\ +\ H_2O_2 \rightarrow E\ (Fe^{IV}\ =\ O,\ R^{\bullet+})\ +\ H_2O \tag{1}$$

$$\text{Compound I}$$

$$E\ (Fe^{IV}\ =\ O,\ R^{\bullet+})\ +\ S_{red} \rightarrow E\ (Fe^{IV}\ =\ O,\ R)\ +\ S_{ox} \tag{2}$$

$$\text{Compound II}$$

$$E\ (Fe^{IV}\ =\ O,\ R)\ +\ S_{red} \rightarrow E\ (Fe^{III},\ R)\ +\ S_{ox}\ +\ H_2O \tag{3}$$

where E, R, S_{red}, and S_{ox} represent the enzyme, site of cation radical, reducing substrate, and oxidized substrate, respectively.

Alternatively, Compound I can undergo a single two-electron reduction back to the ground state. Halides and pseudohalides are used as two-electron reducing substrates by both EPO and MPO Compound I, forming potent antimicrobicidal oxidants, hypohalous acids.

C. Peroxidases and Formation of Halogenating Oxidants

Members of the mammalian peroxidase superfamily all share the unique ability to catalyze the two-electron peroxidation of halides forming potent halogenating intermediates: halogens (X_2), hypohalous acids (HOX), and their conjugate bases, hypohalites (OX^-) (80–82) (Fig. 1):

$$H_2O_2 + X^- + H^+ \rightarrow HOX + H_2O \tag{4}$$

where X is SCN, Br, Cl.

The halide substrate preference of each mammalian peroxidase differs. At normal plasma levels of halides and pseudohalides (100 mM Cl^-, 20–150 μM Br^-, 19–69 μM SCN^-, and <1 μMI^-) (83,84), SCN^- and Br^- are preferred substrates for EPO (80–82,85), while Cl^- is preferred by MPO. The unique ability of leukocyte peroxidases like MPO and EPO to halogenate biological targets through formation of reactive halogenating species has been exploited as a tool for identifying sites of oxidative modification of proteins and tissues mediated by these enzymes. Halogenated products serve as excellent molecular markers for EPO- and MPO-dependent oxidative modification in vivo as there are no other known pathways in humans that result in covalent incorporation of Br or Cl atoms into biomolecules (Fig. 1).

This chapter is organized according to reaction pathways and biochemistry defined for EPO and MPO, as outlined in Figure 1. We will discuss each reaction

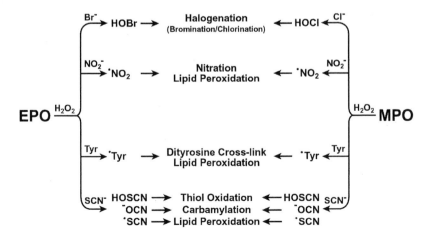

Figure 1 Scheme demonstrating oxidation pathways that may participate in asthma and remodeling of airways. (From Refs. 68,72–76,78,79,82,93,96–98,112,131.)

pathway mediated by the peroxidase, followed by the data currently available supporting a role for peroxidases in catalyzing these reactions in asthmatic lung and airways.

EPO and MPO as Enzymatic Catalysts of Oxidative Damage in Asthma: Halogenation

EPO-mediated oxidation of Br^- yields the potent brominating oxidant HOBr (hypobromous acid), a species with bactericidal, viricidal, and cytotoxic properties (80,81). Br^- is ubiquitous in humans and is present in virtually all biological fluids at ~50–100 μM (83,86). The selective preference of EPO for Br^- as substrate is unique among human peroxidases (80,81,87,88). At least 35% of the oxygen consumed by eosinophils stimulated in vitro in the presence of plasma levels of halides is directed toward generation of potent brominating species (81). HOBr induces characteristic tissue injury and symptoms of asthma in models of the disease (11–20, 89–91). Since EPO is the only human enzyme known that selectively generates reactive brominating species under physiological concentrations of halides, we hypothesized that brominated products may serve as "molecular fingerprints" to identify sites of EPO-mediated oxidative damage (Fig. 1). In prior studies, we similarly exploited the unique ability of MPO to generate reactive chlorinating oxidants like HOCl to demonstrate that atherosclerotic vessels and other sites of inflammation are sites of MPO-mediated oxidation (reviewed in Ref. 92). 3-Chlorotyrosine was identified as a stable specific product formed by modification of proteins by MPO-generated chlorinating oxidants (93,94). Recent studies with MPO knockout (KO) mice and multiple models of inflammation confirm the specificity of chlorotyrosine as a molecular fingerprint for MPO-mediated protein oxidation (79,95).

To identify stable brominated products, both proteins and free amino acids were exposed to either HOBr or purified EPO in the presence of H_2O_2 and plasma levels of Br^- (a HOBr-generating system). Using HPLC with on-line electrospray ionization mass spectrometry (LC/ESI/MS) and multinuclear NMR, 3-bromotyrosine and 3,5-dibromotyrosine were identified as stable markers of EPO-catalyzed oxidation (96). Studies with purified EPO vs. MPO revealed the specificity of bromotyrosine as a molecular marker for EPO-catalyzed oxidation of proteins (96), and studies with isolated human eosinophils vs. neutrophils confirmed the specificity of bromotyrosine as a marker for eosinophil-mediated oxidative damage (82). Recent studies with EPO KO mice and murine models of asthma (79,97) and other models of eosinophilic inflammation (79) all confirm the specificity of protein-bound bromotyrosine as a product of EPO-mediated oxidation (i.e., while significant levels of bromotyrosine are formed in wild-type mice, none has yet been detectable in EPO KO mice).

The first direct evidence that EPO-generated brominating oxidants participate in inflammatory injury during asthma was demonstrated in asthmatic subjects following segmental allergen challenge. Stable isotope dilution gas chromatography-mass spectrometry (GC-MS) was used to monitor bromotyrosine formation (82). Bromotyrosine levels were noted to be an order of magnitude higher in proteins within

BAL recovered from allergen-challenged segments of mild asthmatic subjects, compared to either normal saline-challenged subsegments of asthmatics or allergen-challenged subsegments of nonasthmatic nonatopic controls. These studies also provided the first direct evidence of a role for MPO-generating chlorinating oxidants in oxidative modification of lung and airways proteins in allergic asthma. Significant (~twofold) elevations in chlorotyrosine were noted in proteins recovered from allergen-challenged subsegments from asthmatic subjects (Fig. 1). More recently, bromotyrosine levels were shown to be dramatically elevated (nearly 100-fold) in BAL proteins from subjects with severe asthma admitted to the intensive care unit with respiratory failure (73). In these same subjects, significant increases (~threefold) in MPO-generated chlorotyrosine were noted. Collectively, these results show that eosinophils and neutrophils promote protein oxidative damage in both allergic asthma and severe asthma via formation of reactive halogen species (Fig. 1). These findings support a role for EPO and MPO in promoting oxidative injury during inflammation in asthmatic airways.

The demonstration that brominating and chlorinating oxidants participate in oxidative damage within airways of asthmatics raises the question of what other modifications are mediated by halogenating oxidants. Aromatic halogenation occurs in low yield compared to oxidation of many alternative targets (98,99). HOBr and HOCl react extremely rapidly with the thioethers like methionine, resulting in formation of methionine sulfoxide as the initial product. Free and protein-bound thiol residues, such as cysteine, are readily oxidized to disulfide forms. Interaction of halogenating oxidants with primary amines such as the Nε-amino moiety of lysine residues results in rapid formation of N-mono-haloamines and N-di-haloamines. These reactive species still retain the capacity to oxidize thiols and thioethers. In the case of N-mono-bromoamines and N-di-bromoamines, efficient halogenation of tyrosine still occurs (96). This property has the effect of prolonging the relative half-life of brominating oxidants, resulting in the conveyance of brominating equivalents into stable C-Br bonds on protein tyrosine residues, a chemical reactivity that should make bromotyrosine a better overall molecular marker for oxidative damage by EPO-generated brominating oxidants. EPO-generated HOBr is also able to form other oxidative insults, such as hydroxyl radical through interaction of HOBr with $O_2^{\cdot-}$ (100,101), and prior studies suggest EPO can form electronically excited oxygen in the $^1\Delta_g$ state (singlet oxygen) through interaction of HOBr with H_2O_2 (102,103). The physiological importance of these pathways in asthma is not yet established.

EPO and MPO as Enzymatic Catalysts of Oxidative Damage in Asthma: Nitration

Eosinophil recruitment and enhanced production of NO are characteristic features of asthma (4,104–107). Consequently, it had long been suspected that NO-derived oxidants might participate in cellular injury in inflamed airways in asthma. Immunohistochemical studies using antibodies to nitrotyrosine, a stable product of protein oxidation by NO-derived oxidants (108,109), were first used to demonstrate a role for NO-derived oxidants in asthma. Enhanced staining in lungs and airways of subjects with *status asthmaticus* was reported. Subsequent immunolocalization studies revealed eosinophils as major cellular sources for nitrotyrosine formation in asthmatic airways (73). Definitive evidence of protein modification through nitration in asthma was recently reported where mass spectrometry–based quantification demonstrated 10-fold increases in nitrotyrosine content in proteins recovered from airways of subjects with severe asthma compared to nonasthmatic controls (73). Thus, reactive nitrogen species represent an additional pathway for inflammatory injury in asthma, and eosinophils appear to play a central role in these reactions.

EPO has recently been shown to serve as a major enzymatic source of NO-derived oxidants and nitrotyrosine formation in allergic asthma. EPO has been shown to effectively use physiological levels of nitrite (NO_2^-), a major end product of NO metabolism, as co-substrate to nitrate free and protein-bound tyrosyl residues (72). EPO-mediated aromatic nitration occurs in high yield and is a preferred reaction for EPO in the presence of multiple competing co-substrates. Studies with isolated human eosinophils demonstrate that the cells are capable of generating NO-derived oxidants by at least two distinct pathways—the EPO-H_2O_2-NO_2^- system and $ONOO^-$. At physiologically relevant rates of NO production, the preferred pathway for nitrotyrosine formation is via EPO (73). The relative contributions of the EPO vs. $ONOO^-$ pathways for nitrotyrosine formation in allergic asthma were revealed in studies with EPO KO mice. Using EPO KO mice and an aeroallergen challenge model of asthma, a dominant role for EPO in nitrotyrosine formation was shown since 70% of nitrotyrosine formed in lungs of mice following allergen challenge was attributable to EPO (79). The relative contribution of MPO to protein nitration via a similar mechanism seems plausible since, like EPO, MPO can utilize NO_2^- as substrate to form nitrotyrosine (74,110–112). A role for MPO in formation of NO-derived oxidants in asthma has not yet been reported.

The chemical nature of the nitrating intermediate(s) formed during peroxidase-catalyzed oxidation of NO_2^- has recently been examined. Identifying the oxidizing intermediate involved in peroxidase catalyzed nitrotyrosine formation is important in the potential design of antioxidant or inhibitor strategies aimed at preventing inflammatory injury by NO-derived oxidants. Rapid kinetics studies suggested that the one-electron oxidation product of NO_2^-, nitrogen dioxide ($^\cdot NO_2$), was the primary reactive intermediate formed during MPO catalysis (113). This has now been confirmed for both MPO and EPO by direct detection of $^\cdot NO_2$ in headspace gas above reaction mixtures containing peroxidase and physiological levels of H_2O and NO_2^- (79). A possible role for EPO and MPO in oxidation of NO_2^- through a two-electron oxidation reaction yielding peroxynitrite has also been suggested (114) and recent data support the possibility of formation of a heme-bound $ONOO^-$ intermediate as a minor product (79). The relative contribution of this species to tissue injury in asthmatic airways in unknown, but the acidic pH of airway lining fluid in asthma (115) increases the likelihood of its participation since protonation of the distal histidine in the active site of peroxidases (pKa $\sim$ 4.5) results in its release and oxidation of targets (79).

EPO and MPO as Enzymatic Catalysts of Oxidative Damage in Asthma: Dityrosine Cross-Link

The amino acid tyrosine is itself readily oxidized through loss of its phenolic hydrogen atom, generating tyrosyl radical, a long-lived species that is resonance stabilized by delocalization of the radical around the phenolic ring. Radical-radical addition reactions between a pair of tyrosyl radicals results in formation of stable cross-links that are acid and protease resistant. Numerous examples of such peroxidase-catalyzed reactions exist in biology, such as formation of cork in plants by lignin peroxidases or formation of a protease-resistant coat during egg fertilization, preventing polyspermia (116,117). MPO-generated tyrosyl radical and phenolic addition products of tyrosyl radical (o,o′-dityrosine, isodityrosine, pulcherosine, and trityrosine) have been reported in vitro and in vivo (118,119). Further, the mechanism of aromatic nitration reactions mediated by peroxidase H_2O_2-NO_2^- systems is consistent with formation of a tyrosyl radical intermediate, which then couples with $^{\bullet}NO_2$ to form nitrotyrosine (113,120). The ability of both eosinophils and EPO to generate tyrosyl radical addition products like dityrosine has recently been reported (72,73). In unpublished studies, we have confirmed enrichment of the protein cross-link dityrosine in breath condensates of subjects with mild asthma compared to nonasthmatic controls (S. L. Hazen, 2002).

EPO and MPO as Enzymatic Catalysts of Oxidative Damage in Asthma: Carbamylation

A preferred substrate for EPO, and to a lesser extent MPO, is the pseudohalide thiocyanate (SCN^-). Thiocyanate is termed a pseudohalide because it reacts like a halide in several peroxidase-catalyzed reactions in vitro. The thiocyanate anion is abundant on mucosal surfaces, where it may serve as an in vivo substrate for EPO and LPO as part of host defenses. In recent studies, the proximate oxidation products of SCN^- that accumulate in buffer were determined using multinuclear NMR, mass spectrometry, and chemical characterization studies: hypothiocyanous acid, HOSCN, and cyanate (OCN^-) were identified (121). While the preference of EPO for thiocyanate is highest among the plasma halides, the oxidizing species produced, HOSCN, is a relatively weak oxidizing agent that primarily targets thiol oxidation. Cyanate is not an oxidant but is nonetheless chemically reactive and promotes protein modification through carbamylation of nucleophilic residues (122). Direct demonstration that proteins are carbamylated in asthmatic airways has yet to be reported. In addition to the two-electron oxidation product HOSCN, recent studies suggest that MPO may also use SCN^- as substrate via a one-electron oxidation reaction yielding thiocyanyl radical (Fig. 1). Whether EPO catalyzes similar reactions with SCN^- is unclear.

While thiocyanate is a preferred substrate for EPO and MPO, in plasma its concentrations and availability dictate its use as a co-substrate. Thiocynate levels are primarily dependent upon diet, with cruciferous fruits and vegetables being highest in content. An alternative source is via mainstream tobacco smoke; consequently, smokers can have significantly elevated levels of thiocyanate in plasma. EPO uses thiocyanate in preference to bromide. However, when SCN^- levels are low and limiting, EPO uses alternative substrates such as Br^-, resulting in formation of more potent (and damaging) oxidants like HOBr. Thus, it has been suggested that thiocyanate ingestion may mitigate inflammatory injury in asthma and may represent a novel form of anti-inflammatory therapy (121). It is thus noteworthy that epidemiological studies have suggested that diets rich in broccoli and onions, vegetables particularly rich in SCN^-, are linked to decreased prevalence of asthma (123). Direct experimental testing of this hypothesis is needed.

IV. Potential Physiological Impact of EPO- and MPO-Mediated Oxidation in Asthma

A role for viral and bacterial pathogens as triggers of asthma exacerbation is well recognized. The leukocytes recruited to combat the invading pathogens will wage chemical warfare as a means of incapacitating the microbe through production of reactive oxidants and diffusible radical species via the peroxidase-H_2O_2 systems outlined above. The reactive nature of these intermediates contributes to their capacity to promote inflammatory injury, both acute and chronic, within inflamed lungs and airways of asthmatic subjects. However, one might ask: What are the biological processes that are impacted upon by peroxidase-generated oxidants? Put another way: What role do peroxidases play in the pathogenesis of asthma?

A. Potential Physiological Impact of EPO- and MPO-Mediated Oxidation in Asthma: Mice Aren't Men

The simple answer to this question is that we do not yet know. Initial efforts to determine the role of EPO in asthma relied upon EPO KO mice and the ovalbumin challenge model of asthma. Remarkably, no phenotype could be noted (97). However, further characterization of the model revealed that mouse eosinophils fail to promote oxidative damage of lung and airways at the level observed in humans (Fig 2). Based upon these data and recent studies using the mouse as a model system for allergic pulmonary disease, it is now believed that eosinophil degranulation may not occur in most allergen challenge protocols with mice (124). For example, in contrast to what occurs in humans, eosinophils recruited to mouse lungs remain intact, with no electron microscopic evidence of degranulation in the airway (125–128). Thus, eosinophil recruitment alone within a murine model system cannot be used as an indicator of EPO-dependent oxidative injury in vivo. Rather, EPO-mediated oxidative damage requires concomitant degranulation of eosinophils and production of H_2O_2 by a respiratory burst. These studies also suggest that exploration of the role of EPO-mediated oxidation pathways in vivo within mice will require use of an alternative model of pulmonary inflammation—ones where significant eosinophil degranulation and EPO-mediated oxidative injury is observed, such as that monitored by formation of bromotyrosine.

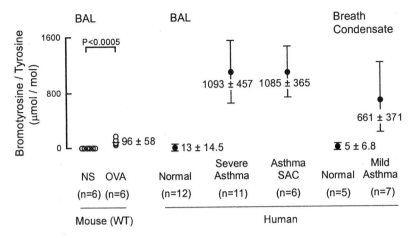

Figure 2 Bromotyrosine levels in BAL protein from allergen-sensitized/aerosolize-challenged mice are 10-fold lower than levels observed in asthma patients. Data shown are for mouse and human BAL protein levels of bromotyrosine 48 hours following allergen challenge. Breath condensate data is from moderate asthmatic subjects (S. L. Hazen, unpublished). WLAC, whole lung allergen challenge; SAC, segmental allergen challenge. (From Refs. 73,82,97.)

B. Potential Physiological Impact of EPO- and MPO-Mediated Oxidation in Asthma: Formation of Bioactive Lipid Oxidation Products

While stable products of protein oxidative modification formed by distinct mechanisms have severed as "molecular fingerprints" to demonstrate which pathways are operational in vivo, their role in the pathogenesis of asthma remains uncertain. Clearly, oxidative modifications of protein tyrosine residues that participate in signaling pathways have the potential to modulate kinase/phosphatase cascades. However, to date, a role of peroxidase-mediated tyrosine oxidation in regulating these processes has not yet been shown. An alternative mechanism where peroxidase-generated oxidants likely participate is via formation of lipid-derived signaling molecules. The lipophilic nature of many of the oxidants formed, combined with their facile ability to initiate lipid peroxidation, suggests that peroxidases may serve as a major source of bioactive eicosanoids and other bioactive lipid oxidation products in vivo. For example, MPO-generated $^{\cdot}NO_2$ and tyrosyl radical have been shown to serve as mechanisms for initiating lipid peroxidation, and isolated neutrophils and monocytes have been shown capable of generating fatty acid, phospholipid, and sterol oxidation products via these pathways (77,78,112,129,130). Recent mass spectrometry–based studies examining the effects of neutrophil activation in plasma using leukocytes isolated from normal and MPO-deficient subjects strongly support a primary role for MPO as a physiological catalyst for lipid peroxidation in vivo at sites of acute inflammation (129). The primary co-substrates in plasma that MPO may utilize to initiate lipid oxidation were also recently determined and shown to include NO_2^-, tyrosine, and SCN^- (129). Given the recent demonstrations that EPO is particularly facile at generating $^\cdot NO_2$ compared to MPO (72,79), a role for EPO in generation of bioactive lipid oxidation products in asthmatic airways seems likely. Further research in this area is warranted.

C. Potential Physiological Impact of EPO- and MPO-Mediated Oxidation in Asthma: Serving as a Catalytic Sink for NO

Mammalian peroxidases were recently shown to utilize NO as a physiological substrate, resulting in its rapid consumption (131). Compounds I and II of EPO, MPO, and LPO were all shown to effectively use NO as a substrate, even in the presence of superoxide and competing alternative co-substrates like plasma levels of halides (75,76,131). LPO is present at high levels in tracheal lining fluid in the airways (52), and EPO levels are markedly enriched in airways of asthmatic patients. Consequently, it has been proposed that peroxidases may serve as a catalytic sink for NO, thereby limiting its bioavailability and function at sites of inflammation, such as in inflamed asthmatic airways. Recent organ chamber studies support this potential role, as NO-dependent bronchodilation of preconstricted tracheal rings was reversibly inhibited by catalytic levels of EPO, LPO, and MPO (75). Further, direct spectroscopic and rapid kinetics studies defining NO interactions with mammalian peroxidases support a facile reaction between peroxidases and NO (75,131). The ability of peroxidases to attenuate bronchodilation may have important implications in the development of asthma. Bronchospasm is a characteristic feature of asthma, suggesting a deficiency of bronchodilator action of NO in tissue. It is tempting to speculate that peroxidases contribute to bronchconstriction by consuming NO in airway lining fluid during the late asthmatic response. An effect of peroxidases in vivo in airway hyperactivity and bronchospasm has not yet been documented.

D. Potential Physiological Impact of EPO- and MPO-Mediated Oxidation in Asthma: Airways Remodeling

Airway inflammation appears to be intimately linked to airways remodeling (recently reviewed in Refs. 107,132–134). A consequence of chronic inflammatory processes is damage and injury. In addition to persistence of inflammatory cells, characteristic features include structural changes in the airways, such as increased wall thickness and permanent reduction in airways caliber. Basement membrane alterations and thickening are often observed, along with enhanced extracellular matrix deposition. These features collectively enhance resistance to airflow, particularly during bronchial constriction and hyperresponsiveness. While asthma is defined by reversible obstructive airways disease, a major clinical consequence of the ultrastructural alterations of remodeling often includes development of an irreversible component of the airways obstruction. Thus, many asthmatic subjects develop evidence of residual airways obstruction (135–139), which may be detected in symptomatic patients (140), as well as months after cessation of asthmatic symptoms in asymptomatic patients (135,140,141).

Another prominent feature associated with remodeling is loss of elastic recoil and lung elasticity and, consequently, increased work of breathing (142–146). The etiology of this is not known but appears to be related to an intrinsic abnormality, such as through ultrastructural changes to matrix during remodeling (144). A prevailing view of the remodeling process is that chronic repairs of injured tissues by replacement with various parenchymal cells, and recurrent regeneration of connective tissues, can lead eventually to fibrosis and scar formation (147). A role for oxidative modifications, particularly formation of protein cross-links by leukocyte-mediated reactions, has not been examined.

Oxidative damage by peroxidases likely contributes to several features of airway remodeling. MPO and EPO both generate tyrosyl radical and thus can form protein cross-links. It seems logical to speculate that a consequence of such modifications is loss of elastic recoil. Fibrotic changes that occur in chronic asthma may also in part be due to the activation of multiple protease cascades, an activity known for MPO. MPO-generated oxidants have been linked to activation of matrix metalloproteases, elastase, and oxidative inactivation of tissue inhibitors of matrix metalloproteases, α_1-antitrypsin and plasminogen activator inhibitor 1 (39–49). Thus, peroxidase activity in asthmatic airways may contribute to oxidative cross-linking, loss of elasticity, and other cumulative effects in the remodeling process.

V. Where Does the Future Lie in Peroxidases and Asthma?

This chapter has attempted to summarize the recent and rapid progress made in characterizing the chemical processes mediated by peroxidases that occur in lungs and airways during asthma, as well as speculations about their potential contributions to the disease process. Studies examining the role of peroxidases in oxidative injury and inflammation in asthma are still in their infancy. Consequently, much more needs to be done. Studies aimed at elucidating whether peroxidases contribute to the pathogenesis of asthma or merely generate oxidative products that can serve as markers of inflammation are of particular importance.

Peroxidase-catalyzed oxidation of targets in asthmatic airways opens numerous avenues for future research, but perhaps most importantly in the areas of diagnostics and therapeutics. There currently are no practical methods for monitoring the degree of airways inflammation in asthma, a process that is critically linked to the development of irreversible injury and airway remodeling in chronic asthma. The specificity of bromotyrosine as a unique molecular fingerprint of eosinophilic inflammation, combined with its stability, unusual structure, and dramatic elevations during asthma, suggested that this product might be measured systemically and serve as a noninvasive mechanism for monitoring airway inflammation. The ability to detect serial levels of oxidation products in plasma or urine opens new vistas towards monitoring treatments of asthma. Bromotyrosine is readily detected in blood and urine of subjects with asthma. Further, elevated levels are observed at time of exacerbation, such as that leading to presentation at an emergency department, and subse-

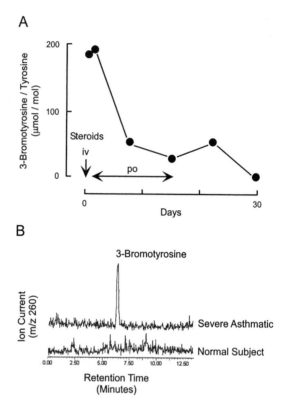

Figure 3 (A) Serum bromotyrosine levels were determined in a subject over time following presentation to the emergency department. The subject was hospitalized and received a course of parenteral corticosteroids, followed by an oral tapered dose as indicated. (B) Detection of bromotyrosine in urine of the same asthmatic subject by high-performance liquid chromatography with online electrospray ionization mass spectrometry.

quent decline following institution of therapy (Fig. 3). We therefore speculate that levels of bromotyrosine may serve as a novel mechanism for monitoring severity of disease as well as the anti-inflammatory response of therapy in an individual. Research in this exciting area is ongoing.

With the realization that leukocyte peroxidase contributes through multiple mechanisms to oxidative injury in asthma, the potential use of peroxidase inhibitors as a novel form of therapy in asthma seems warranted. It is therefore of interest that peroxidase inhibitors are not yet commercially available. Development of this novel class of anti-inflammatory agent is sorely needed.

References

1. Gleich GJ, Ottesen EA, Leiferman KM, Ackerman SJ. Eosinophils and human disease. Int Arch Allergy Appl Immunol 1989; 88:59–62.

2. Wardlaw AJ. Eosinophils in the 1990s: new perspectives on their role in health and disease. Postgrad Med J 1994; 70(826):536–552.
3. Horwitz R, Busse WW. Inflammation and asthma. Clin Chest Med 1995; 16:583–602.
4. Bousquet J, Jeffery PK, Busse WW, Johnson M, Vignola AM. Asthma. From broncho-constriction to airways inflammation and remodeling. Am J Respir Crit Care Med 2000; 161:1720–1745.
5. Hamann KJ, Barker RL, Ten RM, Gleich GJ. The molecular biology of eosinophil granule proteins. Int Arch Allergy Appl Immunol 1991; 94:202–209.
6. Cardell BS, Pearson RBS. Death in asthmatics. Thorax 1959; 14:341–352.
7. Wardlaw AJ, Dunnette S, Gleich GJ, Collins JV, Kay AB. Eosinophils and mast cells in bronchoalveolar lavage fluid and mild asthma: Relationship to bronchial hyperactivity. Am Rev Respir Dis 1988; 137:62–69.
8. Griffin E, Hakansson L, Formgren H, Jorgensen K, Peterson C, Venge P. Blood eosinophil number and activity in relation to lung function in patients with asthma and with eosinophilia. J Allergy Clin Immunol 1991; 87:548–557.
9. Bousquet J, Van Vyve T, Chanez P, Enander I, Michel FB, Godard P. Cells and mediators in bronchoalveolar lavage in asthmatic patients: The example of eosinophilic inflammation. Allergy 1993; 48(17 suppl):70–75.
10. Sanz ML, Parra A, Prieto I, Dieguez I, Oehling AK. Serum eosinophil peroxidase (EPO) levels in asthmatic patients. Allergy 1997; 52:417–422.
11. Durack DT, Sumi SM, Klebanoff SJ. Neurotoxicity of human eosinophils. Proc Natl Acad Sci USA 1997; 76:1443–1447.
12. Davis WB, Fells GA, Sun XH, Gadek JE, Venet A, Crystal RG. Eosinophilmediated injury to lung parenchymal cells and interstitial matrix. J Clin Invest 1984; 74:269–278.
13. Ayars GH, Altman LC, Gleicy GJ, Loegering DA, Baker CB. Eosinophil- and eosinophil granule-mediated pneumocyte injury. J Allergy Clin Immunol 1985; 76:595–603.
14. Laitinen LA, Heino M, Laitinen A, Kava T, Haahtela T. Damage of the airway epithelium and bronchial reactivity in patients with asthma. Am Rev Respir Dis 1985; 131:599–606.
15. Agosti JM, Altman LC, Ayars GH, Loegering DA, Gleich GJ, Klebanoff SJ. The injurious effect of eosinophil peroxidase, hydrogen peroxide, and halides on pneumocytes in vitro. J Allergy Clin Immunol 1987; 79:496–504.
16. Yoshikawa S, Kayes SG, Parker, JC. Eosinophils increase lung microvascular permeability via the peroxidase-hydrogen peroxide-halide system. Bronchoconstriction and vasoconstriction unaffected by eosinophil peroxidase Am Rev Respir Dis 1993; 147:914–920.
17. Minnicozzi M, Duran WN, Gleich GJ, Egan RW. Eosinophil granule proteins increase microvascular macromolecular transport in the hamster cheek pouch. J Immunol 1994; 153:2664–2670.
18. Brottman GM, Regelmann WE, Slungaard A, Wangensteen OD. Effect of eosinophil peroxidase on airway epithelial permeability in the guinea pig. Pediatr Pulmonol 1996; 21:159–166.
19. Hirata A, Motojima S, Fukuda T, Makino S. Damage to respiratory epithelium by guinea-pig eosinophils stimulated with IgG-coated Sepharose beads. Clin Exp Allergy 1996; 26:848–858.
20. Blythe DI, Pedrick MS, Savage TJ, Hessel EM, Fattah D. Lung inflammation and epithelial changes in a murine model of atopic asthma. Am J Respir Cell Mol Biol 1996; 14:425–438.

21. Spector AA, Gordon JA, Moore SA. Hydroxyeicosatetraenoic acids (HETEs). Prog Lipid Res 1988; 27:272–323.
22. Dakle'n SE, Hedquist P, Hammarstrom S, Sammelsson B. Leukotrienes are potent constrictors of human bronchi. Nature 1980; 288:484–486.
23. Shaw RJ, Walsh GM, Cromwell O, Moqbel R, Spry CJF, Kay AB. Activated human eosinophils generate SRS-A leukotrienes following physiological (IgG dependent) stimulation. Nature 1985; 316:150–152.
24. Cuss FM, Dixon CMS, Barnes PJ. Effects of inhaled platelet activating factor on pulmonary function and bronchial responsiveness in man. Lancet 1986; 2:189–192.
25. Campbell HD, Tucker WQ, Hort Y, Martinson ME, Mayo G, Clutterbuck EJ, Sanderson CJ, Young IG. Molecular cloning, nucleotide sequence, and expression of the gene encoding human eosinophil differentiation factor (interleukin 5). Proc Natl Acad Sci USA 1987; 84:6629–6633.
26. Lecki MJ, ten Brinke A, Khan J, Diamant Z, O'Connor BJ, Walls CM, Mathur AK, Cowley HC, Chung KF, Djukanovic R, Hansel TT, Holgate ST, Sterk PJ, Barnes PJ. Effects of an interleukin-5 blocking monoclonal antibody on eosinophils, airway hyper-responsiveness, and the late asthmatic response. Lancet 2000; 356:2144–2148.
27. Samoszuk MK, Nguyen V, Gluzman I, Pham JH. Occult deposition of eosinophil peroxidase in a subset of human breast carcinomas. Am J Pathol 1996; 148:701–706.
28. Samoszuk MK, Anderson AL, Ramzi E, Wang F, Braunstein P, Lutsky J, Majmundar H, Slater LM. Radioimmunodetection of Hodgkin's disease and non-Hodgkin's lymphomas with monoclonal antibody to eosinophil peroxidase. J Nucl Med 1993; 84:1246–1253.
29. Fahy J, Liu J, Wong H, Boushey A. Cellular and biochemical analysis of induced sputum from asthmatic and from healthy subjects. Am Rev Respir Dis 1993; 147:1126–1131.
30. Lacoste JY, Bousquet J, Chanez P, Van Vyve T, Simony-Lafontaine J, Lequeu N, Vic P, Enander I, Godard P, Michel FB. Eosinophilic and neutrophilic inflammation in asthma, chronic bronchitis, and chronic obstructive pulmonary disease. J Allergy Clin Immunol 1993; 92:537–548.
31. Bradley BL, Azzawi M, Jacobson M, Assoufi B, Collins V, Irani AM, Schwartz LB, Durham SR, Jeffrey PK, Kay AB. Eosinophils, T-lymphocytes, mast cells, neutrophils, and macrophages in bronchial biopsy specimens from atopic subjects with asthma: Comparison with biopsy specimens from atopic subjects without asthma and normal control subjects and relationship to bronchial hyperresponsiveness. J Allergy Clin Immunol 1991; 88:661–674.
32. Koh YY, Dupuis R, Pollice M, Albertine KH, Fish JE, Peters SR. Neutrophils recruited to the lungs of humans by segmental antigen challenge display a reduced chemotactic response to leukotriene B4. Am J Respir Cell Mol Biol 1993; 8:493–499.
33. Motefort S, Gratziou C, Goulding D, Polosa R, Haskard DO, Howarth PH. Bronchial biopsy evidence for leukocyte infiltration and upregulation of leukocyte-endothelial cell adhesion molecules 6 hours after local allergen challenge of sensitized asthmatic airways. J Clin Invest 1994; 93:1411–1421.
34. Sur S, Crotty TB, Kephart GM, Hyma BA, Colby TV, Reed CE, Hunt LW, Gleich GJ. Sudden-onset fatal asthma: a distinct entity with a few eosinophils and relatively more neutrophils in the airway submucosa? Am Rev Respir Dis 1993; 148:713–719.
35. Carroll NS, Carello S, Cooke C, James A. Airway structure and inflammatory cells in fatal attacks of asthma. Eur Respir J 1996; 9:709–715.

36. Martin RJ, Cicutto LC, Smith HR, Ballard RD, Szefler SJ. Airways inflammation in nocturnal asthma. Am Rev Respir Dis 1991; 143:351–357.
37. Foresi A, Bertorelli G, Pesci A, Chetta A, Olivieri D. Inflammatory markers in bronchoalveolar lavage and in bronchial biopsy in asthma during remission. Chest 1990; 98:528–535.
38. Tanizaki Y, Kitani H, Mufune T, Mitsunobu F, Kajimoto K, Sugimoto K. Effects of glucocorticoids on humoral and cellular immunity and on airway inflammation in patients with steroid-dependent intractable asthma. J Asthma 1993; 80:485–492.
39. Chu HW, Trudeau JB, Balzar S, Wenzel SE. Peripheral blood and airway tissue expression of transforming growth factor beta by neutrophils in asthmatic subjects and normal control subjects. J Allergy Clin Immunol 2000; 106:1115–1123.
40. Kelly EA, Busse WW, Jarjour NN. Increased matrix metalloproteinase-9 in the airway after allergen challenge. Am J Respir Crit Care Med 2000; 162:1157–1161.
41. Meerschaert J, Kelly EA, Mosher DF, Busse WW, Jarjour NN. Segmental antigen challenge increases fibronectin in brochoalveolar lavage fluid. Am J Respir Crit Care Med 1999; 159:619–625.
42. Vignola AM, Riccobono L, Mirabella A, Profita M, Chanez P, Bellia V, Mautino G, D'accardi P, Bousquet J, Bonsignore G. Sputum metalloproteinase-9/tissue inhibitor of metalloproteinase-1 ration correlates with airflow obstruction in asthma and chronic bronchitis. Am J Respir Crit Care Med 1998; 158:1945–1950.
43. Vignola AM, Bonanno A, Mirabella A, Riccobono L, Mirabella F, Profita M, Bellia V, Bousquet J, Bonsignore G. Increased levels of elastase and alpha1-antitrypsin in sputum of asthmatic patients. Am J Respir Crit Care Med 1998; 157:505–511.
44. Fu X, Kassim SY, Parks WC, Heinecke JW. Hypochlorous acid oxygenates the cysteine switch domain of pro-matrilysin (MMP-7): a mechanism for matrix metalloproteinase activation and atherosclerotic plaque rupture by myeloperoxidase. J Biol Chem 2001; 276:41279–41287.
45. Shabani F, McNeil J, Tippett L. The oxidative inactivation of tissue inhibitor of metalloproteinase-1 (TIMP-1) by hypochlorous acid (HOCl) is suppressed by anti-rheumatic drugs. Free Radic Res 1998; 28:115–123.
46. Zaslow MC, Clark RA, Stone PJ, Calore JD, Snider GL, Franzblau C. Human neutrophil elastase does not bind to alpha 1-protease inhibitor that has been exposed to activated human neutrophils. Am Rev Respir Dis 1983; 128:434–439.
47. Campbell EJ, Senior RM, McDonald JA, Cox DL. Proteolysis by neutrophils. Relative importance of cell-substrate contact and oxidative inactivation of proteinase inhibitors in vitro. J Clin Invest 1982; 70:845–852.
48. Clark RA, Stone PJ, El Hag A, Calore JD, Franzblau C. Myeloperoxidase-catalyzed inactivation of alpha 1-protease inhibitor by human neutrophils. J Biol Chem 1981; 256:3348–3353.
49. Lawrence DA, Loskutoff DJ. Inactivation of plasminogen activator inhibitor by oxidants. Biochemistry 1986; 25:6351–6353.
50. Holt PG, Macaubas C, Stumbles PA, Sly PD. The role of allergy in the development of asthma. Nature 1999; 25:12–17.
51. Gleich GJ, Ottesen EA, Leiferman KM, Ackerman SJ. Eosinophils and human disease. Int Arch Allergy Appl Immunol 1989; 88:59–62.
52. Salathe M, Holderby M, Forteza R, Abraham WM, Wanner A, Conner GE. Isolation and characterization of a peroxidase from the airway. Am J Respir Cell Mol Biol 1997; 17:97–105.
53. Rothenberg ME. Eosinophilia. N Engl J Med 1998; 338:1592–1600.

54. Klebanoff SJ, Clark RA. The neutrophil: function and clinical disorders. In: The Neutrophil: Function and Clinical Disorders. Amsterdam: Elsevier/North Holland Biomedical Press, 1978:447–451.

55. Everse J, Everse KE, Grisham MB. Peroxidases in Chemistry and Biology. Vol. I. Boca Raton, FL: CRC Press, 1991.

56. Spry CJ. F. Eosinophils. A Comprehensive Review and Guide to the Medical Literature. Oxford: Oxford University Press, 1988.

57. Klebanoff SJ. Oxygen metabolism and the toxic properties of phagocytes. Ann Intern Med 1980; 93:480–489.

58. Babior BM. Oxygen-dependent microbial killing by phagocytes. N Engl J Med 1978; 298:659–663.

59. Klebanoff SJ, Locksley RM, Jong EC, Rosen H. Oxidative response of phagocytes to parasite invasion. Ciba Found Symp 1983; 99:92–112.

60. Babior BM, Kipnes RS, Curnutte JT. Biological defense mechanisms. The production by leukocytes of superoxide, a potential bactericidal agent. J Clin Invest 1973; 52: 741–744.

61. Jong EC, Henderson WR, Klebanoff SJ. Bactericidal activity of eosinophil peroxidase. J Immunol 1980; 124:1378–1382.

62. Segal BH, Leto TL, Gallin JI, Malech HL, Holland SM. Genetic, biochemical, and clinical features of chronic granulomatous disease. Medicine 2000; 79:170–200.

63. DeChatelet LR, Shirley PS, McPhail LC, Huntley CC, Muss HB, Bass DA. Oxidative metabolism of the human eosinophil. Blood 1977; 50:525–535.

64. Slungaard A, Vercellotti GM, Walker G, Nelson RD, Jacob HS. Tumor necrosis factor alpha/cachectin stimulates eosinophil oxidant production and toxicity towards human endothelium. J Exp Med 1990; 171:2025–2041.

65. Someya A, Nishijima K, Nunoi H, Irie S, Nagaoka I. Study on the superoxide-producing enzyme of eosinophils and neutrophils—comparison of the NADPH oxidase components. Arch Biochem Biophys 1997; 345:207–213.

66. Migler R, DeChatelet LR. Human eosinophilic peroxidase: biochemical characterization. Biochem Med 1978; 19:16–26.

67. Olsen RL, Little C. Purification and some properties of myeloperoxidase and eosinophil peroxidase from human blood. Biochem J 1983; 209:781–787.

68. Mitra S, Slungaard A, Hazen SL. Eosinophil peroxidase and the origins of protein oxidation in asthma. Redox Rep 2000; 5:215–224.

69. Horton MA, Larson KA, Lee JJ, Lee NA. Cloning of the murine eosinophil peroxidase gene (mEPO): characterization of a conserved subgroup of mammalian hematopoietic peroxidases. J Leukocyte Biol 1996; 60:285–294.

70. Oxvig C, Thomsen AR, Overgaard MT, Sorensen ES, Hojrup P, Bjerrum MJ, Gleich GJ, Sottrup-Jensen L. Biochemical evidence for heme linkage through esters with Asp-93 and Glu-241 in human eosinophil peroxidase. J Biol Chem 1999; 74:16953–16958.

71. Heinecke JW, Li W, Francis GA, Goldstein JA. Tyrosyl radical generated by myeloperoxidase catalyzes the oxidative cross-linking of proteins. J Clin Invest 1993; 91: 2866–2872.

72. Wu W, Chen Y, Hazen SL. Eosinophil peroxidase nitrates protein tyrosyl residues: implications for oxidative damage by nitrating intermediates in eosinophilic inflammatory disorders. J Biol Chem 1999; 274:25933–25944.

73. MacPherson JC, Comhair SA, Erzurum SC, Klein DF, Lipscomb MF, Kavuru MS, Samoszuk M, Hazen SL. Eosinophils are a major source of NO-derived oxidants in

severe asthma: characterization of pathways available to eosinophils for generating reactive nitrogen species. J Immunol 2001; 166:5763–5772.

74. Podrez EA, Schmidt D, Hoff H, Hazen SL. Myeloperoxidase-generated reactive nitrogen species convert LDL into an atherogenic form in vitro, J Clin Invest 1999; 103: 1547–1560.

75. Abu-Soud HM, Khassawneh M, Sohn J, Murray P, Haxhiu MA, Hazen SL. Peroxidases inhibit nitric oxide (NO) dependent bronchodilation: development of a model describing NO-peroxidase interactions. Biochemistry 2001; 40:11866–11875.

76. Abu-Soud H, Hazen SL. Nitric oxide modulates the catalytic activity of myeloperoxidase. J Biol Chem 2000; 275:5425–5430.

77. Savenkova ML, Mueller DM, Heinecke JW. Tyrosyl radical generated by myeloperoxidase is a physiological catalyst for the initiation of lipid peroxidation in low density lipoprotein. J Biol Chem 1994; 12(269):20394–20400.

78. Schmitt D, Shen Z, Zhang R, Colles SM, Wu W, Chen Y, Chisolm GM, Hazen SI, Leukocytes utilize myeloperoxidase-generated nitrating intermediates as physiological catalysts for the generation of biologically active oxidized lipids and sterols in serum. Biochemistry 1999; 38:16904–16915.

79. Brennan, M.-L., Wu W, Fu X, Shen Z, Song, W. Frost H, Vadseth C, Narine L, Lenkiewicz E, Borchers MT, Lusis AJ, Lee JJ, Lee NA, Abu-Soud HM, Ischiropoulos H, Hazen SL. A tale of two controversies: i) Defining the role of peroxidases in nitrotyrosine formation in vivo using eosinophil peroxidase and myeloperoxidase deficient mice; and ii) Defining the nature of peroxidase-generated reactive nitrogen species. J Biol Chem 2002; 277:17415–17427.

80. Weiss SJ, Test ST, Eckmann CM, Ross D, Regiani S. Brominating oxidants generated by human eosinophils. Science 1986; 234:200–203.

81. Mayeno AN, Curran AJ, Roberts RL, Foote CS. Eosinophils preferentially use bromide to generate halogenating agents. J Biol Chem 1989; 264:5660–5668.

82. Wu W, Samoszuk M. Comhair S, Thomassen MJ, Farver C, Dweik R, Kavuru M, Erzurum SC, Hazen SL. Eosinophils generate brominating oxidants in allergen-induced asthma. J Clin Invest 2000; 105:1455–1463.

83. Linder M. In: Nutritional Biochemistry and Metabolism. New York: Elsevier, 1992: 98–128.

84. Teitz, NW. Drugs: therapeutic and toxic. In: Burtis CA, Ashwood ER, eds. *Teitz Textbook of Clinical Chemistry*. Philadelphia: W.B. Saunders Co., 1999:1097.

85. Slungaard A, Mahoney JR, Jr. Thiocyanate is the major substrate for eosinophil peroxidase in physiologic fluids. Implications for cytotoxicity. J Biol Chem 1991; 266: 4903–4910.

86. Nielsen FH. In: Mertz W, ed. Trace Elements in Human and Animal Nutrition. Vol. 2, 5th ed. New York: Academic Press, 1986:426–430.

87. Agner K. Structure and Function of Oxidation-Reduction Enzymes. New York: Pergamon Press, 1972:329–335.

88. Harrison JE, Schultz J. Studies on the chlorinating activity of myeloperoxidase. J Biol Chem 1976; 251:1371–1374.

89. Pretolani M, Ruffie C, Joseph D, Campos MG, Church MK, Lefort J, Vargaftig BB. Role of eosinophil activation in the bronchial reactivity of allergic guinea pigs. Am J Respir Crit Care Med 1994; 149:1167–1174.

90. Samoszuk MK, Nguyen V, Thomas CT, Jacobson DM. Effects of sonicated eosinophils on the in vitro sensitivity of human lymphoma cells to glucose oxidase. Cancer Res 1994; 54:2650–2653.

91. Hamann KJ, Strek ME, Baranowski SL, Munoz NM, Williams FS, White SR, Vita A, Leff AR. Effects of activated eosinophils cultured from human umbilical cord blood on guinea pig trachealis. Am J Physiol 1993; 265:301–307.

92. Podrez EA, Abu-Soud HM. Myeloperoxidase-generated oxidants and atherosclerosis. Free Rad Biol Med 2000; 28:1717–1725.

93. Hazen SL, Heinecke JW. 3-Chlorotyrosine, a specific marker of myeloperoxidase-catalyzed oxidation, is markedly elevated in low density lipoprotein isolated from human atherosclerotic intima. J Clin Invest 1997; 99:2075–2081.

94. Domigan NM, Charlton TS, Duncan MW, Winterbourn CC, Kettle AJ. Chlorination of tyrosyl residues in peptides by myeloperoxidase and human neutrophils. J Biol Chem 1995; 270:16542–16548.

95. Brennan ML, Anderson M, Shih D, Qu X, Wang X, Mehta A, Lim L, Shi W, Hazen SL, Jacob J, Crowley J, Heinecke JW, Lusis AJ. Increased atherosclerosis in myeloperoxidase-deficient mice. J Clin Invest 2001; 107:419–430.

96. Wu W, d'Avignon A, Chen Y, Hazen SL. 3-Bromotyrosine and 3,5-dibromotyrosine are major products of protein oxidation by eosinophil peroxidase: potential markers for eosinophil-dependent tissue injury in vivo. Biochemistry 1999; 38:3538–3548.

97. Denzler KL, Borchers M, Crosby JR, Cieslewicz G, Hines EM, Justice JP, Cormier S, Lindenberger K, Song W, Wu W, Hazen SL, Gleich G, Lee JJ, Lee NA. Extensive eosinophil degranulation and peroxidase-mediated oxidation of airway proteins do not occur in a mouse ovalbumin-challenge model of pulmonary inflammation. J Immunol 2001; 167:1672–1782.

98. Hazen SL, Hsu FF, Gaut JP, Crowley JR, Heinecke JW. Modification of proteins and lipids by myeloperoxidase. Methods Enzymol 1999; 300:88–105.

99. Winterbourn CC, Vissers MC, Kettle AJ. Myeloperoxidase. Curr Opin Hematol 2000; 7:53–58.

100. Shen A, Wu W, Hazen SL. Leukocytes oxidatively damage DNA, RNA and the nucleotide pool through halide-dependent formation of hydroxyl radical. Biochemistry 2000; 39:5474–5482.

101. McCormick ML, Roeder TL, Railsback MA, Britigan BE. Eosinophil peroxidase-dependent hydroxyl radical generation by human eosinophils. J Biol Chem 1994; 269: 27914–27919.

102. Kanofsky JR, Hoogland H, Wever R, Weis SJ. Singlet oxygen production by human eosinophils. J Biol Chem 1988; 263:9692–9696.

103. Krinsky NI. Singlet excited oxygen as a mediator of the antibacterial action of leukocytes. Science 1974; 186:363–365.

104. Barnes PJ. Nitric oxide and asthma. Res Immunol 1995; 146:698–702.

105. Ashutosh K. Nitric oxide and asthma: a review. Curr Opin Pulm Med 2000; 6:21–25.

106. Guo FH, Comhair SA, Zheng S, Dweik RA, Eissa NT, Thomassen MJ, Calhoun W, Erzurum SC. Molecular mechanisms of increased nitric oxide (NO) in asthma: evidence for transcriptional and post-translational regulation of NO synthesis. J Immunol 2000; 164:5970–5980.

107. Bousquet J, Jeffery PK, Busse WW, Johnson M, Vignola AM. Asthma. From bonchoconstriction to airways inflammation and remodeling. Am J Respir Crit Care Med 2000; 161:17200–17245.

108. Saleh D, Ernst P, Lim S, Barnes PJ, Giaid A. Increased formation of the potent oxidant peroxynitrite in the airways of asthmatic patients is associated with induction of nitric oxide synthase: effect of inhaled glucocorticoid. FASEB J 1998; 12:929–937.

109. Kaminsky DA, Mitchell J, Carroll N, James A, Soultanakis R, Janssen Y. Nitrotyrosine formation in the airways and lung parenchyma of patients with asthma. J Allergy Clin Immunol 1999; 104:747–754.

110. Van der Vliet A, Eiserich JP, Halliwell B, Cross CE. Formation of reactive nitrogen species during peroxidase-catalyzed oxidation of nitrite. A potential additional mechanism of nitric oxide-dependent toxicity. J Biol Chem 1997; 272:7617–7625.

111. Eiserich JP, Hristova M, Cross CE, Jones AD, Freeman BA, Halliwell B, van der Vliet A. Formation of nitric oxide-derived inflammatory oxidants by myeloperoxidase in neutrophils. Nature 1998; 391:393–397.

112. Hazen SL, Zhang R, Wu W, Podrez EA, Shen Z, MacPhearson J, Schmitt D, Mitra SN, Chen Y, Cohen P, Hoff HF, Abu-Soud HM. Formation of nitric oxide-derived oxidants by myeloperoxidase in monocytes: pathways for monocyte-mediated protein nitration and lipid peroxidation in vivo. Circ Res 1999; 85:950–958.

113. Burner U, Furtmuller PG, Kettle AJ, Koppenol WH, Obinger C. Mechanism of reaction of myeloperoxidase with nitrite. J Biol Chem 2000; 275:20597–205601.

114. Sampson JB, Ye Y, Rosen H, Beckman JS. Myeloperoxidase and horseradish peroxidase catalyze tyrosine nitration in proteins from nitrite and hydrogen peroxide. Arch Biochem Biophys 1998; 356:207–213.

115. Hunt JF, Fang K, Malik R, Snyder A, Malhotra N, Platts-Mills TA, Gaston B. Endogenous airway acidification. Implications for asthma pathophysiology. Am J Respir Crit Care Med 2000; 161:694–699.

116. Hall HG. Hardening of the sea urchin fertilization envelope by peroxidase-catalyzed phenolic coupling of tyrosines. Cell 1978; 15:343–355.

117. Wallace G, Fry SC. Phenolic components of the plant cell wall. Int Rev Cytol 1994; 151:229–267.

118. Leeuwenburgh C, Rasmussen JE, Hsu FF, Mueller DM, Pennathur S, Heinecke JW. Mass spectrometric quantification of markers for protein oxidation by tyrosyl radical, copper, and hydroxyl radical in low density lipoprotein isolated from human atherosclerotic plaques. J Biol Chem 1997; 272:3520–3526.

119. Jacob JS, Cistola DP, Hsu FF, Muzaffar S, Mueller DM, Hazen SL, Heinecke JW. Human phagocytes employ the myeloperoxidase-hydrogen peroxide system to synthesize dityrosine, trityrosine, pulcherosine, and isodityrosine by a tyrosyl radical-dependent pathway. J Biol Chem 1996; 271:19950–19956.

120. van Dalen CJ, Winterbourn CC, Senthilmohan R, Kettle AJ. Nitrite as a substrate and inhibitor of myeloperoxidase. Implications for nitration and hypochlorous acid production at sites of inflammation. J Biol Chem 2000; 275:11638–11644.

121. Arlandson M, Decker T, Roongta VA, Bonilla L, Mayo KH, MacPherson JC, Hazen SL, Slungaard A. Eosinophil peroxidase oxidation of thiocyanate. Characterization of major reaction products and a potential sulfhydryl-targeted cytotoxicity system. J Biol Chem 2001; 276:215–224.

122. Stark GR. Reactions of cyanate with functional groups of proteins. IV. Intertness of aliphatic hydroxyl groups. Formation of carbamyl- and acylhydantoins. Biochemistry 1965; 4:2363–2367.

123. Dorsch W, Adam O, Weber J, Ziegeltrum T. Antiasthmatic effects of onion extracts—detection of benzyl- and other isothiocyanates (mustard oils) as antiasthmatic compounds of plant origin. Eur J Pharmacol 1984; 107:17–24.

124. Stelts D, Egan RW, Falcone A, Garlisi CG, Gleich GJ, Kruetner W, Kung TT, Nahrebne DK, Chapman RW, Minnicozzi M. Eosinophils retain their granule major basic protein

in a murine model of allergic pulmonary inflammation. Am J Respir Cell Mol Biol 1998; 18:463–470.

125. Persson CG, Erjefalt JS. Ultimate activation of eosinophils in vivo: lysis and release of clusters of free eosinophil granules (Cfegs). Thorax 1997; 52:569–574.

126. Egesten A, Calafat J, Janssen H, Knol EF, Malm J, Persson T. Granules of human eosinophilic leukocytes and their mobilization. Clin Exp Allergy 2001; 81:1173–1188.

127. Malm-Erjefalt M, Persson CG, Erjefalt JS. Degranulation status of airway tissue eosinophils in mouse models of allergic airway inflammation. Am J Respir Cell Mol Biol 2001; 24:352–359.

128. Stelts D, Egan RW, Falcone A, Garlisi CG, Gleich GJ, Kreutner W, Kung TT, Nahrebne DK, Chapman RW, Minnicozzi M. Eosinophils retain their granule major basic protein in a murine model of allergic pulmonary inflammation. Am J Respir Cell Mol Biol 1998; 18:463–470.

129. Zhang R, Shen Z, Nauseef WM, Hazen SL. The role of myeloperoxidase in the initiation of lipid peroxidation in plasma as studied in neutrophils isolated from myeloperoxidase deficient subjects: Systematic approach to the identification and characterization of multiple diffusible endogenous substrates for myeloperoxidase in plasma. Blood 2002; 99:1802–1810.

130. Podrez EA, Febbraio M, Sheibani N, Schmitt D, Silverstein R, Hajjar DP, Cohen PA, Frazier WA, Hoff HF. Hazen SL. The macrophage scavenger receptor CD36 is the major receptor for LDL recognition following modification by monocyte-generated reactive nitrogen species. J Clin Invest 2000; 105:1095–1108.

131. Abu-Soud H, Hazen SL. Nitric oxide is a physiological substrate for mammalian peroxidases. J Biol Chem 2000; 275:37524–37532.

132. Vignola AM, Kips J, Bousquet J. Tissue remodeling as a feature of persistent asthma. J Allergy Clin Immunol 2000; 105:1041–1053.

133. Fish JE, Peters SP. Airway remodeling and persistent airway obstruction in asthma. J Allergy Clin Immunol 1999; 104:509–516.

134. Boushey H. Targets for asthma therapy. Allerg Immunol (Paris) 2000; 9:336–341.

135. Brown PJ, Greville JW, Finucane KE. Asthma and irreversible airflow obstruction. Thorax 1984; 39:131–136.

136. Greenough A, Loftus BG, Pool J, Price JF. Abnormalities of lung mechanics in young asthmatic children. Thorax 1987; 42:500–505.

137. Connolly MJ, Avery AJ, Walters EH, Hendrick DJ. The relationship between bronchial responsiveness to methacholine and bronchial responsiveness to histamine in asthmatic subjects. Pulm Pharmacol 1988; 1:53–58.

138. Boulet LP, Turcotte H, Brochu A. Persistence of airway obstruction and hyperresponsiveness in subjects with asthma remission. Chest 1994; 105:1024–1031.

139. Hudon C, Turcotte H, Laviolette M, Carrier G, Boulet LP. Characteristics of bronchial asthma with incomplete reversibility of airflow obstruction. Ann Allerg Asth Immun 1997; 78:195–202.

140. Cade J, Pain M. Pulmonary function during clinical remission of asthma: How reversible is asthma? Aust NZ J Med 1973; 3:545–551.

141. Ferguson AC. Persisting airway obstruction in asymptomatic children with asthma with normal peak expiratory flow rates. J Allergy Clin Immunol 1988; 82:19–22.

142. Cade J. Lung mechanics during provocation of asthma. Clin Sci 1971; 40:381–386.

143. Colebatch H, Finucane K, Smith M. Pulmonary conductance and elastic recoil in asthma and emphysema. J Appl Physiol 1973; 34:143–153.

144. McCarthy DS, Sigurdson M. Lung elastic recoil and reduced airflow in clinically stable asthma. Thorax 1980; 35:298–302.
145. Woolcock A, Read J. The static elastic properties of the lung in asthma. Am Rev Respir Dis 1968; 98:788–794.
146. Zapletal A, Desmond KJ, Demizio D, Coates AL. Lung recoil and the determination of airflow limitation in cystic fibrosis and asthma. Pediatr Pulmonol 1993; 15:13–18.
147. Rennard SI. Repair mechanisms in asthma. J Allergy Clin Immunol 1996; 98: 5S78–S286.

19

Chemokines in Allergic Airway Inflammation

RAFEUL ALAM

National Jewish Medical and Research Center
Denver, Colorado, U.S.A.

I. Introduction

Chemokines are a newly identified group of chemotactic cytokines that induce directed cellular locomotion (reviewed in Refs. 1, 2) and are involved in homing of immune and inflammatory cells. Some chemokines have additional activity, but the chemotactic activity is the functional hallmark. All of them have molecular weights in the range of 8–12 kDa. Like most cytokines, chemokines are pleiotropic. Their receptors belong to the heptahelical (seven transmembrane spanning) G-protein–coupled receptor superfamily. Many of the receptors bind more than one ligand. Consequently, chemokines have extensive overlapping functions.

II. Classification

Nearly 50 chemokines have been cloned and their activity defined (Table 1) (see also the Internet site http://cytokine.medic.kumamoto-u.ac.jp/). All chemokines have

Partially adapted from Middleton E, et al., eds. Allergy: Principles and Practice. St. Louis: Mosby-Year Book, Inc., 1998:124–136.

Table 1 CXC Chemokine Ligands

CXC chemokine receptor	CXC chemokine ligands	CC chemokine receptors	CC chemokine ligands
CXCR1	CXCL6 (GCP-2), CXCL8 (IL-8)	CCR1	CCL3 (MIP-1α), CCL5 (RANTES), CCL7 (MCP-3)
CXCR2	CXCL1-3 (Gro-α,β,γ), CXCL5 (ENA-78), CXCL6 (GCP-2), CXCL8 (IL-8)	CCR2	CCL2 (MCP-1), CCL7 (MCP-3), CCL8 (MCP-2), CCL12 (MCP-5), CCL13 (MCP-4)
CXCR3	CXCL9 (Mig), CXCL10 (IP10), CXCL11 (ITAC)	CCR3	CCL5 (RANTES), CCL7 (MCP-3), CCL8 (MCP-2), CCL11 (eotaxin-1), CCL13 (MCP-4), CCL24 (eotaxin-2), CCL26 (eotaxin-3)
CXCR4	CXCL12 (SDF-1)	CCR4	CCL17 (TARC), CCL22 (MDC)
CXCR5	CXCL13 (BCA-1/BLC)	CCR5	CCL3 (MIP-1α), CCL4 (MIP-1β), CCL5 (RANTES)
CXCR6	CXCL16	CCR6	CCL20 (LARC/MIP3α)
		CCR7	CCL19 (MIP-3β/ELC), CCL21 (SLC)
		CCR8	CCL1 (I-309)
		CCR9	CCL2 (MCP-1), CCL3-4 (MIP-1α,β)
		CCR10	CCL20 (LAC), CCL21 SLC)
		CCR11	CCL2 (MCP-1), CCL7 (MCP-3), CCL8 (MCP-2), CCL11 (eotaxin-1), CCL12 (MCP-5), CCL13 (MCP-4),

Abbreviations: CCF-18, CC chemokine F-18; CTAP, connective tissue-activating peptide; ENA, epidermal cell–derived neutrophil chemotactic activity; GCP, granulocyte chemotactic protein; Gro, growth factor–related oncogene; HCC, hemofiltrate-derived CC chemokine; IP-10, inducible protein-10; LIX, LPS-induced CXC chemokine; MCP, monocyte chemotactic peptide; Mig, monokine induced with gamma-interferon; MIP, macrophage inflammatory protein; MRP, MIP-related protein; NAP, neutrophil-activating peptide; PBP, platelet basic protein; CCL5 (RANTES), regulated upon activation in normal T cells expressed and secreted; SDF, stromal cell–derived factor.

Acronyms: C10: MRP-1(MIP-related protein-1); Gro: MIP-2, melanocyte growth-stimulating activity (MGSA), cytokine-induced neutrophil chemoattractant (CINC, rat homolog); I309: TCA-3 (T-cell activation gene-3, mouse homolog); IL-8: KC (mouse homolog); MCP-1: monocyte chemotactic and activating factor (MCAF), JE (mouse homolog); MCP-3: fibroblast-induced cytokine (FIC), MARC; SDF-1: pre-B-cell growth-stimulating factor (PBSF).

Table 2 Structural Basis for Chemokine Classification[a]

Chemokine	**CXC (α)**		
IL-8	AVLPRSAKELR **CQC** IKTYSKPFHPKFIKELRVIESGPH	**C**	ANT..
GROα	ASVATELR **CQC** LQT-LQGIHPKNIQSVNVKSPGPH	**C**	AQT..
IP10	VPLSRTVR **CTC** ISISNQPVNPRSLEKLEIIPASQF	**C**	PRV..
	C-C (β)		
MCP-1	QPDAINAPVT **C-C** YNFTNRKISVQRLASY-RRITSSK	**C**	PKE..
RANTES	SPYSSDT-TP **C-C** FAYIARPLPRABIKEY—FYTSGK	**C**	SNP..
MIP-1α	ASLAADTPTA **C-C** FSYTSRQIPQNFIADY—FETSSQ	**C**	SKP..
Lymphotactin	**C (γ)**		
	EGVGTEVLEESS **C** VNLQTQRLPVQKIKTYIIWEG...		
Fractalkine	**CXXXC (CX3C)**		
	QHHGVTK **CNITC** SKMTSKIPVALLIHY-QQNQAS **C** GKR..		

[a] Chemokines have conserved N-terminal cysteine residues that form a specific pattern (CXC, CC, C, or CX3C). This pattern is the basis of their classification.

three to four conserved cysteine residues (Table 2). One family has two N-terminal cysteine (C) residues separated by one nonconserved amino acid residue. This family is called the CXC (X = any amino acid) family, occasionally referred to as the α chemokine family. The second family has two N-terminal conserved cysteine residues in juxtaposition (the CC or β chemokine family). The third family has a single cysteine residue in the conserved position (the C or γ chemokine family). The fourth family is significantly different from the three previous families. Fractalkine, the first cloned member of this family, has a complex structure. Fractalkine is a membrane-anchored protein. It has an N-terminal chemokine-like sequence followed by a mucin-like glycosylated stalk and a transmembrane region. The two N-terminal conserved cysteine residues are separated by three nonconserved residues and has been called the CX3C family. All CC, CXC, and C chemokines primarily exist as secreted soluble proteins. One exception is the recently cloned CXCL16 (3), which exists as a membrane-bound and as a soluble protein.

III. Structure

The nuclear magnetic resonance (NMR) and crystallographic structures of CXCL8 (IL-8), CCL4 (MIP-1β) and CCL5 (RANTES) have been resolved (4–6). Both CC and CXC chemokines share common structural features. They have a C-terminal α helix followed by a β-pleated sheet and a loose N-terminal strand. The CC chemokines have an extended N-terminal strand as compared to the CXC chemokines. The similarity in three-dimensional (3-D) structure perhaps explains the functional overlap among the chemokines.

IV. Cellular Sources

Chemokines are produced by a variety of cells. All leukocytes and platelets secrete chemokines, with the exception of fractalkine, a CX3C chemokine, which is produced by nonhematopoietic cells. Many tissue cells synthesize high quantities of chemokines. Virtually any nucleated cell that has been studied produces chemokines. Some of the important chemokine-producing tissue cells are epithelial cells, fibroblasts, macrophages, mast cells, keratinocytes, and endothelial cells. Epithelial cells have been shown to be the dominant producers of CCL2 (MCP-1), CCL5 (RANTES), CCL7 (MCP-3), CCLI1 (eotaxin-1), CCL26 (eotaxin-3), CCL28 (MEC, or mucosa-associated epithelial chemokine), CXCL14 (BRAK, or breast and kidney chemokine) and other chemokines in airway inflammation (7–11). Some chemokines such as CCL17 (thymus and activation-regulated chemokine), CCL18 (DC-CK1, or dendritic cell chemokine-1), CCL19 (ELC, or Epstein-Barr virus–induced receptor ligand chemokine), CCL21 (SLC, or secondary lymphoid tissue chemokine), CCL25 (TECK, or thymus-expressed chemokine), and CXCL13 (BCA-1, or B-cell–activating chemokine-1) are produced primarily in lymphoid tissues. Cells produce chemokines in response to a variety of factors, including viruses, bacteria, allergens/antigens, parasites, cytokines (e.g., IL-1, IFNs, TNF-α), oxidative stress, complement factors (e.g., C5a), and mediators (e.g., LTB4). Th2-type cytokines such as IL-4 and IL-13 stimulate airway epithelial production of eosinophil-active chemokines, e.g., CCL11 (eotaxin-1), whereas Th1-type cytokines (e.g., IFN-γ) stimulates IP-10, Mig, and ITAC production (11,12), although the principle may vary depending on the source of epithelium and presence of other cofactors. The induction of chemokine mRNA occurs very rapidly, within 2–3 hours after the stimulation of cells. For this reason many investigators call them immediate early response genes.

V. Chemokine Receptors

Six CXC chemokine receptors (CXCR1–6) 11 CC chemokine receptors (CCR1–11), and one CX3C chemokine receptor (CX3CR1) have been cloned and characterized, thus far (Table 1) (Ref. 1). All chemokine receptors belong to the seven transmembrane-spanning G-protein–coupled receptor superfamily. Most receptors are promiscuous and bind more than one ligand, which may explain the overlapping function of many chemokines. Chemokine receptors are expressed on cells either constitutively or upon specific stimulation. Most chemokine receptors are expressed on cells at a relatively low number (1,000–20,000/cell). CCR3 is expressed on eosinophils in relatively high numbers (40,000–50,000 cell). In addition to the seven cloned receptors, the Duffy antigen that is present on red blood cells and many other cells nonspecifically binds many chemokines. The significance of this interaction is not clear, but it may serve as an anti-inflammatory mechanism.

   The chemokine receptors are coupled to Gi type Gα subunits. Stimulation of the receptors induces the association of Gα subunit with GTP and dissociation from the complex of $\beta\gamma$ subunits. The Gα and the $\beta\gamma$ subunits independently activate a series of downstream signaling pathways, including phospholipase Cβ, PI-3 kinase-γ, and tyrosine kinases (reviewed in Refs. 14, 15). The activation of phospholipase Cβ leads to the elevation of Ca^{2+}. Both the calcium signaling and PI-3 kinase-γ are linked to cellular motility and degranulation (16,17). Chemokines activates Pyk2, FAK, and members of the Src family tyrosine kinases (e.g., Hck). The activation of the latter kinases is mediated by β-arrestin, which plays an important role in chemokine-induced neutrophil degranulation (18). Pyk2 and FAK are involved in leukocyte adhesion (19). Src-type tyrosine kinases signal through the p21 family of G proteins (Ras, Rho, Rac) and leads to the activation of MAP kinases. In agreement with the foregoing, chemokines have been show to activate the G proteins Rho and Rac and the MAP kinases ERK1/2 and p38 (20–22). The foregoing signaling molecules play an essential role in eosinophil chemotaxis and adhesion. Chemokine signaling leads to a change in adhesion molecule avidity for its ligands. CC chemokines increase the avidity of β2 integrins but decrease the avidity of β1 integrins (23,24).

VI. Biological Activity of Chemokines

The major functions of chemokines are shown in Figure 1. As mentioned previously, chemotaxis is the most important function of chemokines. Chemokines cause chemotaxis of cells during inflammation, immune response, embryogenesis, regeneration of tissue, and metastasis. Other currently identified functions of chemokines include activation of inflammatory cells, antiviral immunity, immunoregulation, control of hematopoiesis, angiogenesis, and other tissue cell growth and metabolism. The elucidation of novel functions of chemokines is an actively explored field of research, and many more important functions may be unraveled in the near future.

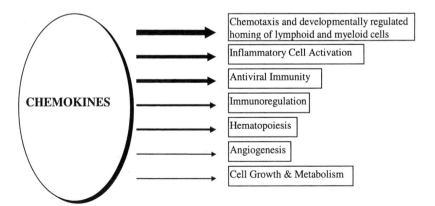

Figure 1 Major functions of chemokines. The width of the arrows indicates the importance of the function.

A. Effect on Immune Cell Development

Appropriate migration and homing of immune cells plays a crucial role in T- and B-cell development. Chemokines are critically involved in this process. CXCR4 (SDF-1 receptor) knockout mice show a dramatic decrease in B-cell and myeloid cell progenitors in hematopoietic organs (25), suggesting that CXCL12 (SDF-1) plays a pivotal role in the generation of B cells and normal myelopoiesis. Immature B cells typically express CCR9 and respond to CCL25 (TECK). As they mature, they lose CCR9 and begin to express CXCR5 and CXCR6 and become responsive to CXCL13 (BCA-1) and CCL20 (MIP-3α), respectively (26; reviewed in Ref. 27). The latter cytokines are important to appropriate homing of mature B cells in peripheral lymph nodes and Peyer's patches. Mature B cells also express CCR7, which is also instrumental in proper homing of B cells.

Chemokines profoundly modulate thymopoiesis and T-cell maturation in thymus. Many chemokines are constitutively but differentially expressed in thymic microenvironments. Like immature B cells, immature cortical thymocytes (e.g., CD4CD8 double-positive T cells) express CCR9 and migrate in response to CCL25 (TECK) (reviewed in Ref. 28). As they mature, they transiently express CCR4 and respond to CCL17 (TARC) and CCL22 (MDC). This transition occurs in the late cortical to early medullary stage of thymopoiesis. Upon further maturation (transition from double-positive to single-positive T cell) they lose CCR9 but begin to express CCR7. Single-positive T cells (e.g., CD4 +) respond to CCR7 ligands—CCL19 (MIP-3β) and CCL21 (SLC)—which allow them to emigrate from the thymic medulla and home into peripheral lymph nodes (29,30). It is interesting that the expression of CXCR4 and responsiveness to CXCL12 (SDF-1) is maintained throughout all developmental phases of T cells. The expression of receptors on differentiating and mature T cells and their migratory response to chemokines are depicted in Figure 2.

B. Effect on T-Helper Cell Differentiation

CCL2 (MCP1)-/- mice show diminished IL-4 and IL-5 production but normal IFN-γ production, suggesting that CCL2 influences T-helper cell differentiation in vivo (31). The major receptor for CCL2 is CCR2. Unexpectedly, CCR2-/- mice show the opposite effect, i.e., decreased IFN-γ production and increased Th2 cytokines and IgE production (32). The latter suggests that CCR2 signals for Th1 differentiation. It is likely that CCL2 signals through another unidentified receptor that signals for Th2 differentiation. Alternatively, the effect of CCL2 is indirect through other cytokines and/or chemokines. Unlike CCL2, CCL3 (MIP-1α) and CCL4 (MIP-1β) seem to promote Th1 cells. CCL3-deficient mice have increased susceptibility to viral infections due to reduced recruitment of inflammatory cells and delayed viral clearance (33). CCR6-/- mice show reduced Th2 differentiation, IgE production, and eosinophilic inflammation (34). CCR6 is expressed on dendritic cells, T cells, and B cells, but the exact mechanism by which CCR6 and its ligand CCL20 (MIP-3α) exert this effect is unknown. CCR8-/- mice also demonstrate an inability to mount a Th2-type eosinophilic inflammation in the airways (35). However, unlike CCR6-/-

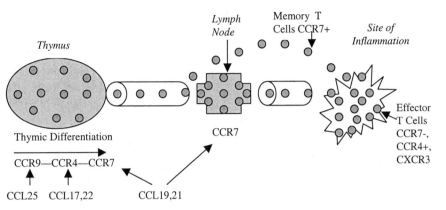

Figure 2 Chemokine regulation of T-cell development. Chemokine receptors are differentially expressed during various stages of T-cell development and maturation. The expression of these receptors determines their response to appropriate chemokines and homing to specific sites and organs.

mice, these mice have no problems with Th2 differentiation per se. Splenic lymphocytes from CCR6-/- mice normally differentiate into Th2 cells. The lack of airway Th2 inflammation is likely due to the impairment of Th2 homing mechanism.

Differentiated Th1 and Th2 cells display select chemokine receptors (Fig. 3). Th1 cells express CCR5, CXCR3, and CXCR6, whereas Th2 cells express CCR4, CCR8, and to a lesser extent CCR3 (36,37). The specificity of expression of these receptors on Th1 and Th2 cells is not absolute, and there are reports of overlap. For example, CCR4 is also expressed on skin-homing Th1 cells. In agreement with preferential expression of certain chemokine receptors, their respective ligands are preferentially detected in Th1 and Th2 inflammatory conditions. The CXCR3 ligand CXCL10 (IP10) is abundantly produced at sites of delayed hypersensitivity reactions in viral infections or in autoimmune diseases (e.g., multiple sclerosis) (39). On the other hand, increased levels of CCR3 ligands (eotaxins and others) are detected in Th2-type allergic inflammation (40,41). Naive T cells typically express CXCR4 and CCR7. Upon interaction with antigen-presenting cells, T cells undergo clonal proliferation, differentiating into T-effector and T-memory cells. T-memory cells continue to express CCR7, but T-effector cells cease to express them. The latter cell type begins to express differentiation and/or function associated chemokines such as CCR4 and CXCR3 (64).

The chemotactic response of circulating T cells has been extensively studied. CCL3 (MIP-1)α selectively attracts CD4 + T cells, whereas CCL4 (MIP-1β) is predominantly chemotactic for CD8 + T cells (42). CCL5 (RANTES) selectively attracts memory subtype CD45RO + CD4 + T cells (43). T cells express very little mRNA for CC chemokine receptors at the basal level. The expression is increased upon stimulation with IL-2 and to a lower extent, IL-12, IL-4, and IL-10. Studies

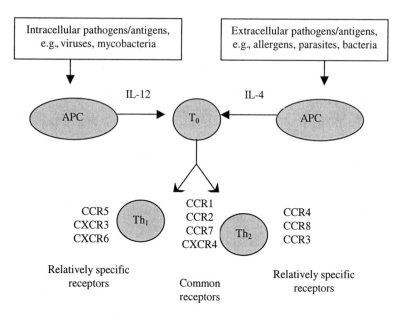

Figure 3 Chemokine receptor expression profile of functionally differentiated T-helper cells. Common receptors are expressed on both T_0 and differentiated T-helper cells.

with T-helper clones show that naïve T cells display migratory response to CCL1, 2, 3, 4 and CXCL12. In contrast, Th1 clones show chemotactic response mostly to CCL2, 3, 4 and CXCL10 12, whereas Th2 clones respond to CCL1, 2, 3, 11 and CXCL8 (44).

C. Effect on Dendritic Cells

Dendritic cells play a key role in immune response. Immature dendritic cells have a distinct repertoire of chemokine receptor expression (reviewed in Ref. 45). Blood-derived CD11c + dendritic cells express CCR2, whereas monocyte-derived dendritic cells express CCR1 and CCR5. Langerhans cells preferentially express CCR6. The immature dendritic cells capture antigens in the mucosa and then migrate into draining lymph nodes. During this period they transform into antigen-presenting cells, begin to express CCR7, a typical lymphoid tissue homing receptor, and are capable of delivering co-stimulatory signals to T cells. The CCR7 ligands CCL19 and CCL21 guide them into the T-dependent areas of lymph nodes. In addition to CCR7, CCR6 has been shown to be critical for homing of myeloid dendritic cells to Peyer's patches. Activated dendritic cells attract naïve T cells by secreting CCL18 (dendritic cell chemokine-1). They also secrete CCL19 and 21, which may attract additional dendritic cells and memory T cells.

D. Effect on Leukocytes and Other Cells

Neutrophils

Most CXC chemokines have chemotactic activity for neutrophils (46,47). CXCL8 (IL-8) is the best example of this activity and is considered the most potent chemotactic factor for polymorphonuclear leukocytes (PMN) (46). It is also a potent activator of PMN. Its biological activity begins at nanomolar concentrations. It causes the secretion of granular enzymes such as myeloperoxidase, β-glucuronidase, elastase, and gelatinase. It induces the production and secretion of LTB4 and oxygen radicals. Further, it stimulates PMN for phagocytosis. CXCL8 has weak histamine-releasing activity, especially for IL-3–primed basophils (48).

Basophils and Mast Cells

MCPs (CCL2,7,8,13), CCL3 (MIP-1α), and CCL5 (RANTES) are chemotactic for basophils (49,50). CCL2, 7, 8, 13 (MCPs) (50–53), CCL11 (eotaxin-1) (54), CCL3 (MIP-1α) (49), CCL5 (RANTES) (55), and CXCL4 (SDF-1) (56) activate basophils and cause histamine and leukotriene secretion. CCL2 (MCP-1) is one of the most potent basophil-activating molecules, and its histamine-releasing activity is comparable to that of C5a and anti-IgE antibody. Some CC chemokines such as CCL3 (MIP-1α) (49, 57) and CCL2 (MCP-1) (58,59) activate mast cells.

Eosinophils

Eosinophils are critical participants of allergic reactions. Their mechanism of chemotaxis and activation is of major interest. CCL3 (MIP-1α) (60), CCL5 (RANTES) (60–62), CCL7 (MCP-3) (50), CCL8 (MCP-2), CCL11 (eotaxin-1, frequently referred to as eotaxin) (63), CCL13 (MCP-4) (54), CCL24 (eotaxin-2) (64), CCL26 (eotaxin-3) (65), CCL20 (MIP-3α/LARC) (66), and CXCL4 (SDF-1) (67) are chemotactic for eosinophils. The chemokines induce transendothelial migration of eosinophils (68). The receptors for the foregoing chemokines transduce Ca^{2+} signals in eosinophils. Interestingly, only the CCR3 ligands but not others (CCL3, CXCL4) induce eosinophil degranulation (69). They cause release of eosinophil cationic protein and superoxide and make them hypodense (62).

The expression of chemokine receptors on leukocytes is a dynamic process and appears to change depending upon environmental milieu. Recently differentiated and circulating leukocytes express a typical set of receptors. For example, recently differentiated eosinophils express CCR1, CCR3, and to lesser extent CXCR4. However, cytokine-primed eosinophils from inflammatory sites express additional receptors including CCR2, CCR4, CCR5, and CXCR1. Basophils, neutrophils, and monocytes also undergo a similar process (Fig. 4).

VII. Activity In Vivo

The function of many chemokines has been studied in vivo in various animal models, including humans. CXCL8 (IL-8) causes an influx of neutrophils when injected

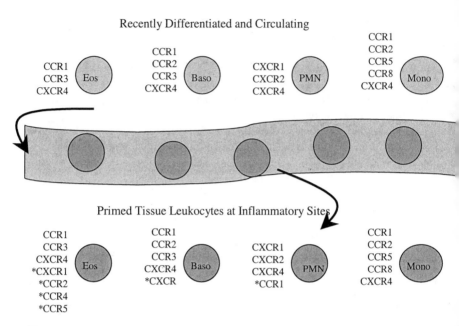

Figure 4 Expression of chemokine receptors on circulating and primed leukocytes. Eos, eosinophil; Baso, basophil; PMN, polymorphonuclear leukocyte; Mono, monocyte.* Indicates a newly expressed receptor.

intradermally (70). The instillation of CXCL8 (IL-8) by itself onto the nasal mucosa of volunteers does not elicit an inflammatory response and clinical symptoms. However, repeated doses of CXCL8 (IL-8) following a single intranasal application of histamine cause progressive influx of neutrophils into the nasal mucosa over a 4-hour observation period (71). Interestingly, nasal resistance increases within the first 90 minutes and then returns to normal despite the progressive increase in neutrophilic influx. The increase in PMN is associated with symptoms of nasal blockage and sore throat. Rhinorrhea, sneezing, nasal itching, and pain are not increased by CXCL8 (IL-8).

The injection of CCL5 (RANTES) into human (72) and dog skin (73) causes an eosinophil-rich inflammation. Further, there is an influx of lymphocytes and monocytes. The instillation of CCL5 (RANTES) into the nose of human allergic volunteers has interesting effects (74). When seasonal allergic patients are studied out of season, CCL5 (RANTES) causes a moderate but significant chemotaxis of eosinophils, basophils, and lymphocytes into the nasal mucosa. The chemotactic effects of CCL5 (RANTES) on eosinophils and other inflammatory cells is much more pronounced when the nasal mucosa is primed with allergens 24 hours earlier. CCL5 (RANTES) induces significant influx of eosinophils, basophils, and lympho-cytes reaching a peak at 4 hours and lasting more than 24 hours. It is possible that the allergen challenge helps CCL5 (RANTES) penetrate better into the mucosa

However, another explanation is that the allergens induce the production of some growth factors (e.g., IL-5), which then primes eosinophils for a heightened response to CCL5 (RANTES). The latter possibility has recently been addressed in a study wherein the injection of CCL11 (eotaxin-1) into guinea pig skin by itself caused minimal inflammation with eosinophils. However, if the animals were first primed with intravenous IL-5, the eosinophilic inflammatory response to CCL11 (eotaxin-1) was much more pronounced (75).

To summarize, both in vitro and in vivo studies suggest that the CXC chemokines predominantly target PMN, whereas the CC chemokines prefer monocytes, eosinophils, and basophils. From this profile of target leukocytes, one may deduce that the CXC chemokines are likely to play an important role in PMN-driven inflammatory processes such as bacterial infections, rheumatoid arthritis, psoriasis, oxidative stress-induced injuries (e.g., infarction), etc. In contrast, the CC chemokines are likely to participate in monocyte-, eosinophil-, and basophil-rich inflammatory processes such as viral and parasitic infections, type I and IV hypersensitivity diseases (e.g., atopic diseases, sarcoidosis), and multiple sclerosis. Many diseases have mixed cellular infiltrates (e.g., hypersensitivity pneumonitis), and it is likely that both chemokine families are involved in these diseases.

VIII. Knockout Models of Chemokines

CCR2-/- mice show decreased production of IFN-γ and increased Th2 cytokines and IgE production (32). The results suggest a role for CCR2 ligands (MCPs) in Th1 immune response. CCL11 (eotaxin-1) knockout mice have reduced early (8 hours post–allergen challenge) eosinophilic inflammation during the late-phase allergic reaction but have normal eosinophilic response at 24 hours (76). As expected, CCR3-/- mice show blunted eosinophilic response (50% reduction) in an asthma model but surprisingly display increased airway reactivity (77). As mentioned previously, CCR6 (34) and CCR8 (35) knockout mice show increased Th2 polarization. However, their mechanism of Th2 induction is different. Chemokines affect the function of lung interstitial cells including fibroblasts and myofibroblasts. Thus, they have the potential for influencing airway remodeling in chronic allergic inflammation. Very little information about this subject is currently available. One study shows that airway remodeling is absent in CCR1-/- mice, suggesting a role for CCR1 ligands (RANTES and MIP-1α and β) in airway remodeling (78). The effect of null mutation of various CC chemokine receptors on eosinophilic inflammation, Th2 development, and airway reactivity is shown in Table 3.

IX. Clinical Relevance

This section will be mostly devoted to the involvement of chemokines in allergic inflammation. Chemokines play an important role in other forms of inflammation. A detailed review of the involvement of chemokines in other inflammatory responses

Table 3 Allergy Phenotype of Chemokine Receptor Null Mutations

Knockout receptor	Ligands	Eosinophilic inflammation	Th2	Overall immunity	Airway hyperreactivity
CCR1	MIP-1α, MIP-1δ, RANTES, MCP-3	No effect	No effect	Specific defects	No effect
CCR2	MCP-1–5	↑	↑	Th1↓	Unknown
CCR3	Eotaxins, MCP-2–4, RANTES	↓	No effect		Increased
CCR4	TARC, MDC	Unchanged	Unchanged	LPS↓	Unknown
CCR5	MIP-1αβ, RANTES	Unchanged	Unchanged	Th1↓	Unknown
CCR6	LARC, MIP-3α	↓	Systemic unchanged Local ↓	Specific defects	Unknown
CCR7	SLC, MIP-3β	Unknown	Unknown	Depleted Lymph nodes	Unknown
CCR8	I-309, TARC, MIP-1β	↓	↓	Specific defects	Unknown
CCR9	MIP-1αβ, MCP-1, MCP-5	Unknown	Unknown	Unknown	Unknown
CCR10	SLC, LARC, BLC-1, Eskine	Unknown	Unknown	Unknown	Unknown
CCR11	MCP-1 to 5, eotaxin	Unknown	Unknown	Unknown	Unknown
CX3CR	Fractalkine	Unknown	Unknown	Delayed allograft rejection	Unknown

is beyond the scope of this chapter. Some recent reviews cover the involvement of chemokines in allergic and other clinical conditions (77).

A. Allergic Rhinitis

The involvement of chemokines in allergic rhinitis has been studied in a number of protocols. In one study an allergen challenge was performed in patients who developed a biphasic allergic response (Fig. 5). In this model, the allergen challenge increased the recovery of CCL2 (MCP-1), CCL3 (MIP-1α), CCL5 (RANTES), and CXCL8 (IL-8) (79,80). Each of the chemokines had distinct kinetics of appearance. CCL2 (MCP-1) appeared late and continued to increase throughout the observation

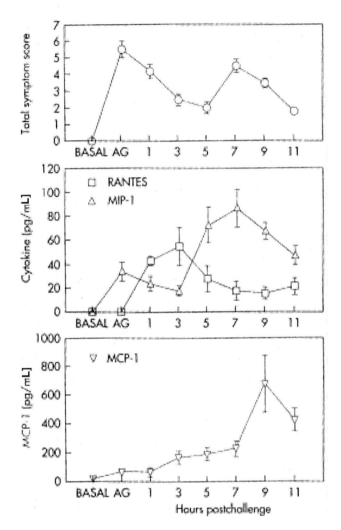

Figure 5 The recovery of chemokines from nasal secretions following an allergen challenge. Ten patients with allergic rhinitis were intranasally challenged with relevant allergens (AG). Composite symptom scores demonstrated an immediate followed by a late phase reaction. Chemokines were measured in nasal secretions every 2 hours by ELISA. (Adapted from Ref. 79.)

period. CCL3 (MIP-1α) had a biphasic response with an initial peak in the immediate-phase reaction and the second peak during the late-phase reaction. CCL5 (RANTES) peaked at 3 hours after the allergen challenge and preceded the development of the late-phase reaction. The appearance of CCL5 (RANTES) before the late-phase reaction may imply a causative effect. In contrast, the increase in CCL2

(MCP-1) after the peak of the late-phase reaction may imply an epiphenomenon or a homeostatic recovery mechanism. The early peak of CCL3 (MIP-1α) within 1 hour after the allergen challenge may point to the mast cell origin of the chemokine during the immediate-phase reaction.

In the same study the treatment of patients with topical beclomethasone dipropionate resulted in a significant reduction in the chemokine secretion into the nasal mucosa. The results suggest that topical glucocorticoids are potent inhibitors of chemokine production in vivo. Further, the inhibition of chemokine synthesis may contribute to the anti-inflammatory effects of topical glucocorticoids. In recent studies the expression of CCL5 (RANTES) in the nasal mucosa following an allergen challenge was investigated using biopsy specimens (81,82). There was an increased expression of mRNA as well as CCL5 (RANTES) protein in the nasal mucosa 4 hours after the allergen challenge (81). Interestingly, eosinophils were the dominant source of CCL5 (RANTES) in the nasal mucosa. The other cells that produced CCL5 (RANTES) included monocytes, mast cells, and lymphocytes. This study suggests that eosinophils may set up a positive feedback mechanism through the elaboration of CCL5 (RANTES).

In another study the recovery of CCL2 (MCP-1) from nasal secretions was investigated before and during natural exposure to the ragweed allergens in the allergy season (83). There was a significant increase in the levels of CCL2 (MCP-1) during the ragweed season. Interestingly, CXCL8 (IL-8) level decreased at the same time in symptomatic patients.

B. Bronchial Asthma

Several studies demonstrated the presence of chemokines in the airway mucosa or bronchoalveolar lavage fluid from allergic asthmatic patients. The airway epithelial cells from asthmatic patients but not normal controls expressed CCL2 (MCP-1) as determined by immunocytochemical staining of biopsy specimens (8). In another study the concentration of four different chemokines—CCL2 (MCP-1), CCL3 (MIP-1α), CCL5 (RANTES), and CXCL8 (IL-8)—was investigated in the lavage fluid from mild to moderate asthmatic patients and healthy controls (84). There was a significant elevation of CCL5 (RANTES), CCL2 (MCP-1), and CCL3 (MIP-1α) in the lavage fluid from asthmatic patients (Fig. 6). Further, the BAL cells expressed mRNA for the above chemokines as well as for CCL7 (MCP-3). The BAL fluid from asthmatic patients had eosinophil chemotactic activity in vitro, which was abolished by antibodies against CCL5 (RANTES) and CCL7 (MCP-3). The presence of increased amounts of CCL3 (MIP-1α) and CCL5 (RANTES) in the BAL fluid from asthmatic patients was confirmed in other studies (85–88). Biopsy studies from asthmatic patients confirmed the presence of eotaxin-1, eotaxin-2 (Fig. 7), MCP-3, and MCP-4 in the airways (40,41,89,90). Increased expression of eotaxin-1 and MCP-4 was also detected in small airways from asthmatic patients (91). T cells play a crucial role in the pathogenesis of asthma. In one study the expression of chemokine receptors on lung T cells from asthmatic and control subjects was studied. T cells from both study groups primarily expressed CXCR3, CXCR4, and CCR5. There

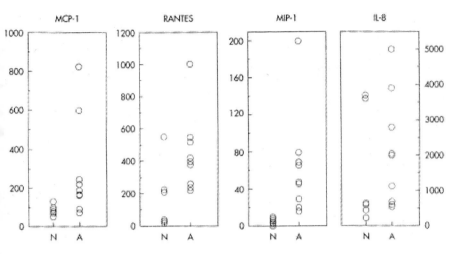

Figure 6 Measurement of MCP-1, CCL5 (RANTES), MIP-1α, and CXCL8 (IL-8) in the BAL fluid by ELISA. BAL fluid from nine asthmatic patients (A) and six normals (N) was concentrated 10 times and used in the ELISA. The difference between asthmatic patients and normal subjects is significant ($p < 0.04$) for MCP-1, CCL5 (RANTES), and MIP-1α, but not for CXCL8 (IL-8). (From Ref. 84.)

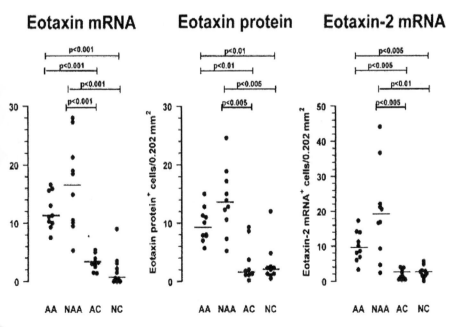

Figure 7 Expression of eotaxin-1 (CCL-11) and eotaxin-2 (CCL24) in biopsy samples from allergic asthmatics (AA), nonallergic asthmatics (NAA), allergic controls (AC), and nonallergic controls (NC). (From Ref. 90.)

was no difference between the study groups (92). An allergen challenge causes recruitment of new T cells into the airways of asthmatic patients. In another study the expression of chemokine receptors on infiltrating T cells following an allergen challenge was examined. Endobronchial biopsies from allergen-challenged asthmatic patients show that most infiltrating T cells express CCR4 but not CCR3 (93). Further, nearly 28% of the CCR4+ T cells also express CCR8.

The production of chemokines was investigated in occupational asthma due to diisocyanates. Mononuclear cells from symptomatic patients showed increased production of CCL2 (MCP-1) in response to diisocyanate stimulation, which correlated with the presence of histamine-releasing factors (94). Mononuclear cells from workers that were exposed to diisocyanates but did not develop occupational asthma did not show this augmented response. The production of CCL5 (RANTES) was not increased in these patients. Since the incidence of diisocyanate-specific IgE antibody is very low in this group of occupational asthma, chemokines such as CCL2 (MCP-1) may play an important role in the pathogenesis of occupational asthma.

It has been speculated that chemokine gene polymorphism is linked to the pathogenesis of asthma. However, the literature in this area has been controversial. The CCR deletion mutation (CCR5-delta 32 polymorphism) was claimed to reduce the risk for asthma (95). However, two subsequent studies failed to confirm this observation (96,97). Similarly a RANTES polymorphism (the 403 G-A promoter polymorphism) was found to be associated with atopy and asthma in one study (98) but was disputed by another study (99). The latter study reported an association of the 2518G polymorphism of the promoter region of MCP-1 with asthma. Recently, a threonine 23 variant of eotaxin has been claimed to be associated with reduced eosinophil count and higher levels of lung function in asthmatic patients (100). The discrepancy of the results is likely due to inadequacy of the study populations.

To summarize, CC chemokines such as CCL2 (MCP-1), CCL3 (MIP-1α), CCL5 (RANTES), CCL7 (MCP-3), CCL11 (eotaxin-1), and CCL26 (eotaxin-3) appear to be produced in high quantities at the site of allergic inflammation. Interestingly, airway epithelial cells may be the major source of the CC chemokines. Since an allergic reaction is an allergen-specific response, it is likely that an IgE-mediated secretion of mediators from mast cells (macrophages, eosinophils?) stimulates the epithelial cell production of CC chemokines. The CC chemokines in combination with other mast cell–derived cytokines then initiate a cascade of events that leads to the development of allergic inflammation.

X. Conclusions

There has been an explosion of information about chemokines, their receptors, and their biological activity in recent years. It has become clear that chemokines play a crucial role in homing of immune cells in various organs. Further, migration of immune cells to inflammatory sites is critically dependent upon chemokine production. Although chemokines are broadly characterized by redundancy, in-depth studies demonstrate that each chemokine has a specific function that is not overcome

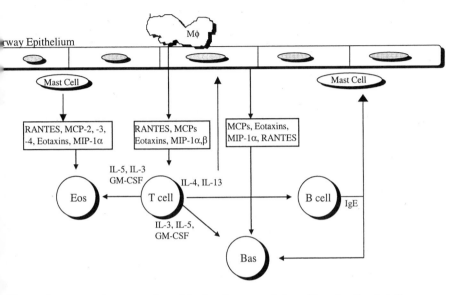

Figure 8   Schematic presentation of the involvement of chemokines in allergic inflammation.

by other chemokines. Many classic inflammatory cytokines such as IL-1, TNF-α, and interferons cause inflammation via the induction of chemokines. Inflammatory and regulatory cytokines in conjunction with chemokines form a complex communicating network among the resident and infiltrating cells that results in allergic inflammation (Fig. 8). Thus, a better understanding of their participation in inflammatory diseases will help design superior anti-inflammatory modalities in the future. Some chemokine receptors and their ligands are involved in chemotaxis and activation of cells that typically infiltrate the sites of allergic reactions. For this reason chemokine receptors such as CCR3, CCR4, CCR8, and their ligands have become the central focus of research in many laboratories. The challenge for the future is to develop novel antagonists against these chemokines and their receptors in a bid to block eosinophilic inflammation and airway hyperreactivity.

References

1. Mackay CR. Chemokines: immunology's high impact factors. Nat Immunol 2001; 2(2):95–101.
2. Luster AD. Chemokines—chemotactic cytokines that mediate inflammation. N Engl J Med 1998; 338(7):436–445.

3. Matloubian M, David A, Engel S, Ryan JE, Cyster JG. A transmembrane CXC chemokine is a ligand for HIV-coreceptor Bonzo. Nat Immunol 2000; 1(4):298–304.
4. Shaw JP, Kryger G, Cleasby A, et al. Crystallization and preliminary x-ray diffraction studies of human RANTES. J Mol Biol 1994; 242:589–590.
5. Clore GM, Gronenborn AM. Three-dimensional structures of α and β chemokines FASEBJ 1995; 9:57–62.
6. Chung CW, Cooke RM, Proudfoot AE, et al. The three-dimensional solution structure of RANTES. Biochemistry 1995; 34:9307–9314.
7. Kwon OJ, Jose PJ, Robbins RA, et al. Glucocorticoid inhiibition of RANTES expression in human lung epithelial cells. Am J Respir Cell Mol Biol 1995; 12:488–496.
8. Sousa AR, Lane SJ, Nakhosteen JA, et al. Increased expression of the monocyte chemoattractant protein-1 in bronchial tissue from asthmatic subjects. Am J Respir Cell Mol Biol 194; 10:142–147.
9. Saito T, Deskin RW, Casola A, et al. Respiratory syncytial virus induces selective production of the chemokine RANTES by upper airway epithelial cells. J Infect Dis 1997; 175:497–504.
10. Stafford S, Li H, Bravo R, et al. Monocyte chemotactic protein-3 in eosinophilic inflammation of the airways and the inhibitory effects of an anti-MCP-3 antibody. J Immunol 158:4953–4960, 1997.
11. Michalec L, Choudhury BK, Postlewait E, Wild JS, Alam R, Lett-Brown MA, Sur S CCL7 and CXC10 orchestrate oxidative stress-induced neutrophilic lung inflammation J Immunol 2001 (in press).
12. Li L, Xia Y, Nguyen A, Lai YH, Feng L, Mosmann TR, Lo D. Effects of Th2 cytokines on chemokine expression in the lung: IL-13 potently induces eotaxin expression by airway epithelial cells. J Immunol 1999; 162(5):2477–2487.
13. Sauty A, Dziejman M, Taha RA, Iarossi AS, Neote K, Garcia-Zepeda EA, Hamid Q Luster AD. The T cell-specific CXC chemokines IP-10, Mig, and I-TAC are expressed by activated human bronchial epithelial cells. J Immunol 1999; 162(6):3549–3558.
14. Wu D, LaRosa GJ, Simon MI. G protein-coupled signal transduction pathways for interleukin-8. Science 1993; 261:101.
15. Thelen M. Dancing to the tune of chemokines. Nature Immunol. 2001; 2:129–134.
16. Li Z, Jiang H, Xie W, Zhang Z, Smrcka AV, Wu D. Roles of PLC-beta2 and -beta3 and PI3K gamma in chemoattractant-mediated signal transduction. Science 2000 287(5455):1046–1049.
17. Hirsch E, Katanaev VL, Garlanda C, Azzolino O, Pirola L, Silengo L, Sozzani S Mantovani A, Altruda F, Wymann MP. Central role for G protein-coupled phosphoinositide 3-kinase gamma in inflammation. Science 2000; 287(5455):1049–1053.
18. Barlic J, Andrews JD, Kelvin AA, Bosinger SE, DeVries ME, Xu L, Dobransky T Feldman RD, Ferguson SS, Kelvin DJ. Regulation of tyrosine kinase activation and granule release through beta-arrestin by CXCRI. Nat Immunol 2000; 1(3):227–233.
19. Bacon KB, Szabo MC, Yssel H, et al. RANTES induces tyrosine kinase activity of stably complexed p125FAK and ZAP-70 in human T cells. J Exp Med 1996; 184 873–882.
20. Laudanna C, Campbell JJ, Butcher EC. Role of Rho in chemoattractantactivated leukocyte adhesion through integrins. Science 1996; 271:981–983.
21. Adachi T, Vita R, Sannohe S, Stafford S, Alam R, Kayaba H, Chihara J. The functional role of Rho and ROCK in eotaxin signaling of eosinophils. J Immunol 2001; 167 4609–4615.

22. Kampen G, Stafford S, Adachi T, Jinquan T, Quan S, Grant JA, Skov P, Poulsen L, Alam R. Eotaxin induces degranulation and chemotaxis of eosinophils through the activation of ERK2 and p38 mitogen-activated protein kinases. Blood 2000; 95: 1911–1917.

23. Carr MW, Alon R, Springer TA. The CC chemokine MCP-1 differentially modulates the avidity of beta 1 and beta 2 integrins on T lymphocytes. Immunity 1996; 4:179–187.

24. Tachimoto H, Burdick MM, Hudson SA, Kikuchi M, Konstantopoulos K, Bochner BS. CCR3-active chemokines promote rapid detachment of eosinophils from VCAM-1 in vitro. J Immunol 2000; 165(5):2748–2754.

25. Nagasawa T, Hirota S, Tachibana K, et al. Defects of B cell lymphopoiesis and bone-marrow myelopoiesis in mice lacking the CXC chemokine PBSF/SDF-1. Nature 1996; 382:635–638.

26. Forster R, Schubel A, Breitfeld D, Kremmer E, Renner-Muller I, Wolf E, Lipp M. CCR7 coordinates the primary immune response by establishing functional microenvironments in secondary lymphoid organs. Cell 1999; 99(1):23–33.

27. Moser B, Loetscher P. Lymphocyte traffic control by chemokines. Nature Immunol 2001; 2:123–128.

28. Luther SA. and Cyster JG. Chemokines as regulators of T cell differentiation. Nature Immunol 2001; 2:102–107.

29. Randolph DA, Huang G, Carruthers CJ, Bromley LE, Chaplin DD. The role of CCR7 in TH1 and TH2 cell localization and delivery of B cell help in vivo. Science 1999; 286(5447):2159–2162.

30. Campbell JJ, Pan J, Butcher EC. Developmental switches in chemokine responses during T cell maturation. J Immunol 1999; 163(5):2353–2357.

31. Gu L, Tseng S, Horner RM, Tam C, Loda M, Rollins BJ. Control of TH2 polarization by the chemokine monocyte chemoattractant protein-1. Nature 2000; 404(6776):407–411.

32. Warmington KS, Boring L, Ruth JH, Sonstein J, Hogaboam CM, Curtis JL, Kunkel SL, Charo IR, Chensue SW. Effect of C-C chemokine receptor 2 (CCR2) knockout on type-2 (schistosomal antigen-elicited) pulmonary granuloma formation: analysis of cellular recruitment and cytokine responses. Am J Pathol 1999; 154(5):1407–1416.

33. Domachowske JB, Bonville CA, Gao JL, Murphy PM, Easton AJ, Rosenberg HF. The chemokine macrophage-inflammatory protein-1alpha and its receptor CCR1 control pulmonary inflammation and antiviral host defense in paramyxovirus infection. J Immunol 2000; 165(5):2677–2682.

34. Lukacs NW, Prosser DM, Wiekowski M, Lira SA, Cook DN. Requirement for the chemokine receptor CCR6 in allergic pulmonary inflammation. J Exp Med 2001; 194(4):551–555.

35. Chensue SW, Lukacs NW, Yang TY, Shang X, Frait KA, Kunkel SL, Kung T, Wiekowski MT, Hedrick JA, Cook DN, Zingoni A, Narula SK, Zlotnik A, Barrat FJ, O'Garra A, Napolitano M, Lira SA. Aberrant in vivo T helper type 2 cell response and impaired eosinophil recruitment in CC chemokine receptor 8 knockout mice. J Exp Med 2001; 193(5):573–584.

36. Sallusto F, Lenig D, Mackay CR, Lanzavecchia A. Flexible programs of chemokine receptor expression on human polarized T helper 1 and 2 lymphocytes. J Exp Med 1998; 187(6):875–883.

37. Bonecchi R, Bianchi G, Bordignon PP, D'Ambrosio D, Lang R, Borsatti A, Sozzani S, Allavena P, Gray PA, Mantovani A, Sinigaglia F. Differential expression of chemokine receptors and chemotactic responsiveness of type 1 T helper cells (Th1s) and Th2s. J Exp Med 1998; 187(1):129–134.

38. Sebastiani S, Allavena P, Albanesi C, Nasorri F, Bianchi G, Traidl C, Sozzani S, Girolomoni G, Cavani A. Chemokine receptor expression and function in CD4 + T lymphocytes with regulatory activity. J Immunol 2001; 166(2):996–1002.

39. Sorensen TL, Tani M, Jensen J, Pierce V, Lucchinetti C, Folcik VA, Qin S, Rottman J, Sellebjerg F, Strieter RM, Frederiksen JL, Ransohoff RM. Expression of specific chemokines and chemokine receptors in the central nervous system of multiple sclerosis patients. J Clin Invest 1999:103(6):807–815.

40. Lilly CM, Nakamura H, Belostotsky OI, Haley KJ, Garcia-Zepeda EA, Luster AD, Israel E. Eotaxin expression after segmental allergen challenge in subjects with atopic asthma. Am J Respir Crit Care Med 2001 63(7):1669–175.

41. Berkman N, Ohnona S, Chung FK, Breuer R. Eotaxin-3 but not eotaxin gene expression is upregulated in asthmatics 24 hours after allergen challenge. Am J Respir Cell Mol Biol 2001; 24(6):682–687.

42. Taub DD, Conlon K, Lloyd AR, et al. Preferential migration of activated CD4 + and CD8 + T cells in response to MIP-1α and MIP-1β. Science 1993; 260:355.

43. Schall TJ, Bacon K, Camp RDR, et al. Human macrophage inflammatory protein α (MIP-1α) and MIP-1β chemokines attract distinct populations of lymphocytes. J Exp Med 1993; 177:1821–1825.

44. Sebastiani S, Allavena P, Albanesi C, Nasorri F, Bianchi G, Traidl C, Sozzani S, Girolomoni G, Cavani A. Chemokine receptor expression and function in CD4 + T lymphocytes with regulatory activity. J Immunol 2001; 166(2):996–1002.

45. Lanzavecchia A, Sallusto F. Regulation of T cell immunity by dendritic cells. Cell 2001; 106(3):263–266.

46. Baggiolini M, Walz A, Kunkel SL. Neutrophil-activating peptide-1/interleukin 8, a novel cytokine that activates neutrophils. J Clin Invest 1989; 84:1045–1049.

47. Walz A, Dewald B, von Tscharner V, Baggiolini M. Effects of the neutrophil-activating peptide NAP-2, platelet basic protein, connective tissue-activating peptide III, and platelet factor 4 on human neutrophils. J Exp Med 1989; 170:1745–1750.

48. Dahinden C, Kurimoto Y, De Weck AL, et al. The neutrophil-activating peptide NAF/NAP-1 induces histamine and leukotriene release by interleukin 3-primed basophils. J Exp Med 1989; 170:1787–1792.

49. Alam R, Forsythe PA, Stafford S, et al. Macrophage inflammatory protein-1α activates basophils and mast cells. J Exp Med 1992; 176:781–786.

50. Dahinden CA, Geiser T, Brunner T, et al. Monocyte chemotactic protein 3 is a most effective basophil- and eosinophil-activating chemokine. J Exp Med 1994; 179 751–756.

51. Alam R, Lett-Brown MA, Forsythe PA, et al. Monocyte chemotactic and activating factor is a potent histamine-releasing factor for basophils. J Clin Invest 1992; 89 723–728.

52. Kuna P, Redigari P, Schall TJ, et al. Monocyte chemotactic and activating factor is a potent histamine-releasing factor for human basophils. J Exp Med 1992; 175:489–493

53. Alam R, Forsythe P, Stafford S, et al. Monocyte chemotactic protein-2, monocyte chemotactic protein-3 and fibroblast-induced cytokine. J Immunol 1994; 153:3155.

54. Uguccioni M, Mackay CR, Ochensberger B, Loetscher P, Rhis S, LaRosa GJ, Rao P, Ponath PD, Baggiolini M, Dahinden CA. High expression of the chemokine receptor CCR3 in human blood basophils. Role in activation by eotaxin, MCP-4, and other chemokines. J Clin Invest 1997; 100(5):1137–1143.

55. Kuna P, Reddigari S, Schall T, et al. RANTES, a monocyte and T lymphocyte chemotactic cytokine releases histamine from human basophils. J Immunol 1992; 149 636–642.

56. Jinquan T, Jacobi HH, Jing C, Reimert CM, Quan S, Dissing S, Poulsen LK, Skov PS. Chemokine stromal cell-derived factor 1alpha activates basophils by means of CXCR4. J Allergy Clin Immunol 2000; 106(2):313–320.

57. Hartmann K, Beiglbock F, Czarnetzki BM, et al. Effect of CC chemokines on mediator release from human skin mast cells and basophils. Int Arch All Immunol 1995; 108: 224–230.

58. Conti P, Boucher W, Letourneau R, et al. Monocyte chemotactic protein-1 provokes mast cell aggregation and ^{3}H-5HT release. Immunology 1995; 86:434–440.

59. Campbell EM, Charo IF, Kunkel SL, Strieter RM, Boring L, Gosling J, Lukacs NW. Monocyte chemoattractant protein-1 mediates cockroach allergen-induced bronchial hyperreactivity in normal but not CCR2-/- mice: the role of mast cells. J Immunol 1999; 163(4):2160–2167.

60. Rot A, Krieger M, Brunner T, et al. RANTES and macrophage inflammatory protein 1α induce the migration and activation of normal human eosinophil granulocytes. J Exp Med 1992; 176:1489–1495.

61. Kameyoshi Y, Dorschner A, Mallet AI, et al. Cytokine RANTES released by thrombin-stimulated platelets is a potent attractant for human eosinophils. J Exp Med 1992; 176: 587–592.

62. Alam R, Stafford S, Forsythe P, et al. RANTES is a chemotactic and activating factor for eosinophils. J Immunol 193; 150:3442–3447.

63. Jose PJ, Griffiths-Johnson DA, Collins PD, et al. Eotaxin: a potent eosinophil chemoattractant cytokine detected in a guinea pig model of allergic airways inflammation. J Exp Med 1994; 179:881–887.

64. Forssmann U, Uguccioni M, Loetscher P, Dahinden CA, Langen H, Thelen M, Baggiolini M. Eotaxin-2, a novel CC chemokine that is selective for the chemokine receptor CCR3, and acts like eotaxin on human eosinophil and basophil leukocytes. J Exp Med 1997; 185(12):2171–2176.

65. Kitaura M, Suzuki N, Imai T, Takagi S, Suzuki R, Nakajima T, Hirai K, Nomiyama H, Yoshie O. Molecular cloning of a novel human CC chemokine (Eotaxin-3) that is a functional ligand of CC chemokine receptor 3. J Biol Chem 1999; 274.

66. Sullivan SK, McGrath DA, Liao F, Boehme SA, Farber JM, Bacon KB. MIP-3alpha induces human eosinophil migration and activation of the mitogen-activated protein kinases (p42/p44 MAPK). J Leukoc Biol 1999; 66(4):674–682.

67. Nagase H, Miyamasu M, Yamaguchi M, Fujisawa T, Ohta K, Yamamoto K, Morita Y, Hirai K. Expression of CXCR4 in eosinophils: functional analyses and cytokine-mediated regulation. J Immunol 2000; 164(11):5935–5943.

68. Ebisawa M, Yamada T, Bickel C, et al. Eosinophil transendothelial migration induced by cytokines. J Immunol 1994; 153:2153.

69. Fujisawa T, Kato Y, Nagase H, Atsuta J, Terada A, Iguchi K, Kamiya H, Morita Y, Kitaura M, Kawasaki H, Yoshie O, Hirai K. Chemokines induce eosinophil degranulation through CCR-3. J Allergy Clin Immunol 2000; 106(3):507–513.

70. Colditz I, Zwahlen R, Dewald B, et al. In vivo inflammatory activity of neutrophil activating factor, a novel chemotactic peptide derived from human monocytes. Am J Pathol 1989; 134:755–760.

71. Douglas JA, Dhami D, Gurr CE, et al. Influence of IL-8 challenge in the nasal mucosa in atopic and nonatopic subjects. Am J Respir Crit Care Med 1994; 150:1108–1113.

72. Beck L, Stellato C, Dalke S, et al. Cutaneous injection of RANTES causes eosinophil recruitment; comparison of nonallergic and allergic human subjects (abstr). J Allergy Clin Immunol 1996; 97:425.

73. Meurer R, Van Riper G, Feeney W, et al. Formation of eosinophilic and monocytic intradermal inflammatory sites in the dog by injection of human RANTES but not human monocyte chemoattractant protein 1, human macrophage inflammatory protein 1α, or human interleukin 8. J Exp Med 1993; 178:1913–1921.

74. Kuna P, Alam R, Ruta U, et al. RANTES induces nasal mucosal inflammation rich in eosinophils, basophils and lymphocytes in vivo. Am Rev Respir Crit Care Med 1998; 157:873–879.

75. Collins PD, Marleau S, Griffiths-Johnson DA, et al. Cooperation between interleukin-5 and the chemokine eotaxin to induce eosinophil accumulation in vivo. J Exp Med 1995; 182:1169–1174.

76. Rothenberg ME, MacLean JA, Pearlman E, Luster AD, Leder P. Targeted disruption of the chemokine eotaxin partially reduces antigen-induced tissue eosinophilia. J Exp Med 1997; 185(4):785–790.

77. Gerard C, Rollins BJ. Chemokines and diseases. Nature Immunol 2001; 2:108–115.

78. Blease K, Mehrad B, Standiford TJ, Lukacs NW, Kunkel SL, Chensue SW, Lu B, Gerard CJ, Hogaboam CM. Airway remodeling is absent in CCR1-/- mice during chronic fungal allergic airway disease. J Immunol 2000; 165(3):1564–1572.

79. Sim TC, Reece LM, Hilsmeier KA, et al. Secretion of chemokines and other cytokines in allergen-induced nasal responses: inhibition by topical steroid treatment. Am J Respir Crit Care Med 1995; 152:927–933.

80. Weido AJ, Reece LM, Alam R, et al. Intranasal fluticasone propionate inhibits the recovery of chemokines and other cytokines in nasal secretions in allergen-induced rhinitis. Ann Allergy Asthma Immunol 1996; 77:407–415.

81. Rajakulasingam K, Hamid Q, O'Brien F, et al. RANTES in human allergen-induced rhinitis. Am J Respir Crit Care Med 1997; 155:696–703.

82. KleinJan A, Dijkstra MD, Boks SS, Severijnen LA, Mulder PG, Fokkens WJ. Increase in IL-8, IL-10, IL-13, and RANTES mRNA levels (in situ hybridization) in the nasal mucosa after nasal allergen provocation. J Allergy Clin Immunol 1999; 103:441–450.

83. Kuna P, Lazarovich M, Kaplan AP. Chemokines in seasonal allergic rhinitis. J Allergy Clin Immunol 1996; 97:104–112.

84. Alam R, York J, Boyars M, et al. Increased MCP-1, RANTES, and MIP-1 in bronchoalveolar lavage in allergic asthmatic patients. Am J Respir Crit Care Med 1996; 153: 1398–1404.

85. Teran LM, Noso, N, Carroll M, et al. Eosinophil recruitment following allergen challenge is associated with the release of the chemokine RANTES into asthmatic airways. J Immunol 1996; 157:1806–1812.

86. Venge J, Lampinen M, Hakansson L, et al. Identification of IL-5 and RANTES as the major eosinophil chemoattractants in the asthmatic lung. J Allergy Clin Immunol 1996; 97:1110–1115.

87. Sur S, Kita H, Gleich GI, et al. Eosinophil recruitment is associated with IL-5, but not with RANTES, twenty four after allergen challenge. J Allergy Clin Immunol 1996; 97:1272–1278.

88. Tillie-Leblond I, Hammad H, Desurmont S, Pugin J, Wallaert B, Tonnel AB, Gosset P. CC chemokines and interleukin-5 in bronchial lavage fluid from patients with status asthmaticus. Potential implication in eosinophil recruitment. Am J Respir Crit Care Med 2000; 162(2 Pt 1):586–592.

89. Lamkhioued B, Garcia-Zepeda EA, Abi-Younes S, Nakamura H, Jedrzkiewicz S, Wagner L, Renzi PM, Allakhverdi Z, Lilly C, Hamid Q, Luster AD. Monocyte chemoattractant protein (MCP)-4 expression in the airways of patients with asthma. Induction in

epithelial cells and mononuclear cells by proinflammatory cytokines. Am J Respir Crit Care Med 2000; 162(2 Pt 1):723–732.

90. Ying S, Meng Q, Zeibecoglou K, Robinson DS, Macfarlane A, Humbert M, Kay AB. Eosinophil chemotactic chemokines (eotaxin, eotaxin-2, RANTES, monocyte chemoattractant protein-3 (MCP-3), and MCP-4), and C-C chemokine receptor 3 expression in bronchial biopsies from atopic and nonatopic (Intrinsic) asthmatics. J Immunol 1999; 163(11):6321–6329.

91. Taha RA, Minshall EM, Miotto D, Shimbara A, Luster A, Hogg JC, Hamid QA. Eotaxin and monocyte chemotactic protein-4 mRNA expression in small airways of asthmatic and nonasthmatic individuals. J Allergy Clin Immunol 1999; 103(3 Pt 1): 476–483.

92. Campbell JJ, Brightling CE, Symon FA, Qin S, Murphy KE, Hodge M, Andrew DP, Wu L, Butcher EC, Wardlaw AJ. Expression of chemokine receptors by lung T cells from normal and asthmatic subjects. J Immunol 2001; 166(4):2842–2848.

93. Panina-Bordignon P, Papi A, Mariani M, Di Lucia P, Casoni G, Bellettato C, Buonsanti C, Miotto D, Mapp C, Villa A, Arrigoni G, Fabbri LM, Sinigaglia F. The C-C chemokine receptors CCR4 and CCR8 identify airway T cells of allergen-challenged atopic asthmatics. J Clin Invest 2001; 107(11):1357–1364.

94. Lummus ZL, Alam R, Bernstein JA, et al. Characterization of histamine-releasing factors in diisocyanate-induced occupational asthma. Toxicol 1996; 111:191–206.

95. Hall IP, Wheatley A, Christie G, McDougall C, Hubbard R, Helms PJ. Association of CCR5 delta32 with reduced risk of asthma. Lancet 1999; 354(9186):1264–1265.

96. Mitchell TJ, Walley AJ, Pease JE, Venables PJ, Wiltshire S, Williams TJ, Cookson WO. Delta 32 deletion of CCR5 gene and association with asthma or atopy. Lancet 2000; 356(9240):1491–1492.

97. Sandford AJ, Zhu S, Bai TR, Fitzgerald JM, Pare PD. The role of the C-C chemokine receptor-5 Delta32 polymorphism in asthma and in the production of regulated on activation, normal T cells expressed and secreted. J Allergy Clin Immunol 2001; 108(1): 69–73.

98. Fryer AA, Spiteri MA, Bianco A, Hepple M, Jones PW, Strange RC, Makki R, Tavernier G, Smilie FI, Custovic A, Woodcock AA, Ollier WE, Hajeer AH. The −403 G→A promoter polymorphism in the RANTES gene is associated with atopy and asthma. Genes Immun 2000; 1(8):509–514.

99. Szalai C, Kozma GT, Nagy A, Bojszko A, Krikovszky D, Szabo T, Falus A. Polymorphism in the gene regulatory region of MCP-1 is associated with asthma susceptibility and severity. J Allergy Clin Immunol 2001; 108(3):375–381.

100. Nakamura H, Luster AD, Nakamura T, In KH, Sonna LA, Deykin A, Israel E, Drazen JM, Lilly CM. Variant eotaxin: Its effects on the asthma phenotype. J Allergy Clin Immunol 2001; 108(6):946–953.

20

Role of the Eotaxin Subfamily of Chemokines in Allergic Eosinophilic Inflammation

NIVES ZIMMERMANN and MARC E. ROTHENBERG

Cincinnati Children's Hospital Medical Center
Cincinnati, Ohio, U.S.A.

I. Introduction

One of the hallmarks of asthma is the accumulation of an abnormally large number of leukocytes, including eosinophils, neutrophils, lymphocytes, basophils, and macrophages, in the lung (1). There is now substantial evidence that inflammatory cells are major effector cells in the pathogenesis of asthma. Of particular interest, eosinophil accumulation in the tissue is a hallmark feature of allergic disorders. Therefore, understanding the mechanisms by which leukocytes accumulate is a fundamental question very relevant to allergic diseases. Another characteristic of allergic inflammation is the activation of leukocytes resulting in the release of biologically active mediators, such as histamine from mast cells and basophils. It is now apparent that chemokines are potent leukocyte chemoattractants, cellular activating factors, histamine-releasing factors, and regulators of homeostatic immunity, making them particularly important in the pathogenesis of allergic inflammation (2). In this regard, chemokines are attractive new therapeutic targets for the treatment of allergic disease. This article will focus on recently emerging data on the importance of chemokines, especially the eosinophil-selective eotaxin subfamily of chemokines, and their receptors in allergic inflammation as well as on the potential for pharmacologically targeting these pathways.

II. Chemokine Family

Chemokines constitute a large family of chemotactic cytokines that has been divided into four groups, designated CXC, CC, C, and CX3C, depending upon the spacing of conserved cysteines (where X is any amino acid) (Fig. 1). The CXC and CC groups, in contrast to the C and CX3C chemokines, contain many members and have been studied in the greatest detail. The CXC chemokines mainly target neutrophils, whereas the CC chemokines target a variety of cell types, including macrophages, eosinophils, and basophils. Due to the complexity of the system, a new nomenclature has recently been proposed (3). This nomenclature is based on the chemokine receptor nomenclature currently used, which uses CC, CXC, XC, or CX3C (to designate the chemokine group) followed by R (for receptor) and then a number. The new chemokine nomenclature substitutes the R with L (for ligand), and the number is derived from the one already assigned to the gene encoding the chemokine from the SCY (small secreted cytokine) nomenclature. Thus, a given gene has the same number as its protein ligand (for example, the gene encoding eotaxin-1 is SCYA11 and the chemokine is referred to as CCL11). Table 1 summarizes the chemokine family utilizing this nomenclature.

This review will concentrate on CC chemokines since the members of this family primarily stimulate the movement of cells associated with allergic responses (including eosinophils, basophils, T cells, and monocytes). Particular focus will be on the eotaxin subfamily of chemokines since these chemokines target eosinophils, cells considered to be principal participants in a variety of allergic disorders. CC chemokines are divided into several structural subgroups including a group composed of the macrophage chemoattractant proteins (MCPs) and eotaxin (also known as eotaxin-1) (4) (Fig. 1). The MCP/eotaxin subfamily of chemokines shares structural and functional features and has been strongly implicated in asthma and other allergic diseases. The four human MCP proteins (− 1, − 2, − 3, − 4) share ~65%

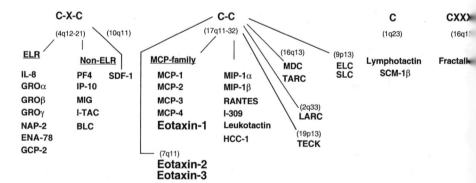

Figure 1 Human chemokine family. The chromosomal position in the human genome is indicated in parentheses.

Table 1 Chemokine Ligands

Systematic name	Human ligand	Mouse ligand[a]
CXC family		
CXCL1	GROα/MGSA-α	GRO/KC?
CXCL2	GROβ/MGSA-β	GRO/KC?
CXCL3	GROγ/MGSA-γ	GRO/KC?
CXCL4	PF4	PF4
CXCL5	ENA-78	LIX?
CXCL6	GCP-2	Ckα-3
CXCL7	NAP-2	—
CXCL8	IL-8	—
CXCL9	Mig	Mig
CXCL10	IP-10	IP-10
CXCL11	I-TAC	—
CXCL12	SDF-1α/β	SDF-1
CXCL13	BLC/BCA-1	BLC/BCA-1
CXCL14	BRAK/bolekine	BRAK
CXCL15	—	Lungkine
CXCL16	SR-PSOX	—
CC family		
CCL1	I-309	TCA-3, P500
CCL2	MCP-1/MCAF	JE?
CCL3	MIP-1α/LD78α	MIP-1α
CCL4	MIP-1β	MIP-1β
CCL5	RANTES	RANTES
CCL6	—	C10, MRP-1
CCL7	MCP-3	MARC?
CCL8	MCP-2	MCP-2?
CCL9/10	—	MRP-2, CCF18, MIP-1γ
CCL11	Eotaxin	Eotaxin
CCL12	—	MCP-5
CCL13	MCP-4	—
CCL14	HCC-1	—
CCL15	HCC-2/Lkn-1/MIP-1δ	—
CCL16	HCC-4/LEC	LCC-1
CCL17	TARC	TARC
CCL18	DC-CK1/PARC/AMAC-1	—
CCL19	MIP-3β/ELC/exodus-3	MIP-3β/ELC/exodus-3
CCL20	MIP-3α/LARC/exodus-1	MIP-3α/LARC/exodus-1
CCL21	6Ckine/SLC/exodus-2	6Ckine/SLC/exodus-2/TCA-4
CCL22	MDC/STCP-1	ABCD-1
CCL23	MPIF-1	—
CCL24	MPIF-2/Eotaxin-2	Eotaxin-2
CCL25	TECK	TECK
CCL26	Eotaxin-3	—
CCL27	CTACK/ILC	ALP/CTACK/ILC/ESkine
CCL28	MEC	MEC
C family		
XCL1	Lymphotactin/SCM-1α/ATAC	Lymphotactin
XCL2	SCM-1β	—
CX3C family		
CX3CL1	Fractalkine	Neurotactin

[a]A question mark indicates that the mouse and human homologues are ambiguous. A dash indicates that the homologue has not been identified. The shading highlights members of the eotaxin subfamily.

amino acid identity. In addition, eotaxin-1 also shares ~65% amino acid identity with the MCP proteins. Comparison of the amino acid sequences has revealed some striking similarities and differences in this family of chemokines. For example, all members of this family have a highly conserved 23-amino-acid leader sequence. In addition to the four conserved cysteines, several other residues are highly conserved between all members of the family, such as the serine-tyrosine residues between the second and third cysteines and the region around the fourth cysteine (4). In contrast to the majority of the MCPs, eotaxin-1 and murine MCP-3 contain one- to five-amino-acid gaps resulting in a shorter amino terminus preceding the first cysteine in the mature protein. Recently, human and murine eotaxin-2 and human eotaxin-3 have been cloned (5–9). Although eotaxin-2 and eotaxin-3 share only ~35% amino acid identity with eotaxin-1 and the MCP proteins, a phylogenetic tree analysis has placed them in the MCP branch of CC chemokines (8).

A. Three-Dimensional Structure

Although members of the different chemokine subfamilies have only weak homology and display nonoverlapping receptor binding, investigations solving the three-dimensional structure of chemokines have revealed that they share the same basic characteristics (10–14). A disordered amino terminus is linked to the rest of the molecule by the two amino-terminal cysteines. This is followed by an extended loop that leads into three antiparallel β-pleated sheets, termed β1, β2, and β3, which provides a flat base over which the carboxy-terminal α-helix lies. For instance, even though eotaxin-1, −2, and −3 share only 35–41% sequence identity, the three β-strands and the α-helix superimpose well. Figure 2 shows an overlay of the structures of eotaxin-1, eotaxin-2, RANTES, MCP-3, vMIP-II, MCP-1, and eotaxin-3.

B. Genomic Organization

Chemokines have a conserved intron-exon structure generally organized into 3 exons and 2 introns (15–18). For example, in the MCP/eotaxin-1 subfamily, the positions of the splice sites within the codons is conserved, suggesting that this subfamily arose from a common ancestral gene. In support of this concept, related chemokines are located in a similar chromosomal position (Fig. 1), suggesting that chemokine diversity may be the product of gene duplication. For example, most CXC chemokines are located on human chromosome 4q in two separate clusters: CXC chemokines that mainly act on neutrophils (through receptors CXCR1 and CXCR2) are clustered at 4q12–13, while those highly specific for T lymphocytes [ligands of CXCR3, such as monokine induced by interferon gamma (MIG), 10 kDa interferon-inducible protein (IP-10) and interferon-inducible T cell alpha chemoattractant (I-TAC)] are located in a separate minicluster at 4q21. Additionally, most CC chemokines are located on human chromosome 17q11–32. The MCPs and eotaxin-1 were found to be contained on the same yeast artificial chromosome clone containing human chromosome 17q11 (19). According to the National Center for Biotechnology Information (NCBI, *www.ncbi.nlm.nih.gov*), 11 of the CC chemokine genes are

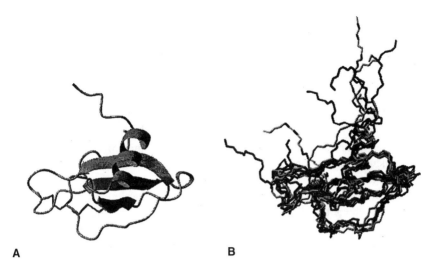

Figure 2 Structures of eosinophil chemokines. (A) Structure of eotaxin-3. Note the carboxy-terminal α-helix and the three β-pleated sheets. (B) Structures of eotaxin-1 (blue), eotaxin-2 (green), RANTES (cyan), MCP-3 (yellow), vMIP-II (orange) and MCP-1 (magenta) are superimposed onto eotaxin-3 (red). (Modified from Ref. 60.)

clustered within 2 Mbp on human chromosome 17q11. In distinction to other CC chemokines, eotaxin-2 and eotaxin-3 have been mapped to human 7q11.23 (8,20).

C. Regulation of Chemokine Production and Activity

The main stimuli for secretion of chemokines are the early pro-inflammatory cytokines, such as interleukin (IL)-1 and tumor necrosis factor alpha (TNF-α), bacterial products such as lipopolysaccharide (LPS), and viral infection (21–23). In addition, products of both Th1 and Th2 cells, interferon-gamma (IFN-γ) and IL-4, respectively, can also induce the production of chemokines independently and in synergy with IL-1 and TNF-α. In addition, IL-13 appears to be the main stimulus for eotaxin-1 mRNA and protein production in vivo (24). While there are many similarities in the regulation of chemokines, important differences that may have implications for asthma are beginning to be appreciated. For example, in the healthy lung, epithelial cells are the primary source of chemokines; however, in the inflamed lung infiltrating cells within the submucosa are a major cellular source of chemokines (25). Furthermore, the induced expression of eotaxin-1 and MCP-4 by TNF-α or IL-1 treatment of epithelial cells is suppressed by the steroid dexamethasone (26). This may be relevant to the clinical effectiveness of inhaled glucocorticoids at decreasing the eosinophil-rich inflammatory exudate characteristically seen in the respiratory tract of individuals with asthma. Recent studies have shown that the selectivity and production of chemokines can be regulated by a concentration-dependent mechanism.

For example, TNF-α is a potent inducer of a variety of chemokines including RANTES (regulated upon activation, normal T-cell expressed and secreted), MCP-4, and eotaxin-1. However, the level of TNF-α required to activate RANTES production (>100 U/mL) is 100-fold higher than required to activate MCP-4 and eotaxin-1 production (23,26,27). Various proinflammatory mediators also possess the ability to regulate chemokine production by modulation in a cell-specific manner. For example, IL-3 activates eotaxin-1 production in eosinophils (22) and IgE cross-linking activates mast cells to produce MCP-3 (28).

Chemokines also undergo substantial post-translational modification, which can influence their biological activity and function. For example, the CXC chemokines connective tissue-activating peptide (CTAP)-III, β-thromboglobulin, and neutrophil-activating protein-2 (NAP-2) arise from the amino-terminal processing of a common precursor platelet basic protein. Furthermore, mature chemokines may also undergo enzymatic modification, which results in the generation of chemokine derivatives with unique receptor usage and functional activity. For example, cleavage of the first two amino acids of RANTES by dipeptidyl peptidase IV (CD26) results in a truncated form of RANTES, which loses its functional activity on CCR1, but retains it on CCR5 (29). Additionally, modification of eotaxin-1 by CD26 results in a truncated eotaxin-1 that is not capable of transmitting positive signals through CCR3, but can desensitize the receptor to subsequent signaling by intact eotaxin-1 (30). Interestingly, infectious organisms appear to have developed pathways to metabolize chemokines. For example, products of the parasite *Necator americanus* enzymatically inactivate eotaxin-1 (31). This process may be a mechanism to curtail antihelminth immunity (31).

D. Chemokine Promoter Analysis

Analysis of the 5′-flanking regions of most chemokines reveals several conserved regulatory elements that may explain the observed regulation of the chemokine genes by cytokines and glucocorticoids (17,32). Of note, nuclear factor (NF)-κB, glucocorticoid response element (GRE), gamma-interferon response element (γIRE), Sp1, and E2A-binding site motifs are well conserved in both human and mouse chemokine promoters. For example, the eotaxin-1 promoter in mice and humans has NF-κB and signal transducer and activator of transcription (STAT)-6 sequences; mutation of the NFκB and STAT-6 site impairs eotaxin-1 promoter activity in response to TNF-α and IL-4, respectively (33). Furthermore, in vivo analysis revealed that IL-4–induced expression of eotaxin-1 and eotaxin-2 is STAT-6 dependent (7). NF-κB is a nuclear factor that is activated following stimulation of cells with various immunological agents, such as LPS, IL-1, and TNF-α. NF-κB has been shown to be important for the transcriptional activation of selected chemokines. For example, a single NF-κB–binding site is essential for TNF-α- and IL-1–induced expression of the MCP-1 (34) and growth-regulated oncogene-α (GROα) (35) genes and LPS-induced expression of the macrophage inflammatory protein (MIP)-2 gene (36). GRE mediates glucocorticoid regulation of transcription (37). Interestingly, IL-5, an eosinophil-specific growth and differentiation factor, and the chemokine IL-8 also contain a GRE sequence in their promoters. Furthermore, deletion analysis of the GRE from the IL-8 promoter revealed that this element participated in dexamethasone suppression of IL-8 expression (38). In vitro, the glucocorticoid budesonide inhibits eotaxin-1 promoter-driven reporter gene activity and accelerates the decay of eotaxin-1 mRNA (39). These studies indicate that glucocorticoids inhibit chemokine expression through multiple mechanisms of action. Finally, Bcl-6 appears to be a repressor of the transcription of several chemokines in vitro, including MCP-1, MCP-3, and macrophage inflammatory protein-related protein (MRP)-1 (40). This correlates in vivo with the STAT-6–independent Th2-type inflammation found in Bcl-6–deficient mice, providing a potential novel mechanism for the regulation of Th2-type inflammation.

III. Chemokine Receptor Family

Chemokines induce leukocyte migration and activation by binding to specific G protein–coupled seven-transmembrane–spanning cell surface receptors (GPCR) (41). Although chemokine receptors are similar to many GPCRs, they have unique structural motifs such as the amino acid sequence DRYLAIV in the second intracellular domain (41,42). Five CXCR receptors have been identified, referred to as CXCR1–5, and 11 human CC chemokine receptor genes have been cloned, known as CCR1 through CCR11. The chemokine and leukocyte selectivity of chemokine receptors overlap extensively; a given leukocyte often expresses multiple chemokine receptors, and more than one chemokine typically binds to the same receptor (Fig. 3). For example, monocytes express the CC chemokine receptors CCR1, CCR2, CCR4, and CCR5; eosinophils express mainly CCR1 and CCR3; and basophils express CCR1, CCR2, and CCR3. All of the MCP proteins characterized to date are ligands for CCR2. In addition MCP-2, −3, and −4 are also ligands for CCR3. In contrast, the eotaxin chemokines signal only through CCR3.

Further complexity is added in that chemokine receptors can be constitutively expressed on some cells, whereas they are inducible on others. For example, CCR1 and CCR2 are constitutively expressed on monocytes, but are only expressed on lymphocytes following IL-2 stimulation (43,44). Activated lymphocytes are then responsive to multiple CC chemokines that utilize these receptors, including the MCPs. In addition, some constitutive receptors can be downmodulated by biological response modifiers. For example, IL-10 modifies the activity of CCR1, CCR2, and CCR5 on dendritic cells and monocytes (45). Normally, dendritic cells mature in response to inflammatory stimuli and shift from expressing CCR1, CCR2, and CCR5 to CCR7 expression. However, IL-10 blocks the chemokine receptor switch. Importantly, while CCR1, CCR2, and CCR5 remain detectable on the cell surface and bind appropriate ligands, they do not signal in calcium mobilization and chemotaxis assays. Thus, IL-10 converts chemokine receptors to functional decoy receptors, thereby serving a downregulatory function.

Chemokines have two main sites for interaction with their receptors: one in the amino-terminal region and the other in the exposed loop of the backbone between

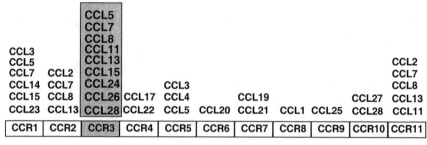

Figure 3   Ligands for CC (A) and CXC (B) receptor families.

the second and third cysteine (46). Site-directed mutagenesis has indicated that the loop region is important for receptor binding, while the amino-terminus is important for receptor activation (47–49). Based on these observations, a "two-step" model has been proposed for chemokine receptor activation (48,50–52). In the first step, the loop region of the chemokine binds to the amino-terminal region of the receptor. In the second step, the amino terminus of the chemokine binds to a second site on the receptor, presumably located between or close to the transmembrane helices, inducing a conformational change of the receptor and consequent transmembrane signaling. In addition to mutagenesis studies, the first step of this model is supported by observations of direct interaction of the CXC chemokine IL-8, the CX3C chemokine fractalkine, and CC chemokines eotaxin-1, eotaxin-2, and MCP-1 with peptides corresponding to the N-terminal regions of their respective receptors (14,49,53–55). Significant insight into chemokine-chemokine receptor interactions comes from comparative structural studies of specific receptor binding and nonbinding ligands. For instance, the structural comparison between six chemokine agonists of CCR3 (eotaxin-1, eotaxin-2, eotaxin-3, RANTES, MCP-3, and vMIP-II) compared to the non-CCR3 agonist MCP-1 has revealed interesting findings (13,52,56–60). Subtle yet significant differences between MCP-1 and CCR3 ligands include (1) the finding of more positive electrostatic potentials at the proposed receptor-binding surfaces of the CCR3 ligands; (2) the tighter turn between the $\beta2$ and $\beta3$ strands for MCP-1, which helps to define the putative receptor-binding groove; and (3) the N-terminal half of the α-helix, which may interact with the receptor N-terminus, is shifted slightly in MCP-1 (60). These data should facilitate rational design of receptor inhibitors.

A. Eosinophil Chemokine Receptors

Because eosinophilia is a hallmark feature of allergic inflammation, a large body of research has focused on the analysis of chemokine receptors and signaling pathways on eosinophils. Eosinophils from most healthy donors express CCR3 at the highest level (4,61,62) and have significantly lower levels of CCR1 (Fig. 4). Consistent with the expression of CCR1 and CCR3, eosinophils respond to MIP-1α, RANTES, MCP-2, MCP-3, MCP-4, eotaxin-1, eotaxin-2, eotaxin-3, and CCL28. Leukotactin (HCC2) has been demonstrated to be a ligand for CCR1 and CCR3, but its activity on eosinophils has not yet been reported (63,64). CCR3 appears to function as the predominant eosinophil chemokine receptor since CCR3 ligands are generally more potent eosinophil chemoattractants. Furthermore, an inhibitory monoclonal antibody specific for CCR3 blocks the activity of RANTES, a chemokine that could signal through CCR1 or CCR3 in eosinophils (65). Additionally, cytokine-primed human eosinophils respond to IL-8 (66) and eosinophils have the capacity to express CXCR2, the low-affinity IL-8 receptor, when they are cultured in IL-5 (65) (Fig. 4). IL-5 also primes eosinophils to respond to CCR3 ligands (67). The mechanism by which IL-5 primes the response of eosinophils to chemotactic signals remains to be elucidated, since IL-5 does not merely increase the expression

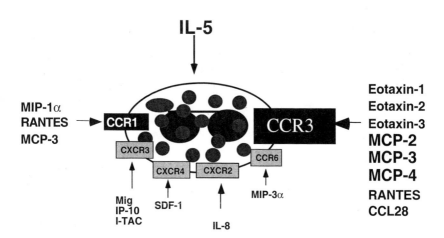

Figure 4 Eosinophil chemokine receptors and some of their ligands. The main chemokine receptors on eosinophils (CCR1 and CCR3) are depicted with black rectangles. Other chemokine receptors present on eosinophil subpopulations or under select conditions are shown in gray rectangles. Representative corresponding ligands are shown. IL-5 is also indicated since this chemokine primes eosinophils to respond to chemokines.

of CCR3 on mature eosinophils. Lastly, eosinophils have recently been shown to express or respond to ligands of CCR6, CXCR3, and CXCR4 (68–70). For instance, eosinophils isolated from allergic donors responded to MIP-3α in chemotaxis and calcium mobilization assays; FACS analysis reveals that ~20% of eosinophils express low levels of CCR6 (Fig. 4). Importantly, eosinophils isolated from nonallergic donors fail to respond to MIP-3α (68). In contrast, 50% of eosinophils from nonallergic donors express CXCR3 by FACS analysis, and these cells respond in functional assays. Interestingly, IL-2 is capable of upregulating CXCR3 on the nonexpressing eosinophils and IL-10 completely downregulates the receptor on cells already expressing CXCR3 (70). Additionally, eosinophils isolated from nonallergic donors express CXCR4 on their surface following incubation in vitro for 24 hours at 37°C. Importantly, incubation of eosinophils in the presence of IL-4 or IL-5 inhibits the increase in CXCR4 expression (69). Additionally, dexamethasone specifically upregulates the expression of CXCR4 on eosinophils (71) and cells expressing CXCR4 respond in functional assays to stromal cell derived factor-1 alpha (SDF-1α), the ligand for CXCR4. The significance of these chemokine receptors in eosinophil accumulation in health and disease remains to be elucidated.

B. Signal Transduction

Chemokine receptor signal transduction mechanisms have not been extensively examined, and most studies have been conducted in nonhematopoietic cells transfected with chemokine receptors (41). Chemokine receptors are, for the most part, inhibited by pertussis toxin, indicating that they are primarily coupled to Gi proteins (41). However, in freshly isolated cells, such as neutrophils and eosinophils, and in an eosinophilic cell line, direct inhibition of adenylate cyclase activity has not been routinely observed (72,73). Receptor activation leads to a cascade of intracellular signaling events leading to activation of phosphatidylinositol-specific phospholipase C, protein kinase C, small GTPases, Src-related tyrosine kinases, phosphatidylinositol-3-OH kinases, and protein kinase B. Phospholipase C delivers two secondary messengers, inositol-1,4,5-triphosphate, which releases intracellular calcium, and diacylglycerol, which activates protein kinase C. Multiple phosphorylation events are triggered by chemokines. Phosphatidylinositol-3-OH kinase can be activated by the βγ subunit of G proteins, small GTPases or Src-related tyrosine kinases. Phosphorylation of the tyrosine kinase RAFTK (related adhesion focal tyrosine kinase), a member of the focal adhesion kinase family, has been shown to be induced by signaling through CCR5 (74). Recently, mitogen-activated protein kinases have also been shown to be phosphorylated and activated within 1 minute after exposure of eosinophils to CCR3 ligands (75,76). This activation was required for eotaxin-1–induced eosinophil chemotaxis, actin polymerization, and degranulation (75,76). Additionally, Src-family kinases Hck and c-Fgr have been shown to associate with CCR3 following eotaxin-1 stimulation (77). In addition to triggering intracellular events, engagement with ligand induces rapid chemokine receptor internalization. For example, in human eosinophils, following only 15 minutes of exposure to eotaxin-1 or RANTES, CCR3 expression is reduced to only 20–40% of the original level. Internalized CCR3 enters an early endosome compartment shared with the transferrin receptor and is subsequently recycled or targeted to the lysozyme for protein degradation. Interestingly, chronic exposure to RANTES results in prolonged receptor internalization for at least 18 hours (78). Ligand-induced internalization of most chemokine receptors occurs independent of calcium transients, G-protein coupling, and protein kinase C, indicating a different mechanism compared with induction of chemotaxis. Thus, chemokine receptor internalization may provide a mechanism for chemokines to also halt leukocyte trafficking in vivo. Recently, the cytokine IL-3, but not IL-5 and GM-CSF, has been shown to induce internalization of CCR3 on eosinophils (79). The significance of this non–ligand-induced internalization remains to be determined.

C. Genetic Organization and Polymorphisms in Chemokine Receptors

The genes for CCR1 through 5 are located on human chromosome 3p21–24. Specifically, CCR1, 2, 3, and 5 are clustered on 3p21 within about 300 kb (80). Similar to other chemoattractant receptor genes, CCR genes are composed of a single coding exon, and the 5′-untranslated region is separated by at least one large intron (41). Several chemokine receptors, including CXCR2, CCR5, and CCR3, have a complex genomic organization with multiple 5′-untranslated exons differentially used by alternative splicing and/or usage of different promoters (81–83). For instance, the CCR3 gene consists of four exons that give rise to multiple mRNA species by alternative splicing (Fig. 5). Exon 1 is present in all transcripts, whereas exon 2 or 3 is present at low frequency (<10%). The function of the untranslated exons is related to transcription. For example, exon 1 of CCR3 acts as an enhancer for the endogenous promoter (83). The open reading frame of the human CCR3 gene (exon 4) is polymorphic and contains five nucleotide variants (Fig. 6); two of these encode for an amino acid substitution. One variant (G824A, allele frequency = 0.01) encodes for a change of arginine to glutamine in position 275 of the protein; this is a nonconservative amino acid change in the third extracellular domain of the receptor, a region implicated in ligand binding to CCR3 (84). Stratification of DNA samples into a population with asthma suggested no change in this allele's frequency, but the frequency may change in other inflammatory conditions (85). Another polymorphism (T1052C, allele frequency = 0.005) encodes for a leucine-to-proline substitution at position 351 in the serine/threonine-rich cytoplasmic tail (85). This occurs in a putative G-protein–coupled receptor kinase (GRK)-2 phosphorylation site and therefore may have consequences on receptor signaling. A recent study reported an additional genetic polymorphism (C218S) found at low frequency (0.001) (86). The promoter region and exon 1 have also been screened for polymorphisms. Surprisingly, only one polymorphism was found in 19 tested individuals. This mutation, C-37T, disrupts a CREB (cAMP response element–binding protein) DNA-binding consensus sequence and may effect CCR3 transcription regulation (83). Genetic polymorphisms have been found in other chemokine receptors and appear to have an effect on human disease. For instance, chemokine receptors were identified as

genomic DNA

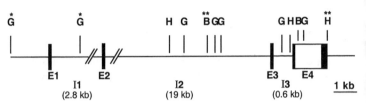

mRNA processing

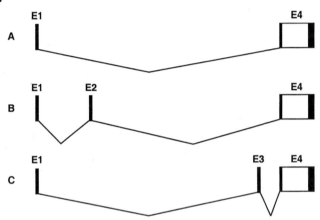

Figure 5 Genomic organization and mRNA processing of the CCR3 gene. A schematic diagram of the organization of the CCR3 gene is shown. The translated DNA area is depicted as an open rectangle and untranslated DNA is shown as shaded rectangles. Restriction enzymes are labeled as follows: G, Bgl II; B, Bam HI, and H, Hind III. Exons are labeled as E1 through E4; introns as I1 through I3. DNA fragments flanked by a single asterisk (*) and double asterisk (**) were fully sequenced (Genbank accession numbers AF237380, U51241, and AF237381). Below are the corresponding mRNA species: (A) Majority of mRNA species contain only exons 1 and 4; (B and C) usage of exon 1 with exons 2 or 3, respectively. (Adapted from Ref. 83.)

co-receptors for the entry of HIV-1 into cells (87). While CXCR4 serves as a co-receptor for T-cell–trophic HIV strains, CCR5 can function as a co-receptor for macrophage (M)-trophic strains of the virus. CCR2b and CCR3 also serve as receptors for some M-trophic strains, and administration of a CCR3-specific ligand such as eotaxin-1 blocks the entry of selected strains of HIV-1 into cells in vitro (88). Interestingly, genetic polymorphisms in the CCR2 and CCR5 gene confer protection from HIV infection (89–93). Interestingly, a small study has suggested that individuals carrying the CCR5Δ32 polymorphism may be protected from developing asthma (94). Thus, chemokine receptors contain several genetic variations that may have consequences in disease processes.

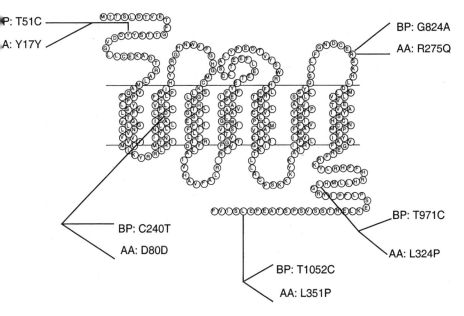

P: T51C
A: Y17Y

BP: G824A
AA: R275Q

BP: C240T
AA: D80D

BP: T971C
AA: L324P

BP: T1052C
AA: L351P

Figure 6 Polymorphisms found in CCR3. Five nucleotide polymorphisms, and their respective amino acid positions, found in the open reading frame of the CCR3 gene are indicated in a schematic molecule. BP, base pair; AA, amino acid.

IV. Chemokine- and Chemokine Receptor Gene–Deficient Mice

Research utilizing chemokine and chemokine-receptor gene disruptions have substantially contributed to the current understanding of the pleiotropic functions of these molecules. A summary of chemokine gene-targeted mice is presented in Table 2. The first chemokine gene deletion to be reported was the targeted disruption of the MIP-1α chemokine (95). Mice deficient in MIP-1α had a marked impairment in inflammatory responses following virus-induced myocarditis and pneumonitis. This demonstrates the essential role for MIP-1α in the development of antiviral immunity. The SDF-1 gene was the second chemokine to be gene targeted in mice (96). This targeted disruption resulted in embryonic lethality due to the surprising essential role of SDF-1 in cardiac development. Immunological analysis of embryonic blood also revealed defects in hematopoiesis in these animals (96). Eotaxin-1 was the third chemokine gene to be deleted from mice (97). As discussed below, eotaxin-1–deficient mice had an impairment in the early recruitment of eosinophils to the lung following allergen challenge. Additionally, they had a marked deficiency in the levels of tissue eosinophils indicating the critical importance of eotaxin-1 as a homeostatic chemokine that regulates eosinophil homing to nonhematopoietic tissues (98). MCP-1–deficient mice were developed and found to have a marked im-

Table 2   Phenotype of Chemokine Gene–Deleted Mice

Chemokine	Phenotype
MIP-1α	Impaired inflammatory responses to viral infections
SDF-1	Embryonic lethality due to impaired cardiac development and defects in hematopoiesis
Eotaxin-1	Impaired early recruitment of eosinophils to the lung following allergen challenge
	Reduced levels of eosinophils in tissues at baseline
	Protection from gastrointestinal allergy
MCP-1	Impaired macrophage recruitment
	Th1/Th2 imbalance
Lungkine	Impaired neutrophil recruitment into the airspace and increased susceptibility to *Klebsiella pneumoniae* infection

pairment in macrophage recruitment in response to peritoneal injection of thioglyco-late (99). Additionally, they had an imbalance in Th1 versus Th2 cytokines. Recently, lungkine-deficient mice have been generated and demonstrated to have increased susceptibility to *Klebsiella pneumoniae* infection, which correlated with reduced neutrophil recruitment into the airway (100).

Several chemokine receptors have been genetically deleted (Table 3). The first chemokine receptor to be gene-deleted in mice was the low-affinity receptor for IL-8 (CXCR2) (101). These mice had no overt abnormalities, but they had an impairment in neutrophil recruitment in response to thioglycolate. Additionally, they had a surprising increase in myelopoiesis and marked lymphadenopathy due to B-cell expansion when housed in conventional animal facilities. The second chemokine receptor to be gene-targeted was CXCR5 (102). These gene-deleted mice lacked inguinal lymph nodes and possessed markedly reduced and abnormal Peyer's patches. Furthermore, the migration of B lymphocytes into the spleen was abnormal, resulting in no functional germinal centers in these mice. These results indicated the critical role of CXCR5 in B-cell homing into lymphoid compartments. Next, CCR1- and CCR2-deficient mice have been generated (103–105). CCR1-deficient mice have dysregulated trafficking of mature leukocytes into hematopoietic tissues during both steady states and inflammatory conditions. Additionally, mature neutrophils in these mice failed to respond to MIP-1α, indicating that the predominant receptor for MIP-1α in neutrophils was CCR1. CCR1-deficient mice have impaired clearance of *Aspergillus fumigatus* that appears to result from an imbalanced Th1 response compared to a Th2 response in wild-type mice. These mice suggest that chemokines and their receptors have a role in inducing the type of immune response (Th1 vs. Th2). CCR2-deficient mice develop normally and have no impairment in hematopoiesis. However, they failed to clear the intracellular pathogen *Listeria monocytogenes* and to recruit macrophages into the peritoneum in response to thio-glycolate (104,105). Recently, both CCR1- and CCR2-deficient mice have been

Table 3 Chemokine Receptor Gene–Deleted Mice

Chemokine receptor	Phenotype
CXCR2	Splenomegaly, bone marrow myeloid hyperplasia, neutrophilia, and an increase in B cells (these abnormalities do not develop in germ-free facilities) Delayed wound healing Impaired resistance to multiple microbial pathogens
CXCR3	Delayed or absent allograft rejection
CXCR4	Lethal phenotype with hematopoietic and cardiac defects
CXCR5	Lack inguinal lymph nodes and reduced or abnormal Peyer's patches Lack of functional germinal centers
CCR1	Impaired neutrophil-mediated host defense mechanisms Dysregulation of Th1/Th2 balance Reduced airway remodeling in asthma model
CCR2	Failure to clear infection by *Listeria monocytogenes* Failure to recruit macrophages into the peritoneum in response to thioglycolate Variable effect in asthma model
CCR4	Decreased mortality in LPS-induced endotoxic shock
CCR5	Reduce clearance of *Listeria monocytogenes* Enhanced delayed-type hypersensitivity (DTH) reaction and increased humoral responses
CCR6	Absence of CD11c positive dendritic cells in the subepithelial dome of the Peyer's patches. Impaired humoral responses Increased T cell populations within the intestinal mucosa
CCR7	Reduced trafficking of T cells to lymph nodes
CCR8	Impaired Th2 responses (reduced production of Th2 cytokines and diminished eosinophilia) No effect on Th1 immune responses
DARC	Exaggerated response to endotoxin with significantly increased inflammatory infiltrates in lung and liver
CX3CR1	Protection from transplant rejection. Reduction in the number of NK cells in the graft

tested in allergic airway inflammation models. In a model of eosinophilic inflammation of the lungs in response to *A. fumigatus*, CCR1-deficient animals were found to have significantly fewer goblet cells and subepithelial fibrosis implicating CCR1 in airway remodeling (106). In the same model, CCR2-deficient animals exhibited an increase in eosinophils and lymphocytes in the airways, serum IgE, Th2 cytokines, and Th2-induced chemokines, airway hyperresponsiveness, and fibrosis compared to wild-type mice (107). However, in an ovalbumin-induced model of allergic airway inflammation, CCR2-deficient mice displayed no difference in pulmonary eosinophilia, Th2 cytokine levels, and airway hyperresponsiveness compared to wild-type mice (108). CCR8-deficient mice have been developed and tested in models of Th2 immune responses, such as *Schistosoma mansoni* soluble egg antigen–induced granuloma formation as well as OVA and cockroach antigen–induced allergic airway inflammation. In these mice, Th2 immune responses were defective with impaired Th2 cytokine production and reduced eosinophilia, while the Th1 response to *Mycobacterium bovis* purified protein derivative was unaffected (109). Additionally, gene targeting of CXCR4 resulted in a lethal phenotype with hematopoietic and cardiac defects reminiscent of those observed in SDF-1–targeted mice (110,111). Recently, CCR4-, CCR5-, CCR6-, CCR7-, CXCR3-, DARC (Duffy antigen/receptor for chemokines), and CX3CR1-deficient mice were generated and displayed various immunological defects (Table 3) (112–118). For instance, the CCR4-deficient mice displayed decreased mortality in LPS-induced endotoxic shock. While humans carrying the CCR5Δ32 polymorphism appear to be healthy despite their lack of CCR5 expression, mice deficient in CCR5 display reduced clearance of *Listeria monocytogenes*, enhanced delayed-type hypersensitivity (DTH) reactions, and increased humoral responses. CCR6- and CCR7-deficient mice display defects in T-cell and dendritic cell trafficking, as discussed below. Finally, CXCR3- and CX3CR1-deficient animals present with delayed or absent allograft rejection. The role of these defects in allergic airway inflammation remains to be elucidated.

Taken together, these studies indicate that despite the large number of chemokines and their receptors, there is likely to be a nonredundant role for each individual molecule. Similar gene targeting approaches will provide essential information regarding the complexity and importance of chemokines and their receptors in allergic and other inflammatory states.

V. Pleiotropic Functions of Chemokines in Allergic Responses

Chemokines have been implicated in diverse functions, and the significance of these results as related to allergy will be reviewed (Table 4).

Table 4 Pleiotropic Effects of Chemokines in Allergic Diseases

Cellular activation[a]
Chemoattraction[a]
Airway hyperreactivity
Histamine release
Modulation of dendritic cell function
Modulation of lymphocyte function
Regulation of hematopoiesis[a]
Regulation of homeostatic immunity[a]

[a] This property has been demonstrated for the eotaxin chemokines.

A. Chemoattraction

The interaction between leukocytes in the circulation and endothelial cells lining blood vessels is a complex network of signaling events regulating trafficking of particular leukocyte subsets (119). The interaction is mediated by a multistep process that involves (1) leukocyte rolling (mediated by endothelial selectin and specific leukocyte ligands), (2) rapid activation of leukocyte integrins, (3) firm adhesion to endothelial ligands through activated integrins, and (4) transmigration of leukocytes through the endothelial layer. Chemokines have a central role in the modulation of this multistep process by activating both the leukocyte and the endothelium and by increasing leukocyte integrin and adhesion molecule interaction affinity. The rapidity of the chemokine-mediated signaling events in this multistep process (seconds to minutes) is important for leukocytes, which dynamically roll through venules. Thus, the multistep chemokine signaling cascade must occur rapidly to allow for the leukocyte to reduce rolling velocity, mediate adherence, and extravasate into tissues in response to a chemokine gradient. In addition to mediating leukocyte movement from the bloodstream into tissues, chemokines utilize similar steps to mediate leukocyte-directed motion across other tissue barriers such as respiratory epithelium.

ELR (Glu-Leu-Arg) containing CXC chemokines (e.g., IL-8) are mainly chemoattractive for neutrophils, while non-ELR CXC chemokines (e.g., IP-10) chemoattract selected populations of lymphocytes. CC chemokines are active on a variety of leukocytes including dendritic cells, monocytes, basophils, lymphocytes, and eosinophils. As their names imply, all MCPs have strong chemoattractive activity for monocytes. However, they display partially overlapping chemoattractant activity on basophils and eosinophils. For example, MCP-2, MCP-3, and MCP-4 have basophil and eosinophil chemoattractive activity, but MCP-1 is only active on basophils. In distinction to the MCPs, eotaxin-1 has limited activity on macrophages, whereas it is a potent eosinophil and basophil chemoattractant (4,120). Interestingly, eotaxin-1 is a competitive antagonist for CCR2 and may therefore downregulate chemokine-induced trafficking and functional activation of CCR2 + macrophages and dendritic cells (121). The entire MCP/eotaxin family has variable lymphocyte chemoattractive activity. Administration of eotaxin-1 intranasally or subcutaneously revealed that eotaxin-1 induced a rapid selective tissue accumulation of eosinophils in murine lung or skin, respectively, in the presence of high levels of IL-5, an eosinophil growth and activating cytokine (using IL-5 transgenic mice) (122). Cooperativity between eotaxin-1 and IL-5 in promoting tissue eosinophilia has been reported by several groups (123,124). IL-5 collaborates with eotaxin-1 in promoting tissue eosinophilia by increasing the pool of circulating eosinophils (by stimulating eosinophilopoiesis and bone marrow release) and priming eosinophils to have enhanced responsiveness to eotaxin-1. Additionally, synergy between eotaxin-1 and the lipid mediator 5-oxo-6,8,11,14-eicosatetraenoic acid in inducing eosinophil chemotaxis has been demonstrated (125). Although eotaxin-1 has been demonstrated to have activity on basophils in vitro, all administration studies in vivo have shown a selective eosinophil accumulation in guinea pigs (126), mice (122), and monkeys (127). This indicates that eotaxin-1's predominant role in leukocyte recruitment in vivo is restricted to eosinophils. It remains possible that eotaxin-1 may promote the cellular accumulation of noneosinophils in vivo if the appropriate second signal is present. For example, eotaxin-1 may promote basophil accumulation if coadministered with IL-3. The ability of two cytokines (IL-5 and eotaxin-1) that are relatively eosinophil-selective to cooperate in promoting tissue eosinophilia offers a molecular explanation for the occurrence of selective tissue eosinophilia in human allergic diseases.

B. Cellular Activation

In addition to promoting leukocyte accumulation, chemokines are potent cell activators. After binding to the appropriate G-protein–linked seven-transmembrane-spanning receptor, chemokines elicit transient intracellular calcium flux, actin polymerization, oxidative burst with release of superoxide free radicals, the exocytosis of secondary granule constituents, and increased avidity of integrins for their adhesion molecules (128–130). For example, in basophils, chemokine-induced cellular activation results in degranulation with the release of histamine and the de novo generation of leukotriene C4 (22,131,132). Basophil activation by chemokines requires cellular priming with IL-3, IL-5, or granulocyte-monocyte colony-stimulating factor (GM-CSF) for the maximal effect of each chemokine. Although all MCPs can induce histamine release in cytokine-primed basophils, there is marked variability between individual basophil donors. MCP-1 appears to be the most potent secretagogue for basophils, whereas eotaxin-1 is weak. In eosinophils, CCR3 ligands induce degranulation and this effect is amplified when cells are primed with IL-5 (133–135).

C. Hematopoiesis

In addition to being involved in leukocyte accumulation during inflammatory reactions, chemokines also have a role in regulating baseline hematopoiesis. These functions include (1) chemotaxis of hematopoietic progenitor cells (HPC); (2) suppression and enhancement activity on HPC proliferation and differentiation; and (3) mobilization of HPCs to the peripheral blood (reviewed in Ref. 136). For example, SDF-1, a CXC chemokine, is critical for B-cell lymphopoiesis and bone marrow myelopoiesis, as demonstrated by gene targeting (96). Furthermore, eotaxin-1 has been shown to directly stimulate the release of eosinophilic progenitor cells and mature eosinophils from the bone marrow (137). Eotaxin-1 synergizes with stem cell factor in stimulating yolk sac development into mast cells in vitro (138) and has been shown to function as a GM-CSF following allergic challenge in the lung (139). In contrast, eotaxin-2 suppresses the colony formation of high proliferative potential colony-forming cells (HPP-CFC), which represent multipotential hematopoietic progenitors (5).

D. Homeostatic Role

Chemokines have an important role in baseline leukocyte trafficking during development, differentiation, and immune surveillance (140,141). For example, several chemokines including thymus-expressed chemokine (TECK), SDF-1, secondary lymphoid organ chemokine (SLC), liver and activation regulated chemokine (LARC), and dendritic cell–derived CC chemokine (DC-CK-1) and eotaxin-1 have been shown to be constitutively expressed at high levels in a broad range of tissues including the thymus, lymph nodes, and gastrointestinal tract (142,143). Individual chemokines may also have multifunctional roles, modulating both cellular trafficking and differentiation. For example, SDF-1 has been shown to regulate B-cell trafficking into lymphoid organs and to also be crucial for B-cell development and differentiation (96). Recent studies in CXCR5-deficient mice suggest that chemokines also have a role in lymph organ architecture and compartmentalization. As described above, CXCR5-deficient mice are characterized by defective formation of primary and secondary follicles and germinal centers in the spleen and other lymphoid follicles (102). T-cell trafficking into lymph nodes is also dependent on chemokines, specifically SLC and ELC (Epstein-Barr virus–induced molecule ligand chemokine) and their receptor CCR7. SLC is expressed by high endothelial venules (HEV), which are the site of T-lymphocyte entry into lymph nodes. Both SLC and ELC are expressed by stromal cells within T-cell areas of lymph nodes, spleen, and Peyer's patches. The role for SLC and ELC in T-cell migration into lymph nodes was suggested by the observation that mice bearing a spontaneous mutation, *plt* (paucity of lymph node T cells), have markedly reduced or absent SLC and ELC expression and have defective T-cell trafficking into lymph nodes as well as severely disturbed organization of cells in the T-cell areas (144,145). This was further supported by the demonstration that lymph nodes in CCR7-deficient mice have significantly reduced T cells (116). Recent studies have characterized a subset of T cells that express the B-cell chemokine receptor CXCR5 and home to B-cell zones of lymphoid tissues (146–148). Interestingly, the function of these T cells, called follicular B-helper T cells or T_{FH}, appears to be providing help to B cells for antibody production. Collectively, these studies suggest that chemokines have an important role in B- and T-cell trafficking into lymph nodes and the structural organization of lymphoid tissues.

The role of chemokines in homeostatic leukocyte trafficking has important implications in allergic states since the leukocytes involved in allergic responses (e.g., mast cells and eosinophils) primarily reside in tissue locations rather than hematopoietic organs. The eosinophil selective chemokine eotaxin-1 is constitutively expressed in a variety of tissues especially mucosal tissues wherein eosinophils normally reside (25,149). Furthermore, mice deficient in eotaxin-1 have a selective and marked reduction of tissue eosinophils in the gastrointestinal tract and thymus (98,150). This underscores the critical role of chemokines in establishing the location of allergic inflammatory cells at baseline.

E. Role in Allergen Uptake, Processing, and Presentation by Dendritic Cells

A central question in allergy research is to understand the mechanism for initial allergen recognition in mucosal surfaces. Tissue resident dendritic cells are believed to have a fundamental role in this process since they are able to efficiently take up, process, and deliver antigens to lymphoid tissues. The migration pattern of dendritic cells is complex and is thought to involve a coordinated chemokine signaling network. Dendritic cell progenitors from the bone marrow migrate into nonlymphoid tissues, where they develop into immature dendritic cells that have an active role in antigen uptake and processing. Antigen stimulation and the production of inflammatory cytokines promote the differentiation of immature "processing-stage" dendritic cells into mature presenting dendritic cells and mobilizes these cells. This promotes trafficking from the periphery to regional lymph nodes via afferent lymphatics. Upon reaching the lymph nodes, dendritic cells home to T-cell–rich regions, where they present the processed antigen to naive T cells and generate an antigen-specific primary T-cell response. As part of the maturation process, immature dendritic cells upregulate the expression of CCR7 and become responsive to ELC and SLC, chemokines responsible for their trafficking to lymph nodes. At the same time, they decrease the expression of CCR1, CCR2, and CCR5—the receptors for inflammatory chemokines (151–153). However, it is becoming apparent that there may be differences between distinct subsets of dendritic cells. For instance, in mice lacking CCR6, myeloid-derived dendritic cells (expressing CD11b and CD11c) are absent from the subepithelial dome of Peyer's patches. Additionally, these mice have impaired humoral immune responses and increased T-cell populations within the intestinal mucosa (117). Although the role of dendritic cells and the chemokines that regulate their trafficking in allergic responses has not been extensively evaluated, these processes are likely to have fundamental implications in understanding allergic responses. Recent studies indicate that dendritic cells are required for the development of eosinophilic airway inflammation in response to inhaled antigen (154). Importantly, adoptive transfer of antigen-pulsed dendritic cells has been shown to be sufficient for the induction of Th2 responses and eosinophilic airway inflammation in response to inhaled antigen (155).

F. Effector Function in Elicitation of End-Organ Damage

Chronic allergic inflammation is associated with end-organ damage, including tissue remodeling and airway hyperreactivity (156,157). Chemokines have been shown to participate, directly and indirectly, in the pathogenesis of tissue damage by multiple mechanisms. For example, direct administration of selected chemokines to pulmonary tissue (e.g., MCP-1) in vivo is sufficient for the induction of rapid airway hyperreactivity (156,157). This effect may be mediated by a combination of processes including activation of allergic inflammatory cells (e.g., basophils) and by direct effects on structural tissue cells. Chemokines have also been shown to participate in wound healing and tissue remodeling since they can have direct effects on angiogenesis (140).

G. Modulation of T-Cell Immune Responses

Recently there has been rapid progress in understanding the effects of chemokines on T-lymphocyte biology (141). T lymphocytes have been shown to express a majority of chemokine receptors, thus making them potentially responsive to a large number of different chemokines. Characterization of chemokine receptor expression has shown that T lymphocytes display a dynamic expression pattern of chemokine receptors, and it is the differential expression of receptors during T lymphocyte maturation and differentiation that is thought to allow for individual chemokine specific functionality on T lymphocytes (141). As mentioned previously, CCR7 plays an important role in trafficking of naïve T cells into lymph nodes (158). Upon activation, T cells may express an array of chemokine receptors including CCR1, CCR2, CCR5, CXCR1, and CXCR4. They thus become sensitive to inflammatory chemokines including MIP-1α, MIP-1β, MCP-3, and RANTES, which are thought to mediate T-cell trafficking to sites of inflammation (159). Additionally, specific subsets of memory T cells can be distinguished based on their expression of CCR7 and the propensity to migrate into lymph nodes (160). Chemokines have an important role in the induction of inflammatory responses and are also central in selecting the type of immune response (Th1 vs. Th2). During bacterial or viral infections IP-10, MIG, IL-8, and I-TAC production correlates with the presence of CD4+ Th1-type T cells. In contrast during allergic inflammatory responses, eotaxin-1, RANTES, MCP-2, MCP-3, and MCP-4 are induced, and the majority of the CD4+ T lymphocytes are of the Th2-type phenotype. Characterization of chemokine receptor expression on T lymphocytes suggests that this may be explained by the expression of CXCR3 and CCR5 predominantly on Th1-type T cells, whereas CCR3, CCR4, and CCR8 have been associated with Th2-type T cells. Additionally, Th1 and Th2 cells secrete distinct chemokines (161). In mice, Th1 cells preferentially secrete RANTES and lymphotactin, whereas Th2 cells secrete monocyte-derived chemokine (MDC) and thymus-derived chemotactic agent (TCA)-3. Interestingly, supernatants from Th2 cells preferentially attract Th2 cells. These data suggest that the presence of specific patterns of chemokine receptors on T-cell subsets predicts which subset will be preferentially accumulated at sites of inflammation. Alternatively, chemokines may directly influence the differentiation of naïve T cells to the Th1 or Th2 phenotype. MIP-1α and MCP-1 have been described as capable of inducing the differentiation of Th1 and Th2 cells (162), and MCP-1–deficient mice have defective Th2 responses (163). Consistent with this, animals deficient in Bcl-6, a transcriptional repressor described above, express high levels of chemokines, including MCP-1, and suffer from systemic Th2-type inflammation (40).

VI. Chemokines in Animal Models of Allergy

A. Animal Models

The importance of eosinophils in the pathogenesis of airway damage has been an active area of research in animals (164). Most studies utilize a model of eosinophilic pulmonary inflammation that is induced by challenging sensitized animals with antigen exposure in the lung. Although no one model mimics all the features of the human disease, they have been useful in dissecting the mechanisms required for the induction of allergic inflammation (165–167). These models involve sensitization of animals with systemic doses of antigen, typically ovalbumin (OVA), in the presence of an adjuvant such as alum. While the use of an adjuvant is not necessary, it enhances the magnitude of the IgG1, IgE, and cellular responses. Following sensitization, the animals are mucosally exposed to antigen by direct intranasal application of antigen to anesthetized animals or by aerosolization of the antigen to conscious animals via a nebulizer. Alternatively, unsensitized animals are exposed to repeated doses of mucosal antigen, which induces sensitization and allergic inflammation. In each of these models, antigen challenge leads to a marked accumulation of inflammatory leukocytes in the lung primarily composed of eosinophils, lymphocytes, and, to a lesser extent, neutrophils. Most studies in guinea pigs and mice have shown that eosinophils and IL-5 are required for the induction of airway hyperresponsiveness; however, the mere presence of eosinophils in the airway does not always lead to hyperresponsiveness (168–171). This indicates that other signals in addition to those provided by IL-5, such as chemokines, are likely to be responsible for eosinophil-mediated tissue damage (172). A smaller set of experiments has clearly shown that pathways independent of eosinophils for the induction of allergic airway inflammation can also be operational (173,174). Recent studies have indicated that IL-13 is sufficient to induce many of the pathophysiological processes associated with asthma and, interestingly, IL-13 is a potent activator of chemokine expression (24,175–177). We have demonstrated that IL-13–induced eosinophil recruitment to the lung, but not mucus production, is IL-5 and eotaxin-1 dependent (178).

Models of allergic airway inflammation have proven useful for the study of chemokines. In fact, eotaxin-1 was initially discovered as the chief chemoattractive activity released into the bronchoalveolar lavage fluid in a guinea pig model of allergic airway disease (126). These models have demonstrated rapid induction of chemokine mRNA expression following allergen challenge. For example, following OVA sensitization and challenge, eotaxin-1 mRNA increased at 3 hours in guinea pigs; in mice, eotaxin-1 peaked at 3–6 hours after OVA, but remained elevated for at least 48 hours (179). Additionally, the MCPs have been demonstrated to be induced by OVA and remain elevated between 3 to 48 hours after antigen challenge (4). Likewise, repeated exposure of animals to intranasal *A. fumigatus* antigen resulted in ~60-fold increase in eotaxin-1 lung mRNA at 18 hours after the last antigen dose compared to saline-treated animals (4).

T lymphocytes have been demonstrated to be essential for the induction of eosinophilic allergic airway inflammation (164,180,181). Antigen-specific CD4 + Th2 lymphocytes play a central role in eosinophil recruitment, as depletion of these cells (181,182) or their secreted products (IL-4 and IL-5) (169,180,183,184) significantly reduces pulmonary eosinophilia. The mechanism by which T cells assist in the recruitment of eosinophils to the lung in these models is not completely understood. As discussed earlier, T-cell products such as IL-5 cooperate with eotaxin-1 in vivo. Treatment of allergen-challenged mice with a monoclonal antibody against CD3 inhibited eotaxin-1, but not MIP-1α mRNA induction, and significantly reduced eosinophil accumulation in the lung (179). In addition, antigen-specific antibody responses and mast cell degranulation following antigen challenge in sensitized mice were not affected by T-cell elimination (179). Thus, mast cell degranulation alone is not sufficient for the induction of eotaxin-1 and pulmonary eosinophilia. These findings suggest that selective chemokines such as eotaxin-1 may be molecular links between antigen-specific T-cell activation and the recruitment of eosinophils into the airways.

B. Role of Chemokines in Allergy Models

Multiple studies have demonstrated that a variety of chemokines are strongly induced in models of allergic inflammation and in human allergic disorders, but few studies have determined the relative importance of one chemokine over another in promoting the pathological events. Determining the significance of each chemokine has important implications for the design of therapeutic intervention aimed at blocking chemokine activity and suggests whether therapy should target individual chemokines or particular chemokine receptors. Because members of the chemokine family have apparent in vitro redundancy, it might be expected that no one chemokine would provide a critical signal for cell recruitment. However, a variety of approaches including antibody neutralization experiments and gene targeting have shown nonredundant specific roles for selected chemokines in allergic diseases. For example, eotaxin-1 gene–deficient mice have been shown to have an impairment in the recruitment of eosinophils during the early part of the late phase response in the lung and cornea in experimental models of asthma and keratitis (97). Additionally, employment of neutralizing antibodies against RANTES, MIP-1α, MCP-1, MCP-5, and eotaxin-1 have indicated the individual importance of each of these chemokines in the development and regional localization of inflammatory cells during allergen-induced pulmonary inflammation and airway hyperreactivity (157). For instance, neutralization of eotaxin-1 reduced eosinophil infiltration and airway hyperresponsiveness transiently after each allergen challenge, while neutralization of MCP-5 abolished airway hyperresponsiveness by altering the trafficking of eosinophils through the lung interstitium. In contrast, neutralization of MCP-1 blocked the development of airway hyperresponsiveness even though eosinophil recruitment was unchanged in these mice (157). Taken together, these studies suggest that pharmacological therapy that targets chemokine and/or chemokine receptor pathways involved in allergic inflammation is a promising therapeutic strategy.

VII. Evidence for the Role of Chemokines in Patients with Asthma

Allergic diseases are thought to be polygenic diseases, with multiple genes contributing to the pathogenesis of the disease. In support of the complex polygenic nature of allergic diseases, genetic linkage analysis has identified multiple different candidate genes including the high-affinity IgE receptor, IL-4 receptor alpha chain, a locus that maps near the IL-4 and IL-5 cytokine gene cluster on chromosome 5q31–32, and, most relevant for this review, a locus that maps near the CC chemokine locus on chromosome 17q11.2 (185–192). Additionally, the occurrence of eosinophilia in atopics has been genetically mapped to a locus near the class I genes of the major histocompatability complex on chromosome 6. Finally, a familial form of the idiopathic hypereosinophilic syndrome with autosomal dominant inheritance has been genetically linked to the cytokine locus on chromosome 5q32 (193,194). Clinical and experimental investigations have shown that epithelial cells from bronchial biopsy specimens have an increased expression level of several chemokines including eotaxin-1 and MCPs (67,195). In support of these findings, the concentration of MCP-1, MCP-4, MIP-1α, RANTES, IL-8, and eotaxin-1 in the bronchoalveolar fluid is elevated in patients with mild asthma (196). Furthermore, an endobronchial challenge with allergen results in an increase in the level of chemokines in the bronchoalveolar lavage fluid. The chemoattractant activity of the lavage fluid from patients with asthma is partially inhibited by antibodies against RANTES, MCP-3, MCP-4, and eotaxin-1 (67). For example, a combination of antibodies against eotaxin-1, MCP-4, and RANTES inhibits ∼50% of the eosinophil chemotactic activity in the bronchoalveolar fluid (67). In a clinical study, an association between the plasma concentration of eotaxin-1 and the incidence of asthma and reduced lung function was established (197). Experimental induction of cutaneous and pulmonary late phase responses in humans has revealed that eotaxin-1 is induced early (6 h) and correlates with early eosinophil recruitment; in contrast, eotaxin-2 and MCP-4 correlate with eosinophil accumulation at 24 hours (198,199). In a similar study, eotaxin-1 and eotaxin-2 mRNA were found to be increased in patients with asthma as compared to normal controls; however, there was no further increase following allergen challenge (200). In contrast, eotaxin-3 mRNA was dramatically enhanced 24 hours after allergen challenge (200). Together, these studies indicate the importance of chemokines in the pathogenesis of airway inflammation in humans.

Polymorphisms in individual chemokines and chemokine receptor genes are likely to influence the course of asthma. As noted earlier, CCR5Δ32 appears to protect against asthma (94). Additionally, a polymorphism in the RANTES promoter (G → A at position −401) appears to have an effect on atopic dermatitis (201). The polymorphism confers higher transcriptional activity and a new GATA transcription binding site. Additionally, it is associated with increased susceptibility to atopic dermatitis since the proportion of individuals carrying the mutant allele is higher in children with atopic dermatitis. Furthermore, the polymorphism has a higher frequency in individuals of African descent compared to Caucasian subjects and has recently been associated with increased susceptibility to both asthma and atopy since the proportion of individuals carrying the mutant allele is higher in atopic and nonatopic asthma patients (202). Additionally, the polymorphism is associated with increased aeroallergen skin test positivity and homozygosity is associated with increased risk of airway obstruction.

From a variety of clinical and experimental human studies the following generalizations can be made: (1) the mRNA and protein for selected chemokines (such as MCPs and eotaxin-1) are constitutively expressed in pulmonary tissue and primarily derived from epithelial cells; (2) allergen challenge in atopic and nonatopic asthmatics promotes an increase in both protein and mRNA for selected chemokines (such as the eotaxin subfamily and MCP-4) as compared with saline challenge; (3) during pulmonary inflammation, macrophages and to a lesser extent eosinophils and lymphocytes localized to the subepithelial layer are significant sources of chemokines; (4) allergen-induced chemokine expression during experimental late phase responses reveal kinetic correlation between individual chemokines and infiltrating cell types; and (5) genetic polymorphisms in chemokines and their receptors are likely to influence disease risk and phenotype.

VIII. Therapeutic Approach to Interfering with Chemokines

One of the actions of glucocorticoids is to inhibit the transcription and/or stability of chemokine mRNA. However, the ideal pharmaceutical agent would interfere with the selective function of critical chemokines and/or their receptors in the pathophysiology of asthma but not in protective immune responses. CCR3 represents such a potential target since preliminary studies indicate that it is likely to be critically involved in allergic inflammation and antagonizing CCR3 would selectively target eosinophils, basophils, and Th2 cells. While benefits of targeting eosinophils may be questioned with the results from preliminary clinical trials of antibody blockade of IL-5 in mild asthmatics (203), activity on Th2 cells may be important since these cells contribute to airway hyperresponsiveness. Additionally, CCR4 and CCR8 may be potential targets since both are reported to be Th2-specific and involved in the recruitment of Th2 cells in allergic inflammation (109,204). CCR8 represents a potentially attractive target since recent studies with CCR8-deficient mice have shown impaired antigen-driven Th2 responses and pulmonary eosinophilia (109). The impact of CCR3 targeting on physiological responses should also be considered. However, the cells that mainly express CCR3 (such as eosinophils and basophils) do not appear to have essential physiological roles, so targeting these cells would be unlikely to result in significant immunosuppression. The role of CCR3 in Th2 cells and other cell types that may express this receptor is not fully understood. However, the impact of antagonists on physiological homeostasis will need to be evaluated.

Chemokine and/or chemokine receptor inhibition has thus been an active area of research. Studies have also been fueled by the finding that natural chemokine receptor mutations block the HIV co-receptor function of selected chemokine receptors (such as CCR2 and CCR5), suggesting that pharmaceutical targeting of chemokine receptors is a promising strategy for treatment of HIV infection (89,93). There are several potential approaches for blockade of chemokines and their receptors (Table 5). One approach is to develop humanized monoclonal antibodies against chemokines and/or their receptors, an approach already validated in animal models (205). Specifically, an antibody directed against CCR3 would offer an advantage over antibodies against chemokines, since actions of multiple chemokines through a single receptor would be affected. An antibody against human CCR3, designated 7B11, has been validated as a potent binding and functional antagonist in vitro (206). However, rodent-derived antibodies, such as 7B11, would have to be humanized before clinical trials are conducted. Another approach involves developing receptor antagonists based on chemokine protein modifications. One such agent has been derived by the addition of a single methionine to the amino terminus of RANTES

Table 5   Therapeutic Approaches to Inhibiting Chemokines and Their Receptors

Humanized monoclonal antibodies against chemokines and/or their receptors[a]
Induction of receptor desensitization and/or internalization[a]
Receptor antagonists[a]
Small-molecule receptor inhibitors[a]
Signal transduction inhibitors
Transcriptional inhibitors
   Antisense oligonucleotides
   Transcription factor inhibitors

[a] This property has been demonstrated for the eotaxin chemokines and/or CCR3.

(designated Met-RANTES; Serono) (207,208). This agent acts as a strong competitive inhibitor of CCR1, CCR3, and CCR5. In vivo studies have demonstrated significant reduction in eosinophil numbers following Met-RANTES administration in a murine model of allergic airway inflammation (209). The success of protein antagonists has already been recognized by viruses, some of which have developed their

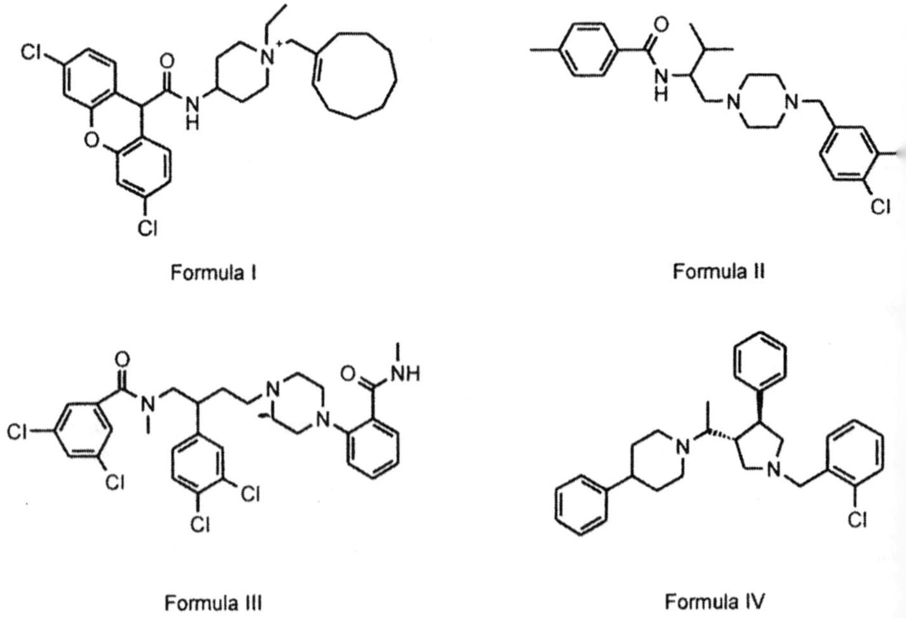

Formula I   Formula II

Formula III   Formula IV

Figure 7   Chemical structure of CCR3 antagonists. Representative chemical structures of CCR3 antagonists from Banyu Pharmaceuticals (Formula I), Hoffmann-La Roche (Formula II), and Merck (Formulas III and IV). (From Ref. 215.)

own chemokine antagonists. For example, the human herpes simplex virus-8 genome encodes for two chemokine-related proteins, and one of these, vMIP-II, is a potent broad-spectrum antagonist against both CXC and CC chemokine receptors (210,211). Another example is a potent CCR8 antagonist encoded by the poxvirus molluscum contagiosum, termed MC148 (212). Additionally, small molecule inhibitors of chemokine receptors have recently been described and display potent inhibition at nanomolar concentrations in vitro (213,214). Three companies (Banyu Pharmaceuticals, Hoffmann-La Roche, and Merck) have reported the development of small molecule CCR3 antagonists (Fig. 7) (215,216). These compounds share the presence of a hydrophobic group some distance away from a basic nitrogen group. It has been postulated that the basic nitrogen group interacts with a key anionic residue in or near the seven-transmembrane region of the receptor, as found with antagonists of the monoamine receptors, which are seven-transmembrane-spanning receptors. However, no in vivo data are yet available.

An additional approach to inhibiting chemokines can be induction of prolonged desensitization to chemokine stimulation (217). It may be possible to induce cellular desensitization by promoting chemokine receptor internalization (78). Alternatively, the transcription or translation of specific chemokines or chemokine receptors could be blocked. For example, antisense oligonucleotides and transcription factor inhibitors specifically designed to interact with regulatory regions in the CCR3 gene (83) may have clinical utility. A more detailed understanding of the regulation of chemokine and chemokine receptor genes is necessary for the development of these approaches.

IX. Summary

Over the last decade, chemokines, in particular the eotaxin subfamily, have emerged as cytokines likely to be important in the regulation of allergic inflammation. A combination of mouse and human studies has been used to define the role of chemokines in allergic diseases and their potential as therapeutic targets. Through the use of targeted gene deletion and neutralizing antibodies, the role of individual chemokines in mouse models of inflammation has begun to be determined. Furthermore, murine studies have been used to understand the regulation of chemokine expression in vivo. These murine studies have been correlated with human studies aimed at determining which chemokines are relevant to distinct human disease processes such as asthma.

While we are in the early phase of this type of analysis and there has only been a partial identification of the molecules involved in allergic inflammation, some principles are emerging. First, chemokines collaborate with other cytokines in the generation of eosinophil-rich inflammatory exudates. This involves increasing the pool of circulating leukocytes, upregulation of particular adhesion molecules, and increasing a leukocyte's responsiveness to chemokines. So while the eotaxin chemokines may be induced in many situations where TNF-α and IL-1 are present, it is only in those situations where IL-5 is coproduced (IL-4 and IL-13 associated processes) that significant pathological tissue eosinophilia occurs. Second, several chemokines appear to contribute to eosinophil recruitment in allergic inflammation in the lung. For example, the human genome contains three eosinophil-selective chemokines (eotaxin-1, eotaxin-2, eotaxin-3) and gene-targeting eotaxin-1 has only a partial effect on allergen-induced lung inflammation. Likewise, in bronchoalveolar lavage fluid from patients with asthma, eotaxin-1 and MCP-4 contribute to the eosinophil chemotactic activity. Third, the partially overlapping activity of these chemokines in allergic inflammation is explained by the coexpression of multiple chemokines in allergic tissue and the fact that each recruited inflammatory cell expresses multiple promiscuous chemokine receptors. Fourth, we have seen that the role of chemokines varies in different tissues and during baseline or inflammatory states. So while the role of the eotaxin subfamily of chemokines in the lung may be partially overlapping with other cytokines; in the gastrointestinal tract, eotaxin-1 has a more dominant role (98,150,218). This suggests that targeting allergic diseases of the lung may be best accomplished with more broad-spectrum agents (anti-CCR3 agents), whereas allergic diseases in the gastrointestinal tract may be amenable to antieotaxin therapeutics.

In conclusion, chemokines, especially the eotaxin subfamily, have now emerged as potentially critical cytokines involved in the pathogenesis of allergic airway inflammation. This has provided the rationale for increased scientific investigation in the field and for the development of antichemokine and anti–chemokine receptor therapeutics. The challenge for the future will be to understand the role of each chemokine, chemokine receptor, and their polymorphic variants in the pathophysiology of allergic diseases. Once this is accomplished, neutralization of chemokine function is likely to have therapeutic value in the treatment of allergic diseases. However, the ultimate proof of these principles awaits the testing of these therapeutics in human, which may not be too far in the future.

Acknowledgments

The editorial assistance of Andrea Lippelman is appreciated. This work was supported in part by NIH grant R01 AI42242 (to M.E.R.), a grant from the Human Frontier Science Program (to M.E.R.), and the American Heart Association Scientist Development Grant (to N.Z.). N.Z. is a Parker B. Francis fellow in pulmonary research. This manuscript was largely adopted and updated from our previous reviews (219,220).

References

1.   Bousquet J, Chanez P, Lacoste JY, Barneon G, Ghavanian N, Enander I, Venge P, Ahlstedt S, Simony-Lafontaine J, Godard P, Michel FB. Eosinophilic inflammation in asthma. N Engl J Med 1990; 323:1033–1039.
2.   Baggiolini M, Dahinden CA. CC chemokines in allergic inflammation. Immunol Today 1994; 15:127–133.

3. Zlotnik A, Yoshie O. Chemokines: a new classification system and their role in immunity. Immunity 2000; 12:121–127.

4. Luster AD, Rothenberg ME. Role of monocyte chemoattractant protein and eotaxin subfamily of chemokines in allergic inflammation. J Leukoc Biol 1997; 62:620–633.

5. Patel VP, Kreider BL, Li H, Leung K, Salcedo T, Nardelli B, Pippalla V, Gentz S, Thotakura R, Parmelee D, Gentz R, Garotta G. Molecular and functional characterization of two novel human C-C chemokines as inhibitors of two distinct classes of myeloid progenitors. J Exp Med 1997; 185:1163–1172.

6. Forssmann U, Uguccioni M, Loetscher P, Dahinden CA, Langen H, Thelen M, Baggiolini M. Eotaxin-2, a novel CC chemokine that is selective for the chemokine receptor CCR3, and acts like eotaxin on human eosinophil and basophil leukocytes. J Exp Med 1997; 185:2171–2176.

7. Zimmermann N, Hogan SP, Mishra A, Brandt EB, Bodette TR, Pope SM, Finkelman FD, Rothenberg ME. Murine eotaxin-2: a constitutive eosinophil chemokine induced by allergen challenge and IL-4 overexpression. J Immunol 2000; 165:5839–5846.

8. Kitaura M, Suzuki N, Imai T, Takagi S, Suzuki R, Nakajima T, Hirai K, Nomiyama H, Yoshie O. Molecular cloning of a novel human CC chemokine (eotaxin-3) that is a functional ligand of CC chemokine receptor 3. J Biol Chem 1999; 274:27975–27980.

9. Shinkai A, Yoshisue H, Koike M, Shoji E, Nakagawa S, Saito A, Takeda T, Imabeppu S, Kato Y, Hanai N, Anazawa H, Kuga T, Nishi T. A novel human CC chemokine, eotaxin-3, which is expressed in IL-4-stimulated vascular endothelial cells, exhibits potent activity toward eosinophils. J Immunol 1999; 163:1602–1610.

10. Clore GM, Gronenborn AM. Three-dimensional structures of alpha and beta chemokines. FASEB J 1995; 9:57–62.

11. Lodi PJ, Garrett DS, Kuszewski J, Tsang ML, Weatherbee JA, Leonard WJ, Gronenborn AM, Clore GM. High-resolution solution structure of the beta chemokine hMIP-1 beta by multidimensional NMR. Science 1994; 263:1762–1767.

12. Handel TM, Domaille PJ. Heteronuclear (1H, 13C, 15N) NMR assignments and solution structure of the monocyte chemoattractant protein-1 (MCP-1) dimer. Biochemistry 1996; 35:6569–6584.

13. Stone MJ, Mayer KL. Three-dimensional structure of chemokines. In: Rothenberg ME, ed. Chemokines in Allergic Diseases. New York: Marcel Dekker, 1999:67–94.

14. Mayer KL, Stone MJ. NMR solution structure and receptor peptide binding of the CC chemokine eotaxin-2. Biochemistry 2000; 39:8382–8395.

15. Rothenberg ME, Luster AD, Leder P. Murine eotaxin: an eosinophil chemoattractant inducible in endothelial cells and in interleukin 4-induced tumor suppression. Proc Natl Acad Sci USA 1995; 92:8960–8964.

16. Garcia-Zepeda EA, Combadiere CC, Rothenberg ME, Sarafi MN, Lavigne F, Hamid Q, Murphy PM, Luster AD. Human monocyte chemoattractant protein (MCP)-4: a novel CC chemokine with activities on monocytes, eosinophils, and basophils induced in allergic and non-allergic inflammation that signals through the CC chemokine receptors CKR-2 and -3. J Immunol 1996; 157:5613–5626.

17. Garcia-Zepeda EA, Rothenberg ME, Weremowicz S, Sarafi MN, Morton CC, Luster AD. Genomic organization, complete sequence, and chromosomal location of the gene for human eotaxin (SCYA11), an eosinophil-specific CC chemokine. Genomics 1997; 41:471–476.

18. Coillie EV, Fiten P, Nomiyama H, Sakaki Y, Miura R, Yoshie O, Damme JV, Opdenakker G. The human MCP-2 Gene (Scya8): cloning, sequence analysis, tissue expression,

and assignment to the CC chemokine contig on chromosome 17q11.2. Genomics 1997; 40:323–331.

19. Naruse K, Ueno M, Satoh T, Nomiyama H, Tei H, Takeda M, Ledbetter DH, Coillie EV, Opdenakker G, Gunge N, Sakaki Y, Iio M, Miura R. A YAC contig of the human CC chemokine genes clustered on chromosome 17q11.2. Genomics 1996; 34:236–240.

20. Nomiyama H, Osborne LR, Imai T, Kusuda J, Miura R, Tsui LC, Yoshie O. Assignment of the human CC chemokine MPIF-2/eotaxin-2 (SCYA24) to chromosome 7q11.23. Genomics 1998; 49:339–340.

21. Proost P, Wuyts A, Van Damme J. Human monocyte chemotactic proteins-2 and -3: structural and functional comparison with MCP-1. J Leukoc Biol 1996; 59:67–74.

22. Garcia-Zepeda EA, Rothenberg ME, Ownbey RT, Celestin J, Leder P, Luster AD. Human eotaxin is a specific chemoattractant for eosinophil cells and provides a new mechanism to explain tissue eosinophilia. Nature Med 1996; 2:449–456.

23. Stellato C, Collins P, Ponath PD, Soler D, Newman W, La RG, Li H, White J, Schwiebert LM, Bickel C, Liu M, Bochner BS, Williams T, Schleimer RP. Production of the novel C-C chemokine MCP-4 by airway cells and comparison of its biological activity to other C-C chemokines. J Clin Invest 1997; 99:926–936.

24. Li L, Xia Y, Nguyen A, Lai YH, Feng L, Mosmann TR, Lo D. Effects of Th2 cytokines on chemokine expression in the lung: IL-13 potently induces eotaxin expression by airway epithelial cells. J Immunol 1999; 162:2477–2487.

25. Minshall E, Cameron L, Levigne F, Hamilos D, Rothenberg M, Luster A, Hamid Q. Eotaxin mRNA expression in chronic sinusitis and allergen-induced nasal responses in seasonal allergic rhinitis. Am J Respir Cell Mol Biol 1997; 17:683–690.

26. Lilly CM, Nakamura H, Kesselman H, Nagler-Anderson C, Asano K, Garcia-Zepeda EA, Rothenberg ME, Drazen JM, Luster AD. Expression of eotaxin by human lung epithelial cells: induction by cytokines and inhibition by glucocorticoids. J Clin Invest 1997; 99:1767–1773.

27. Kulmburg PA, Huber NE, Scheer BJ, Wrann M, Baumruker T. Immunoglobulin E plus antigen challenge induces a novel intercrine/chemokine in mouse mast cells. J Exp Med 1992; 176:1773–1778.

28. Burd PR, Rogers HW, Gordon JR, Martin CA, Jayaraman S, Wilson SD, Dvorak AM, Galli SJ, Dorf ME. Interleukin 3-dependent and -independent mast cells stimulated with IgE and antigen express multiple cytokines. J Exp Med 1989; 170:245–257.

29. Oravecz T, Pall M, Roderiquez G, Gorrell MD, Ditto M, Nguyen NY, Boykins R, Unsworth E, Norcross MA. Regulation of the receptor specificity and function of the chemokine RANTES (regulated on activation, normal T cell expressed and secreted) by dipeptidyl peptidase IV (CD26)-mediated cleavage. J Exp Med 1997; 186:1865–1872.

30. Struyf S, Proost P, Schols D, De Clercq E, Opdenakker G, Lenaerts JP, Detheux M, Parmentier M, De Meester I, Scharp S, Van Damme J. CD26/dipeptidyl-peptidase IV down-regulates the eosinophil chemotactic potency, but not the anti-HIV activity of human eotaxin by affecting its interaction with CC chemokine receptor 3. J Immunol 1999; 162:4903–4909.

31. Culley FJ, Brown A, Conroy DM, Sabroe I, Pritchard DI, Williams TJ. Eotaxin is specifically cleaved by hookworm metalloproteases preventing its action in vitro and in vivo. J Immunol 2000; 165:6447–6453.

32. Nelson PJ, Kim HT, Manning WC, Goralski TJ, Krensky AM. Genomic organization and transcriptional regulation of the RANTES chemokine gene. J Immunol 1993; 151: 2601–2612.

33. Matsukura S, Stellato C, Plitt JR, Bickel C, Miura K, Georas SN, Casolaro V, Schleimer RP. Activation of eotaxin gene transcription by NF-kappa B and STAT6 in human airway epithelial cells. J Immunol 1999; 163:6876–6883.

34. Ueda A, Okuda K, Ohno S, Shirai A, Igarashi T, Matsunaga K, Fukushima J, Kawamoto S, Ishigatsubo Y, Okubo T. NF-kappa B and Sp1 regulate transcription of the human monocyte chemoattractant protein-1 gene. J Immunol 1994; 153:2052–2063.

35. Anisowicz A, Messineo M, Lee SW, Sager R. An NF-kappa B-like transcription factor mediates IL-1/TNF-alpha induction of gro in human fibroblasts. J Immunol 1991; 147: 520–527.

36. Widmer U, Manogue KR, Cerami A, Sherry B. Genomic cloning and promoter analysis of macrophage inflammatory protein (MIP)-2, MIP-1 alpha, and MIP-1 beta, members of the chemokine superfamily of proinflammatory cytokines. J Immunol 1993; 150: 4996–5012.

37. Beato M. Gene regulation by steroid hormones. Cell 1989; 56:335–344.

38. Mukaida N, Gussella GL, Kasahara T, Ko Y, Zachariae CO, Kawai T, Matsushima K. Molecular analysis of the inhibition of interleukin-8 production by dexamethasone in a human fibrosarcoma cell line. Immunology 1992; 75:674–679.

39. Stellato C, Matsukura S, Fal A, White J, Beck LA, Proud D, Schleimer RP. Differential regulation of epithelial-derived C-C chemokine expression by IL-4 and the glucocorticoid budesonide. J Immunol 1999; 163:5624–5632.

40. Toney LM, Cattoretti G, Graf JA, Merghoub T, Pandolfi PP, Dalla-Favera R, Ye BH, Dent AL. BCL-6 regulates chemokine gene transcription in macrophages. Nature Immunol 2000; 1:214–220.

41. Murphy PM. The molecular biology of leukocyte chemoattractant receptors. Annu Rev Immunol 1994; 12:593–633.

42. Gerard C, Gerard NP. The pro-inflammatory seven-transmembrane segment receptors of the leukocyte. Curr Opin Immunol 1994; 6:140–145.

43. Loetscher P, Seitz M, Baggiolini M, Moser B. Interleukin-2 regulates CC chemokine receptor expression and chemotactic responsiveness in T lymphocytes. J Exp Med 1996; 184:569–577.

44. Loetscher M, Gerber B, Loetscher P, Jones SA, Piali L, Clark-Lewis I, Baggiolini M, Moser B. Chemokine receptor specific for IP10 and mig: structure, function, and expression in activated T-lymphocytes. J Exp Med 1996; 184:963–969.

45. D'Amico G, Frascaroli G, Bianchi G, Transidico P, Doni A, Vecchi A, Sozzani S, Allavena P, Mantovani A. Uncoupling of inflammatory chemokine receptors by IL-10: generation of functional decoys. Nature Immunol 2000; 1:387–391.

46. Clark-Lewis I, Kim KS, Rajarathnam K, Gong JH, Dewald B, Moser B, Baggiolini M, Sykes BD. Structure-activity relationships of chemokines. J Leukoc Biol 1995; 57: 703–711.

47. Hebert CA, Vitangcol RV, Baker JB. Scanning mutagenesis of interleukin-8 identifies a cluster of residues required for receptor binding. J Biol Chem 1991; 266:18989–18994.

48. Crump MP, Gong JH, Loetscher P, Rajarathnam K, Amara A, Arenzana-Seisdedos F, Virelizier JL, Baggiolini M, Sykes BD, Clark-Lewis I. Solution structure and basis for functional activity of stromal cell-derived factor-1; dissociation of CXCR4 activation from binding and inhibition of HIV-1. EMBO J 1997; 16:6996–7007.

49. Hemmerich S, Paavola C, Bloom A, Bhakta S, Freedman R, Grunberger D, Krstenansky J, Lee S, McCarley D, Mulkins M, Wong B, Pease J, Mizoue L, Mirzadegan T, Polsky I, Thompson K, Handel TM, Jarnagin K. Identification of residues in the monocyte

chemotactic protein-1 that contact the MCP-1 receptor, CCR2. Biochemistry 1999; 38:13013–13025.

50. Siciliano SJ, Rollins TE, DeMartino J, Konteatis Z, Malkowitz L, Van Riper G, Bondy S, Rosen H, Springer MS. Two-site binding of C5a by its receptor: an alternative binding paradigm for G protein-coupled receptors. Proc Natl Acad Sci USA 1994; 91: 1214–1218.

51. Wells TNC, Guyecoulin F, Bacon KB. Peptides from the amino-terminus of Rantes cause chemotaxis of human T-lymphocytes. Biochem Biophys Res Commun 1995; 211:100–105.

52. Crump MP, Rajarathnam K, Kim KS, Clark-Lewis I, Sykes BD. Solution structure of eotaxin, a chemokine that selectively recruits eosinophils in allergic inflammation. J Biol Chem 1998; 273:22471–22479.

53. Clubb RT, Omichinski JG, Clore GM, Gronenborn AM. Mapping the binding surface of interleukin-8 complexes with an N-terminal fragment of the type 1 human interleukin-8 receptor. FEBS Lett 1994; 338:93–97.

54. Mizoue LS, Bazan JF, Johnson EC, Handel TM. Solution structure and dynamics of the CX3C chemokine domain of fractalkine and its interaction with an N-terminal fragment of CX3CR1. Biochemistry 1999; 38:1402–1414.

55. Ye J, Kohli LL, Stone MJ. Characterization of binding between the chemokine eotaxin and peptides derived from the chemokine receptor CCR3. J Biol Chem 2000; 275: 27250–27257.

56. Chung CW, Cooke RM, Proudfoot AEI, Wells TN. C. The three-dimensional solution structure of RANTES. Biochemistry 1995; 34:9307–9314.

57. Skelton NJ, Aspiras F, Ogez J, Schall TJ. Proton NMR assignments and solution conformation of RANTES, a chemokine of the C-C type. Biochemistry 1995; 34: 5329–5342.

58. Kim KS, Rajarathnam K, Clark-Lewis I, Sykes BD. Structural characterization of a monomeric chemokine: monocyte chemoattractant protein-3. FEBS Lett 1996; 395: 277–282.

59. Liwang AC, Wang ZX, Sun Y, Peiper SC, Liwang PJ. The solution structure of the anti-HIV chemokine vMIP-II. Protein Sci 1999; 8:2270–2280.

60. Ye J, Mayer KL, Mayer MR, Stone MJ. NMR solution structure and backbone dynamics of the CC chemokine eotaxin-3. Biochemistry 2001; 40:7820–7831.

61. Ponath PD, Qin S, Post TW, Wang J, Wu L, Gerard NP, Newman W, Gerard C, Mackay CR. Molecular cloning and characterization of a human eotaxin receptor expressed selectively on eosinophils. J Exp Med 1996; 183:2437–2448.

62. Daugherty BL, Siciliano SJ, DeMartino JA, Malkowitz L, Sirotina A, Springer MS. Cloning, expression, and characterization of the human eosinophil eotaxin receptor. J Exp Med 1996; 183:2349–2354.

63. Youn BS, Zhang SM, Lee EK, Park DH, Broxmeyer HE, Murphy PM, Locati M, Pease JE, Kim KK, Antol K, Kwon BS. Molecular cloning of leukotactin-1: a novel human beta-chemokine, a chemoattractant for neutrophils, monocytes, and lympho-cytes, and a potent agonist at CC chemokine receptors 1 and 3. J Immunol 1997; 159: 5201–5205.

64. Zhang S, Youn BS, Gao JL, Murphy PM, Kwon BS. Differential effects of leukotactin-1 and macrophage inflammatory protein-1alpha on neutrophils mediated by CCR1. J Immunol 1999; 162:4938–4942.

65. Heath H, Qin SX, Rao P, Wu LJ, Larosa G, Kassam N, Ponath PD, Mackay CR. Chemokine receptor usage by human eosinophils-the importance of CCR3 demon-strated using an antagonistic monoclonal antibody. J Clin Invest 1997; 99:178–184.

66. Warringa RAJ, Koenderman L, Kok PTM, Kreukniet J, Bruijnzeel PL. B. Modulation and induction of eosinophil chemotaxis by granulocyte-macrophage colony-stimulating factor and interleukin-3. Blood 1991; 77:2694–2700.

67. Lamkhioued B, Renzi PM, Abi-Younes S, Garcia-Zepeda EA, Allakhverdi Z, Ghaffar O, Rothenberg ME, Luster AD, Hamid Q. Increased expression of eotaxin in bronchoalveolar lavage and airways of asthmatics contributes to the chemotaxis of eosinophils to the site of inflammation. J Immunol 1997; 159:4593–4601.

68. Sullivan SK, McGrath DA, Liao F, Boehme SA, Farber JM, Bacon KB. MIP-3 alpha induces human eosinophil migration and activation of the mitogen-activated protein kinases (p42/p44 MAPK). J Leukoc Biol 1999; 66:674–682.

69. Nagase H, Miyamasu M, Yamaguchi M, Fujisawa T, Ohta K, Yamamoto K, Morita Y, Hirai K. Expression of CXCR4 in eosinophils: functional analyses and cytokine-mediated regulation. J Immunol 2000; 164:5935–5943.

70. Jinquan T, Jing C, Jacobi HH, Reimert CM, Millner A, Quan S, Hansen JB, Dissing S, Malling HJ, Skov PS, Poulsen LK. CXCR3 expression and activation of eosinophils: role of IFN-gamma-inducible protein-10 and monokine induced by IFN-gamma. J Immunol 2000; 165:1548–1556.

71. Nagase H, Miyamasu M, Yamaguchi M, Kawasaki H, Ohta K, Yamamoto K, Morita Y, Hirai K. Glucocorticoids preferentially upregulate functional CXCR4 expression in eosinophils. J Allergy Clin Immunol 2000; 106:1132–1139.

72. Uhing RJ, Gettys TW, Tomhave E, Synderman R, Didsbury JR. Differential regulation of cAMP by endogenous versus transfected formylpeptide chemoattractant receptors: implications for Gi-coupled receptor signalling. Biochem Biophys Res Commun 1992; 183:1033–1039.

73. Zimmermann N, Daugherty BL, Stark JM, Rothenberg ME. Molecular analysis of CCR-3 events in eosinophilic cells. J Immunol 2000; 164:1055–1064.

74. Ganju RK, Dutt P, Wu L, Newman W, Avraham H, Avraham S, Groopman JE. Beta-chemokine receptor CCR5 signals via the novel tyrosine kinase RAFTK. Blood 1998; 91:791–797.

75. Boehme SA, Sullivan SK, Crowe PD, Santos M, Conlon PJ, Sriramarao P, Bacon KB. Activation of mitogen-activated protein kinase regulates eotaxin-induced eosinophil migration. J Immunol 1999; 163:1611–1618.

76. Kampen GT, Stafford S, Adachi T, Jinquan T, Quan S, Grant JA, Skov PS, Poulsen LK, Alam R. Eotaxin induces degranulation and chemotaxis of eosinophils through the activation of ERK2 and p38 mitogen-activated protein kinases. Blood 2000; 95: 1911–1917.

77. El-Shazly A, Yamaguchi N, Masuyama K, Suda T, Ishikawa T. Novel association of the src family kinases, hck and c-fgr, with CCR3 receptor stimulation: a possible mechanism for eotaxin-induced human eosinophil chemotaxis. Biochem Biophys Res Commun 1999; 264:163–170.

78. Zimmermann N, Conkright JJ, Rothenberg ME. CC chemokine receptor-3 undergoes prolonged ligand-induced internalization. J Biol Chem 1999; 274:12611–12618.

79. Dulkys Y, Kluthe C, Buschermohle T, Barg I, Knoss S, Kapp A, Proudfoot AE, Elsner J. IL-3 induces down-regulation of CCR3 protein and mRNA in human eosinophils. J Immunol 2001; 167:3443–3453.

80. Daugherty BL, Springer MS. The beta-chemokine receptor genes CCR1 (CMKBR1), CCR2 (CMKBR2), and CCR3 (CMKBR3) cluster within 285 kb on human chromosome 3p21. Genomics 1997; 41:294–295.

81. Ahuja SK, Shetty A, Tiffany HL, Murphy PM. Comparison of the genomic organization and promoter function for human interleukin-8 receptors A and B. J Biol Chem 1994; 269:26381–26389.

82. Mummidi S, Ahuja SS, McDaniel BL, Ahuja SK. The human CC chemokine receptor 5 (CCR5) gene. Multiple transcripts with 5′-end heterogeneity, dual promoter usage, and evidence for polymorphisms within the regulatory regions and noncoding exons. J Biol Chem 1997; 272:30662–30671.

83. Zimmermann N, Daugherty BL, Kavanaugh JL, El-Awar FY, Moulton EA, Rothenberg ME. Analysis of the CC chemokine receptor 3 gene reveals a complex 5′ exon organization, a functional role for untranslated exon 1, and a broadly active promoter with eosinophil-selective elements. Blood 2000; 96:2346–2354.

84. Pease JE, Wang J, Ponath PD, Murphy PM. The N-terminal extracellular segments of the chemokine receptors CCR1 and CCR3 are determinants for MIP-1 alpha and eotaxin binding, respectively, but a second domain is essential for efficient receptor activation. J Biol Chem 1998; 273:19972–19976.

85. Zimmermann N, Bernstein JA, Rothenberg ME. Polymorphisms in the human CC chemokine receptor-3 gene. Biochim Biophys Acta 1998; 1442:170–176.

86. Kato H, Tsuchiya N, Izumi S, Miyamasu M, Nakajima T, Kawasaki H, Hirai K, Tokunaga K. New variations of human CC-chemokine receptors CCR3 and CCR4. Genes Immun 1999; 1:97–104.

87. Bates P. Chemokine receptors and HIV-1: an attractive pair? Cell 1996; 86:1–3.

88. Choe H, Farzan M, Sun Y, Sullivan N, Rollins B, Ponath PD, Wu LJ, Mackay CR, Larosa G, Newman W, Gerard N, Gerard C, Sodroski J. The beta-chemokine receptors CCR3 and CCR5 facilitate infection by primary HIV-1 isolates. Cell 1996; 85: 1135–1148.

89. Dean M, Carrington M, Winkler C, Huttley GA, Smith MW, Allikmets R, Goedert JJ, Buchbinder SP, Vittinghoff E, Gomperts E, Donfield S, Flahov D, Kaslow R, Saah A, Rinaldo C, Detels R, O'Brien SJ. Genetic restriction of HIV-1 infection and progression to AIDS by a deletion allele of the CKR5 structural gene. Hemophilia Growth and Development Study, Multicenter AIDS Cohort Study, Multicenter Hemophilia Cohort Study, San Francisco City Cohort, ALIVE Study. Science 1996; 273: 1856–1862.

90. Liu R, Paxton WA, Choe S, Ceradini D, Martin SR, Horuk R, MacDonald ME, Stuhlmann H, Koup RA, Landau NR. Homozygous defect in HIV-1 coreceptor accounts for resistance of some multiply-exposed individuals to HIV-1 infection. Cell 1996; 86:367–377.

91. Samson M, Soularue P, Vassart G, Parmentier M. The genes encoding the human CC-chemokine receptors CC-CKR1 to CC-CKR5 (CMKBR1–CMKBR5) are clustered in the p21.3–p24 region of chromosome 3. Genomics 1996; 36:522–526.

92. Quillent C, Oberlin E, Braun J, Rousset D, Gonzalez-Canali G, Metais P, Montagier L, Virelizier J, Arenzana-Seisdedos F, Beretta A. HIV-1-resistance phenotype conferred by combination of two separate inherited mutations of CCR-5 gene. Lancet 1998; 351:14–18.

93. Smith MW, Dean M, Carrington M, Winkler C, Huttley GA, Lomb DA, Goedert JJ, O'Brien TR, Jacobson LP, Kaslow R, Buchbinder S, Vittinghoff E, Vlahov D, Hoots K, Kilgartner MW, O'Brien SJ. Contrasting genetic influence of CCR2 and CCR5 variants on HIV-1 infection and disease progression. Hemophilia Growth and Development Study (HGDS), Multicenter AIDS Cohort Study (MACS), Multicenter Hemo-

philia Cohort Study (MHCS), San Francisco City Cohort (SFCC), ALIVE Study. Science 1997; 277:959–965.

94. Gerard C, Rollins BJ. Chemokines and disease. Nature Immunol 2001; 2:108–115.
95. Cook DN, Beck MA, Coffman TM, Kirby SL, Sheridan JF, Pragnell IB, Smithies O. Requirement of MIP-1 alpha for an inflammatory response to viral infection. Science 1995; 269:1583–1585.
96. Nagasawa T, Hirota S, Tachibana K, Takakura N, Nishikawa S, Kitamura Y, Yoshida N, Kikutani H, Kishimoto T. Defects of B-cell lymphopoiesis and bone-marrow myelopoiesis in mice lacking the CXC chemokine PBSF/SDF-1. Nature 1996; 382:635–638.
97. Rothenberg ME, MacLean JA, Pearlman E, Luster AD, Leder P. Targeted disruption of the chemokine eotaxin partially reduces antigen-induced tissue eosinophilia. J Exp Med 1997; 185:785–790.
98. Matthews AN, Friend DS, Zimmermann N, Sarafi MN, Luster AD, Pearlman E, Wert SE, Rothenberg ME. Eotaxin is required for the baseline level of tissue eosinophils. Proc Natl Acad Sci USA 1998; 95:6273–6278.
99. Lu B, Rutledge BJ, Gu L, Fiorillo J, Lukacs NW, Kunkel SL, North R, Gerard C, Rollins BJ. Abnormalities in monocyte recruitment and cytokine expression in monocyte chemoattractant protein 1-deficient mice. J Exp Med 1998; 187:601–608.
100. Chen SC, Mehrad B, Deng JC, Vassileva G, Manfra DJ, Cook DN, Wiekowski MT, Zlotnik A, Standiford TJ, Lira SA. Impaired pulmonary host defense in mice lacking expression of the CXC chemokine lungkine. J Immunol 2001; 166:3362–3368.
101. Cacalano G, Lee J, Kikly K, Ryan AM, Pitts-Meek S, Hultgren B, Wood WI, Moore MW. Neutrophil and B cell expansion in mice that lack the murine IL-8 receptor homolog. Science 1994; 265:682–684.
102. Forster R, Mattis AE, Kremmer E, Wolf E, Brem G, Lipp M. A putative chemokine receptor, BLR1, directs B cell migration to defined lymphoid organs and specific anatomic compartments of the spleen. Cell 1996; 87:1037–1047.
103. Gao JL, Wynn TA, Chang Y, Lee EJ, Broxmeyer HE, Cooper S, Tiffany HL, Westphal H, Kwon-Chung J, Murphy PM. Impaired host defense, hematopoiesis, granulomatous inflammation and type 1-type 2 cytokine balance in mice lacking CC chemokine receptor 1. J Exp Med 1997; 185:1959–1968.
104. Boring L, Gosling J, Chensue SW, Kunkel SL, Farese RV, Jr., Broxmeyer HE, Charo IF. Impaired monocyte migration and reduced type 1 (Th1) cytokine responses in CC chemokine receptor 2 knockout mice. J Clin Invest 1997; 100:2552–2561.
105. Kurihara T, Warr G, Loy J, Bravo R. Defects in macrophage recruitment and host defense in mice lacking the CCR2 chemokine receptor. J Exp Med 1997; 186: 1757–1762.
106. Blease K, Mehrad B, Standiford TJ, Lukacs NW, Kunkel SL, Chensue SW, Lu B, Gerard CJ, Hogaboam CM. Airway remodeling is absent in CCR1-/- mice during chronic fungal allergic airway disease. J Immunol 2000; 165:1564–1572.
107. Blease K, Mehrad B, Standiford TJ, Lukacs NW, Gosling J, Boring L, Charo IF, Kunkel SL, Hogaboam CM. Enhanced pulmonary allergic responses to aspergillus in CCR2-/- mice. J Immunol 2000; 165:2603–2611.
108. MacLean JA, De Sanctis GT, Ackerman KG, Drazen JM, Sauty A, DeHaan E, Green FH, Charo IF, Luster AD. CC chemokine receptor-2 is not essential for the development of antigen-induced pulmonary eosinophilia and airway hyperresponsiveness. J Immunol 2000; 165:6568–6575.
109. Chensue SW, Lukacs NW, Yang TY, Shang X, Frait KA, Kunkel SL, Kung T, Wiekowski MT, Hedrick JA, Cook DN, Zingoni A, Narula SK, Zlotnick A, Barrat FJ, O'Garra

A, Napolitano M, Lira SA. Aberrant in vivo T helper type 2 cell response and impaired eosinophil recruitment in cc chemokine receptor 8 knockout mice. J Exp Med 2001; 193:573–584.

110. Zou YR, Kottmann AH, Kuroda M, Taniuchi I, Littman DR. Function of the chemokine receptor CXCR4 in haematopoiesis and in cerebellar development. Nature 1998; 393: 595–599.

111. Tachibana K, Hirota S, Iizasa H, Yoshida H, Kawabata K, Kataoka Y, Kitamura Y, Matsushima K, Yoshida N, Nishikawa S, Kishimoto T, Nagasawa T. The chemokine receptor CXCR4 is essential for vascularization of the gastrointestinal tract. Nature 1998; 393:591–594.

112. Zhou Y, Kurihara T, Ryseck RP, Yang Y, Ryan C, Loy J, Warr G, Bravo R. Impaired macrophage function and enhanced T cell-dependent immune response in mice lacking CCR5, the mouse homologue of the major HIV-1 coreceptor. J Immunol 1998; 160: 4018–4025.

113. Chvatchko Y, Hoogewerf AJ, Meyer A, Alouani S, Juillard P, Buser R, Conquet F, Proudfoot AE, Wells TN, Power CA. A key role for CC chemokine receptor 4 in lipopolysaccharide-induced endotoxic shock. J Exp Med 2000; 191:1755–1764.

114. Dawson TC, Lentsch AB, Wang Z, Cowhig JE, Rot A, Maeda N, Peiper SC. Exaggerated response to endotoxin in mice lacking the Duffy antigen/receptor for chemokines (DARC). Blood 2000; 96:1681–1684.

115. Hancock WW, Lu B, Gao W, Csizmadia V, Faia K, King JA, Smiley ST, Ling M, Gerard NP, Gerard C. Requirement of the chemokine receptor CXCR3 for acute allograft rejection. J Exp Med 2000; 192:1515–1520.

116. Forster R, Schubel A, Breitfeld D, Kremmer E, Renner-Muller I, Wolf E, Lipp M. CCR7 coordinates the primary immune response by establishing functional microenvironments in secondary lymphoid organs. Cell 1999; 99:23–33.

117. Cook DN, Prosser DM, Forster R, Zhang J, Kuklin NA, Abbondanzo SJ, Niu XD, Chen SC, Manfra DJ, Wiekowski MT, Sullivan LM, Smith SR, Greenberg HB, Narula SK, Lipp M, Lira SA. CCR6 mediates dendritic cell localization, lymphocyte homeostasis, and immune responses in mucosal tissue. Immunity 2000; 12:495–503.

118. Haskell CA, Hancock WW, Salant DJ, Gao W, Csizmadia V, Peters W, Faia K, Fituri O, Rottman JB, Charo IF. Targeted deletion of CX(3)CR1 reveals a role for fractalkine in cardiac allograft rejection. J Clin Invest 2001; 108:679–688.

119. Butcher EC. Leukocyte-endothelial cell recognition: three (or more) steps to specificity and diversity. Cell 1991; 67:1033–1036.

120. Yamada H, Hirai K, Miyamasu M, Iikura M, Misaki Y, Shoji S, Takaishi T, Kasahara T, Morita Y, Ito K. Eotaxin is a potent chemotaxin for human basophils. Biochem Biophys Res Commun 1997; 231:365–368.

121. Ogilvie P, Bardi G, Clark-Lewis I, Baggiolini M, Uguccioni M. Eotaxin is a natural antagonist for CCR2 and an agonist for CCR5. Blood 2001; 97:1920–1924.

122. Rothenberg ME, Ownbey R, Mehlhop PD, Loiselle PM, Van de Rijn M, Bonventre JV, Oettgen HC, Leder P, Luster AD. Eotaxin triggers eosinophil-selective chemotaxis and calcium flux via a distinct receptor and induces pulmonary eosinophilia in the presence of interleukin 5 in mice. Molec Med 1996; 2:334–348.

123. Collins PD, Marleau S, Griffiths-Johnson DA, Jose PJ, Williams TJ. Cooperation between interleukin-5 and the chemokine eotaxin to induce eosinophil accumulation in vivo. J Exp Med 1995; 182:1169–1174.

124. Mould AW, Matthaei KI, Young IG, Foster PS. Relationship between interleukin-5 and eotaxin in regulating blood and tissue eosinophilia in mice. J Clin Invest 1997; 99:1064–1071.

125. Powell WS, Ahmed S, Gravel S, Rokach J. Eotaxin and RANTES enhance 5-oxo-6,8,11,14-eicosatetraenoic acid-induced eosinophil chemotaxis. J Allergy Clin Immunol 2001; 107:272–278.

126. Jose PJ, Griffiths-Johnson DA, Collins PD, Walsh DT, Moqbel R, Totty NF, Truong O, Hsuan JJ, Williams TJ. Eotaxin: a potent eosinophil chemoattractant cytokine detected in a guinea pig model of allergic airways inflammation. J Exp Med 1994; 179: 881–887.

127. Ponath PD, Qin SX, Ringler DJ, Clark-Lewis I, Wang J, Kassam N, Smith H, Shi XJ, Gonzalo JA, Newman W, Gutierrez-Ramos JC, Mackay CR. Cloning of the human eosinophil chemoattractant, eotaxin-expression, receptor binding, and functional properties suggest a mechanism for the selective recruitment of eosinophils. J Clin Invest 1996; 97:604–612.

128. Bischoff SC, Krieger M, Brunner T, Dahinden CA. Monocyte chemotactic protein 1 is a potent activator of human basophils. J Exp Med 1992; 175:1271–1275.

129. Dahinden CA, Geiser T, Brunner T, Vontscharner V, Caput D, Ferrara P, Minty A, Baggiolini M. Monocyte chemotactic protein 3 is a most effective basophil- and eosinophil-activating chemokine. J Exp Med 1994; 179:751–756.

130. Elsner J, Hochstetter R, Kimmig D, Kapp A. Human eotaxin represents a potent activator of the respiratory burst of human eosinophils. Eur J Immunol 1996; 26:1919–1925.

131. Alam R, Lett-Brown MA, Forsythe PA, Anderson-Walters DJ, Kenamore C, Kormos C, Grant JA. Monocyte chemotactic and activating factor is a potent histamine-releasing factor for basophils. J Clin Invest 1992; 89:723–728.

132. Alam R, Forsythe P, Stafford S, Heinrich J, Bravo R, Proost P, Van Damme J. Monocyte chemotactic protein-2, monocyte chemotactic protein-3, and fibroblast-induced cytokine. Three new chemokines induce chemotaxis and activation of basophils. J Immunol 1994; 153:3155–3159.

133. Alam R, Stafford S, Forsythe P, Harrison R, Faubion D, Lett-Brown MA, Grant JA. RANTES is a chemotactic and activating factor for human eosinophils. J Immunol 1993; 150:3442–3448.

134. El-Shazly A, Masuyama K, Nakano K, Eura M, Samejima Y, Ishikawa T. Human eotaxin induces eosinophil-derived neurotoxin release from normal human eosinophils. Int Arch Allergy Immunol 1998; 117(suppl 1):55–58.

135. Fujisawa T, Kato Y, Nagase H, Atsuta J, Terada A, Iguchi K, Kamiya H, Morita Y, Kitaura M, Kawasaki H, Yoshie O, Hirai K. Chemokines induce eosinophil degranulation through CCR-3. J Allergy Clin Immunol 2000; 106:507–513.

136. Kim CH, Broxmeyer HE. Chemokines for immature blood cells: effects on migration, proliferation, and differentiation. In: Rothenberg ME, ed. Chemokines in Allergic Diseases. New York: Marcel Dekker 1999:227–262.

137. Palframan RT, Collins PD, Williams TJ, Rankin SM. Eotaxin induces a rapid release of eosinophils and their progenitors from the bone marrow. Blood 1998; 91:2240–2248.

138. Quackenbush EJ, Aguirre V, Wershil BK, Gutierrez-Ramos JC. Eotaxin influences the development of embryonic hematopoietic progenitors in the mouse. J Leukoc Biol 1997; 62:661–666.

139. Peled A, Gonzalo JA, Lloyd C, Gutierrrez-Ramos JC. The chemotactic cytokine eotaxin acts as a granulocyte-macrophage colony-stimulating factor during lung inflammation. Blood 1998; 91:1909–1916.

140. Luster AD. Chemokines-chemotactic cytokines that mediate inflammation. N Engl J Med 1998; 338:436–445.

141. Rollins BJ. Chemokines. Blood 1997; 90:909–928.

142. Hromas R, Kim CH, Klemsz M, Krathwohl M, Fife K, Cooper S, Schnizlein BC, Broxmeyer HE. Isolation and characterization of Exodus-2, a novel C-C chemokine with a unique 37-amino acid carboxyl-terminal extension. J Immunol 1997; 159: 2554–2558.

143. Imai T, Baba M, Nishimura M, Kakizaki M, Takagi S, Yoshie O. The T cell-directed CC chemokine TARC is a highly specific biological ligand for CC chemokine receptor 4. J Biol Chem 1997; 272:15036–15042.

144. Gunn MD, Kyuwa S, Tam C, Kakiuchi T, Matsuzawa A, Williams LT, Nakano H. Mice lacking expression of secondary lymphoid organ chemokine have defects in lymphocyte homing and dendritic cell localization. J Exp Med 1999; 189:451–460.

145. Luther SA, Tang HL, Hyman PL, Farr AG, Cyster JG. Coexpression of the chemokines ELC and SLC by T zone stromal cells and deletion of the ELC gene in the plt/plt mouse. Proc Natl Acad Sci USA 2000; 97:12694–12699.

146. Kim CH, Rott LS, Clark-Lewis I, Campbell DJ, Wu L, Butcher EC. Subspecialization of CXCR5 + T cells: B helper activity is focused in a germinal center-localized subset of CXCR5 + T cells. J Exp Med 2001; 193:1373–1381.

147. Schaerli P, Willimann K, Lang AB, Lipp M, Loetscher P, Moser B. CXC chemokine receptor 5 expression defines follicular homing T cells with B cell helper function. J Exp Med 2000; 192:1553–1562.

148. Breitfeld D, Ohl L, Kremmer E, Ellwart J, Sallusto F, Lipp M, Forster R. Follicular B helper T cells express CXC chemokine receptor 5, localize to B cell follicles, and support immunoglobulin production. J Exp Med 2000; 192:1545–1552.

149. Stahl J, Cook E, Rothenberg ME, Graziano FM. Epithelial cells are a major cellular source of eotaxin mRNA in the guinea pig lung. J Allergy Clin Immunol 1997; 97: 403a.

150. Mishra A, Hogan SP, Lee JJ, Foster PS, Rothenberg ME. Fundamental signals that regulate eosinophil homing to the gastrointestinal tract. J Clin Invest 1999; 103: 1719–1727.

151. Sallusto F, Schaerli P, Loetscher P, Schaniel C, Lenig D, Mackay CR, Qin S, Lanzavecchia A. Rapid and coordinated switch in chemokine receptor expression during dendritic cell maturation. Eur J Immunol 1998; 28:2760–2769.

152. Sozzani S, Luini W, Borsatti A, Polentarutti N, Zhou D, Piemonti L, D'Amico G, Power CA, Wells TN, Gobbi M, Allavena P, Mantovani A. Receptor expression and responsiveness of human dendritic cells to a defined set of CC and CXC chemokines. J Immunol 1997; 159:1993–2000.

153. Dieu-Nosjean MC, Vicari A, Lebecque S, Caux C. Regulation of dendritic cell trafficking: a process that involves the participation of selective chemokines. J Leukoc Biol 1999; 66:252–262.

154. Lambrecht BN, Salomon B, Klatzmann D, Pauwels RA. Dendritic cells are required for the development of chronic eosinophilic airway inflammation in response to inhaled antigen in sensitized mice. J Immunol 1998; 160:4090–4097.

155. Lambrecht BN, De Veerman M, Coyle AJ, Gutierrez-Ramos JC, Thielemans K, Pauwels RA. Myeloid dendritic cells induce Th2 responses to inhaled antigen, leading to eosinophilic airway inflammation. J Clin Invest 2000; 106:551–559.

156. Lukacs NW, Strieter RM, Warmington K, Lincoln P, Chensue SW, Kunkel SL. Differential recruitment of leukocyte populations and alteration of airway hyperreactivity by C-C family chemokines in allergic airway inflammation. J Immunol 1997; 158: 4398–4404.

157. Gonzalo JA, Lloyd CM, Wen D, Albar JP, Wells TNC, Proudfoot A, Martinez AC, Dorf M, Bjerke T, Coyle AJ, Gutierrez-Ramos JC. The coordinated action of CC chemokines in the lung orchestrates allergic inflammation and airway hyperresponsiveness. J Exp Med 1998; 188:157–167.

158. Gunn MD, Tangemann K, Tam C, Cyster JG, Rosen SD, Williams LT. A chemokine expressed in lymphoid high endothelial venules promotes the adhesion and chemotaxis of naive T lymphocytes. Proc Natl Acad Sci USA 1998; 95:258–263.

159. Ward SG, Bacon K, Westwick J. Chemokines and T lymphocytes: more than an attraction. Immunity 1998; 9:1–11.

160. Sallusto F, Lenig D, Forster R, Lipp M, Lanzavecchia A. Two subsets of memory T lymphocytes with distinct homing potentials and effector functions. Nature 1999; 401: 708–712.

161. Zhang S, Lukacs NW, Lawless VA, Kunkel SL, Kaplan MH. Cutting edge: differential expression of chemokines in Th1 and Th2 cells is dependent on Stat6 but not Stat4. J Immunol 2000; 165:10–14.

162. Karpus WJ, Kennedy KJ. MIP-1alpha and MCP-1 differentially regulate acute and relapsing autoimmune encephalomyelitis as well as Th1/Th2 lymphocyte differentiation. J Leukoc Biol 1997; 62:681–687.

163. Gu L, Tseng S, Horner RM, Tam C, Loda M, Rollins BJ. Control of TH2 polarization by the chemokine monocyte chemoattractant protein-1. Nature 2000; 404:407–411.

164. Hogan SP, Mould AW, Young JM, Rothenberg ME, Ramsay AJ, Matthaei K, Young IG, Foster PS. Cellular and molecular regulation of eosinophil trafficking to the lung. Immunol Cell Biol 1998; 76:454–460.

165. Dunn CJ, Elliott GA, Oostveen JA, Richards IM. Development of a prolonged eosinophil-rich inflammatory leukocyte infiltration in the guinea-pig asthmatic response to ovalbumin inhalation. Am Rev Respir Dis 1988; 137:541–547.

166. Wegner CD, Gundel RH, Reilly P, Haynes N, Letts LG, Rothlein R. Intercellular adhesion molecule-1 (ICAM-1) in the pathogenesis of asthma. Science 1990; 247: 456–459.

167. Renz H, Smith HR, Henson JE, Ray BS, Irvin CG, Gelfand EW. Aerosolized antigen exposure without adjuvant causes increased IgE production and increased airway responsiveness in the mouse. J Allergy Clin Immunol 1992; 89:1127–1138.

168. Chand N, Harrison JE, Rooney S, Pillar J, Jakubicki R, Nolan K, Diamantis W, Sofia RD. Anti-IL-5 monoclonal antibody inhibits allergic late phase bronchial eosinophilia in guinea pigs: a therapeutic approach. Eur J Pharmacol 1992; 211:121–123.

169. Foster PS, Hogan SP, Ramsay AJ, Matthaei KI, Young IG. Interleukin 5 deficiency abolishes eosinophilia, airways hyperreactivity, and lung damage in a mouse asthma model. J Exp Med 1996; 183:195–201.

170. Lefort J, Bachelet CM, Leduc D, Vargaftig BB. Effect of antigen provocation of IL-5 transgenic mice on eosinophil mobilization and bronchial hyperresponsiveness. J Allergy Clin Immunol 1996; 97:788–799.

171. Lilly CM, Chapman RW, Sehring SJ, Mauser PJ, Egan RW, Drazen JM. Effects of interleukin 5-induced pulmonary eosinophilia on airway reactivity in the guinea pig. Am J Physiol 1996; 270:L368–375.

172. Drazen JM, Arm JP, Austen KF. Sorting out the cytokines of asthma. J Exp Med 1996; 183:1–5.

173. Corry DB, Folkesson ML, Warnock DJ, Erle DJ, Matthay MA, Wiener-Kronish JP, Locksley RC. Interleukin 4, but not interleukin 5 or eosinophils, is required in a murine model of acute airway hyperreactivity. J Exp Med 1996; 183:109–117.

174. Hogan SP, Matthaei KI, Young JM, Koskinen A, Young IG, Foster PS. A novel T cell-regulated mechanism modulating allergen-induced airways hyperreactivity in BALB/c mice independently of IL-4 and IL-5. J Immunol 1998; 161:1501–1509.

175. Wills-Karp M, Luyimbazi J, Xu X, Schofield B, Neben TY, Karp CL, Donaldson DD. Interleukin-13: central mediator of allergic asthma. Science 1998; 282:2258–2261.

176. Chiaramonte MG, Schopf LR, Neben TY, Cheever AW, Donaldson DD, Wynn TA. IL-13 is a key regulatory cytokine for Th2 cell-mediated pulmonary granuloma formation and IgE responses induced by Schistosoma mansoni eggs. J Immunol 1999; 162: 920–930.

177. Grunig G, Warnock M, Wakil AE, Venkayya R, Brombacher F, Rennick DM, Sheppard D, Mohrs M, Donaldson DD, Locksley RM, Corry DB. Requirement for IL-13 independently of IL-4 in experimental asthma. Science 1998; 282:2261–2263.

178. Pope SM, Brandt EB, Mishra A, Hogan SP, Zimmermann N, Matthaei KI, Foster PS, Rothenberg ME. Interleukin-13 induces eosinophil recruitment to the lung by an IL-5 and eotaxin dependent mechanism. J Allergy Clin Immunol 2001; 108:594–601.

179. MacLean JA, Ownbey R, Luster AD. T cell-dependent regulation of eotaxin in antigen-induced pulmonary eosinophila. J Exp Med 1996; 184:1461–1469.

180. Nakajima H, Iwamoto I, Tomoe S, Matsumura R, Tomioka H, Takatsu K, Yoshida S. CD4 + T-lymphocytes and interleukin-5 mediate antigen-induced eosinophil infiltration into the mouse trachea. Am Rev Respir Dis 1992; 146:374–377.

181. Gavett SH, Chen X, Finkelman F, Wills-Karp M. Depletion of murine CD4 + T lymphocytes prevent antigen-induced airway hyperreactivity and pulmonary eosinophilia. Am J Respir Cell Mol Biol 1994; 10:587–593.

182. Garlisi CG, Falcone A, Kung TT, Stelts D, Pennline KJ, Beavis AJ, Smith SR, Egan RW, Umland SP. T cells are necessary for Th2 cytokine production and eosinophil accumulation in airways of antigen-challenged allergic mice. Clin Immunol Immunopathol 1995; 75:75–83.

183. Iwamoto I, Tomoe S, Tomioka H, Takatsu K, Yoshida S. Role of CD4 + T lymphocytes and interleukin-5 in antigen-induced eosinophil recruitment into the site of cutaneous late-phase reaction in mice. J Leukoc Biol 1992; 52:572–578.

184. Lukacs NW, Strieter RM, Chensue SW, Kunkel SL. Interleukin-4-dependent pulmonary eosinophil infiltration in a murine model of asthma. Am J Respir Cell Mol Biol 1994; 10:526–532.

185. Marsh DG, Hsu SH, Roebber M. HLA-Dw2: a genetic marker for human immune response to short pollen allergen Ra5. I. Response resulting primarily from antigenic exposure. J Exp Med 1982; 155:1439–1451.

186. Reihaus E, Innis M, MacIntyre N, Liggett SB. Mutations in the gene encoding for the beta 2-adrenergic receptor in normal and asthmatic subjects. Am J Respir Cell Mol Biol 1993; 8:334–339.

187. Young RP, Dekker JW, Wordsworth BP. HLA-DR and HLA-DP genotypes and immunoglobulin E responses to common major allergens. Clin Exp Allergy 1994; 24: 431–439.

188. Shirakawa T, Li A, Dubowitz M, Dekker JM, Shaw AE, Faux JA, Ra C, Cookson W, Hopkin JM. Association between atopy and variants of the β subunit of the high-affinity IgE receptor. Nature Genet 1994; 7:125–129.

189. Meyers DA, Postma DS, Panhuysen CI, Xu J, Amelung PJ, Levitt RC, Bleecker ER. Evidence for a locus regulating total serum IgE levels mapping to chromosome 5. Genomics 1994; 23:464–470.

190. Postma DS, Bleecker ER, Amelung PJ, Holroyd KJ, Xu J, Panhuysen CI, Meyers DA, Levitt RC. Genetic susceptibility to asthma—bronchial hyperresponsiveness coinherited with a major gene for atopy. N Engl J Med 1995; 333:894–900.

191. Hershey GK, Friedrich MF, Esswein LA, Thomas ML, Chatila TA. Association of atopy with gain-of-function mutation in the interleukin-4 receptor alpha chain. N Engl J Med 1997; 337:1720–1725.

192. Nickel R, Barnes KC, Sengler CA, Casolaro V, Freidhoff LR, Weber P, Naidu RP, Caraballo L, Ehrlich E, Plitt J, Schleimer RP, Huang SK, Beaty T. Evidence for linkage of chemokine polymorphisms to asthma in populations of African descent. J Allergy Clin Immunol 1999; 103:S174.

193. Lin AY, Nutman TB, Kaslow D, Mulvihill JJ, Fontaine L, White BJ, Knutsen T, Theil KS, Raghuprasad PK, Goldstein AM, Tucker MA. Familial eosinophilia: clinical and laboratory results on a U.S. kindred. Am J Med Genet 1998; 76:229–237.

194. Rioux JD, Stone VA, Daly MJ, Cargill M, Green T, Nguyen H, Nutman T, Zimmerman PA, Tucker MA, Hudson T, Goldstein AM, Lander E, Lin AY. Familial eosinophilia maps to the cytokine gene cluster on human chromosomal region 5q31–q33. Am J Hum Genet 1998; 63:1086–1094.

195. Ying S, Robinson DS, Meng Q, Rottman J, Kennedy R, Ringler DJ, Mackay CR, Daugherty BL, Springer MS, Durham SR, Williams TJ, Kay AB. Enhanced expression of eotaxin and CCR3 mRNA and protein in atopic asthma. Association with airway hyperresponsiveness and predominant co-localization of mRNA to bronchial epithelial and endothelial cells. Eur J Immunol 1997; 27:3507–3516.

196. Alam R, York J, Boyars M, Stafford S, Grant JA, Lee J, Forsythe P, Sim T, Ida N. Increased MCP-1, RANTES, and MIP-1alpha in bronchoalveolar lavage fluid of allergic asthmatic patients. Am J Respir Crit Care Med 1996; 153:1398–1404.

197. Lilly CM, Woodruff PG, Camargo CA, Jr., Nakamura H, Drazen JM, Nadel ES, Hanrahan JP. Elevated plasma eotaxin levels in patients with acute asthma. J Allergy Clin Immunol 1999; 104:786–790.

198. Ying S, Meng Q, Zeibecoglou K, Robinson DS, Macfarlane A, Humbert M, Kay AB. Eosinophil chemotactic chemokines (eotaxin, eotaxin-2, RANTES, monocyte chemoattractant protein-3 (MCP-3), and MCP-4), and C-C chemokine receptor 3 expression in bronchial biopsies from atopic and nonatopic (intrinsic) asthmatics. J Immunol 1999; 163:6321–6329.

199. Ying S, Robinson DS, Meng Q, Barata LT, McEuen AR, Buckley MG, Walls AF, Askenase PW, Kay AB. C-C chemokines in allergen-induced late-phase cutaneous responses in atopic subjects: association of eotaxin with early 6-hour eosinophils, and of eotaxin-2 and monocyte chemoattractant protein-4 with the later 24-hour tissue eosinophilia, and relationship to basophils and other C-C chemokines (monocyte chemoattractant protein-3 and RANTES). J Immunol 1999; 163:3976–3984.

200. Berkman N, Ohnona S, Chung FK, Breuer R. Eotaxin-3 but not eotaxin gene expression is upregulated in asthmatics 24 hours after allergen challenge. Am J Respir Cell Mol Biol 2001; 24:682–687.

201. Nickel RG, Casolaro V, Wahn U, Beyer K, Barnes KC, Plunkett BS, Freidhoff LR, Sengler C, Plitt JR, Schleimer RP, Caraballo L, Naidu RP, Levett PN, Beaty TH, Huang SK. Atopic dermatitis is associated with a functional mutation in the promoter of the C-C chemokine RANTES. J Immunol 2000; 164:1612–1616.

202. Fryer AA, Spiteri MA, Bianco A, Hepple M, Jones PW, Strange RC, Makki R, Tavernier G, Smilie FI, Custovic A, Woodcock AA, Ollier WE, Hajeer AH. The −403

G—>A promoter polymorphism in the RANTES gene is associated with atopy and asthma. Genes Immun 2000; 1:509–514.

203. Leckie MJ, ten Brinke A, Khan J, Diamant Z, O'Connor BJ, Walls CM, Mathur AK, Cowley HC, Chung KF, Djukanovic R, Hansel TT, Holgate ST, Sterk PJ, Barnes PJ. Effects of an interleukin-5 blocking monoclonal antibody on eosinophils, airway hyperresponsiveness, and the late asthmatic response. Lancet 2000; 356:2144–2148.

204. Lloyd CM, Delaney T, Nguyen T, Tian J, Martinez AC, Coyle AJ, Gutierrez-Ramos JC. CC chemokine receptor (CCR)3/eotaxin is followed by CCR4/monocyte-derived chemokine in mediating pulmonary T helper lymphocyte type 2 recruitment after serial antigen challenge in vivo. J Exp Med 2000; 191:265–274.

205. Sabroe I, Conroy DM, Gerard NP, Li Y, Collins PD, Post TW, Jose PJ, Williams TJ, Gerard CJ, Ponath PD. Cloning and characterization of the guinea pig eosinophil eotaxin receptor, C-C chemokine receptor-3: blockade using a monoclonal antibody in vivo. J Immunol 1998; 161:6139–6147.

206. Heath H, Qin S, Rao P, Wu L, LaRosa G, Kassam N, Ponath PD, Mackay CR. Chemokine receptor usage by human eosinophils. The importance of CCR3 demonstrated using an antagonistic monoclonal antibody. J Clin Invest 1997; 99:178–184.

207. Proudfoot AE, Power CA, Hoogewerf AJ, Montjovent MO, Borlat F, Offord RE, Wells TN. Extension of recombinant human RANTES by the retention of the initiating methionine produces a potent antagonist. J Biol Chem 1996; 271:2599–2603.

208. Elsner J, Petering H, Hochstetter R, Kimmig D, Wells TN, Kapp A, Proudfoot AE. The CC chemokine antagonist Met-RANTES inhibits eosinophil effector functions through the chemokine receptors CCR1 and CCR3. Eur J Immunol 1997; 27: 2892–2898.

209. Kips J, Palmans E, Proudfoot A, et al. The effect of Met-RANTES on the allergeninduced airway eosinophilia in an in vivo mouse model. Am J Respir Crit Care Med 1997; 155:A733.

210. Moore PS, Boshoff C, Weiss RA, Chang Y. Molecular mimicry of human cytokine and cytokine response pathway genes by KSHV. Science 1996; 274:1739–1744.

211. Kledal TN, Rosenkilde MM, Coulin F, Simmons G, Johnsen AH, Alouani S, Power CA, Luttichau HR, Gerstoft J, Clapham PR, Clark-Lewis I, Wells TNC, Schwartz TW. A broad-spectrum chemokine antagonist encoded by Kaposi's sarcoma-associated herpesvirus. Science 1997; 277:1656–1659.

212. Luttichau HR, Stine J, Boesen TP, Johnsen AH, Chantry D, Gerstoft J, Schwartz TW. A highly selective CC chemokine receptor (CCR)8 antagonist encoded by the poxvirus molluscum contagiosum. J Exp Med 2000; 191:171–180.

213. White JR, Lee JM, Young PR, Hertzberg RP, Jurewicz AJ, Chaikin MA, Widdowson K, Foley JJ, Martin LD, Griswold DE, Sarau HM. Identification of a potent, selective non-peptide CXCR2 antagonist that inhibits interleukin-8-induced neutrophil migration. J Biol Chem 1998; 273:10095–10098.

214. Hesselgesser J, Ng HP, Liang M, Zheng W, May K, Bauman JG, Monahan S, Islam I, Wei GP, Ghannam A, Taub DD, Rosser M, Snider RM, Morrissey MM, Perez HD, Horuk R. Identification and characterization of small molecule functional antagonists of the CCR1 chemokine receptor. J Biol Chem 1998; 273:15687–15692.

215. Bertrand CP, Ponath PD. CCR3 blockade as a new therapy for asthma. Expert Opin Investig Drugs 2000; 9:43–52.

216. Sabroe I, Peck MJ, Van Keulen BJ, Jorritsma A, Simmons G, Clapham PR, Williams TJ, Pease JE. A small molecule antagonist of chemokine receptors CCR1 and CCR3.

Potent inhibition of eosinophil function and CCR3-mediated HIV-1 entry. J Biol Chem 2000; 275:25985–25992.

217. Rutledge BJ, Rayburn H, Rosenberg R, North RJ, Gladue RP, Corless CL, Rollins BJ. High level monocyte chemoattractant protein-1 expression in transgenic mice increases their susceptibility to intracellular pathogens. J Immunol 1995; 155:4838–4843.

218. Hogan SP, Mishra A, Brandt EB, Foster PS, Rothenberg ME. A critical role for eotaxin in experimental oral antigen-induced eosinophilic gastrointestinal allergy. Proc Natl Acad Sci USA 2000; 97:6681–6686.

219. Rothenberg ME, Zimmermann N, Mishra A, Brandt E, Birkenberger LA, Hogan SP, Foster PS. Chemokines and chemokine receptors: their role in allergic airway disease. J Clin Immunol 1999; 19:250–265.

220. Zimmermann N, Rothenberg ME. Therapeutic targeting of chemokines and chemokine receptors. In: Agosti J, Sheffer AL, eds. Biotherapeutic Approaches to Asthma. New York: Marcel Dekker, Inc., 2001:167–209.

21

Interleukin-4 and Interleukin-13 in Human and Experimental Asthma

DAVID B. CORRY

Baylor College of Medicine
Houston, Texas, U.S.A.

I. Introduction

The last several years have contributed explosively to our understanding of the pathogenesis of experimental asthma. Coincidentally, a previous generation of human and experimental studies has culminated in a series of ambitious asthma clinical trials that aim to interrupt disease by inhibiting key inflammatory pathways. The results of these trials have been less than extraordinary (1–4), suggesting that, at least during established disease, inflammatory molecules such as interleukin 4 (IL-4), immunoglobulin E (IgE), and IL-5 may not be as critical as once believed. The more recent murine studies now propose that distinct inflammatory molecules and rather different pathogenic mechanisms may underlie allergic asthma. What are these new asthma mediators and disease pathways, and are their prospects for therapeutic targeting any brighter than those previously identified? I will first consider new findings that implicate the cytokines IL-4 and IL-13 and their related signaling pathway in experimental asthma. In the final part of this chapter I discuss the prospects of future therapies based on this unique family of molecules.

II. Inflammation and Airway Obstruction in Human Asthma

The major clinical endpoints in asthma—death, dyspnea, and cough—are strongly related to, and likely caused by, airway obstruction. Indeed, mortality from asthma is largely due to asphyxiation (5). Airway obstruction in asthma consists of at least three components: (1) airway hyperresponsiveness (AHR), defined as an enhanced constrictive response to provocative challenge with cholinergic agonists, (2) physical obstruction due to mucus and other debris, and (3) airway remodeling due to fibrosis, which is believed to contribute to both the rapid decline in lung function and fixed, irreversible airway obstruction observed in some patients with chronic disease (6–9).

There now exists a large body of literature linking airway obstruction in asthma to local and systemic inflammation. The term "allergic" is often used interchangeably with "atopic" in referring to asthma patients, both generally referring to serum IgE reactivity, either elevated total levels or the presence of antigen-specific IgE against one or more well-defined allergens. Asthma patients are often broadly categorized as either atopic or nonatopic (corresponding roughly to extrinsic and intrinsic asthma subpopulations). However, serum IgE is a poor general indicator of immune activation, allergic or otherwise. This is probably due to many factors, not least of which is that antigen-specific assays are only as good as the defined antigens available to test against and the list of known and readily available antigens for serum IgE testing is very far from complete. In addition, the regulation of serum IgE is complex and circulating IgE only represents a fraction of the total that is made. Most IgE is probably secreted into lumenal structures such as the airway and gut, suggesting that sampling of fluid from these organs would identify far more asthma patients with allergic reactivity (10).

In addition to IgE reactivity, asthma patients also demonstrate elevated blood levels of eosinophils, activated lymphocytes including CD4+ T cells and B cells (11), mast cells, and predominant type 2 cytokines, including IL-4, IL-5, IL-9, and IL-13, from sputum, bronchoalveolar lavage (BAL), and airway biopsy specimens (12–18). These studies are particularly noteworthy because whereas not all asthma patients display serum IgE reactivity or blood eosinophilia, lung and airway-specific assays more consistently reveal evidence of local inflammation. Most dramatically, autopsy series of patients dying of asthma have demonstrated a more potent degree of airway inflammation compared even to biopsy specimens, particularly occlusive airway impaction due to inflammatory cells and mucus and intense peribronchovascular inflammation (19–21). Together, these studies document that inflammation, especially allergic inflammation of the lung, is intimately associated with asthma.

III. Overview of Asthma Pathogenesis

There is widespread agreement in experimental literature, and considerable support from human studies, that T cells mediate airway obstruction either directly or indirectly, particularly T_H2 cells that secrete type 2 cytokines (22–29). How T_H2 cells and other components of allergic inflammation induce airway obstruction is classically described in terms of Type I hypersensitivity (Fig. 1). According to this mechanism, T_H2-secreted cytokines activate and/or recruit various effector cells to the lung, including B cells that produce IgE and mast cells expressing the high-affinity IgE receptor, FcεRI. Antigen-specific IgE captured on the surface of mast cells

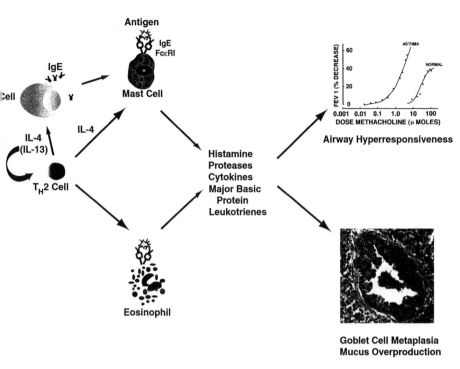

Figure 1 IL-4 and IL-13 in afferent immunity and Type I hypersensitivity. IL-4 is the principal cytokine-activating T_H2 cells (likely through an autocrine mechanism as indicated) and B cells to produce IgE, but is also a growth factor for mast cells. To a minor extent, IL-13 may also participate in Th2 activation and IgE secretion. When IgE captured by FcεRI is crosslinked by antigen, FcεRI-bearing cells such as eosinophils and mast cells are activated to release mediators such as histamine, leukotrienes, and other substances. These secondary inflammatory molecules are believed to induce the canonical features of allergic airway obstruction: exaggerated airway contractility in response to provocative agents such as methacholine (airway hyperresponsiveness) and goblet cell metaplasia of the airways with mucus overproduction. The photomicrograph depicts a highly metaplastic medium sized airway partially obstructed with mucus from an antigen-challenged mouse ($\times 600$).

is crosslinked upon subsequent exposure to antigen, causing release of preformed mediators and other substances from mast cells, but perhaps also eosinophils. These secondary mediators of inflammation, including histamine, proteases, leukotrienes, cytokines, and others, subsequently induce airway obstruction and other features of asthma.

It is likely that forms of asthma exist that bear no relation to allergic mechanisms, particularly those in which the small airways have been permanently damaged through nonimmune mechanisms such as toxic gas inhalation, hyperoxia-related bronchiolitis, and perhaps childhood viral infections. Nonetheless, available data indicate that the vast majority of asthma patients, including those with the most severe, life-threatening forms of disease, have concomitant allergic reactivity as defined by a variety of parameters. The following discussion will therefore review the experimental evidence linking allergic mechanisms directly to the pathophysiology of airway obstruction in asthma. Although a variety of mechanisms have been shown, two are intimately tied to the cytokines IL-4 and IL-13 and will be emphasized here. The potential contributions of IL-5 and eosinophils will be reviewed elsewhere in this book.

IV. IL-4 and IL-13 in Experimental Asthma

IL-4 and IL-13 function very differently depending on the phase of the immune response under consideration. For purposes of this review, these immune phases are twofold. Afferent immunity refers to the inductive phase of the immune response in which T and B cells undergo developmental maturation following initial encounter with antigen and in response to essential signals derived from the local immune environment (Fig. 1). Efferent, or effector, immunity refers to the effects mediated by mature T and B cells (Fig. 2). As will be developed below, IL-4 is far more

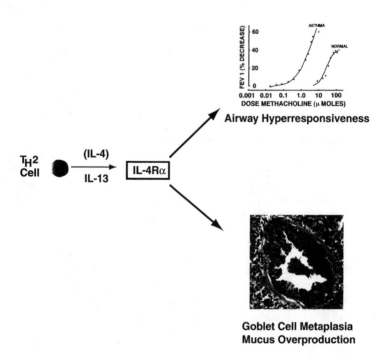

Airway Hyperresponsiveness

Goblet Cell Metaplasia
Mucus Overproduction

Figure 2   IL-4 and IL-13 in effector immunity. The second major mechanism described to underlie experimental asthma also involves T_H2 cells, but with IL-4 and IL-13 participating more directly in disease. Here, however, IL-13 is much more important than IL-4, inducing through IL-4Rα the same features of airway obstruction.

important in afferent immunity, whereas IL-13 is the more relevant molecule during effector immunity.

A. T-Cell Development

T_H2 cells participate importantly in allergic conditions, either directly or by supplying signals essential for secondary allergic effector cells such as mast cells and eosinophils. Abundant data strongly implicate IL-4 as a principal mediator of T_H2 development as without this seminally important cytokine T_H2 cells do not develop following antigen challenge (26,27,30,31). IL-4–independent pathways for T_H2 development do exist but with uncertain relevance to allergic disease (32,33). A potential role for IL-13 in T_H2 activation is suggested by the observation that human T cells express a functional IL-13 receptor (34) capable of transducing the transcription factor signal (signal transducer and activation of transcription 6; STAT6) important for T_H2 development (35). Although T cells are themselves important sources of IL-13, other cells, including NK cells and mast cells/basophils, also secrete this cytokine and may participate in early IL-13–dependent signaling events (36,37). Human alveolar macrophages are another potential source of IL-13, with obvious relevance to asthma (38).

Additional data from mice support a role for IL-13 in T_H2 cell development. Naive T cells prepared from IL-13–deficient mice show impaired T_H2 cytokine secretion when cultured in vitro (39). Instead, these cells secrete interferon gamma (IFN-γ) and resist type 2 cytokine production even when cultured with excess IL-4 and IL-13. However, when provoked with strong allergens such as intestinal helminths, IL-13–deficient mice demonstrate equivalent or superior T_H2 responses compared to wild-type mice. More recent studies confirm that allergen-specific T_H2 responses, including IL-4 production, proceed unhindered in the genetic absence of IL-13 (40). Together, these studies suggest that IL-13 plays little or no significant role in influencing T_H2 effector commitment; rather, during antigen challenge this function is mediated almost exclusively through IL-4.

B. B-Cell Development and IgE Secretion

IL-13 is sufficient to elicit IgE secretion from cultured human, but not murine, B cells independently of IL-4 (41). The lack of effect on murine cells remains unexplained but is unlikely to be due to lack of expression of IL-13–specific receptor subunits (42,43). Additional studies in mice deficient in IL-4, the alpha chain of the IL-4 receptor (IL-4Rα), and STAT6 confirm the importance of this receptor signaling pathway but suggest an independently greater contribution of IL-4 compared to IL-13 in mediating IgE secretion (35,44–46). It should be noted, however, that an IL-4–independent pathway exists for IgE secretion, although again this finding is uncertain with regard to allergic disease (47).

Both transgenic and cytokine-deficient mice reveal evidence that IL-13 may contribute in vivo to IgE responses. Relative to wild-type, transgenic mice that constitutively express IL-13 show markedly elevated baseline IgE levels that vary directly with the level of transgene expression (48). The effect is independent of

IL-4 as elevated IgE levels were still observed after crossing IL-13 transgenic mice to an IL-4–deficient background. Further, IL-13–deficient mice show baseline IgE levels below those of wild-type littermates and reduced total IgE responses following immunization with a conventional antigen (39). Antigen-specific IgE and IgG1 levels from IL-13-/-mice are only 50% those of wild-type mice but are abrogated in the combined absence of IL-4 and IL-13 (40,49). Further, neutralization of IL-13 during challenge with strong allergens such as *Schistosoma* eggs also results in significantly reduced IgE titers (50). However, the reduced IgE-secreting potential of IL-13–deficient mice can be overcome by a more complex allergic challenge such as an intestinal parasite (*Nippostrongylus brasiliensis*) (39), suggesting perhaps that lack of IL-13 only delays IgE responses or that IL-13–dependent effects are antigen specific. Thus, similar to its role in T_H2 development, IL-13 appears to promote IgE secretion independently of IL-4, although this effect is weak and ultimately not required for robust IgE responses.

C. Mast Cell Development

Together with stem cell factor, IL-3, and IL-9, IL-4 is an important growth factor for tissue mast cells present in the gut and lung (51–53). IL-13 potentially modulates mast cell activation but is less potent than IL-4 in this regard (54). Conversely, mast cells are a potentially important source of IL-13 and IL-4 during inflammation (37,55–57).

D. Effector Immune Responses

Whereas the IL-4–and IL-13–dependent features of the asthma phenotype discussed above relate primarily to afferent immunity distinct from the lung, the more clinically relevant features of asthma, especially airway obstruction and mucus overproduction, relate exclusively to the airways and effector immunity. Here too, IL-4 and IL-13 both play important roles, but IL-13 has been clearly shown to be the more critical effector molecule. The importance of IL-13 in the murine lung, and the distinction between IL-13 from IL-4, has been shown using several approaches. IL-4–deficient mice challenged with antigen show a severe defect in T_H2 generation and the asthma phenotype (26,27, 29,58–61). However, an even more profound defect in the asthma phenotype, in which disease is essentially abrogated, is observed in mice deficient in IL-4Rα, which is shared between the IL-4 and IL-13 receptor complexes (29,62). This phenotype is essentially the same as mice simultaneously deficient in IL-4 and IL-13 and persists even when T-helper cell developmental defects, which are the result of the genetic absence of IL-4Rα, are accounted for (40,49). Further, IL-4–deficient T cells conditioned to produce all other T_H2 cytokines are capable of inducing airway hyperresponsiveness but not airway eosinophilia (62). Together these data indicate that especially airway obstruction is induced during established T_H2 immunity by one or more secreted T-cell products other than IL-4 and that one of the likely candidates is IL-13.

The importance of IL-13 was subsequently confirmed in experiments in which IL-13 was specifically neutralized using a defined inhibitor, soluble IL-13 receptor alpha 2 (sIL-13Rα2), a soluble version of one of the IL-13 receptor chains. This synthetic inhibitor binds to and neutralizes IL-13 but not IL-4 (29,40,63). sIL-13Rα2 substantially reduces all aspects of the asthma phenotype if given during established inflammation, but does not completely reverse disease. In comparison, neutralization of IL-4 during established airway inflammation has no effect aside from a minor reduction in airway eosinophil recruitment (26). Either IL-4 or IL-13 administered intranasally to mice is sufficient to induce airway hyperresponsiveness and mucus overproduction to levels seen in antigen challenged wild-type mice, although IL-13 is more potent in this regard (29). Together, these data indicate that during established T_H2 immunity, both IL-4 and IL-13 contribute to the asthma phenotype, but IL-13 is the more important cytokine (Fig. 2) (64).

Although not yet clearly shown, it is likely that differences in configurations of the distinct IL-4 and IL-13 receptor complexes account for the differences in biological activity of these cytokines. This concept is supported by the finding that IL-4 can induce all of the murine asthma phenotype in the complete absence of IL-13, perhaps indicating upregulation of IL-4–specific receptor subunits under these conditions (61). However, regardless of the more relevant ligand, allergic airway obstruction shows a marked dependency on IL-4Rα (29) (see below).

E. The IL-4 and IL-13 Receptors

Considerable controversy exists regarding the composition of the IL-4 and IL-13 receptors. Based on numerous studies in primarily hematopoietic cells, the complete IL-4 receptor is thought to consist of IL-4Rα and the gamma chain of the IL-2 receptor (common gamma chain; γ_c) (65). However, additional studies show that γ_c is not essential for IL-4 signaling in all tissue (42,65–68). Far less is certain about the composition of the IL-13 receptor. Almost all studies support an essential role for IL-4Rα in IL-13 signaling, but two additional IL-13 receptor chains have been discovered that may participate singly, together, or individually combined with γ_c to form a complete IL-13 receptor. These additional IL-13 receptor subunits are IL-13Rα1 and IL-13Rα2 (42,67–80). Considerably less is known about the tissue distribution and regulation of both IL-4 and IL-13 receptor subunits.

As discussed above, mice deficient in IL-4Rα develop essentially none of the canonical features of asthma following antigen challenge, nor can they be induced to have an asthma phenotype even after administration of IL-4, IL-13, and T_H2 cells with antigen (29). Similarly, wild-type mice given a blocking antibody to IL-4Rα during antigen challenge show marked attenuation of the asthma phenotype (81). Together, these studies confirm the importance of IL-4 and IL-13 and their receptor signaling pathway in experimental asthma. Redundant mechanisms exist by which airway obstruction is induced in the allergic setting, but this redundancy is confined to the IL-4/IL-13 system described. The challenge in the design of future asthma therapies is to fully account for the potentially overlapping functions of IL-4 and IL-13.

V. IL-4 and IL-13 in Human Asthma

As described earlier, both IL-4 and IL-13 are found in the airways of asthmatic humans. Evidence that these molecules may be important in disease is suggested primarily by genetic studies. Polymorphisms in the IL-4 and IL-13 promoters and genes have recently been identified and are associated with an elevated risk of allergic asthma or increased serum IgE titers (82–85). Additional polymorphisms in the extracellular and intracytoplasmic domains of IL-4Rα are also associated with asthma (86–88), with one allelic variant having an especially strong correlation and exhibiting a possible gene dose effect in a prospectively analyzed asthma population (89). Although these studies do not demonstrate a definite role for IL-4 or IL-13 in human asthma, some of the polymorphisms may serve as potentially useful biomarkers of disease.

VI. Prospects for Drug Development

Although the studies cited above are suggestive, there are no data that unequivocally establish important roles for either IL-4 or IL-13 in human asthma. Consequently, there are currently no asthma therapies that specifically target the IL-4/IL-13/IL-4Rα signaling complex. However, even if IL-4 and IL-13 are shown to have as important a role in human as in murine asthma, such information is insufficient for designing new therapies. This issue is particularly relevant considering the unique circumstances that govern the pathophysiology of experimental asthma, especially the biological overlap between IL-4 and IL-13. Although experimentally IL-13 is the dominant cytokine mediating AHR and mucus overproduction, there is concern that chronic neutralization of IL-13 may paradoxically have little, or perhaps diminishing, effect in humans. This paradoxical response, if observed, is understood by the fact that the asthma phenotype may become entirely dependent on IL-4 in the absence of IL-13 (61). The interchangeability of IL-4 and IL-13 perhaps explains why soluble IL-4Rα, which neutralizes IL-4 but not IL-13, has little effect on airway physiological parameters either experimentally or when given to asthma patients (4). There are no data from humans indicating that IL-4 and IL-13 are regulated in a substantially different manner compared to their murine counterparts. Thus, an important lesson from these experimental studies is that if IL-13 or IL-4 is to be targeted as a potential therapy for asthma, one should not be neutralized and the other ignored; they should be targeted together. One approach for this is to co-administer neutralizing agents specific for each cytokine, but this complicates therapy at the risk of increased adverse effects compared with monotherapy.

A more efficient means for targeting IL-4 and IL-13 is to neutralize IL-4Rα. The critical role for this receptor signaling chain in mediating the biological effects of both cytokines suggests that its blockade may be highly efficacious in diseases such as asthma. Nonetheless, a full understanding of the IL-4 and IL-13 receptors has been elusive, and the possibility that asthma-like disease may emerge even in the absence of significant IL-4Rα activity, especially with chronic exposure to allergen, remains a possibility. The risk of aberrant signaling events may be avoided by neutralizing STAT6 instead of IL-4Rα, perhaps using gene therapy approaches that target only the lung. However, reliable means for targeting transcription factors in vivo have yet to be demonstrated, and recent adverse outcomes seem to make gene therapy a distant prospect at this time. Thus, for the moment, more traditional means of targeting IL-4Rα, perhaps using humanized monoclonal antibodies or small blocking molecules, appear to be the most reasonable choices for neutralizing the IL-4/IL-13 signaling pathway.

As with any new therapy, safety is an important issue that warrants consideration here. Some IL-4/IL-13–based allergic responses are beneficial and are required for resolution of experimental parasitic infestations. Although such infections are uncommon in modern societies, it would be unwise to assume that systemic blockade of IL-4/IL-13 would have no serious sequelae, especially regarding infection control. Fortunately, the lung offers the distinct advantage that pharmaceuticals may be delivered directly through respiratory aerosols. Where technically and economically feasible, this approach is preferable to systemic delivery except, as is sometimes the case with corticosteroids, when delivery through the respiratory tract unacceptably limits drug dosage. There are no parasitic infestations of the respiratory tract or other known lung homeostatic requirements for the IL-4/IL-13/IL-4Rα signaling pathway. Therefore, local blockade of this pathway may be very safe, but only well-designed clinical trials can determine this with certainty.

Because anti-IL-4/IL-13 therapies do not actually address the underlying cause of disease, the T_H2 cell, a concern with such approaches is that abrupt withdrawal of treatment may lead to rapid recurrence of disease. Withdrawal of other asthma drugs such as corticosteroids and leukotriene modifiers is further associated with rare, life-threatening complications such as vasculitis (Churg-Strauss syndrome) (90). Future therapies based on IL-4/IL-13 blockade may not necessarily be associated with such complications, but this possibility should be considered as part of any clinical trial and during posttrial surveillance.

References

1. Leckie MJ, ten Brinke A, Khan J, et al. Effects of an interleukin-5 blocking monoclonal antibody on eosinophils, airway hyper-responsiveness, and the late asthmatic response. Lancet 2000; 356:2144–2148.
2. Bryan SA, O'Connor BJ, Matti S, et al. Effects of recombinant human interleukin-12 on eosinophils, airway hyper-responsiveness, and the late asthmatic response. Lancet 2000; 356:2149–2153.
3. Busse W, Corren J, Lanier BQ, et al. Omalizumab, anti-IgE recombinant humanized monoclonal antibody, for the treatment of severe allergic asthma. J Allergy Clin Immunol 2001; 108:184–190.
4. Borish LC, Nelson HS, Corren J, et al. Efficacy of soluble IL-4 receptor for the treatment of adults with asthma. J Allergy Clin Immunol 2001; 107:963–970.

5. Molfino NA, Nannini LJ, Martelli AN, Slutsky AS. Respiratory arrest in near-fatal asthma. N Engl J Med 1991; 324:285–288.
6. Van Schayck CP, Dompleing E, Van Herwaarden CL, Wever AM, Van Weel C. Interacting effects of atopy and bronchial hyperresponsiveness on the annual decline in lung function and the exacerbation rate in asthma. Am Rev Respir Dis 1991; 144:1297–1301.
7. Pare PD, Bai TR, Roberts CR. The structural and functional consequences of chronic allergic inflammation of the airways. Ciba Found Symp 1997; 206:71–86; discussion 86–89, 106–110.
8. Brown PJ, Greville HW, Finucane KE. Asthma and irreversible airflow obstruction. Thorax 1984; 39:131–136.
9. Backman KS, Greenberger PA, Patterson R. Airways obstruction in patients with long-term asthma consistent with "irreversible asthma." Chest 1997; 112:1234–1240.
10. Corry DB, Kheradmand F. Induction and regulation of the IgE response. Nature 1999; 402:B18–23.
11. Kidney JC, Wong AG, Efthimiadis A, et al. Elevated B cells in sputum of asthmatics. Close correlation with eosinophils. Am J Respir Crit Care Med 1996; 153:540–544.
12. Robinson DS, Hamid Q, Ying S, et al. Predominant TH2-like bronchoalveolar T-lymphocyte population in atopic asthma. N Engl J Med 1992; 326:298–304.
13. Synek M, Beasley R, Frew AJ, et al. Cellular infiltration of the airways in asthma of varying severity. Am J Respir Crit Care Med 1996; 154:224–230.
14. Kraft M, Djukanovic R, Wilson S, Holgate ST, Martin RJ. Alveolar tissue inflammation in asthma. Am J Respir Crit Care Med 1996; 154:1505–1510.
15. Ying S, Humbert M, Barkans J, et al. Expression of IL-4 and IL-5 mRNA and protein product by CD4 + and CD8 + T cells, eosinophils, and mast cells in bronchial biopsies obtained from atopic and nonatopic (intrinsic) asthmatics. J Immunol 1997; 158: 3539–3544.
16. Humbert M, Durham SR, Ying S, et al. IL-4 and IL-5 mRNA and protein in bronchial biopsies from patients with atopic and nonatopic asthma: evidence against "intrinsic" asthma being a distinct immunopathologic entity. Am J Respir Crit Care Med 1996; 154:1497–1504.
17. Gratziou C, Carroll M, Montefort S, Teran L, Howarth PH, Holgate ST. Inflammatory and T-cell profile of asthmatic airways 6 hours after local allergen provocation. Am J Respir Crit Care Med 1996; 153:515–520.
18. Bradley BL, Azzawi M, Jacobson M, et al. Eosinophils, T-lymphocytes, mast cells, neutrophils, and macrophages in bronchial biopsy specimens from atopic subjects with asthma: comparison with biopsy specimens from atopic subjects without asthma and normal control subjects and relationship to bronchial hyperresponsiveness. J Allergy Clin Immunol 1991; 88:661–674.
19. Shimura S, Andoh Y, Haraguchi M, Shirato K. Continuity of airway goblet cells and intraluminal mucus in the airways of patients with bronchial asthma. Eur Respir J 1996; 9:1395–1401.
20. Aikawa T, Shimura S, Sasaki H, Ebina M, Takishima T. Marked goblet cell hyperplasia with mucus accumulation in the airways of patients who died of severe acute asthma attack. Chest 1992; 101:916–921.
21. Hogg JC. The pathology of asthma. Apmis 1997; 105:735–745.
22. Busse WW, Coffman RL, Gelfand EW, Kay AB, Rosenwasser LJ. Mechanisms of persistent airway inflammation in asthma. A role for T cells and T-cell products. Am J Respir Crit Care Med 1995; 152:388–393.

23. Krinzman SJ, De Sanctis GT, Cernadas M, et al. Inhibition of T cell costimulation abrogates airway hyperresponsiveness in a murine model. J Clin Invest 1996; 98: 2693–2699.

24. Van Oosterhout AJ, Hofstra CL, Shields R, et al. Murine CTLA4-IgG treatment inhibits airway eosinophilia and hyperresponsiveness and attenuates IgE upregulation in a murine model of allergic asthma. Am J Respir Cell Mol Biol 1997; 17:386–392.

25. Gavett SH, Chen X, Finkelman F, Wills-Karp M. Depletion of murine CD4 + T lymphocytes prevents antigen-induced airway hyperreactivity and pulmonary eosinophilia. Am J Respir Cell Mol Biol 1994; 10:587–593.

26. Corry DB, Folkesson HG, Warnock ML, et al. Interleukin 4, but not interleukin 5 or eosinophils, is required in a murine model of acute airway hyperreactivity. J Exp Med 1996; 183:109–117.

27. Corry DB, Grunig G, Hadeiba H, et al. Requirements for allergen-induced airway hyperreactivity in T and B cell-deficient mice. Mol Med 1998; 4:344–355.

28. Watanabe A, Mishima H, Kotsimbos TC, et al. Adoptively transferred late allergic airway responses are associated with Th2-type cytokines in the rat. Am J Respir Cell Mol Biol 1997; 16:69–74.

29. Grunig G, Warnock M, Wakil AE, et al. Requirement for IL-13 independently of IL-4 in experimental asthma. Science 1998; 282:2261–2263.

30. Kopf M, Le GG, Bachmann M, Lamers MC, Bluethmann H, Kohler G. Disruption of the murine IL-4 gene blocks Th2 cytokine responses. Nature 1993; 362:245–248.

31. Kamogawa Y, Minasi LE, Carding SR, Bottomly K, Flavell RA. The relationship of IL-4- and IFNγ-producing T cells studied by lineage ablation of IL-4-producing cells. Cell 1993; 75:985–995.

32. Noben-Trauth N, Shultz LD, Brombacher F, Urban JF, Jr., Gu H, Paul WE. An interleukin 4 (IL-4)-independent pathway for CD + T cell IL-4 production is revealed in IL-4 receptor-deficient mice. Proc Natl Acad Sci USA 1997; 94:10838–10843.

33. Dent AL, Hu-Li J, Paul WE, Staudt LM. T helper type 2 inflammatory disease in the absence of interleukin 4 and transcription factor STAT6. Proc Natl Acad Sci USA 1998; 95:13823–13828.

34. Gauchat JF, Schlagenhauf E, Feng NP, et al. A novel 4-kb interleukin-13 receptor alpha mRNA expressed in human B, T, and endothelial cells encoding an alternate type-II interleukin-4/interleukin-13 receptor. Eur J Immunol 1997; 27:971–978.

35. Kaplan MH, Schindler U, Smiley ST, Grusby MJ. Stat6 is required for mediating responses to IL-4 and for development of Th2 cells. Immunity 1996; 4:313–319.

36. Hoshino T, Winkler-Pickett RT, Mason AT, Ortaldo JR, Young HA. IL-13 production by NK cells: IL-13-producing NK and T cells are present in vivo in the absence of IFN-gamma. J Immunol 1999; 162:51–59.

37. Burd PR, Thompson WC, Max EE, Mills FC. Activated mast cells produce interleukin 13. J Exp Med 1995; 181:1373–1380.

38. Hancock A, Armstrong L, Gama R, Millar A. Production of interleukin 13 by alveolar macrophages from normal and fibrotic lung. Am J Respir Cell Mol Biol 1998; 18: 60–65.

39. McKenzie GJ, Emson CL, Bell SE, et al. Impaired development of Th2 cells in IL-13-deficient mice. Immunity 1998; 9:423–432.

40. Walter DM, Mcintire JJ, Berry G, et al. Critical role for IL-13 in the development of allergen-induced airway hyperreactivity. J Immunol 2001; 167:4668–4675.

41. Zurawski G, de Vries JE. Interleukin 13, an interleukin 4-like cytokine that acts on monocytes and B cells, but not on T cells. Immunol Today 1994; 15:19–26.

42. Hilton DJ, Zhang JG, Metcalf D, Alexander WS, Nicola NA, Willson TA. Cloning and characterization of a binding subunit of the interleukin 13 receptor that is also a component of the interleukin 4 receptor. Proc Natl Acad Sci USA 1996; 93:497–501.

43. Donaldson DD, Whitters MJ, Fitz L, et al. The murine IL-13Rα2: molecular cloning, characterization and comparison with murine IL-13Rα1. J Immunol 1998; 161: 2317–2324.

44. Shimoda K, van Deursen J, Sangster MY, et al. Lack of IL-4-induced Th2 response and IgE class switching in mice with disrupted Stat6 gene. Nature 1996; 380:630–633.

45. Kuhn R, Rajewsky K, Muller W. Generation and analysis of interleukin-4 deficient mice. Science 1991; 254:707–710.

46. Grunewald SM, Werthmann A, Schnarr B, et al. An antagonistic IL-4 mutant prevents type I allergy in the mouse: inhibition of the IL-4/IL-13 receptor system completely abrogates humoral immune response to allergen and development of allergic symptoms in vivo. J Immunol 1998; 160:4004–4009.

47. Morawetz RA, Gabriele L, Rizzo LV, et al. Interleukin (IL)-4-independent immunoglobulin class switch to immunoglobulin (Ig)E in the mouse. J Exp Med 1996; 184: 1651–1661.

48. Emson CL, Bell SE, Jones A, Wisden W, McKenzie AN. Interleukin (IL)-4-independent induction of immunoglobulin (Ig)E, and perturbation of T cell development in transgenic mice expressing IL-13. J Exp Med 1998; 188:399–404.

49. McKenzie GJ, Fallon PG, Emson CL, Grencis RK, McKenzie AN. Simultaneous disruption of interleukin (IL)-4 and IL-13 defines individual roles in T helper cell type 2-mediated responses. J Exp Med 1999; 189:1565–1572.

50. Chiaramonte MG, Schopf LR, Neben TY, Cheever AW, Donaldson DD, Wynn TA. IL-13 is a key regulatory cytokine for Th2 cell-mediated pulmonary granuloma formation and IgE responses induced by Schistosoma mansoni eggs. J Immunol 1999; 162: 920–930.

51. Madden KB, Urban JF, Jr., Ziltener HJ, Schrader JW, Finkelman FD, Katona IM. Antibodies to IL-3 and IL-4 suppress helminth-induced intestinal mastocytosis. J Immunol 1991; 147:1387–1391.

52. Temann UA, Geba GP, Rankin JA, Flavell RA. Expression of interleukin 9 in the lungs of transgenic mice causes airway inflammation, mast cell hyperplasia, and bronchial hyperresponsiveness. J Exp Med 1998; 188:1307–1320.

53. Renauld JC, Kermouni A, Vink A, Louahed J, Van Snick J. Interleukin-9 and its receptor: involvement in mast cell differentiation and T cell oncogenesis. J Leukoc Biol 1995; 57:353–360.

54. Nilsson G, Nilsson K. Effects of interleukin (IL)-13 on immediate-early response gene expression, phenotype and differentiation of human mast cells. Comparison with IL-4. Eur J Immunol 1995; 25:870–873.

55. Seder RA, Paul WE, Ben SS, et al. Production of interleukin-4 and other cytokines following stimulation of mast cell lines and in vivo mast cells/basophils. Int Arch All Appl Immunol 1991; 94:137–140.

56. Bradding P, Roberts JA, Britten KM, et al. Interleukin-4, -5, and -6 and tumor necrosis factor-alpha in normal and asthmatic airways: evidence for the human mast cell as a source of these cytokines. Am J Respir Cell Mol Biol 1994; 10:471–480.

57. Bradding P, Feather IH, Howarth PH, et al. Interleukin 4 is localized to and released by human mast cells. J Exp Med 1992; 176:1381–1386.

58. Hogan SP, Mould A, Kikutani H, Ramsay AJ, Foster PS. Aeroallergen-induced eosinophilic inflammation, lung damage, and airways hyperreactivity in mice can occur inde-

pendently of IL-4 and allergen-specific immunoglobulins. J Clin Invest 1997; 99: 1329–1339.

59. Brusselle G, Kips J, Joos G, Bluethmann H, Pauwels R. Allergen-induced airway inflammation and bronchial responsiveness in wild-type and interleukin-4-deficient mice. Am J Respir Cell Mol Biol 1995; 12:254–259.

60. Hogan SP, Matthaei KI, Young JM, Koskinen A, Young IG, Foster PS. A novel T cell-regulated mechanism modulating allergen-induced airways hyperreactivity in BALB/c mice independently of IL-4 and IL-5. J Immunol 1998; 161:1501–1509.

61. Webb DC, McKenzie AN, Koskinen AM, Yang M, Mattes J, Foster PS. Integrated signals between IL-13, IL-4, and IL-5 regulate airways hyperreactivity. J Immunol 2000; 165:108–113.

62. Cohn L, Tepper JS, Bottomly K. IL-4-independent induction of airway hyperresponsiveness by Th2, but not Th1, cells. J Immunol 1998; 161:3813–3816.

63. Wills-Karp M, Luyimbazi J, Xu X, et al. Interleukin-13: central mediator of allergic asthma. Science 1998; 282:2258–2261.

64. Corry DB, IL-13 in allergy: home at last. Curr Opin Immunol 1999; 11:610–614.

65. Nelms K, Keegan AD, Zamorano J, Ryan JJ, Paul WE. The IL-4 receptor: signaling mechanisms and biologic functions. Annu Rev Immunol 1999; 17:701–738.

66. Chomarat P, Banchereau J. An update on interleukin-4 and its receptor. Eur Cytokine Netw 1997; 8:333–344.

67. Miloux B, Laurent P, Bonnin O, et al. Cloning of the human IL-13R alpha1 chain and reconstitution with the IL4R alpha of a functional IL-4/IL-13 receptor complex. FEBS Lett 1997; 401:163–166.

68. Palmer-Crocker RL, Hughes CC, Pober JS. IL-4 and IL-13 activate the JAK2 tyrosine kinase and Stat6 in cultured human vascular endothelial cells through a common pathway that does not involve the gamma c chain. J Clin Invest 1996; 98:604–609.

69. Callard RE, Matthews DJ, Hibbert L. IL-4 and IL-13 receptors: are they one and the same? Immunol Today 1996; 17:108–110.

70. Kotowicz K, Callard RE, Friedrich K, Matthews DJ, Klein N. Biological activity of IL-4 and IL-13 on human endothelial cells: functional evidence that both cytokines act through the same receptor. Int Immunol 1996; 8:1915–1925.

71. Murata T, Obiri NI, Puri RK. Human ovarian-carcinoma cell lines express IL-4 and IL-13 receptors: comparison between IL-4- and IL-13-induced signal transduction. Int J Cancer 1997; 70:230–240.

72. Murata T, Obiri NI, Debinski W, Puri RK. Structure of IL-13 receptor: analysis of subunit composition in cancer and immune cells. Biochem Biophys Res Commun 1997; 238:90–94.

73. Murata T, Noguchi PD, Puri RK. IL-13 induces phosphorylation and activation of JAK2 Janus kinase in human colon carcinoma cell lines: similarities between IL-4 and IL-13 signaling. J Immunol 1996; 156:2972–2978.

74. Murata T, Puri RK. Comparison of IL-13- and IL-4-induced signaling in EBV-immortalized human B cells. Cell Immunol 1997; 175:33–40.

75. Murata T, Taguchi J, Puri RK. Interleukin-13 receptor alpha' but not alpha chain: a functional component of interleukin-4 receptors. Blood 1998; 91:3884–3891.

76. Obiri NI, Debinski W, Leonard WJ, Puri RK. Receptor for interleukin 13. Interaction with interleukin 4 by a mechanism that does not involve the common gamma chain shared by receptors for interleukins 2, 4, 7, 9, and 15. J Biol Chem 1995; 270:8797–8804.

77. Obiri NI, Murata T, Debinski W, Puri RK. Modulation of interleukin (IL)-13 binding and signaling by the gamma c chain of the IL-2 receptor. J Biol Chem 1997; 272: 20251–20258.

78. Obiri NI, Leland P, Murata T, Debinski W, Puri RK. The IL-13 receptor structure differs on various cell types and may share more than one component with IL-4 receptor. J Immunol 1997; 158:756–764.

79. Vita N, Lefort S, Laurent P, Caput D, Ferrara P. Characterization and comparison of the interleukin 13 receptor with the interleukin 4 receptor on several cell types. J Biol Chem 1995; 270:3512–3517.

80. Zhang JG, Hilton DJ, Willson TA, et al. Identification, purification, and characterization of a soluble interleukin (IL)-13-binding protein. Evidence that it is distinct from the cloned II-13 receptor and II-4 receptor alpha-chains. J Biol Chem 1997; 272:9474–9480.

81. Gavett SH, O'Hearn DJ, Karp CL, et al. Interleukin-4 receptor blockade prevents airway responses induced by antigen challenge in mice. Am J Physiol 1997; 272:L253–261.

82. van der Pouw Kraan TC, van Veen A, Boeije LC, et al. An IL-13 promoter polymorphism associated with increased risk of allergic asthma. Genes Immun 1999; 1:61–65.

83. Graves PE, Kabesch M, Halonen M, et al. A cluster of seven tightly linked polymorphisms in the IL-13 gene is associated with total serum IgE levels in three populations of white children. J Allergy Clin Immunol 2000; 105:506–513.

84. Suzuki I, Hizawa N, Yamaguchi E, Kawakami Y. Association between a C + 33T polymorphism in the IL-4 promoter region and total serum IgE levels. Clin Exp Allergy 2000; 30:1746–1749.

85. Chouchane L, Sfar I, Bousaffara R, El Kamel A, Sfar MT, Ismail A. A repeat polymorphism in interleukin-4 gene is highly associated with specific clinical phenotypes of asthma. Int Arch Allergy Immunol 1999; 120:50–55.

86. Mitsuyasu H, Yanagihara Y, Mao XQ, et al. Cutting edge: dominant effect of Ile50Val variant of the human IL-4 receptor alpha-chain in IgE synthesis. J Immunol 1999; 162: 1227–1231.

87. Hershey GK, Friedrich MF, Esswein LA, Thomas ML, Chatila TA. The association of atopy with a gain-of-function mutation in the alpha subunit of the interleukin-4 receptor. N Engl J Med 1997; 337:1720–1725.

88. Takabayashi A, Ihara K, Sasaki Y, et al. Childhood atopic asthma: positive association with a polymorphism of IL-4 receptor alpha gene but not with that of IL-4 promoter of Fc epsilon receptor I beta gene. Exp Clin Immunogen 2000; 17:63–70.

89. Rosa-Rosa L, Zimmermann N, Bernstein JA, Rothenberg ME, Khurana Hershey GK. The R576 IL-4 receptor alpha allele correlates with asthma severity. J Allergy Clin Immunol 1999; 104:1008–1014.

90. Weller PF, Plaut M, Taggart V, Trontell A. The relationship of asthma therapy and Churg-Strauss syndrome: NIH workshop summary report. J Allergy Clin Immunol 2001; 108:175–183.

22

Interleukin-5 and Eosinophils as Therapeutic Targets for the Treatment of Asthma

PAUL S. FOSTER

John Curtin School of Medical Research
Australian National University
Canberra, Australia

I. Introduction

Inflammation of the airway mucosa and submucosa is thought to play a major role in the pathogenesis of asthma (1,2). Although the inflammatory response is complex, airway CD4+ Th2-type lymphocytes (Th2 cells), mast cells, basophils, and eosinophils appear to be the primary effector cells that orchestrate the clinical manifestations of disease. In particular, the infiltration of the airways by Th2 cells and eosinophils are predominant features of the late-phase asthmatic response. Indeed, the hallmark features of allergic asthma: elevated serum immunoglobulin E (IgE), mucus hypersecretion, eosinophilia, and enhanced bronchial reactivity [airways hyperreactivity (AHR)] to nonspecific spasmogenic stimuli have all been linked to the effector functions of Th2 cytokines [e.g., interleukin(IL)-4,-5,-9,-10, and -13] (2). Importantly, it is these pathogenic processes that are thought to promote airways obstruction in asthma, which predisposes to wheezing, shortness of breath, and life-threatening limitations in airflow. Although the etiology and pathophysiology of asthma are complex, a central paradigm in asthma pathogenesis has emerged whereby Th2 cells regulate disease processes through the recruitment and activation of eosinophils in the allergic lung. In this model, Th2 cells, through the secretion of IL-5, regulate eosinophil recruitment to the lung and thereby pathogenic processes that predispose to the development of airways obstruction and AHR.

Eosinophilic inflammation is a hallmark feature of both allergic and nonallergic asthma, and there is a large body of clinical and experimental data that implicates this granulocyte as a central player in pathogenesis (3–12). Eosinophils and their products in the allergic lung correlate with severity and exacerbations of disease. Furthermore, physiological studies have shown that the inflammatory mediators secreted by eosinophils can induce a number of pathological features of asthma. In particular, eosinophil granular proteins have been show to damage the respiratory epithelium and also promote AHR. The strong association of eosinophils with asthma pathogenesis has identified molecules that regulate eosinophil function (development, migration, activation, and survival) as key therapeutic targets for the treatment of asthma. Of all the factors identified to regulate eosinophil function the cytokine IL-5, which is predominantly secreted from Th2 cells, demonstrates the most specificity. Although IL-5 is a key regulator of many aspects of eosinophil function, it is becoming increasingly obvious that pathways also operate independently of this cytokine to regulate eosinophil development and migration to the allergic lung. In this chapter the role of IL-5 in asthma and in the regulation of eosinophil function in models of Th2-driven allergic lung disease will be discussed. We also address the emerging concept that eosinophils may not be central mediators of asthma but are bystander cells recruited to the airways in response to aberrant Th2-cell activation.

II. IL-5-Regulated Eosinophilia as Key Pathogenic Mechanisms in Asthma

A. The Paradigm of IL-5, Eosinophils, and Asthma

The model that IL-5-regulated eosinophilia plays a central role in the pathogenesis of asthma is based on extensive clinical and experimental investigations that show a strong correlation between eosinophils, their secreted products, and IL-5 with severity and exacerbation of disease (6,7,9–22). Once recruited to sites of allergic inflammation, eosinophils become activated and are thought to induce disease through the release of proinflammatory molecules and granular proteins (3,4). In particular, there is evidence that eosinophilic products damage the respiratory epithelium and induce AHR (5–8). Eosinophils release a wide range of proinflammatory mediators (cytokines, lipid mediators, and granular proteins) that have the potential to initiate and exacerbate the inflammatory response, induce damage to the respiratory epithelium, and promote AHR. Notably, granular proteins such as major basic protein are highly toxic to the respiratory epithelium and have been show to alter muscarinic receptor function and promote AHR (23,24).

Increased numbers of eosinophil and basophil colony-forming units (progenitor cells) are also found in the blood of allergic individuals, and elevated numbers correlate with exacerbation of disease (25–32). Thus, severity and exacerbations of allergic disease are directly linked to eosinophil regulatory pathways.

Although the trafficking of eosinophils into tissues is regulated by a multiplicity of cytokines, chemokines, adhesion molecules, and lipid mediators (33) (all of which have been implicated to some degree in allergic disease), the eosinophil paradigm identifies IL-5-regulated eosinophilia as a central pathogenic pathway. This primarily stems from investigations that show elevated levels of IL-5 and cells expressing mRNA for this cytokine in the blood and lung secretions of asthmatics (9,12–20). Moreover, after allergen-induced late phase asthmatic responses, increased levels of IL-5 in the lung correlate with the degree of eosinophilic inflammation (7,9,12–20). In addition, IL-5 has very specific biological activities in relation to the regulation of eosinophil function (development, differentiation, activation, survival, and movement) and is a critical molecular switch for the induction of eosinophilia in the blood and bone marrow (11,34,35). Furthermore, inhibition of IL-5 function in animal models of asthma often results in attenuation of hallmark features of disease, in particular eosinophilia and AHR (10,11, 36–39). Thus, the specificity of IL-5 for eosinophil-regulated processes and the proposed role for this granulocyte in pathogenesis has identified IL-5 as an important therapeutic target for the resolution of disease.

III. Regulation of Eosinophil Function by IL-5

The mechanisms that underpin eosinophil development and movement are complex (33). Recruitment of eosinophils to sites of allergic inflammation may be potentially regulated by a range of inflammatory cytokines [IL-1β, IL-3, IL-4, IL-9, IL-13, granulocyte-macrophage colony-stimulating factor (GM-CSF) and tumor necrosis factor α], chemokines (RANTES, monocyte chemoattractant proteins, macrophage inflammatory proteins, and the eotaxin family) and lipid mediators (platelet-activating factor and leukotriene B_4) (33). Often, IL-5 is incorrectly reported as being the critical molecular switch for the development and migration of eosinophils. From our investigations the critical role for IL-5 appears to be in the induction of eosinophilia in the bone marrow and the rapid migration of eosinophils from this compartment to the blood. This function amplifies eosinophil accumulation and inflammation at sites of allergic disease. Notably, eosinophils fully differentiate independently of IL-5, and although eosinophil trafficking is significantly attenuated in the absence of IL-5, other mechanisms operate independently of this cytokine to promote the accumulation of eosinophils in the allergic lung. In the following sections we will provide some insights into the role of IL-5 in eosinophil biology under basal (baseline) conditions and during allergic inflammation.

A. Role of IL-5 in Eosinophil Development, Mobilization, and Homing to Tissues

There is a sustainable body of literature that has demonstrated the central importance of IL-5 in the development, differentiation, activation, and survival of eosinophils (34). Collectively, these investigations have led to the concept/paradigm (in part, due to the cellular specificity of the actions of IL-5) that eosinophils cannot develop or adequately function in the absence of IL-5. However, these conclusions have been primarily drawn from in vitro experimental systems where the delivery of factors to culture medium is strictly controlled (34,40–43). Thus, the concept of IL-

5 being essential rather than an important cofactor for eosinophil function may not be warranted.

We have extensively characterized IL-5-deficient (IL-5$^{-/-}$) mice at baseline and under allergic inflammatory conditions (11,44–47). Under baseline conditions mature eosinophils are found in the bone marrow and in blood and tissues (albeit significantly reduced in the circulation), indicating that IL-5 is not essential for eosinophil differentiation, maturation, survival, or subsequent migration from the bone marrow (48). IL-3 and GM-CSF are known to prime progenitor cells for IL-5 responsiveness, and all three cytokines employ the β-common chain to transduce signals (34). However, although IL-5, IL-3, and GM-CSF all contribute to eosinopoiesis, mature eosinophils are found in the bone marrow of mice deficient in these factors or in common components of their receptor signaling systems (β-common chain) (11,49). This demonstrates the presence of alternative, as yet unidentified pathways that regulate eosinophil differentiation and maturation. Furthermore, a rapid blood eosinophilia can also be induced in naive IL-5$^{-/-}$ mice by the intravenous instillation of the eosinophil specific chemokine eotaxin, indicating that these cells are functional and can migrate in response to specific chemotactic stimuli (47).

By contrast to wild-type littermates, allergic IL-5$^{-/-}$ mice (systemically sensitized to allergen) do not generate eosinophilia in the blood or bone marrow compartments in response to allergen provocation of the lung (aeroallergen challenge), and this greatly reduces the level of eosinophils recruited to the airways (11,45,46). However, since basal levels of eosinophils are still produced in IL-5$^{-/-}$ mice, residual tissue eosinophilia persists (albeit profoundly reduced) in the allergic airways of these mice (11,46). The production of IL-5 by recombinant vaccinia virus (rVV-IL-5) instilled into the airways of allergic IL-5$^{-/-}$ mice completely restores aeroallergen-induced eosinophilia in the bone marrow, blood, and lung to levels normally observed in allergic wild-type mice (11). Notably, in similar studies the transient expression of IL-5 in the lungs of naive IL-5$^{-/-}$ mice by rVV-IL-5 does not induce eosinophilia in these compartments, indicating that additional factors are required to amplify the IL-5 signal for eosinopoiesis and migration (11). The importance of signals derived from Th2 cells in eliciting these additional signals in association with IL-5 for the mechanisms underlying eosinophilia is highlighted in experiments in which we adoptively transferred wild-type Th2 cells (IL-5–producing) to aeroallergen-challenged naive or allergic IL-5$^{-/-}$ mice (45). Under both conditions (naive or sensitized) the transfer of Th2 cells in conjunction with the delivery of allergen to the lung resulted in the induction of bone marrow, blood, and airways eosinophilia and the characteristic pathological features of allergic lung disease (45). Thus, Th2 cells provide the additional signals that underpin eosinopoiesis and migration.

The adoptive transfer of wild-type or IL-5$^{-/-}$ eosinophils to the blood of allergic IL-5$^{-/-}$ mice during aeroallergen challenge also increases the number of eosinophils recruited to the airways, indicating that IL-5 does not play an obligatory role in the homing of this leukocyte to the allergic lung (48). Furthermore, it is these homing mechanisms that may underpin tissue accumulation independently of IL-5.

Our results suggest that the critical roles for IL-5 are in the expansion of the eosinophil pool in the bone marrow and in the induction of blood eosinophilia in response to allergic stimulation. IL-5 also amplifies tissue recruitment of this leukocyte in response to locally derived chemotactic signals by increasing the circulating pool of eosinophils. This cytokine also participates in the maintenance of baseline levels of eosinophils in the blood and tissues. However, additional factors that are under the control of Th2 cells regulate eosinophil homing to sites of allergic disease and amplify eosinopoiesis.

B. IL-5-Regulated Tissue Eosinophilia and Regulation of AHR in Experimental Models

IL-5-regulated eosinophilic inflammation has been associated and dissociated from the induction of AHR in animal models of allergic airways inflammation. In these experimental models of asthma, inhibition of the actions of IL-5 consistently suppresses pulmonary eosinophilia in response to allergen inhalation, but this effect does not always correlate with a reduction of AHR (10,11,38,39,46,50–55). Indeed, this dichotomy is highlighted by findings from our laboratory where allergic IL-5 $^{-/-}$ mice of the C57BL/6 strain (11) do not develop allergen-induced AHR, while BALB/c mice develop enhanced reactivity independently of this factor (46). What mechanism could potentially underlie these different responses?

Careful dissection of all anti-IL-5 studies in allergic disease models shows that eosinophils have resided in the allergic lung at some time before the measurement of lung function (AHR) or are still present (albeit in reduced numbers) at the time of analyses (see above references). For example, although we and others have observed that eosinophil trafficking to the allergic lung is profoundly attenuated in IL-5 $^{-/-}$ mice or those treated with anti-IL-5 antibodies in comparison to wild-type responses, a marked residual tissue eosinophilia can persist in these mice after allergen inhalation (10,11,38,46,50,51). Importantly, this residual tissue eosinophilia in allergic mice is significantly greater than that observed in naive nonallergic controls (48). Furthermore, we have observed that the degree of residual tissue eosinophilia is under genetic regulation as this pool was 10 to 100-fold greater in the BALB/c strain (where AHR persists) in comparison to the C57BL/6 strain (where airways reactivity was abolished) in the absence of IL-5 (11,46). Thus, anti-IL-5 treatment does not completely inhibit the accumulation of eosinophils in the allergic lung, and this cell may therefore still contribute to pathogenesis. Interestingly, tissue eosinophilia (albeit reduced) is also a predominant feature of IL-5 $^{-/-}$ mice with allergic inflammation of the gastrointestinal tract (56) and the lung infected with *Toxocara canis* (57). Eosinophils also fluctuate normally (albeit reduced levels) in the uterus of IL-5 $^{-/-}$ mice during the estrus cycle (58). We have also shown that chronic delivery of antigen to the lung of allergic IL-5 $^{-/-}$ mice results in focal accumulation of eosinophils to the airway mucosa (unpublished data).

Notably, a blood eosinophilia is not always a feature of disorders characterized by the accumulation of this cell in diseased tissues (4). For example, patients with gastroesophageal reflux have eosinophilia in the esophagus but rarely have elevated levels of this cell, and only a subset of patients with asthma have both peripheral blood and tissue eosinophilia (4). Thus, the contribution of IL-5 to pathogenesis may be more important where a substantial blood eosinophilia is required to maintain tissue levels of this cell and diseases progression.

C. Proinflammatory Role of IL-5 and Non-Eosinophil Targets

Although IL-5 has been primarily thought of as a key regulator of eosinophil function, it was first identified as a terminal differentiation factor for B lymphocytes (59). In limited studies, IL-5 has also been implicated in regulating cytotoxic lymphocyte development, promoting AHR by directly acting on smooth muscle cells and through the release of tachykinins from nerves (59,60). Thus, in studies where IL-5 but not eosinophils are dissociated from the induction of AHR, these pathways may be operative in the abnormal response. We have also observed in IL-5$^{-/-}$ mice that although eosinophil trafficking is profoundly impaired, the recruitment of lymphocytes to the lung compartment is also significantly attenuated. Indeed this effect is more pronounced in allergic IL-5$^{-/-}$ C57BL/6 mice, which do not develop antigen-induced AHR by comparison to the BALB/c strain that develop enhanced reactivity independently of this cytokine. Recently, we have also shown (unpublished) that IL-5 deficiency results in lower levels of IL-13 production in the allergic lung. Interestingly, in allergic IL-5$^{-/-}$ mice the level correlates with the absence (C57BL/6 mice) or persistence (BALB/c mice) of AHR. Thus, IL-5 is proinflammatory and potentially regulating cytokine function at the level of the T cell. It is unlikely that IL-5 can directly influence the lymphocyte pool but may regulate T-cell responses through eosinophils. In this regard, we and others have recently show that eosinophils can modulate CD4$^+$ T cell function. Eosinophils in the allergic lung can present antigen and traffic to local lymph nodes where they co-localize with T cells, and this granulocyte can induce proliferation and cytokine secretion from Th2 cells (61,62). Eosinophils are also known to secrete a wide range of T-cell growth and chemotactic factors. Thus, evidence is emerging that eosinophils may not only act as terminal effector cells, but also actively modulate allergic inflammation by amplifying the type 2 cytokine response. IL-5 plays an import role in these processes by regulating eosinophil accumulation in the allergic lung. It is important to note that of the Th2 cytokines (e.g., IL-13 and IL-4) we have investigated in models of allergic airways disease, IL-5 is the most proinflammatory. Absence of IL-13 and/or IL-4 may attenuate aspects of pathogenesis, but inflammation is still a pronounced feature of the allergic lung.

IV. Recruitment of Eosinophils into Tissues Independently of IL-5

Recently we investigated the possibility that local chemokine systems can operate independently of IL-5 to recruit eosinophils into the allergic lung. Of particular interest in allergic inflammation is the role of the eotaxin, because of its demonstrated potency and selectivity for eosinophil recruitment in experimental models and its strong clinical association with disease in humans (47,63–68).

A. Role of Eotaxin

Of the factors implicated in regulating eosinophil migration, we have observed a unique interplay between eotaxin and IL-5 for the selective recruitment of this cell into tissues (47,69). We transiently expressed (over 4 days) IL-5 and/or eotaxin in the airways of naive mice by the delivery of rVV vectors encoding these factors (69). Expression of eotaxin or IL-5 induced a selective airways eosinophilia that was markedly potentiated by concomitantly increasing the number of circulating eosinophils by pulsing intravenously with IL-5. Furthermore, co-expression of these cytokines in the airways resulted in the synergistic amplification of the number of eosinophils recruited to the airways. Notably, gene transfer of either cytokine alone or in combination to the lung failed to induce a blood eosinophilia. However, intravenous delivery of recombinant IL-5 induced a rapid and pronounced blood eosinophilia with a subsequent decrease in bone marrow levels of this leukocyte (47). Although lung expression of IL-5 and eotaxin can induce pulmonary eosinophilia, the failure of this compartmentalized expression to induce a blood eosinophilia, while still promoting tissue accumulation, suggests that there is a substantial extramedullary pool of eosinophils that can be recruited to the airways in response to specific chemotactic stimuli (47,69).

Although IL-5 is an important cofactor for eotaxin-induced eosinophilia, we have also observed that this chemokine can regulate eosinophil migration independently of IL-5 (47,48,69). Injection of eotaxin into the blood of IL-5$^{-/-}$ mice results in a rapid induction of blood eosinophilia (47). We have also shown that eotaxin plays a more predominant role in regulating eosinophil recruitment to sites of allergic inflammation of the gastrointestinal tract by contrast with IL-5 (56).

B. Eosinophil Migration in IL-5 and Eotaxin-Deficient Mice

To investigate the possibility that eotaxin contributes to eosinophil accumulation and disease progression in the absence of IL-5, we generated BALB/c mice deficient in both IL-5 and eotaxin (IL-5/eotaxin$^{-/-}$) in an attempt to completely inhibit the recruitment of this cell to the allergic lung. Although tissue eosinophilia was markedly attenuated in the absence of IL-5 or eotaxin alone, by comparison to allergic wild-type mice, significant numbers of eosinophils were still recruited to the airways compartment (eosinophil numbers in eotaxin-/- are similar to those seen in IL-5$^{-/-}$ mice) (48). However, peripheral eosinophilia (blood and bone marrow) was attenuated only in the absence of IL-5 (48). By contrast, in allergic mice deficient in both molecules (eotaxin/IL-5$^{-/-}$), not only was peripheral eosinophilia abolished, but tissue numbers of this cell were reduced to the levels seen in nonallergic wild-type mice (48) (unpublished observation). Notably, only in the absence of both eotaxin and IL-5 was AHR abolished (unpublished observation). Thus, IL-5 and eotaxin cooperate to selectively regulate tissue eosinophilia, and there is a direct correlation between the number of tissue-dwelling eosinophils and the induction of AHR to cholinergic stimuli in the allergic lung.

These studies indicate that pathways operated by local chemokine systems (in particular those that operate CCR3, the eotaxin receptor) play an important role in regulating the recruitment of eosinophils into tissues independently of IL-5 and that this mechanism is linked to the induction of disease. The mechanism also operates in the absence of a blood eosinophilia. These studies highlight that, under allergic inflammatory conditions, eosinophilia may be differentially regulated and that the central importance of individual eosinophil regulatory molecules to pathogenesis is variable.

Recently, the expression of eotaxin was shown to be regulated by IL-13 (70,71). Importantly, IL-13 has been identified as a potential key regulator of the pathogenesis of asthma. This cytokine is present in respiratory secretions and expressed in T cells from asthmatics (72–74). Additionally, IL-13 is a potent regulator of bronchoconstriction, mucus hypersecretion, and eosinophilia in mouse models of asthma and experimental AHR (75–78). Recently, we also demonstrated, by the delivery of recombinant protein to the airways of naive mice, that IL-13 employs both IL-5 and eotaxin to induce eosinophilia (79). These data suggest that the molecules (IL-5, IL-13, and eotaxin) may cooperate to regulate certain aspects of the asthma phenotype. It is tempting to speculate that IL-13 secreted from Th2 cells may induce eotaxin and eosinophilia and promote disease independently of IL-5.

C. Eotaxin and Eosinophil Progenitors

While inflammatory signals derived from the lung induce eosinopoiesis in the bone marrow and the subsequent recruitment of mature eosinophils to the airways, evidence is accumulating that allergen provocation of the airways also promotes the migration of eosinophil progenitor cells to the lung compartment (25,26,28,32). Cytokines elaborated from resident inflammatory cells or airway cells are thought to locally induce differentiation of these lineage-committed progenitor cells to mature effector cells. Production of eosinophil-active cytokines IL-3, GM-CSF, and IL-5 may also increase the life span of eosinophils at sites of inflammation. These cytokines are all found upregulated in the allergic lung (12). Thus, two mechanisms potently exist to promote the accumulation of mature eosinophils in the lung during allergic responses: one localized to the bone marrow compartment and the other at the site of inflammation.

A role for eosinophil progenitors in the allergic inflammatory cascade is partly based on the observations that these cells are elevated in the blood of atopic individuals after seasonal exposure to allergens and that circulating numbers often correlate with the exacerbation and resolution of clinical asthma (25–27,29,31). Furthermore, allergen challenge of atopic asthmatics results in the specific upregulation of eosinophil progenitors in the bone marrow and blood (30,32). Investigations in canine and mouse models of allergic lung disease have also provided experimental evidence for a role of bone marrow myloid progenitors in allergen induced AHR (28,31,80).

The migration of eosinophils and their progenitors from the bone marrow are regulated by eotaxin, while IL-5 appears to exclusively regulate the efflux of differentiated cells (68). The lower abundance of eosinophils in the blood of allergic IL-5$^{-/-}$ mice may mask the development of a marked eosinophilia in response to eotaxin. Further, it is likely that once eosinophils and/or progenitors enter the circulation in IL-5$^{-/-}$ mice in response to eotaxin, they are rapidly sequestered into the allergic lung.

It is tempting to speculate that in the absence of IL-5 and a blood eosinophilia (IL-5$^{-/-}$ mice) that eotaxin (CCR3)–operated pathways regulate the recruitment of eosinophils and their progenitors to the allergic lung and, in association with Th2-derived eosinophil differentiation factors (IL-3 and GM-CSF), promote local tissue eosinophilia. Thus, targeting both eotaxin (or local chemokine systems) and IL-5-operated pathways may be required to adequately resolve tissue eosinophilia and AHR in asthma. However, a recent clinical trial that employed a humanized monoclonal antibody to IL-5 (hmAb-IL-5) has questioned the role of eosinophils in mediating the late-asthmatic response and inducing airway hyperresponsiveness in response to controlled allergen inhalation (81).

V. Clinical Trials with Humanized IL-5 Monoclonal Antibodies

A recent clinical trial with hmAb-IL-5 in conjunction with the dogma that IL-5 is the critical regulator of eosinophil development and migration has led to the growing concept that eosinophils do not participate in disease pathogenesis. Administration of hmAb-IL-5 limited eosinophil migration into the lung but failed to inhibit the development of allergen-induced AHR. In limited studies, eosinophils have also been dissociated from the induction of AHR in asthma (82–85). However, a closer examination of Leckie et al. (81) has raised questions as to whether this study had the methodological power to either support or refute the concept that eosinophils play an important role in the mechanisms predisposing to allergen-induced changes in airways function (86). Although hmAb-IL-5 treatment reduced eosinophil numbers in the blood and sputum, the lack of effect of treatment on allergen induced changes in lung function are ambiguous (86). For example, the investigators failed to demonstrate significant changes in allergen-induced AHR to histamine (the spasmogen employed in this study) during the baseline period or after placebo treatment, and the sample size and the methodological approach to assessing changes in AHR may have been inadequate to draw firm statistical outcomes (86).

In conjunction with this analysis we would also like to highlight that eosinophil trafficking is a complex process (33) and that although IL-5 is a key regulator of eosinophil function, there is more than one way to get this granulocyte into allergic tissues. We have shown that eosinophils can accumulate in allergic tissues independently of IL-5 (46,56,57). Indeed, analysis of eosinophil numbers in allergen-challenged patients that received either the low or high dose of hmAb-IL-5 show that although they are significantly reduced, this cell still persists in the lung (sputum). Furthermore, while measurement of eosinophil numbers in the blood may be indicative of the efficacy of hmAb-IL-5, it does not provide information on whether or not these cells are accumulating in the lung. It should be remembered that blood eosinophilia is not a feature of all disorders characterized by the accumulation of eosinophils in tissues and only a subset of patients with asthma have both peripheral blood and tissue eosinophilia (4). Furthermore, a fall in blood eosinophil numbers below baseline may reflect inhibition of efflux from the bone marrow as well as sequestration into tissues. Indeed, blood eosinophil levels in allergen-challenged allergic IL-5$^{-/-}$ mice are lower than those observed in naive wild-type mice, yet appreciable amounts (albeit significantly decreased in comparison to wild-type responses) of eosinophil accumulate independently of this cytokine in the allergic lung and gastrointestinal tract (46,48,56,57). Furthermore, measurement of eosinophil levels in respiratory secretions under conditions where eosinophil regulatory pathways have been impaired is not always indicative of the numbers of this cell in lung tissues (87). Often eosinophils in IL-5–depleted mice are present in the tissue even though they are almost absent from bronchial lavage fluid. Mechanisms that regulate the spatial and temporal aspects of eosinophil migration from blood to tissue compartments and then into the airways lumen may be differentially controlled (87). It should also be highlighted that eosinophils have resided in the allergic lungs of these asthmatic individuals at some time before the initiation of the investigations with hmAb-IL-5 (81). Thus, the study by Leckie should not be used by commentators to exclude IL-5 and/or eosinophils in the mechanism of disease initiation, progression, or exacerbation.

VI. Conclusion

IL-5 plays a central role in the regulation of eosinophil recruitment to sites of allergic disease and as a critical molecular switch for eosinophilia. Importantly, in the absence of IL-5, inflammation per se is also significantly attenuated. However, in IL-5$^{-/-}$ mice mature eosinophils persist and have the ability to traffic to sites of allergen deposition. Moreover, a direct correlation exists between the number of eosinophils residing in tissues independently of IL-5 and the induction of airways hyperresponsiveness. Thus, eosinophil accumulation into allergic tissues should not be viewed as a process that is exclusively regulated by IL-5. We speculate that under allergic inflammatory conditions, eosinophilia may be differentially regulated and that the central importance of individual eosinophil regulatory molecules to pathogenesis is variable. The contribution of IL-5 and IL-5–independent mechanisms for the recruitment of eosinophils into tissues in various allergic inflammatory disorders must be considered in therapeutic strategies designed to identify the role eosinophils in the induction, progression, or exacerbation of disease.

References

1. Bochner BS, Undem BJ, Lichtenstein LM. Immunological aspects of allergic asthma. Annu Rev Immunol 1994; 12:295.
2. Wills-Karp M. Immunological basis of antigen-induced airways hyperresponsiveness. Ann Rev Immunol 1999; 17:255.
3. Gleich GJ. The eosinophil and bronchial asthma: current understanding. J Allergy Clin Immunol 1990; 85:422.

4. Rothenberg ME. Eosinophilia. N Engl J Med 1998; 338:1592.

5. Gleich GJ, Frigas E, Loegering DA, Wassom DL, Steinmuller D. Cytotoxic properties of the eosinophil major basic protein. J Immunol 1979; 123:2925.

6. Gleich GJ, Flavahan NA, Fujisawa T, Vanhoutte PM. The eosinophil as a mediator of damage to respiratory epithelium: a model for bronchial hyperreactivity. J Allergy Clin Immunol 1988; 81:776.

7. Gleich GJ, Adolphson C. Bronchial hyperreactivity and eosinophil granule proteins. Agents Actions Suppl 1993; 43:223.

8. Sedgwick JB, Vrtis RF, Gourley MF. 1993; Busse WW. Stimulus-dependent differences in superoxide anion generation by normal human eosinophils and neutrophils. J Allergy Clin Immunol 1988; 81:876.

9. Hamid Q, Azzawi M, Ying S, Moqbel R, Wardlaw AJ, Corrigan CJ, Bradley B, Durham SR, Collins JV, Jeffery PK, et al. Expression of mRNA for interleukin-5 in mucosal bronchial biopsies from asthma. J Clin Invest 1991; 87:1541.

10. Hamelmann E, Oshiba A, Loader J, Larsen GL, Gleich G, Lee J, Gelfand EW. Antiinterleukin-5 antibody prevents airway hyperresponsiveness in a murine model of airway sensitization. Am J Respir Crit Care Med 1997; 155:819.

11. Foster PS, Hogan SP, Ramsay AJ, Matthaei KI, Young IG. Interleukin-5 deficiency abolishes eosinophilia, airways hyperreactivity, and lung damage in a mouse asthma model [see comments]. J Exp Med 1996; 183:195.

12. Robinson DS, Hamid Q, Ying S, Tsicopoulos A, Barkans J, Bentley AM, Corrigan C, Durham SR, Kay AB. Predominant TH2-like bronchoalveolar T-lymphocyte population in atopic asthma. N Engl Med 1992; 326:298.

13. Azzawi, M, Bradley B, Jeffery PK, Frew AJ, Wardlaw AJ, Knowles G, Assoufi B, Collins JV, Durham S, Kay AB. Identification of activated T lymphocytes and eosinophils in bronchial biopsies in stable atopic asthma. Am Rev Respir Dis 1990; 142:1407.

14. Azzawi M, Johnston PW, Majumdar S, Kay AB, Jeffery PK. T lymphocytes and activated eosinophils in airway mucosa in fatal asthma and cystic fibrosis. Am Rev Respir Dis 1992; 145:1477.

15. Bentley AM, Menz G, Storz C, Robinson DS, Bradley B, Jeffery PK, Durham SR, Kay AB. Identification of T lymphocytes, macrophages, and activated eosinophils in the bronchial mucosa in intrinsic asthma. Relationship to symptoms and bronchial responsiveness. Am Rev Respir Dis 1992; 146:500.

16. Bentley AM, Meng Q, Robinson DS, Hamid Q, Kay AB, Durham SR. Increases in activated T lymphocytes, eosinophils, and cytokine mRNA expression for interleukin-5 and granulocyte/macrophage colony-stimulating factor in bronchial biopsies after allergen inhalation challenge in atopic asthmatics. Am J Respir Cell Mol Biol 1993; 8:35.

17. Sur S, Gleich GJ, Swanson MC, Bartemes KR, Broide DH. Eosinophilic inflammation is associated with elevation of interleukin-5 in the airways of patients with spontaneous symptomatic asthma. J Allergy Clin Immunol 1995; 96:661.

18. Sur, S, Gleich GJ, Offord KP, Swanson MC, Ohnishi T, Martin LB, Wagner JM, Weiler DA, Hunt LW. Allergen challenge in asthma: association of eosinophils and lymphocytes with interleukin-5. Allergy 1995; 50:891.

19. Jarjour NN, Calhoun WJ, Kelly EA, Gleich GJ, Schwartz LB, Busse WW. The immediate and late allergic response to segmental bronchopulmonary provocation in asthma. Am J Respir Crit Care Med 1997; 155:1515.

20. Robinson D, Hamid Q, Bentley A, Ying S, Kay AB. and Durham SR. Activation of CD4 + T cells, increased TH2-type cytokine mRNA expression, and eosinophil recruit-

ment in bronchoalveolar lavage after allergen inhalation challenge in patients with atopic asthma. J Allergy Clin Immunol 1993; 92:313.

21. Flavahan NA, Slifman NR, Gleich GJ, Vanhoutte PM. Human eosinophil major basic protein causes hyperreactivity of respiratory smooth muscle. Role of the epithelium. Am Rev Respir Dis 1988; 138:685.

22. Seminario MC, Gleich GJ. The role of eosinophils in the pathogenesis of asthma. Curr Opin Immunol 1994; 6:860.

23. Jacoby DB, Costello RM, Fryer AD. Eosinophil recruitment to the airway nerves. J Allergy Clin Immunol 2001; 107:211.

24. Jacoby DB, Gleich GJ, Fryer AD. Human eosinophil major basic protein is an endogenous allosteric antagonist at the inhibitory muscarinic M2 receptor. J Clin Invest 1993; 91:1314.

25. Gibson PG, Dolovich J, Girgis-Gabardo A, Morris MM, Anderson M, Hargreave FE, Denburg JA. The inflammatory response in asthma exacerbation: changes in circulating eosinophils, basophils and their progenitors. Clin Exp Allergy 1990; 20:661.

26. Gibson PG, Manning PJ, O'Byrne PM, Girgis-Gabardo A, Dolovich J, Denburg JA, Hargreave FE. Allergen-induced asthmatic responses. Relationship between increases in airway responsiveness and increases in circulating eosinophils, basophils, and their progenitors. Am Rev Respir Dis 1991; 143:331.

27. Wood LJ, Inman MD, Watson RM, Foley R, Denburg JA, O'Byrne PM. Changes in bone marrow inflammatory cell progenitors after inhaled allergen in asthmatic subjects. Am J Respir Crit Care Med 1998; 157:99.

28. Inman MD, Ellis R, Wattie J, Denburg JA, O'Byrne PM. Allergen-induced increase in airway responsiveness, airway eosinophilia, and bone-marrow eosinophil progenitors in mice. Am J Respir Cell Mol Biol 1999; 21:473.

29. Otsuka H, Dolovich J, Befus D, Bienenstock J, Denburg J. Peripheral blood basophils, basophil progenitors, and nasal metachromatic cells in allergic rhinitis. Am Rev Respir Dis 1986; 133:757.

30. Sehmi R, Wood LJ, Watson R, Foley R, Hamid Q, O'Byrne PM, Denburg JA. Allergen-induced increases in IL-5 receptor alpha-subunit expression on bone marrow-derived CD34+ cells from asthmatic subjects. A novel marker of progenitor cell commitment towards eosinophilic differentiation. J Clin Invest 1997; 100:2466.

31. Wood LJ, Inman MD, Denburg JA, O'Byrne PM. Allergen challenge increases cell traffic between bone marrow and lung. Am J Respir Cell Mol Biol 1998; 18:759.

32. Denburg JA, Wood L, Gauvreau G, Sehmi R, Inman MD, O'Byrne PM. Bone marrow contribution to eosinophilic inflammation. Mem Inst Oswaldo Cruz 1997; 92:33.

33. Hogan SP, Mould AW, Young JM, Rothenberg ME, Ramsay AJ, Matthaei K, Young IG, Foster PS. Cellular and molecular regulation of eosinophil trafficking to the lung. Immunol Cell Biol 1998; 76:454.

34. Sanderson CJ, Campbell HD. and Young IG. Molecular and cellular biology of eosinophil differentiation factor (interleukin-5) and its effects on human and mouse B cells. Immunol Rev 1988; 102:29.

35. Coffman RL, Seymour BW, Hudak S, Jackson J, Rennick D. Antibody to interleukin-5 inhibits helminth-induced eosinophilia in mice. Science 1989; 245:308.

36. Hamelmann E, Takeda K, Haczku A, Cieslewicz G, Shultz L, Hamid Q, Xing Z, Gauldie J, Gelfand EW. Interleukin (IL)-5 but not immunoglobulin E reconstitutes airway inflammation and airway hyperresponsiveness in IL-4-deficient mice. Am J Respir Cell Mol Biol 2000; 23:327.

37. Hamelmann E, Takeda K, Schwarze J, Vella AT, Irvin CG, Gelfand EW. Development of eosinophilic airway inflammation and airway hyperresponsiveness requires interleukin-5 but not immunoglobulin E or B lymphocytes. Am J Respir Cell Mol Biol 1999; 21: 480.

38. Iwama T, Nagai H, Tsuruoka N, Koda A. Effect of murine recombinant interleukin-5 on bronchial reactivity in guinea-pigs. Clin-Exp-Allergy 1993; 23:32.

39. Mauser PJ, Pitman A, Witt A, Fernandez X, Zurcher J, Kung T, Jones H, Watnick AS, Egan RW, Kreutner W, et al. Inhibitory effect of the TRFK-5 anti-IL-5 antibody in a guinea pig model of asthma. Am Rev Respir Dis 1993; 148:1623.

40. Clutterbuck EJ, Hirst EM, Sanderson CJ. Human interleukin-5 (IL-5) regulates the production of eosinophils in human bone marrow cultures: comparison and interaction with IL-1, IL-3, IL-6, and GMCSF. Blood 1989; 73:1504.

41. Campbell HD, Tucker WQ, Hort Y, Martinson ME, Mayo G, Clutterbuck EJ, Sanderson CJ, Young IG. Molecular cloning, nucleotide sequence, and expression of the gene encoding human eosinophil differentiation factor (interleukin 5). Proc Natl Acad Sci USA 1987; 84:6629.

42. Lopez AF, Sanderson CJ, Gamble JR, Campbell HD, Young IG, Vadas MA. Recombinant human interleukin 5 is a selective activator of human eosinophil function. J Exp Med 1988; 167:219.

43. Yamaguchi Y, Hayashi Y, Sugama Y, Miura Y, Kasahara T, Kitamura S, Torisu M, Mita S, Tominaga A, Takatsu K. Highly purified murine interleukin 5 (IL-5) stimulates eosinophil function and prolongs in vitro survival. IL-5 as an eosinophil chemotactic factor. J Exp Med 1988; 167:1737.

44. Kopf M, Brombacher F, Hodgkin PD, Ramsay AJ, Milbourne EA, Dai WJ, Ovington KS, Behm CA, Kohler G, Young IG, Matthaei KI. IL-5-deficient mice have a developmental defect in CD5+ B-1 cells and lack eosinophilia but have normal antibody and cytotoxic T cell responses. Immunity 1996; 4:15.

45. Hogan SP, Koskinen A, Matthaei KI, Young IG, Foster PS. Interleukin-5-producing CD4+ T cells play a pivotal role in aeroallergen-induced eosinophilia, bronchial hyperreactivity, and lung damage in mice. Am J Respir Crit Care Med 1998; 157:210.

46. Hogan SP, Matthaei KI, Young JM, Koskinen A, Young IG, Foster PS. A novel T cell-regulated mechanism modulating allergen-induced airways hyperreactivity in BALB/c mice independently of IL-4 and IL-5. J Immunol 1998; 161:1501.

47. Mould AW, Matthaei KI, Young IG, Foster PS. Relationship between interleukin-5 and eotaxin in regulating blood and tissue eosinophilia in mice. J Clin Invest 1997; 99:1064.

48. Foster PS, Mould AW, Yang M, Mackenzie J, Mattes J, Hogan SP, Mahalingam S, McKenzie AN, Rothenberg ME, Young IG, Matthaei KI, Webb DC. Elemental signals regulating eosinophil accumulation in the lung. Immunol Rev 2001; 179:173.

49. Nishinakamura R, Miyajima A, Mee PJ, Tybulewicz VL, Murray R. Hematopoiesis in mice lacking the entire granulocyte-macrophage colony-stimulating factor/interleukin-3/interleukin-5 functions. Blood 1996; 88:2458.

50. Corry DB, Folkesson HG, Warnock ML, Erle DJ, Matthay MA, Wiener-Kronish JP, Locksley RM. Interleukin 4, but not interleukin 5 or eosinophils, is required in a murine model of acute airway hyperreactivity [see comments] [published erratum appears in J Exp Med 1997 May 5_5(9):1715]. J Exp Med 1996; 183:109.

51. Nagai H, Yamaguchi S, Inagaki N, Tsuruoka N, Hitoshi Y, Takatsu K. Effect of anti-IL-5 monoclonal antibody on allergic bronchial eosinophilia and airway hyperresponsiveness in mice. Life Sci 1993; 53:L243.

52. Tournoy KG, Kips JC, Schou C, Pauwels RA. Airway eosinophilia is not a requirement for allergen-induced airway hyperresponsiveness. Clin Exp Allergy 2000; 30:79.

53. Tournoy KG, Kips JC, Pauwels RA. The allergen-induced airway hyperresponsiveness in a human-mouse chimera model of asthma is T cell and IL-4 and IL-5 dependent. J Immunol 2001; 166:6982.

54. Karras JG, McGraw K, McKay RA, Cooper SR, Lerner D, Lu T, Walker C, Dean NM, Monia BP. Inhibition of antigen-induced eosinophilia and late phase airway hyperresponsiveness by an IL-5 antisense oligonucleotide in mouse models of asthma. J Immunol 2000; 164:5409.

55. Shardonofsky FR, Venzor J, 3rd, Barrios R, Leong KP, Huston DP. Therapeutic efficacy of an anti-IL-5 monoclonal antibody delivered into the respiratory tract in a murine model of asthma. J Allergy Clin Immunol 1999; 104:215.

56. Hogan SP, Mishra A, Brandt EB, Royalty MP, Pope SM, Zimmermann N, Foster PS, Rothenberg ME. A pathological function for eotaxin and eosinophils in eosinophilic gastrointestinal inflammation. Nat Immunol 2001; 2:353.

57. Takamoto M, Ovington KS, Behm CA, Sugane K, Young IG, Matthaei KI. Eosinophilia, parasite burden and lung damage in *Toxocara canis* infection in C57B1/6 mice genetically deficient in IL-5. Immunology 1997; 90:511.

58. Robertson SA, Mau VJ, Young IG, Matthaei KI. Uterine eosinophils and reproductive performance in interleukin 5-deficient mice. J Reprod Fertil 2000; 120:423.

59. Takatsu K, Takaki S, Hitoshi Y. Interleukin-5 and its receptor system: implications in the immune system and inflammation. Adv Immunol 1994; 57:145.

60. Kraneveld AD, Nijkamp FP, Van Oosterhout AJ. Role for neurokinin-2 receptor in interleukin-5-induced airway hyperresponsiveness but not eosinophilia in guinea pigs. Am J Respir Crit Care Med 1997; 156:367.

61. Shi HZ, Humbles A, Gerard C, Jin Z, Weller PF. Lymph node trafficking and antigen presentation by endobronchial eosinophils. J Clin Invest 2000; 105:945.

62. MacKenzie JR, Mattes J, Dent LA, Foster PS. Eosinophils promote allergic disease of the lung by regulating CD4(+) Th2 lymphocyte function. J Immunol 2001; 167:3146.

63. Jose PJ, Griffiths Johnson DA, Collins PD, Walsh DT, Moqbel R, Totty NF, Truong O, Hsuan JJ, Williams TJ. Eotaxin: a potent eosinophil chemoattractant cytokine detected in a guinea pig model of allergic airways inflammation. J Exp Med 1994; 179:881.

64. Ying S, Robinson DS, Meng Q, Rottman J, Kennedy R, Ringler DJ, Mackay CR, Daugherty BL, Springer MS, Durham SR, Williams TJ, Kay AB. Enhanced expression of eotaxin and CCR3 mRNA and protein in atopic asthma. Association with airway hyperresponsiveness and predominant co-localization of eotaxin mRNA to bronchial epithelial and endothelial cells. Eur J Immunol 1997; 27:3507.

65. Rothenberg ME, MacLean JA, Pearlman E, Luster AD, Leder P. Targeted disruption of the chemokine eotaxin partially reduces antigen-induced tissue eosinophilia. J Exp Med 1997; 185:785.

66. Lamkhioued B, Renzi PM, Abi-Younes S, Garcia-Zepada EA, Allakhverdi Z, Ghaffar O, Rothenberg MD, Luster AD, Hamid Q. Increased expression of eotaxin in bronchoalveolar lavage and airways of asthmatics contributes to the chemotaxis of eosinophils to the site of inflammation. J Immunol 1997; 159:4593.

67. Lilly CM, Nakamura H, Kesselman H, Nagler-Anderson C, Asano K, Garcia-Zepeda EA, Rothenberg ME, Drazen JM, Luster AD. Expression of eotaxin by human lung epithelial cells: induction by cytokines and inhibition by glucocorticoids. J Clin Invest 1997; 99:1767.

68. Palframan RT, Collins PD, Williams TJ, Rankin SM, Eotaxin induces a rapid release of eosinophils and their progenitors from the bone marrow. Blood 1998; 91:2240.

69. Mould AW, Ramsay AJ, Matthaei KI, Young IG, Rothenberg ME, Foster PS. The effect of IL-5 and eotaxin expression in the lung on eosinophil trafficking and degranulation and the induction of bronchial hyperreactivity. J Immunol 2000; 164:2142.

70. Li L, Xia Y, Nguyen A, Feng L, Lo D. Th2-induced eotaxin expression and eosinophilia coexist with Th1 responses at the effector stage of lung inflammation. J Immunol 1998; 161:3128.

71. Li L, Xia Y, Nguyen A, Lai YH, Feng L, Mosmann TR, Lo D. Effects of Th2 cytokines on chemokine expression in the lung: IL-13 potently induces eotaxin expression by airway epithelial cells. J Immunol 1999; 162:2477.

72. Huang SK, Xiao HQ, Kleine-Tebbe J, Paciotti G, Marsh DG, Lichtenstein LM, Liu MC. IL-13 expression at the sites of allergen challenge in patients with asthma. J Immunol 1995; 155:2688.

73. Kroegel C, Julius P, Matthys H, Virchow JC, Jr., Luttmann W. Endobronchial secretion of interleukin-13 following local allergen challenge in atopic asthma: relationship to interleukin-4 and eosinophil counts. Eur Respir J 1996; 9:899.

74. Humbert M, Durham SR, Kimmitt P, Powell N, Assoufi B, Pfister R, Menz G, Kay AB, Corrigan CJ. Elevated expression of messenger ribonucleic acid encoding IL-13 in the bronchial mucosa of atopic and nonatopic subjects with asthma. J Allergy Clin Immunol 1997; 99:657.

75. Grunig G, Warnock M, Wakil AE, Venkayya R, Brombacher F, Rennick DM, Sheppard D, Mohrs M, Donaldson DD, Locksley RM, Corry DB, Requirement for IL-13 independently of IL-4 in experimental asthma [see comments]. Science 1998; 282:2261.

76. Wills-Karp M, Luyimbazi J, Xu X, Schofield B, Neben TY, Karp CL, Donaldson DD. Interleukin-13: central mediator of allergic asthma [see comments]. Science 1998; 282:2258.

77. Mattes J, Yang M, Siqueira A, Clark K, MacKenzie J, McKenzie AN, Webb DC, Matthaei KI, Foster PS. IL-13 induces airways hyperreactivity independently of the il-4ralpha chain in the allergic lung. J Immunol 2001; 167:1683.

78. Zhu Z, Homer RJ, Wang Z, Chen Q, Geba GP, Wang J, Zhang Y, Elias JA. Pulmonary expression of interleukin-13 causes inflammation, mucus hypersecretion, subepithelial fibrosis, physiologic abnormalities, and eotaxin production. J Clin Invest 1999; 103:779.

79. Pope SM, Brandt EB, Mishra A, Hogan SP, Zimmermann N, Matthaei KI, Foster PS, Rothenberg ME. IL-13 induces eosinophil recruitment into the lung by an IL-5- and eotaxin-dependent mechanism. J Allergy Clin Immunol 2001; 108:594.

80. Gaspar Elsas MI, Joseph D, Elsas PX, Vargaftig BB. Rapid increase in bone-marrow eosinophil production and responses to eosinopoietic interleukins triggered by intranasal allergen challenge. Am J Respir Cell Mol Biol 1997; 17:404.

81. Leckie MJ, ten Brinke A, Khan J, Diamant Z, O'Connor BJ, Walls CM, Mathur AK, Cowley HC, Chung KF, Djukanovic R, Hansel TT, Holgate ST, Sterk PJ, Barnes PJ. Effects of an interleukin-5 blocking monoclonal antibody on eosinophils, airway hyperresponsiveness, and the late asthmatic response. Lancet 2000; 356:2144.

82. Beasley R, Roche WR, Roberts JA, Holgate ST. Cellular events in the bronchi in mild asthma and after bronchial provocation. Am Rev Respir Dis 1989; 139:806.

83. Djukanovic R, Wilson JW, Britten KM, Wilson SJ, Walls AF, Roche WR, Howarth PH, Holgate ST. Quantitation of mast cells and eosinophils in the bronchial mucosa of

symptomatic atopic asthmatics and healthy control subjects using immunohistochemistry [see comments]. Am Rev Respir Dis 1990; 142:863.

84. Ishida K, Thomson RJ, Beattie LL, Wiggs B, Schellenberg RR. Inhibition of antigen-induced airway hyperresponsiveness, but not acute hypoxia nor airway eosinophilia, by an antagonist of platelet-activating factor. J Immunol 1990; 144:3907.

85. McFadden ER, Jr. Asthma: morphologic-physiologic interactions. Am J Respir Crit Care Med 1994; 150:S23.

86. O'Byrne PM, Inman MD, Parameswaran K. The trials and tribulations of IL-5, eosinophils, and allergic asthma. J Allergy Clin Immunol 2001; 108:503.

87. Webb DC, McKenzie AN, Koskinen AM, Yang M, Mattes J, Foster PS. Integrated signals between IL-13, IL-4, and IL-5 regulate airways hyperreactivity. J Immunol 2000; 165:108.

23

Modulating the Interleukin-5 Response in Asthma

JENNIFER C. HUANG, MARGARITA MARTINEZ-MOCZYGEMBA,
ANTHONY P. NGUYEN, and DAVID P. HUSTON

Baylor College of Medicine
Houston, Texas, U.S.A.

I. Introduction: Rationale for Targeting IL-5

Over the past decade, scientific advances have greatly enhanced our understanding of the cellular, molecular, and genetic mechanisms of allergy and asthma and have enabled identification of disease-specific targets for therapeutic intervention. The eosinophil is a highly specialized effector cell that has long been thought to play a central role in atopy and asthma. In allergic asthmatics, peripheral blood eosinophil counts rise within 24 hours of allergen challenge, and eosinophilic infiltration of the lungs is a hallmark of the late phase asthmatic response (1). Eosinophilic granule proteins, such as eosinophilic cationic protein (ECP), major basic protein (MBP), and eosinophilic peroxidase (EPO), are cytotoxic to the bronchial epithelium, and eosinophil-derived leukotrienes are potent bronchospastic agents (2).

Eosinophil physiology is critically dependent on interleukin-5 (IL-5). IL-5 is a Th2-derived hematopoietic cytokine with highly specific bioactivity as a regulator of eosinophil differentiation and survival (1). Several lines of evidence implicate IL-5 as an important mediator driving the eosinophilic inflammation and pathophysiology of asthma (Table 1). Levels of IL-5, Th2 cells, and eosinophils are all increased in the bronchoalveolar lavage (BAL) fluid of humans with atopic asthma and correlate with disease severity (3,4). Th2 cells and eosinophils are also found in increased numbers in biopsies of bronchial mucosa from these subjects (5,6). Finally, exoge-

Table 1 IL-5 and Asthma: Clinical Studies

IL-5 in BAL fluid
Th2 cells in BAL fluid
Th2 cells in bronchial mucosa
Eosinophils in BAL fluid
Eosinophils in bronchial mucosa
Inhaled IL-5 causes bronchial hyperreactivity and sputum eosinophilia
IL-5 mAb decreases blood and sputum eosinophils

nously inhaled IL-5 induces not only sputum eosinophilia, but also airway hyperreactivity (AHR) (7), while administration of anti-IL-5 monoclonal antibodies (mAb) decreases the number of eosinophils in the sputum and peripheral blood of human subjects (8).

The human data are supported by extensive data derived from animal models (Table 2). T-cell–deficient or–depleted mice that are unable to produce IL-5 fail to develop pulmonary eosinophilia in response to allergen challenge (9). In addition, both pulmonary eosinophilia and airway hyperresponsiveness fail to develop in IL-5 knockout mice, but are restored by vector-directed IL-5 gene expression in the lungs (10). Furthermore, transgenic mice overexpressing IL-5 in the lungs develop AHR and eosinophilic inflammation characteristic of asthma even in the absence of allergen sensitization (11). The intrinsic AHR in these transgenic mice is dependent on CD4 T cells and CD49d (α4-integrin)–mediated signaling (12). Numerous studies have also demonstrated that neutralizing mAb against IL-5 effectively inhibit pulmonary eosinophilia and AHR in murine, guinea pig, and primate models of airway hyperreactivity (13–18). Taken together, these data suggest a direct and critical role for IL-5 as a mediator not only of allergic inflammation, but also of AHR.

However, biological systems and disease processes are rarely so simple, and other studies have produced conflicting data. For instance, in some studies, IL-4

Table 2 IL-5 and Asthma: Animal Studies

Mast cell deficiency (WW^V) delays antigen-induced pulmonary eosinophilia
T-cell deficiency or depletion prevents antigen-induced pulmonary eosinophilia
IL-5 gene disruption prevents antigen-induced pulmonary eosinophilia and bronchial hyperreactivity
Vector-directed lung expression of IL-5 in IL-5 knockouts restores antigen-induced pulmonary eosinophilia and bronchial hyperreactivity
IL-5 transgene expression by bronchial endothelial cells induced pulmonary eosinophilia and bronchial hyperreactivity in the absence of antigen
IL-5 mAb prevents antigen-induced pulmonary eosinophilia and bronchial hyperreactivity
Vaccine-induced autologous anti-IL-5 antibodies reduce antigen-induced pulmonary inflammation and bronchial hyperreactivity

and IL-13, rather than IL-5, have been implicated as key players in the development of the murine asthma phenotype (19–21). The role of IL-5 in the pathophysiology of asthma has also been challenged by results from murine models in which the allergen challenge protocols were prolonged to induce chronic asthma with histological changes closely resembling the airway remodeling seen in human asthma, as well as eosinophilic inflammation and AHR (22–24). In one study, mice were sensitized with an intraperitoneal injection of *Schistosoma mansoni* eggs, then rechallenged at days 7 and 14 with soluble egg antigen delivered directly to the airways. In this model, an anti-IL-5 mAb (TRFK-5), administered on day 18 (4 days after the last allergen challenge) dramatically inhibited BAL eosinophilia, but did not prevent AHR (22). More recently, a murine model of chronic asthma was reported in which ovalbumin-sensitized mice were exposed to low concentrations of aerosolized allergen over a period of 6 weeks (23). Wild-type animals developed AHR as well as chronic pulmonary inflammation. However, when IL-5 knockout mice were exposed to this same protocol, the characteristic eosinophilic inflammatory infiltrate and AHR failed to develop, although airway remodeling was observed (24). A dissociation between airway eosinophils and AHR was also observed following anti-IL-5 mAb administration in the cynomolgus monkey model of chronic asthma (25). In aggregate, these results suggest that eosinophilic inflammation and AHR may develop through distinct and possibly overlapping pathophysiological mechanisms and that they may be differentially regulated.

The incongruity between eosinophilic inflammation and airway symptoms has now also been seen in human subjects. Leckie and colleagues conducted a randomized, double-blind, placebo-controlled pilot trial assessing the activity of a single intravenous infusion of an anti-IL-5 mAb (mepolizumab, SB240563), in young men with mild allergic asthma (8). At a dose of 10 mg/kg of body weight, both peripheral blood and sputum eosinophils were significantly lower in treated subjects up to 30 days from the time of infusion. Furthermore, subjects treated with the mAb failed to display the allergen-induced rise in peripheral blood eosinophils normally seen in atopic individuals within 24 hours of allergen challenge. Improvement in laboratory parameters, however, did not translate into demonstrable improvement of clinical symptoms or lung mechanics, since AHR, as measured by histamine challenge 8 and 29 days following mAb infusion, remained unchanged in both placebo and treated subjects. Although this pilot study challenged the argument that IL-5 is required for AHR, further review of the data indicates that such a conclusion is difficult to support (26).

Of particular concern in analyzing the data was the highly variable AHR to histamine after allergen challenge at baseline for subjects in each treatment arm, as well as the highly variable allergen-induced AHR among the placebo treatment subjects. Such variability limits the capacity to adequately power for detection of significant differences between each study arm. Furthermore, the sample size of 8 subjects in each arm of the study may not have been adequate to power the detection of significant differences among treatment options. Hence, larger randomized crossover studies that include intrasubject and intersubject analyses of AHR will be required to determine the potential for efficacy on AHR by neutralizing IL-5.

These conflicting data on the role of IL-5 in AHR create a challenging conundrum and have raised concern as to the rationale for pursuing this cytokine as a target for therapeutic intervention. With over 25 cytokines and numerous cells types having been implicated in the pathophysiology of asthma, clearly IL-5 is not the sole player (27). Nonetheless, despite the incongruity of evidence for the impact of IL-5 on AHR, IL-5 is clearly necessary for the differentiation and survival of eosinophils, and the correlation of IL-5 and eosinophils as hallmarks of asthma provide a strong impetus for continued study. Through a detailed understanding of the biology of IL-5, the rationale and the most appropriate strategies for the therapeutic targeting of this cytokine in asthma and atopy will be elucidated.

II. IL-5 Biology

IL-5 is produced primarily by activated Th2 cells and mast cells, and eosinophils are an autocrine source of IL-5 (28) (Fig. 1). Recent studies have implicated the

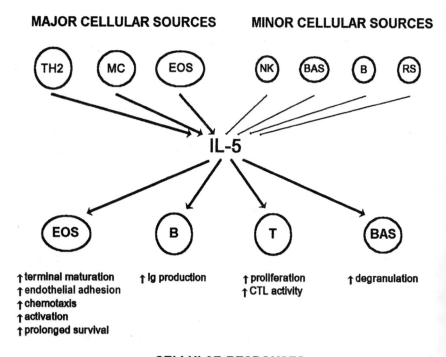

Figure 1 IL-5 paradigm for eosinophilic inflammation. The major sources of IL-5 are type 2 helper T cells (TH2) stimulated by antigen (Ag) presented by antigen-presenting cells (APC), mast cells (MC) stimulated by Ag crosslinking of cell surface IgE, and eosinophils (EOS), which are the cell type most affected by IL-5.

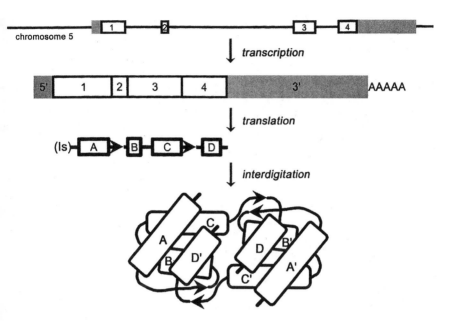

Figure 2 Expression of IL-5. The IL-5 gene is located on human chromosome 5 and consists of 4 exons (1–4). Spliced IL-5 mRNA contains, in addition to its coding sequence, 5'- and 3'-untranslated tails containing regulatory sequences. The block diagram below the spliced transcript represents the translated secondary structures of IL-5 aligned with the appropriate mRNA coding regions. Rectangles represent alpha-helixes (A–D), arrowheads represent beta-strands, lines represent random loop structures, and (Is) stands for the leader sequence. Two IL-5 monomers then interdigitate to form native IL-5, in which the D helix of each monomer is shared with the A–C helices of the other monomer.

transcription factor GATA-3 as the master regulator of Th2 cytokine production (29), and GATA-3 has been shown in vitro to play a crucial role in the expression of IL-5 by Th2 cells (30). In asthmatic subjects, GATA-3 and IL-5 mRNA are significantly increased in a large proportion of T lymphocytes (31).

IL-5 is a 115-amino-acid member of the short-chain helical bundle family of cytokines. Other closely related members of this structural family include IL-3 and GM-CSF. IL-5 is unusual among such cytokines in that it exists not as a monomer, but as an interdigitating homodimer that forms a pair of four α-helical bundle motifs, with the D helix of each monomer shared with the A–C helices of the other (32) (Fig. 2). Although the native IL-5 monomer is not functional, a biologically active IL-5 monomer has been engineered, thereby demonstrating fully functional receptor domains within each of the helical bundle motifs of native IL-5 (33).

The IL-5 receptor is a heterodimer comprised of a ligand specific binding subunit, IL-5Rα, and a common signaling subunit, βc, which is shared by IL-5, IL-3, and GM-CSF (34). IL-5Rα binds IL-5 with weak affinity and interacts with IL-

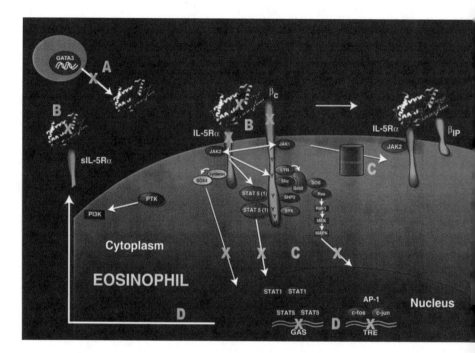

Figure 3   Regulation of IL-5. Production of IL-5 is regulated by the transcription factor GATA 3. The specific receptor for IL-5 is IL-5Rα. Upon IL-5 binding to transmembrane IL-5Rα, the βc receptor is engaged, resulting in transphosphorylation of JAK2 and JAK1. Activated JAK2 then phosphorylates residues in the βc cytoplasmic domain, leading to activation of the signal transduction pathways mediated by STAT5, Ras/MAPK, and PI3K. Termination of IL-5 signaling is mediated in part by ubiquitin-dependent proteasome degradation of the βc cytoplasmic domain. A soluble isoform of IL-5Rα (sIL-5Rα) can bind and neutralize IL-5. (A) Inhibition of IL-5 production; (B) inhibition of IL-5 by neutralization of IL-5, prevention of IL-5 binding to IL-5Rα, or prevention of IL-5 engaging βc; (C) inhibition of signal transduction or accelerated termination of signaling; (D) inhibition of transcription or enhanced production of sIL-5Rα.

5 in a 1:1 stoichiometry (35). βc is unable to bind IL-5 alone; however, recruitment of βc by the IL-5/IL-5Rα complex results in a high-affinity complex capable of intracellular signal transduction (34). Although recent reports suggest that βc may exist as a homodimer on the cell surface, the exact stoichiometry of interaction between IL-5, IL-5Rα, and βc is unresolved (36,37).

Receptor activation (Fig. 3) involves phosphorylation of seven tyrosine residues and one serine residue on the cytoplasmic domain of βc (38), with subsequent activation of the Jak/STAT5, Ras/MAPK, and PI3K/PKC pathways (39). Signaling is rapidly terminated by proteasome cleavage of the cytoplasmic tail of βc, as well as other negative regulators of signal transduction (40). A recent report indicates that IL-5Rα also plays a direct role in signaling through the association of its cytoplasmic tail with the adaptor protein, syntenin, with subsequent activation of the transcription factor Sox-4 (41). Regulation of IL-5 activity may also occur through a soluble receptor isoform, sIL-5Rα (34). The full-length transmembrane form of IL-5Rα is produced as an alternatively spliced product of the mRNA transcript. Translation of the unspliced message results in the soluble isoform (42). The exact biological function of sIL-5Rα is unknown, but recombinant sIL-5Rα acts in vitro as a weak antagonist in ligand binding and cell proliferation assays (43).

Mutational analysis and epitope mapping have defined specific regions of the IL-5 molecule that are important for receptor engagement (Fig. 4). The IL-5Rα binding domain is centered at the interface of loops 1 and 3 and the carboxy terminus of helix D (44,45). In particular, a cluster of charged residues at positions 88–92 of loop 3 (also known as the CD loop) are critical for interaction with IL-5Rα (46). Mutants in which the charged residue at Glu89 or Arg91 is replaced by a neutral alanine showed marked reductions in binding activity (47). Wu and colleagues have reported a single chain variant of IL-5 in which retention of a single positively

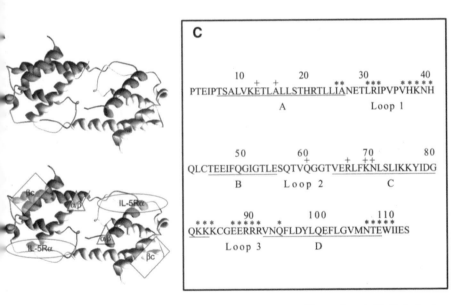

Figure 4 IL-5 functional domains. (A) The ribbon structure of homodimeric IL-5, derived from the crystal coordinates of the crystal structure. (B) Regions of the IL-5 conformational structure involved in receptor engagement are overlaid on the paired helical bundle motifs. Each of the helical bundle motifs has an IL-5Rα (α)-binding domain and a βc (β)-binding domain and a region that may affect both IL-5Rα- and βc-binding domain (β/α). (C) Each monomer of IL-5 contains 115 amino acids. Residues in helixes A–D are underlined. Residues potentially involved in binding to IL-5Rα are denoted by*. Residues potentially involved in binding to βc are denoted by +.

charged arginine residue at position 90 seems to confer IL-5Rα binding activity equivalent to almost 40% of wild-type activity (48). Taken together, the data suggest that the absolute amino acid composition of the receptor binding epitope is less important than the net charge distribution and that different domains exist for receptor binding and activation.

Similar charge distribution principles have been observed in studies of the βc binding domain. βc binding is centered at the A helix, located at the distal corners of each half of the IL-5 homodimer (44). The anionic Glu13, in particular, has been implicated as critical for receptor activation (45). Another glutamate at position 110 was originally thought to be involved in IL-5Rα binding (45–47), but is likely to be more important for receptor activation (49,50).

III. Antagonism of IL-5 Production

In designing a molecular strategy for targeting IL-5, the most logical approach begins at the level of production. Indeed, corticosteroids, a mainstay of treatment in allergy and inflammation, exert their immunomodulatory effects at least partially through the downregulation of cytokines such as IL-2, IL-4, and IL-5 (51). Such downregulation of IL-5 production is mediated, at least in part, by inhibiting the inducible binding of the nuclear factor of activated T cells (NFAT-c) from binding to the IL-5 promotor regulatory element II (52). However, a major concern for using corticosteroids in asthma therapy is their pleotropic and often undesirable physiological side effects. Similarly, other broad range immunomodulators such as FK506 and cyclosporin A, while efficacious in downregulating IL-5 production, exert numerous additional effects that limit their therapeutic utility for asthma (53,54). In recent years, researchers have endeavored to identify agents with a more restricted range of action. Several groups have targeted the transcription factor GATA-3 as a means of modulating Th2 responses in a murine model of asthma. When GATA-3 dominant negative transgenic mice were sensitized to allergen, the typical pulmonary eosinophilia, airway mucus secretion, and IgE production were all attenuated (55). IL-4, IL-5, and IL-13 production were also suppressed. Local blockade of GATA-3 expression in lung cells has also been accomplished in a murine model of asthma using an antisense oligonucleotide against GATA-3 mRNA (56). The oligonucleotide treatment decreased airway eosinophils, Th2 cytokine production, and AHR.

Mori and colleagues have identified a class of compounds, the polynactins, which specifically and efficiently suppresses IL-5 production by human T cells in vitro (57). Transcriptional regulation of IL-5 occurs through a 515-base-pair promoter (58) and appears to involve transcription factors distinct from those regulating IL-2 and IL-4 gene transcription (59). In unpublished data, Mori and colleagues have reported that OM-01, a polynactin compound, suppresses transcription of a reporter gene construct fused to the 5'-promoter region of the IL-5 gene. In vivo studies have shown that nonactin, another member of the polynactin family, greatly attenuates the late phase infiltration (48 hours post–allergen challenge) of eosinophils into the lungs of sensitized mice (60).

IV. Anti-IL-5 Antibodies

As elucidation of the transcriptional regulation of IL-5 continues, therapeutic strategies employing antibody-mediated antagonism of IL-5 have progressed rapidly. Neutralizing mAb to IL-5 function by occupying sterically blocking the IL-5Rα or βc binding sites, thus blocking interaction between the cytokine and receptor complex (61). A number of animal studies have demonstrated the therapeutic potential of mAbs against IL-5 in asthma, as discussed in the introduction. If anti-IL-5 mAb therapy is efficacious in asthma, the potential for respiratory delivery of the antibody may be therapeutically advantageous (18). Systemic delivery of anti-IL-5 mAb has been the traditional protocol for treatment studies in animal models of asthma (13–18) and the limited human trials (8). However, recent evidence indicates that systemic delivery of anti-IL-5 mAb may not be sufficient to eliminate eosinophils from the lung, despite the marked decrease in peripheral blood and airway eosinophils (8). Although the rationale for systemic delivery of anti-IL-5 mAb was to affect bone marrow eosinophilopoiesis, which it did, the rationale for targeting the lung postulates that eosinophilopoiesis also occurs outside the bone marrow, such as in the lung itself. Support for this latter rationale comes from IL-5 transgenic mice in which the IL-5 transgene is under the control of a tissue-specific promotor and the limitation of eosinophil-mediated tissue pathology to the tissue expressing the IL-5 transgene, despite spillover of the IL-5 into the circulation and consequent peripheral blood eosinophilia (62). Shardonofsky et al. (18) have provided evidence that respiratory delivery is efficacious in attenuating AHR, airway eosinophilia, and lung inflammation in a murine model of asthma, as shown in Figs. 4 to 6. Additional studies in human subjects will be necessary to determine the ultimate benefit of this treatment approach.

An alternative to exogenous anti-IL-5 antibodies is the vaccine induction of a transient endogenous polyclonal antibody response to IL-5. Proof of concept for this approach was recently reported using an IL-5 construct engineered with a sequence derived from tetanus toxoid that was inserted into the lop 1 sequence of IL-5 to yield a protein containing a promiscuous foreign helper T-cell epitope (63). The endogenous anti-IL-5 antibody response to the engineered protein lasted for 1–2 months in mice and reduced the development of pulmonary inflammation and AHR in the ovalbumin model of asthma. The efficacy of this approach in established disease remains to be demonstrated. Nonetheless, this strategy represents a novel approach to vaccine induction of an autoimmune response to IL-5 that equates to the autologous production of humanized anti-IL-5 antibodies.

Interference with the action of IL-5 is not limited to antibody therapy. Min and colleagues (64) have reported that isoflavonoids derived from the *Sophora japonica* plant disrupt the effects of IL-5, inhibiting proliferation of an IL-5-dependent cell line in vitro.

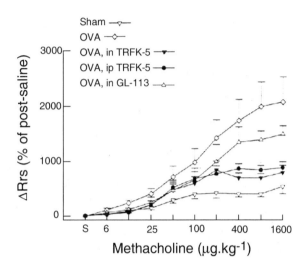

Figure 5 Comparison of systemic versus respiratory delivery of anti-IL-5 mAb therapy on AHR in a murine model of asthma. Data are expressed as the means ± SEM of methacholine dose–airway response relationships using Rrs as an index of airway caliber from sham—sensitized or ovalbumin (OVA)—sensitized mice treated either intranasally or intraperitoneally (ip) with the anti-IL-5 mAb TRFK-5 or the isotype control mAb GL-113. Intranasal therapy was as effective as systemic anti-IL-5 mAb therapy. (From Ref. 18.)

V. IL-5 Receptor Antagonists

A. IL-5 Mutants

Another potential strategy for therapeutic intervention of IL-5 bioactivity is through the development of IL-5 mutants that can bind and occupy IL-5Rα, but are unable to engage and signal through βc. As discussed above, a cluster of charged residues ([88]EERRR[92]) located on loop 3 (CD loop) forms the critical motif for IL-5Rα interactions, while the βc binding domain is centered at glutamate 13 of helix A (Fig. 7). Computer modeling programs predict dramatic alterations in the positive charge fields comprising the βc engagement domain when the anionic Glu13 that maintains the native charge field conformation is mutated to either a neutral or cationic residue. Indeed, substitution of a lysine at position 13 results in an IL-5 mutant (E13K) with antagonistic properties (65). E13K is able to bind IL-5Rα with similar affinity to wild-type IL-5 and causes dose-dependent inhibition of proliferation and βc tyrosine phosphorylation in an IL-5-dependent cell line, TF1, when administered in competition with native IL-5. The antagonistic properties of E13K, however, are not absolute (66); it can act as a partial agonist of TF1 proliferation when administered in the absence of native IL-5 (67). These findings indicate that additional residues are involved in receptor activation. Mutagenesis studies of another glutamate at position 110 suggest that this residue, while originally thought to be involved in IL-5Rα

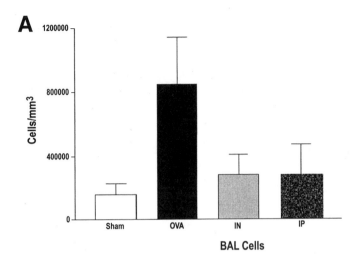

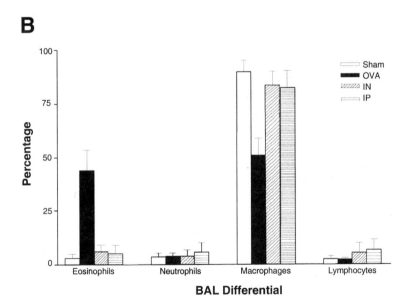

Figure 6 Comparison of systemic versus respiratory delivery of anti-IL-5 mAb therapy on leukocytes in bronchoalveolar fluid (BAL) in a murine model of asthma. Data are expressed as the number of leukocytes (A) and leukocyte differential (B) in BAL of sham-sensitized versus ovalbumin (OVA)-sensitized mice treated intranasally or intraperitoneally (ip) with the anti-IL-5 mAb TRFK-5 or the isotype control mAb GL-113. Intranasal therapy was as effective as systemic anti-IL-5 mAb therapy. Intranasal anti-IL-5 mAb therapy was more effective than intraperitoneally administered anti-IL-5 mAb in reducing the eosinophils in the lung parenchyma (data not shown). (From Ref. 18.)

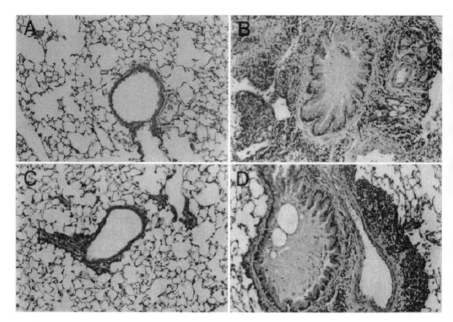

Figure 7 Comparison of systemic versus respiratory delivery of anti-IL-5 mAb therapy on lung histopathology in a murine model of asthma. (A) Lung section from a sham-sensitized and challenged mouse shows no inflammatory changes. (B) Lung section from an ovalbumin-sensitized mouse. Inflammatory cells, including eosinophils, macrophages, and lymphocytes, infiltrate the interstitium and adventitia of a bronchiole. The latter contains debris within its lumen. (C) Lung section from an ovalbumin-sensitized mouse treated intranasally with an anti-IL-5 mAb (TRFK-5). The magnitude of the peribronchiolar inflammatory cellular infiltrate is substantially decreased relative to that observed in the ovalbumin-sensitized and challenged mouse that received no mAb treatment (B). (D) Lung section from an ovalbumin-sensitized and challenged mouse treated intranasally with an isotype-matched control mAb (GL-113). A bronchiole whose lumen is filled with mucus is encased by a dense inflammatory infiltrate similar to that seen in ovalbumin-sensitized and challenged mice that received no mAb treatment (B). Lungs were fixed after bronchoalveolar lavage was performed. (Hematoxylin and eosin stain; original magnification, ×70). (From Ref. 8.)

binding (45–47), actually plays a critical role in receptor activation along with Glu13 by contributing to the βc-engaging charge field conformation (49,50).

Identification of residues involved in receptor binding and activation have enabled the rational design of additional IL-5 mutants that retain binding activity, but are unable to induce signaling, thereby serving as functional antagonists. Plugariu and colleagues have recently reported two monomeric double mutants of IL-5 (50). The first was constructed with alanine substitutions at both residues thought to be critical for βc binding, Glu13 and Glu110. The second employs an alternate sequence for the IL-5Rα binding epitope ([88]SLRGG[92]) and a tryptophan substitution at Glu110 (E110W). The monomeric double mutants bound to IL-5Rα with only slightly lower affinity than nonmutated monomeric IL-5, but neither mutant was able to induce TF1 proliferation. Computer modeling should enable the identification of additional residues which may contribute to the charge field of the βc binding domain.

B. IL-5Rα Antagonists

An alternative strategy for developing competitive antagonist molecules that bind IL-5Rα but are unable to bind and signal through βc is to use molecules that target the IL-5Rα to prevent the binding of IL-5. An oligopeptide sequence based on the CD loop of IL-5 and containing the [88]EERRR[92] motif may act to occupy IL-5Rα sites while lacking the structural capability to engage βc. Such a molecule may offer marked advantages over IL-5 mutants, which contain novel epitopes potentially capable of eliciting an immune response. However, as discussed earlier, the amino acid sequence of the receptor binding epitope is likely less important than the three-dimensional conformation and charge field of the binding region. Indeed, England and colleagues have used random libraries to identify a peptide antagonist of IL-5Rα, which is active not as a linear peptide but as a disulfide-linked homodimer (68). Though the nature of the interaction between this peptide and the IL-5 receptor has not yet been elucidated, the data suggest that engagement of IL-5Rα requires specific three-dimensional spatial and charge factors.

Lach-Trifilieff and colleagues have targeted IL-5Rα by using antisense oligonucleotides to modulate expression of both the transmembrane and soluble isoforms of the receptor (69). The oligonucleotides effectively inhibited eosinophilopoiesis from murine fetal liver cells in vitro. Both blood and tissue eosinophilia in an in vivo murine model of ragweed-induced allergic peritonitis were also attenuated.

Limited studies have addressed the therapeutic potential of monoclonal antibodies against IL-5Rα. In mice, administration of a mAb against IL-5Rα effectively inhibited the peripheral blood eosinophilia normally seen following injection of IL-5 (70). The mAb also normalized the hypereosinophilia seen in IL-5 transgenic mice. Anti-IL-5Rα has not been tried in models of asthma or eosinophilic inflammation. The data suggest, however, that this strategy may be useful either as a primary or adjunctive approach to intervention of IL-5-mediated disease.

C. βc Antagonists

As an alternative to targeting the IL-5Rα subunit, the common β subunit may also be targeted for intervention. βc is the crucial signaling subunit shared by the IL-5, IL-3, and GM-CSF receptor complexes. The cytokine/receptor α complexes share overlapping binding sites on βc, which have been mapped to the B-C and F-G loops of the membrane proximal domain of βc (71).

Sun et al. have developed a murine mAb, which recognizes and antagonizes the ligand binding region of βc (71). Both the intact mAb and its F_{ab} fragment effectively antagonized binding of IL-5, IL-3, and GM-CSF to human eosinophils. Eosinophilopoiesis from human bone marrow progenitors and cytokine-induced survival of peripheral blood eosinophils were also inhibited in a dose-dependent fashion in vitro. The clinical utility of anti-βc mAbs, however, is uncertain. Though IL-5,

IL-3, and GM-CSF may all contribute to eosinophilopoesis, caution is warranted in targeting βc as a therapeutic intervention for asthma. IL-3 and GM-CSF are highly pleotropic, serving as hematopoietic mediators for a number of cell lines. Antagonism of βc may therefore result in dysregulation of important physiological processes. Indeed, βc knockout mice have abnormal surfactant metabolism and develop a peculiar pulmonary pathology with characteristics of pulmonary alveolar proteinosis (72–74). Targeted disruption of IL-5 through antagonism of IL-5Rα may prove to be a safer approach to asthma therapy.

VI. Regulation of IL-5 Signal Transduction

Formation of the high-affinity IL-5/IL-5Rα/βc complex results in activation of signaling pathways mediated through both the α and β receptor subunits. The IL-5Rα/syntenin/Sox-4 cascade was recently reported (25). Although the functional significance of this pathway has yet to be characterized, elucidation of this pathway and other IL-5Rα–mediated cascades may provide novel molecular targets for therapeutic strategies designed specifically to interfere with IL-5-mediated signal transduction.

βc activates three major intracellular signaling pathways: a PTK/PI3 kinase pathway, Jak2/STAT5 pathway, and a Lyn kinase/Ras/MAP kinase pathway (39). The Jak kinases are a pleotropic family of proteins that mediate signaling for a broad range of cytokines. In contrast, Lyn kinase functions in a more restricted fashion. It is constitutively bound to a membrane proximal motif on the cytoplasmic domain of βc. Ligation of βc by the IL-5/IL-5Rα complex results in Lyn tyrosine phosphorylation, which subsequently activates a downstream Ras/MAP kinase cascade. This cascade culminates in activation of c-fos and c-jun, transcription factors important in promoting proliferation of IL-5-responsive cells (39).

Adachi and colleagues recently developed a 15-amino-acid stearated lipopeptide, which functions as a competitive inhibitor of Lyn binding to βc, thereby disrupting the Ras/MAPK cascade (75). The peptide sequence was based on the amino acid sequence of the Lyn kinase binding site of βc. The lipid-conjugated peptide is internalized into cells and prevents the constitutive association of Lyn with βc in vitro. Ligand-induced tyrosine phosphorylation of Lyn and a number of other intracellular proteins is also inhibited. Furthermore, the lipopeptide significantly reduced eosinophil differentiation from murine bone marrow stem cells and attenuated the anti-apoptotic effect of IL-5 on the survival of mature eosinophils. In vivo, bronchial administration of the peptide resulted in a reduction in pulmonary eosinophilic infiltration in allergen-challenged mice. The effects of the lipopeptide appear to be restricted to eosinophils, since B-cell proliferation and histamine release from basophils appeared to be unaffected in vitro.

The Jak2/STAT5 pathway may also serve as a target for intervention of IL-5-induced cell activation. Activation of the Jak2/STAT5 signal transduction pathway results in homodimerization of STAT5 monomers by their SH2 domains. The homodimeric complex translocates to the nucleus and binds to specific enhancer sequences known as GAS elements (gamma-activated sequences) in the promoter regions of relevant genes. Genes activated through the Jak2/STAT5 pathway are important for differentiation and proliferation in IL-5-responsive cells (39). The JAKs, however, are a pleotropic family of kinases that mediate signaling for a broad range of cytokines. Interference with this pathway may disrupt a number of important physiological responses.

Microarray analysis of eosinophil mRNA has been used to identify candidate genes activated by IL-5 signaling that governs eosinophil apoptosis (76). Four genes were identified: Pim-1, DSP-5, CD24, and SLP76. Of these, Pim-1 and SLP76 were relatively tissue restricted to eosinophils, making them potential small molecule targets for modulating eosinophil survival. A better understanding of the IL-5-specific functions of this pathway are needed in order to identify the ideal targets for intervention.

Mechanisms that terminate IL-5 signaling are also attractive therapeutic targets. Such regulators of signaling include kinases, phosphatases, suppressors of cytokine synthesis (SOCS), and inhibitors of nuclear binding factor. However, recent evidence suggests that proteasome degradation of the signaling domain of βc may be the predominant mechanism for rapid termination of IL-5, as well as IL-3 and GM-CSF signaling (40). Importantly, the proteasomal regulation of βc signaling serves as a mechanism of heterotypic desensitization of all of the βc-engaging cytokines and may be a novel mechanism for heterotypic desensitization of shared cytokine receptor signaling.

VII. Regulation of IL-5-Induced Gene Transcription and Splicing

Therapeutic intervention may also be targeted at the furthest downstream site of IL-5 action, gene transcription. As discussed above, signaling pathways activated in IL-5-responsive cells culminate in activation of a number of transcription factors, including the STAT5 homodimer, c-fos and c-jun. Activation results in modulation of a broad range of genes involved in differentiation, proliferation, and survival. One possible mechanism of IL-5 action is that of autocrine regulation of levels of IL-5 receptor expression on IL-5-responsive cells (77). Recent efforts have been made to dissect and elucidate the mechanisms of gene action on eosinophilopoiesis and IL-5 receptor modulation. In one report, *all-trans*-retinoic acid (ATRA) selectively inhibited the differentiation of eosinophils and basophils from human bone marrow progenitors and cord blood CD34+ cells in vitro. In cultured CD34+ cells, expression of the membrane-bound IL-5Rα subunit was also attenuated by ATRA in a dose-dependent fashion, while sIL-5Rα expression was increased. The effects of ATRA appeared to be restricted to the eosinophil/basophil lineage (77). These preliminary results suggest a mechanism for the selective modulation of IL-5Rα expression in hematopoietic progenitors.

Downregulation of membrane-bound IL-5Rα with concomitant upregulation of its soluble receptor isoform may provide a selective mechanism to attenuate the body's response to high levels of circulating IL-5 induced by allergic inflammation. However, the exact mechanisms for IL-5-induced gene regulation on stem cell differentiation and IL-5Rα gene transcription or splicing of message remain ambiguous.

VIII. IL-5 and Eosinophils in Asthma: Time for a New Paradigm?

While recent advances in molecular techniques have enabled rapid progression of research on potential therapeutic strategies to antagonize IL-5, the conundrum regarding the importance of IL-5 in the pathophysiology of asthma remains unresolved. What are the roles of IL-5 and eosinophils in mediating allergic inflammation and asthma, and how beneficial will IL-5 targeted therapies ultimately prove to be in asthma?

An accurate understanding of the role of IL-5 in asthma may require a new paradigm that embraces the temporal and dynamic nature of disease processes. The body exists in a constant state of evolution as it responds and adapts to various endogenous and exogenous stressors. Physiological adaptations to disease may modify an organism's response to various therapeutic interventions over time. Hormone-replacement therapy, for instance, is most effective in preventing osteoporosis in the early stages of menopause, when the body has not yet adapted to a long-term low estrogen state (78). In a similar fashion, unique changes in structural, cellular, or soluble factors may modulate the temporal or spatial impact of various cytokines over the natural history of a disease.

In chronic asthma, airway remodeling and subepithelial fibrosis invariably develop over time (26). The gradual development of airway remodeling may explain the conflicting data collected in studies targeting IL-5. Most animal systems provide a relatively acute model of asthma. Animals are usually sensitized with allergen no more than days or weeks prior to allergen challenge and experimental intervention. However, human subjects have usually suffered from some degree of allergic asthma for many years prior to experimental intervention. Adaptive remodeling of the airways in response to chronic inflammation may alter the human subject's response to various cellular and soluble effectors, including IL-5 (Fig. 8). Early in the disease process, IL-5 may very well play a prominent role not only in promoting blood and tissue eosinophilia, but also in exacerbating the clinical symptoms of AHR as eosinophils release bronchospastic leukotrienes and cytotoxic granule proteins.

Potentially, the eosinophil's phagocytic and antigen-presenting activities may further serve as an important means of perpetuating pulmonary inflammation through ongoing recruitment of inflammatory cells (Fig. 8). Such an antigen-presenting function would represent yet further diversity for the role of eosinophils in the pathophysiology of allergic asthma. Over time, however, the airways may develop subepithelial fibrosis as a consequence of the chronic inflammation and tissue damage. IL-5 is at least partially responsible for this airway remodeling, as anti-IL-5 mAb (TRFK-5) administered at the time of allergen challenge can attenuate airway subepithelial

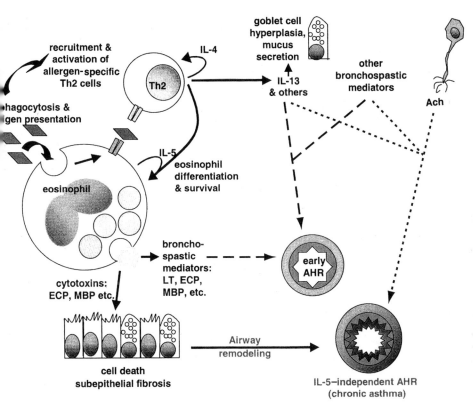

Figure 8 Proposed mechanisms for IL-5 and eosinophil involvement in asthma pathophysiology. Dashed arrows represent mechanisms of AHR operative during the early stages of asthmatic disease, with eosinophil-derived bronchospastic agents playing a major role. At this stage, eosinophils may also release cytotoxic granule proteins. As cell death, fibrosis, and airway remodeling ensue, airway sensitivity to various bronchospastic mediators is altered, with IL-5/eosinophil-independent mechanisms taking on a more prominent role over time (dotted arrows). IL-13, for example, is not only a potent inducer of goblet cell hyperplasia and mucus secretion, it also acts as a bronchoconstrictor. IL-5 and eosinophils may continue to play an important role in chronic asthma pathophysiology, through the phagocytic and antigen-presenting (APC) functions of the eosinophil. As APCs, eosinophils may amplify and perpetuate airway inflammation through ongoing recruitment and activation of allergen-specific Th2 cells. Eosinophils may also perpetuate airway damage through ongoing toxic degranulation. These ongoing processes are indicated by solid arrows. Abbreviations: acetylcholine (Ach), airway hyperreactivity (AHR), eosinophilic cationic protein (ECP), major basic protein (MBP), leukotriene (LT).

fibrosis in sensitized mice (79). Thus, IL-5- and eosinophil-mediated bronchospasm likely occur in conjunction with eosinophil initiated inflammation and fibrosis in the early stages of asthma.

In later stages, however, as remodeling and fibrosis progress, the effects of IL-5 and eosinophils may become dissociated from the clinical symptoms of asthma (Fig. 8). Ongoing antigen exposure could continue to result in eosinophil-mediated activation of Th2 cells, and therefore continued production of IL-5, with consequent persistence of blood and tissue eosinophilia. However, the airway remodeling, induced at least in part by the initial inflammatory effects of IL-5-derived eosinophils, may now limit the actual clinical impact of IL-5 on AHR. While eosinophils may continue to act as antigen-presenting cells and perpetuate inflammation, IL-5-independent mechanisms of AHR may now take on a more prominent role. In this model, therapeutic antagonism of IL-5 may best be employed at the earliest stages of disease, prior to the development of any extensive airway remodeling.

An alternative or perhaps simultaneous physiological role for eosinophils during an inflammatory response to antigens is as a downregulating cell. For example, eosinophils can produce IL-12, a potent cytokine for directing the differentiation of T cells to a TH1 cytokine phenotype (80). In addition, eosinophils express the IL-12 receptor. Furthermore, IL-12 is pro-apoptotic for eosinophils, and this effect is abrogated by IL-5 (81). Differences in IL-12 and IL-5 expression by eosinophils among asthmatics and nonasthmatics (80) raises the possibility that dysregulation of these cytokines may be relevant to persistent eosinophilic inflammation and the pathogenesis of asthma.

IX. Conclusion

The exact role of IL-5 in allergic asthma remains unresolved. It is clear that IL-5 is but one of many factors contributing to the pathophysiology of asthma and that the necessity of IL-5 and eosinophils for AHR may change over the natural history of the disease. Although antagonism solely of IL-5 may not be the cure-all solution for asthma, it is difficult to imagine that this cytokine and the consequent eosinophilic inflammation are not pathophysiologically important. Just as expecting any one molecule to be the total basis for asthma is naïve, dismissing IL-5 as an irrelevant molecule in asthma ignores compelling evidence to the contrary. The intellectual challenge is to predict and define the paradigm that accurately explains the role of IL-5 and eosinophils in asthma. Perhaps IL-5 will need to be targeted in concert with other molecules, such as exotoxin, as was suggested in a recent report from the 2001 International Eosinophil Society (82). Future therapies will likely be both multifaceted and temporally directed, targeting different mediators at different points of action and at different points in time, thereby enabling highly specific, individualized, and efficacious treatments for asthma sufferers.

Acknowledgments

The authors appreciate the secretarial assistance of Ms. Anna Wirt and Tammy Kocurek in the preparation of this manuscript. Support was provided in part by grants from the NIH (AI36936 and AI07496), the Cullen Foundation, the Trammell Foundation, the Mendenhall Foundation, and the Howard Hughes Medical Institute (Medical Student Research Fellowship).

References

1. Wardlaw AJ, Brightling C, Green R, Woltmann G, Pavord I. Eosinophils in asthma and other allergic diseases. Br Med Bull 56:985–1003.
2. Coyle AJ, Ackerman SJ, Irvin CG, Cationic proteins induce airway hyperresponsiveness dependent on charge interactions. Am Rev Respir Dis 1993; 147:896–900.
3. Robinson DS, Hamid Q, Ying S, Tsicopoulos A, Barkans J, Bentley AM, Corrigan C, Durham SR, Kay AB. Predominant Th2 like bronchoalveolar T lymphocyte population in atopic asthma. N Engl J Med 1992; 326:298–302.
4. Walker C, Kaegi MK, Braun P, Blaser K. Activated T cells and eosinophilia in bronchoalveolar lavages from subjects with asthma correlate with disease severity. J Allergy Clin Immunol 1991; 88:835–942.
5. Bradley BL, Azzawi M, Jacobson M, Assoufi B, Collins JV, Irani AM, Schwartz LB, Durham SR, Jeffrey PK, Kay AB. Eosinophils, T lymphocytes, mast cells, neutrophils, and macrophages in bronchial biopsy specimens from atopic subjects with asthma: comparison with biopsy specimens from atopic subjects without asthma and normal control subjects and relationship to bronchial hyperrepsonsiveness. J Allergy Clin Immunol 1991; 88:661–674.
6. Azzawi M, Bradley B, Jeffrey PK, Frew AJ, Wardlaw AJ, Knowles G, Assoufi B, Collins JV, Durham S, Kay AB. Identification of activated T lymphocytes and eosinophils in bronchial biopsies in stable atopic asthma. Am Rev Respir Dis 1990; 142:1407–1413.
7. Shi HZ, Xiao CQ, Zhong D, Qin SM, Liu Y, Liang GR, Xu H, Chen YQ, Long XM, Xie ZF. Effect of inhaled interleukin 5 on airway hyperreactivity and eosinophilia in asthmatics. Am J Respir Crit Care Med 1998; 157:204–209.
8. Leckie MJ, ten Brinke A, Khan J, Diamant Z, O'Connor BJ, Walls CM, Mathur AK, Cowley HC, Chung KF, Djukanovic R, Hansel TT, Holgate ST, Sterk PJ, Barnes PJ. Effects of an interleukin-5 blocking monoclonal antibody on eosinophils, airway hyperresponsiveness, and the late asthmatic response. Lancet 2000; 356:2144–2148.
9. Corry D, Grunig G, Habeiba H, Kurup VP, Warnock ML, Sheppard D, Rennick DM, Locksley RM. Requirements for allergen-induced airway hyperreactivity in T and B cell-deficient mice. Mol Med 1998; 4:344–355.
10. Foster PS, Hogan SP, Ramsay AJ, Matthaei KI, Young IG. Interleukin 5 deficiency abolishes eosinophilia, airway hyperreactivity, and lung damage in a mouse asthma model. J Exp Med 1996; 183:195–201.
11. Lee JJ, McGarry MP, Farmer SC, Denzler KL, Larson KA, Carrigan PE, Brenneise IE, Horton MA, Hazku A, Gelfand EW, Leikauf GD, Lee NA. Interleukin-5 expression in the lung epithelium of transgenic mice leads to pulmonary changes pathognomonic of asthma. J Exp Med 1997; 185:2143–2156.
12. Borchers MT, Crosby J, Justice P, Farmer S, Hines E, Lee JJ, Lee NA. Intrinsic AHR in IL-5 transgenic mice is dependent on CD4(+) cells and CD49d-mediated signaling. Am J Physiol Lung Cell Mol Physiol 2001; 281(3):L653–659.
13. Mauser PJ, Pitman AM, Witt A, Fernandez X, Zurcher J, Kung T, Jones H, Watnick AS, Egan RW, Kreutner W. Inhibitory effect of the TRFK-5 anti-IL-5 antibody in a guinea pig model of asthma. Am Rev Respir Dis 1993; 148:1623–1627.

14. Mauser PJ, Pitman AM, Fernandez X, Foran KS, Adams GK, Kreutner W, Egan RW, Chapman RW. Effects of an antibody to interleukin 5 in a monkey model of asthma. Am J Respir Crit Care Med 1995; 152:467–472.

15. Kung TT, Seltes DM, Zurcher JA, Adams GK, Egan RW, Kreutner W, Watnick AS, Jones H, Chapman RW. Involvement of IL-5 in a murine model of allergic pulmonary inflammation: prophylactic and therapeutic effect of an anti-IL-5 antibody. Am J Respir Cell Mol Biol 1995; 13:360–365.

16. Hamelmann E, Oshiba A, Loader J, Larsen GL, Glech G, Lee J, Gelfand EW. Anti-interleukin 5 antibody prevents airway hyperresponsiveness in a murine model of airway sensitization. Am J Respir Crit Care Med 1997; 155:819–825.

17. Van Oosterhout AJM, Van Ark I, Folkerts G, Van der Linde HJ, Savelkoul HFG, Verheyen KCP, Nijkamp FP. Antibody to interleukin 5 inhibits virus induced airway hyperresponsiveness to histamine in guinea pigs. Am J Respir Crit Care Med 1995; 151:177–183.

18. Shardonofsky FR, Venzor J, Barrios R, Leong KP, Huston DP. Therapeutic efficacy of an anti-IL-5 monoclonal antibody delivered into the respiratory tract in a murine model of asthma. J Allergy Clin Immunol 1999; 104:215–221.

19. Corry DB, Folkesson HG, Warnock ML, Eile DJ, Matthay MA, Werner-Kronish JP, Locksley RM. Interleukin 4, but not interleukin 5 or eosinophils, is required in a murine model of acute airway hyperreactivity. J Exp Med 1996; 183:109–117.

20. Wills-Karp M, Luyimbazi J, Xu X, Schofield B, Neben T, Karp C, Donaldson D. Interleukin-13: central mediator of allergic asthma. Science 1998; 282:2258–2261.

21. Grunig G, Warnock M, Wakil A, Venkayya R, Brombacher F, Rennick D, Sheppard D, Mohrs M, Donaldson D, Locksley R, Corry D. Science 1998; 282:2261–2263.

22. Mathur M, Herman K, Li X, Qin Y, Weinstock J, Elliott D, Monahan J, Padrid P. TRFK-5 reverses established airway eosinophilia but not established hyperresponsiveness in a murine model of chronic asthma. Am J Respir Crit Care Med 1999; 159:580–587.

23. Temelkovski J, Hogan SP, Shepherd DP, Foster PS, Kumar R. An improved model of asthma: selective airway inflammation, epithelial lesions and increased methacholine responsiveness following chronic exposure to aerosolized allergen. Thorax 1998; 53: 849–856.

24. Foster PS, Ming Y, Matthei KI, Young IG, Temelkovski J, Kumar R. Dissociation of inflammatory and epithelial responses in a murine model of chronic asthma. Lab Invest 2000; 80:655–662.

25. Hart TK, Cook R, Zia-Amirhosseini P, Minthorn E, Sellers T, Maleef BE, Eustis S, Schwartz LW, Tsui P, Appelbaum ER, Martin EC, Bugelski PJ, and Herzyk DJ, Preclinical efficacy and safety of mepolizumab (SB-240563), a humanized monoclonal antibody to IL-5, in cynomolgus monkeys. J Allergy Clin Immunol 2001; 108:250–257.

26. O'Byrne PM, Inman MD, Parameswaran K. The trials and tribulations of IL-5, eosinophils, and allergic asthma. J Allergy Clin Immunol 2001; 108(4):503–508.

27. Busse WW, Lemanske R. Advances in immunology: asthma. N Engl J Med 2001; 344: 350–362.

28. Plaut M, Pierce JH, Watson CJ, Hanley-Hyde J, Nordan RP, Paul WE. Mast cell lines produce lymphokines in response to cross linkage of Fc epsilon RI or to calcium ionophores. Nature 1989; 339:64–67.

29. Zheng WP, Flavell RA. The transcription factor GATA-3 is necessary and sufficient for Th2 cytokine gene expression in CD4 T cells. Cell 1997; 89:587–596.

30. Zhang DH, Cohn L, Ray P, Bottomly K, Ray A. Transcription factor GATA-3 is differentially expressed in murine Th1 and Th2 cells and controls Th2 specific expression of the interleukin 5 gene. J Biol Chem 1997; 272:21597–21603.

31. Nakamura Y, Ghaffar O, Olivenstein R, Taha RA, Soussi-Gounni A, Zhang DH, Ray A, Hamid Q. Gene expression of the GATA-3 transcription factor is increased in atopic asthma. J Allergy Clin Immunol 1999; 103:215–222.

32. Rozwarski D, Gronenborn A, Clore GM, Bazan J, Bohm A, Wlodawer A, Hatada M, Karplus P. Structural comparisons among the short-chain helical cytokines. Structure 1994; 2:159–173.

33. Dickason RR, Huston DP. Creation of a biologically active interleukin-5 monomer. Nature 1996; 379:652–655.

34. Tavernier J, Devos R, Cornelis S, Tuypens T, Van der Heyden J, Fiers A, Plaetnick G. A human high affinity interleukin-5 receptor (IL-5R) is composed of an IL5-specific α chain and a β chain shared with the receptor for GM-CSF. Cell 1991; 66:1175–1184.

35. Li J, Cook R, Doyle M, Hensley P, McNulty D, Chaiken I. Monomeric isomers of human interleukin-5 show that 1:1 receptor recruitment is sufficient for function. Proc Natl Acad Sci USA 1997; 94:6694–6699.

36. Carr P, Gustin S, Church A, Murphy JM, Ford S, Mann D, Woltring D, Walker I, Ollis D, Young I. Structure of the complete extracellular domain of the common β subunit of the human GM-CSF, IL-3, and IL-5 receptors reveals a novel dimer configuration. Cell 2001; 104:291–300.

37. Muto A, Watanabe S, Miyajima A, Yokota T and Arai K. The β subunit of the human granulocyte-macrophage colony-stimulating factor receptor forms a homodimer and is activated via association with the α subunit. J Exp Med 1996; 183:1911–1916.

38. DeGroot RP, Coffer P, Koenderman L. Regulation of proliferation, differntiation and survival by the IL-3/IL-5/GM-CSF receptor family. Cell Signal 1998; 8:12–18.

39. Adachi T, Alam R. The mechanism of IL-5 signal transduction. Am J Physiol 1998; 275:C623–633.

40. Martinez-Moczygemba M, Huston DP. Proteasome regulation of βc signaling reveals a novel mechanism for cytokine receptor heterotypic desensitization. J Clin Invest 2001; 108(12):1797–1806.

41. Geijsen N, Uings I, Cornelieke P, Armstrong J, McKinnon M, Raaijmakers J, Lammers J, Koenderman L, Coffer PJ. Cytokine-specific transcriptional regulation through an IL-5Rα interacting protein. Science 2001; 293:1136–1138.

42. Tavernier J, Tuypens T, Plaetnick G, Verhee A, Fiers W, Devos R. Molecular basis of the membrane-anchored and two soluble isoforms of the human interteukin-5 receptor α subunit. Proc Natl Acad Sci USA 1998; 89:7041–7045.

43. Monahan J, Siegel N, Keith R, Caparon M, Christine L, Comptom R, Cusik S, Hirsch J, Huynh M, Devine C, Polazzi J, Rangwala S, Tsai B, Portanova J. Attenuation of IL-5 mediated signal transduction, eosinophil survival and inflammatory mediator release by a soluble human IL-5 receptor. J Immunol 1997; 159:4024–2034.

44. Dickason RR, Huston MM, Huston DP. Delineation of IL-5 domains predicted to engage the IL-5 receptor complex. J Immunol 1996; 156:1030–1037.

45. Graber P, Proudfoot AE, Talabot F, Bernard A, McKinnon M, Banks M, Fattah D, Solari R, Peitsch MC, Wells TN. Identification of key charged residues of human interleukin-5 in receptor binding and cellular activation. J Biol Chem 1995; 270:15762–15769.

46. Morton T, Li J, Cook R, Chaiken I. Mutagenesis in the C-terminal region of human interleukin-5 reveals a central patch for receptor α chain recognition. Proc Natl Acad Sci USA 1995; 92:10879–10883.

47. Tavernier J, Tuypens AV, Plaetnick RD, Heyden JV, Guisez Y, Oefner C. Identification of receptor-binding domains on human interleukin 5 and design of an interleukin 5-derived receptor antagonist. Proc Natl Acad Sci USA 1995; 92:5194–5198.

48. Wu SJ, Li J, Tsui P, Cook R, Zhang W, Hu Y, Canziani G, Chaiken I. Randomization of the receptor α chain recruitment epitope reveals a functional interleukin 5 with charge depletion in the CD loop. J Biol Chem 1999; 274:20479–20488.

49. Wu SJ, Tambyraja R, Zhang W, Zahn S, Godillot AP, Chaiken I. Epitope randomization redefines the functional role of glutamic acid 110 in interleukin-5 receptor activation. J Biol Chem 2000; 275:7351–7358.

50. Plugariu CG, Wu SJ, Zhang W, Chaiken I. Multisite mutagenesis of interleukin 5 differentiates sites for receptor recognition and receptor activation. Biochemistry 2000; 39: 14939–14949.

51. Schleimer RP, Bochner BS. The effects of glucocorticoids on human eosinophils. J Allergy Clin Immunol 1994; 94:1202–1213.

52. Quan A, McCall MN, Sewell WA. Dexamethasone inhibits the binding of nuclear factors to the IL-5 promoter in human CD4 + T cells. J Allergy Clin Immunol 2001; 108(3): 340–348.

53. Mori AM, Suko Y, Nishizaki G, Matsuzaki G, Okudaira H. Regulation of IL-5 production by peripheral blood mononuclear cells from atopic patients with FK506, cyclosporin A and glucocorticoid. Int Arch Allergy Immunol 1994; 104:32–35.

54. Mori A, Suko M, Nishizaki Y, Akinuma O, Kobayashi S, Matsuzaki G, Yamamoto K, Ito K, Tsuruoka N, Okudaira H. IL-5 production by CD4 + T cells of asthmatic patients is suppressed by glucocorticoids and the immunosuppressants FK506 and cyclosporin A. Int Immunol 1995; 7:449–457.

55. Zhang DH, Yang L, Cohn L, Parkyn L, Homer R, Ray P, Ray A. Inhibition of allergic inflammation in a murine model of asthma by expression of a dominant negative mutant of GATA-3. Immunity 1999; 11:473–482.

56. Finotto S, De Sanctis GT, Lehr HA, Herz U, Buerke M, Schipp M, Bartsch B, Atreya R, Schmitt E, Galle PR, Renz H, Neurath MF. Treatment of allergic airway inflammation and hyperresponsiveness by antisense-induced local blockade of GATA-3 expression. J Exp Med 2001; 193:1247–1260.

57. Mori A, Kaminuma O, Suko M, Mikami T, Nishizaki Y, Ohmura T, Hoshino A, Asakura Y, Miyazawa K, Ando T, Okumura Y, Yamamoto K, Okudaira H. Cellular and molecular mechanisms of IL-5 synthesis in atopic disease: a study with allergen specific human helper T cells. J Allergy Clin Immunol 1997; 100:S56–64.

58. Ogawa K, Kaminuma O, Kikkawa K, Akiyama K, Mori K. IL-5 Synthesis by T cells of allergic subjects is regulated at the transcriptional level. Int Arch Allergy Immunol 2000; 122:S63–66.

59. Mori A, Kaminuma O, Mikami T, Inoue S, Okumura Y, Akiyama K, Okudaira H. Transcriptional control of the IL-5 gene by human helper T cells: IL-5 synthesis is regulated independently from IL-2 or IL-4 synthesis. J Allergy Clin Immunol 1999; 103:S429–436.

60. Mori A, Kaminuma O, Ogawa K, Nakata A, Egan RW, Akiyama K, Okudaira H. Control of IL-5 production by human helper T cells as a treatment for eosinophilic inflammation: comparison of in vitro and in vivo effects between selective and nonselective cytokine synthesis inhibitors. J Allergy Clin Immunol 2000; 106:S58–64.

61. Lee NA, McGarry MP, Larson KA, Horton MA, Kristensen AB, Lee JJ. Expression of IL-5 in thymocytes/T cells leads to the development of a massive eosinophilia, extramedullary eosinophilopoiesis, and unique histopathologies. J Immunol 1997; 158(3): 1332–1344.

62. Zhang J, Kuvelkar R, Murgolo N, Taremi S, Chou CC, Wang P, Billah MM, Egan RW. Mapping and characterization of the epitope(s) of Sch 55700, a humanized mAb, that inhibits human IL-5. Int Immunol 1999; 11:1935–1943.

63. Hertz M, Mahalingam S, Dalum I, Klysner S, Mattes J, Neisig A, Mouritsen S, Foster PS, Gautam A. Active vaccination against IL-5 bypasses immunological tolerance and ameliorates experimental asthma. J Immunol 2001; 167:3792–3799.

64. Min B, Oh SR, Lee HK, Takatsu K, Chang IM, Min KR, Kim Y. Sophoricoside analogs as the IL-5 inhibitors from Sophora japonica. Planta Med 1999; 65:408–412.

65. McKinnon M, Page K, Uings IJ, Banks M, Fattah D, Proudfoot AE, Graber P, Arod C, Fish R, Wells TC. Solari R. An interleukin 5 mutant distinguishes between two functional responses in human eosinophils. J Exp Med 1997; 186:121–129.

66. Edgerton MD, Graber P, Willard D, Consler T, McKinnon M, Uings I, Arod CY, Borlat F, Fish R, Peitsch MC, Wells TN, Proudfoot AE. Spatial orientation of the alpha and beta-c receptor chain binding sites on monomeric human interleukin-5 constructs. J Biol Chem 1997; 272:20611–20618.

67. Nguyen A, Tavana G, Moore JP, Martinez-Moczygemba M, Huston DP. Engineering novel therapeutic antagonists of interleukin-5 bioactivity and signaling. J Allergy Clin Immunol 2001; 107:S325.

68. England BP, Balasubramanian P, Uings I, Bethell S, Chen MJ, Schatz PJ, Yin Q, Chen YF, Whitehorn EA, Tsavealer A, Martens CL, Barrett RW, McKinnon M. A potent dimeric peptide antagonist of interleukin-5 that binds two interleukin-5 receptor α chains. Proc Natl Acad Sci USA 2000; 97:6862–6867.

69. Lach-Trifilieff E, McKay RA, Monia BP, Karras JG, Walker C. In vitro and in vivo inhibition of interleukin (IL)-5 mediated eosinopoiesis by murine IL-5Rα antisense oligonucleotide. Am J Respir Cell Mol Biol 2001; 24:116–122.

70. Hitoshi Y, Yamaguchi N, Korenaga M, Mita S, Tominaga A, Takatsu K. In vivo administration of antibody to murine IL-5 receptor inhibits eosinophilia of IL-5 transgenic mice. Int Immunol 1991; 3:135–139.

71. Sun Q, Jones K, McClure B, Cambareri B, Zacharakis B, Iverson PO, Stomski F, Woodcock JM, Bagley CJ, D'Andrea R, Lopez AF. Simultaneous antagonism of interleukin-5, GM-CSF, and interleukin-3 stimulation of human eosinophils by targeting the common cytokine binding site of their receptors. Blood 1999; 94:1943–1951.

72. Robb L, Drinkwater CC, Metcalf D, Li R, Kontgen F, Nicola NA, Begley CG. Hematopoietic and lung abnormalities in mice with a null mutation of the common beta subunit of the receptors for granulocyte-macrophage colony stimulating factor and interleukins 3 and 5. Proc Natl Acad Sci USA 1995; 92:9565–9569.

73. Dranoff G, Crawford AD, Sadelain M, Ream B, Rashid A, Bronson RT, Dickerson GR, Bachurski CJ, Mark EL, Whitsett JA, Mulligan RC. Involvement of granulocyte macrophage colony stimulating factor in pulmonary homeostasis. Science 1994; 264:713–716.

74. Nishinakamura R, Nakayama N, Hirabayashi T, Inoue T, Aud D, McNeil T, Azuma S, Yoshida S, Toyoda Y, Arai K, Miyajima A, Murray R. Mice deficient for the IL-3/GM-CSF/IL-5 beta c receptor exhibit lung pathology and impaired immune response, while beta IL3 receptor deficient mice are normal. Immunity 1995; 2:211–222.

75. Adachi T, Stafford S, Sur S, Alam R. A novel lyn-binding peptide inhibitor blocks eosinophil differentiation, survival, and airway eosinophilic inflammation. J Immunol 1999; 163:939–946.

76. Temple R, Allen E, Fordham J, Phipps S, Schneider H-C., Lindauer K, Hayes I, Lockey J, Pollock K, Jupp R. Microarray analysis of eosinophils reveals a number of candidate survival and apoptosis genes. Am J Respir Cell Mol Biol 2001; 25:425–433.

77. Denburg JA, Sehmi R, Upham J. Regulation of IL-5 receptor on eosinophil progenitors in allergic inflammation: role of retinoic acid. Int Arch Allergy Immunol 2001; 124:246–248.

78. Manson JE, Martin K. Postmenopausal hormone replacement therapy. N Engl J Med 2001; 345:34–40.
79. Blyth DI, Wharton TF, Pedrick MS, Savage TJ, Sanjar S. Airway subepithelial fibrosis in a murine model of atopic asthma: suppression by dexamethasone or anti-interleukin 5 antibody. Am J Respir Cell Mol Biol 2000; 23:241–246.
80. Nutku E, Gounni AS, Olivenstein R, Hamid Q. Evidence for expression of eosinophil-associated IL-12 messenger RNA and immunoreactivity in bronchial asthma. J Allergy Clin Immunol 2000; 106(2):288–292.
81. Nutku E, Zhuang Q, Soussi-Gounni A, Aris F, Mazer BD, Hamid Q. Functional expression of IL-12 receptor by human eosinophils: IL-12 promotes eosinophil apoptosis. J Immunol 2001; 167(2):1039–1046.
82. Lacy P, Weller PF, Moqbel R. A report from the International Eosinophil Society: eosinophils in a tug of war. J Allergy Clin Immunol 2001; 108:895–900.

24

The Role of Interleukin-9 in Allergic Inflammation of Asthma

ULLA-ANGELA TEMANN and RICHARD A. FLAVELL

Howard Hughes Medical Institute
Yale University School of Medicine
New Haven, Connecticut, U.S.A.

I. Introduction

Airway inflammation is thought to play a central role in the pathogenesis of allergic asthma (1). However, the precise roles that different inflammatory cells and mediators play in the development of pathological and physiological changes seen in the lungs of asthmatics are still not understood. Various inflammatory cell types, including T cells, B cells, eosinophils, macrophages, and mast cells, are involved in the complex immune response in the airway (2). In particular, activated CD4+ T cells of the Th2 subset seem to play a major role in the initiation and maintenance of allergic inflammation (3). Production of cytokines like interleukin (IL)-4, IL-5, IL-9, IL-10, and IL-13 by Th2 cells is believed to be implicated in the development of asthmatic features, including lung eosinophilia, mucus hypersecretion, mast cell hyperplasia, and bronchial hyperresponsiveness. This chapter will focus on one of these Th2-type cytokines, IL-9, and its potential role in allergic inflammation in asthma.

IL-9 was originally discovered as a growth factor for a subset of murine T-cell clones (4,5). Subsequently, more activities of IL-9 or various cell types including mast cells, hematopoietic progenitors, B cells, eosinophils, neutrophils, and airway epithelial cells have been described during the last decade (6–16).

II. IL-9 in Asthma

A potential physiological role of IL-9 in asthma remained unexplored until recently, when several genetic linkage studies and in vivo experiments in humans and in mice implied the involvement of IL-9 in the pathophysiology of allergic asthma. Genetic susceptibility to human asthma is thought to be multigenic (17, 18). Biological variability in allergic and inflammatory response and the recognition of the importance of cytokines in this process have stimulated the analysis of candidate genes for genetic variability in structure and function. Although the gene(s) predisposing to asthma and its accompanying features like atopy, increased serum IgE levels, and bronchial hyperresponsiveness have not yet identified, various genetic studies in humans have linked these characteristics to chromosome 5q31-q35 (19,20), a chromosomal region that contains several genes thought to be involved in bronchial inflammation associated with asthma (21,22). The human IL-9 gene has been shown to reside within this region, known as the Th2 cytokine gene cluster, closely linked to genes encoding IL-3, IL-4, IL-5, IL-13, and GM-CSF. The mouse IL-9 gene, however, has been localized on chromosome 13 (23), separated from the Th2 cytokine gene cluster on chromosome 11. Both human and mouse genes encoding IL-9 exhibit similar genomic organization and are composed of 5 exons and 4 introns spanning approximately 4 kb (24). Several specific binding sequences for transcription factors including activator of protein 1 (AP-1), AP-2, IFN-regulating factor 1, and NF-κB have been identified in the 5′-flanking region of both the human and murine IL-9 gene (21,24). The product of each of these genes is a 14 kDa glycoprotein. The mature form consists of 144 amino acids along with a signal sequence of 18 amino acids. The homology between human and mouse IL-9 is 69% at the nucleotide level and 55% at the amino acid level (24).

The first indications of an involvement of IL-9 in the pathology of human asthma resulted from genetic linkage studies in humans focusing on the identification of important loci that contribute to the development of allergic asthma or asthma-associated phenotypes like bronchial hyperresponsiveness, atopy, or increased serum IgE levels. Early studies reported linkage of increased serum IgE levels with markers on chromosome 5q, in particular 5q31.1, which contains the Th2 cytokine gene cluster, including IL-9 (20,25). Shortly thereafter, bronchial hyperresponsiveness was mapped to a region on chromosome 5q31-q33 (26). Finally, two independent studies linked asthma and serum total IgE to the IL-9 locus on chromosome 5q31–q33 (19,27), pointing to the IL-9 gene as one candidate gene relevant for the development of allergic asthma. In addition, two promoter polymorphisms in the human IL-9 gene have been identified that might effect genetic regulation and therefore influence susceptibility to develop allergic asthma.

Recently, the human IL-9 receptor gene locus, located in the Xq/Yq pseudoautosomal region (28), has been implicated in determining susceptibility to bronchial hyperresponsiveness and asthma (29). Interestingly, the mouse IL-9R gene locus was mapped on chromosome 11 and is therefore autosomal in mice (28).

Strong support for an important role of IL-9 in the pathology of allergic asthma came also from genetic studies in mice. Strain-specific differences in bronchial responses were linked to a region on mouse chromosome 13 that is syntenic with the human chromosomal region 5q31-q33 and contains the IL-9 gene (30). These data were further substantiated by the finding that bronchial hyporesponsiveness was correlated with greatly reduced IL-9 mRNA and protein levels. Although no genetic variations between the IL-9 genes from hypo-and hyperresponsive strains could be identified, a genetic alteration at a strain-specific locus effecting IL-9 gene expression could not be excluded. Based on these results and the pleiotropic functions of the cytokine, IL-9 was suggested as a candidate gene for asthma (30).

Important information on the physiological effects of IL-9 in relation to a potential role in the pathology of allergic asthma was provided by analysis of transgenic mice that overexpressed this cytokine, either systemically (31) or specifically within the lungs (32). Lung-specific expression of IL-9 resulted in lymphocytic and eosinophilic lung inflammation, airway epithelial cell hypertrophy with mucus overproduction, mast cell hyperplasia, and subepithelial fibrosis. Lung-specific IL-9 transgenic mice also demonstrated airway hyperresponsiveness to inhaled methacholine (32). Therefore, the overexpression of IL-9 resulted in impressive pathological and physiological changes in the lungs similar to those seen in asthmatic patients. Intraepithelial mastocytosis was also observed in transgenic mice overexpressing IL-9 systemically, sustaining a role for IL-9 in mast cell differentiation and proliferation (33). Moreover, following lung challenge with antigen, these mice displayed enhanced eosinophilic airway inflammation, elevated serum total IgE, and airway hyperresponsiveness compared to challenged nontransgenic control mice, providing additional support for a significant contribution of IL-9 to the pathogenesis of allergic asthma (34).

The complex phenotype observed in the lungs of IL-9 transgenic mice has made it difficult to differentiate the direct and indirect effects of IL-9 on lung pathology. The generation of IL-9–deficient mice has facilitated studies to analyze distinct contributions of IL-9 to allergen-specific responses in the lung (35). In vivo experiments using a pulmonary granuloma model established that IL-9 was essential for a rapid and robust generation of goblet cell hyperplasia and mastocytosis in a primary response to lung challenge, adding more evidence of an important function of IL-9 in mucus production and mast cell hyperplasia. Surprisingly, no participation in lung eosinophilia in this model was observed, since IL-9–deficient mice were able to mount a strong eosinophilic reaction in response to lung challenge, comparable to that observed in control mice (35). However, the exact requirements of IL-9 in murine models of allergic asthma using IL-9–deficient mice have not been defined so far, and results might differ from lung disease models involving parasites.

III. Cellular Sources of IL-9

A. T Lymphocytes

The major cellular source of IL-9, as demonstrated in vitro and in vivo, are T cells, prominently that of the CD4 + Th2 subset (36–39). These results agree with in vivo data received from asthmatic subjects where the major cells expressing IL-9 mRNA were identified as CD3+ T cells (40). In studies using human peripheral T cells, expression of IL-9 was detectable in CD4+ T cells after stimulation with potent mitogens such as PHA or anti-CD3 in vitro (24). IL-9 expression was delayed after T-cell activation, indicating that secondary signals were required in this process. Initially, IL-2 was identified as a major element controlling IL-9 production in human T cells (41). However, further studies revealed that a cascade of cytokines, namely IL-2, IL-4, and IL-10, were involved in IL-9 expression following T-cell activation. Specifically, IL-2 was required for IL-4 production, a combination of IL-2 and IL-4 for IL-10 production, and finally a combination of IL-4 and IL-10 for IL-9 production (42). This result suggested that IL-9 expression is a late event during Th2 responses that follows the production of other effector cytokines.

An important role of IL-2 in the regulation of IL-9 expression in T cells was confirmed in murine systems (43). The use of activated CD4+ T cells from IL-2–deficient mice revealed that IL-2 is essential for IL-9 production by T cells in vitro (43). In addition, TGF-β1 was found to significantly stimulate the production of IL-9, which was further enhanced by the addition of IL-4 or inhibited by IFN-γ. However, in contrast to in vitro activated human T cells, induction of IL-9 in murine T cells was not dependent on IL-4 but required this cytokine for optimal in vitro production (43,44). Contrasting with in vitro experiments, IL-4-independent and IL-4-dependent pathways for IL-9 expression in T cells have been demonstrated. In vivo immunization of mice with soluble antigens revealed IL-4-independent expression of IL-9 in murine CD4+ T cells (44), since IL-9 expression was not affected in IL-4-deficient mice (44). Using IL-4-sufficient mice in these experiments, IL-9 expression preceded that of IL-4, indicating that IL-9 could also be an early effector cytokine during a Th2 response under certain conditions. In addition, IL-9 expression was significantly reduced in IL-10-deficient mice, indicating an involvement of IL-10 in IL-9 production in murine T cells. In contrast, in vivo experiments involving parasite infections showed the existence of an IL-4-dependent pathway for IL-9 expression (37). IL-9 expression of in vitro restimulated lymph node and spleen cell cultures of *Leishmania major*–infected BALB/c mice was suppressed by in vivo anti-IL-4 treatment (37). Further, IL-9 production after in vitro restimulation of lymph node cells from mice infected with *Nippostrongylus brasiliensis* was dramatically decreased (45). However, there might still exist regulatory mechanisms other than those involving cytokines like IL-2, IL-4, and IL-10 that could be involved in IL-9 expression. It has been reported that IL-1, rather than IL-2, could serve as a secondary signal for IL-9 production by activated T cells in vitro (46).

B. Mast Cells and Eosinophils

Several recent reports have revealed that production of IL-9 may not be restricted to T cells. IL-9 expression had been detected in mast cells and eosinophils, both important effector cells in human asthma (40,47).

Mast cells are known to be important mediator-secreting cells in the asthmatic airway. Upon activation by IgE/antigen-complexes, they produce, besides mediators such as histamine, leukotriens, and prostaglandins, a wide variety of chemokines, growth factors, and multifunctional cytokines that may enhance allergic inflammation. The range of cytokines expressed by mast cells includes IL-3, IL-4, IL-5, IL-6, IL-10, IL-13, and TNF-α (48). Recently, IL-9 was found to be produced by activated mast cells (47). In primary mouse bone marrow–derived mast cells activated with ionomycin or IgE/antigen-complex, IL-9 expression was upregulated by IL-1 along with other cytokines such as IL-3, IL-5, IL-6, and TNF-α (47). This production of IL-9 was further enhanced by the addition of c-kit ligand (KL) or IL-10, both factors known to promote mast cell growth and differentiation (49,50). These effects of KL and IL-10 might be of physiological importance in asthma since both factors are produced by bronchial epithelial cells and might therefore promote the production of cytokines by mast cells during asthmatic reactions (51,52).

It has been reported that the presence of lipopolysaccharide (LPS) can enhance the production of IL-9 concurrently with IL-13 in activated murine bone marrow–derived mast cells. Co-activation of mast cells by LPS resulted in NF-κB activation. It was shown that IL-9 expression was driven by NF-κB via three newly identified sites for NF-κB in the IL-9 promoter (53). These observations indicate that LPS originating from gram-negative bacteria during infections could act as a stimulator of cytokine expression by already activated mast cells and therefore exacerbate a preexistent inflammation. Interestingly, it has been described that inhalation of endotoxin by asthmatic patients or bacterial infections could trigger inflammatory and bronchial responses (54,55). In conclusion, these findings indicate that IL-9 derived from mast cells during the early asthmatic response might play an important role in the late phase of asthmatic reactions.

Eosinophilia is one hallmark of atopic diseases, including asthma (56). Eosinophils have been commonly studied as effector cells during allergic responses by releasing a wide variety of granule proteins, reactive oxygen species, and lipid mediators. However, it has become more obvious that these cells may also play an active role in regulation and potentiation of an immune response through their ability to produce multifunctional cytokines such as IL-2, IL-4, IL-5, IL-10, IL-13, IFN-γ, TNF-α, and TGF-β (57,58). Indications for eosinophils as a source for IL-9 came first from studies using in situ hybridization and immunocytochemistry that identified eosinophils as one of the cell types expressing IL-9 in asthmatic tissue (40). Further studies revealed that expression of IL-9 was also detectable in human peripheral blood eosinophils from asthmatic subjects. Stimulation of cultured peripheral blood eosinophils with TNF-α and IL-1β up regulated the production and release of IL-9 (59). It was suggested that the release of IL-9 by eosinophils might be involved in enhancing the local production of chemokines by IL-9 for the recruitment of inflammatory cells to the site of allergic inflammation.

IV. Effects of IL-9 on Inflammatory Cells Relevant to Allergic Asthma

A. IL-9 Receptor Expression and Signal Transduction

The effects of IL-9 on various cell types are mediated by the IL-9 receptor (IL-9R), which consists of a ligand-specific α chain (IL-9Rα) and IL-2 receptor (IL-2R) γ

chain. The IL-2R γ chain, normally referred to as the common γ chain (γc chain), is shared by receptors for IL-2, IL-4, IL-7, IL-9, and IL-15 (60). The IL-9Rα is IL-9 specific and responsible for its binding. Both IL-9Rα and γc chain are members of the hematopoietin receptor superfamily, based on sharing a similar four–α-helical bundle structure (61). IL-9 effects are mediated through the activation of the JAK (Janus kinase)-STAT (signal transducer and activator of transcription) pathway (62). IL-9 activates two JAK tyrosine kinases, JAK1 and JAK3, preassociated with IL-9Rα and γ c chain, respectively. These kinases are responsible for the activation of STAT1, STAT3, and STAT5 transcription factors by IL-9 (62). These factors play a key role in cytokine intracellular signaling and are essential for most IL-9 activities investigated so far, such as cell differentiation, regulation of proliferation, and inhibition of apoptosis (62–64).

Analysis of human bronchial biopsy specimens coupled chronic airway inflammation in asthmatics with increased IL-9R expression (40,65). Although there was no difference in IL-9R expression on the level of mRNA expression determined by in situ hybridization between asthmatic and control subjects, IL-9R immunoreactivity in asthmatic tissue was significantly increased (40). In an independent study, IL-9R expression was detected by RT-PCR in airway epithelial cells and bronchoalveolar lavage cells from asthmatic but not control individuals (65). Further evidence implicating IL-9R in allergic asthma came from the analysis of receptor transcripts isolated from human peripheral blood mononuclear cells (66). A splice variant was identified that codes for a nonfunctional cell surface receptor, which may have a potential role in downregulating IL-9 signaling in effector cells. Importantly, this IL-9R splice variant was more prevalent in a group of healthy subjects than in the allergic and/or asthmatic group (66).

B. T Lymphocytes

It is well established that T cells, especially CD4 + cells of the Th2 subset, play an important role in the induction and maintenance of the allergic inflammation in human asthma (67). However, a biological role of IL-9 for T cells relevant to asthma remains undefined. Originally, IL-9 was described as a cytokine that allowed the antigen-independent proliferation of murine T-helper cell clones (5,68). But IL-9 does not function as a general T-cell growth factor since freshly isolated murine T cells appeared to be unresponsive to IL-9 even in the presence of phorbol myristate acetate (PMA) (4). However, IL-9 is a strong stimulator of in vitro cell proliferation for murine thymic lymphomas (69) and is even able to protect these cells from dexamethasone-induced apoptosis (70). Moreover, consistent with these in vitro observations, systemic overexpression of IL-9 in transgenic mice resulted in a high susceptibility to develop thymic lymphomas but did not affect normal T-cell development (31). Of great importance was the recent finding using a fetal-thymus-organ-culture (FTOC) system that blocking the signaling of IL-9 through the IL-9Rα chain resulted in a dramatic reduction in the number of developed human T cells (71). Further, addition of IL-9 to FTOC increased T-cell numbers in general. From these data it was proposed that IL-9Rα signaling is critical for optimal survival, growth, and differentiation during early stages of intrathymic T-cell development (71) However, IL-9-deficient mice did not show any changes in the T-cell subpopulations of the thymus, suggesting that if IL-9 plays a role in T-cell development, alternative pathways must function in its absence in mice (35).

C. B Lymphocytes

The most obvious role of B cells in asthma is the generation of IgE and IgG antibodies. The effect of IL-9 on B cells was first studied using human peripheral B cells. It is well established that IL-4 stimulation can trigger IgE release by human peripheral blood lymphocytes, but a similar effect was not observed for IL-9. However, IL-9 enhanced IgE and IgG production induced by suboptimal doses of IL-4 (9). A direct effect of IL-9 on B cells was suggested since IL-9 also potentiated the IL-4-induced IgE production in purified CD20+ B cells upon costimulation with irradiated EL4 murine T cells (9). In an independent study it was found that neutralizing anti-IL-9 antibodies inhibited the IL-7 induced increase of IgE production in human peripheral blood mononuclear cells mediated by IL-4 (72). The potentiating effect of IL-9 appeared to be associated with an increase in the number of IgE-producing cells (9), an observation also reported for murine systems (73), although an enhancing effect on immunoglobulin (Ig) synthesis could not be excluded. In the mouse, effects similar to that in humans for IL-9 on B cells were reported (73). The IL-4–Induced release of IgE and IgG1 from LPS-primed B cells was enhanced by IL-9, while IL-9 alone did not have any effect (73). In vivo, transgenic mice overexpressing IL-9 systemically showed increased serum levels of all Ig isotypes, including IgE and IgG1 (74). In addition, an expansion of lymphocytes of the B-1 subpopulation was found in peritoneal and pleuropericardial cavities and in the blood. Most of these expanded B-1 cells belonged to the B-1b subset (IgM$^+$Mac-1$^+$ CD5$^-$), and it was suggested that this cell type might be directly or indirectly involved in antibody responses in IL-9 transgenic mice. Dramatically increased serum IgE levels were also reported in IL-9 transgenic mice after lung challenge with antigen compared to control mice (34). Furthermore, lung-specific expression of IL-9 also resulted in accumulation of B cells in the lung (32), but this was not associated with elevated serum Ig levels of any type (U.-A. Temann, unpublished observation). However, if these observations taken together reflect a direct effect of IL-9 on the B-cell population, in transgenic mice this remains to be evaluated, since antigen-specific responses in mice deficient for IL-9 were not altered by the absence of IL-9 expression (35). Finally, there is as yet no evidence that IL-9 might influence in vivo B-cell populations and Ig production during inflammatory responses in human asthma.

D. Mast Cells

Mast cells are important in immediate allergic responses and acute bronchoconstriction in asthma. Cross-linking of allergen-specific IgE bound to high-affinity receptors FcεRI on the surface of mast cells by antigen leads to activation and secretion of a wide variety of mediators causing direct bronchoconstriction and enhancement of airway inflammation (75,76). The number of mast cells is increased in the airways of asthmatics, and they often exhibit signs of degranulation (77). The activity of IL-9 on mast cells was discovered in experiments showing that IL-9 supported the growth of bone marrow–derived mast cell lines in vitro and induced secretion of IL-6 by these cells (11,78). Stimulation of murine primary bone marrow–derived mast cells by IL-9 in combination with c-kit ligand enhanced their survival and led to phenotypic changes by inducing the accumulation of transcripts for two mast cell proteases, mMCP-1 and mMCP-2 (79). IL-9 also induced granzyme B expression in two different mast cell lines, suggesting that IL-9 might play a key role in mast cell differentiation by regulating the expression of mast cell-specific proteases (80). The effects of IL-9 on mast cell proliferation and differentiation were supported by studies with transgenic mice overexpressing IL-9 (32,33). Lung-specific expression of IL-9 caused mast cell hyperplasia in the airway epithelium of transgenic mice (32). This development of mast cells seemed to be a direct effect of IL-9, since mast cell hyperplasia had not been described in transgenic mice expression other Th2 type cytokines, IL-4, IL-5, IL-6, or IL-13, selectively within their lungs (81–84). Further, intraepithelial mast cells were found in the upper airways and the intestinal tract from IL-9 transgenic mice expressing IL-9 systemically (33). These mast cells were characterized by a mixed phenotype showing strong positive staining for safranin and expression of mouse mast cell proteases mMCP-4 and mMCP-5, typical for connective-tissue type mast cells, as well as expression of mMCP-1 and mMCP-2, typical for mucosal mast cells (33). This phenotype was similar to that induced in in vitro cultured mast cells in the presence of c-kit ligand and IL-9 (79). It could be speculated from these observations that mast cells are recruited to, or proliferate and differentiate in, the airways of asthmatics as a consequence of local IL-9 production by activated Th2 lymphocytes.

E. Eosinophils

Airway eosinophilia is a predominant feature of allergic asthma, and elevated numbers of eosinophils often correlate with disease severity (85). Eosinophils are believed to contribute to the pathophysiology of asthma through release of granule proteins, reactive oxygen metabolites, and multifunctional cytokines, which results in tissue damage and changes in airway structure and function (86). It has been shown that IL-5 is one of the most important cytokines for eosinophils by promoting differentiation, maturation, and survival of human and murine eosinophils (87). Recently, several reports have proposed an involvement of IL-9 in the development of lung eosinophilia. Transgenic mice, overexpressing IL-9 selectively within the lungs, showed impressive eosinophilia (32). Similar observations were reported following intratracheal installation of IL-9 in naive mice (88). That IL-9 might promote eosinophilia was also demonstrated by lung challenge of IL-9 transgenic mice with antigen resulting in enhanced eosinophilic airway inflammation compared to challenged control mice (34). In contrast, studies with IL-9-deficient mice have shown that expression of IL-9 is not essential for the development of eosinophilia using a pulmonary granuloma model (35). But these data do not exclude a potential function of IL-9 in intensifying an already ongoing eosinophilic reaction. Recently it was shown that intratracheal instillation of IL-9 in mice resulted in increased levels of IL-5 receptor α (IL-5Rα) in the lung, linking IL-9 to the actions of IL-5 in eosinophilic responses (88). Evidence for a direct effect of IL-9 on eosinophils was provided by the detection of IL-9Rα expression by human peripheral blood eosinophils (10). Further, IL-9 stimulated eosinophilic development in human CD34+ cord blood cells cultured in the presence of IL-3 and IL-5 and induced alone the expression of IL-5Rα (10). However, blockade of IL-5 during lung-specific, inducible expression of IL-9 in transgenic mice dramatically reduced the number of eosinophils in the lung, demonstrating that IL-9 was not able to directly induce lung eosinophilia in the absence of IL-5 (89). A possible mechanism by which IL-9 might act on eosinophilia in allergic asthma could, however, involve increased responsiveness of eosinophils to IL-5 induced differentiation, maturation, and survival via IL-5Rα upregulation.

F. Neutrophils

Although polymorphonuclear neutrophilis (PMNs) have been described in the human bronchial wall of both allergic and nonallergic subjects (90), their role in the pathogenesis of asthma remains undefined. Neutrophils have been primarily viewed as a phagocytic cell in host defense and IgG-mediated humoral immune responses, but they also produce a variety of inflammatory mediators, including cytokines, growth factors, and chemokines (91,92). Recently, it has become apparent that these express many cytokine and chemokine receptors, such as IL-4, IL-13, GM-CSF, and IL-8, indicating the ability of neutrophils to respond to stimuli typically implicated in allergic responses (93–96). In addition, expression of IL-9Rα had been established by RT-PCR in freshly isolated human peripheral blood PMNs from asthmatic patients and normal controls, as well as in bronchoalveolar lavage (BAL)-derived PMNs from asthmatic patients (6). A more heterogeneous expression of IL-9Rα protein on the surface of PMNs was detected by FACS; however, a significant difference was found between IL-9Rα and PMNs from asthmatic subjects and controls. This suggested that the expression of IL-9Rα was under regulatory control. Subsequently, it was shown that IL-9 induced production and release of IL-8 from human PMNs isolated from asthmatics in a dose-dependent manner (6). These effects of IL-9 on IL-8 release could be suppressed by the addition of anti-IL-9 antibodies, but this had no effect on GM-CSF–induced IL-8 release. IL-8 has been previously shown to be a chemotactic factor for T cells, eosinophils, and basophils (97). These data imply that IL-9 might be involved in chemokine production and recruitment of inflammatory cells.

G. Airway Epithelial Cells

A characteristic feature of asthma is mucin overproduction, a condition that contributes to airway obstruction. The exact mechanisms underlying the induction of mucin in airway epithelial cells are poorly understood but are thought to be associated with mediators of chronic inflammation. Recently, interest has focused on the roles of

Th2 cell–derived cytokines, among them IL-9, in regulating mucus production in the airway. In vivo, overexpression of IL-9 in transgenic mice caused airway epithelial cell hypertrophy with mucus accumulation (14,32). Expression studies showed that two mucin genes, MUC2 and MUC5AC, were expressed in the lung in response to IL-9 (14). Similar results were obtained when IL-9 was directly administered to the airways (14). IL-9 induction of mucin was also confirmed in human primary lung cultures and a pulmonary epithelial cell line, NCI-H292 (13,14). MUC2 and MUC5AC expression was upregulated when cultured in the presence of IL-9, providing further evidence for a direct effect of IL-9 on mucin production. Consistent with these data was the finding that lavage fluid from asthmatic subjects or allergen-challenged dogs stimulated mucin (MUC5AC) synthesis in cultured airway epithelial cells. The addition of anti-IL-9 antibodies to the dog airway fluid inhibited the mucin-stimulating activity identifying IL-9 as one major factor contributing to mucin production (13). However, studies with inducible, lung-specific IL-9 transgenic mice demonstrated that induction of mucus production in airway epithelial cells by IL-9 expression was dependent on IL-13 (89). These results may suggest that more than one cytokine might be involved in mucus production in the airways.

The airway epithelium is believed to play an important role during inflammation in the lung by producing a variety of cytokines and chemokines. The effect of IL-9 on airway epithelial cells promoting chemokine production has been investigated in vivo and in vitro. IL-9 transgenic mice showed upregulation of several chemokines, including eotaxin, MIP-1α, MCP-1, -3, and -5, in their lungs (8). In vitro, the addition of IL-9 the primary lung cultures or human lung epithelial cell lines also resulted in upregulation of a subset of these chemokines demonstrating the direct activity of IL-9 on airway epithelial cells. The stimulatory effect on chemokine production in lung epithelial cells might be one of the mechanisms by which IL-9 induces lung inflammation in transgenic mice and possibly the lungs of allergic asthmatics.

V. Concluding Remarks

It has been shown that IL-9 is expressed by Th2-type lymphocytes, mast cells, and eosinophils, all of them important effector cells in the pathology of human asthma. Furthermore, in vitro and in vivo data have provided evidence that IL-9 has multiple effects on various cell types involved in allergic inflammation, including T cells, B cells, mast cells, eosinophils, neutrophils, and airway epithelial cells. These data combined with those obtained from genetic linkage studies provide substantial support for a complex and important role of IL-9 in the pathology of human asthma. Therefore, IL-9 itself or a component of its signaling pathway might be a possible target for therapeutic invention in human asthma. However, the blockade of IL-9 directly or its signaling pathway during allergic inflammation in animal models of asthma has not yet been reported. Future animal studies will therefore first have to reveal the efficacy of any potential therapeutic modality based on the understanding of the aspects of IL-9 and its signaling pathway relevant to the development of allergic inflammation.

References

1. Holgate ST. The inflammatory basis of asthma and its implications for drug treatment. Clin Exp Allergy 1996; 26(suppl 4):1–4.
2. Lukacs NW, Stricter RM, Kunkel SL. Leukocyte infiltration in allergic airway inflammation. Am J Respir Cell Mol Biol 1995; 13:1–6.
3. Robinson DS, Hamid Q, Ying S, et al. Predominant TH2-like bronchoalveolar T-lymphocyte population in atopic asthma. N Engl J Med 1992; 326:298–304.
4. Schmitt E, Van Brandwijk R, Van Snick J, Siebold B, Rude E. TCGF III/P40 is produced by naive murine CD4 + T cells but is not a general T cell growth factor. Eur J Immunol 1989; 19:2167–2170.
5. Uyttenhove C, Simpson RJ, Van Snick J. Functional and structural characterization of P40, a mouse glycoprotein with T-cell growth factor activity. Proc Natl Acad Sci USA 1988; 85:6934–6938.
6. Abdelilah S, Latifa K, Esra N, et al. Functional expression of IL-9 receptor by human neutrophils from asthmatic donors: role in IL-8 release. J Immunol 2001; 166: 2768–2774.
7. Donahue RE, Yang YC, Clark SC. Human P40 T-cell growth factor (interleukin-9) supports erythroid colony formation. Blood 1990; 75:2271–2275.
8. Dong Q, Louahed J, Vink A, et al. IL-9 induces chemokine expression in lung epithelial cells and baseline airway eosinophilia in transgenic mice. Eur J Immunol 1999; 29: 2130–2139.
9. Dugas B, Renauld JC, Pene J, et al. Interleukin-9 potentiates the interleukin-4-induced immunoglobulin (IgG, IgM and IgE) production by normal human B lymphocytes. Eur J Immunol 1993; 23:1687–1692.
10. Gounni AS, Gregory B, Nutku E, et al. Interleukin-9 enhances interleukin-5 receptor expression, differentiation, and survival of human eosinophils. Blood 2000; 96: 2163–2171.
11. Hultner L, Moeller J. Mast cell growth-enhancing activity (MEA) stimulates interleukin 6 production in a mouse bone marrow-derived mast cell line and a malignant subline. Exp Hematol 1990; 18:873–877.
12. Little FF, Cruikshank WW, Center DM. Il-9 stimulates release of chemotactic factors from human bronchial epithelial cells. Am J Respir Cell Mol Biol 2001; 25:347–352.
13. Longphre M, Li D, Gallup M, et al. Allergen-induced IL-9 directly stimulates mucin transcription in respiratory epithelial cells. J Clin Invest 1999; 104:1375–1382.
14. Louahed J, Toda M, Jen J, et al. Interleukin-9 upregulates mucus expression in the airways. Am J Respir Cell Mol Biol 2000; 22:649–656.
15. Louahed J, Zhou Y, Maloy WL, et al. Interleukin 9 promotes influx and local maturation of eosinophils. Blood 2001; 97:1035–1042.
16. Williams DE, Morrissey PJ, Mochizuki DY, et al. T-cell growth factor P40 promotes the proliferation of myeloid cell lines and enhances erythroid burst formation by normal murine bone marrow cells in vitro. Blood 1990; 76:906–911.
17. A genome-wide search for asthma susceptibility loci in ethnically diverse populations. The Collaborative Study on the Genetics of Asthma (CSGA). Nat Genet 1997; 15: 389–392.
18. Morton NE. Major loci for atopy? Clin Exp Allergy 1992; 22:1041–1043.
19. Doull IJ, Lawrence S, Watson M, et al. Allelic association of gene markers on chromosomes 5q and 11q with atopy and bronchial hyperresponsiveness. Am J Respir Crit Care Med 1996; 153:1280–1284.

20. Marsh DG, Neely JD, Breazeale DR, et al. Linkage analysis of IL4 and other chromosome 5q31.1 markers and total serum immunoglobulin E concentrations. Science 1994; 264:1152–1156.

21. Kelleher K, Bean K, Clark SC, et al. Human interleukin-9: genomic sequence, chromosomal location, and sequences essential for its expression in human T-cell leukemia virus (HTLV)-I-transformed human T cells. Blood 1991; 77:1436–1441.

22. van Leeuwen BH, Martinson ME, Webb GC, Young IG. Molecular organization of the cytokine gene cluster, involving the human IL-3, IL-4, IL-5, and GM-CSF genes, on human chromosome 5. Blood 1989; 73:1142–1148.

23. Mock BA, Krall M, Kozak CA, et al. IL9 maps to mouse chromosome 13 and human chromosome 5. Immunogenetics 1990; 31:265–270.

24. Renauld JC, Goethals A, Houssiau F, Merz H, Van Roost E, Van Snick J. Human P40/IL-9. Expression in activated CD4+ T cells, genomic organization, and comparison with the mouse gene. J Immunol 1990; 144:4235–4241.

25. Meyers DA, Postma DS, Panhuysen CI, et al. Evidence for a locus regulating total serum IgE levels mapping to chromosome 5. Genomics 1994; 23:464–470.

26. Postma DS, Bleecker ER, Amelung PJ, et al. Genetic susceptibility to asthma—bronchial hyperresponsiveness coinherited with a major gene for atopy. N Engl J Med 1995; 333: 894–900.

27. Noguchi E, Shibasaki M, Arinami T, et al. Evidence for linkage between asthma/atopy in childhood and chromosome 5q31–q33 in a Japanese population. Am J Respir Crit Care Med 1997; 156:1390–1393.

28. Vermeesch JR, Petit P, Kermouni A, Renauld JC, Van Den Berghe H, Marynen P. The IL-9 receptor gene, located in the Xq/Yq pseudoautosomal region, has an autosomal origin, escapes X inactivation and is expressed from the Y. Hum Mol Genet 1997; 6: 1–8.

29. Holroyd KJ, Martinati LC, Trabetti E, et al. Asthma and bronchial hyperresponsiveness linked to the XY long arm pseudoautosomal region. Genomics 1998; 52:233–235.

30. Nicolaides NC, Holroyd KJ, Ewart SL, et al. Interleukin 9: a candidate gene for asthma. Proc Natl Acad Sci USA 1997; 94:13175–13180.

31. Renauld JC, van der Lugt N, Vink A, et al. Thymic lymphomas in interleukin 9 transgenic mice. Oncogene 1994; 9:1327–1332.

32. Temann UA, Geba GP, Rankin JA, Flavell RA. Expression of interleukin 9 in the lungs of transgenic mice causes airway inflammation, mast cell hyperplasia, and bronchial hyperresponsiveness. J Exp Med 1998; 188:1307–1320.

33. Godfraind C, Louahed J, Faulkner H, et al. Intraepithelial infiltration by mast cells with both connective tissue- type and mucosal-type characteristics in gut, trachea, and kidneys of IL-9 transgenic mice. J Immunol 1998; 160:3989–3996.

34. McLane MP, Haczku A, van de Rijn M, et al. Interleukin-9 promotes allergen-induced eosinophilic inflammation and airway hyperresponsiveness in transgenic mice. Am J Respir Cell Mol Biol 1998; 19:713–720.

35. Townsend JM, Fallon GP, Matthews JD, Smith P, Jolin EH, McKenzie NA. IL-9-deficient mice establish fundamental roles for IL-9 in pulmonary mastocytosis and goblet cell hyperplasia but not T cell development. Immunity 2000; 13:573–583.

36. Else KJ, Hultner L, Grencis RK. Cellular immune responses to the murine nematode parasite *Trichuris muris*. II. Differential induction of TH-cell subsets in resistant versus susceptible mice. Immunology 1992; 75:232–237.

37. Gessner A, Blum H, Rollinghoff M. Differential regulation of IL-9-expression after infection with Leishmania major in susceptible and resistant mice. Immunobiology 1993; 189:419–435.

38. Grencis RK, Hultner L, Else KJ. Host protective immunity to *Trichinella spiralis* in mice: activation of Th cell subsets and lymphokine secretion in mice expressing different response phenotypes. Immunology 1991; 74:329–332.

39. Svetic A, Madden KB, Zhou XD, et al. A primary intestinal helminthic infection rapidly induces a gut- associated elevation of Th2-associated cytokines and IL-3. J Immunol 1993; 150:3434–3441.

40. Shimbara A, Christodoulopoulos P, Soussi-Gounni A, et al. IL-9 and its receptor in allergic and nonallergic lung disease: increased expression in asthma. J Allergy Clin Immunol 2000; 105:108–115.

41. Houssiau FA, Renauld JC, Fibbe WE, Van Snick J. IL-2 dependence of IL-9 expression in human T lymphocytes. J Immunol 1992; 148:3147–3151.

42. Houssiau FA, Schandene L, Stevens M, et al. A cascade of cytokines is responsible for IL-9 expression in human T cells. Involvement of IL-2, IL-4, and IL-10. J Immunol 1995; 154:2624–2630.

43. Schmitt E, Germann T, Goedert S, et al. IL-9 production of naive CD4 + T cells depends on IL-2, is synergistically enhanced by a combination of TGF-beta and IL-4, and is inhibited by IFN-gamma. J Immunol 1994; 153:3989–3996.

44. Monteyne P, Renauld JC, Van Broeck J, Dunne DW, Brombacher F, Coutelier JP. IL-4-independent regulation of in vivo IL-9 expression. J Immunol 1997; 159:2616–2623.

45. Kopf M, Le Gros G, Bachmann M, Lamers MC, Bluethmann H, Kohler G. Disruption of the murine IL-4 gene blocks Th2 cytokine responses. Nature 1993; 362:245–248.

46. Schmitt E, Beuscher HU, Huels C, et al. IL-1 serves as a secondary signal for IL-9 expression. J Immunol 1991; 147:3848–3854.

47. Hultner L, Kolsch S, Stassen M, et al. In activated mast cells, IL-1 up-regulates the production of several Th2-related cytokines including IL-9. J Immunol 2000; 164: 5556–5563.

48. Holgate ST. The role of mast cells and basophils in inflammation. Clin Exp Allergy 2000; 30(suppl 1):28–32.

49. Nocka K, Buck J, Levi E, Besmer P. Candidate ligand for the c-kit transmembrane kinase receptor: KL, a fibroblast derived growth factor stimulates mast cells and erythroid progenitors. EMBO J 1990; 9:3287–3294.

50. Thompson-Snipes L, Dhar V, Bond MW, Mosmann TR, Moore KW, Rennick DM. Interleukin 10: a novel stimulatory factor for mast cells and their progenitors. J Exp Med 1991; 173:507–510.

51. Bonfield TL, Konstan MW, Burfeind P, Panuska JR, Hilliard JB, Berger M. Normal bronchial epithelial cells constitutively produce the anti- inflammatory cytokine interleukin-10, which is downregulated in cystic fibrosis. Am J Respir Cell Mol Biol 1995; 13: 257–261.

52. Wen LP, Fahrni JA, Matsui S, Rosen GD. Airway epithelial cells produce stem cell factor. Biochim Biophys Acta 1996; 1314:183–186.

53. Stassen M, Muller C, Arnold M, et al. IL-9 and IL-13 production by activated mast cells is strongly enhanced in the presence of lipopolysaccharide: NF-kappa B is decisively involved in the expression of IL-9. J Immunol 2001; 166:4391–4398.

54. Michel O, Ginanni R, Le Bon B, Content J, Duchateau J, Sergysels R. Inflammatory response to acute inhalation of endotoxin in asthmatic patients. Am Rev Respir Dis 1992; 146:352–357.

55. Oehling AK. Bacterial infection as an important triggering factor in bronchial asthma. J Investig Allergol Clin Immunol 1999; 9:6–13.

56. Seminario MC, Gleich GJ. The role of eosinophils in the pathogenesis of asthma. Curr Opin Immunol 1994; 6:860–864.
57. Woerly G, Roger N, Loiseau S, Capron M. Expression of Th1 and Th2 immunoregulatory cytokines by human eosinophils. Int Arch Allergy Immunol 1999; 118:95–97.
58. Wong DT, Elovic A, Matossian K, et al. Eosinophils from patients with blood eosinophilia express transforming growth factor beta 1. Blood 1991; 78:2702–2707.
59. Gounni AS, Nutku E, Koussih L, et al. IL-9 expression by human eosinophils: regulation by IL-1beta and TNF-alpha. J Allergy Clin Immunol 2000; 106:460–466.
60. Demoulin JB, Renauld JC. Interleukin 9 and its receptor: an overview of structure and function. Int Rev Immunol 1998; 16:345–364.
61. Idzerda RL, March CJ, Mosley B, et al. Human interleukin 4 receptor confers biological responsiveness and defines a novel receptor superfamily. J Exp Med 1990; 171:861–873.
62. Demoulin JB, Uyttenhove C, Van Roost E, et al. A single tyrosine of the interleukin-9 (IL-9) receptor is required for STAT activation, antiapoptotic activity, and growth regulation by IL-9. Mol Cell Biol 1996; 16:4710–4716.
63. Demoulin JB, Van Roost E, Stevens M, Groner B, Renauld JC. Distinct roles for STAT1, STAT3, and STAT5 in differentiation gene induction and apoptosis inhibition by interleukin-9. J Biol Chem 1999; 274:25855–25861.
64. Leonard WJ, O'Shea JJ. Jaks and STATs: biological implications. Annu Rev Immunol 1998; 16:293–322.
65. Bhathena PR, Comhair SA, Holroyd KJ, Erzurum SC. Interleukin-9 receptor expression in asthmatic airways In vivo. Lung 2000; 178:149–160.
66. Grasso L, Huang M, Sullivan CD, et al. Molecular analysis of human interleukin-9 receptor transcripts in peripheral blood mononuclear cells. Identification of a splice variant encoding for a nonfunctional cell surface receptor. J Biol Chem 1998; 273: 24016–24024.
67. Busse WW, Coffman RL, Gelfand EW, Kay AB, Rosenwasser LJ. Mechanisms of persistent airway inflammation in asthma. A role for T cells and T-cell products. Am J Respir Crit Care Med 1995; 152:388–393.
68. Van Snick J, Goethals A, Renauld JC, et al. Cloning and characterization of a cDNA for a new mouse T cell growth factor (P40). J Exp Med 1989; 169:363–368.
69. Vink A, Renauld JC, Warnier G, Van Snick J. Interleukin-9 stimulates in vitro growth of mouse thymic lymphomas. Eur J Immunol 1993; 23:1134–1138.
70. Renauld JC, Vink A, Louahed J, Van Snick J. Interleukin-9 is a major anti-apoptotic factor for thymic lymphomas. Blood 1995; 85:1300–1305.
71. De Smedt M, Verhasselt B, Kerre T, et al. Signals from the IL-9 receptor are critical for the early stages of human intrathymic T cell development. J Immunol 2000; 164: 1761–1767.
72. Jeannin P, Delneste Y, Lecoanet-Henchoz S, Gretener D, Bonnefoy JY. Interleukin-7 (IL-7) enhances class switching to IgE and IgG4 in the presence of T cells via IL-9 and sCD23. Blood 1998; 91:1355–1361.
73. Petit-Frere C, Dugas B, Braquet P, Mencia-Huerta JM. Interleukin-9 potentiates the interleukin-4-induced IgE and IgG1 release from murine B lymphocytes. Immunology 1993; 79:146–151.
74. Vink A, Warnier G, Brombacher F, Renauld JC. Interleukin 9-induced in vivo expansion of the B-1 lymphocyte population. J Exp Med 1999; 189:1413–1423.
75. Broide DH, Gleich GJ, Cuomo AJ, et al. Evidence of ongoing mast cell and eosinophil degranulation in symptomatic asthma airway. J Allergy Clin Immunol 1991; 88: 637–648.

76. Schleimer RP, MacGlashan DW, Jr., Peters SP, Pinckard RN, Adkinson NF, Jr., Lichtenstein LM. Characterization of inflammatory mediator release from purified human lung mast cells. Am Rev Respir Dis 1986; 133:614–617.

77. Van Overveld FJ, Houben LA, Schmitz du Moulin FE, Bruijnzeel PL, Raaijmakers JA, Terpstra GK. Mast cell heterogeneity in human lung tissue. Clin Sci (Colch) 1989; 77: 297–304.

78. Hultner L, Druez C, Moeller J, et al. Mast cell growth-enhancing activity (MEA) is structurally related and functionally identical to the novel mouse T cell growth factor P40/TCGFIII (interleukin 9). Eur J Immunol 1990; 20:1413–1416.

79. Eklund KK, Ghildyal N, Austen KF, Stevens RL. Induction by IL-9 and suppression by IL-3 and IL-4 of the levels of chromosome 14-derived transcripts that encode late-expressed mouse mast cell proteases. J Immunol 1993; 151:4266–4273.

80. Louahed J, Kermouni A, Van Snick J, Renauld JC. IL-9 induces expression of granzymes and high-affinity IgE receptor in murine T helper clones. J Immunol 1995; 154: 5061–5070.

81. DiCosmo BF, Geba GP, Picarella D, et al. Airway epithelial cell expression of interleukin-6 in transgenic mice. Uncoupling of airway inflammation and bronchial hyperreactivity. J Clin Invest 1994; 94:2028–2035.

82. Lee JJ, McGarry MP, Farmer SC, et al. Interleukin-5 expression in the lung epithelium of transgenic mice leads to pulmonary changes pathognomonic of asthma. J Exp Med 1997; 185:2143–2156.

83. Rankin JA, Picarella DE, Geba GP, et al. Phenotypic and physiologic characterization of transgenic mice expressing interleukin 4 in the lung: lymphocytic and eosinophilic inflammation without airway hyperreactivity. Proc Natl Acad Sci USA 1996; 93: 7821–7825.

84. Zhu Z, Homer RJ, Wang Z, et al. Pulmonary expression of interleukin-13 causes inflammation, mucus hypersecretion, subepithelial fibrosis, physiologic abnormalities, and eotaxin production. J Clin Invest 1999; 103:779–788.

85. Walker C, Kaegi MK, Braun P, Blaser K. Activated T cells and eosinophilia in bronchoalveolar lavages from subjects with asthma correlated with disease severity. J Allergy Clin Immunol 1991; 88:935–942.

86. Lee NA, Gelfand EW, Lee JJ. Pulmonary T cells and eosinophils: coconspirators or independent triggers of allergic respiratory pathology? J Allergy Clin Immunol 2001; 107:945–957.

87. Hamelmann E, Gelfand EW. IL-5-induced airway eosinophilia—the key to asthma? Immunol Rev 2001; 179:182–191.

88. Levitt RC, McLane MP, MacDonald D, et al. IL-9 pathway in asthma: new therapeutic targets for allergic inflammatory disorders. J Allergy Clin Immunol 1999; 103: S485–491.

89. Temann UA, Ray P, Flavell RA. Pulmonary overexpression of IL-9 induces Th2 cytokine expression, leading to immune pathology. J Clin Invest 2002; 109:29–39.

90. Bradley BL, Azzawi M, Jacobson M, et al. Eosinophils, T-lymphocytes, mast cells, neutrophils, and macrophages in bronchial biopsy specimens from atopic subjects with asthma: comparison with biopsy specimens from atopic subjects without asthma and normal control subjects and relationship to bronchial hyperresponsiveness. J Allergy Clin Immunol 1991; 88:661–674.

91. Cassatella MA. The production of cytokines by polymorphonuclear neutrophils. Immunol Today 1995; 16:21–26.

92. Lloyd AR, Oppenheim JJ. Poly's lament: the neglected role of the polymorphonuclear neutrophil in the afferent limb of the immune response. Immunol Today 1992; 13: 169–172.

93. Dale DC, Liles WC, Llewellyn C, Price TH. Effects of granulocyte-macrophage colony-stimulating factor (GM-CSF) on neutrophil kinetics and function in normal human volunteers. Am J Hematol 1998; 57:7–15.

94. Girard D, Paquin R, Beaulieu AD. Responsiveness of human neutrophils to interleukin-4: induction of cytoskeletal rearrangements, de novo protein synthesis and delay of apoptosis. Biochem J 1997; 325:147–153.

95. Girard D, Boiani N, Beaulieu AD. Human neutrophils express the interleukin-15 receptor alpha chain (IL-15Ralpha) but not the IL-9Ralpha component. Clin Immunol Immunopathol 1998; 88:232–240.

96. Manna SK, Bhattacharya C, Gupta SK, Samanta AK. Regulation of interleukin-8 receptor expression in human polymorphonuclear neutrophils. Mol Immunol 1995; 32: 883–893.

97. Baggiolini M, Moser B, Clark-Lewis I. Interleukin-8 and related chemotactic cytokines. The Giles Filley Lecture. Chest 1994; 105:95S–98S.

25

Epithelial Production of IL-12 p80 During Viral Infection and Asthma Supports an Altered Paradigm for Airway Inflammation

MICHAEL J. WALTER and MICHAEL J. HOLTZMAN

Washington University School of Medicine
St. Louis, Missouri, U.S.A.

I. Introduction

The concept that airway inflammation leads to airway disease has led to a widening search for the types of inflammatory cells and mediators that might be responsible for abnormal airway function. It has not yet been possible to integrate all of this information into a single model for the development of airway inflammation and remodeling, but a useful framework has been based on the behavior of the adaptive immune system. In that paradigm, an exaggeration of T helper type 2 (Th2) over Th1 responses to allergic and nonallergic stimuli leads to airway inflammatory disease, especially asthma. In this review, we summarize alternative evidence that the innate immune system, typified by actions of airway epithelial cells and macrophages, may also be specially programmed for antiviral defense and abnormally programmed in inflammatory disease. In that regard, we concentrate on recent studies of specific IL-12 family members as a product of airway epithelial cells and a mediator of macrophage function. We also introduce evidence that abnormalities in epithelial programming may be inducible by paramyxoviral infection and, with the proper genetic background, may persist indefinitely. Taken together, we propose a new model that highlights specific interactions between epithelial, viral, and allergic (Epi-Vir-All) components and so better explains the basis for airway immunity, inflammation, and remodeling in response to viral infection and the development of long-term disease phenotypes typical of asthma and other hypersecretory airway diseases.

This chapter is divided into seven major sections. The next section provides the background for our proposal that airway epithelial cells are specially programmed for host defense and abnormally programmed in airway inflammatory diseases such as asthma, focusing on studies of cell adhesion molecule expression via Jak/Stat signaling and chemokine expression via mRNA stabilization. The third section provides the background for the biological properties of the IL-12 family members. The fourth section presents the newly defined capacity of airway epithelial cells to generate biologically significant levels of IL-12 family members (i.e., IL-12 p80) and the capacity of these products to mediate airway inflammation in a mouse model of viral bronchiolitis and in human subjects with asthma. The fifth section reviews the efficacy of blocking the action of IL-12 family members in this setting and identifies future strategies for achieving this type of blockade. The sixth section places the work on IL-12 into the context that airway epithelial cells contain a network of immune-response genes that are programmed for anti-viral defense and may be reprogrammed in asthma. That section also presents a model for how the epithelial gene network might interact with the Th1/Th2 balance to cause airway inflammation in asthma and introduces the possibility that this same gene network may also underlie persistent abnormalities in airway epithelial mucosal behavior found in chronic airway disease. The final section summarizes the chapter.

II. Background on Airway Epithelial Function

We have proposed (since 1983) that epithelial cells lining the airway surface (i.e., airway epithelial cells) provide critical signals for immune cell influx and activation and that epithelial–immune cell interaction is a critical feature of airway inflammation and hyperreactivity (1,2). This concept was similar to one (now fairly well established) that the innate immune system provides signals to the adaptive immune system about the origin of antigens and the type of response to be induced (3). However, the role of the epithelium has turned out to be much broader than originally suspected. As outlined below and summarized recently (4–6), we have learned that airway epithelial cells are extensively and specially programmed to respond to inhaled agents in complex pathways that breach innate and adaptive responses. Furthermore, these same cells may be reprogrammed in the setting of disease in ways that may contribute to airway inflammation and remodeling.

The initial evidence that airway epithelial cells took an active role in the immune response came from observations of the pattern of immune cell traffic in experimental models of airway inflammation. In particular, the accumulation of immune cells in the epithelium suggested that the epithelium was the source of chemotactic factors directing immune cell migration from the subepithelial vascular compartment to the airway lumen (1). These in vivo observations were eventually extended to studies of airway epithelial cell monolayers and resulted in a model for a two-step area code to regulate transepithelial movement of immune cells (7–10).

The two steps were primarily encoded by genes for a cell adhesion molecule (typified by ICAM-1) and a chemoattractant (typified by RANTES). The pattern of cellular presentation for each of these mediators, i.e., circumferential distribution of ICAM-1 and polarized secretion of RANTES, was distinct for airway epithelial cells and was specially adapted to mediate ablumenal-to-lumenal movement of immune cells (Fig. 1).

These studies indicated that epithelial function depended quantitatively on the level of gene expression. Accordingly, we next studied the mechanisms that control epithelial immune-response gene expression, using ICAM-1 and RANTES as prototypes. Work on the ICAM-1 system identified a specific IFN-γ-driven Jak/Stat 1 signaling pathway that relied on regulation at the transcriptional level (7,11–14).

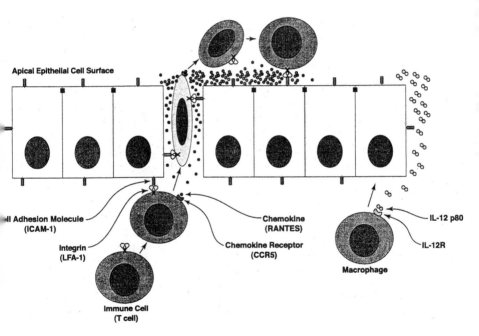

Figure 1 Molecular interactions that mediate immune cell adhesion to airway epithelial cells, transepithelial cell migration, and retention at the airway lumen. Critical steps include: (1) initial integrin (e.g., LFA-1) binding to cell adhesion molecule (e.g., ICAM-1) on the basolateral epithelial cell surface; (2) subsequent β-chemokine receptor (e.g., CCR5) binding to chemokine (e.g., RANTES) and migration along the chemical gradient for RANTES, which is secreted preferentially to the apical epithelial cell surface; and (3) renewed LFA-1 binding to ICAM-1 for retention and/or migration along the apical cell surface. Examples for cell adhesion molecules and chemokine and their receptors are most applicable to mononuclear cell traffic. Ongoing work indicates that additional recruitment of macrophages may depend on epithelial release of IL-12 p80 and binding to its cognate receptor, i.e. IL-12Rβ1. (Modified from Ref. 4.)

This work further indicated that ICAM-1 was representative of an epithelial gene network that was tied to Jak/STAT signaling and was particularly engineered for antiviral host defense (4,14,15). Additional work on the RANTES system indicated that epithelial gene expression was also directly inducible by viral replication, thereby bypassing the need for immune cell–derived products such as IFN-γ (16). Moreover, the mechanism for viral induction in airway epithelial cells was distinct from proposals that it depended on Toll-like receptors (TLRs) and NF-κB signaling that was also driven by nonreplicating virus (17,18). Rather, in the case of airway epithelial cells and paramyxoviruses, optimal responses of host genes also depended on viral replication and consequent effects at the posttranscriptional level, e.g., mRNA stabilization (16). Taken together, the work on isolated airway epithelial cells defined a subset of epithelial immune-response genes programmed for antiviral defense under distinct transcriptional and posttranscriptional controls.

In concert with these in vitro studies, we also aimed to test whether epithelial gene networks were functional in vivo. As described further below (see Sec. IV), we developed a mouse model of viral bronchiolitis that allowed for studies relevant to epithelial-dependent immune function. The mouse model (by design) offers an opportunity for defining the genetic basis for virus-inducible factors that control cell death and proliferation and the role of these factors in mediating airway immunity, inflammation, remodeling, and hyperreactivity. The effects of paramyxoviruses appeared particularly relevant, based on the epidemiological evidence that members of the Paramyxoviradae family (especially respiratory syncytial and parainfluenza viruses) were more closely associated with recurrent wheezing and asthma in young children. Preliminary results indicate that the profile of epithelial gene expression is similar in vivo and in vitro. For example, ICAM-1, RANTES, and Stat1 are similarly induced in both systems (19). Furthermore, ongoing work indicates that loss of epithelial gene function causes significant alterations in host defense as well (20–22) (J. Tyner, N. Kajiwara, O. Uchida, and M. Holtzman, unpublished). However, one of the most informative findings from this system has been the discovery of new pathways for epithelial-dependent immunity, inflammation, and remodeling, including our work on the IL-12 system.

While we expected some correlation between studies of epithelial behavior in isolated cell and animal model systems, we did not know what the behavior of these pathways would be like in human subjects with airway disease. As described further below (see Sec. VI), we found that epithelial immune-response pathways were invariably activated in subjects with asthma. In some cases, e.g., ICAM-1 and Stat1, we found activation of signaling pathways even in well-controlled subjects treated with glucocorticoids (23). In other cases, e.g., RANTES, we found increased gene expression that was responsive to glucocorticoid treatment and was correlated with airway inflammation, hyperreactivity, and obstruction (10) (M. Castro and M. Holtzman, unpublished). Taken together, the data suggest emerging paradigm for mucosal immunity and inflammation in which the epithelial cell is necessary for normal host defense and chronically pressured to a different phenotype for inflammatory disease. This paradigm set the stage for our studies of IL-12.

III. Background on IL-12 Biology

IL-12 family members consist of glycoproteins encoded by four independently regulated genes: IL-12 p40, IL-12 p35, Ebstein-Barr virus–induced gene 3 (EBI3), and IL-12 p19. Due to heterodimeric partnering, the family includes six secreted proteins: IL-12 (a p40/p35 heterodimer often designated p70), IL-12 p80 (a p40/p40 homodimer), EBI3/p35 (an EIB3/p35 heterodimer), EBI3 (an EIB3 monomer), IL-23 (a p40/p19 heterodimer), and p40 monomer (Table 1). Human IL-12 p40 and EBI3 protein are members of the type I cytokine receptor (hematopoietin receptor) family and share 27% homology, whereas p35 and p19 are closely related members of the long-chain α-helical cytokine family (24,25). Neither human nor murine IL-12 p35 and p19 are secreted in the absence of p40, and immunomodulatory or inflammatory properties of p40 monomer or EBI3 have not been defined (24–27). The properties of other family members are reviewed in this section.

A. IL-12

IL-12, also known as natural killer cell stimulatory factor (NKSF), cytotoxic lymphocyte maturation factor (CLMF), and IL-12 p70, was originally identified by its capacity to stimulate IFN-γ production by T cells, augment natural killer (NK) cell–mediated cytotoxicity and enhance lymphocyte proliferation (28,29). Subsequent molecular cloning indicates that IL-12 consists of two disulfide-linked glycoproteins encoded by the IL-12 p40 and p35 genes (26,27). These genes are independently and differentially regulated during IL-12 production from immune cells. Thus, IL-12 production often depends on induction of IL-12 p40 expression in the context of constitutive p35 expression (30). IL-12 evokes potent immune and inflammatory

Table 1   Characteristics of IL-12 Family Members

Family member	Protein components	IL-12 receptor	Receptor affinity (human/mouse)[a]	Biological function
IL-12	p40/p35	β1 and β2	4–7/2–3	IFN-γ secretion from NK/T cells; CD4+ Th1 cell differentiation
p80	p40/p40	β1	20–70/1–2	IL-12 antagonism; macrophage chemotaxis
p40	p40	β1	400–700/ 25–100	ND
EBI3/p35	EBI3/p35	ND	ND	ND
EB13	EBI3	ND	ND	ND
IL-23	p19/p35	β1 and IL-23R	ND	Memory T cell proliferation; IFN-γ secretion from T cells

ND = not determined.
[a]Values represent inhibitory concentration 50% (IC$_{50}$) in ng/mL.

responses by promoting CD4 + Th1 cell differentiation and enhancing IFN-γ production (31–40). Depending on the type of antigen challenge, IL-12 may or may not be required for the development of an appropriate Th1 response to microbial pathogens. For example, IL-12 is required for the development of a Th1 response to *Leishmania major*, *Mycobacterium tuberculosis*, *Histoplasma capsulatum*, *Salmonella*, and *Klebsiella pneumoniae* (38–48). By contrast, IL-12 is not required for the response to certain viral pathogens, such as lymphocytic choriomeningitis virus, vesicular stomatitis virus, mouse hepatitis virus, or, as discussed below, mouse parainfluenza virus (49–51). IL-12 is also unnecessary for the response to allogeneic transplant tissue (52). In the context of a Th1 response, exogenously administered IL-12 can provide protection or cause inflammation depending on the microbial challenge and administration regimens (44,45, 53–61).

Additional studies have demonstrated the influence of IL-12 during the Th2 response to allergen. For example, IL-12 administration concurrent with allergen sensitization or challenge prevents airway hyperreactivity, eosinophil recruitment, and IL-4 and IL-5 production while it increases IFN-γ production (62–65). In addition, IL-12 blockade with neutralizing mAb at the time of allergen challenge allowed for the development of a Th2 response in otherwise resistant C3H mice and increased the response in sensitive A/J mice (66). Ovalbumin-challenged p40-null mice often develop an enhanced Th2 response with increased airway, peripheral blood, and bone marrow eosinophils and increased IL-4 and IgE concentrations (67,68), although this effect is not found in all studies (69).

The role of IL-12 in asthma pathogenesis has not been clearly defined. IL-12 treatment of mild asthmatic subjects caused decreases in peripheral blood and sputum eosinophilia but failed to alter airway reactivity to histamine or inhaled antigen (70). An additional study found decreased IL-12 p40 mRNA levels in mild asthmatic subjects at baseline and increased levels following glucocorticoid treatment (71). Furthermore, the increase in IL-12 p40 mRNA correlated with increases in FEV_1. However, specific levels of IL-12 family members were not determined in this study, so the contribution of other members, particularly IL-12 p80, was not defined.

B. IL-12 p80

IL-12 p80 is a covalently linked p40 homodimer and can function as a competitive antagonist for IL-12 binding. In this capacity, IL-12 p80 can effectively block IL-12–dependent IFN-γ production and proliferation of lymphocytes as well as NK cell activity (72–75). Other transgenic mice with IL-12 p40 and p80 overexpression in the liver exhibit a blunted Th1 immune response to *Plasmodium berghei* (76). In some systems, however, IL-12 p80 may exhibit biological activity even in the absence of IL-12 (77,78). Transgenic mice that selectively overexpress IL-12 p40 and p80 in the basal epithelial cells of the skin develop inappropriate accumulation of immune cells within the epidermal and dermal layers and skin lesions that appear similar to ones found in eczema (79). In that regard, IL-12 p80 may function at least in vitro as a macrophage chemoattractant agent (80) and can induce iNOS expression and activate NF-κB in isolated mouse peritoneal macrophages and microglial cells

(81). Similarly, exogenously administered IL-12 p80 can inhibit endotoxin-induced IFN-γ production and decrease mortality (73,75). Overexpression of IL-12 p40 in a subcutaneous bladder cancer model using adenoviral gene transfer has promoted tumor progression (82), and subcutaneous delivery of IL-12 p40 expressing rat hepatoma cells has resulted in tumor regression (80). Although the basis for the differences in biological effects of IL-12 p80 on immune function and cancer progress are still uncertain, each of these reports suggest that IL-12 p80 may cause effects that are separate from its role as an IL-12 antagonist. As developed further in the next section, epithelial production of IL12 p80 is increased in viral and asthmatic inflammation and specifically contributes to the macrophage component in these conditions.

C. EBI3/p35

EBI3/p35 is a noncovalently linked EBI3/p35 heterodimer with production levels that depend primarily on induction of EBI3 expression. Although this pattern of regulation for EBI3 is similar the one for IL-12 p40, the expression of EBI3 exhibits a broader distribution among cell types. Thus, expression is found in macrophages (within the spleen, tonsil, and colonic tissue from subjects with ulcerative colitis) as well as synciotrophoblasts and extravillous trophoblasts. EBI3/p35 heterodimers are present in whole cell placental extracts, and immunohistochemical colocalization of EBI3 and p35 protein occurs in placental cells. However, EBI3/p35 heterodimer has not been found in primary-culture placental extracts or serum from pregnant women, making its biological function in this setting uncertain (24,83–85). Perhaps more relevant to the present discussion of IL-12 function in the airway, EBI3 mRNA has not been detectable in lungs of normal human subjects, although its possible expression under other conditions remains uncertain.

D. IL-23

IL-23 is a heterodimer composed of covalently linked p19 and p40 subunits and is secreted by dendritic cells. The compound exerts overlapping as well as distinct activities with IL-12. For example, IL-23 and IL-12 can both induce IFN-γ secretion and proliferation in phytohemaglutinin-stimulated T lymphoblasts as well as CD45RO+ memory T cells, but only IL-23 induces proliferation of CD4+CD45Rb^{low} memory T cells (25). Transgenic mice that overexpress p19 develop a phenotype characterized by low body weight, neutrophilia, infertility, systemic inflammation manifested as lymphocyte and macrophage accumulation in multiple organs (including the lung), and early death (86).

IV. Epithelial IL-12 p80 in Viral and Asthmatic Inflammation

As noted above, airway epithelial cells appear specially programmed for expression of immune-response genes, and this programming is typified by IFN-γ–driven Jak/

Stat regulation of the ICAM-1 gene. To better determine how this epithelial system operates in vivo, we analyzed its behavior in mouse models that allow for in vitro versus in vivo comparison and genetic modification. In particular, we are able to compare the behavior of epithelial cells isolated from the mouse airway to the characteristics of mouse airway function in vivo. These experimental comparisons indicated that TNF-α induction of epithelial ICAM-1 required sequential induction of IL-12 and IFN-γ and, unexpectedly, localized IL-12 production to airway epithelial cells (51). These findings indicated that airway epithelial cells may express other signatures of the Th1 pathway (in addition to IFN-γ–driven signal transduction). The findings also raised the possibility that other Th1-linked events may be activated in the epithelium during viral infection and in asthma. We therefore set out to test each of these possibilities using a mouse model of viral bronchiolitis and a standardized protocol for human subjects with asthma.

A. Studies in Mice

Results from murine models of airway inflammation have been reported on numerous occasions and reviewed by us and others (15,87–89). In the present context, we aimed to develop a mouse model to better determine how the airway epithelial system operates in vivo and to subject the system to genetic modification. Because the epithelial system is programmed for antiviral defense, we also aimed for a model with high fidelity to viral bronchiolitis in humans. While RSV is often used for studies of human airway epithelial cells and human subjects, based on its link to childhood asthma, this virus does not cause a similar type of bronchiolitis in the mouse. For that reason, we chose another Paramyxoviridae family member, mouse parainfluenza type I or Sendai virus, based on its capacity as a natural pathogen in rodents to cause top-down infection leading from the nose to the bronchi to the bronchioles to the alveoli. By limiting the inoculum, infection is limited to the airways and so resembles the pathology and pathophysiology of the human condition (20,21,51,90). This pathogenesis is the same as observed in human subjects with paramyxoviral infection and so offers an appropriate model for analysis. Sendai virus also infects isolated human airway epithelial cells, presumably because the allantoic fluid medium provides the Clara cell tryptase that is ordinarily provided by the rodent airway. Thus, heterologous cell systems can be used to validate fidelity to RSV behavior when possible. This section summarizes our initial experience with this model for first identifying gene expression that is prominently inducible in airway epithelial cells during paramyxoviral infection and then determining the response in same-strain mice with targeted mutagenesis of these genes.

Viral Infection Induces IL-12 p40 Expression in Airway Epithelial Cells

In other systems IL-12 is selectively produced by immune cells, especially antigen-presenting cells, and production depends on induction of the IL-12 p40 subunit in the context of constitutive p35 expression (30). However, when we submitted tracheal and lung tissue from TNF-α-treated mice to immunohistochemistry, we found that airway epithelial cells were the predominant site of induction of IL-12 p40 expression. We also found constitutive IL-12 p35 expression in airway epithelial as well as other parenchymal and immune cells. To next determine whether a more natural stimulus of airway inflammation might cause similar upregulation of IL-12 p40 expression, we examined the response to a moderate inoculum of Sendai virus. This inoculum (5000 EID_{50}) causes reversible bronchiolitis with transient epithelial expression of viral protein and mononuclear cell influx that is limited to the adjacent bronchovascular tissue compartment. In this setting we found that induction of IL-12 p40 was again localized to airway epithelial cells, rather than adjacent mononuclear cells, and was colocalized (temporally and spatially) with viral protein expression while constitutive expression of IL-12 p35 remained unchanged in all cell populations (51). Thus, airway epithelial cells (rather than immune cells) appear to be the major cellular source for IL-12 p40 production during airway inflammatory conditions initiated by TNF-α administration or respiratory viral infection.

As noted above, IL-12 production is often (but not always) limited by production of IL-12 p40, so we expected these measurements to track together (as was the case for TNF-α-stimulation experiments). Indeed, this appeared to be the case at early times after viral inoculation when concentrations of IL-12 p40 were relatively low (50 pg/mL) and similar to the range that we observed for TNF-α-stimulation experiments. In addition, however, at later times after SdV inoculation, we observed a marked increase in IL-12 p40 relative to IL-12 levels, so that the ratio of IL-12 p40/p70 was in excess of 75:1. Western blots of BAL fluid indicated that a significant proportion of IL-12 p40 existed as the IL-12 p40 homodimer (designated IL-12 p80).

Increased Mortality and Persistent Airway Inflammation in IL-12 p35–Deficient Mice Following Viral Infection

To define the roles for IL-12 and IL-12 p40 homodimer production during viral bronchitis, we compared wild-type mice to mice rendered deficient in IL-12 p35 (but still capable of IL-12 p40 and p80 generation) versus mice deficient in IL-12 p40 (and so incapable of generating IL-12 or functional IL-12 p40). Following viral inoculation at 5000 EID_{50} we found a trend towards greater weight loss in the p35-deficient animals, and at 50,0000 EID_{50} we observed an increased mortality rate and a persistent viral pneumonia in IL-12 p35 (−/−) mice compared to wild-type and IL-12 p40 (−/−) mice. We found no difference in susceptibility to infection between wild-type and IL-12 p40 (−/−) mice and no differences in viral persistence or histological features of viral pneumonia between these two groups of mice. Similarly, we found no difference in IFN-γ levels in BAL fluid in the presence or absence of IL-12 or IL-12 p40, indicating that Sendai virus infection triggers IFN-γ production pathways that do not depend on IL-12 but may instead depend on IFN-α/β (91). Even if there were differences in IFN-γ production, however, we have also found that IFN-γ (−/−) mice exhibit no increase in susceptibility in this model (20). In these same groups of mice, we found concomitant virus-inducible release of TNF-α, suggesting (as noted above) that TNF-α may help drive IL-12 p40 gene expression in this setting.

IL-12 p40 Overproduction in the p35-Deficient Mouse Causes Airway Macrophage Accumulation

The selective increase in mortality rate for the IL-12 p35 ($-/-$) mice indicated that IL-12 p40 exerts a biological function in the absence of IL-12. Furthermore, postmortem histopathology indicated that organ abnormalities were confined to the lung. To better define the mechanism for how IL-12 p40 expression (in the absence of IL-12) may lead to increased morbidity from viral infection, we next determined the lung levels of IL-12 p40 under these conditions. We found that the increased mortality was associated with increased levels of IL-12 p40 in BAL fluid (Fig. 2A) and serum (data not shown) relative to wild-type mice. These findings indicated that IL-12 and/or IL-12 p35 may prevent overexpression of IL-12 p40 (i.e., negative

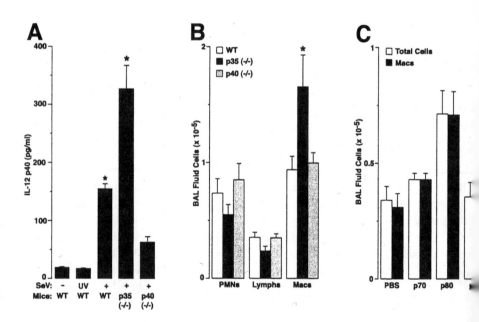

Figure 2 Evidence of IL-12 p40 generation and macrophage recruitment in viral bronchiolitis (A,B) and cytokine administration (C). (A,B) Wild-type (WT) and p35 ($-/-$) mice were inoculated with Sendai virus (SeV) or UV-inactivated virus (SeV-UV), and BAL fluid was analyzed for p40 levels and cell counts. Values represent mean ± SEM ($n = 4$), and a significant difference from the wild-type cohort is indicated by (*). (C) C57BL/6J mice underwent intratracheal injection of PBS vehicle (PBS), IL-12 p70, IL-12 p80, or IL-12 p40 (40 μg/kg). At 18 h after treatment, BAL fluid was analyzed for total cells and macrophages. Values represent mean ± SEM ($n = 3$), and a significant difference from the PBS cohort is indicated by (*). (Modified from Ref. 51.)

feedback). We note that the persistence of low levels of p40 in p40-null mice is likely due to the generation of a nonfunctional p40 fragment as described previously (38), since we observed viral induction of this fragment at least at the mRNA level by RT-PCR. By contrast, IL-12 p80 exhibits selective macrophage chemoattractant activity in vitro and in vivo (80). Consistent with this observation, we detected a selective enrichment in macrophages in BAL fluid (Fig. 2B) and accumulation of macrophages in bronchial and bronchiolar epithelium in IL-12 p35-deficient mice that overproduce IL-12 p80. Quantitation of tissue macrophages more precisely supported these findings. Moreover, as further discussed in Sec. V, neutralization of IL-12 p40 and p80 (by treatment with anti-IL-12 p40 mAb) prevented the enhanced macrophage accumulation in the BAL fluid and reversed the increased mortality in IL-12 p35–deficient mice. Taken together, it appears that epithelial overexpression of IL-12 p80 may cause macrophage accumulation and so contribute to airway inflammation and consequent morbidity during viral bronchitis.

B. Studies in Human Subjects

The results in mice suggest that overexpression of IL-12 p40 by the airway epithelium may lead to airway inflammation. As noted above, we have suggested that abnormal programming of epithelial immune-response genes may serve as a basis for airway inflammation due to asthma (10,23). Accordingly, we next determined the level of IL-12 p40 and p35 expression in endobronchial biopsies and IL-12 and IL-12 p40 levels in BAL fluid obtained from normal versus asthma or chronic bronchitis subjects. In endobronchial biopsies, we found that airway epithelial cell IL-12 p40 expression was present in each of seven asthmatic but none of seven normal or eight chronic bronchitis subjects, whereas IL-12 p40 expression was constitutively expressed in airway epithelial, parenchymal, and inflammatory cells from all groups of subjects (51). In addition, we found that increased epithelial IL-12 p40 expression in asthmatic subjects resulted in increased BAL fluid IL-12 p40 (but not IL-12 p70) concentrations that was unaltered by the concomitant administration of glucocorticoids (Fig. 3A, B). Additional experiments using a glucocorticoid-withdrawal protocol to compare 6 asthmatic subjects to themselves with and without glucocorticoid treatment confirmed the lack of correlation between treatment status and IL-12 p40 levels in BAL fluid (20.5 $\pm$ 8.5 pg/mL and 31.4 = 8.0 pg/mL with and without treatment, respectively; $p > 0.05$). Further analysis of BAL fluid samples indicated that IL-12 p40 appeared to be expressed predominantly as the homodimer (although background in concentrated BAL fluid is necessarily increased) and to correlate with macrophage accumulation (Fig. 3C). The asthmatic BAL fluid IL-12 p40/p70 ratio was elevated relative to normal subjects at a level (mean ratio of 221 $\pm$ 86) similar to the one found in viral bronchitis. Taken together, these data indicate that airway epithelial IL-12 p40 overexpression (particularly as the homodimer) may similarly contribute to airway inflammation in asthmatic subjects as it does during viral infection.

C. IL-12 p80 as a Chemotaxin for Macrophages

To define the relationship between IL-12 p40 and p80 expression and airway macrophage accumulation, we determined the capacity of IL-12 family members to act

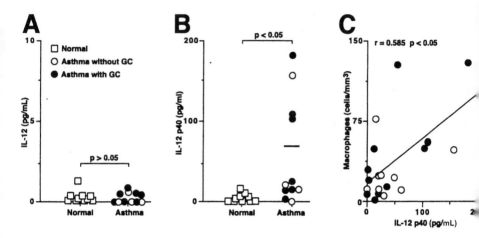

Figure 3 IL-12 p80 expression and macrophage accumulation in asthmatic subjects. (A,B) BAL fluid from 10 normal, 4 asthmatic (treated without glucocorticoids), and 7 asthmatic subjects (treated with glucocorticoids) was concentrated 35-fold and used for duplicate measurements of IL-12 p70 and p40 by ELISA. Bold lines represent mean value and *p*-values (by independent-groups *t*-test) are indicated. (C) Levels of asthmatic BAL fluid p40 concentration are correlated with macrophage accumulation (cells/mm^3), *r* equals correlation coefficient, and *p*-value (by *t*-test for correlation) is indicated. (Modified from Ref. 51.)

as macrophage chemoattractants in vivo and in vitro. For in vivo experiments, we instilled cytokines into the airway of mice and monitored BAL fluid cell counts. We found that intratracheal administration of IL-12 p80 but not IL-12 or p40 caused significant increases in the number of macrophages in BAL fluid (Fig. 2C). For in vitro experiments, we monitored chemotactic responses of thioglycolate-elicited peritoneal macrophages using modified-Boyden chambers. These studies also demonstrated that IL-12 p80 but not IL-12 or p40 caused a concentration-dependent increase in macrophage movement that was nearly equivalent to macrophage chemoattractants such as f-met-leu-phe (fMLP) and and the chemokine JE (the mouse equivalent to human MCP-1) (M. Walter unpublished observations). Furthermore, macrophage migration occurred only in the presence of an established gradient for IL-12 p80, indicative of chemotaxis rather than chemokinesis. Initial studies indicate that p80-induced chemotaxis is blocked by anti-IL-12 receptor β1 (IL-12Rβ1) antibody and in IL-12Rβ1–deficient mice (M. Walter, unpublished observations). Taken together, the findings establish epithelial-derived IL-12 p80 as a biologically active chemoattractant for macrophages via IL-12Rβ1 signaling.

V. IL-12 p80 as a Therapeutic Target in Airway Inflammation

The association of increased IL-12 p80 levels with postviral and asthmatic inflammation has prompted experiments aimed at blocking p80 activity in the setting of airway inflammation. Accordingly, we performed IL-12 p80 neutralization experiments utilizing a schedule of intraperitoneal anti-p40 mAb that accomplished effective IL-12 p40 blockade in BAL fluid for 96 hours (51). As predicted, neutralization of IL-12 p80 and IL-12 p40 resulted in a survival advantage in p35-deficient mice (from 12% survival after treatment with control IgG to 22% with anti-IL-12 p40 mAb compared with 25% in wild-type mice treated with IgG) (Fig. 4). Furthermore, this treatment prevented macrophage accumulation in BAL fluid. We note, however, that all cohorts exhibit higher mortality rates when injected with mAb, IgG, or PBS vehicle compared with uninjected mice, likely reflecting the added stress of intraperitoneal injection procedures during viral bronchopneumonia. Nonetheless, IL-12 p80 blockade during conditions associated with IL-12 p80 overexpression resulted in beneficial anti-inflammatory properties manifested as improved survival and decreased airway macrophage accumulation. These experiments suggest that

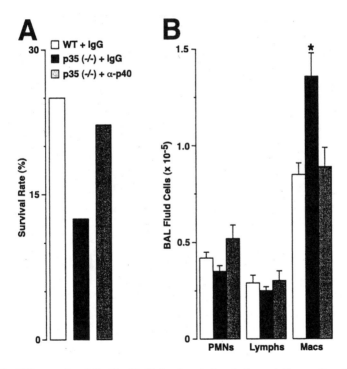

Figure 4 Efficacy of anti-IL-12 p40 Ab in virus-induced airway inflammation. (A) Wild-type (WT) and p35 ($-/-$) mice were inoculated with SdV and treated with rat IgG or rat anti-p40 IgG on days 2 and 6 and monitored for survival ($n = 9$–12 in each group). (B) The same conditions were used, and at post inoculation day 7, BAL fluid cell counts were determined. Values represent mean $\pm$ SEM ($n = 4$), and a significant difference from the wild-type plus IgG is indicated by (*). (Modified from Ref. 51.)

IL-12 p80 is a therapeutic target of airway inflammation for additional disease states associated with p80 overexpression, such as asthma.

A successful therapeutic regimen will correct pathophysiological abnormalities with minimal toxicity. In the particular context of treating asthma, the regimen should prevent airway inflammation while preserving immunity. In the present context, the goal would be to selectively normalize IL-12 p80 levels. This goal is technically challenging, however, since the p40 component is common to IL-12 and IL-23 as well as IL-12 p80. Although nonselective p40 blockade was beneficial in p35-deficient mice during viral bronchiolitis, it is still possible that nonselective blockade of p40 in other settings will immunocompromise the host. Additional studies are underway to determine whether IL-12 p40 blockade will also benefit wild-type mice. More specific strategies include identifying or generating an anti-p80 antibody that does not recognize IL-12 or IL-23. In that regard, it may prove useful to develop an antibody that recognizes the p40-p40 disulfide linked region. It may also be worthwhile to downregulate IL-12 p80 generation, e.g., by modification of a p80-dependent disulfide isomerase, or to increase p80 breakdown to p40 monomers, e.g., by reducing p80 disulfide linkage. Each of these strategies may generate elevated p40 monomer concentrations, but this event should cause few consequences since the biological activity of p40 does not appear to be significant. Further studies of p40 monomer function will be needed to be certain that this is the case.

Additional approaches to downregulating IL-12 p80 action in the airway include targeting p80-dependent signaling pathways or the cellular responses to these pathways. As noted above, an IL-12Rβ1–blocking strategy (e.g., using an anti-IL-12Rβ1 antibody) may inhibit p80-dependent chemotaxis. Because IL-12Rβ1 receptor chain also mediates IL-12 and IL-23 signaling, the effect of blockade may be less specific in vivo. Here again, specific blockade may be achieved by developing antibodies or other reagents that selectively block IL-12 p80/IL-12Rβ1 interaction. Further studies are needed to identify the intracellular proteins that mediate p80-dependent intracellular signaling and any additional macrophage functions, e.g., phagocytosis, oxidative burst, and antigen presentation, that may be linked to p80 signaling and may further promote inflammation.

VI. Implications for Asthma Pathogenesis

Evidence of immune abnormalities and excessive airway inflammation has driven an attempt to define the types of inflammatory cells and mediators that might be responsible for abnormal airway function in asthma. Cell types implicated in the development of asthmatic airway inflammation include immune cells as well as parenchymal cells. Cell-cell interactions are attributed to classes of mediators that include lipids, proteases, peptides, glycoproteins, and cytokines. Similar to the case for allergic rhinitis, the leading scheme for integrating this information has been based on the classification of the adaptive immune system, and especially the responses of Th cells. In this scheme, CD4 + T-cell-dependent responses are classified into Th1 or Th2. Th1 cells characteristically mediate delayed-type hypersensitivity reactions and selectively produce IL-2 and IFN-γ, whereas Th2 cells promote B-cell-dependent humoral immunity and selectively produce IL-4. Thus, as noted above, Th2 reactions may underlie the airway hyperreactivity and inflammation characteristic of the late-response to allergen inhalation and so account for the over-production of Th2-derived cytokines that is characteristic of allergic rhinitis and asthma (92,93).

The traditional proposal for asthma pathogenesis (often designated the Th2 hypothesis) is therefore similar to the one for allergic rhinitis and other allergic disease (6). Each scheme is based on a relative increase in Th2 cellular responses in combination with a decrease in Th1 responses (often linked to the so-called hygiene hypothesis whereby fewer infections lead to a less robust Th1 system). The consequent alteration in cytokine milieu, with excess Th2 products (e.g., IL-4, IL-5, and IL-13) and decreased Th1 products (e.g., IFN-γ and IL-12), is predicted to drive the asthma phenotype (as modeled in Fig. 5). Evidence for such a shift in the Th1/Th2 balance derives from studies of asthma in cellular and murine models, where T-helper-cell polarization and allergen-dependence of Th2 responses are most clearly defined and from human studies that profile cytokine production and immune cell infiltrate. Thus, in the murine system, IL-4, IL-5, IL-9, and IL-13 promote Th2 cell differentiation and B-cell-dependent IgE production, tissue eosinophilia, mucous cell hyperplasia, and airway hyperreactivity (94–97). Furthermore, these responses are downregulated by Th1 cytokines such as IFN-γ and IL-12 (62,98). In humans, asthma is tied to this paradigm by association with atopy and increased production of IgE and Th2 cell cytokines, as well as genetic linkage to polymorphisms in the IgE receptor, IL-4, IL-4 receptor, and IL-13 genes (93,99–101). Similarly, eosinophils and mast cells are characteristic of upper and lower airway inflammation (92,102,103) and may act as critical effector cells at least under some circumstances (104,105).

How then can a Th2-polarized response account for asthma that is also triggered by exposure to nonallergic stimuli (especially respiratory viruses) that would ordinarily trigger a Th1 response? Based on the likelihood that Th2-skewed responses may develop in this setting as well (106–108), it is possible that a Th2-dominant response may mediate inflammation and hyperreactivity in response to nonallergic stimuli as well (see Fig. 5). However, this dichotomous view of the immune response may not be completely accurate, since there is often ambiguity in the type of Th response triggered by most stimuli as well as significant cross-regulation between the two types of responses (88). In fact, recent studies in mice using adoptive transfer with Th1 and Th2 cells have indicated that Th1 cells may even be required for allergic inflammation (109–111). Presumably, this Th1 involvement is based on superior trafficking ability of these cells into (airway) tissue compared to Th2 counterparts and the consequent establishment of an inflammatory milieu that is conductive to Th2 recruitment during allergen exposure (Fig. 5B). Respiratory viruses might then influence allergic inflammation by increasing Th1 activity and so also be able to increase subsequent allergic inflammation.

Each of these traditional proposals for asthma pathogenesis relies on the possibility that excessive production of Th2 cytokines is responsible for driving the asthma

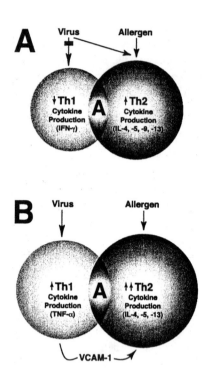

Figure 5   Scheme for the role of the airway immune response in the development of asthmatic airway inflammation. (A) Decreases in virus-driven production of Th1 cytokines (e.g., IFN-γ) and increases in allergen-dependent production of Th2 cytokines (e.g., IL-4, IL-5, IL-9, and IL-13) are characteristic of asthma (designated as "A"). This Th2-skewed setting thereby provides for flares of the disease driven either by virus infection (with a functional blockade in the normal Th1 response and a concomitant shift to an increase in the Th2 response) or by allergen (with an increase in the Th2 response). (B) A modified scheme based on an increased activity of both Th1 and Th2 responses. In this case, pathogen-activated Th1 cells in the airway tissue generate factors (e.g., TNF-α) that mediate subsequent recruitment of Th2 cells (e.g., via VCAM-1) that provide a setting for enhanced allergen responsiveness. (Modified from Ref. 110.)

phenotype. However, several lines of evidence in model systems and in humans raise questions for the Th2 hypothesis as a sole explanation for asthma. First, as noted above, asthma and allergy do not correlate completely in human subjects. Subjects with allergy do not always develop asthma, and subjects with asthma do not have an absolute requirement for developing allergy. In fact, endpoints of the asthmatic phenotype, such as airway hyperreactivity and mucus production, may develop without IgE production and eosinophil influx in experimental models and in asthmatic subjects (88,95,112,113). Second, the Th1 response and the antiviral response in general are incompletely characterized in human airways, and much of the commentary about these responses is extrapolated from experimental models or observations of tissues other than the airway. In addition, the possible primary role of viral infection in causing, as well as triggering, asthma is poorly characterized. Thus, the relationship between RSV bronchiolitis and the subsequent development of childhood asthma still needs to be defined. Third, in model systems and in humans, the Th2 hypothesis is confined to the adaptive immune response and so does not account for components of the innate immune system (e.g., airway epithelial cells) that may take an active and critical role in airway inflammation. Because of these uncertainties, we have questioned whether other aspects of immunity and inflammation might also be critical for the pathogenesis of airway disease. In particular, we aimed to develop a model that better accounted for the dissociation between the development of allergy and asthma in many subjects and was based on a more precise appraisal of the Th1 system and the innate immune response in the airway.

One particular deficiency of the Th2 hypothesis is that it does not account for the possibility that the airway epithelial cells may act as active sentinels of innate immunity, and so, like other components of the innate immune system, may provide critical signals to the adaptive immune system. In fact, studies of airway epithelial cells over the past 20 years now indicate that they are specially programmed to mediate host defense and are abnormally programmed in airway disease (reviewed in Ref. 5). In the case of host defense, studies proceeded from a relatively simple scheme for leukocyte recruitment (based on cell adhesion and chemoattraction) to one that depends on the coordinated expression of a network of epithelial immune-response genes under distinct transcriptional and posttranscriptional controls. The transcriptional program depends primarily on interferon-Jak/Stat signaling while posttranscriptional regulation uses a distinct RNA-protein interaction that is responsive directly to viral replication (7–9,11,12,14,16).

Perhaps even more striking is that the same pathways that appear appropriate for antiviral immunity are also activated in asthma even in the apparent absence of viral infection. For example, selective activation of Stat1 in the airway epithelium is an invariant feature of asthma (23). Since Stat1 activation is not dependent on cytokine (i.e., IFN-γ) production in this setting, the findings point to a signaling abnormality, likely in the upstream kinases or downstream phosphatases that regulate Stat1 phosphorylation/activation status. Other epithelial behavior typical of the anti-paramyxoviral response is also found in asthmatic subjects. Thus, epithelial IL-12 p40 is expressed in a pattern that resembles the response to experimental paramyxoviral infection (51). These epithelial programs are activated in subjects with asthma despite symptomatic control with glucocorticoid treatment. However, other programs are activated in asthmatic subjects with exacerbations following withdrawal of glucocorticoid treatment. Thus, increased expression of epithelial RANTES may be found in these subjects and correlates with increases in symptoms, inflammation, and airway obstruction and hyperreactivity (10) (M. Castro and M.J. Holtzman, unpublished observations).

To integrate these concepts and so better explain the pathogenesis of airway inflammatory disease, we have revised the model for the role of the airway immune response in asthma. The revised model accounts for how an alternative Th1-oriented epithelial network may act in combination with an enhanced Th2 response, and the combination of epithelial, viral, and allergic components led to its designation as an Epi-Vir-All paradigm (Fig. 6). In this scheme, increases in epithelial antiviral signals (e.g., Stat1 activation and IL-12 p40 expression) and allergen-driven production of Th2 cytokines (e.g., IL-4, IL-5, IL-9, and IL-13) are characteristic of subjects with asthma under stable conditions during treatment with inhaled glucocorticoids. Further increases in epithelial signaling (driven by viral infection) or Th2 cytokine production (driven by further allergen exposure) would develop in subjects with asthma during a flare of the disease. In addition, increased levels of Stat1 activity may mediate a hypersensitive Th1-type response in the airway. At least in vitro, persistent Stat1 activation leads to exaggerated Stat1-dependent gene expression in response to normal levels of stimulation (Y. Zhang, and M. J. Holtzman, unpublished observations). In addition, flares of the disease are closely associated with induction of RANTES gene expression. This system, which appears to be regulated at the

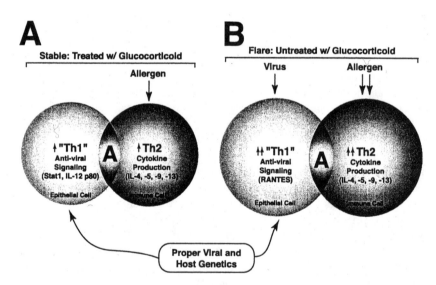

Figure 6 Revised model for the role of the airway immune response in the development of airway inflammation and remodeling. (A) Increases in epithelial antiviral signals (e.g., Stat1 activation and IL-12 p40 expression) and allergen-driven production of Th2 cytokines (e.g., IL-4, IL-5, and IL-13) are characteristic of subjects with asthma (designated as an "A") studied under stable conditions during treatment with inhaled glucocorticoids. (B) Further increases in epithelial signaling (driven by viral infection) or Th2 cytokine production (driven by further allergen exposure) may develop in subjects with asthma studied during a flare without glucocorticoid treatment. The abnormality in epithelial cell behavior may depend on specific genetic properties of the virus as well as proper genetic background of the host. The combination of epithelial, viral, and allergic components led to designation of this pathogenesis model as an Epi-Vir-All paradigm. (Modified from Ref. 5.)

posttranscriptional level during viral infection, may rely on a similar regulatory mechanism in asthmatic flares.

Each of these possibilities begs the question as to how the abnormality in epithelial cell behavior originally develops in asthma. In that context, we questioned whether the antiviral response could persist, and if so, how? In fact, a relationship between viral infection and the development of chronic inflammatory disease has been proposed for diverse clinical syndromes, but the basis for this relationship is often uncertain. In the particular context of asthma, paramyxoviral infections are the leading cause of lower respiratory tract illness in infants and young children (114,115). In addition, children with clinically significant viral bronchiolitis appear to be marked for the subsequent development of a chronic wheezing illness that is independent of allergy (116–118). Presumably paramyxoviral infection triggers a switch to an abnormal host response, since paramyxoviruses (or other respiratory RNA viruses) are not thought to persist in airway tissue as a cause of chronic respiratory disease (119). With or without viral persistence, however, the role of specific host factors in the development of chronic wheezing or lifelong asthma has not been determined. In ongoing work, we have observed that transient paramyxoviral infection causes not only acute but also chronic manifestations of the asthma phenotype in some genetic backgrounds (M. Walter, J. Morton, E. Agapov, and M. Holtzman, unpublished observations). Initial observations were obtained in a mouse model of viral bronchiolitis, but the same phenotypic markers appear in human subjects with asthma (J. Morton, M. Castro, and M. Holtzman, unpublished observations). Taken together, the findings raise the exciting possibility that asthma may not only be characterized by a persistent antiviral response but may even be caused by such a response. Further studies of this system using inbred mice will allow for molecular definition of genetic susceptibility and then extension to studies of human subjects.

VII. Summary

The role of the epithelium has evolved from a relatively simple scheme for mediating leukocyte recruitment to one that depends on the coordinated expression of a network of epithelial immune-response genes coordinated for host defense under distinct transcriptional and posttranscriptional controls. The transcriptional program is typified by an interferon-driven Jak/Stat signaling pathway, while posttranscriptional regulation uses RNA-protein interactions that are responsive directly to viral replication. Respiratory viruses ordinarily interact with this Th1-style gene network in a battle of host defense versus immune subversion, but the same network is also activated in asthma even in the absence of overt viral infection. Thus, the barrier epithelial cell population appears specially programmed for normal host defense but abnormally programmed in inflammatory airway disease. Consistent with this concept, we have used a new model of viral bronchiolitis to show that epithelial expression of IL-12 p80 may help mediate postviral inflammation that is characterized by macrophage recruitment to the airway. Similar events are found in asthmatic subjects. Together, this information defines IL-12 p80 as a new therapeutic target in these conditions. Recent results in the same model and in human subjects also indicate that airway epithelial cells may be reprogrammed for permanent proliferation and skewed mucus cell differentiation by asthmagenic RNA viruses that cause effects even after viral clearance. This alteration in the epithelial repair process exhibits genetic susceptibility and so appears analogous to abnormal mucosal phenotypes in asthma and other hypersecretory diseases. These concepts can be integrated into a scheme that incorporates epithelial, viral, and allergic components (designated an Epi-Vir-All paradigm) for a more complete explanation of the pathogenesis of airway disease. By extension, the same epithelial network is a target for therapy in airway disease and for improving host defense against respiratory viruses.

Acknowledgments

Our work was supported by the National Institutes of Health (Heart, Lung, and Blood Institute), the Martin Schaeffer Fund, and the Alan A. and Edith L. Wolff Charitable Trust.

References

1. Holtzman MJ, Fabbri LM, O'Byrne PM, Gold BD, Aizawa H, Walters EH, Alpert SE, Nadel JA. Importance of airway inflammation for hyperresponsiveness induced by ozone in dogs. Am Rev Respir Dis 1983; 127:686–690.
2. Holtzman MJ, Fabbri LM, Skoogh B-E, O'Byrne PM, Walters EH, Aizawa H, Nadel JA. Time course of airway hyperresponsiveness induced by ozone in dogs. J Appl Physiol 1983; 55:1232–1236.
3. Medzhitov R, Janeway CA, Jr. An ancient system of host defense. Curr Opin Immunol 1998; 10:12–15.
4. Holtzman MJ, Castro M, Look DC, O'Sullivan M, Walter MJ. Regulation of epithelial-leukocyte interaction and epithelial immune-response genes. In: Busse WW, Holgate ST, eds. Asthma and Rhinitis. Cambridge, MA: Blackwell Scientific, 2000:784–800.
5. Holtzman MJ, Morton JD, Shornick LP, Tyner JW, O'Sullivan MP, Antao A, Lo M, Castro M, Walter MJ. Immunity, inflammation, and remodeling in the airway epithelial barrier: the epithelial-viral-allergic (epi-vir-all) paradigm. Physiol Rev 2002; 82:19–46.
6. Grayson MH, Holtzman MJ. Lessons from allergic rhinitis versus asthma pathogenesis and treatment. Immunol Allergy Clin N Am 2002; 22: in press.
7. Look DC, Keller BT, Rapp SR, Holtzman MJ. Selective induction of intercellular adhesion molecule-1 by interferon-γ in human airway epithelial cells. Am J Physiol 1992; 263:L79–L87.
8. Nakajima S, Look DC, Roswit WT, Bragdon MJ, Holtzman MJ. Selective differences in vascular endothelial- vs. airway epithelial-T cell adhesion mechanisms. Am J Physiol 1994; 267:L422–L432.
9. Nakajima S, Roswit WT, Look DC, Holtzman MJ. A hierarchy for integrin expression and adhesiveness among T cell subsets that is linked to TCR gene usage and emphasizes V$\delta1^+$ $\gamma\delta$ T cell adherence and tissue retention. J Immunol 1995; 155:1117–1131.

10. Taguchi M, Sampath D, Koga T, Castro M, Look DC, Nakajima S, Holtzman MJ. Patterns for RANTES secretion and intercellular adhesion molecule-1 expression mediate transepithelial T cell traffic based on analyses in vitro and in vivo. J Exp Med 1998; 187:1927–1940.

11. Look DC, Pelletier MR, Holtzman MJ. Selective interaction of a subset of interferon-γ response element binding proteins with the intercellular adhesion molecule-1 (ICAM-1) gene promoter controls the pattern of expression on epithelial cells. J Biol Chem 1994; 269:8952–8958.

12. Look DC, Pelletier MR, Tidwell RM, Roswit WT, Holtzman MJ. Stat1 depends on transcriptional synergy with Sp1. J Biol Chem 1995; 270:30264–30267.

13. Walter MJ, Look DC, Tidwell RM, Roswit WT, Holtzman MJ. Targeted inhibition of interferon-γ-dependent ICAM-1 expression using dominant-negative Stat1. J Biol Chem 1997; 272:28582–28589.

14. Look DC, Roswit WT, Frick AG, Gris-Alevy Y, Dickhaus DM, Walter MJ, Holtzman MJ. Direct suppression of Stat1 function during adenoviral infection. Immunity 1998; 9:871–880.

15. Holtzman MJ, Look DC, Sampath D, Castro M, Koga T, Walter MJ. Control of epithelial immune-response genes and implications for airway immunity and inflammation. Proc Assoc Am Phys 1998; 110:1–11.

16. Koga T, Sardina E, Tidwell RM, Pelletier MR, Look DC, Holtzman MJ. Virus-inducible expression of a host chemokine gene relies on replication-linked mRNA stabilization. Proc Natl Acad Sci USA 1999; 96:5680–5685.

17. Thanos D, Maniatis T. Virus induction of human IFNβ gene expression requires the assembly of an enhanceosome. Cell 1995; 83:1091–1100.

18. Kurt-Jones EA, Popova L, Kwinn L, et al. Pattern recognition receptors TLR4 and CD14 mediate response to respiratory syncytial virus. Nat Immunol 2000; 1:398–401.

19. Walter MJ, Kajiwara N, Sampath D, Rucker J, Holtzman MJ. Induction of epithelial immune-response genes in a mouse model of viral bronchitis and hyperreactivity. FASEB J 1998; 12:A1453.

20. Walter MJ, Kajiwara N, Sampath D, Rucker J, Xia D, Holtzman MJ. Epithelial immune-response gene expression during viral bronchitis and hyperreactivity in wild-type and IFN-γ-deficient mice. Am J Respir Crit Care Med 1999; 159:A437.

21. Walter MJ, Kajiwara N, Holtzman MJ. Diminished airway inflammation and hyperreactivity in ICAM-1-deficient mice during primary viral bronchitis. Am J Respir Crit Care Med 2000; 161:A778.

22. Shornick LP, Briner DM, Lo MS, and Holtzman MJ. Role of Stat1 in defense against respiratory viruses. Proc Keystone Symp Mol Aspects Viral Immun 2001; 56.

23. Sampath D, Castro M, Look DC, Holtzman MJ. Constitutive activation of an epithelial signal transducer and activator of transcription (Stat1) pathway in asthma. J Clin Invest 1999; 103:1353–1361.

24. Devergne O, Hummel M, Koeppen H, Le Beau M, Nathanson E, Kieff E, Birkenbach M. A novel interleukin-12 p40 related protein induced by latent Epstein-Barr virus infection in B lymphocytes. J Virol 1996; 70:1143–1153.

25. Oppmann B, Lesley R, Blom B, et al. Novel p19 protein engages IL-12p40 to form a cytokine, IL-23, with biologic activities similar as well as distinct from IL-12. Immunity 2000; 13:715–725.

26. Wolf SF, Temple PA, Kobayashi M, et al. Cloning of cDNA for natural killer cell stimulatory factor, a heterodimer cytokine with multiple biologic effects on T and natural killer cells. J Immunol 1991; 146:3074–3081.

27. Gubler U, Chua AO, Schoenhaut DS, et al. Coexpression of two distinct genes is required to generate secreted bioactive cytotoxic lymphocyte maturation factor. Proc Natl Acad Sci USA 1991; 88:4143–4147.

28. Kobayashi M, Fitz L, Ryan M, et al. Identification and purification of natural killer cell stimulatory factor (NKSF), a cytokine with multiple biologic effects on human lymphocytes. J Exp Med 1989; 170:827–845.

29. Stern AS, Podlaski FJ, Hulmes JD, et al. Purification to homogeneity and partial characterization of cytotoxic lymphocyte maturation factor from human B-lymphoblastoid cells. Proc Natl Acad Sci USA 1990; 87:6808–6812.

30. Trinchieri G, Scott P. Interleukin-12: basic principles and clinical applications. Curr Topics Microbiol Immunol 1999; 238:57–78.

31. Hsieh CS, Macatonia SE, Tripp CS, Wolf SF, O'Garra A, Murphy KM. Development of TH1 CD4$^+$ T cells through IL-12 produced by *Listeria*-induced macrophages. Science 1993; 260:547–554.

32. Manetti R, Parronchi P, Giudizi MG, Piccinni MP, Maggi E, Trinchieri G, Romagnani S. Natural killer cell stimulatory factor (interleukin 12 [IL-12]) induces T helper type 1 (TH1)-specific immune responses and inhibits the development of IL-4-producing Th cells. J Exp Med 1993; 177:1199–1204.

33. Giese NA, Gazzinelli RT, Actor JK, Morawetz RA, Sarzotti M, Morse HC. Retrovirus-elicited interleukin-12 and tumor necrosis factor-α as inducers of interferon-γ-mediated pathology in mouse AIDS. Immunol 1996; 87:467–474.

34. Halpern MD, Kurlander RJ, Pisetsky DS. Bacterial DNA induces murine interferon-γ production by stimulation of interleukin-12 and tumor necrosis factor-α. Cell Immunol 1996; 167:72–78.

35. Tripp CS, Wolf SF, Unanue ER. Interleukin 12 and tumor necrosis factor α are costimulators of interferon γ production by natural killer cells in severe combined immunodeficiency mice with listeriosis, and interleukin 10 is a physiologic antagonist. Proc Natl Acad Sci USA 1993; 90:3725–3729.

36. Morris SC, Madden KB, Adamovicz JJ, Gause WC, Hubbard BR, Gately MK, Finkelman FD. Effects of IL-12 on in vivo cytokine gene expression and Ig isotype selection. J Immunol 1994; 152:1047–1056.

37. Car BD, Eng VM, Schnyder B, et al. Role of interferon-γ in interleukin 12-induced pathology in mice. Am J Pathol 1995; 147:1693–1707.

38. Magram J, Connaughton SE, Warrier RR, et al. IL-12-deficient mice are defective in IFN-γ production and type 1 cytokine responses. Immunity 1996; 4:471–481.

39. Mattner F, Magram J, Ferrante J, Launois P, Di Padova K, Behin R, Gately MK, Louis JA, Alber G. Genetically resistant mice lacking interleukin-12 are susceptible to infection with *Leishmania major* and mount a polarized Th2 cell response. Eur J Immunol 1996; 26:1553–1559.

40. Altare F, Durandy A, Lammas D, et al. Impairment of mycobacterial immunity in human interleukin-12 receptor deficiency. Science 1998; 280:1432–1435.

41. Wu C, Ferrante J, Gately MK, Magram J. Characterization of IL-12 receptor β1 chain (IL-12Rβ1)-deficient mice: IL-12Rβ1 is an essential component of the functional mouse IL-12 receptor. J Immunol 1997; 159:1658–1665.

42. de Jong RD, Altare F, Haagen I, et al. Severe mycobacterial and *Salmonella* infections in interleukin-12 receptor deficient patients. Science 1998; 280:1435–1438.

43. Decken K, Kohler G, Palmer-Lehman K, Wunderlin A, Mattner F, Magram J, Gately MK, Alber G. Interleukin-12 is essential for a protective Th1 response in mice infected with *Cryptococcus neoformans*. Infect Immun 1998; 66:4994–5000.

44. Flynn JL, Goldstein MM, Triebold KJ, Sypek J, Wolf S, Bloom BR. IL-12 increases resistance of BALB/c mice to *Mycobacterium tuberculosis* infection. J Immunol 1995; 155:2515–2524.

45. Stevenson MM, Tam MF, Wolf SF, Sher A. IL-12-induced protection against blood-stage *Plasmodium chabaudi* requires IFN-γ and TNF-α and occurs via a nitric oxide-dependent mechanism. J Immunol 1995; 155:2545–2556.

46. Greenberger MJ, Kunkel SL, Strieter RM, et al. IL-12 gene therapy protects mice in lethal *Klebsiella* pneumonia. J Immunol 1996; 157:3006–3012.

47. Zhou P, Sieve MC, Bennett J, Kwon-Chung K, Tewari RP, Gazzinelli RT, Sher A, Seder R. IL-12 prevents mortality in mice infected with *Histoplasma capsulatum* through induction of IFN-γ. J Immunol 1995; 155:785–795.

48. Gazzinelli RT, Hieny S, Wynn TA, Wolf S, Sher A. Interleukin 12 is required for the T-lymphocyte-independent induction of interferon-γ by an intracellular parasite and induces resistance in T-cell deficient hosts. Proc Natl Acad Sci USA 1993; 90: 6115–6119.

49. Schijns VECJ, Haagmans BL, Wierda CMH, Kruithof B, Heijnen AFM, Alber G, Horzinek MC. Mice lacking IL-12 develop polarized Th1 cells during viral infection. J Immunol 1998; 160:3958–3964.

50. Oxenius A, Karrer U, Zinkernagel RM, Hengartner H. IL-12 is not required for induction of type 1 cytokine responses in viral infections. J Immunol 1999; 162:965–973.

51. Walter MJ, Kajiwara N, Karanja P, Castro M, Holtzman MJ. IL-12 p40 production by barrier epithelial cells during airway inflammation. J Exp Med 2001; 193:339–352.

52. Piccotti JR, Chan SY, Ferrantee J, Magram J, Eichwald EJ, Bishop DK. Alloantigen-reactive Th1 development in IL-12-deficient mice. J Immunol 1998; 160:1132–1138.

53. Heinzel FP, Schoenhaut DS, Rerko RM, Rosser LE, Gately MK. Recombinant interleukin 12 cures mice infected with *Leishmania major*. J Exp Med 1993; 177:1505–1509.

54. Sypek JP, Chung CL, Mayor SEH, Subramanyam JM, Goldman SJ, Sieburth DS, Wolf SF, Schaub RG. Resolution of cutaneous leishmaniasis: interleukin 12 initiates a protective T helper type 1 immune response. J Exp Med 1993; 177:1797–1802.

55. Bi Z, Quandt P, Komatsu T, Barna M, Reiss CS. IL-12 promotes enhanced recovery from vesicular stomatitis virus infection of the central nervous system. J Immunol 1995; 155:5684–5689.

56. Ozmen L, Aguet M, Trinchieri G, Garotta G. The in vivo antiviral activity of interleukin-12 is mediated by gamma interferon. J Virol 1995; 69:8147–8150.

57. Schijns VECJ, Wierda CMH, van Hoeji M, Horzinek MC. Exacerbated viral hepatitis in IFN-γ receptor-deficient mice not suppressed by IL-12. J Immunol 1996; 157: 815–821.

58. Komatsu T, Reiss C. IFN-γ is not required in the IL-12 response to vesicular stomatitis virus infection of the olfactory bulb. J Immunol 1997; 159:3444–3452.

59. Carr JA, Rogerson J, Mulqueen MJ, Roberts NA, Booth RFG. Interleukin-12 exhibits potent antiviral activity in experimental herpesvirus infections. J Virol 1997; 71: 7799–7803.

60. van den Broek M, Bachmann MF, Kohler G, Barner M, Escher R, Zinkernagel R, Kopf M. IL-4 and IL-10 antagonize IL-12-mediated protection against acute vaccinia virus infection with a limited role of IFN-γ and nitric oxide synthetase 2. J Immunol 2000; 164:371–378.

61. Orange JS, Wolf SF, Biron CA. Effects of IL-12 on the response and susceptibility to experimental viral infections. J Immunol 1994; 152:1253–1264.

62. Gavett SH, O'Hearn DJ, Li X, Huang S-K, Finkelman FD, Wills-Karp M. Interleukin 12 inhibits antigen-induced airway hyperresponsiveness, inflammation, and Th2 cytokine expression in mice. J Exp Med 1995; 182:1527–1536.

63. Kips JC, Bursselle GJ, Joos GF, Peleman RA, Tavernier JH, Devos RR, Pauwels RA. Interleukin-12 inhibits antigen-induced airway hyperresponsiveness in mice. Am J Resp Crit Care Med 1996; 153:535–539.

64. Iwamoto I, Kumano K, Kasai M, Kurasawa K, Nakao A. Interleukin-12 prevents antigen-induced eosinophil recruitment into mouse airways. Am J Resp Crit Care Med 1996; 154:1257–1260.

65. Schwartz J, Hemelmann E, Cieslewicz G, Tomkinson A, Joetham A, Bradley K, Gelfand EW. Local treatment with IL-12 is an effective inhibitor of airway hyperresponsiveness and lung eosinophilia after airway challenge in sensitized mice. J Allergy Clin Immunol 1998; 102:86–93.

66. Keane-Myers A, Wysocka M, Trinchieri G, Wills-Karp M. Resistance to antigen-induced airway hyperresponsiveness requires endogenous production of IL-12. J Immunol 1998; 161:919–926.

67. Gately MK, Renzetti LM, Magram J, Stern AS, Adorini L, Gubler U, Presky DH. The interleukin-12/interleukin-12-receptor system: role in normal and pathologic immune responses. Annu Rev Immunol 1998; 16:495–521.

68. Zhao LL, Linden A, Sjostrand M, Cui ZH, Lotvall J. IL-12 regulates bone marrow eosinophilia and airway eotaxin levels induced by airway allergen exposure. Allergy 2000; 55:749–756.

69. Wang S, Fan Y, Han X, Yang J, Bilenki L, Yang X. IL-12-dependent vascular cell adhesion molecule-1 expression contributes to airway eosinophilic inflammation in a mouse model of asthma-like reaction. J Immunol 2001; 166:2741–2749.

70. Bryan SA, O'Connor BJ, Matti S, et al. Effects of recombinant human interleukin-12 on eosinophils, airway hyperresponsiveness, and the late asthmatic response. Lancet 2000; 356:2149–2153.

71. Naseer T, Minshall EM, Leung DYM, Laberge S, Ernst P, Martin RJ, Hamid Q. Expression of IL-12 and IL-13 mRNA in asthma and their modulation in response to steroid therapy. Am J Respir Crit Care Med 1997; 155:845–851.

72. Gillessen S, Carvajal D, Ling P, et al. Mouse interleukin-12 (IL-12) p40 homodimer: a potent IL-12 antagonist. Eur J Immunol 1995; 25:200–206.

73. Heinzel FP, Hujer AM, Ahmed FN, Rerko RM. In vivo production and function of IL-12 p40 homodimers. J Immunol 1997; 158:4381–4388.

74. Wang X, Wilkinson VI, Podlaski FJ, Wu C, Stern AS, Presky DH, Magram J. Characterization of mouse interleukin-12 p40 homodimer binding to the interleukin-12 receptor subunits. Eur J Immunol 1999; 29:2007–2013.

75. Mattner F, Ozmen L, Podlaski F, Wilkinson VL, Presky DH, Gately MK, Alber G. Treatment with homodimeric interleukin-1 (IL-12) p40 protects mice from IL-12-dependent shock but not from tumor necrosis factor alpha-dependent shock. Infection Immunity 1997; 65:4734–4737.

76. Yoshimoto T, Wang C-R, Yoneto T, Waki S, Sunaga S, Komagata Y, Mitsuyama M, Miyazaki J, Nariuchi H. Reduced T helper 1 responses in IL-12 p40 transgenic mice. J Immunol 1998; 160:588–594.

77. Lehmann J, Bellman S, Werner C, Schroder R, Schutze N, Alber G. IL-12 p40-dependent agonistic effects on the development of protective innate and adaptive immunity against *Salmonella enteritidis*. J Immunol 2001; 167:5304–5315.

78. Carr J, Rogerson JA, Mulqueen MJ, Roberts NA, Nash AA. The role of endogenous interleukin-12 in resistance to murine cytomegalovirus (MCMV) infection and a novel action for endogenous IL-12 p40. J Interferon Cytokine Res 1999; 19:1145–1152.

79. Kopp T, Kieffer D, Rot A, Strommer S, Stingl G, Kupper TS. Inflammatory skin disease in K14/p40 transgenic mice: evidence for interleukin-12-like activities of p40. J Invest Dermatol 2001; 117:618–626.

80. Ha SJ, Lee CH, Lee SB, Kim. CM, Jang KL, Shin HS, Sung YC. A novel function of IL-12 p40 as a chemotactic molecule for macrophages. J Immunol 1999; 163: 2902–2908.

81. Pahan K, Sheikh FG, Liu X, Hilger S, McKinney M, Petro TM. Induction of nitric-oxide synthase and activation of NF-κB by interleukin-12 p40 in microglial cells. J Biol Chem 2001; 276:7899–7905.

82. Chen L, Chen D, Block E, O'Donnell M, Kufe DW, Clinton SK. Eradication of murine bladder carcinoma by intratumor injection of a bicistronic adenoviral vector carrying cDNAs for the IL-12 heterodimer and its inhibition by the IL-12 p40 subunit homodimer. J Immunol 1997; 159:351–359.

83. Devergne O, Birkenbach M, Kieff E. Epstein-Barr virus-induced gene 3 and the p35 subunit of interleukin 12 form a novel heterodimeric hematopoietin. Proc Natl Acad Sci USA 1997; 94:12041–12046.

84. Christ AD, Stevens AC, Koeppen H, Walsh S, Omata F, Devergne O, Birkenbach M, Blumberg RS. An interleukin 12-related cytokine is up-regulated in ulcerative colitis but not Crohn's disease. Gastroenterology 1998; 115:307–313.

85. Devergne O, Coulomb-L'Hermine A, Capel F, Moussa M, Capron F. Expression of Epstein-Barr virus-induced gene 3, an interleukin-12 p40-related molecule, throughout human pregnancy. Am J Pathol 2001; 159:1763–1776.

86. Wiekowski MT, Leach MW, Evans EW, et al. Ubiquitous transgenic expression of the IL-23 subunit p19 induces multiorgan inflammation, runting, infertility, and premature death. J Immunol 2001; 166:7563–7570.

87. Drazen JM, Arm JP, Austen KF. Sorting out the cytokines of asthma. J Exp Med 1996; 183:1–5.

88. Holtzman MJ, Sampath D, Castro M, Look DC, Jayaraman S. The one-two of T helper cells: does interferon-γ knockout the Th2 hypothesis for asthma? Am J Respir Cell Mol Biol 1996; 14:316–318.

89. Holtzman MJ, Look DC, Iademarco MF, Dean DC, Sampath D, Castro M. Asthma. In: Jameson JL, ed. Principles of Molecular Medicine. Totawa, NJ: Humana Press, 1998:319–327.

90. Walter MJ, Kajiwara N, Xia D, Holtzman MJ. Early-phase innate immunity and late-phase remodeling of the epithelium during primary viral bronchitis and hyprreactivity. J Invest Med 1999; 47:256A.

91. Cousens LP, Peterson R, Hsu S, Dorner A, Altman JD, Ahmed R, Biron CA. Two roads diverged: interferon α/β- and interleukin 12-mediated pathways in promoting T cell interferon γ responses during viral infection. J Exp Med 1999; 189:1315–1327.

92. Poston RN, Chanez P, Lacoste JY, Litchfield T, Lee TH, Bousquet J. Immunohisto-chemical characterization of the cellular infiltration in asthmatic bronchi. Am Rev Respir Dis 1992; 145:918–921.

93. Ying S, Durham SR, Corrigan CJ, Hamid Q, Kay AB. Phenotype of cells expressing mRNA for TH2-type (interleukin 4 and interleukin 5) and TH1-type (interleukin 2 and interferon γ) cytokines in bronchoalveolar lavage and bronchial biopsies from atopic asthmatic and normal control subjects. Am J Respir Cell Mol Biol 1995; 12:477–487.

94. Coyle AJ. Interleukin-4 is required for the induction of lung Th2 mucosal immunity. Am J Respir Cell Mol Biol 1995; 13:54–59.

95. Wills-Karp M, Luyimbazi J, Xu X, Schofield B, Neben TY, Karp CL, Donaldson DD. Interleukin-13: central mediator of allergic asthma. Science 1998; 282:2258–2261.

96. Grunig G, Warnock M, Wakil AE, et al. Requirement for IL-13 independently of IL-4 in experimental asthma. Science 1998; 282:2261–2263.

97. Webb DC, McKenzie ANJ, Koskinen AML, Yang M, Mattes J, Foster PS. Integrated signals between IL-13, IL-4, and IL-5 regulate airways hyperreactivity. J Immunol 2000; 165:108–113.

98. Lack G, Bradley KL, Hamelmann E, Renz H, Loader J, Leung DYM, Larsen GL, Gelfand EW. Nebulized IFN-γ inhibits the development of secondary allergic responses in mice. J Immunol 1996; 157:1432–1439.

99. Burrows B, Martinez FD, Halonen M, Barbee RA, Cline MG. Association of asthma with serum IgE levels and skin-test reactivity to allergens. N Engl J Med 1989; 320: 271–277.

100. Kay AB. Allergy and allergic diseases. N Engl J Med 2001; 344:30–37.

101. Ober C, Moffatt MF. Contributing factors to the pathobiology. The genetics of asthma. Clin Chest Med 2000; 21:245–261.

102. Broide DH, Gleich GJ, Cuomo AJ, Coburn DA, Federman EC, Schwartz LB, Wasserman SI. Evidence of ongoing mast cell and eosinophil activation in symptomatic asthma airway. J Allergy Clin Immunol 1991; 88:637–648.

103. Bentley A, Jacobson M, Cumberworth V, Barkans J, Moqbel R, Schwartz L, Irani A, Kay A, Durham S. Immunohistology of the nasal mucosa in seasonal allergic rhinitis: increases in activated eosinophils and epithelial mast cells. J Allergy Clin Immunol 1992; 89:877–883.

104. Williams CMM, Galli SJ. Mast cells can amplify airway reactivity and features of chronic inflammation in an asthma model in mice. J Exp Med 2000; 192:455–462.

105. Bandeira-Melo C, Herbst A, Weller PF. Eotaxins. Contributing to the diversity of eosinophil recruitment and activation. Am J Respir Cell Mol Biol 2001; 24:653–657.

106. Coyle AJ, Erard F, Bertrand C, Walti S, Pircher H, Le Gros G. Virus-specific CD8⁺ cells can switch to interleukin 5 production and induce airway eosinophilia. J Exp Med 1995; 181:1229–1233.

107. Srikiatkhachorn A, Braciale TJ. Virus-specific CD8⁺ T lymphocytes downregulate T helper cell type 2 cytokine secretion and pulmonary eosinophilia during experimental murine respiratory syncytial virus infection. J Exp Med 1997; 186:421–432.

108. Johnson TR, Johnson JE, Roberts SR, Wertz GW, Parker RA, Graham BS. Priming with secreted glycoprotein G of respiratory syncytial virus (RSV) augments interleukin-5 production and tissue eosinophilia after RSV challenge. J Virol 1998; 72:2871–2880.

109. Randolph DA, Stephens R, Carruthers CJL, Chaplin DD. Cooperation between Th1 and Th2 cells in a murine model of eosinophilic airway inflammation. J Clin Invest 1999; 104:1021–1029.

110. Castro M, Walter MJ, Chaplin DD, Holtzman MJ. Could asthma worsen by stimulating the T helper type 1 (Th1) response? Am J Respir Cell Mol Biol 2000; 22:143–146.

111. Hansen G, Berry G, DeKruyff R, Umetsu D. Allergen-specific Th1 cells fail to counterbalance Th2 cell-induced airway hyperreactivity but cause severe airway inflammation. J Clin Invest 1999; 103:175–183.

112. Melhop PD, van de Rijn M, Goldberg AB, Brewer JP, Kurup VP, Martin TR, Oettgen HC. Allergen-induced bronchial hyperreactivity and eosinophilic inflammation occur

in the absence of IgE in a mouse model of asthma. Proc Natl Acad Sci USA 1997; 94:1344–1349.

113. Hogan SP, Mould A, Kikutani H, Ramsay AJ, Foster PS. Aeroallergen-induced eosinophilic inflammation, lung damage, and airways hyperreactivity in mice can occur independently of IL-4 and allergen-specific immunoglobulins. J Clin Invest 1997; 99: 1329–1339.

114. Collins PL, Chanock RM, McIntosh K. Parainfluenza viruses. In: Fields BN, Knipe DM, Howley PM, eds. Fields Virology. Philadelphia: Lippincott-Raven, 1996: 1205–1241.

115. Domachowske JB, Rosenberg HF. Respiratory syncytial virus infection: immune response, immunopathogenesis, and treatment. Clin Microbiol Rev 1999; 12:298–309.

116. Pattemore PK, Johnston SL, Bardin PG. Viruses as precipitants of asthma symptoms. I. Epidemiology. Clin Exp Allergy 1992; 22:325–336.

117. Sigurs N, Bjarnason R, Sigurbergsson F, Kjellman B, Bjorksten B. Asthma and immunoglobulin E antibodies after respiratory syncytial virus bronchiolitis: a prospective cohort study with matched controls. Pediatrics 1995; 95:500–505.

118. Stein RT, Sherrill D, Morgan WJ, Holberg CJ, Halonen M, Taussig LM, Wright AL, Martinez FD. Respiratory syncytial virus in early life and risk of wheeze and allergy by age 13 years. Lancet 1999; 345:541–545.

119. Ahmed R, Morrison LA, Knipe DM. Persistence of viruses. In: Fields BN, Knipe DM, Howley PM, eds. Fields Virology. Philadelphia: Lippincott Williams & Wilkins, 1996: 219–249.

26

Interleukin-16 and Airway Hyperresponsiveness in Asthma

FRÉDÉRIC F. LITTLE, WILLIAM W. CRUIKSHANK, and DAVID M. CENTER

Boston University School of Medicine
Boston, Massachusetts, U.S.A.

I. Introduction

In the early 1980s, Cruikshank and Center described T-lymphocyte chemoattractant activity in the supernatants of concanavalin-A–stimulated peripheral blood lymphocytes (1,2). The major T-cell chemoattractant activity from these supernatants was characterized and later designated interleukin-16 (IL-16), previously termed lymphocyte chemoattractant factor (LCF). While initially found to be the product of antigen-, mitogen- (concanavalin A), and histamine-stimulated CD8 + T cells, IL-16 has since been identified in CD4 + T cells (3), B cells (4), eosinophils (5), mast cells (6), dendritic cells (7), fibroblasts (8), and epithelial cells of the upper and lower airways (9,10) and gastrointestinal tract (11).

Because of its selective chemotactic activity for CD4 + cells, early studies in humans sought to determine a relationship between the expression of IL-16 and atopic symptoms. IL-16 is present in the bronchoalveolar lavage (BAL) fluid of atopic asthmatics within 6 hours after segmental bronchoprovocation with allergen (12) or histamine (13). Of the many possible cellular sources for IL-16, IL-16 mRNA and protein is most prominently present in the bronchial and nasal epithelia of atopic asthmatics and rhinitics (9,10), respectively, and is further induced following antigen exposure (14). These observations in humans led to animal studies designed to determine if IL-16 plays a pathogenic role in allergic airway inflammation.

As in humans, the bronchial epithelium of mice sensitized and aerosol-challenged with ovalbumin (OVA) expresses high levels of IL-16 compared to unsensitized or saline-challenged sensitized controls, and bioactive IL-16 is present in the BAL of OVA-challenged, sensitized mice (15). However, studies employing IL-16 null mice and wild-type type mice treated with IL-16 suggest that rather than playing a proinflammatory role in allergic inflammation as a result of its T-cell chemoattractant properties, the major effect of IL-16 in the airways is to downregulate antigen-driven T_H2 cell–mediated inflammation. These experiments indicate that IL-16 plays an immunomodulatory role with respect to immune activation of T lymphocytes, while retaining the ability to be chemotactic to these cells. These studies are consistent with the in vitro observations that IL-16 renders T cells unresponsive to alloantigen (MLR) or antigen stimulation and markedly inhibits T-cell receptor–dependent T_H2 cytokine secretion from T cells of atopic individuals.

Following an outline of the molecular and cell biology of IL-16, we will review the key evidence leading to the current understanding of IL-16's role in allergic airway inflammation. Finally, the therapeutic implications and advances in this regard will be presented.

II. Background

A. Interleukin-16 Protein Biology

IL-16 is synthesized either as a 1233-amino-acid precursor (in brain) or as a 631-amino-acid precursor comprising the C-terminal 631 amino acids of the neuronal form. Both forms are cleaved into two fragments by caspase-3 (16,17). While caspase-3 activity is classically associated with cell apoptosis, we have identified that caspase-3 activation and processing of IL-16 can be independent of T-cell apoptosis (18,19). The precursor form of the 1233-amino-acid brain form contains four PDZ domains and has been demonstrated to interact with ion channels (17). In T cells, the ~60 kDa N-terminal product of caspase-3 cleavage contains 2 PDZ domains and a dual phosphorylation regulated nuclear localization sequence permitting translocation to the nucleus, where it has cell-cycle regulatory properties that will not be reviewed in this chapter (20,21). The 121-amino-acid carboxy-terminal product of caspase-3 cleavage retains the key CD4-binding ability and consequent T-cell chemotactic and immunomodulatory properties (22,23). The majority of this bioactive C-terminus peptide is comprised of a PDZ domain with a core GLGF sequence at Gly41 though the significance of this region is unclear. There is low homology between the originally described PDZ domain containing proteins and IL-16; NMR spectroscopy has revealed that the core GLGF region is partially occluded by a tryptophan residue (20). While there is evidence that IL-16 autoaggregates into homotetramers (23), the role of the PDZ domain in this process has not been established. Autoaggregation is essential for bioactivity and occurs intracellularly before secretion. Like IL-1, IL-16 does not contain a signal secretory peptide. The pathway for secretion is unknown.

The most C-terminal 16 amino acids are essential for bioactivity of aggregated IL-16 homotetramers. This has been demonstrated by the ability of peptides derived from the distal 16 amino acid sequence to inhibit native IL-16/CD4 interaction and subsequent chemotactic activity (24). In addition, monoclonal antibodies generated against the distal C-terminus fully inhibit IL-16's T-cell attractant properties. Mutational analyses of IL-16 have determined four amino acids (^{106}RRKS^{109}) to be critical for bioactivity (24). The localization of CD4 binding to this region of IL-16 has led to the exploration of potential therapeutics based on peptides derived from this region. There is a high degree of sequence and functional homology of IL-16 from all species (e.g., human, simian, and murine) (25–27). There is >98% sequence homology between simian and human secreted IL-16 and 82% homology between human and murine IL-16. Both murine and simian IL-16 are chemotactic to human T cells with a similar dose-response relationship as human IL-16. Conversely, monoclonal antibodies generated to secreted human IL-16 can be used to affinity purify as well as neutralize the bioactivity of murine IL-16. The conserved protein structure and biological actions of IL-16 across species not only implies a conserved evolutionary function but also bears on the determination of compounds assayed in different models as potential therapeutic targets.

B. Interleukin-16 Gene Structure

The IL-16 gene is a single copy gene that maps to human chromosome 15.26.1–3, and chromosome 7 D2–D3 in the mouse (28,27). The entire gene stretches over 20 kilobases and encodes for two forms of the precursor molecule, synthesized by alternative splicing. A larger 1233-amino-acid precursor form is expressed exclusively in the brain (17). It has an unknown number of exons. The T-cell form of human IL-16, which is also the form expressed in mast cells, eosinophils, fibroblasts, dendritic cells, and epithelial cells, will be the sole topic of this review. The gene contains 7 exons, of which the first is noncoding, and results in a 2.6 kb mRNA species (27). Studies on the secretion of IL-16 have revealed that the proximal promoter is TATA-less yet contains two CAAT box-like motifs and three GA-binding protein transcription factor binding site consensus sequences, one of which lies in the 5′ UTR (29). These putative sites have been found to be transcriptionally active. We have identified several single nucleotide polymorphisms (SNPs) at −155, −295, −399, and −524 base pairs upstream from the transcriptional start site, beyond the proximal CAAT motifs and GABP consensus sites (W. W. Cruikshank, unpublished observation, 2000). One of these polymorphisms, the −295 T→C, has been further characterized in the Japanese and Thai populations, and found to have an allelic frequency of approximately 22% and 18%, respectively (30). Because IL-16 inhibits HIV-1 replication, and high levels are associated with lack of progression to AIDS, these investigators looked for differences in susceptibility to HIV-1 infection. There was no difference in the prevalence of HIV-1 infection between those with or without the SNP-containing genotype, but this might be expected as IL-16 does not inhibit HIV-1 infection, it inhibits viral replication. The relevance of the IL-16-−295C and other SNPs in the IL-16 promoter are being investigated for their association with asthma severity. Preliminary studies suggest that pro-IL-16 is constitutively transcribed in T cells with equal abundance in the presence of $-295C$ or $-295T$; however, the expression of pro-IL-16 in airway epithelium (which is inducible) may be based on the presence of the $-295C$ SNP (D. M. Center, unpublished observation, 2000).

Beyond initial studies in an immortalized human T-cell line, the transcriptional regulation of IL-16 has not been fully characterized. By contrast, the nature of IL-16 message production in different cell types has been examined in detail. All immune cells that have been studied generate constitutive mRNA, namely CD4 + and CD8 + T cells (3), eosinophils (5), mast cells (6), and dendritic cells (31). By contrast, nonimmune cells such as airway epithelial cells must be induced to transcribe IL-16 message. With the notable exception of CD8 + T cells, caspase-3 activation is a major regulator of IL-16 release in all cells that constitutively express mRNA and protein. CD8 + T cells appear to contain cleaved, aggregated bioactive IL-16 that is released within hours following stimulation by histamine or serotonin via H2 or S2 receptors, respectively (32,33). Stimulation of CD4 + or CD8 + T-cells with antigen, phorbol ester/calcium ionophore, or anti-CD3/CD28 antibodies fails to induce IL-16 message in cells that constitutively transcribe IL-16 (19). It is likely that the stimuli responsible for IL-16 release in non–T-cells result in new transcription and translation and posttranslational cleavage by activated caspase-3. The significance of airway epithelium as a major source of IL-16 in allergic inflammation is addressed in a later section.

C. Association Between IL-16 and CD4

The major and most extensively studied receptor for IL-16 is CD4. Murine L3T4-T-cell hybridomas are not chemotactic to IL-16; this function is gained by transfection of human CD4 cDNA and resultant surface expression (34,35). Second messenger activation is evidenced by a rise in intracellular Ca^{2+} and inositol (1,4,5)-trisphosphate (IP_3) within minutes after IL-16 stimulation. Neither these intracellular events nor chemotaxis were observed in cells transfected with mutant CD4 lacking a cytoplasmic tail and stimulated with IL-16 (35). All cells with a well-described effector response to IL-16 express surface CD4, including T lymphocytes, eosinophils, dendritic cells, monocytes, and neuronal cells. The reported responsiveness of blood monocytes from CD4 $-/-$ mice (36) and from CD4 $-$ Langherhans cells (37) suggests that IL-16 may signal through alternate pathways in the absence of CD4 or that there may be a co-receptor for IL-16.

Further evidence of the importance of CD4 as the major receptor for IL-16 is derived from experiments that demonstrate a physical association between the two molecules. IL-16 can be identified when biological fluids containing IL-16 are subjected to recombinant soluble CD4 (rsCD4) affinity chromatography (23). Binding of anti-CD4 Ab (OKT4) to CD4 + T lymphocytes is displaced by IL-16 (38). In addition, IL-16 can be identified by Western analysis following immunoprecipitation of rIL-16 with anti-CD4-protein A/Sepharose (23,22).

IL-16 has a distinct binding site on CD4 from other CD4 ligands, including HIV gp120 and MHC class II antigens (39). IL-16 associates with CD4 in its D4 domain, which resides closest to the cell surface and has been identified as the region responsible for autoaggregation and facilitation of TCR-CD3 activation (40,41). Pretreatment of T cells with $F(ab)_2$ fragments of OKT4 antibody, which is directed against this domain of CD4, prevent typical IL-16–induced responses (23). By contrast, antibodies directed against epitopes in the D1 and D2 domains (OKT4a, Leu-3a) do not inhibit IL-16 effects. The precise binding sites on CD4 for IL-16 have been mapped by peptide inhibition and CD4 mutagenesis studies (22). The IL-16 binding region is comprised of two 6-amino-acid stretches that form a groove in the tertiary structure of the D4 region. The location of IL-16's binding site(s) in this region bears directly on its ability to inhibit aspects of CD3-TCR–mediated T-cell activation by antigen or that induced by a mixed lymphocyte reaction (MLR). The implications of this and its potential relevance to novel therapeutic approaches for asthmatic inflammation will be discussed later.

D. Cellular Response to IL-16

CD4 ligation with IL-16 leads to a sequence of cellular responses that are well described (35). Following ligation of CD4 by IL-16, activation of the *src*-related tyrosine kinase $p56^{lck}$ by coupling to the intracytoplasmic tail of CD4 occurs followed by increases in intracellular Ca^{2+}, IP_3, and activation of PI-3 kinase. This first response leads to autocatalytic activity of $p56^{lck}$ with tyrosine phosphorylation. While the catalytic activity of $p56^{lck}$ is not necessary to mediate T-cell chemoattraction, the adaptor function of $p56^{lck}$ coupling to PI-3 kinase is required. Point mutations in key intracytoplasmic regions of CD4 necessary for CD4-$p56^{lck}$ association abrogate the T-cell chemotactic response to IL-16 (35). Cells expressing these mutations retain migratory responses to other chemoattractants. The chemotactic response also appears independent of the rise in Ca^{2+} and IP_3 turnover. It is likely that these two latter signals and the enzymatic activity of $p56^{lck}$ are required for IL-16–induced expression of CD25, but this has not been proven. These findings imply that there are multiple CD4-associated signals induced by IL-16 that lead separately to lymphocyte migration and selective gene expression.

IL-16 inhibits the MLR (38) and anti-CD3–induced TcR-dependent proliferation and cytokine synthesis (42). Thus, as a consequence of being bound by IL-16, CD4 can function to transduce signals sufficient to induce T-cell chemotaxis, cell cycle progression, and expression of IL-2Rα and β, while CD4's facilitation of antigen recognition function is inhibited. Incubation of T cells for 1 hour (insufficient to directly affect IL-2Rα expression) inhibits anti-CD3–induced IL-2Rα expression, and IL-16 treatment prior to TCR stimulation with antigen or anti-CD3 inhibits T-cell proliferation (42). In that regard, T cells isolated from transwell chambers after chemotaxis to IL-16 are unresponsive to TCR stimulation (W. W. Cruikshank, unpublished observation, 2001). Furthermore, IL-16 inhibits both TCR-mediated Fas expression and antigen-induced cell death. All of these phenomena are reversible within 24 hours.

In a microenvironment with high concentrations of IL-16, it is likely that CD4 autoaggregation is prevented, as is its functional participation in the CD3-

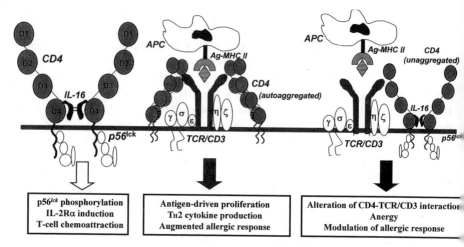

Figure 1 Proposed role of IL-16 in CD4-mediated pathways of T-lymphocyte activation. In the absence of antigen, IL-16 oligomers bind CD4 in the D4 region, causing a complex steric relationship that leads to coupling and autophosphorylation of p56^{lck} activation of PI-3 kinase, rises in intracellular Ca^{2+} and IP3; not shown) with subsequent induction of IL-2Rα, and chemotaxis (left). In the presence of antigen/MHC II (center), TCR/CD3-mediated cell activation is facilitated by autoaggregated CD4 of a different steric conformation than that bound by IL-16, leading to antigen-driven proliferation and cytokine production that augments the allergic response. In the presence of IL-16 (right), CD4 aggregation and facilitation of TCR/CD3 activation by antigen/MHC II is altered, causing anergy and modulation of antigen-driven responses.

TCR–mediated immune response to antigen in the context of MHC II (Fig. 1). These considerations are of direct relevance to the role of epithelial-derived IL-16 in modulating T-cell immune activation in general and specifically in allergic airway inflammation and AHR.

III. Immunobiology of Interleukin-16 and Airway Inflammation

A. Biological Activities of IL-16

In vitro IL-16 was initially described as a chemoattractant for CD4+ T cells at a half-maximal effective dose (ED$_{50}$) of ~10^{-11} M (23). In fact, it is chemotactic for all CD4+ cells, including eosinophils, monocytes, and dendritic cells. IL-16 stimulation of CD4+ T cells also results in upregulation of the IL-2Rα and β receptors (37). These cells are then responsive to IL-2- or IL-15–induced proliferation. IL-16 also has a direct effect on the production of proinflammatory cytokines from monocytes. In response to IL-16 stimulation, monocytes produce TNF-α, IL-1β, IL-6, and IL-15 (43) and T cells generate IL-3 and GM-CSF (44). Eosinophils increase synthesis of lipid inflammatory mediators including LTC4. In addition, IL-16 stimulation of T cells induces IFN-γ mRNA as detected by RT-PCR (M. V. Mashikian, unpublished observation, 1999). IFN-γ protein is not detected in the supernatants, however, until the cells receive a secondary stimulus such as IL-2. A more recent finding indicates that IL-16 stimulation of T cells results in a transient refractory period wherein the T cells are unresponsive to antigenic stimulation. These cells fail to proliferate or express Fas (CD90) in response to antigen or anti-CD3 stimulation (42). This effect of IL-16 could have several ramifications in vivo. Induction of T-cell anergy and Fas expression could potentially translate into a reduction in antigen-induced cell death, thereby resulting in more CD4+ T cells at sites of inflammation. In order for these cells to participate in the inflammatory process, they would have to be responsive to other stimuli. In vitro studies have indicated that CD4+ T cells exposed to IL-16 are still responsive to stimuli such as TGF-β and IL-1β, in addition to IL-2 and IL-15. Alternatively, T-cell anergy induced by IL-16 could result in a significant decrease in antigen-driven inflammation. T cells stimulated by IL-16 would not be responsive to antigenic stimulation, and therefore initiating steps for inflammation would be inhibited.

As a further consequence to inhibition of TCR-induced T-cell proliferation, IL-16 stimulation results in a significant decrease in IL-4 and IL-5 secretion by T cells (45). This effect has been demonstrated both for human peripheral blood and murine lymph node T cells. The effect on IFN-γ production, however, was not that of inhibition but rather augmentation (45). The mechanism for this effect has not been elucidated but does suggest a differential effect by IL-16 on T_H1 versus T_H2 T cells. As discussed above, IL-16 stimulation of CD4+ T cells results in the induction of IFN-γ mRNA, but a secondary signal is required for elaboration of secreted protein. It is feasible that the signal transmitted by the TCR, in the presence of IL-16, is insufficient for induction of T-cell activation, but is sufficient to induce IFN-γ synthesis following IL-16 priming. The implication of these findings is that under conditions of antigenic stimulation, the presence of IL-16 likely alters the T_{H1}/T_H2 ratio, promoting a T_H1 cytokine phenotype.

The process by which IL-16 can regulate T-cell receptor signaling and T-cell activation resides predominantly in its interaction with CD4. Liu et al. determined that IL-16 binds and signals by associating with the proximal portion of the D4 domain of CD4 (22). This region, defined by amino acids Typ[355] to Leu[366], is also the region where CD4 autoaggregates during antigenic stimulation. Autoaggregation by CD4 appears to be essential for complete complex formation with the TCR and MHC class II, facilitating efficient TCR signaling. Disruption of CD4 aggregation results in insufficient TCR signaling and incomplete T-cell activation. The regulatory role of CD4 on TCR signaling was first identified in 1985 using anti-CD4 antibodies (46). A natural ligand for CD4, IL-16 is capable of regulating TCR stimulation by binding to the aggregation site on CD4, thus preventing CD4 autoaggregation. An IL-16–derived peptide based on the bioactive sequence has been synthesized and assessed for its ability to alter CD4 aggregation. The peptide functions similarly to IL-16 protein in its ability to inhibit TCR signaling and cell activation. The potential therapeutic application for this peptide will be addressed later.

In addition to acting as a coreceptor for the TCR, there is an intimate connection between CD4 and several of the chemokine receptors. CCR5 is constitutively associated with CD4, and CXCR4 can be induced to associate with CD4 following binding of the envelope glycoprotein for HIV-1, gp120. Wang et al. (47) first reported that ligation of CD4 by gp120 induces CCR5 unresponsiveness. The effect was later found to exist for CXCR4 (47). Along those lines, we have reported that IL-16 stimulation of T cells also results in receptor cross-desensitization for both CCR5 and CXCR4 (48,49). The mechanism for this effect is different for each chemokine receptor as deactivation of CCR5 requires enzymatic activity of the *src* kinase family member p56^{lck}, via SH1, while deactivation of CXCR4 does not involve the SH1 domain, but is dependent on signaling through the SH3 domain of p56^{lck}. By regulating T-cell recruitment induced by certain chemokines, the presence of IL-16, at sites of inflammation, could significantly influence development of the inflammatory process. The effect of IL-16 on a number of other chemokine receptors as well as the in vivo effect on chemokine-induced cell recruitment is currently being investigated.

B. IL-16 in Inflammation

IL-16 protein and message have been detected in tissues from a variety of different disease states with no particular bias towards either T_H1- or T_H2-mediated diseases. Increased serum IL-16 levels have been associated with disease activity in patients with systemic lupus erythematosus (SLE) (50,51), cutaneous T-cell lymphoma (52,53), cancer (54), and rheumatoid arthritis (RA) (55–57). In addition, immunohistochemical staining of sarcoidosis-associated granulomas from the lymph node and lung reveals high levels of IL-16 staining, with greatest prevalence in the perivascular areas of lymphocyte accumulation (58). In patients with Crohn's disease, colonic tissue sections show increased IL-16 protein and message compared to uninvolved colonic tissues from the same patients or normal controls (11,59,60).

The role of IL-16 in the pathogenesis of inflammation appears to vary depending upon the organ involved. In an animal model of Crohn's disease, for example, treatment with neutralizing concentrations of anti-IL-16 antibody significantly reduced all parameters of inflammation (11). Similarly, using an animal model of delayed-type hypersensitivity, Yoshimoto et al. demonstrated that anti-IL-16 antibody treatment significantly reduced CD4 + cell recruitment and granuloma formation in murine footpads (61). While these experiments clearly support a pro-inflammatory role for IL-16, other animal models have identified a different role for IL-16. Klimiuk et al. reported that in a murine model of rheumatoid arthritis, mice treated with IL-16 protein demonstrated decreased cellular infiltrate and inflammation in explanted synovial RA tissue (62). Along these lines, Kageyama et al. reported that the level and time course for elevated expression of IL-16 protein in synovial fluid obtained from RA patients is not consistent with pro-inflammatory effects (63). These findings suggest that under different inflammatory conditions, IL-16 can participate as either a pro-inflammatory or an immunomodulatory cytokine.

C. Detection and Association of IL-16 with Asthmatic Inflammation

The disease that has received the most attention to date in regards to in vivo biological activities of IL-16 is allergic asthma. A number of studies have been conducted investigating the potential role of IL-16 in human disease as well as in animal models. With the understanding that IL-16's bioactivity was restricted to CD4+ cells, identifying a role for IL-16 in inflammation initially focused on diseases characterized by CD4+ infiltrates. Asthma was the first disease to be directly associated with IL-16 production. Bellini et al. identified IL-16 in cultures of histamine-stimulated primary epithelial cells obtained from asthmatics, but not from normal nonatopic individuals (64). The cells were stimulated with histamine and cell supernatants determined to have IL-16 bioactivity.

These observations were extended by Mashikian et al. (13) in studies where asthmatic individuals underwent subsegmental histamine challenge. Following histamine challenge, the BAL fluid obtained from asthmatics, but not nonasthmatics, contained significantly elevated levels of IL-16 protein and bioactivity. Similar results were reported when asthmatic individuals were challenged with specific antigen (12). No IL-16 is detected in the BAL fluid from asthmatics without prior antigenic or histamine challenge. In both studies the presence of IL-16 was detected relatively rapidly, peaking by 4 hours following challenge, a time point that precedes detection of a number chemokines and T-cell influx. IL-16 protein is still detected in the BAL fluid 24 hours postchallenge in antigen-challenged asthmatics (65). IL-16 could not be detected in normals or atopic nonasthmatic individuals challenged with histamine, indicating selective production of IL-16 in association with asthma rather than as a result of general inflammation. When biopsies obtained from asthmatics were assessed for IL-16 mRNA and protein by in situ hybridization and immunohistochemical staining, IL-16 message and protein were detected in the airway epithelium and infiltrating CD4+ cells (10,66). There was a significant correlation between the amount of protein and message with the number of infiltrating CD4+ cells. Nonasthmatics have little detectable IL-16 protein and message, either before or after antigen or histamine airway challenge.

D. Major Cell Source of IL-16 in Asthmatic Inflammation

A number of cell types involved in the asthmatic response have been shown to be potential sources of IL-16. As mentioned earlier, most immune cells, such as T cells, macrophages, eosinophils, mast cells, and dendritic cells, have either constitutive or inducible IL-16 message and protein. The "nonimmune" epithelial cells and fibroblasts (8) have also been shown to produce IL-16 message and protein following stimulation. In regards to asthma, recent data from a number of different labs now suggest that much of the immune cell influx and activation is orchestrated by the airway epithelial cell. Based on immunohistochemical staining, it appears that this cell type is also a source of IL-16 (67). Lung biopsies obtained from asthmatic individuals reveal a number of IL-16+ T cells, but most of the detected IL-16 protein

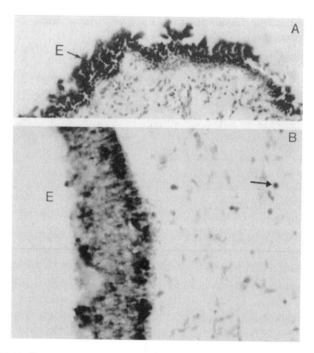

Figure 2 Epithelium as major source of IL-16 in allergic bronchial inflammation. (A) Immunohistochemical staining for IL-16 of bronchial biopsies of atopic asthmatics reveals that the epithelium (E) is the predominant source of IL-16, which appears black in this reproduction (100×). (B) IL-16+ mononuclear cells in the subepithelial layer (*arrow*) (400×). (From Ref. 10.)

is contained within the epithelium (Fig. 2) (10). The observations that histamine stimulation of cultured airway epithelial cells from asthmatics results in IL-16 production along with the ability of histamine to induce IL-16 production in vivo suggests that the epithelium is the major cell source of IL-16 in asthma. While CD8+ T cells are present in the lung, the low numbers detected would make it unlikely that they are a major source.

There is no evidence thus far that histamine stimulation results in de novo synthesis of IL-16 or activation of caspase-3 enzymatic activity in primary epithelial cells. Arima et al. have demonstrated that histamine stimulation of the BEAS-2B epithelial cell line induces IL-16 message and protein synthesis (67), but this effect is not observed in primary human epithelial cells or other airway epithelial cell lines such as HBE4-E6/E7 or A549. The ability of histamine to induce the presence of IL-16 in the BAL fluid of challenged asthmatics but not nonasthmatics indicates not only that epithelial cells contain histamine receptors, but also that histamine is acting as a secretagogue rather than inducing de novo synthesis. This is consistent with the findings that while IL-16 protein is easily detected in the epithelium of asthmatics, neither IL-16 protein nor bioactivity is detected in the BAL fluid until after histamine challenge. Factors that induce epithelial cells to synthesize and store IL-16 in vivo have not been clearly defined. In vitro studies have suggested that TNF-α (67,68) and IL-9 (69) stimulation induces IL-16 synthesis and secretion. We have determined that stimulation with low doses of TNF-α (approximately 1 pg/mL) results in synthesis but not secretion of IL-16 protein. Subsequent stimulation by histamine or serotonin then facilitates secretion (F. F. Little, 2002, in press). Interestingly, IL-16 can be detected in the airway epithelium of mice that have been intraperitoneally sensitized with OVA but that have not as yet received airway OVA challenge (15). Prior to airway challenge IL-16 is not detected in the BAL fluid. This suggests that factors generated during sensitization are capable of inducing IL-16 synthesis and storage. The T_H2 cytokines IL-9 and IL-13 are candidates for the induction of expression of IL-16, as IL-9 alone is sufficient to induce IL-16 mRNA, protein synthesis, and secretion (69). This phenomenon is markedly enhanced by co-stimulation with IL-13 (F. F. Little, unpublished observation). Following airway aerosol challenge with antigen, IL-16 expression is markedly unregulated, perhaps by a combination to T_H2 cytokines, TNF-α, and histamine.

IV. Therapeutic Considerations

A. IL-16 in Animal Models of Airway Inflammation

The in vitro and in vivo studies in humans have identified abundant IL-16 expression in airway epithelium, but have failed to identify a role for the protein in the pathogenic process. Animal studies in mice have been more illustrative and surprising. Despite the fact that IL-16 was initially identified as a chemoattractant factor selective for CD4 + T cells and is chemotactic for all CD4 + cells including eosinphils, monocytes, and dendritic cells, a causal relationship between the presence of CD4 + cells and IL-16 in the airways has not been established. Along these lines, we have recently reproduced the OVA sensitization/aerosol challenge model in IL-16 null mice, backbred to BALB/c for comparison with other studies. Surprisingly, these animals demonstrate markedly greater airway inflammation characterized by cellular influx of T cells and eosinophils when compared to IL-16–expressing littermates. The effects on AHR were similarly increased to 170% compared with OVA-challenged littermate controls (W. W. Cruikshank and F. F. Little, unpublished observation, 2001). Along these lines, exogenous rmuIL-16 delivered either by aerosolization or intratracheal injection during the challenge phase of the model eliminates the inflammatory infiltrate and AHR. When regional lymph node T cells from these IL-16–treated animals were isolated and cultured in the presence of OVA, generation of the T_H2 cytokines IL-4 and IL-5 was selectively inhibited, while synthesis of T_H1 cytokines remained intact (J. J. de Bie, 2002, in press). Lymph node T cells derived from control animals demonstrated normal production of both T_H1 and T_H2 cytokines. These findings are consistent with the hypothesis that in the IL-16-/- mouse there is a lack of an endogenous negative regulatory effect, while with the addition of elevated levels of exogenous IL-16, given in the proper time sequence, lung CD4 + T cells are rendered unresponsive to antigen-induced responses.

In another model of airway inflammation induced by constitutive transgenic overexpression of IL-13, concomitant transgenic overexpression of IL-16 targeted to airway epithelial cells diminishes immune cell recruitment and airway inflammation approximately 25% at all time points; and IL-16/IL-13 Tg + / + live 30–40% longer than IL-13 Tg + littermates (G. Chupp, personal communication, 2000). The mechanism for IL-16 interference in IL-13–mediated inflammation in the absence of antigenic stimulation is unknown, but presumably relates to the ability of IL-16 to inhibit CD4 + T-cell–mediated phenomena that are independent of the T-cell receptor. IL-9 Tg + mice also spontaneously develop airway inflammation and AHR (70). When these mice are treated with exogenous IL-16 for 7–10 days following onset of increased airway hyperreactivity, a marked decrease in airway is detected (F. F.

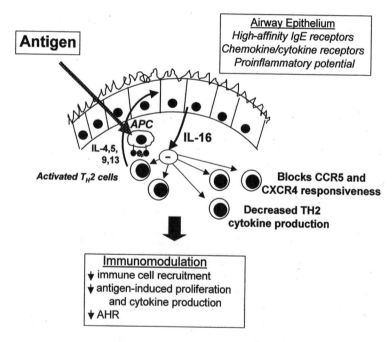

Figure 3 Model of the immunomodulatory function of IL-16 in allergic airway inflammation. Environmental allergenic antigen is processed and presented in the context of MHC II by epithelial dendritic (antigen presenting) cells (APC), eliciting differentiation of CD4 + T lymphocytes in an atopic individual to the T_H2 phenotype. The T_H2 cytokines IL-4, 5, 9, and 13 produced by activated T_H2 cells directly stimulate airway epithelial cells to produce several cytokines and chemokines, including IL-16. In turn, IL-16 downregulates the T-cell–mediated allergic response by causing T-cell anergy, decreased cytokine production, and chemokine receptor desensitization. The factors that regulate of IL-16 synthesis and release, and therefore the degree of immunomodulation, are incompletely understood.

Little, unpublished observation, 2001). For both of these models reduction in immune cell recruitment to the lung in the presence of IL-16 may relate to the ability of IL-16 to induce chemotactic cross-desensitization for chemokines that utilize CCR5 and CXCR4. Therefore, chemokines such as RANTES, MIP-1α, and MIP1-β would be affected. Taken together, the data suggest that IL-16 can reduce airway inflammation induced by antigenic stimulation as well as by altering signaling events that are downstream of antigen activation.

B. Potential Therapeutic Applications for IL-16

The in vivo studies indicate that elevated levels of IL-16 protein in the lung attenuates the asthmatic response. A model for the immunomodulatory effect of IL-16 consequent to epithelial stimulation by T_H2 cytokines is depicted in Figure 3. The mechanism for this effect is centered around the ability of IL-16 to bind to CD4 in the same region in which CD4 autoaggregates during T-lymphocyte activation. A logical extension of this line of thought would be that any peptide capable of binding to this region would have the capacity to limit T-cell activation and subsequent T-cell–dependent inflammation. As mentioned earlier, we have generated an IL-16 peptide based on the bioactive region of IL-16. This peptide has no agonistic activity but is capable of neutralizing IL-16 bioactivity and, more importantly, inhibiting T-cell activation induced by antigenic stimulation or in a MLR. When administered by aerosol this peptide has proven to be as effective as whole IL-16 protein in reducing AHR and inflammation in a murine model of allergic asthma (Fig. 4) (71;

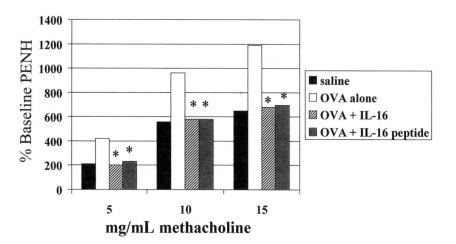

Figure 4 Effect of IL-16 and IL-16–derived peptide on airway reactivity in a murine model of asthma. Ovalbumin-sensitized mice were aerosol challenged with saline, OVA, OVA + IL-16, or OVA + IL-16 peptide, and airway reactivity to aerosolized methacholine at different concentrations was assessed. Results are expressed as mean percent airway resistance (PENH) of unchallenged animals. Both IL-16 and IL-16 peptide significantly attenuated OVA-induced airway hyperresponsiveness. *$p < 0.05$ compared to mice challenged with OVA alone.

J. J. de Bie, 2002, in press). This peptide, which is 16 amino acids in length and highly hydrophilic, is more readily soluble in aqueous solutions than whole IL-16 protein. The size and solubility characteristics make the IL-16 peptide a more attractive candidate for the treatment of asthma. These data suggest that the use of the IL-16 peptide may represent a novel modality for asthma therapy, the feasibility of which awaits clinical trials.

References

1. Center DM, Berman JS, Kornfeld H, Theodore AC, Cruikshank WW. The lymphocyte chemoattractant factor. J Lab Clin Med 1995; 125:167–172.
2. Cruikshank WW, Center DM. Modulation of lymphocyte migration by human lymphokines. II. Purification of a lymphotactic factor (LCF). J Immunol 1982; 128:2569–2574.
3. Chupp GL, Wright EA, Wu D, Vallen-Mashikian M, Cruikshank WW, Center DM, Kornfeld H, Berman JS. Tissue and T cell distribution of precursor and mature IL-16. J Immunol 1998; 161:3114–3119.
4. Kaser A, Dunzendorfer S, Offner FA, Ludwiczek O, Enrich B, Koch RO, Cruikshank WW, Wiedermann CJ, Tilg H. B lymphocyte-derived IL-16 attracts dendritic cells and Th cells. J Immunol 2000; 165:2474–2480.
5. Lim KG, Wan HC, Bozza PT, Resnick MB, Wong DT, Cruikshank WW, Kornfeld H, Center DM, Weller PF. Human eosinophils elaborate the lymphocyte chemoattractants. IL-16 (lymphocyte chemoattractant factor) and RANTES. J Immunol 1996; 156: 2566–2570.
6. Rumsaeng V, Cruikshank WW, Foster B, Prussin C, Kirshenbaum AS, Davis TA, Kornfeld H, Center DM, Metcalfe DD. Human mast cells produce the CD4 + T lymphocyte chemoattractant factor, IL-16. J Immunol 1997; 159:2904–2910.
7. Blaschke V, Reich K, Blaschke S, Zipprich S, Neumann C. Rapid quantitation of proinflammatory and chemoattractant cytokine expression in small tissue samples and monocyte-derived dendritic cells: validation of a new real-time RT-PCR technology. J Immunol Methods 2000; 246:79–90.
8. Sciaky D, Brazer W, Center DM, Cruikshank WW, Smith TJ. Cultured human fibroblasts express constitutive IL-16 mRNA: cytokine induction of active IL-16 protein synthesis through a caspase-3-dependent mechanism. J Immunol 2000; 164:3806–3814.
9. Laberge S, Durham SR, Ghaffar O, Rak S, Center DM, Jacobson M, Hamid Q. Expression of IL-16 in allergen-induced late-phase nasal responses and relation to topical glucocorticosteroid treatment. J Allergy Clin Immunol 1997; 100:569–574.
10. Laberge S, Ernst P, Ghaffar O, Cruikshank WW, Kornfeld H, Center DM, Hamid Q. Increased expression of interleukin-16 in bronchial mucosa of subjects with atopic asthma. Am J Respir Cell Mol Biol 1997; 17:193–202.
11. Keates AC, Castagliuolo I, Cruikshank WW, Qiu B, Arseneau KO, Brazer W, Kelly CP. Interleukin 16 is up-regulated in Crohn's disease and participates in TNBS colitis in mice. Gastroenterology 2000; 119:972–982.
12. Cruikshank WW, Long A, Tarpy RE, Kornfeld H, Carroll MP, Teran L, Holgate ST, Center DM. Early identification of interleukin-16 (lymphocyte chemoattractant factor) and macrophage inflammatory protein 1 alpha (MIP1 alpha) in bronchoalveolar lavage fluid of antigen-challenged asthmatics. Am J Respir Cell Mol Biol 1995; 13:738–747.
13. Mashikian MV, Tarpy RE, Saukkonen JJ, Lim KG, Fine GD, Cruikshank WW, Center DM. Identification of IL-16 as the lymphocyte chemotactic activity in the bronchoal-

veolar lavage fluid of histamine-challenged asthmatic patients. J Allergy Clin Immunol 1998; 101:786–792.

14. Pullerits T, Linden A, Malmhall C, Lotvall J. Effect of seasonal allergen exposure on mucosal IL-16 and CD4+ cells in patients with allergic rhinitis. Allergy 2001; 56: 871–877.

15. Hessel EM, Cruikshank WW, Van A, JJ de Bie I, Van Esch B, Hofman G, Nijkamp FP, Center DM, van Oosterhout AJ. Involvement of IL-16 in the induction of airway hyper-responsiveness and up-regulation of IgE in a murine model of allergic asthma. J Immunol 1998; 160:2998–3005.

16. Zhang Y, Center DM, Wu DM, Cruikshank WW, Yuan J, Andrews DW, Kornfeld H. Processing and activation of pro-interleukin-16 by caspase-3. J Biol Chem 1998; 273: 1144–1149.

17. Kurschner C, Yuzaki M. Neuronal interleukin-16 (NIL-16): a dual function PDZ domain protein. J Neurosci 1999; 19:7770–7780.

18. Ludwiczek O, Kaser A, Koch RO, Vogel W, Cruikshank WW, Tilg H. Activation of caspase-3 by interferon alpha causes interleukin-16 secretion but fails to modulate activation induced cell death. Eur Cytokine Netw 2001; 12:478–486.

19. Wu DM, Zhang Y, Parada NA, Kornfeld H, Nicoll J, Center DM, Cruikshank WW. Processing and release of IL-16 from CD4+ but not CD8+ T cells is activation dependent. J Immunol 1999; 162:1287–1293.

20. Muhlhahn P, Zweckstetter M, Georgescu J, Ciosto C, Renner C, Lanzendorfer M, Lang K, Ambrosius D, Baier M, Kurth R, Holak TA. Structure of interleukin 16 resembles a PDZ domain with an occluded peptide binding site. Nat Struct Biol 1998; 5:682–686.

21. Zhang Y, Kornfeld H, Cruikshank WW, Kim S, Reardon CC, Center DM. Nuclear translocation of the N-terminal prodomain of interleukin-16. J Biol Chem 2001; 276: 1299–1303.

22. Liu Y, Cruikshank WW, O'Loughlin T, O'Reilly P, Center DM, Kornfeld H. Identification of a CD4 domain required for interleukin-16 binding and lymphocyte activation. J Biol Chem 1999; 274:23387–23395.

23. Cruikshank WW, Center DM, Nisar N, Wu M, Natke B, Theodore AC, Kornfeld H. Molecular and functional analysis of a lymphocyte chemoattractant factor: association of biologic function with CD4 expression. Proc Natl Acad Sci USA 1994; 91:5109–5113.

24. Nicoll J, Cruikshank WW, Brazer W, Liu Y, Center DM, Kornfeld H. Identification of domains in IL-16 critical for biological activity. J Immunol 1999; 163:1827–1832.

25. Keane J, Nicoll J, Kim S, Wu DM, Cruikshank WW, Brazer W, Natke B, Zhang Y, Center DM, Kornfeld H. Conservation of structure and function between human and murine IL-16. J Immunol 1998; 160:5945–5954.

26. Bannert N, Adler HS, Werner A, Baier M, Kurth R. Molecular cloning and sequence analysis of interleukin 16 from nonhuman primates and from the mouse. Immunogenetics 1998; 47:390–397.

27. Bannert N, Kurth R, Baier M. The gene encoding mouse interleukin-16 consists of seven exons and maps to chromosome 7 D2-D3. Immunogenetics 1999; 49:704–706.

28. Kim HS. Assignment of human interleukin 16 (IL 16) to chromosome 15q26.3 by radiation hybrid mapping. Cytogenet Cell Genet 1999; 84:93.

29. Bannert N, Avots A, Baier M, Serfling E, Kurth R. GA-binding protein factors, in concert with the coactivator CREB binding protein/p300, control the induction of the interleukin 16 promoter in T lymphocytes. Proc Natl Acad Sci USA 1999; 96: 1541–1546.

30. Nakayama EE, Wasi C, Ajisawa A, Iwamoto A, Shioda T. A new polymorphism in the promoter region of the human interleukin-16 (IL-16) gene. Genes Immun 2000; 1: 293–294.

31. Kaser A, Dunzendorfer S, Offner FA, Ryan T, Schwabegger A, Cruikshank WW, Wiedermann CJ, Tilg H. A role for IL-16 in the cross-talk between dendritic cells and T cells. J Immunol 1999; 163:3232–3238.

32. Laberge S, Cruikshank WW, Kornfeld H, Center DM. Histamine-induced secretion of lymphocyte chemoattractant factor from CD8 + T cells is independent of transcription and translation. Evidence for constitutive protein synthesis and storage. J Immunol 1995; 155:2902–2910.

33. Laberge S, Cruikshank WW, Beer DJ, Center DM. Secretion of IL-16 (lymphocyte chemoattractant factor) from serotonin-stimulated CD8 + T cells in vitro. J Immunol 1996; 156:310–315.

34. Cruikshank WW, Greenstein JL, Theodore AC, Center DM. Lymphocyte chemoattractant factor induces CD4-dependent intracytoplasmic signaling in lymphocytes. J Immunol 1991; 146:2928–2934.

35. Ryan TC, Cruikshank WW, Kornfeld H, Collins TL, Center DM. The CD4-associated tyrosine kinase p56lck is required for lymphocyte chemoattractant factor-induced T lymphocyte migration. J Biol Chem 1995; 270:17081–17086.

36. Mathy NL, Bannert N, Norley SG, Kurth R. Cutting edge: CD4 is not required for the functional activity of IL-16. J Immunol 2000; 164:4429–4432.

37. Stoitzner P, Ratzinger G, Koch F, Janke K, Scholler T, Kaser A, Tilg H, Cruikshank WW, Fritsch P, Romani N. Interleukin-16 supports the migration of Langerhans cells, partly in a CD4-independent way. J Invest Dermatol 2001; 116:641–649.

38. Theodore AC, Center DM, Nicoll J, Fine G, Kornfeld H, Cruikshank WW. CD4 ligand IL-16 inhibits the mixed lymphocyte reaction. J Immunol 1996; 157:1958–1964.

39. Yang J, Liu CQ. Interaction between human interleukin-16 and CD4 receptor of HIV-1. Acta Pharmacol Sin 2000; 21:547–553.

40. Wu H, Kwong PD, Hendrickson WA. Dimeric association and segmental variability in the structure of human CD4. Nature 1997; 387:527–530.

41. Gratton S, Haughn L, Sekaly RP, Julius M. The extracellular domain of CD4 regulates the initiation of T cell activation. Mol Immunol 2000; 37:213–219.

42. Cruikshank WW, Lim K, Theodore AC, Cook J, Fine G, Weller PF, Center DM. IL-16 inhibition of CD3-dependent lymphocyte activation and proliferation. J Immunol 1996; 157:5240–5248.

43. Mathy NL, Scheuer W, Lanzendorfer M, Honold K, Ambrosius D, Norley S, Kurth R. Interleukin-16 stimulates the expression and production of pro-inflammatory cytokines by human monocytes. Immunology 2000; 100:63–69.

44. Parada NA, Center DM, Kornfeld H, Rodriguez WL, Cook J, Vallen M, Cruikshank WW. Synergistic activation of CD4 + T cells by IL-16 and IL-2. J Immunol 1998; 160: 2115–2120.

45. Pinsonneault S, El Bassam S, Mazer B, Cruikshank WW, Laberge S. IL-16 inhibits IL-5 production by antigen-stimulated T cells in atopic subjects. J Allergy Clin Immunol 2001; 107:477–482.

46. Bank I, Chess L. Perturbation of the T4 molecule transmits a negative signal to T cells. J Exp Med 1985; 162:1294–1303.

47. Wang JM, Ueda H, Howard OM, Grimm MC, Chertov O, Gong X, Gong W, Resau JH, Broder CC, Evans G, Arthur LO, Ruscetti FW, Oppenheim JJ. HIV-1 envelope

gp120 inhibits the monocyte response to chemokines through CD4 signal-dependent chemokine receptor down-regulation. J Immunol 1998; 161:4309–4317.

48. Mashikian MV, Ryan TC, Seman A, Brazer W, Center DM, Cruikshank WW. Reciprocal desensitization of CCR5 and CD4 is mediated by IL-16 and macrophage-inflammatory protein-1 beta, respectively. J Immunol 1999; 163:3123–3130.

49. Van Drenth C, Jenkins A, Ledwich L, Ryan TC, Mashikian MV, Brazer W, Center DM, Cruikshank WW. Desensitization of CXC chemokine receptor 4, mediated by IL-16/CD4, is independent of p561ck enzymatic activity. J Immunol 2000; 165:6356–6363.

50. Sekigawa I, Matsushita M, Lee S, Maeda N, Ogasawara H, Kaneko H, Iida N, Hashimoto H. A possible pathogenic role of CD8 + T cells and their derived cytokine, IL-16, in SLE. Autoimmunity 2000; 33:37–44.

51. Lee S, Kaneko H, Sekigawa I, Tokano Y, Takasaki Y, Hashimoto H. Circulating interleukin-16 in systemic lupus erythematosus. Br J Rheumatol 1998; 37:1334–1337.

52. Asadullah K, Haeussler-Quade A, Gellrich S, Hanneken S, Hansen-Hagge TE, Docke WD, Volk HD, Sterry W. IL-15 and IL-16 overexpression in cutaneous T-cell lymphomas: stage-dependent increase in mycosis fungoides progression. Exp Dermatol 2000; 9:248–251.

53. Blaschke V, Reich K, Middel P, Letschert M, Sachse F, Harwix S, Neumann C. Expression of the CD4 + cell-specific chemoattractant interleukin-16 in mycosis fungoides. J Invest Dermatol 1999; 113:658–663.

54. Kovacs E. The serum levels of IL-12 and IL-16 in cancer patients. Relation to the tumour stage and previous therapy. Biomed Pharmacother 2001; 55:111–116.

55. Kaufmann J, Franke S, Kientsch-Engel R, Oelzner P, Hein G, Stein G. Correlation of circulating interleukin 16 with proinflammatory cytokines in patients with rheumatoid arthritis. Rheumatology (Oxford) 2001; 40:474–475.

56. Blaschke S, Schulz H, Schwarz G, Blaschke V, Muller GA, Reuss-Borst M. Interleukin 16 expression in relation to disease activity in rheumatoid arthritis. J Rheumatol 2001; 28:12–21.

57. Kageyama Y, Ozeki T, Suzuki M, Ichikawa T, Miura T, Miyamoto S, Machida A, Nagano A. Interleukin-16 in synovial fluids from cases of various types of arthritis. Joint Bone Spine 2000; 67:188–193.

58. Cappelli G, Volpe P, Sanduzzi A, Sacchi A, Colizzi V, Mariani F. Human macrophage gamma interferon decreases gene expression but not replication of *Mycobacterium tuberculosis*: analysis of the host-pathogen reciprocal influence on transcription in a comparison of strains H37Rv and CMT97. Infect Immun 2001; 69:7262–7270.

59. Middel P, Reich K, Polzien F, Blaschke V, Hemmerlein B, Herms J, Korabiowska M, Radzun HJ. Interleukin 16 expression and phenotype of interleukin 16 producing cells in Crohn's disease. Gut 2001; 49:795–803.

60. Seegert D, Rosenstiel P, Pfahler H, Pfefferkorn P, Nikolaus S, Schreiber S. Increased expression of IL-16 in inflammatory bowel disease. Gut 2001; 48:326–332.

61. Yoshimoto T, Wang CR, Yoneto T, Matsuzawa A, Cruikshank WW, Nariuchi H. Role of IL-16 in delayed-type hypersensitivity reaction. Blood 2000; 95:2869–2874.

62. Klimiuk PA, Goronzy JJ, Weyand CM. IL-16 as an anti-inflammatory cytokine in rheumatoid synovitis. J Immunol 1999; 162:4293–4299.

63. Kageyama Y, Ozeki T, Suzuki M, Ichikawa T, Miura T, Miyamoto S, Machida A, Nagano A. Interleukin-16 in synovial fluids from cases of various types of arthritis. Joint Bone Spine 2000; 67:188–193.

64. Bellini A, Yoshimura H, Vittori E, Marini M, Mattoli S. Bronchial epithelial cells of patients with asthma release chemoattractant factors for T lymphocytes. J Allergy Clin Immunol 1993; 92:412–424.

65. Krug N, Cruikshank WW, Tschernig T, Erpenbeck VJ, Balke K, Hohlfeld JM, Center DM, Fabel H. Interleukin 16 and T-cell chemoattractant activity in bronchoalveolar lavage 24 hours after allergen challenge in asthma. Am J Respir Crit Care Med 2000; 162:105–111.

66. Laberge S, Pinsonneault S, Varga EM, Till SJ, Nouri-Aria K, Jacobson M, Cruikshank WW, Center DM, Hamid Q, Durham SR. Increased expression of IL-16 immunoreactivity in bronchial mucosa after segmental allergen challenge in patients with asthma. J Allergy Clin Immunol 2000; 106:293–301.

67. Arima M, Plitt J, Stellato C, Bickel C, Motojima S, Makino S, Fukuda T, Schleimer RP. Expression of interleukin-16 by human epithelial cells. Inhibition by dexamethasone. Am J Respir Cell Mol Biol 1999; 21:684–692.

68. Cheng G, Ueda T, Eda F, Arima M, Yoshida N, Fukuda T. A549 cells can express interleukin-16 and stimulate eosinophil chemotaxis. Am J Respir Cell Mol Biol 2001; 25:212–218.

69. Little FF, Cruikshank WW, Center DM. Il-9 stimulates release of chemotactic factors from human bronchial epithelial cells. Am J Respir Cell Mol Biol 2001; 25:347–352.

70. Temann UA, Geba GP, Rankin JA, Flavell RA. Expression of interleukin 9 in the lungs of transgenic mice causes airway inflammation, mast cell hyperplasia, and bronchial hyperresponsiveness. J Exp Med 1998; 188:1307–1320.

71. de Bie JJ, Henricks PA, Cruikshank WW, Hofman G, Nijkamp FP, van Oosterhout AJ. Effect of interleukin-16-blocking peptide on parameters of allergic asthma in a murine model. Eur J Pharmacol 1999; 383:189–196.

27

Modulation of the Allergic Response
The Role of IL-18

DAVID M. WALTER

Roche Bioscience
Palo Alto, California

ROSEMARIE H. DeKRUYFF and
DALE T. UMETSU

Stanford University
Stanford, California, U.S.A.

I. Introduction

Interleukin-18 (IL-18) is a recently characterized cytokine belonging to the IL-1 cytokine family that has important and complex effects in regulating immune responses. In the lung, IL-18 critically controls pulmonary homeostasis. Following bacterial and viral infection it is produced by a wide variety of cells, including dendritic cells, macrophages, as well as airway and intestinal epithelial cells (1–5). IL-18 is produced early during innate immune responses and critically affects subsequent adaptive immune responses, enhancing either Th1 or Th2 cytokine production, depending on specific circumstances. IL-18 was discovered initially as a potent IFN-γ-inducing factor, and was initially classified as a Th1 cytokine with antiallergic activity and strong activity in host defense against infection with intracellular pathogens (6–8). However, IL-18 can under some circumstances also induce Th2 cytokine production, particularly in the absence of IL-12, and therefore possesses allergy-promoting activity. In this chapter we will review the immunobiology of IL-18 and its capacity to modulate respiratory immune responses and asthma.

II. Structure of IL-18

As a member of the IL-1 cytokine family, IL-18 shares structural homology with IL-1. It is synthesized as an inactive precursor and requires cleavage by caspase-1

(ICE) for activity (8–11). The precursor of human IL-18 is synthesized as a 193-amino-acid protein with an observed molecular weight of 24 kDa, and once activated, IL-18 has an observed molecular weight of 18 kDa (9). Recent reports also suggest that pro-IL-18 can be activated by alternative cleavage enzymes such as proteinase 3, a serine protease released by activated neutrophils (12), or by a Fas/Fas ligand-associated pathway (13). While most cytokines are expressed after cell activation, some cells produce IL-18 constitutively, though cell activation clearly increases the secretion of active IL-18. This may be due to the structure of the IL-18 gene, which contains seven exons as well as two promoters, located in the first two noncoding exons (14). IL-18 expression that is under control of the promoter upstream of exon 2 is constitutive, while IL-18 expression that is under control of the promoter upstream of exon 1 is upregulated by factors such as lipopolysaccharide (LPS). Unlike most cytokines, IL-18 does not use promoters containing TATA boxes; rather it uses TATA-less and G + C poor type promoters that are commonly used in many cell types (1). The promoter type may explain the wide variety of cells that express IL-18, comprising both immune and nonimmune cells. Immune cells that express IL-18 include dendritic cells and macrophages (2,5,6,15), while nonimmune cells that produce IL-18 include airway and intestinal epithelial cells, keratinocytes, osteoblasts, astrocytes, and microglial cells (3–5,16,17). Macrophages (Kupffer cells, splenic macrophages, alveolar macrophages) produce active IL-18 only after immunological stimulation, for example, with bacterial or viral infection (18–20), although dendritic cells produce some active IL-18 constitutively. Keratinocytes and epithelial cells secrete low levels of inactive IL-18 constitutively, but exposure to contact allergens (2) results in the production of active IL-18.

III. IL-18 Receptor

IL-18 and IL-12 have been shown to synergistically induce IFN-γ production in T cells and natural killer (NK) cells. This synergy is due, in part, to the ability of IL-12 to upregulate IL-18Rα expression in naïve T cells and the reciprocal ability of IL-18 to upregulate production of IL-12Rα2 (21,22). Two different IL-18 receptors have been identified, IL-18Rα and IL-18Rβ, which together function as the high-affinity IL-18 receptor. IL-18Rα was first purified and characterized by Torigoe et al. from the human Hodgkin's disease cell line L428 using a monoclonal antibody against a cell surface protein that blocked IL-18 binding (23). IL-18 binds with low affinity to IL-18Rα, with a dissociation constant (Kd) reported in the range of 18–45 nmol/L (23,24). IL-18 binds with high affinity to the functional IL-18 receptor dimer complex, which consists of IL-18Rα, (the ligand-binding subunit), and IL-18Rβ, the signal-transducing subunit (25). Because the cytoplasmic tail of IL-18R and IL-1R are similar to each other and to Toll receptor family members, it is not surprising that they share signal transduction pathway elements (26,27). Studies in knockout mice have elucidated the requirement for various proteins in the IL-18R complex

(28). The IL-18Rα and IL-18Rβ receptor complex recruits MyD88, an adapter protein involved in Toll receptor signaling, to the cell membrane cluster, which then recruits IRAK and TRAF-6 followed by the activation of NIK and IKK (29–31). This results in the degradation of IκB, NFκB translocation into the nucleus, and in cell activation, including enhanced IL-2 gene expression by T cells (32). IL-18 signaling may also proceed via mitogen-activated protein kinase (MAPK) pathways. In this pathway, IL-18 signaling activates the src kinase p56lck and protein tyrosine kinase in Th1 cells and in NK cells, resulting in expansion of these cell types (21,33,34).

IV. Biological Function of IL-18

A. IL-18 Enhances Th2 Immune Responses

IL-18 is a pleotropic cytokine, such that under certain circumstances IL-18 greatly enhances Th2 responses and promotes allergic inflammatory responses in mice and humans, but under other circumstances IL-18 greatly enhances Th1-driven responses. Although the primary role of IL-18 in vivo may be to amplify Th1 responses and cell-mediated immunity, its paradoxical role in enhancing Th2 responses in experimental systems is well documented, but difficult to explain.

B. Induction of IL-4, IL-13

IL-18 was initially characterized as a potent inducer of IFN-γ production, but in vitro studies by Hoshino et al. showed that IL-18 in combination with anti-CD3 mAb, induced IL-4, IL-10, and IL-13 production, and increased expression of CD40L in NK and T cells (35,36). This may be partly due to the fact that naïve T cells express low levels of IL-18Rα, which results in production of IL-13 and GM-CSF upon stimulation with IL-18. Moreover, incubation of naïve CD4+ T cells with IL-18 and IL-2 without TCR engagement and in the absence of IL-12 resulted in production of IL-13 and IL-4. Continued stimulation with anti-CD3 mAb resulted in Th2 polarization and in the induction of IgE synthesis by bystander B cells (37). In addition, IL-18 increased the capacity of basophils to produce IL-4, IL-13, and histamine in vitro and in helminth-infected mice (38). Thus, IL-18, in the absence of IL-12, selectively stimulates the development of Th2 responses. This may explain the fact that patients with lepromatous leprosy, which is a Th2-polarized disease, have significantly higher serum IL-18 than patients with tuberculoid leprosy, a Th1-polarized situation, and suggests that IL-18 has the potential (in the absence of IL-12) to play a role in the pathogenesis of allergic disorders. Consistent with this idea, investigators demonstrated that intraperitoneal administration of very high doses of IL-18 in conjunction with allergic sensitization and allergen challenge resulted in increased IL-4 and IL-5 production from splenocytes cultured with allergen (39) and in increased serum levels of IL-13, IL-4, and IFN-γ in a CD4+ cell–dependent manner (37,40). Others have also found that NK T cells are the main target for IL-

18-induced IL-4 production, with IL-18 enhancing both the production of IL-4 and the number of IL-4 + cells among NK T cells (41).

C. Induction of IgE

One of the hallmarks of an allergic response is the production of IgE in response to sensitization with allergen. Administration of IL-18 intraperitoneally in either naïve or sensitized mice leads to increased levels of serum IgE (36,39). Similar paradoxical effects have been associated with IL-12, which under some circumstances can enhance IL-4, IL-10, and IgE production (41–43). The IL-18–induced IgE production appears to be dependent on IL-4 and STAT6, but not on IL-13 (37). In addition, both Caspase-1 overexpressing transgenic mice and IL-18 overexpressing transgenic mice have high serum levels of IL-18 and elevated serum levels of IgE and IgG1 (37,40). When the Caspase-1 transgenic mice were crossed with IL-18–deficient mice, the resulting Caspase-1–transgenic, IL-18–deficient mice had no detectable serum IL-18 and low serum levels of IgE (37), indicating that the increased levels of IgE was dependent on the presence of IL-18.

D. Induction of Eotaxin

Consistent with the Th2 biasing effects of IL-18, administration of IL-18 was found to enhance allergen-induced eosinophil recruitment into the airways of sensitized mice, perhaps by increasing levels of TNF-α or eotaxin (39,44,45). Eotaxin is a chemokine that was originally isolated from the bronchoalveolar lavage (BAL) fluid of guinea pigs as a potent chemoattractant for eosinophils, as well as basophils and Th2 lymphocytes. The release of eotaxin in the lungs of asthmatics from a variety of cells recruits eosinophils into the lungs and is in part responsible for the characteristic eosinophilia that has been associated with allergic asthma (46–49). Eotaxin was induced with very high doses of IL-18, suggesting that the eosinophil-enhancing effects of IL-18 might be due to a pharmacological rather than physiological effect of IL-18 or may be due to the relative absence of IL-12 activity.

E. IL-18 in Human Asthma and Atopic Dermatitis

In human studies, higher levels of serum IL-18 were found in patients with acute asthma compared to patients with stable asthma and healthy controls. These high levels of IL-18 in the acute asthma patients decreased after medical treatment for the symptoms of asthma, and serum levels of IL-18 in stable asthmatics were found to be similar to those of healthy controls (50). While serum levels of IL-18 in patients with acute asthma were similar to those with sarcoidosis, a Th1-deviated disease, serum levels of IFN-γ were significantly elevated and correlated with IL-18 levels only in patients with pulmonary sarcoidosis (50). This suggests that IL-18 production in asthma is paradoxically increased and, in the absence of IFN-γ production, may indeed contribute to disease pathogenesis. However, expression of IL-18 protein in airway epithelial cells was found to be reduced in patients with asthma compared to that of healthy individuals, while epithelial cell production of IL-18 was greatest in tissue from patients with sarcoidosis (51). Consistent with these studies, mononuclear cells from patients with asthma or with atopic dermatitis were found to produce higher levels of IL-18 but lower levels of IFN-γ than cells from nonallergic controls (52). Although histamine, released during the acute asthma attack, can induce IL-18 production (53), these studies suggest that IL-18 contributes to disease pathogenesis in asthma and atopic dermatitis, as it does in mycobacteria infection, where patients with Th2-deviated lepromatous leprosy develop higher serum levels of IL-18 compared to patients with the Th1-deviated tuberculoid leprosy (37).

F. IL-18 and IL-12 Synergistically Induce Th1 Responses

While in some systems IL-18 enhances Th2 cytokine production and promotes airway eosinophilia, there is a great deal of evidence generated in other systems demonstrating that IL-18 potently induces IFN-γ production and the development of Th1 cells and effectively prevents airway hyperreactivity and allergy. IL-18 induces IFN-γ production in activated T cells 10-fold more effectively than IL-12 (6) and can induce IFN-γ synthesis in the absence of T-cell receptor signaling. However, IL-18 cannot induce IFN-γ production in naïve T cells or in Th2 cells, because naïve T cells and Th2 cells express very low levels of the high-affinity receptor for IL-18 (21,54). In addition, in the absence of IFN-γ, and particularly in the presence of IL-4, the expression of IL-18Rα is downmodulated (55). On the other hand, in the presence of IL-12, the induction of IFN-γ by IL-18 is greatly enhanced (22). The synergy between IL-12 and IL-18 in inducing prolonged production of IFN-γ develops because IL-12 upregulates the expression of IL-18 receptor on the surface of T cells (21,22,56–60), while IL-18 upregulates the expression of the IL-12β2 receptor (21,22,54,61). Therefore, dendritic cells that produce both IL-18 and IL-12, or situations that induce antigen-presenting cells (APC) to produce both cytokines, greatly enhance IFN-γ production in T cells and deviate immune responses toward Th1 (15,60). In contrast to T cells, NK cells constitutively express both the IL-18 receptor and the IL-12Rβ (62) and can respond rapidly to either IL-18 or IL-12 and produce IFN-γ. However, in the absence of IFN-γ, IL-18 induces high levels of IL-13, particularly in NK cells (35). This suggests that the observation of increased serum levels of IL-18 but not of IFN-γ in patients with Th2-biased diseases such as asthma and atopic dermatitis is due to the production of IL-18 in the absence of adequate IL-12 synthesis.

The effectiveness of IL-18 in inducing Th1 polarization results in protection against intracellular infections, such as *Listeria monocytogenes*. Most interestingly, this protection by IL-18 can occur in the absence of IFN-γ production, reinforcing the idea that IL-18, while highly pleiotropic, is primarily a "Th1" cytokine (63,64). IL-18 activates macrophages to produce IFN-γ, TNF-α, and nitric oxide, all of which are critical in cell-mediated immune responses (65).

G. Induction of Th1 Cell Polarization by IL-18 and the Treatment of Asthma

The capacity of IL-18 to induce Th1 polarization, particularly in combination with IL-12, allows IL-18 to be very effective in preventing or reversing the development of Th2-driven diseases such as asthma and allergy. This has been shown in in vitro systems and in in vivo models, which are discussed below.

In mice, when both IL-18 and IL-12 are administered together, they synergistically enhance IFN-γ production (66) and inhibit allergen-induced airway hyperreactivity (AHR) and airway eosinophilia (67). In a mouse model in which mice were sensitized and challenged with ovalbumin (OVA), treatment with neither IL-12 nor IL-18 alone during the challenge period was effective in reducing IgE production, AHR, and airway inflammation. However, combined treatment with IL-12 and IL-18 inhibited antigen-specific Th2-like cell development, IgE upregulation, and AHR. Moreover, coadministration of IL-12 and IL-18 protein results in increased levels of IgG2a in the serum (57,67). This indicated that the synergistic action of IL-12 and IL-18 together was required to prevent Th2-like cell differentiation and inhibit the development of AHR, presumably because IL-12 and IL-18 synergistically increase IFN-γ production, and because IL-12 induces IL-18 receptor expression on Th1 but not Th2 cells (54).

Supporting the idea that IL-18 can inhibit Th2-driven responses is the fact that IL-18–deficient mice develop significant levels of allergen-induced eosinophilia (68). Thus, in IL-18–deficient mice sensitized and challenged with allergen, eosinophilia and pulmonary pathology were much greater than in wild-type littermate controls. In contrast, administration of rIL-18 to IL-18–deficient mice reduced these allergen-induced changes to levels seen in wild-type mice. However, administration of rIL-18 did not affect the IFN-γ level and somewhat enhanced the production of IL-5, suggesting that maximal Th1-inducing effects required the administration of IL-12 as well. Nevertheless, these findings indicate that IL-18 inhibits antigen-specific Th2-biased responses, though in the absence of elevated IL-12 levels these effects are diminished.

H. Administration of IL-18 cDNA with an Adenovirus Vector

The synergistic effect of IL-18 and IL-12 is illustrated by experiments in which IL-18 was administered to mice in the form of cDNA in an adenovirus vector (IL-18: Adv) (69). By delivering IL-18 cDNA into the lungs of mice with the IL-18:Adv vector, IL-18 was not only able to prevent the development of AHR, but also reversed established AHR and converted Th2 cytokine profiles into Th1 profiles (Fig. 1) (69). The ability of IL-18 to both prevent and reverse established AHR was dependent on the induction of IL-12 and IFN-γ synthesis by the vector, since neutralization of IL-12 or of IFN-γ with neutralizing monoclonal antibodies abolished the beneficial effects of the IL-18:Adv vector. These results demonstrated that IL-18, when administered into the respiratory tract with a viral vector that can induce IL-12 production, effectively reduces AHR and replaces an established Th2-biased immune response with a Th1-biased response.

Although IL-18 can reverse established AHR and its associated Th2 response, administration of IL-18 as cDNA in an adenovirus does not result in a normal lung with absence of pulmonary inflammation. Rather, the IL-18:Adv vector induces a Th1-like response in the lung, which although not associated with increased airway

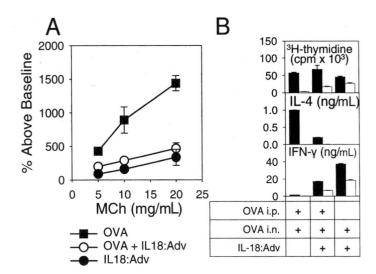

Figure 1 Treatment of mice with intranasal adenovirus expressing IL-18 (IL-18:Adv) can reverse established AHR and convert a Th2 like response in the lungs to a Th1-like response. (A) To determine whether treatment with the IL-18–containing adenovirus could reverse established AHR, mice were first sensitized intraperitoneally (i.p.) and then challenged intranasally (i.n.) with OVA, which induces AHR. The mice were then treated with IL-18-containing adenovirus, followed by further challenges with OVA, to further induce AHR. AHR in response to methacholine challenge was then measured. Only the IL-18-containing adenovirus was capable of reversing established AHR under these conditions, while a control virus expressing luciferase had no effect. (B) After measuring the AHR, bronchial lymph node cells from the treated mice were removed and cultured in the presence of 100 μg/mL OVA (black bars) or medium only (white bars). Measurement of cytokine levels of the cultures cells indicate that IL-18 converted an established Th2 response into a Th1 response. (From Ref. 69.)

reactivity to methacholine, is associated with airway inflammation, consisting primarily of lymphocytes but no eosinophils (Fig. 2C,D) (69). While this Th1-biased immune response effectively reversed even ongoing AHR, its long-term effects of Th1-biased inflammation on pulmonary physiology is not yet clear. In addition, previous studies demonstrated that pure Th1 responses, in the form of classical allergen-specific Th1 cell lines, cannot reverse the effects of pure Th2 cell lines, and that pure Th1 responses may adversely affect airway inflammation and AHR (70–72).

I. Administration of Allergen–IL-18 Fusion cDNA

The effective role of IL-18 and of IL-12 in reducing Th2-biased disease is also demonstrated in studies with allergen–IL-18 fusion cDNA. A DNA vaccination

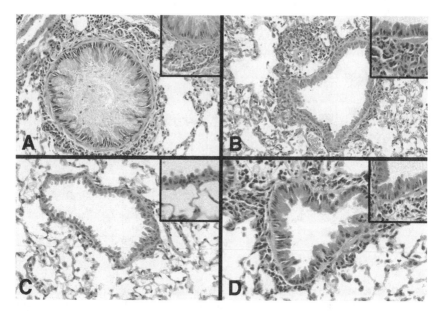

Figure 2 Lung histology of BALB/c mice treated as indicated below. Two days after the last OVA challenge, the lungs were removed and fixed in formalin. The tissue sections were then embedded in paraffin, sectioned at 5 μm, and stained with H&E. (A) Mice treated with luciferase-containing (control) adenovirus and sensitized and challenged with OVA developed AHR with intense airway inflammation and abundant luminal mucus secretions (H&E × 200). (Insert) High-power magnification showing epithelial lining cells with prominent intra-cytoplasmic mucin and collections of eosinophils around the airways (H&E × 400). (B) Mice treated with IL-18-containing adenovirus and sensitized and challenged with OVA did not develop AHR and displayed less intense airway inflammation and the absence of luminal secretions (H&E × 200). (Insert) Low columnar epithelial cells line the airways and contain sparse mucin within the cells. The peribronchiolar and perivascular inflammatory cells are predominantly lymphocytic (H&E × 400). (C) Mice treated with luciferase-containing (control) adenovirus and challenged with OVA without sensitization did not develop AHR and showed normal lung histology (H&E × 200). (Insert) High-powered magnification demonstrating low columnar lining cells and absence of airway inflammation (H&E × 400). (D) Mice treated with IL-18-containing adenovirus and challenged with OVA without sensitization did not develop AHR but developed a mild peribronchiolar inflammatory response, but no airway mucus secretions (H&E × 250). (Insert) The epithelial cells lack abundant intracyto-plasmic mucin, and the inflammatory cells are predominantly mononuclear in composition (H&E × 400). This indicates that IL-18 induces a Th1-driven inflammatory response in the lungs. (From Ref. 69.)

plasmid containing IL-18 cDNA fused with allergen (OVA) cDNA administered intramuscularly protected mice from the subsequent induction of AHR (73). The protection from AHR correlated with increased IFN-γ production and reduced OVA-specific IgE production. The protection appeared to be mediated by IFN-γ and CD8+ cells because treatment of mice with neutralizing anti-IFN-γ mAb or with depleting anti-CD8 mAb abolished the protective effect. Moreover, when mice with established AHR were treated, the OVA–IL-18 plasmid was unique among other cDNA constructs examined (OVA plasmid, IL-18 plasmid) in its capacity to reverse preexisting AHR, reduce allergen-specific IL-4, increase allergen-specific IFN-γ production, and decrease the number of eosinophils in the lungs (Fig. 3). Our studies with allergen–IL-18 cDNA suggest that cDNA vaccination may be clinically effective in the prevention of, and in reversing ongoing, allergic asthma.

Many other studies have demonstrated the effectiveness of genetic vaccination for infectious disease, cancer, or autoimmune disease (74–77). The effectiveness of cDNA vaccines is dependent on the presence of unmethylated CpG motifs present on the vector backbone of the vector (78), which by binding to Toll-like receptor 9 (79) activate MyD88 pathways involved in both the innate and acquired immune systems by inducing the production of IL-12, IL-18, and IFN-γ (80,81). When DNA vaccines containing cDNA for allergen are used for the treatment of allergy (82–86), the CpG motifs in the plasmid, by enhancing IL-18 and IL-12 production, likely contribute to the reduction in Th2-biased responses. In addition to reducing Th2 cytokine production, the IL-18 in combination with IL-12 very effectively reduces IgE production in primed B cells and even induces the production of IFN-γ in B cells (57,67), although in the absence of IL-12, IL-18 enhances IgE production in a CD4+ T cells–, IL-4–, and STAT6-dependent fashion (37). However, although allergen cDNA vaccines can *prevent* the development of Th2-biased responses and AHR, allergen-alone cDNA vaccines (or cytokine cDNA vaccines) have not been effective in *reversing* established AHR. Because fusing IL-18 cDNA to allergen cDNA generates a vaccine plasmid that is effective in reversing established AHR (73), it is likely that overexpression of IL-18 greatly enhances the induction of protective immunity against asthma and allergy.

J. Adjuvant Therapy for the Treatment of Established Allergic Disease

Established allergic disease can be reversed by treatment with conventional allergen immunotherapy, performed by the subcutaneous injection of increasing doses of allergen, resulting in clinical tolerance to subsequent allergen exposure (87,88). However, effective control of symptoms with conventional allergen immunotherapy requires nearly 100 injections over 3–5 years and, in addition, is associated with frequent unpredicted allergic reactions. IL-18, induced along with IL-12 by adjuvants, may serve to enhance the efficiency of allergen-based immunotherapies in reversing the symptoms of asthma and allergy. We will discuss two of these adjuvants that induce IL-18 production, CpG DNA oligonucleotides and heat-killed *Listeria monocytogenes*, in the context of allergen immunotherapy.

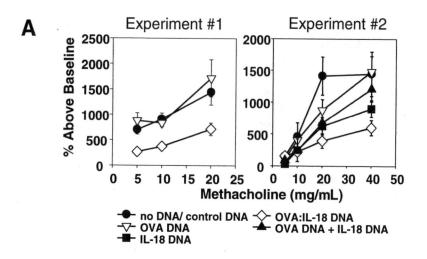

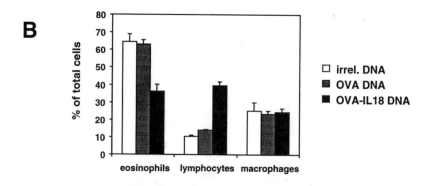

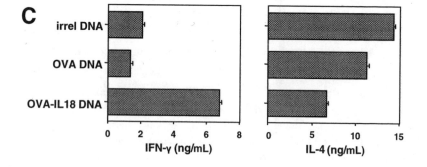

CpG Motifs

CpG oligonucleotides, when administered prior to or with allergen, has been shown to prevent airway hypersensitivity in murine models of asthma (83,89). Moreover, conjugates composed of CpG oligonucleotides covalently linked to antigen have been shown to be 100-fold more efficient in reducing airway eosinophilia, Th2 responses, and AHR than unconjugated mixtures (90). The use of conjugates allows much lower doses of CpG oligonucleotides to be used and focuses the effects on antigen-specific cells. In addition, the precise immune response activated by the CpG oligonucleotides when it binds to Toll-like receptor 9 is not fully understood. Therefore, CpG conjugates may induce the production of multiple cytokines, such as IL-10, as well as IL-18, IL-12, and IFN-γ, which together may modulate Th2-dominated immune responses without provoking a potent pure Th1 response and without inducing Th1-mediated tissue injury. Thus, allergen-CpG constructs may be effective in immunotherapy for asthma and atopic disorders, and clinical trials with these agents are currently underway.

Listeria monocytogenes *as Adjuvant*

L. monocytogenes is a gram-positive facultative intracellular bacteria that elicits strong cell-mediated immune responses and potently stimulates the innate immune system by inducing the production of large quantities of IL-18 (20,63), IL-12, and IL-10. The *Listeria* cell wall component lipoteichoic acid potently induces IL-12 production in macrophages (91). When heat-killed *Listeria* (HKL) is used as an adjuvant with antigen, a complex response that includes antigen-specific Th1-biased immune response is induced, characterized by production of Th1 cytokines and antigen-specific IgG2a antibody (92). Moreover, a single dose of HKL administered with antigen was able to effectively convert Th2-dominated immune responses into responses that protected against the development of AHR. Moreover, the effect of

◄──

Figure 3 (A) Reversal of AHR by OVA–IL-18 DNA vaccination. To determine whether OVA–IL-18 DNA vaccination could reverse established AHR, mice were first sensitized to OVA, which induces AHR. The mice were then immunized with either OVA DNA, IL-18 DNA, or OVA–IL-18 DNA, followed by further challenges with OVA, to further induce AHR. AHR in response to methacholine challenge was then measured, and OVA-IL-18 DNA was the most effective in reversing established AHR. (B) Recruitment of specific cell types into the airways of immunized mice. BAL was performed on the above mice just prior to sacrifice, and the percentages of eosinophils, lymphocytes, and macrophages (identified morphologically) were tabulated. Only OVA–IL-18 DNA–vaccinated mice showed a decrease in eosinophil proportion, along with a rise in lymphocyte proportion of total BAL cells. (C) After measuring their AHR, bronchial lymph node cells from the treated mice were removed and cultured in the presence of 100 μg/mL OVA. Measurement of cytokine levels in the culture supernatants indicated that only OVA–IL-18 DNA–immunized mice showed an appreciable increase in IFN-γ production and decrease in IL-4 production. All results are representative of two different experiments. (From Ref. 86.)

HKL occurred in an allergen-specific manner and was effective in reversing established AHR when given late after allergen sensitization (20,92). HKL as adjuvant also dramatically inhibited airway inflammation, eosinophilia, and mucus production, significantly reduced antigen-specific IgE and IL-4 production, and greatly increased antigen-specific IFN-γ synthesis. More importantly, mice treated with HKL and antigen showed almost normal lung histology, with a minimal lymphocytic infiltration, suggesting that HKL as adjuvant induced a complex immune response that included Th1 cytokines, as well as anti-inflammatory cytokines that reduced airway inflammation and protected against AHR. Consistent with this idea, the inhibitory effect of HKL on AHR depended on the presence of IL-12 and CD8 + T cells as well as on IL-10, TGF-β production, and was associated with IL-18 mRNA expression. These results demonstrate that HKL as an adjuvant for immunotherapy is associated with the induction of IL-18, protects against Th2-dominated immune responses and AHR, and may be clinically effective in the treatment of patients with established asthma and allergic disease.

V. Conclusion

Since its initial discovery and characterization as an IFN-γ inducing cytokine, IL-18 has been shown to play a very complex role in regulating immune responses to antigen. IL-18 is made under a number of different conditions, by a large number of different cell types, including macrophages, dendritic cells, as well as airway and gastrointestinal epithelial cells, keratinocytes, and microglial cells. IL-18 activity is regulated by proteolytic cleavage by caspases, and IL-18 affects both innate and adaptive immunity. The predominant in vivo effects of IL-18, particularly when produced in combination with IL-12, include the induction of IFN-γ production in T cells, B cells, NK cells, and macrophages, Th1 cell polarization, and macrophage activation. On the other hand, when produced in the absence of IL-12, or when administered in high doses, IL-18 can enhance Th2 polarization, NK cell production of IL-13, and B-cell production of IgE. Therapies that enhance production of IL-18 or that involve administration of IL-18 can therefore either promote or reverse Th2-biased responses. However, as our understanding of the full spectrum of effects of IL-18 improves, we will be better able to predict its behavior in affecting both innate and adaptive immunity and better utilize IL-18 to more successfully modulate allergic responses and asthma.

References

1. Nakanishi K, Yoshimoto T, Tsutsui H, Okamura H. Interleukin-18 regulates both Th1 and Th2 responses. Annu Rev Immunol 19:423.
2. Stoll S, Muller G, Kurimoto M, Saloga J, Tanimoto T, Yamauchi H, Okamura J, Knop AH. Enk. Production of IL-18 (IFN-gamma-inducing factor) messenger RNA and functional protein by murine keratinocytes. J Immunol 1997; 159:298.

3. Takeuchi M, Nishizaki Y, Sano O, Ohta T, Ikeda M. Kurimoto. Immunohistochemical and immuno-electron-microscopic detection of interferon-gamma-inducing factor ("interleukin-18") in mouse intestinal epithelial cells. Cell Tissue Res 1997; 289:499.

4. Matsui K, Yoshimoto T, Tsutsui H, Hyodo Y, Hayashi N, Hiroishi K, Kawada N, Okamura H, Nakanishi K, Higashino K. Propionibacterium acnes treatment diminishes CD4+ NK1.1+ T cells but induces type I T cells in the liver by induction of IL-12 and IL-18 production from Kupffer cells. J Immunol 1997; 159:97.

5. Nakanishi K, Yoshimoto T, Tsutsui H, Okamura H. Interleukin-18 is a unique cytokine that stimulates both Th1 and Th2 responses depending on its cytokine milieu. Cytokine Growth Factor Rev 2001; 12:53.

6. Okamura H, Tsutsi H, Komatsu T, Yutsudo M, Hakura A, Tanimoto T, Torigoe K, Okura T, Nukada Y, Hattori K, et al. Cloning of a new cytokine that induces IFN-gamma production by T cells. Nature 1995; 378:88.

7. Okamura H, Nagata K, Komatsu T, Tanimoto T, Nukata Y, Tanabe F, Akita K, Torigoe K, Okura T, Fukuda S, et al. A novel costimulatory factor for gamma interferon induction found in the livers of mice causes endotoxic shock. Infect Immun 1995; 63:3966.

8. Bazan JF, Timans JC, Kastelein RA. A newly defined interleukin-1? Nature 1996; 379: 591.

9. Ushio S, Namba M, Okura T, Hattori K, Nukada Y, Akita K, Tanabe F, Konishi K, Micallef M, Fujii M, Torigoe K, Tanimoto T, Fukuda S, Ikeda M, Okamura H and Kurimoto M. Cloning of the cDNA for human IFN-gamma-inducing factor, expression in *Escherichia coli*, and studies on the biologic activities of the protein. J Immunol 1996; 156:4274.

10. Gu Y, Kuida K, Tsutsui H, Ku G, Hsiao K, Fleming MA, Hayashi N, Higashino K, Okamura H, Nakanishi K, Kurimoto M, Tanimoto T, Flavell RA, Sato V, Harding MW, Livingston DJ, Su MS. Activation of interferon-gamma inducing factor mediated by interleukin-1 beta converting enzyme. Science 1997; 275:206.

11. Ghayur T, Banerjee S, Hugunin M, Butler D, Herzog L, Carter A, Quintal L, Sekut L, Talanian R, Paskind M, Wong W, Kamen R, Tracey D, Allen H. Caspase-1 processes IFN-gamma-inducing factor and regulates LPS-induced IFN-gamma production. Nature 1997; 386:619.

12. Fantuzzi G, Dinarello CA. Interleukin-18 and interleukin-1 beta: two cytokine substrates for ICE (caspase-1). J Clin Immunol 1999; 19:1.

13. Tsutsui H, Kayagaki N, Kuida K, Nakano H, Hayashi N, Takeda K, Matsui K, Kashiwamura S, Hada T, Akira S, Yagita H, Okamura H, Nakanishi K. Caspase-1-independent, Fas/Fas ligand-mediated IL-18 secretion from macrophages causes acute liver injury in mice. Immunity 1999; 11:359.

14. Tone M, Thompson S, Tone Y, Fairchild P, Waldmann H. Regulation of IL-18 (IFN-gamma-inducing factor) gene expression. J Immunol 1997; 159:6156.

15. Stoll S, Jonuleit H, Schmitt E, Muller G, Yamauchi H, Kurimoto M, Knop J, Enk AH. Production of functional IL-18 by different subtypes of murine and human dendritic cells (DC): DC-derived IL-18 enhances IL-12-dependent Th1 development. Eur J Immunol 1998; 28:3231.

16. Udagawa N, Horwood NJ, Elliott J, Mackay A, Owens J, Okamura H, Kurimoto M, Chambers TJ, Martin TJ, Gillespie MT. Interleukin-18 (interferon-gamma-inducing factor) is produced by osteoblasts and acts via granulocyte/macrophage colony-stimulating factor and not via interferon-gamma to inhibit osteoclast formation. J Exp Med 1997; 185:1005.

17. Prinz M, Hanisch UK. Murine microglial cells produce and respond to interleukin-18. J Neurochem 1999; 72:2215.

18. Vankayalapati R, Wizel B, Weis SE, Samten B, Girard WM, Barnes PF. Production of interleukin-18 in human tuberculosis. J Infect Dis 2000; 182:234.

19. Pirhonen J, Sareneva T, Kurimoto M, Julkunen I, Matikainen S. Virus infection activates IL-1 beta and IL-18 production in human macrophages by a caspase-1-dependent pathway. J Immunol 1999; 162:7322.

20. Hansen G, Yeung VP, Berry G, Umetsu DT, DeKruyff RH. Vaccination with heat-killed *Listeria* as adjuvant reverses established allergen-induced airway hyperreactivity and inflammation: role of CD8 + T cells and IL-18. J Immunol 2000; 164:223.

21. Yoshimoto T, Takeda K, Tanaka T, Ohkusu K, Kashiwamura S, Okamura H, Akira S, Nakanishi K. IL-12 up-regulates IL-18 receptor expression on T cells, Th1 cells, and B cells: synergism with IL-18 for IFN-gamma production. J Immunol 1998; 161:3400.

22. Chang JT, Segal BM, Nakanishi K, Okamura H, Shevach EM. The costimulatory effect of IL-18 on the induction of antigen-specific IFN-gamma production by resting T cells is IL-12 dependent and is mediated by up-regulation of the IL-12 receptor beta2 subunit. Eur J Immunol 2000; 30:1113.

23. Torigoe K, Ushio S, Okura T, Kobayashi S, Taniai M, Kunikata T, Murakami T, Sanou O, Kojima H, Fujii M, Ohta T, Ikeda M, Ikegami H, Kurimoto M. Purification and characterization of the human interleukin-18 receptor. J Biol Chem 1997; 272:25737.

24. Boraschi D, Villa L, Volpini G, Bossu P, Censini S, Ghiara P, Scapigliati G, Nencioni L, Bartalini M, Matteucci G, et al. Differential activity of interleukin 1 alpha and interleukin 1 beta in the stimulation of the immune response in vivo. Eur J Immunol 1990; 20: 317.

25. Born TL, Thomassen E, Bird TA, Sims JE. Cloning of a novel receptor subunit, AcPL, required for interleukin-18 signaling. J Biol Chem 1998; 273:29445.

26. O'Neill LA, Dinarello CA. The IL-1 receptor/toll-like receptor superfamily: crucial receptors for inflammation and host defense. Immunol Today 2000; 21:206.

27. Dinarello CA. Biologic basis for interleukin-1 in disease. Blood 1996; 87:2095.

28. Hoshino K, Tsutsui H, Kawai T, Takeda K, Nakanishi K, Takeda Y, Akira S. Cutting edge: generation of IL-18 receptor-deficient mice: evidence for IL-1 receptor-related protein as an essential IL-18 binding receptor. J Immunol 1999; 162:5041.

29. Adachi O, Kawai T, Takeda K, Matsumoto M, Tsutsui H, Sakagami M, Nakanishi K, Akira S. Targeted disruption of the MyD88 gene results in loss of IL-1- and IL-18-mediated function. Immunity 1998; 9:143.

30. Kanakaraj P, Ngo K, Wu Y, Angulo A, Ghazal P, Harris CA, Siekierka JJ, Peterson PA, Fung-Leung WP. Defective interleukin (IL)-18-mediated natural killer and T helper cell type 1 responses in IL-1 receptor-associated kinase (IRAK)-deficient mice. J Exp Med 1999; 189:1129.

31. Thomas JA, Allen JL, Tsen M, Dubnicoff T, Danao J, Liao XC, Cao Z, Wasserman SA. Impaired cytokine signaling in mice lacking the IL-1 receptor-associated kinase. J Immunol 1999; 163:978.

32. Matsumoto S, Tsuji-Takayama K, Aizawa Y, Koide K, Takeuchi M, Ohta T, Kurimoto M. Interleukin-18 activates NF-kappaB in murine T helper type 1 cells. Biochem Biophys Res Commun 1997; 234:454.

33. Tsuji-Takayama K, Matsumoto S, Koide K, Takeuchi M, Ikeda M, Ohta T, Kurimoto M. Interleukin-18 induces activation and association of p56(lck) and MAPK in a murine TH1 clone. Biochem Biophys Res Commun 1997; 237:126.

34. Tomura M, Zhou XY, Maruo S, Ahn HJ, Hamaoka T, Okamura H, Nakanishi K, Tanimoto T, Kurimoto M, Fujiwara H. A critical role for IL-18 in the proliferation and activation of NK1.1+ CD3-cells. J Immunol 1998; 160:4738.

35. Hoshino T, Wiltrout RH, Young HA. IL-18 is a potent coinducer of IL-13 in NK and T cells: a new potential role for IL-18 in modulating the immune response. J Immunol 1999; 162:5070.

36. Hoshino T, Yagita H, Ortaldo JR, Wiltrout RH, Young HA. In vivo administration of IL-18 can induce IgE production through Th2 cytokine induction and up-regulation of CD40 ligand (CD154) expression on CD4+ T cells. Eur J Immunol 2000; 30:1998.

37. Yoshimoto T, Mizutani H, Tsutsui H, Noben-Trauth N, Yamanaka K, Tanaka M, Izumi S, Okamura H, Paul WE, Nakanishi K. IL-18 induction of IgE: dependence on CD4+ T cells, IL-4 and STAT6. Nat Immunol 2000; 1:132.

38. Yoshimoto T, Tsutsui H, Tominaga K, Hoshino K, Okamura H, Akira S, Paul WE, Nakanishi K. IL-18, although antiallergic when administered with IL-12, stimulates IL-4 and histamine release by basophils. Proc Natl Acad Sci USA 1999; 96:13962.

39. Wild JS, Sigounas A, Sur N, Siddiqui MS, Alam R, Kurimoto M, Sur S. IFN-gamma-inducing factor (IL-18) increases allergic sensitization, serum IgE, Th2 cytokines, and airway eosinophilia in a mouse model of allergic asthma. J Immunol 2000; 164:2701.

40. Hoshino T, Kawase Y, Okamoto M, Yokota K, Yoshino K, Yamamura K, Miyazaki J, Young HA, Oizumi K. Cutting edge: IL-18-transgenic mice: in vivo evidence of a broad role for IL-18 in modulating immune function. J Immunol 2001; 166:7014.

41. Leite-De-Moraes MC, Hameg A, Pacilio M, Koezuka Y, Taniguchi M, Van Kaer L, Schneider E, Dy M, Herbelin A. IL-18 enhances IL-4 production by ligand-activated NKT lymphocytes: a pro-Th2 effect of IL-18 exerted through NKT cells. J Immunol 2001; 166:945.

42. Rempel JD, Wang MD, HayGlass KT. Failure of rIL-12 administration to inhibit established IgE responses in vivo is associated with enhanced IL-4 synthesis by non-B/non-T cells. Int Immunol 2000; 12:1025.

43. Germann T, Guckes S, Bongartz M, Dlugonska H, Schmitt E, Kolbe L, Kolsch E, Podlaski FJ, Gately MK, Rude E. Administration of IL-12 during ongoing immune responses fails to permanently suppress and can even enhance the synthesis of antigen-specific IgE. Int Immunol 1995; 7:1649.

44. Kumano K, Nakao A, Nakajima H, Hayashi F, Kurimoto M, Okamura H, Saito Y, Iwamoto I. Interleukin-18 enhances antigen-induced eosinophil recruitment into the mouse airways. Am J Respir Crit Care Med 1999; 160:873.

45. Campbell E, Kunkel SL, Strieter RM, Lukacs NW. Differential roles of IL-18 in allergic airway disease: induction of eotaxin by resident cell populations exacerbates eosinophil accumulation. J Immunol 2000; 164:1096.

46. Li D, Wang D, Griffiths-Johnson DA, Wells TN, Williams TJ, Jose PJ, Jeffery PK. Eotaxin protein and gene expression in guinea-pig lungs: constitutive expression and upregulation after allergen challenge. Eur Respir J 1997; 10:1946.

47. Jose PJ, Adcock IM, Griffiths-Johnson DA, Berkman N, Wells TN, Williams TJ, Power CA. Eotaxin: cloning of an eosinophil chemoattractant cytokine and increased mRNA expression in allergen-challenged guinea-pig lungs. Biochem Biophys Res Commun 1994; 205:788.

48. Jose PJ, Griffiths-Johnson DA, Collins PD, Walsh DT, Moqbel R, Totty NF, Truong O, Hsuan JJ, Williams TJ. Eotaxin: a potent eosinophil chemoattractant cytokine detected in a guinea pig model of allergic airways inflammation. J Exp Med 1994; 179:881.

49. Griffiths-Johnson DA, Collins PD, Rossi AG, Jose PJ, Williams TJ. The chemokine, eotaxin, activates guinea-pig eosinophils in vitro and causes their accumulation into the lung in vivo. Biochem Biophys Res Commun 1993; 197:1167.

50. Tanaka H, Miyazaki N, Oashi K, Teramoto S, Shiratori M, Hashimoto M, Ohmichi M, Abe S. IL-18 might reflect disease activity in mild and moderate asthma exacerbation. J Allergy Clin Immunol 2001; 107:331.

51. Cameron LA, Taha RA, Tsicopoulos A, Kurimoto M, Olivenstein R, Wallaert B, Minshall EM, Hamid QA. Airway epithelium expresses interleukin-18. Eur Respir J 1999; 14:553.

52. El-Mezzein RE, Matsumoto T, Nomiyama H, Miike T. Increased secretion of IL-18 in vitro by peripheral blood mononuclear cells of patients with bronchial asthma and atopic dermatitis. Clin Exp Immunol 2001; 126:193.

53. Kohka H, Nishibori M, Iwagaki H, Nakaya N, Yoshino T, Kobashi K, Saeki K, Tanaka N, Akagi T. Histamine is a potent inducer of IL-18 and IFN-gamma in human peripheral blood mononuclear cells. J Immunol 2000; 164:6640.

54. Xu D, Chan WL, Leung BP, Hunter D, Schulz K, Carter RW, McInnes IB, Robinson JH, Liew FY. Selective expression and functions of interleukin 18 receptor on T helper (Th) type 1 but not Th2 cells. J Exp Med 1998; 188:1485.

55. Smeltz RB, Chen J, Hu-Li J, Shevach EM. Regulation of interleukin (IL)-18 receptor alpha chain expression on CD4(+) T cells during T helper (Th)1/Th2 differentiation. Critical downregulatory role of IL-4. J Exp Med 2001; 194:143.

56. Robinson D, Shibuya K, Mui A, Zonin F, Murphy E, Sana T, Hartley SB, Menon S, Kastelein R, Bazan F, O'Garra A. IGIF does not drive Th1 development but synergizes with IL-12 for interferon-gamma production and activates IRAK and NFkappaB. Immunity 1997; 7:571.

57. Yoshimoto T, Okamura H, Tagawa YI, Iwakura Y, Nakanishi K. Interleukin 18 together with interleukin 12 inhibits IgE production by induction of interferon-gamma production from activated B cells. Proc Natl Acad Sci USA 1997; 94:3948.

58. Yang J, Murphy TL, Ouyang W, Murphy KM. Induction of interferon-gamma production in Th1 CD4+ T cells: evidence for two distinct pathways for promoter activation. Eur J Immunol 1999; 29:548.

59. Tominaga K, Yoshimoto T, Torigoe K, Kurimoto M, Matsui K, Hada T, Okamura H, Nakanishi K. IL-12 synergizes with IL-18 or IL-1beta for IFN-gamma production from human T cells. Int Immunol 2000; 12:151.

60. Fukao T, Matsuda S, Koyasu S. Synergistic effects of IL-4 and IL-18 on IL-12-dependent IFN-gamma production by dendritic cells. J Immunol 2000; 164:64.

61. Shevach EM, Chang JT, Segal BM. The critical role of IL-12 and the IL-12R beta 2 subunit in the generation of pathogenic autoreactive Th1 cells. Springer Semin Immunopathol 1999; 21:249.

62. Hyodo Y, Matsui K, Hayashi N, Tsutsui H, Kashiwamura S, Yamauchi H, Hiroishi K, Takeda K, Tagawa Y, Iwakura Y, Kayagaki N, Kurimoto M, Okamura H, Hada T, Yagita H, Akira S, Nakanishi K, Higashino K. IL-18 up-regulates perforin-mediated NK activity without increasing perforin messenger RNA expression by binding to constitutively expressed IL-18 receptor. J Immunol 1999; 162:1662.

63. Neighbors M, Xu X, Barrat FJ, Ruuls SR, Churakova T, Debets R, Bazan JF, Kastelein RA, Abrams JS, O'Garra A. A critical role for interleukin 18 in primary and memory effector responses to Listeria monocytogenes that extends beyond its effects on interferon gamma production. J Exp Med 2001; 194:343.

64. Swain SL. Interleukin 18: tipping the balance towards a T helper cell 1 response. J Exp Med 2001; 194:F11.
65. Helmby H, Takeda K, Akira S, Grencis RK. Interleukin (IL)-18 promotes the development of chronic gastrointestinal helminth infection by downregulating IL-13. J Exp Med 2001; 194:355.
66. Yoshimoto T, Nagai N, Ohkusu K, Ueda H, Okamura H, Nakanishi K. LPS-stimulated SJL macrophages produce IL-12 and IL-18 that inhibit IgE production in vitro by induction of IFN-gamma production from CD3intIL-2R beta+ T cells. J Immunol 1998; 161:1483.
67. Hofstra CL, Van Ark I, Hofman G, Kool M, Nijkamp FP, Van Oosterhout AJ. Prevention of Th2-like cell responses by coadministration of IL-12 and IL-18 is associated with inhibition of antigen-induced airway hyperresponsiveness, eosinophilia, and serum IgE levels. J Immunol 1998; 161:5054.
68. Kodama T, Matsuyama T, Kuribayashi K, Nishioka Y, Sugita M, Akira S, Nakanishi K, Okamura H. IL-18 deficiency selectively enhances allergen-induced eosinophilia in mice. J Allergy Clin Immunol 2000; 105:45.
69. Walter DM, Wong CP, DeKruyff RH, Berry GJ, Levy S, Umetsu DT. Il-18 gene transfer by adenovirus prevents the development of and reverses established allergen-induced airway hyperreactivity. J Immunol 2001; 166:6392.
70. Hansen G, Berry G, DeKruyff RH, Umetsu DT. Allergen-specific Th1 cells fail to counterbalance Th2 cell-induced airway hyperreactivity but cause severe airway inflammation. J Clin Invest 1999; 103:175.
71. Randolph DA, Stephens R, Carruthers CJ, Chaplin DD. Cooperation between Th1 and Th2 cells in a murine model of eosinophilic airway inflammation. J Clin Invest 1999; 104:1021.
72. Randolph DA, Carruthers CJ, Szabo SJ, Murphy KM, Chaplin DD. Modulation of airway inflammation by passive transfer of allergen-specific Th1 and Th2 cells in a mouse model of asthma. J Immunol 1999; 162:2375.
73. Maecker HT, Hansen G, Walter DM, DeKruyff RH, Levy S, Umetsu DT. Vaccination with allergen-IL-18 fusion DNA protects against, and reverses established, airway hyperreactivity in a murine asthma model. J Immunol 2001; 166:959.
74. Ulmer JB, Donnelly JJ, Parker SE, Rhodes GH, Felgner PL, Dwarki VJ, Gromkowski SH, Deck RR, DeWitt CM, Friedman A, et al. Heterologous protection against influenza by injection of DNA encoding a viral protein. Science 1993; 259:1745.
75. Tascon RE, Colston MJ, Ragno S, Stavropoulos E, Gregory D, Lowrie DB. Vaccination against tuberculosis by DNA injection. Nat Med 1996; 2:888.
76. Syrengelas AD, Chen TT, Levy R. DNA immunization induces protective immunity against B-cell lymphoma. Nat Med 1996; 2:1038.
77. Seder RA, Gurunathan S. DNA vaccines—designer vaccines for the 21st century. N Engl J Med 1999; 341:277.
78. Roman M, Martin-Orozco E, Goodman JS, Nguyen MD, Sato Y, Ronaghy A, Kornbluth RS, Richman DD, Carson DA, Raz E. Immunostimulatory DNA sequences function as T helper-1-promoting adjuvants. Nat Med 1997; 3:849.
79. Hemmi H, Takeuchi O, Kawai T, Kaisho T, Sato S, Sanjo H, Matsumoto M, Hoshino K, Wagner H, Takeda K, Akira S. A Toll-like receptor recognizes bacterial DNA. Nature 2000; 408:740.
80. Messina JP, Gilkeson GS, Pisetsky DS. Stimulation of in vitro murine lymphocyte proliferation by bacterial DNA. J Immunol 1991; 147:1759.

81. Tokunaga T, Yamamoto H, Shimada S, Abe H, Fukuda T, Fujisawa Y, Furutani Y, Yano O, Kataoka T, Sudo T, et al. Antitumor activity of deoxyribonucleic acid fraction from *Mycobacterium bovis* BCG. I. Isolation, physicochemical characterization, and antitumor activity. J Natl Cancer Inst 1984; 72:955.

82. Roy K, Mao HQ, Huang SK, Leong KW. Oral gene delivery with chitosan–DNA nanoparticles generates immunologic protection in a murine model of peanut allergy. Nat Med 1999; 5:387.

83. Broide D, Schwarze J, Tighe H, Gifford T, Nguyen MD, Malek S, Van Uden J, Martin-Orozco E, Gelfand EW, Raz E. Immunostimulatory DNA sequences inhibit IL-5, eosinophilic inflammation, and airway hyperresponsiveness in mice. J Immunol 1998; 161: 7054.

84. Hsu CH, Chua KY, Tao MH, Huang SK, Hsieh KH. Inhibition of specific IgE response in vivo by allergen-gene transfer. Int Immunol 1996; 8:1405.

85. Hsu CH, Chua KY, Tao MH, Lai YL, Wu HD, Huang SK, Hsieh KH. Immunoprophylaxis of allergen-induced immunoglobulin E synthesis and airway hyperresponsiveness in vivo by genetic immunization. Nat Med 1996; 2:540.

86. Raz E, Tighe H, Sato Y, Corr M, Dudler JA, Roman M, Swain SL, Spiegelberg HL, Carson DA. Preferential induction of a Th1 immune response and inhibition of specific IgE antibody formation by plasmid DNA immunization. Proc Natl Acad Sci USA 1996; 93:5141.

87. Bousquet J, Lockey R, Malling HJ, Alvarez-Cuesta E, Canonica GW, Chapman MD, Creticos PJ, Dayer JM, Durham SR, Demoly P, Goldstein RJ, Ishikawa T, Ito K, Kraft D, Lambert PH, Lowenstein H, Muller U, Norman PS, Reisman RE, Valenta R, Valovirta E, Yssel H. Allergen immunotherapy: therapeutic vaccines for allergic diseases. Ann Allergy Asthma Immunol 1998; 81:401.

88. Campbell D, DeKruyff RH, Umetsu DT. Allergen immunotherapy: novel approaches in the management of allergic diseases and asthma. Clin Immunol 2000; 97:193.

89. Kline JN, Waldschmidt TJ, Businga TR, Lemish JE, Weinstock JV, Thorne PS, Krieg AM. Modulation of airway inflammation by CpG oligodeoxynucleotides in a murine model of asthma. J Immunol 1998; 160:2555.

90. Shirota H, Sano K, Kikuchi T, Tamura G, Shirato K. Regulation of murine airway eosinophilia and Th2 cells by antigen-conjugated CpG oligodeoxynucleotides as a novel antigen-specific immunomodulator. J Immunol 2000; 164:5575.

91. Cleveland MG, Gorham JD, Murphy TL, Tuomanen E, Murphy KM. Lipoteichoic acid preparations of gram-positive bacteria induce interleukin-12 through a CD14-dependent pathway. Infect Immun 1996; 64:1906.

92. Yeung VP, Gieni RS, Umetsu DT, DeKruyff RH. Heat-killed *Listeria monocytogenes* as an adjuvant converts established murine Th2-dominated immune responses into Th1-dominated responses. J Immunol 1998; 161:4146.

28

Inhibition of Cytokine Signaling

ARNOB BANERJEE, MIERA B. HARRIS, and PAUL ROTHMAN

College of Physicians and Surgeons
Columbia University
New York, New York, U.S.A.

I. Introduction

The pathways by which cytokines exert their biological effects have been a major focus of research over the past several years. Much of this work has defined the mechanisms by which binding of cytokines to their specific receptors initiates downstream signaling. This work has defined several major signaling pathways initiated by this process. Although the effect of most cytokines is limited in both magnitude and duration, the mechanisms responsible for this limitation have not been well studied. Most limitation of cytokine activity occurs through regulated production of cytokines. In addition, the developmentally regulated expression of cytokine receptors is an important mechanism utilized by the immune system to limit the biological effects of cytokines. More recent attention has been centered on the intracellular mechanisms used to limit cytokine signaling. There are several proposed mechanisms by which cytokine signaling is regulated within the cell. Tyrosine phosphatases can regulate the phosphorylation of various components in the signaling pathway. For example, the recruitment of SHP-1 to cytokine receptors (e.g., erythropoietin) is believed to regulate the duration and/or magnitude of cytokine signaling (1–4). In addition, there is some evidence that the stability of STAT proteins is altered after their activation by the targeting of phosphorylated STATs to the proteosome (5). Finally, PIAS proteins may limit the ability of STATs to bind DNA (6).

In this review, we will focus on two novel mechanisms by which cytokine signaling is regulated. One of these involves members of a newly described family of inhibitory signaling molecules, the suppressor of cytokine signaling, or SOCS, proteins. These proteins appear to be extremely important inhibitors of signaling initiated by many cytokines. We will also review the role of BCL-6, a transcriptional repressor that appears to be a regulator of type 2 (Th2) immune responses through its regulation of IL-4 signaling.

II. IL-4 Signaling

We will briefly review how cytokine signaling is initiated in cells. Because of its importance in controlling allergic immune responses, such as those observed in atopic asthma, we will use IL-4 as a paradigm for other type I and II cytokines. IL-4 is a type I cytokine that is produced by activated Th2 cells, mast cells, and basophils (reviewed in Ref. 7). The ligand-binding chain of the IL-4 receptor (IL-4Rα) is expressed on a wide variety of cell types (8,9). IL-4 plays an important role in the differentiation of T and B lymphocytes, promoting Th2 development in T cells and immunoglobulin class switching to IgE in B cells. B cells and T cells demonstrate enhanced survival when cultured in the presence of IL-4, while introduction of IL-4Rα confers IL-3–dependent cell lines with protection from apoptosis upon cytokine withdrawal (10–12).

IL-4 signaling is initiated by oligomerization of the IL-4 receptor complex. In hematopoeitic cells, this complex consists of the IL-4 receptor α chain and the common γ chain (γC) (13). In nonhematopoeitic cells, IL-4 signals through a complex consisting of IL-4Rα and the IL-13 receptor α1 chain (IL-13Rα1) (14). Subsequent downstream signaling events are mediated by nonreceptor tyrosine kinases constitutively associated with the receptor chains (15). The predominant kinases implicated in the initiation of cytokine signal transduction pathways are Janus family tyrosine kinases (JAKs). Indeed, IL-4Rα has been shown to associate with Jak1, while γC interacts with Jak3 (16–18). IL-4 binding induces the dimerization of the IL-4Rα and γC chains, an event that results in the juxtaposition of the receptor-associated Jak1 and Jak3 kinases, allowing their transphosphorylation and consequent activation. The JAKs then catalyze the phosphorylation of five conserved tyrosine residues found in the cytoplasmic tail of the IL-4Rα chain. These five tyrosines (Y1-Y5) all occur within the context of recognized PTB or SH2 domain-binding motifs, and upon phosphorylation they gain the ability to recruit proteins with these interaction modules, providing additional substrates for the JAKs.

The importance of Y1 in the activation of pathways necessary for IL-4–mediated proliferation and protection from apoptosis has been demonstrated in studies of IL-4Rα truncation mutants and specific point mutations, which replace the tyrosine at Y1 with phenylalanine (Y497F) (19–21). This tyrosine is found within a central NPxY sequence that is a recognized phosphotyrosine binding (PTB) domain–binding site. The phosphorylation has been shown to recruit insulin receptor substrate (IRS)-1 and IRS-2 (also known as 4PS), large phosphoproteins containing

20 potential sites for tyrosine phosphorylation. Among the proteins demonstrated to interact with IRS-1/2 are the p85 regulatory subunit of P13K and the adaptor molecule Grb-2 (22–24). While signaling through Y1 of the IL-4Rα chain promotes cell growth and survival, IL-4–induced gene activation is dependent on signals generated at Y2–Y4 (Y575, Y603, and Y631 of the human receptor) (25). Upon phosphorylation, these tyrosines can serve as docking sites for the SH2 domain of signal transducer and activator of transcription 6 (STAT6) (reviewed in Refs. 26,27). STAT6, in turn, is phosphorylated by Jak1, allowing the homodimerization of STAT6 molecules via a reciprocal SH2-pY interaction. Stat dimerization allows the molecule to enter the nucleus, where it binds a specific motif defined by the sequence TTC(N)$_{3-4}$GAA (26). STAT6-binding elements have been identified in the regulatory regions of several IL-4–responsive genes, including IL-4Rα, MHC class II, CD23, and the immunoglobulin germline ε, γ1 (murine) and γ4 (human) promoters (28–33). Studies of STAT6 −/− mice have confirmed the importance of STAT6 in mediated IL-4-induced transcription. These mice are unable to upregulate MHC class II or CD23b and demonstrate pronounced defects in IgE class switching and TH2 cell differentiation in response to IL-4 (34–36).

III. The Suppressor of Cytokine Signaling Family

The SOCS proteins comprise a recently defined family that has been implicated in the negative regulation of cytokine signaling. The first member of the SOCS family to be cloned was identified in a cDNA subtraction screening assay for genes induced by the membrane proximal portion of the EPO receptor cytoplasmic domain upon receptor ligation (37). As expression of this protein was found to be inducible by several cytokines, it was denoted CIS (cytokine-inducible SH2-containing protein). CIS was shown to associate with both the tyrosine-phosphorylated EPO receptor and the tyrosine-phosphorylated IL-3 receptor and to negatively regulate signaling through these receptors (37,38). Further studies have supported a role for CIS in the negative regulation of STAT5 activation in response to multiple cytokines, including EPO, IL-2, and IL-3 (39). As CIS associates with tyrosine-phosphorylated receptor chains, it is possible that CIS inhibits STAT5 activation by competing with STAT5 for binding sites on activated receptors. It has also been suggested that CIS may act as a scaffold, binding simultaneously to activated receptors and to other negative regulators (40). Studies utilizing transgenic mice expressing CIS under the control of the β-actin promoter have supported an in vivo role for CIS in the regulation of cytokine signal transduction: mice overexpressing CIS are smaller than their wild-type littermates, suggesting the suppression of GH signaling, while the defective development of mammary glands in female transgenic animals indicates an inhibition of prolactin signaling (41). Interestingly, while IL-2–induced STAT5 activation is inhibited in T cells from these mice, LIF-induced STAT3 activation in T cells is not affected, demonstrating the specificity of cytokine signal regulation by CIS. Somewhat surprisingly, mice deficient in CIS do not have any phenotypic differences from wild-type mice (41).

Two years after the cloning of CIS, SOCS-1 was simultaneously cloned by three different groups. One of these groups isolated SOCS-1 in a yeast two hybrid screen using the JH1 domain of JAK2 as bait (42). Another group used a monoclonal antibody directed against a sequence in the SH2 domain of STAT3 (GTFLLRFS) to screen a murine thymus cDNA expression library in an attempt to identify additional members of the STAT family (43). Of the 20 unknown genes isolated in this assay, only 2 had SH2 domains: SOCS-1 and CIS. A third group isolated SOCS-1 using an expression cloning system designed to identify genes that could block the IL-6–induced differentiation of the murine monocytic M1 cell line into macrophages (44). A cDNA library derived from the factor-dependent hematopoietic cell line FDC-P1 was retrovirally infected into M1 cells, and clones that became unresponsive to IL-6 were selected. SOCS-1 was identified in this assay, and a subsequent search of translated nucleic acid databases with the amino acid sequence predicted for SOCS-1 revealed its similarity to CIS and to two other classes of ESTs, leading to the cloning of SOCS-2 AND SOCS-3. These three different groups named the newly cloned molecule JAB, SSI-1, and SOCS-1, respectively (42–44). The SOCS family has also been referred to as the CIS family. In this chapter the SOCS nomenclature will be used for the sake of simplicity.

Of the different SOCS family members, SOCS-1 has been the most extensively studied. Found to interact with JAK2 and inhibit IL-6 signaling at the time of cloning, SOCS-1 was soon shown to be capable of interaction with all four JAK kinases through its SH2 domain and to inhibit their tyrosine kinase activity in vitro (42,43,45). When overexpressed in cell lines, SOCS-1 inhibits STAT activation by multiple cytokines, including IFNα, IFNγ, IL-2, IL-3, IL-4, IL-6, GH, prolactin, Epo, OSM, TSLP, Tpo, and LIF (42,44,46–50). Further overexpression studies have shown that SOCS-1 can also inhibit the activity of Tec and Vav and that it can suppress c-kit–mediated proliferation (51). While in vitro studies have provided many potential functions for SOCS-1, the generation of SOCS-1–deficient mice has helped clarify its physiological role. Mice lacking SOCS-1 exhibit perinatal lethality, dying by 3 weeks of age (52–54). In addition to severe lymphopenia and a moderate granulocytosis, these mice demonstrate fatty degeneration and necrosis of the liver and an infiltration of the lungs, heart, and pancreas by macrophages (53). These defects resemble those seen in wild-type mice given IFNγ as neonates (55). Interestingly, macrophages derived from SOCS-1–deficient bone marrow are hyperresponsive to IFNγ; furthermore, injection of neutralizing anti-IFNγ antibody twice weekly from birth can prevent disease in SOCS-1–deficient mice, thus demonstrating a requirement for IFNγ in the observed perinatal lethality (53). Mice that are doubly deficient in SOCS-1 and IFNγ do not suffer perinatal lethality, further implicating excessive IFNγ signaling in the disease observed in SOCS-1 −/− animals (54). The SOCS-1 −/− phenotype is transferable by injection of SOCS-1–deficient bone marrow into sublethally irradiated JAK3-deficient mice (54).Together with the observation that SOCS-1 deficiency does not result in perinatal lethality in a RAG2 −/− background, these data indicate the involvement of lymphocytes in the generation of the disease seen in SOCS-1 −/− mice (54).

T-cell development is also abnormal in SOCS-1–deficient mice (54). SOCS-1 is expressed in thymocytes, and thymic subset populations are perturbed in SOCS-1 −/− animals; further, peripheral T cells derived from these mice exhibit an activated phenotype. Elevated levels of IFNγ are detected in the serum of SOCS-1 −/− mice, but not in the serum of SOCS-1 −/− RAG2 −/− mice. These results suggest that in addition to a hyperresponsiveness to IFNγ, alterations in T-cell differentiation and the hypersecretion of IFNγ by peripheral T cells may contribute to the early lethality seen in SOCS-1 deficiency.

The study of mice deficient in SOCS-1 has indicated its importance in the regulation of signaling by other cytokines as well. The lymphopenia observed in SOCS-1–deficient mice is thought to be due, in part, to the accelerated apoptosis of lymphocytes derived from these mice secondary to the increased expression of the pro-apoptotic protein Bax (56). Subsequent studies have shown that murine embryonic fibroblasts lacking SOCS-1 are more sensitive to TNF-α–induced cell death than wild-type controls (57). In SOCS-1 −/− IFNγ −/− mice, accelerated lobuloalveolar development in the mammary gland and precocious lactation are seen during pregnancy, suggesting a role for SOCS-1 in the in vivo regulation of prolactin signaling (58). The presence of a single SOCS-1 allele in heterozygous females rescues the lactogenic defect in these mice, providing further evidence supporting a role for SOCS-1 in prolactin signaling. SOCS-1 has also been implicated in the regulation of insulin signaling (59). SOCS-1 −/− mice exhibit abnormally low blood sugar levels, and cells derived from these animals demonstrate a sustained phosphorylation of IRS-1 in response to insulin. IL-4 is yet another cytokine that appears to be regulated by SOCS-1: STAT6 activation by IL-4 is prolonged in SOCS-1–deficient mice (56). Some of the phenotypes seen in SOCS-1 deficiency cannot yet be ascribed to particular cytokines. For example, in contrast to SOCS-1 +/+ IFNγ −/− controls, SOCS-1 −/− IFNγ −/− mice exhibit polycystic kidneys with defective renal tubule organization, pneumonia, accelerated cataract formation, skin ulceration, and a granulomatous disease in the gut (60). A great deal of work remains to elucidate all of the physiological functions of SOCS-1.

In vitro studies have shown that SOCS-2 can inhibit signaling by GH, IL-6, and LIF (61–63). Further studies in cell lines have demonstrated association of SOCS-2 with the IGF-1 receptor (64). Analysis of mice lacking SOCS-2 has supported a role for SOCS-2 in the regulation of signaling by GH and IGF-1. Although indistinguishable from wild-type mice at birth, SOCS-2–deficient mice grow at a faster rate than wild-type littermates, eventually attaining a body weight 40% heavier in males and 20% heavier in females (65). This phenotype is thought to be due to a lack of regulation of the growth hormone/IGF-1 signaling pathway. SOCS-2–deficient mice begin to exhibit accelerated growth at 3–4 weeks of age, which is consistent with the timing of tissue growth hormone receptor expression. While the excessive bone growth seen in these mice resembles that in mice overexpressing growth hormone, their rate of growth and adult body weights more closely resemble those of IGF-1 transgenic mice. Excessive dermal collagen desposition, also seen in SOCS-2–deficient mice, is seen in mice overexpressing either growth hormone or

IGF-1. RNase protection assays demonstrate increased IGF-1 production in multiple organs of SOCS-2–deficient mice.

SOCS-3 has also been implicated in the regulation of cytokine signal transduction. As in the case of SOCS-1, SOCS-3 has been found to inhibit a number of cytokine signaling pathways in vitro, including IL-2, IL-3, IL-4, IL-6, IL-11, GH, prolactin, Epo, LIF, IFNγ, IFNα, CNTF, leptin, and OSM (46,48–50, 61, 66–70). To date, the most significant effect that may be attributed to SOCS-3 in vivo implicates SOCS-3 in the regulation of erythropoiesis. Deletion of SOCS-3 in mice results in embryonic lethality at 12–16 days, apparently secondary to severe erythrocytosis (67). The erythrocytosis is greatest in the abdomen surrounding the fetal liver, which is distorted by the abundance of erythrocytes. Because the cytokine Epo is thought to be the primary stimulator of erythrocyte proliferation, this result supports a role for SOCS-3 in the regulation of Epo signaling. Subsequent experiments have demonstrated that SOCS-3 binds to both the Epo receptor and to JAK2, which is constitutively associated with the cytoplasmic tail of the EPO receptor (71). Overexpression of SOCS-3 blocks the activation of STAT5 by Epo (71). The potential involvement of SOCS-3 in Epo regulation is further supported by the finding that mice expressing a SOCS-3 transgene under control of an H2K MHC class I promoter also exhibit embryonic lethality with a complete lack of fetal liver erythropoiesis (67). Curiously, reconstitution of lethally irradiated wild-type adult mice with fetal liver cells from SOCS-3–deficient embryos does not lead to erythrocytosis (67). In these reconstitution experiments, SOCS-3–deficient fetal liver cells were able to generate grossly normal thymic T-cell populations and splenic B-cell populations. These observations suggest that SOCS-3 function is not important for regulation of erythroid development in adult animals and raise the possibility that an alternate molecule or system with functions similar to those of SOCS-3 may operate in the bone marrow.

The first four members of the SOCS family to be described share two conserved domains: a central SH2 domain and a carboxy-terminal region designated the SOCS box (44). Further searching of DNA databases using the SOCS box amino acid consensus led to the discovery of four additional SOCS family members, which contain both a central SH2 domain and a C-terminal SOCS box, as well as 12 additional proteins with the SOCS box motif (72). Eight of these latter proteins have been separated into the subfamilies WSB, SSB, and ASB, indicating WD-40 repeat–containing proteins, SPRY domain–containing proteins, and ankyrin repeat–containing proteins, respectively. Of the four remaining proteins, two belong to a class of small GTPases and two represent ESTs of unknown structural class.

The functions of SOCS-4, SOCS-5, SOCS-6, and SOCS-7 remain to be determined. These four proteins each have a much larger N-terminal region preceding their SH2 domains when compared to the other family members (72). None of these N-terminal regions contains recognizable motifs except for that of SOCS-7, which contains a putative nuclear localization signal (73). Expression of SOCS-5 can be induced in the livers of mice injected with IL-6. SOCS-5 weakly inhibits signaling by LIF and IL-6 when overexpressed in M1 cells (61,72). A partial cDNA clone of SOCS-7 has been shown to interact with the adaptor molecules Nck and Ash and also with phospholipase C-γ (73). Mice deficient in each of these family members are currently being generated and are expected to shed light on their physiological functions.

IV. SOCS Family Structural Domains

The SOCS family (Fig. 1) is defined by the presence of a central SH2 domain and a C-terminal SOCS box (40,74,75). Analysis of the genomic structure and primary amino acid sequence within the SH2 domain has revealed that pairs of SOCS family members may be more closely related to each other than to other family members (76). These pairs are formed by CIS and SOCS-2, SOCS-1 and SOCS-3, SOCS-4 and SOCS-5, and SOCS-6 and SOCS-7. The importance of the SH2 domain in SOCS protein function has been examined in the cases of SOCS-1 and SOCS-3. Mutational analysis of SOCS-1 has demonstrated the requirement of both the SH2 domain and the 24 amino acids N-terminal to the SH2 domain for suppression of IL-6 signaling (77). The 24 amino acids N-terminal to the SH2 domain have been divided into two functionally distinct regions (45). The 12 residues immediately N-terminal to the SH2 domain are referred to as the extended SH2 subdomain (ESS) and are important in the binding of SOCS-1 to tyrosine phosporylated JAK2. The kinase inhibitory region (KIR) is composed of the 12 residues N-terminal to the ESS and is required for inhibition of cytokine signaling by SOCS-1. SOCS-1 also interacts with, and inhibits, the kinase activity of both JAK1 and JAK2 in LIF-mediated signaling (61). Mutation of arginine 105 of the SOCS-1 SH2 domain to

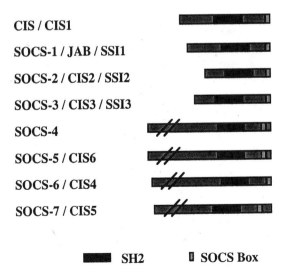

CIS / CIS1

SOCS-1 / JAB / SSI1

SOCS-2 / CIS2 / SSI2

SOCS-3 / CIS3 / SSI3

SOCS-4

SOCS-5 / CIS6

SOCS-6 / CIS4

SOCS-7 / CIS5

▬▬ SH2   ▯ SOCS Box

Figure 1 Domain structure of the SOCS family of proteins. Each of the SOCS family members contains a central SH2 domain and a C-terminal SOCS box.

lysine abolishes the inhibitory activity of SOCS-1 towards LIF signaling, further demonstrating the importance of the SOCS-1 SH2 domain for its function (61).

Although both proteins have been shown to inhibit cytokine signaling, studies have revealed several differences between SOCS-1 and SOCS-3. Interestingly, the introduction of an R71K mutation (corresponding to the R105K mutation described above for SOCS-1) within the SH2 domain of SOCS-3 does not change the ability of SOCS-3 to inhibit LIF-mediated activation of STAT3, in contrast to the effects of the analogous mutation in SOCS-1 (61). Further mutation of the SH2 domain of SOCS-3 is required to attenuate the ability of SOCS-3 to inhibit intracellular signaling; inclusion of the mutations D72E and S73C results in 50% suppression of STAT3 reporter activation, compared with the >90% inhibition of reporter activity seen in transfection assays using wild-type SOCS-3. Thus, while the SH2 domains of both SOCS-1 and SOCS-3 are functionally important, there appears to be a difference in the degree to which the SH2 domains of these proteins are necessary for the SOCS-mediated inhibition of cytokine signal transduction.

Although the precise function of the SOCS box remains unclear, it has been demonstrated to play an important role in signal transduction for at least SOCS-1. Deletion of the SOCS box was first reported to result in much lower expression levels of SOCS-1 in M1 cells (77). Expression levels of SOCS-1 with a SOCS box deletion were restored by treatment of the cells with proteasome inhibitors (77). A subsequent study found that SOCS-1 interaction with the Elongin BC complex prevents the proteasome-dependent degradation of SOCS-1 (78). These studies suggest a role for the SOCS box in stabilizing SOCS-1; however, interaction of the SOCS box of SOCS-1 with Elongin BC was observed to accelerate SOCS-1 degradation in a third study (79). The Elongin BC complex is part of an E3 ubiquitin ligase complex. This complex has also been shown to bind to the von Hippel-Lindau tumor suppressor protein, which contains a sequence conserved in the N-terminal half of all SOCS boxes and induces the degradation of bound hypoxia-inducible factors by the proteasome (79). Similarly, the F-box containing proteins of yeast have also been shown to interact with Elongin BC and to induce the proteasome-mediated intracellular degradation of cyclins.

More recently, Zhang et al. have generated mice with a deletion of the portion of the SOCS-1 gene encoding the SOCS box (80). Studies in these mice have demonstrated the in vivo importance of the SOCS box in the inhibition of IFNγ signaling by SOCS-1. While the SOCS-1 deletion mutant retains the ability to bind to JAK1, the phenotype of the mice is not as severe as that seen in SOCS-1–deficient mice. Like the SOCS-1–deficient mice, the SOCS box deletion mutants die prematurely and have a reduced body weight with inflammatory lesions in skeletal muscle, heart muscle, cornea, pancreas, and dermis. However, the onset of disease is later, and its severity decreased, in mice lacking the SOCS-1–SOCS box when compared to the disease observed in mice lacking SOCS-1 entirely. Survival of mice lacking the SOCS box is intermediate between that of SOCS-1–deficient mice and wild-type mice. The phenotype of mice with the SOCS box deletion has been compared to that of SOCS-1 −/− IFNγ +/− mice. On a molecular level, activation of STAT1 in response to IFNγ is prolonged in the livers of mice deficient in the SOCS box of SOCS-1. Interestingly, the SOCS box deletion mutant protein is expressed at much lower levels than the wild-type SOCS-1 protein in heterozygote mice, supporting a role for the SOCS box and, perhaps, for its interaction with the Elongin BC complex in protein stabilization. It has recently been shown that the von Hippel-Lindau protein is protected from proteosomal degradation by its association with the Elongin BC complex (81).

V. Mechanisms of Inhibition of Cytokine Signaling

At least three different mechanisms have been put forth to explain how SOCS family members inhibit cytokine signaling (summarized in Fig. 2). SOCS-1, both in studies in which it was initially cloned and in subsequent reports, has been shown to interact with all four JAK kinases and to inhibit their tyrosine kinase activity (42,43,45,61). As mentioned earlier, the KIR and ESS domains of SOCS-1, contained within the 24 amino acid residues N-terminal to the SH2 domain, are important in the inhibition of JAK kinase activity (45,77). It has been suggested that this region of 24 amino acids acts as a pseudosubstrate, blocking the access of JAK substrates (45). While SOCS-3 also binds to JAK2, it does so with a much lower affinity than SOCS-1. Similarly, SOCS-3 can inhibit the kinase activity of JAKs but must be expressed at much higher levels than SOCS-1 to achieve the same levels of inhibition (75).

Further evidence that SOCS-1 and SOCS-3 act through different mechanisms has been reported by Nicholson et al. (61). Both SOCS-1 and SOCS-3 can inhibit signaling by the LIF receptor, which activates JAK1, JAK2, and STAT3. Unlike SOCS-1, SOCS-3 does not inhibit the kinase activity of JAK1 or JAK2 when both SOCS-1/3 and JAK1/2 are overexpressed in 293T cells. The ability of SOCS-3 to inhibit IL-6 signaling is dependent on Y759 of gp130, the signal transducing subunit of the IL-6 receptor, and SOCS-3 co-precipitates with a tyrosine-phosphory-lated peptide corresponding to the region surrounding Y759 of gp130 (82). In contrast, SOCS-1 maintains suppression of IL-6 signaling in the absence of Y759 (82). These experiments have shed some light on the differences between SOCS-1 and SOCS-3. While inhibition of cytokine signaling by SOCS-1 is critically dependent on the conserved arginine residue within its SH2 domain and probably does not involve binding to cytokine receptor chains, neither of these elements is true for SOCS-3. In addition to its ability to bind gp130 and inhibit IL-6 signaling, SOCS-3 has been shown to interact with the tyrosine-phosphorylated GH receptor and the activated IL-2Rβ chain and to inhibit signaling by GH and IL-2 (48,66). Interestingly, in the studies on GH signaling, SOCS-3 did not inhibit the kinase activity of JAK2 significantly in 293 cells unless the GH receptor was co-expressed along with SOCS-3. Greater levels of SOCS-3–mediated inhibition of JAK2 kinase activity in this system were seen with increasing levels of GH receptor expression (48). Similarly, in IL-2 signaling, SOCS-3–mediated inhibition of JAK1 kinase activity is maximal in the presence of the IL-2Rβ chain. Another set of recent studies measured the affinity of SOCS-3 for tyrosine-phosphorylated peptides derived from JAKs, STATs, and gp130 (83). Of these, SOCS-3 was found to have a much greater affinity

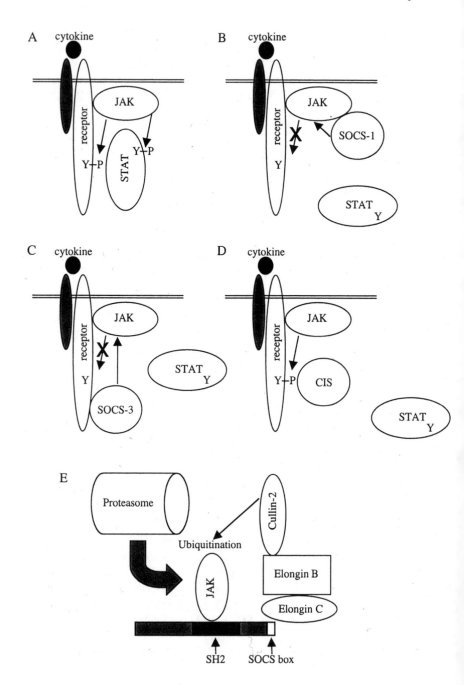

for phospho-peptides derived from the region surrounding Y759 of gp130 than for any of the other peptides. These results suggest that SOCS-3 acts on JAK kinases through association with receptor chains. In spite of this difference in binding partners between SOCS-1 and SOCS-3, the N-terminal domains of both proteins have been shown to be able to block JAK kinase activity. Domain-swapping experiments have demonstrated that the N-terminal domains of SOCS-1 and SOCS-3 are interchangeable (61).

In contrast, CIS is not thought to act through inhibiting JAK kinase activity. Like SOCS-3, CIS has been found to associate with activated cytokine receptors, including the activated IL-3 and EPO receptors (37). CIS binds at Y401 on the Epo receptor, one of the two STAT5-binding sites on this receptor (84). High levels of STAT5 expression overcome the inhibition of Epo signaling by CIS, suggesting that one mechanism by which CIS acts is through competition with STAT5 for access to phosphorylated Y401 (41). The potential for an additional mechanism for CIS-mediated inhibition of Epo signaling remains, as mutation of Y401 of the Epo receptor to phenylalanine does not abolish STAT5 activation by Epo. The activation of STAT5 in this case is thought to occur through Y343 on the Epo receptor, which has not been shown to be a binding site for CIS.

In addition to inhibiting JAK kinase activity and blocking access of STATs to receptor docking sites, a third mechanism by which SOCS proteins may inhibit cytokine signaling involves the targeting of substrates to proteasomal degradation. As discussed earlier, studies of the SOCS box have shown the ability of this domain to interact with the Elongin BC complex. This complex also interacts with cullin-2, which is an E3 ubiquitin ligase (79). In this model of signal regulation, signaling proteins associated with the SOCS molecules, and possibly the SOCS proteins themselves, are ubiquitinated and degraded by the proteasome. Proteasome-mediated

◀——

Figure 2 Mechanisms of inhibiting cytokine signaling. Upon cytokine binding, cytokine receptor chains oligomerize and JAK kinases are activated by auto- and transphosphorylation. The activated JAK kinases proceed to phosphorylate receptor chains, which permit the binding of the SH2 domain of STAT molecules to the tyrosine-phosphorylated receptor. The JAKs then phosphorylate the docked STAT molecules, which then dimerize and translocate to the nucleus to activate transcription (A). One mechanism by which SOCS-1 is thought to inhibit signaling is by binding directly to tyrosine-phosphorylated JAKs via its central SH2 domain and inhibiting JAK kinase activity (B). Current evidence suggests that SOCS-3 binds to tyrosine-phosphorylated cytokine receptor chains rather than to JAK kinases directly (C). Like SOCS-1, SOCS-3 also has the ability to inhibit the activity of JAK kinases via its N-terminal KIR. CIS has been shown to bind to tyrosine-phosphorylated residues on cytokine receptor chains, and is thought to block STAT activation by inhibiting the access of STAT molecules to the activated receptor (D). Another proposed mechanism by which SOCS proteins may inhibit cytokine signaling involves the interaction of the SOCS box with the Elongin BC complex. The complex binds to cullin-2, which acts as an E3 ubiquitin ligase and could ubiquitinate both SOCS molecules and/or other associated proteins (such as JAKs) and lead to their degradation by the proteasome (E).

regulation of cytokine signaling has been previously demonstrated, as activation of STAT5 downstream of Epo or IL-2 signaling is prolonged in the presence of proteasome inhibitors (84,85). Further, a monoubiquitinated form of CIS has been shown to accumulate in the presence of proteasome inhibitors, an observation that supports the hpothesis that SOCS molecules may themselves be regulated by ubiquitination and proteasomal degradation (84).

VI. Regulation of SOCS Expression

Transcripts encoding CIS, SOCS-1, SOCS-2, and SOCS-3 are present in a variety of tissues at low levels. Analysis of mouse tissues has revealed steady-state mRNA levels of CIS in kidney, fat, muscle, liver, hypothalamus, and heart (44). SOCS-1 expression is highly expressed in the thymus, with lower levels of expression in the spleen and lungs. SOCS-2 is expressed in the liver, lungs, and testis, while SOCS-3 expression is seen in the lungs, spleen, and thymus (44). CIS, SOCS-1, SOCS-2, SOCS-3, and SOCS-5 expression can be induced by several different cytokines including IFNγ, Epo, G-CSF, GM-CSF, IL-2, IL-3, IL-4, IL-6, LIF, GH, and prolactin (44,86). Cytokine-inducible expression of SOCS-4, SOCS-6, and SOCS-7 has not been demonstrated to date. The induction of SOCS molecules by cytokines seems to be tissue specific. For example, while GH stimulates expression of CIS, SOCS-2, and SOCS-3 in murine liver, in the murine mammary gland only CIS and SOCS-2 are induced by GH (86). In addition to the tissue specificity of SOCS induction, specific SOCS molecules can be induced by specific cytokines. Stimulation of mouse hypothalamus with CNTF has been shown to induce the expression of SOCS-3, but not CIS, SOCS-1, or SOCS-2 (69,70,87). SOCS-3 is also specifically induced by IL-10 in monocytes and by LPS in macrophages (88,89). However, this level of cytokine specificity is not always seen, as stimulation of murine bone marrow with different cytokines results in induction of multiple SOCS mRNA transcripts. For example, Epo stimulation leads to the upregulation of CIS, SOCS-2, and SOCS-3; stimulation by IL-3 leads to the induction of CIS, SOCS-2, SOCS-3, and (to a lesser degree) SOCS-1; IFNγ stimulation induces CIS, SOCS-1, SOCS-2, and SOCS-3 (44).

STATs have been implicated in the induction of SOCS expression by cytokines. CIS induction in response to IL-3 is repressed in the presence of a dominant negative mutant of STAT5 (90). There are four STAT5-binding sites in the proximal promoter of CIS, which are all required for Epo-mediated activation of the CIS promoter in transient transfection experiments (38). Finally, CIS expression is normally seen in the wild-type mouse ovary, but is absent in mice deficient in both STAT5a and STAT5b (91). Similarly, the SOCS-1 promoter contains binding sites for STAT1, STAT3, and STAT6, and expression of a dominant negative STAT3 mutant in M1 cells blocks induction of SOCS-1 by IL-6 or LIF (43).

The timing of induction by cytokines also varies between different SOCS family members. Injection of GH into mice with subsequent examination of SOCS expression in the liver demonstrates a rapid induction of SOCS-3 mRNA, with expression peaking at 2 hours before returning to base levels (86,92). Early CIS expression patterns appear similar, but an additional broad pulse is observed later in the time course. SOCS-2 expression is induced much more slowly and is of greater duration. Examination of livers derived from mice injected with IL-6 also shows different patterns of expression among different SOCS family members: SOCS-1, SOCS-2, and SOCS-3 are all induced within 20 minutes of stimulation (44); however, SOCS-1 mRNA levels tapers off after 2 hours, SOCS-3 mRNA is greatly reduced after 4 hours and is not seen beyond 12 hours, while SOCS-2 mRNA is still prominent 24 hours after stimulation. CIS expression in this system is also seen within 20 minutes, fading by 4 hours but reappearing at the 12- and 24-hour time points. The timing of SOCS expression also seems to vary by tissue type, as the timing of SOCS-1 and CIS expression in M1 cells is different from that seen in the liver. After stimulation of M1 cells with IL-6, SOCS-1 expression is seen approximately 40 minutes poststimulation, peaking by 2 hours and persisting at low levels for 12 hours (44). In M1 cells stimulated with IL-6, CIS expression is first seen at 1 hour and remains for at least 24 hours.

VII. SOCS Perspectives and Future Directions

SOCS proteins have emerged as important regulators of cytokine signaling. The observation that STATs can mediate SOCS expression reveals a classical feedback loop for the termination of cytokine-stimulated signals. Gene deletion of SOCS-1 and SOCS-3 results in lethality, demonstrating the critical role these molecules play in checking the cellular response to cytokine stimulation. The SOCS family has been the subject of much research over the past 5 years, and many questions still remain. Continued studies of mice deficient in various SOCS family members will lead to further understanding of the physiological role of these molecules, which demonstrate many activities in vitro. The generation of mice deficient in SOCS-4, SOCS-5, SOCS-6, and SOCS-7, along with continued efforts to find binding partners for these proteins, will help to elucidate their function. The ability of SOCS proteins to block cytokine signaling pathways raises the possibility of their clinical utilization in the suppression of inflammation. In this regard, promising results have recently been published demonstrating that injection of recombinant adenovirus carrying SOCS-3 cDNA into ankles of mice with collagen-induced arthritis greatly reduces the severity of the arthritis (93).

VIII. BCL-6 Expression in Normal Tissue
   and Lymphoma

In recent years, the transcriptional repressor BCL-6 has emerged as an important nuclear regulator of the immune response through its modulation of cytokine signal transduction pathways. In addition to its role in the maintainence of the immune system, BCL-6 has been implicated in the regulation of normal cell growth and development: mice homozygous for a deletion of BCL-6 are runted, and recent evidence indicates that overexpression of BCL-6 may either promote or inhibit apoptosis in various cell lines (94–98). Furthermore, DNA chip analysis has identified a number of genes involved in lymphocyte differentiation and cell cycle regulation as targets of repression by BCL-6 (99). The dysregulation of BCL-6 expression is believed to be a critical determinant in the evolution of certain lymphoid malignancies (100–105).

The BCL-6 proto-oncogene encodes a 96–100 kDa phosphoprotein that is normally expressed in a tissue-specific and developmentally regulated manner. Although many tissues express low levels of BCL-6 mRNA, high levels of the BCL-6 protein have been found only in certain B cells and T cells (106). Within the B-cell lineage, BCL-6 is expressed at high levels in mature, germinal center B cells, but not in other B cells or plasma cells (106–108). BCL-6 expression in T cells is limited to cortical thymocytes and a population of CD4+ cells within the germinal center and perifollicular zones of the lymph nodes (106). BCL-6 expression is further regulated in an activation-dependent manner. Signaling through CD40 has been shown to result in a reduction of BCL-6 mRNA levels within B cells, while stimulation through the B-cell receptor induces the proteosome-mediated degradation of the BCL-6 protein (109–111). Given the highly regulated nature of BCL-6 expression in differentiating germinal center cells, it is perhaps not surprising that perturbations of BCL-6 expression are correlated with the development of B-cell lymphomas.

Rearrangement of BCL-6 at chromosome band 3q27 can be detected in 30–40% of diffuse large-cell lymphomas (DLCL) and in 6–14% of follicular lymphomas (FL) (100–105). The translocations affecting the BCL-6 gene are located within a region spanning approximately 4 kb of the promoter and the first exon and result in the juxtaposition of the BCL-6 coding domains downstream of heterologous promoters derived from a number of other chromosomes (112–116). A number of studies have also demonstrated a high frequency of point mutations within 2 kb of the BCL-6 transcriptional initiation site (117–119). These mutations are apparently unrelated to tumorigenesis, as they occur similarly in normal and malignant B-cell populations. Instead, these modifications are consistent with those produced by somatic hypermutation of the IgV loci in germinal center B cells, and likely result from the same mechanism (117,118). However, while the specific mutations generated by this process may not be the direct cause of subsequent cellular transformation, it is possible that the mechanism that targets these loci for alterations of germline structure is ultimately responsible for their frequent involvement in translocations. Rearrangements of BCL-6 lead to the production of chimeric transcripts that encode a wild-type protein, indicating that the functional consequence of these translocations is the deregulation of BCL-6 expression by promoter substitution (116,120). The high frequency of dysregulated BCL-6 expression in these tumors suggests that this oncogene plays an important role in the transformation of human B cells.

IX.   Structure of BCL-6 and PDZ Family Proteins

The BCL-6 gene encodes a polypeptide containing six carboxy-terminal zinc-finger motifs homologous to members of the Krüppel subfamily of zinc-finger proteins

(101,103,121). This domain of BCL-6 has been shown to recognize and bind to specific DNA sequences in vitro (104,122,123). The N-terminal portion of BCL-6 contains a BTB (bric-a-brac/tramtrack/broad-complex)/Zin (zinc-finger N-terminal)/ PDZ (POX/zinc-finger) domain, an evolutionarily conserved motif that has been identified in nearly 50 proteins to date (124–130). Most of these proteins fall into one of two categories, based on the presence of other conserved domains and their predicted functions (reviewed in Ref. 126). The majority of PDZ-domain proteins appear to be transcriptional regulators, containing site-specific zinc-finger DNA-binding domains, as is the case with BCL-6. The second class of PDZ-domain proteins, typified by the *Drosophila* kelch protein, features a C-terminal domain containing six imperfect 50aa repeats, each terminating with a Gly-Gly doublet. This Gly-Gly motif is believed to mediate actin binding and bundling activity (126,131,132).

The PDZ domain itself is an 120-amino-acid motif generally found at the extreme amino terminus of BTB/PDZ proteins. Family members demonstrate extensive homology throughout the length of this hydrophobic domain, with 30–50% conservation of amino acid sequence identity (127,133). Numerous overexpression studies have catalogued the ability of PDZ-containing proteins to form homo- or heterodimers; further, the PDZ domain is suspected to mediate the formation of larger oligomeric structures in vivo (104,127,133–137). The recently solved crystal structure of the PDZ domain of PLZF, a zinc-finger transcription factor implicated in retinoic acid–unresponsive acute promyelocytic leukemia, reveals the PLZF dimer to be considerably more stable than the monomeric form, confirming the multimeric association of the PDZ domain (133,138). The hydrophobic dimerization interface of PLZF-PDZ is extensively distributed throughout the domain and involves approximately 25% of the monomer surface area in a tightly intertwined dimer, as is characteristic for an obligate homodimer (133). Thus, both biochemical and structural studies indicate a role for the PDZ domain in mediating multimeric protein-protein interactions.

X. Transcriptional Regulation by PDZ Family Proteins

Transfection experiments have demonstrated that BCL-6 can act as a transcriptional repressor, and that its ability to mediate repression requires the N-terminal PDZ domain (122, 123,139). These results suggest that BCL-6 modulates transcription not simply through competitive binding, but through a mechanism of active repression dependent on an intact PDZ domain. Members of the DNA-binding class of BTB/ PDZ proteins are believed to have the capacity to modify gene expression on a global and/or local scale. PDZ domain–mediated aggregation of DNA-bound transcription factors may effect long-range changes in higher-order chromatin structure through chromatin condensation or decondensation, resulting in the repression or activation of gene expression (126). This mechanism has been implicated in the chromatin modeling activity of the *Drosophila* proteins GAGA and E(var)3-93D (126,135,140, 141). However, many other PDZ domain–containing proteins, particularly a growing set of mammalian transcriptional repressors, appear to utilize alternative mechanisms in order to achieve a more local regulation of gene expression. One of the more interesting recent developments was the discovery that the PDZ domains of BCL-6, PLZF, and BACH2 are able to mediate heterophilic interactions with multiple components of the histone deacetylase (HDAC) repressor complex, including the SMRT/N-CoR co-repressors (silencing mediator of retinoid and thyroid hormone receptor/nuclear receptor corepressor), BCoR (BCL-6 interacting corepressor, which appears to specifically interact with BCL-6 to the exclusion of other PDZ proteins), mSin3A, and HDAC-1 (142–149). While apparently not a general mechanism of PDZ-mediated repression (150), the ability of some family members to recruit the repressor complex provides a reasonable mechanistic explanation for the dependence of transcriptional repression on the presence of an intact PDZ domain. Current evidence suggests that covalent modification of histones, through either acetylation or phosphorylation, is a mechanism widely used by transcriptional activators in the induction of gene expression (151–154). These changes contribute a net negative charge to histone molecules and are believed to allow the transcriptional machinery increased access to DNA, due to a relaxation of chromatin structure resulting from the reduction in the electrostatic attraction of DNA for the altered nucleosome units. The reversal of these modifications catalyzed through the recruitment of the multisubunit histone deacetylase complex may negatively regulate transcription through induction of a more repressive chromatin structure. Individual components of the PDZ-recruited HDAC complex may have additional roles in promoting repression by interfering with the basal transcription machinery, as has been suggested by the observation that the co-repressors SMRT and N-CoR can interact with the basal factors $TF_{II}B$, $TAF_{II}32$, and $TAF_{II}70$ in a manner that apparently disrupts critical associations between these proteins (145,155).

XI. Chromatin and Cancer

A number of recent reports have demonstrated a causal link between alterations in the normal function of chromatin-modifying complexes and carcinogenesis (156–160). Many of these studies attribute transformation to effects that result in the inappropriate induction of an open chromatin structure, either through the inactivation of a tumor suppressor gene whose normal function is to recruit HDAC in a sequence specific manner, as has been suggested by the discovery of an Rb/E2F/HDAC-1 complex, or by coopting mechanisms established to regulate the function of HAT, as has been demonstrated in the case of E1a (158–162). However, while the recently described PDZ protein APM-1 appears to act as a traditional tumor suppressor (163), BCL-6 and PLZF represent a somewhat different paradigm in which it is the (presumed) overexpression of a transcriptional repressor and the resultant hyperactivation of the histone deacetylase machinery that is implicated in tumorigenesis. It is therefore likely that the role of these PDZ proteins in promoting transformation arises from an ability to inhibit normal differentiation programs, a function that may be appropriate in the context of the germinal center but poses the risk of uncontrolled growth when temporally deregulated.

XII. Lessons from the BCL-6 Knockout Mouse

The role of BCL-6 in tumorigenesis has been inferred from studies linking its deregulation to certain classes of lymphoid malignancies. Little is known, however, regarding the physiological role of this proto-oncogene. The importance of BCL-6 in normal lymphocyte function has been demonstrated in mice in which the gene for BCL-6 is disrupted by homologous recombination (95,97,164). Although these mice produce normal numbers of B and T cells, they fail to form germinal centers or mount T-cell-dependent antibody responses. In addition, many of these mice develop a systemic inflammatory disease characterized by the infiltration of the heart, lung, gut, and skin by eosinophils and IgE+ B cells. These features are indicative of a Th2-polarized inflammatory response, which might result from the inappropriate influence of Th2 cytokines (IL-4, IL-5, IL-6, and IL-13) on immune function. Indeed, in vitro activated T cells isolated from the BCL-6 knockout mouse express higher levels of IL-4, IL-5, and IL-13 than their wild-type counterparts, with no difference in the expression of the Th1 cytokine IFNγ (97). Interestingly, genetic complementation studies in RAG-1 −/−, IgM −/−, and TCRβδ −/− mice demonstrate that a nonlymphoid population is also required for the generation of the inflammatory disease of the BCL-6 −/− mouse (165). These studies also describe a hyper-secretion of MCP-1, MCP-3, and MRP-1 from BCL-6 −/− macrophages that is suppressed upon retroviral introduction of BCL-6. Chemokines are known to have an important role in regulating inflammatory processes; MCP-1, in particular, has been shown to promote IL-4 production by T cells and inhibit the secretion of IL-12 by monocytes. These data, therefore, suggest that dysregulated chemokine expression in myeloid cells may play a role in initiating the inflammatory response of the BCL-6 −/− animal (165).

XIII. BCL-6 Regulation of IL-4-Dependent Signaling Pathways

The striking phenotype of the knockout animal implicates BCL-6 in the normal regulation of the immune system. Given the Th2-type inflammation evident in the BCL-6-deficient mouse, it is likely that this regulation is accomplished at least partly through the modulation of cytokine signal transduction pathways.

While cytokine-mediated signaling events may be regulated at many levels, the ability of BCL-6 to act as a transcriptional repressor suggests that BCL-6 influences these pathways at the level of gene expression. Interestingly, an in vitro defined by binding site for BCL-6 (B6BS: AAAT<u>TCCTAGAAAG</u>CAT) bears marked homology to the TTC(N$_{3-4}$)GAA consensus sequence recognized by STAT proteins, important downstream mediators of cytokine signaling. This observation has led to the hypothesis that BCL-6 is targeted to STAT-responsive genes through the shared recognition of similar binding motifs (95,97,139). The Th2-type nature of the inflammatory disease seen in the BCL-6 −/− mouse suggests a perturbation of IL-4-dependent signaling pathways, directing initial investigations toward the study of genes responsive to this cytokine. These studies demonstrate that BCL-6 can bind to Stat6 sites found in a number of IL-4-responsive genes, but with varying affinity. Furthermore, the IL-4/Stat6–dependent murine germline ε promoter (mIε) has been identified as a physiological target of BCL-6 repression (139). Transcription from mIε is required for subsequent class switching to IgE; the presence of IgE+ B cells in the inflammatory infiltrate of the BCL-6 knockout mouse is consistent with deregulated IgE production in the absence of a natural repressor of IgE class switching. Another less well-characterized potential target of BCL-6 is the murine germline γ1 promoter, an IL-4-responsive site that regulates class switching to IgG1 (139).

Interestingly, while initial reports suggested that CD23 might be regulated by BCL-6, further studies have failed to support this conclusion (97,99,139). These results indicate that BCL-6 represses a subset of Stat6-activated genes, and that its role in the regulation of IL-4-induced responses may be quite specific. Whether this may be attributed to variations in the intrinsic affinity of BCL-6 for the Stat6 sites present in different IL-4-responsive genes or is due to differences in promoter architecture is not yet clear. Evidence indicates, however, that BCL-6–mediated repression is dependent upon its ability to bind cooperatively to multiple promoter elements in a manner that requires an intact PDZ domain (M. Harris and P. Rothman, unpublished). As cooperative systems allow high-affinity binding sites to drive the occupancy of associated weak sites at protein concentrations 10- to 1000-fold lower than would be predicted by characterization of individual sites, it is likely that promoter architecture does in fact play a key role in determining the site selectivity of BCL-6 (166).

XIV. BCL-6 and Atopic Disorders

Elevated IgE production is the hallmark of atopy, a common hereditary predisposition towards the development of hypersensitivity reactions such as asthma and eczema. The generation of atopic responses has been associated, both conceptually and functionally, with the deregulation of signaling pathways downstream of IL-4. Recent studies have demonstrated a linkage between certain IL-4Rα polymorphisms and atopy in isolated populations (167–170). These receptor variants are believed to lead to enhanced STAT6 activation and STAT6-dependent gene expression. An Ile50Val mutation, in particular, has been shown to promote increased STAT6 phosphorylation and increased levels of IL-4–induced CD23 expression and germline ε transcription (168,169).

Regulation of the IgE response by BCL-6 presents a mechanism whereby variations in the expression or function of the repressor may be linked to the development of atopic disorders. In fact, one recent report has demonstrated a correlation between a HindIII polymorphism found in the first intron of BCL-6 and marked atopy in a British population (171). As this polymorphism is located within the 5′-untranslated region of the gene, it is likely that the phenotype associated with this variant results from altered (presumably lower) cellular levels of BCL-6. Further investigation may reveal additional BCL-6 polymorphisms related to the generation of atopic responses. Mutations within the domains responsible for protein-protein and protein-DNA interaction would be expected to affect susceptibility to atopy. It is also tempting to speculate the existence of polymorphisms within Iε that influence the efficiency of BCL-6 binding at the promoter, resulting in a heightened sensitivity towards allergenic stimuli and a resultant atopy. Promoter variations are of particular interest as they would necessarily result in specific defects of BCL-6–mediated transcriptional regulation, rather than the more global defects predicted to result from mutations that alter the structure or function of BCL-6.

XV. Other Targets of BCL-6 Repression

While initial investigation of BCL-6 focused on its ability to repress STAT6-activated gene transcription, many studies have presented convincing evidence that BCL-6 is in fact involved in the regulation of events mediated by cytokines other than IL-4. Analysis of mice doubly deficient in BCL-6 and either the IL-4 receptor or STAT6 reveals that while these mice, like their BCL-6 $-/-$ counterparts, are deficient in the STAT6-dependent process of IgE production, they exhibit much of the same pathology as their BCL-6–deficient littermates—including the eosinophilic infiltration of multiple organ systems (139,172). The chemokines MCP-1, MCP-3, MRP-1, MIP-1α, and IP-10 have been identified as possible targets of BCL-6, providing a potential mechanism for the STAT6-independent initiation of the inflammatory response seen in the BCL-6 $-/-$ STAT6 $-/-$ animals (99,165). BCL-6 has been implicated in the regulation of B-cell terminal differentiation through repression of the STAT3-dependent transcription of Blimp-1, a principal mediator of plasma cell development (173). Other evidence linking BCL-6 to the regulation of normal cell growth and development includes overexpression studies that indicate that BCL-6 may either promote or inhibit apoptosis in various cell lines by repression of BCL-2 family members (94,96,98). Finally, DNA chip analysis has identified a number of genes involved in lymphocyte differentiation and cell cycle regulation that are activated in the absence of BCL-6 (99).

References

1. David M, et al. A nuclear tyrosine phosphatase downregulates interferon-induced gene expression. Mol Cell Biol 1993; 13(12):7515–7521.
2. Haque SJ, et al. Protein-tyrosine phosphatase Shp-1 is a negative regulator of IL-4- and IL-13-dependent signal transduction. J Biol Chem 1998; 273(51):33893–33896.
3. Neel BG. Role of phosphatases in lymphocyte activation. Curr Opin Immunol 1997; 9(3):405–420.
4. Neel BG, Tonks NK. Protein tyrosine phosphatases in signal transduction. Curr Opin Cell Biol, 1997; 9(2):193–204.
5. Kim TK, Maniatis T. Regulation of interferon-gamma-activated STAT1 by the ubiquitin-proteasome pathway. Science, 1996; 273(5282):1717–1719.
6. Liu B, et al. Inhibition of Stat1-mediated gene activation by PIAS1. Proc Natl Acad Sci USA 1998; 95(18):10626–10631.

7. Nelms K, et al. The IL-4 receptor: signaling mechanisms and biologic functions. Annu Rev Immunol 1999; 17:701–738.

8. Lowenthal JW, et al. Up-regulation of interleukin 4 receptor expression on immature (Lyt-2-/L3T4-) thymocytes. J Immunol 1988; 140(2):474–478.

9. Ohara J, Paul WE. Receptors for B-cell stimulatory factor-1 expressed on cells of haematopoietic lineage. Nature 1987; 325(6104):537–540.

10. Zamorano J, et al. IL-4 protects cells from apoptosis via the insulin receptor substrate pathway and a second independent signaling pathway. J Immunol 1996; 157(11): 4926–4934.

11. Hu-Li J, et al. B cell stimulatory factor 1 (interleukin 4) is a potent costimulant for normal resting T lymphocytes. J Exp Med 1987; 165(1):157–172.

12. Dancescu M, et al. Interleukin 4 protects chronic lymphocytic leukemic B cells from death by apoptosis and upregulates Bcl-2 expression. J Exp Med 1992; 176(5): 1319–1326.

13. Russell SM, et al. Interleukin-2 receptor gamma chain: a functional component of the interleukin-4 receptor. Science 1993; 262(5141):1880–1883.

14. Murata T, Taguchi J, Puri RK. Interleukin-13 receptor alpha' but not alpha chain: a functional component of interleukin-4 receptors. Blood 1998; 91(10):3884–3891.

15. Murakami M, et al. Critical cytoplasmic region of the interleukin 6 signal transducer gp130 is conserved in the cytokine receptor family. Proc Natl Acad Sci USA 1991; 88(24):11349–11353.

16. Russell SM, et al. Interaction of IL-2R beta and gamma c chains with Jak1 and Jak3: implications for XSCID and XCID. Science 1994; 266(5187):1042–1045.

17. Murata T, Noguchi PD, Puri RK. IL-13 induces phosphorylation and activation of JAK2 Janus kinase in human colon carcinoma cell lines: similarities between IL-4 and IL-13 signaling. J Immunol 1996; 156(8):2972–2978.

18. Miyazaki T, et al. Functional activation of Jak1 and Jak3 by selective association with IL-2 receptor subunits. Science 1994; 266(5187):1045–1047.

19. Seldin DC, Leder P. Mutational analysis of a critical signaling domain of the human interleukin 4 receptor. Proc Natl Acad Sci USA 1994; 91(6):2140–2144.

20. Keegan AD, et al. An IL-4 receptor region containing an insulin receptor motif is important for IL-4-mediated IRS-1 phosphorylation and cell growth. Cell 1994; 76(5): 811–820.

21. Deutsch HH, et al. Distinct sequence motifs within the cytoplasmic domain of the human IL-4 receptor differentially regulate apoptosis inhibition and cell growth. J Immunol 1995; 154(8):3696–3703.

22. Sun XJ, et al. Role of IRS-2 in insulin and cytokine signalling. Nature 1995; 377(6545): 173–177.

23. Sun XJ, et al. Pleiotropic insulin signals are engaged by multisite phosphorylation of IRS-1. Mol Cell Biol 1993; 13(12):7418–7428.

24. Sun XJ, et al. Structure of the insulin receptor substrate IRS-1 defines a unique signal transduction protein. Nature 1991; 352(6330):73–77.

25. Ryan JJ, et al. Growth and gene expression are predominantly controlled by distinct regions of the human IL-4 receptor. Immunity 1996; 4(2):123–132.

26. Schindler C, Darnell JE, Jr. Transcriptional responses to polypeptide ligands: the JAK-STAT pathway. Annu Rev Biochem 1995; 64:621–651.

27. Leonard WJ, O'Shea JJ, Jaks and STATs: biological implications. Annu Rev Immunol 1998; 16:293–322.

28. Noelle R, et al. Increased expression of Ia antigens on resting B cells: an additional role for B-cell growth factor. Proc Natl Acad Sci USA 1984; 81(19):6149–6153.

29. Ohara J, Paul WE. Up-regulation of interleukin 4/B-cell stimulatory factor 1 receptor expression. Proc Natl Acad Sci USA 1988; 85(21):8221–8225.

30. Vitetta ES, et al. Serological, biochemical, and functional identity of B cell-stimulatory factor 1 and B cell differentiation factor for IgG1. J Exp Med 1985; 162(5):1726–1731.

31. Gascan H, et al. Human B cell clones can be induced to proliferate and to switch to IgE and IgG4 synthesis by interleukin 4 and a signal provided by activated CD4+ T cell clones. J Exp Med 1991; 173(3):747–750.

32. Defrance T, et al. Human recombinant interleukin 4 induces Fc epsilon receptors (CD23) on normal human B lymphocytes. J Exp Med 1987; 165(6):1459–1467.

33. Coffman RL, et al. B cell stimulatory factor-1 enhances the IgE response of lipopolysaccharide-activated B cells. J Immunol 1986; 136(12):4538–4541.

34. Takeda K, et al. Essential role of Stat6 in IL-4 signalling. Nature 1996; 380(6575):627–630.

35. Shimoda K, et al. Lack of IL-4-induced Th2 response and IgE class switching in mice with disrupted Stat6 gene. Nature 1996; 380(6575):630–633.

36. Kaplan MH, et al. Stat6 is required for mediating responses to IL-4 and for development of Th2 cells. Immunity 1996; 4(3):313–319.

37. Yoshimura A, et al. A novel cytokine-inducible gene CIS encodes an SH2-containing protein that binds to tyrosine-phosphorylated interleukin 3 and erythropoietin receptors. Embo J 1995; 14(12):2816–2826.

38. Matsumoto A, et al. CIS, a cytokine inducible SH2 protein, is a target of the JAK-STAT5 pathway and modulates STAT5 activation. Blood 1997; 89(9):3148–3154.

39. Aman MJ, et al. CIS associates with the interleukin-2 receptor beta chain and inhibits interleukin-2-dependent signaling. J Biol Chem 1999; 274(42):30266–30272.

40. Chen XP, Losman JA, Rothman P. SOCS proteins, regulators of intracellular signaling. Immunity 2000; 13(3):287–290.

41. Matsumoto A, et al. Suppression of STAT5 functions in liver, mammary glands, and T cells in cytokine-inducible SH2-containing protein 1 transgenic mice. Mol Cell Biol 1999; 19(9):6396–6407.

42. Endo TA, et al. A new protein containing an SH2 domain that inhibits JAK kinases. Nature 1997; 387(6636):921–924.

43. Naka T, et al. Structure and function of a new STAT-induced STAT inhibitor. Nature 1997; 387(6636):924–929.

44. Starr R, et al. A family of cytokine-inducible inhibitors of signalling. Nature 1997; 387(6636):917–921.

45. Yasukawa H, et al. The JAK-binding protein JAB inhibits Janus tyrosine kinase activity through binding in the activation loop. Embo J 1999; 18(5):1309–1320.

46. Losman JA, et al. Cutting edge: SOCS-1 is a potent inhibitor of IL-4 signal transduction. J Immunol 1999; 162(7):3770–3774.

47. Isaksen DE, et al. Requirement for stat5 in thymic stromal lymphopoietin-mediated signal transduction. J Immunol 1999; 163(11):5971–5977.

48. Hansen JA, et al. Mechanism of inhibition of growth hormone receptor signaling by suppressor of cytokine signaling proteins. Mol Endocrinol 1999; 13(11):1832–1843.

49. Pezet A, et al. Inhibition and restoration of prolactin signal transduction by suppressors of cytokine signaling. J Biol Chem 1999; 274(35):24497–24502.

50. Song MM, Shuai K. The suppressor of cytokine signaling (SOCS) 1 and SOCS3 but not SOCS2 proteins inhibit interferon-mediated antiviral and antiproliferative activities. J Biol Chem 1998; 273(52):35056–35062.

51. Yasukawa H, Sasaki A, Yoshimura A. Negative regulation of cytokine signaling pathways. Annu Rev Immunol 2000; 18:143–164.

52. Starr R, et al. Liver degeneration and lymphoid deficiencies in mice lacking suppressor of cytokine signaling-1. Proc Natl Acad Sci USA 1998; 95(24):14395–14399.

53. Alexander WS, et al. SOCS1 is a critical inhibitor of interferon gamma signaling and prevents the potentially fatal neonatal actions of this cytokine. Cell 1999; 98(5): 597–608.

54. Christophe-Marine JC, et al. SOCS1 deficiency causes a lymphocyte-dependent perinatal lethality. Cell 1999; 98(5):609–616.

55. Gresser I, et al. Electrophoretically pure mouse interferon inhibits growth, induces liver and kidney lesions, and kills suckling mice. Am J Pathol 1981; 102(3):396–402.

56. Naka T, et al. Accelerated apoptosis of lymphocytes by augmented induction of Bax in SSI-1 (STAT-induced STAT inhibitor-1) deficient mice. Proc Natl Acad Sci USA 1998; 95(26):15577–15582.

57. Morita Y, et al. Signals transducers and activators of transcription (STAT)-induced STAT inhibitor-1 (SSI-1)/suppressor of cytokine signaling-1 (SOCS-1) suppresses tumor necrosis factor alpha-induced cell death in fibroblasts. Proc Natl Acad Sci USA, 2000; 97(10):5405–5410.

58. Lindeman GJ, et al. SOCS1 deficiency results in accelerated mammary gland development and rescues lactation in prolactin receptor-deficient mice. Genes Dev 2001; 15(13):1631–1636.

59. Kawazoe Y, et al. Signal transducer and activator of transcription (STAT)-induced STAT inhibitor 1 (SSI-1)/suppressor of cytokine signaling 1 (SOCS1) inhibits insulin signal transduction pathway through modulating insulin receptor substrate 1 (IRS-1) phosphorylation. J Exp Med 2001; 193(2):263–269.

60. Metcalf D, et al. Polycystic kidneys and chronic inflammatory lesions are the delayed consequences of loss of the suppressor of cytokine signaling-1 (SOCS-1). Proc Natl Acad Sci USA 2002; 99(2):943–948.

61. Nicholson SE, et al. Mutational analyses of the SOCS proteins suggest a dual domain requirement but distinct mechanisms for inhibition of LIF and IL-6 signal transduction. Embo J 1999; 18(2):375–385.

62. Minamoto S, et al. Cloning and functional analysis of new members of STAT induced STAT inhibitor (SSI) family: SSI-2 and SSI-3. Biochem Biophys Res Commun 1997; 237(1):79–83.

63. Ram PA, Waxman DJ. SOCS/CIS protein inhibition of growth hormone-stimulated STAT5 signaling by multiple mechanisms. J Biol Chem 1999; 274(50):35553–35561.

64. Dey BR, et al. Interaction of human suppressor of cytokine signaling (SOCS)-2 with the insulin-like growth factor-I receptor. J Biol Chem 1998; 273(37):24095–24101.

65. Metcalf D, et al. Gigantism in mice lacking suppressor of cytokine signalling-2. Nature 2000; 405(6790):1069–1073.

66. Cohney SJ, et al. SOCS-3 is tyrosine phosphorylated in response to interleukin-2 and suppresses STAT5 phosphorylation and lymphocyte proliferation. Mol Cell Biol 1999; 19(7):4980–4988.

67. Christophe-Marine JC, et al. SOCS3 is essential in the regulation of fetal liver erythropoiesis. Cell 1999; 98(5):617–627.

68. Auernhammer CJ, Melmed S. Interleukin-11 stimulates proopiomelanocortin gene expression and adrenocorticotropin secretion in corticotroph cells: evidence for a redundant cytokine network in the hypothalamo-pituitary-adrenal axis. Endocrinology 1999; 140(4):1559–1566.

69. Bjorbaek C, et al. Activation of SOCS-3 messenger ribonucleic acid in the hypothalamus by ciliary neurotrophic factor. Endocrinology 1999; 140(5):2035–2043.
70. Bjorbaek C, et al. The role of SOCS-3 in leptin signaling and leptin resistance. J Biol Chem 1999; 274(42):30059–30065.
71. Sasaki A, et al. CIS3/SOCS-3 suppresses erythropoietin (EPO) signaling by binding the EPO receptor and JAK2. J Biol Chem 2000; 275(38):29338–29347.
72. Hilton DJ, et al. Twenty proteins containing a C-terminal SOCS box form five structural classes. Proc Natl Acad Sci USA 1998; 95(1):114–119.
73. Matuoka K, et al. A novel ligand for an SH3 domain of the adaptor protein Nck bears an SH2 domain and nuclear signaling motifs. Biochem Biophys Res Commun 1997; 239(2):488–492.
74. Krebs DL, Hilton DJ. SOCS: physiological suppressors of cytokine signaling. J Cell Sci 2000; 113(Pt 16):2813–2819.
75. Nicola NA, Greenhalgh CJ. The suppressors of cytokine signaling (SOCS) proteins: important feedback inhibitors of cytokine action. Exp Hematol 2000; 28(10): 1105–1112.
76. Yoshimura A. The CIS/JAB family: novel negative regulators of JAK signaling pathways. Leukemia 1998; 12(12):1851–1857.
77. Narazaki M, et al. Three distinct domains of SSI-1/SOCS-1/JAB protein are required for its suppression of interleukin 6 signaling. Proc Natl Acad Sci USA 1998; 95(22): 13130–13134.
78. Kamura T, et al. The Elongin BC complex interacts with the conserved SOCS-box motif present in members of the SOCS, ras, WD-40 repeat, and ankyrin repeat families. Genes Dev 1998; 12(24):3872–3881.
79. Zhang JG, et al. The conserved SOCS box motif in suppressors of cytokine signaling binds to elongins B and C and may couple bound proteins to proteasomal degradation. Proc Natl Acad Sci USA 1999; 96(5):2071–2076.
80. Zhang JG, et al. The SOCS box of suppressor of cytokine signaling-1 is important for inhibition of cytokine action in vivo. Proc Natl Acad Sci USA 2001; 98(23): 13261–13265.
81. Schoenfeld AR, Davidowitz EJ, Burk RD. Elongin BC complex prevents degradation of von Hippel-Lindau tumor suppressor gene products. Proc Natl Acad Sci USA 2000; 97(15):8507–8512.
82. Schmitz J, et al. SOCS3 exerts its inhibitory function on interleukin-6 signal transduction through the SHP2 recruitment site of gp130. J Biol Chem 2000; 275(17): 12848–12856.
83. Nicholson SE, et al. Suppressor of cytokine signaling-3 preferentially binds to the SHP-2-binding site on the shared cytokine receptor subunit gp130. Proc Natl Acad Sci USA 2000; 97(12):6493–6498.
84. Verdier F, et al. Proteasomes regulate erythropoietin receptor and signal transducer and activator of transcription 5 (STAT5) activation. Possible involvement of the ubiquitinated Cis protein. J Biol Chem 1998; 273(43):28185–28190.
85. Yu CL, Burakoff SJ. Involvement of proteasomes in regulating Jak-STAT pathways upon interleukin-2 stimulation. J Biol Chem 1997; 272(22):14017–14020.
86. Davey HW, et al. STAT5b mediates the GH-induced expression of SOCS-2 and SOCS-3 mRNA in the liver. Mol Cell Endocrinol 1999; 158(1–2):111–116.
87. Bjorbaek C, et al. Identification of SOCS-3 as a potential mediator of central leptin resistance. Mol Cell 1998; 1(4):619–625.

88.   Ito S, et al. Interleukin-10 inhibits expression of both interferon alpha- and interferon gamma-induced genes by suppressing tyrosine phosphorylation of STAT1. Blood 1999; 93(5):1456–1463.

89.   Stoiber D, et al. Lipopolysaccharide induces in macrophages the synthesis of the suppressor of cytokine signaling 3 and suppresses signal transduction in response to the activating factor IFN-gamma. J Immunol 1999; 163(5):2640–2647.

90.   Mui AL, et al. Suppression of interleukin-3-induced gene expression by a C-terminal truncated Stat5: role of Stat5 in proliferation. Embo J 1996; 15(10):2425–2433.

91.   Teglund S, et al. Stat5a and Stat5b proteins have essential and nonessential, or redundant, roles in cytokine responses. Cell 1998; 93(5):841–850.

92.   Adams TE, et al. Growth hormone preferentially induces the rapid, transient expression of SOCS-3, a novel inhibitor of cytokine receptor signaling. J Biol Chem 1998; 273(3): 1285–1287.

93.   Shouda T, et al. Induction of the cytokine signal regulator SOCS3/CIS3 as a therapeutic strategy for treating inflammatory arthritis. J Clin Invest 2001; 108(12):1781–1788.

94.   Yamochi T, et al. Adenovirus-mediated high expression of BCL-6 in CV-1 cells induces apoptotic cell death accompanied by down-regulation of BCL-2 and BCL-X(L). Oncogene 1999; 18(2):487–494.

95.   Ye BH, et al. The BCL-6 proto-oncogene controls germinal-centre formation and Th2-type inflammation. Nat Genet 1997; 16(2):161–170.

96.   Kumagai T, et al. The proto-oncogene Bcl6 inhibits apoptotic cell death in differentiation-induced mouse myogenic cells. Oncogene 1999; 18(2):467–475.

97.   Dent AL, et al. Control of inflammation, cytokine expression, and germinal center formation by BCL-6. Science 1997; 276(5312):589–592.

98.   Albagli O, et al. Overexpressed BCL6 (LAZ3) oncoprotein triggers apoptosis, delays S phase progression and associates with replication foci. Oncogene 1999; 18(36): 5063–5075.

99.   Shaffer AL, et al. BCL-6 represses genes that function in lymphocyte differentiation, inflammation, and cell cycle control. Immunity 2000; 13(2):199–212.

100. Otsuki T, et al. Analysis of LAZ3 (BCL-6) status in B-cell non-Hodgkin's lymphomas: results of rearrangement and gene expression studies and a mutational analysis of coding region sequences. Blood 1995; 85(10):2877–2884.

101. Ye BH, et al. Cloning of bcl-6, the locus involved in chromosome translocations affecting band 3q27 in B-cell lymphoma. Cancer Res 1993; 53(12):2732–2735.

102. Lo Coco F, et al. Rearrangements of the BCL6 gene in diffuse large cell non-Hodgkin's lymphoma. Blood 1994; 83(7):1757–1759.

103. Kerckaert JP, et al. LAZ3, a novel zinc-finger encoding gene, is disrupted by recurring chromosome 3q27 translocations in human lymphomas. Nat Genet 1993; 5(1):66–70.

104. Baron BW, et al. Identification of the gene associated with the recurring chromosomal translocations t(3;14)(q27;q32) and t(3;22)(q27;q11) in B-cell lymphomas. Proc Natl Acad Sci USA 1993; 90(11):5262–5266.

105. Bastard C, et al. LAZ3 rearrangements in non-Hodgkin's lymphoma: correlation with histology, immunophenotype, karyotype, and clinical outcome in 217 patients. Blood 1994; 83(9):2423–2427.

106. Cattoretti G, et al. BCL-6 protein is expressed in germinal-center B cells. Blood 1995; 86(1):45–53.

107. Onizuka T, et al. BCL-6 gene product, a 92- to 98-kD nuclear phosphoprotein, is highly expressed in germinal center B cells and their neoplastic counterparts. Blood 1995; 86(1):28–37.

108. Flenghi L, et al. A specific monoclonal antibody (PG-B6) detects expression of the BCL-6 protein in germinal center B cells. Am J Pathol 1995; 147(2):405–411.

109. Niu H, Ye BH, Dalla-Favera R. Antigen receptor signaling induces MAP kinase-mediated phosphorylation and degradation of the BCL-6 transcription factor. Genes Dev 1998; 12(13):1953–1961.

110. Cattoretti G, et al. Downregulation of BCL-6 gene expression by CD40 and EBV latent membrane protein-1 (LMP1) and its block in lymphoma carrying BCL-6 rearrangements. Blood 1997; 90(Suppl I):175a.

111. Allman D, et al. BCL-6 expression during B-cell activation. Blood 1996; 87(12): 5257–5268.

112. Akasaka T, et al. A recurring translocation, t(3;6)(q27❋1), in non-Hodgkin's lymphoma results in replacement of the 5′ regulatory region of BCL6 with a novel H4 histone gene. Cancer Res 1997; 57(1):7–12.

113. Dallery E, et al. TTF, a gene encoding a novel small G protein, fuses to the lymphoma-associated LAZ3 gene by t(3;4) chromosomal translocation. Oncogene 1995; 10(11): 2171–2178.

114. Galiegue-Zouitina S, et al. Fusion of the LAZ3/BCL6 and BOB1/OBF1 genes by t(3,)(q27; q23) chromosomal translocation. CR Acad Sci III 1995; 318(11):1125–1131.

115. Wlodarska I, et al. Fluorescence in situ hybridization identifies new chromosomal changes involving 3q27 in non-Hodgkin's lymphomas with BCL6/LAZ3 rearrangement. Genes Chromosomes Cancer 1995; 14(1):1–7.

116. Ye BH, et al. Chromosomal translocations cause deregulated BCL6 expression by promoter substitution in B cell lymphoma. Embo J 1995; 14(24):6209–6217.

117. Shen HM, et al. Mutation of BCL-6 gene in normal B cells by the process of somatic hypermutation of Ig genes. Science 1998; 280(5370):1750–1752.

118. Pasqualucci L, et al. BCL-6 mutations in normal germinal center B cells: evidence of somatic hypermutation acting outside Ig loci. Proc Natl Acad Sci USA 1998; 95(20): 11816–11821.

119. Migliazza A, et al. Frequent somatic hypermutation of the 5′ noncoding region of the BCL6 gene in B-cell lymphoma. Proc Natl Acad Sci USA 1995; 92(26):12520–12524.

120. Chen W, et al. Heterologous promoters fused to BCL6 by chromosomal translocations affecting band 3q27 cause its deregulated expression during B-cell differentiation. Blood 1998; 91(2):603–607.

121. Miki T, et al. Gene involved in the 3q27 translocation associated with B-cell lymphoma, BCL5, encodes a Kruppel-like zinc-finger protein. Blood 1994; 83(1):26–32.

122. Seyfert VL, et al. Transcriptional repression by the proto-oncogene BCL-6. Oncogene 1996; 12(11):2331–2342.

123. Chang CC, et al. BCL-6, a PDZ/zinc-finger protein, is a sequence-specific transcriptional repressor. Proc Natl Acad Sci USA 1996; 93(14):6947–6952.

124. Zollman S, et al. The BTB domain, found primarily in zinc finger proteins, defines an evolutionarily conserved family that includes several developmentally regulated genes in *Drosophila*. Proc Natl Acad Sci USA 1994; 91(22):10717–10721.

125. Numoto M, et al. Transcriptional repressor ZF5 identifies a new conserved domain in zinc finger proteins. Nucleic Acids Res 1993; 21(16):3767–3775.

126. Albagli O, et al. The BTB/PDZ domain: a new protein-protein interaction motif common to DNA- and actin-binding proteins. Cell Growth Differ 1995; 6(9):1193–1198.

127. Bardwell VJ, Treisman R. The PDZ domain: a conserved protein-protein interaction motif. Genes Dev 1994; 8(14):1664–1677.

128. Chardin P, et al. The KUP gene, located on human chromosome 14, encodes a protein with two distant zinc fingers. Nucleic Acids Res 1991; 19(7):1431–1436.

129. Chen Z, et al. Fusion between a novel Kruppel-like zinc finger gene and the retinoic acid receptor-alpha locus due to a variant t(11k) translocation associated with acute promyelocytic leukaemia. Embo J 1993; 12(3):1161–1167.

130. DiBello PR, et al. The Drosophila Broad-Complex encodes a family of related proteins containing zinc fingers. Genetics 1991; 129(2):385–397.

131. Way M, et al. Sequence and domain organization of scruin, an actin-cross-linking protein in the acrosomal process of Limulus sperm. J Cell Biol 1995; 128(1–2):51–60.

132. Cooley L, Theurkauf WE. Cytoskeletal functions during *Drosophila* oogenesis. Science 1994; 266(5185):590–596.

133. Ahmad KF, Engel CK, Prive GG. Crystal structure of the BTB domain from PLZF. Proc Natl Acad Sci USA 1998; 95(21):12123–12128.

134. Davies JM, et al. Novel BTB/PDZ domain zinc-finger protein, LRF, is a potential target of the LAZ-3/BCL-6 oncogene. Oncogene 1999; 18(2):365–375.

135. Katsani KR, Hajibagheri MA, Verrijzer CP. Co-operative DNA binding by GAGA transcription factor requires the conserved BTB/PDZ domain and reorganizes promoter topology. Embo J 1999; 18(3):698–708.

136. Numoto M, Yokoro K, Koshi J. ZF5, which is a Kruppel-type transcriptional repressor, requires the zinc finger domain for self-association. Biochem Biophys Res Commun 1999; 256(3):573–578.

137. Kobayashi A, et al. A combinatorial code for gene expression generated by transcription factor Bach2 and MAZR (MAZ-related factor) through the BTB/PDZ domain. Mol Cell Biol 2000; 20(5):1733–1746.

138. Li X, et al. Overexpression, purification, characterization, and crystallization of the BTB/PDZ domain from the PLZF oncoprotein. J Biol Chem 1997; 272(43): 27324–27329.

139. Harris MB, et al. Transcriptional repression of Stat6-dependent interleukin-4-induced genes by BCL-6: specific regulation of iepsilon transcription and immunoglobulin E switching. Mol Cell Biol 1999; 9(10):7264–7275.

140. Raff JW, Kellum R, Alberts B. The Drosophila GAGA transcription factor is associated with specific regions of heterochromatin throughout the cell cycle. Embo J 1994; 13(24):5977–5983.

141. Dorn R, et al. The enhancer of position-effect variegation of Drosophila, E(var)3-93D, codes for a chromatin protein containing a conserved domain common to several transcriptional regulators. Proc Natl Acad Sci USA 1993; 90(23):11376–11380.

142. Dhordain P, et al. Corepressor SMRT binds the BTB/PDZ repressing domain of the LAZ3/BCL6 oncoprotein. Proc Natl Acad Sci USA 1997; 94(20):10762–10767.

143. David G, et al. Histone deacetylase associated with mSin3A mediates repression by the acute promyelocytic leukemia-associated PLZF protein. Oncogene 1998; 16(19): 2549–2556.

144. Muto A, et al. Identification of Bach2 as a B-cell-specific partner for small maf proteins that negatively regulate the immunoglobulin heavy chain gene 3′ enhancer. Embo J 1998; 17(19):5734–5743.

145. Wong CW, Privalsky ML. Transcriptional repression by the SMRT-mSin3 corepressor: multiple interactions, multiple mechanisms, and a potential role for TFIIB. Mol Cell Biol 1998; 18(9):5500–5510.

146. Lin RJ, et al. Role of the histone deacetylase complex in acute promyelocytic leukaemia. Nature 1998; 391(6669):811–814.

147. Huynh KD, et al. BCoR, a novel corepressor involved in BCL-6 repression. Genes Dev 2000; 14(14):1810–1823.
148. Hong SH, et al. SMRT corepressor interacts with PLZF and with the PML-retinoic acid receptor alpha (RARalpha) and PLZF-RARalpha oncoproteins associated with acute promyelocytic leukemia. Proc Natl Acad Sci USA 1997; 94(17):9028–9033.
149. Grignani F, et al. Fusion proteins of the retinoic acid receptor-alpha recruit histone deacetylase in promyelocytic leukaemia. Nature 1998; 391(6669):815–818.
150. Deltour S, Guerardel C, Leprince D. Recruitment of SMRT/N-CoR-mSin3A-HDAC-repressing complexes is not a general mechanism for BTB/PDZ transcriptional repressors: the case of HIC-1 and gammaFBP-B. Proc Natl Acad Sci USA 1999; 96(26): 14831–14836.
151. Sassone-Corsi P, et al. Requirement of Rsk-2 for epidermal growth factor-activated phosphorylation of histone H3. Science 1999; 285(5429):886–891.
152. Struhl K. Histone acetylation and transcriptional regulatory mechanisms. Genes Dev 1998; 12(5):599–606.
153. Mizzen CA, Allis CD. Linking histone acetylation to transcriptional regulation. Cell Mol Life Sci 1998; 54(1):6–20.
154. Hassig CA, Schreiber SL. Nuclear histone acetylases and deacetylases and transcriptional regulation: HATs off to HDACs. Curr Opin Chem Biol 1997; 1(3):300–308.
155. Muscat GE, Burke LJ, Downes M. The corepressor N-CoR and its variants RIP13a and RIP13Delta1 directly interact with the basal transcription factors TFIIB, TAFII32 and TAFII70. Nucleic Acids Res 1998; 26(12):2899–2907.
156. DePinho RA. Transcriptional repression. The cancer-chromatin connection. Nature 1998; 391(6667):533, 535–536.
157. Alland L, et al. Role for N-CoR and histone deacetylase in Sin3-mediated transcriptional repression. Nature 1997; 387(6628):49–55.
158. Brehm A, et al. Retinoblastoma protein recruits histone deacetylase to repress transcription. Nature 1998; 391(6667):597–601.
159. Magnaghi-Jaulin L, et al. Retinoblastoma protein represses transcription by recruiting a histone deacetylase. Nature 1998; 391(6667):601–605.
160. Yang XJ, et al. A p300/CBP-associated factor that competes with the adenoviral oncoprotein E1A. Nature 1996; 382(6589):319–324.
161. Bannister AJ, Kouzarides T. The CBP co-activator is a histone acetyltransferase. Nature 1996; 384(6610):641–643.
162. O'Connor MJ, et al. Characterization of an E1A-CBP interaction defines a novel transcriptional adapter motif (TRAM) in CBP/p300. J Virol 1999; 73(5):3574–3581.
163. Reuter S, et al. APM-1, a novel human gene, identified by aberrant co-transcription with papillomavirus oncogenes in a cervical carcinoma cell line, encodes a BTB/PDZ-zinc finger protein with growth inhibitory activity. Embo J 1998; 17(1):215–222.
164. Fukuda T, et al. Disruption of the Bcl6 gene results in an impaired germinal center formation. J Exp Med 1997; 186(3):439–448.
165. Toney LM, et al. BCL-6 regulates chemokine gene transcription in macrophages. Nat Immunol 2000; 1(3):214–220.
166. Burz DS, et al. Cooperative DNA-binding by Bicoid provides a mechanism for threshold-dependent gene activation in the *Drosophila* embryo. Embo J 1998; 17(20): 5998–6009.
167. Hershey GK, et al. The association of atopy with a gain-of-function mutation in the alpha subunit of the interleukin-4 receptor. N Engl J Med 1997; 337(24):1720–1725.

168. Mitsuyasu H, et al. Ile50Val variant of IL4R alpha upregulates IgE synthesis and associates with atopic asthma. Nat Genet 1998; 19(2):119–120.

169. Mitsuyasu H, et al. Cutting edge: dominant effect of Ile50Val variant of the human IL-4 receptor alpha-chain in IgE synthesis. J Immunol 1999; 162(3):1227–1231.

170. Shirakawa I, et al. Atopy and asthma: genetic variants of IL-4 and IL-13 signalling. Immunol Today 2000; 21(2):60–64.

171. Adra CN, et al. Variants of B cell lymphoma 6 (BCL6) and marked atopy. Clin Genet 1998; 54(4):362–364.

172. Dent AL, et al. T helper type 2 inflammatory disease in the absence of interleukin 4 and transcription factor STAT6. Proc Natl Acad Sci USA 1998; 95(23):13823–13828.

173. Reljic R, et al. Suppression of signal transducer and activator of transcription 3-dependent B lymphocyte terminal differentiation by BCL-6. J Exp Med 2000; 192(12):1841–1848.

29

Eicosanoids as Mediators and Therapeutic Targets in Airway Inflammation

MARC PETERS-GOLDEN

University of Michigan Health System
Ann Arbor, Michigan, U.S.A.

I. Introduction

Arachidonic acid (AA) is a fatty acid constituent of the phospholipids of cell membranes. It is the precursor for a family of bioactive lipids collectively known as *eicosanoids*, the best known of which are leukotrienes (LTs) and prostaglandins (PGs). A low rate of eicosanoid synthesis occurs under basal conditions, but synthesis can be dramatically increased in response to a myriad of stimuli. Generation of eicosanoids and their interactions with cellular receptors result in a host of responses in target cells and tissues that are central to the pathogenesis of asthma. These include effects on inflammatory and immune processes, airway tone and reactivity, mucus secretion, vascular permeability, and events relevant to airway remodeling.

Although eicosanoids have been under investigation for approximately 50 years, a number of important findings have advanced our understanding of these substances during the last decade. These include (1) the molecular characterization of most of the enzymes in the biosynthetic pathways; (2) knowledge of the cell biology and regulation of these enzymes; (3) identification of many of the receptors for these mediators and their consequent signaling pathways; (4) improved means of measuring eicosanoids in vivo; (5) development of transgenic animal models; and (6) the development of pharmacological agents that inhibit the synthesis or actions of eicosanoids with substantial potency and specificity.

This chapter will review the actions of eicosanoids relevant to asthma, the evidence that abnormalities in eicosanoid production are found in asthma, and the therapeutic potential and implications for interventions targeting these mediators.

II. Eicosanoids and Their Synthesis

Although eicosanoid synthesis will be considered in detail elsewhere in this volume, certain key points will be briefly summarized here (see Ref. 1 for review). The initial step in this biosynthetic pathway (see Fig. 1) involves activation of a phospholipase A_2 (PLA_2) enzyme, which hydrolyzes AA from membrane phospholipids. This is generally a consequence of an increase in intracellular calcium, which can be triggered by exogenous substances such as antigen, endotoxin, particulates, oxidants, and xenobiotics, as well as by endogenous factors such as cytokines, proteases, kinins, hormones, and complement. Once liberated, free AA is converted to a variety of oxygenated metabolites by several parallel metabolic pathways. The two best-studied pathways are the cyclooxygenase (COX) and 5-lipoxygenase (5-LO) pathways. The former gives rise to the prostanoids [PGs, prostacyclin (PGI_2) and thromboxane (TxA_2)], while the latter yields the LTs and 5-hydroxyeicosatetraenoic acid (5-HETE). Other lipoxygenase pathways yield additional HETEs as well as lipoxins, while epoxides arise from the actions of cytochrome P450 enzymes.

The COX enzyme converts AA to an unstable intermediate, PGH_2. Subsequent metabolism to the bioactive prostanoids (PGD_2, $PGF_{2\alpha}$, PGE_2, PGI_2, and TxA_2) is carried out by the corresponding synthase (e.g., PGD_2 synthase). The first committed

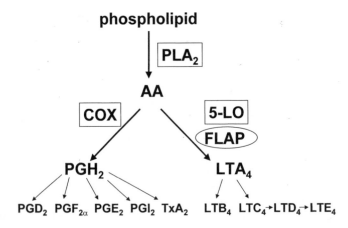

Figure 1   Biosynthetic pathways for the formation of LTs and prostanoids. The distal enzyme responsible for converting PGH_2 to a given prostanoid (not shown) is termed the relevant prostanoid synthase. The distal enzymes responsible for converting LTA_4 to LTB_4 and LTC_4 (not shown) are termed LTA_4 hydrolase and LTC_4 synthase, respectively. (Abbreviations are defined in the text.)

step in LT synthesis is catalyzed by the enzyme 5-LO, acting in concert with its helper protein, 5-LO–activating protein (FLAP); FLAP is thought to act as an AA-binding protein, which optimally "presents" AA to 5-LO. The resultant intermediate LTA_4 can be hydrolyzed by LTA_4 hydrolase to LTB_4 or be conjugated with reduced glutathione to form LTC_4 by the glutathione transferase, LTC_4 synthase. Once secreted from the cell, LTC_4 can be metabolized to LTD_4 and then to LTE_4 by the sequential removal of glutathione's glutamic acid and glycine constituents. Because LTs C_4, D_4, and E_4 have similar biological actions and all retain the cysteine moiety of glutathione, they are often collectively referred to as cysteinyl-LTs; it is these molecules that comprise the biological activity previously known as slow-reacting substance (SRS).

Cellular specificity in the profiles of eicosanoid generation exists. Although both leukocytes and structural cells are capable of prostanoid synthesis, substantial 5-LO expression is confined primarily to leukocytes. Furthermore, while PGE_2 is the major prostanoid product of epithelial cells, fibroblasts, and smooth muscle cells, PGD_2 is the major prostanoid of mast cells. Finally, eosinophils and mast cells synthesize primarily LTC_4, neutrophils synthesize primarily LTB_4, and macrophages synthesize both LTs.

Cells must have the capacity to modulate their potential for eicosanoid synthesis. In fact, most of the eicosanoid-forming enzymes can be regulated in three distinct ways. First, the level of expression of the protein can be enhanced at either transcriptional or translational steps, e.g., by cytokines or growth factors. Second, the catalytic efficiency of existing enzyme molecules can be modulated, either by posttranslational modification (such as phosphorylation by kinases) or by alterations in the level of essential enzyme cofactors such as calcium. Finally, changes in the intracellular localization of some of these proteins can influence their function; for example, activation of PLA_2 and of 5-LO is associated with translocation from a soluble intracellular site to the perinuclear membrane.

One unique feature of eicosanoid synthesis is the rapidity with which it can occur. Since the requisite enzymes are generally expressed constitutively and since stimulus-induced calcium transients necessary to activate AA release (and 5-LO, the only other enzyme in the pathway that requires specific activation) occur within seconds or minutes, eicosanoids can be synthesized and released from source cells within this same time frame. Their generation, therefore, lags behind that of a preformed mediator such as histamine only slightly, but precedes that of typical protein mediators such as cytokines, whose elaboration require new transcription and translation, by hours. However, the fact that eicosanoid synthesis can be further amplified by increases in expression of eicosanoid-forming enzymes also permits sustained generation or delayed bursts of synthesis. Eicosanoids are therefore unique among mediators in their ability to participate in both immediate and delayed phases of various responses.

III. Measuring Eicosanoids

Eicosanoids can be measured in in vitro cell culture systems, in organ cultures, or in vivo. The lipids or their metabolites can be separated by various chromatographic techniques and quantitated by determinations of absorbance or mass, or they can be individually measured using enzyme-linked immunoassays with specific antibodies. Such measurements in vivo have most often been performed using plasma, lung lavage fluid, or urine (2). Recently, these techniques have been extended to measure eicosanoids in expectorated sputum (3) and even in exhaled breath condensate (4). They can also be quantitated in tissue homogenates, e.g., from lung biopsy specimens (5). However, it is clear that the in vivo measurement of eicosanoids is complicated by their propensity to be metabolized by enzymatic or nonenzymatic mechanisms and to be transported among various body compartments. Factors such as these compromise the sensitivity of such measurements. Complementary information can be obtained by quantitating the level of expression of specific eicosanoid-forming proteins (e.g., by immunoblot analysis or by immunohistochemical staining of sections) or messenger RNA (by Northern blot analysis, polymerase chain reaction, or in situ hybridization) in tissues. Finally, the intracellular locale of eicosanoid-forming proteins such as PLA_2 or 5-LO, which is a reflection of their state of activation, can be determined in situ by immunohistochemical staining of tissue sections (5).

IV. Eicosanoid Receptors and Signal Transduction Mechanisms

The biological actions of eicosanoids are generally presumed to be mediated by their binding to specific receptors on target cells. Ligation of these receptors results in the generation of intracellular signals, which, in turn, transduce the biological actions of the lipid mediator. Receptors for most of the major eicosanoids have been characterized using classical pharmacological techniques, and more recently, many have been cloned. These are G-protein-coupled transmembrane receptors similar to those for hormones and chemokines. They are coupled to signal transduction events including activation of protein kinase C and tyrosine kinases, alterations in intracellular calcium concentration, and adenyl cyclase activation. Although these receptors are assumed to be primarily distributed on the plasma membrane, receptors for PGE_2 have also been identified on the nuclear membrane (6). It has recently been discovered that certain eicosanoids can also bind to an alternative type of receptor known as peroxisome proliferator-activated receptors (PPARs) (7). These are intranuclear receptors that also act as transcription factors, regulating the expression of proteins involved in lipid metabolism, inflammation, and cellular proliferation. It is attractive to speculate that interaction with nuclear receptors of either the classic G-protein-coupled or of the PPAR classes may mediate some of the autocrine effects of eicosanoids formed locally at the nucleus.

It is now recognized that receptors for a given eicosanoid can be encoded by multiple genes. This is best exemplified by the receptors for PGE_2 (termed the E prostanoid or EP receptors); four distinct EP receptors are known, with some coupled to adenyl cyclase and others to calcium mobilization (8). More recently, two distinct

Table 1 Eicosanoid Receptors

Receptor	Ligand specificity	Signal transduction
cysLT1	$LTD_4 \gg LTE_4 = LTC_4$	$\uparrow Ca^{2+}$
cysLT2	$LTC_4 = LTD_4 \gg LTE_4$	$\uparrow Ca^{2+}$
BLT1	LTB_4	$\uparrow Ca^{2+}, \downarrow cAMP$
BLT2	$LTB_4 > 12\text{-HETE} > 15\text{-HETE}$	$\uparrow Ca^{2+}, \downarrow cAMP$
EP1	PGE_2	$\uparrow Ca^{2+}$
EP2	PGE_2	$\uparrow cAMP$
EP3	PGE_2	$\downarrow cAMP, \uparrow Ca^{2+}$
EP4	PGE_2	$\uparrow cAMP$
IP	PGE_2	$\uparrow cAMP$
TP	$TxA_2 > PGD_2$	$\downarrow cAMP, \uparrow Ca^{2+}$
DP(1)	PGD_2	$\uparrow cAMP$
CRTH2 (DP2)	PGD_2	$\downarrow cAMP, \uparrow Ca^{2+}$
FP	$PGF_{2\alpha}$	$\uparrow Ca^{2+}$

In general, ligation of receptors that increase intracellular cyclic AMP (cAMP) result in bronchodilatation, vasodilatation, anti-inflammatory effects, and antiproliferative effects. By contrast, ligation of receptors that increase intracellular Ca^{2+} and/or decrease cAMP result in bronchoconstriction, vasoconstriction, pro-inflammatory effects, and pro-proliferative effects.

receptors for cysteinyl-LTs ($cysLT_1$ and $cysLT_2$) have been identified that vary in their specificity for LTC_4 vs. LTD_4 and in their tissue distribution (9,10). Likewise, two receptors for LTB_4 (BLT_1 and BLT_2) with different affinities and tissue distributions have been identified (11,12). It is likely that such complex receptor variety provides a means for functional and cellular specificity in the actions of these potent mediators. The major eicosanoid receptors as well as their ligand specificity and signaling mechanisms are listed in Table 1.

V. Eicosanoid Actions: General Comments

The actions of eicosanoids that have been classically recognized include "macro" level effects on processes such as smooth muscle tone, microvascular permeability, airway mucus secretion, platelet aggregation, and pain. More recently, a host of "novel" actions that reflect more "micro" actions have become appreciated. These include effects on leukocyte recruitment and activation, signal transduction, gene transcription, immune responses, cell proliferation and differentiation, apoptosis, receptor expression, matrix protein synthesis, and antimicrobial defense. These latter effects are quite reminiscent of the pleiotropic effects of cytokines.

Eicosanoids further resemble cytokines in that their actions may be either unique or redundant within their class. Unique actions include the ability of TxA_2 to stimulate and of PGI_2 to inhibit platelet aggregation. Another example is the unique ability of PGE_2 to act in the hypothalamus to cause fever. By contrast, several eicosanoids have the capacity to induce contraction ($PGF_{2\alpha}$, PGD_2, TxA_2, and cysteinyl-LTs) or relaxation (PGE_2 and PGI_2) of airway smooth muscle. Likewise, eosinophil chemotaxis can be elicited by cysteinyl-LTs, LTB_4, the 5-HETE metabolite 5-oxo-eicosatetraenoic acid, and PGD_2.

Finally, another cytokine-like property of eicosanoids is the ability of particular pairs of these mediators to exert opposing actions. The opposing effects of TxA_2 and PGI_2 on platelet aggregation were mentioned above. PGI_2 can also cause vasodilatation, opposing the actions of vasoconstrictors such as $PGF_{2\alpha}$, TxA_2, and cysteinyl-LTs. However, the best example of this yin-yang relationship is provided by the LTs and PGE_2. The LTs (B_4 and/or cysteinyl-LTs) promote airway smooth muscle contraction, leukocyte chemotaxis, leukocyte production of inflammatory mediators such as cytokines and superoxide, humoral and cellular immune function, proliferation of smooth muscle cells and fibroblasts, and collagen synthesis. Although PGE_2 is often thought of as "pro-inflammatory," this reflects its capacity to reproduce classical features of inflammation such as pain, fever, and vasodilatation, rather than its effects on inflammatory, immune, and mesenchymal cells. In fact, PGE_2 causes bronchodilatation and inhibits leukocyte chemotaxis, inflammatory mediator generation, immune function, mesenchymal cell proliferation, and collagen synthesis. These actions will be discussed more fully below.

VI. Cysteinyl-LTs: Koch's Postulates Fulfilled

In the 1930s, antigen-challenged guinea pig lungs were noted to release into the bathing medium a bioactivity that elicited a much more potent and protracted smooth muscle contractile response than histamine, the only spasmogen known at the time. This bioactivity was termed "SRS" (13). In 1960, SRS was reported to be elaborated by the lungs of human asthmatics and was thereafter considered to be an important mediator of bronchoconstriction in asthma (14). Incremental progress from studies carried out by a number of laboratories around the world culminated in 1979 in the elucidation by Murphy and Samuelsson of SRS as a mixture of eicosanoids termed LTs C_4, D_4, and E_4 (15), now termed the cysteinyl-LTs. Samuelsson was the co-recipient of the 1982 Nobel Prize in Physiology or Medicine for this discovery.

The chemical elucidation of SRS permitted investigators to determine if cysteinyl-LTs indeed fulfilled Koch's postulates as mediators of asthma. First, cysteinyl-LTs could be measured in appropriate biological fluids under appropriate circumstances to determine if their generation was associated with asthmatic bronchospasm. Second, they could be synthesized and then tested in vitro and in vivo in order to ascertain if they reproduce the pathophysiological features of asthma. Third, pharmacological agents that interfere with either cysteinyl-LT biosynthesis or actions (collectively known as *LT modifiers* or *anti-LT agents*) could be tested to determine if they abrogate the clinical and pathophysiological features of asthma. The former strategy is exemplified by the 5-LO inhibitor zileuton, and the latter by the cysLT$_1$

receptor antagonists pranlukast, zafirlukast, and montelukast. More recently, genetic strategies such as targeted deletion of specific cysteinyl-LT–synthesizing enzymes or receptors have permitted animal models to provide complementary information about the in vivo roles of these mediators. In the 20 years since the identification of SRS, cysteinyl-LTs have unequivocally been demonstrated to fulfill all of these criteria, implicating them as important mediators of asthma. This key information will be summarized below.

A. Overproduction of Cysteinyl-LTs in Asthma

A large body of information indicates that pulmonary synthesis of cysteinyl-LTs is elevated in patients with asthma. This has been established by measuring levels of these LTs in lung lavage fluid, sputum, exhaled breath condensate, and plasma. Urinary LTE_4 reflects total body biosynthesis, and levels have likewise been shown to be elevated in asthma. Overproduction of cysteinyl-LTs (as compared to nonasthmatic control subjects) has been demonstrated in the baseline state for patients with well-controlled asthma (16). Levels of cysteinyl-LTs have been shown to correlate with asthma severity in some studies (3). Levels have also been shown to increase further following challenge in a laboratory setting with agents or actions that provoke bronchospasm, including exercise (17), antigen inhalation (18), and aspirin administration (19). Of greatest relevance is the fact that naturally occurring exacerbations of asthma are associated with very high levels of cysteinyl-LTs, which return to baseline after several weeks of treatment (20). Thus, cysteinyl-LTs have indeed been detected "at the scene of the crime" in relevant body compartments and in relevant circumstances.

B. Actions of Cysteinyl-LTs Pertinent to the Pathophysiology of Asthma: Classic Actions

Bronchospasm is the hallmark of asthma. The fact that bronchospasm occurred when synthetic cysteinyl-LTs were administered by inhalation to the airways of either normal or asthmatic humans was to be expected (reviewed in Ref. 21). As is true for many of the effects of these substances, LTD_4 was the most potent and LTE_4 the least potent in this regard; this order of potency can now be explained by the agonist specificity at the $cysLT_1$ receptor. On a molar basis, cysteinyl-LTs are the most potent bronchoconstrictor substances known. Their duration of bronchoconstrictor action is also greater than that of histamine. Once an initial dose of an oral anti-LT agent results in therapeutic plasma levels (i.e., within 2 to 3 hours), a modest but statistically significant increase in airflow rates can be demonstrated in well-controlled asthmatics (22). This likely reflects the facts that cysteinyl-LTs are overproduced at baseline in these individuals and that these mediators contribute to their increased bronchial tone. Furthermore, pretreatment with anti-LT agents very effectively abrogates both the immediate and delayed bronchoconstrictor responses to such challenges as exercise (23), antigen inhalation (22), aspirin administration (24), and inhalation of the pollutant sulfur dioxide (25).

Table 2   Pro-Asthmatic Actions of Cysteinyl-LTs

Classic Actions
    Potent and long-lived bronchoconstriction
    Increased BHR
    Increased vascular permeability
    Increased mucus secretion
    Decreased mucus clearance
Novel Actions
    Mediate rhinosinusitis
    Promote eosinophil recruitment and survival
    Amplify generation of inflammatory mediators
    Promote Th2 immune response
    Increase expression of mediator receptors
    Promote systemic immune responses
    β_2-Adrenergic receptor desensitization
    Contribute to airway remodeling responses

Bronchial hyperresponsiveness (BHR) is another hallmark feature of asthma. Inhalation of cysteinyl-LTs increases airway responsiveness to nonspecific broncho-constrictors such as methacholine and histamine in some but not all studies (26). Moreover, administration of anti-LT agents results in a modest reduction in BHR in patients with asthma (27). Finally, BHR was also reduced in antigen-sensitized mice whose 5-LO gene was disrupted, rendering them LT-deficient (28).

Cysteinyl-LTs increase microvascular permeability, thereby contributing to edema of the airway wall, another characteristic feature of asthma. Finally, they increase mucus secretion by airway mucus glands and also inhibit ciliary clearance of mucus, actions that might contribute to the mucus plugging often observed in asthma.

Table 2 summarizes these classic actions of cysteinyl-LTs.

C. Actions of Cysteinyl-LTs Pertinent to the Pathophysiology of Asthma: Novel Actions

Bronchospasm, edema, and mucus plugging are central to the pathophysiology of asthma, and blocking such effects provides a cogent therapeutic rationale for anti-LT agents. However, recent evidence indicates that cysteinyl-LTs also possess a variety of previously unanticipated novel actions that are also pertinent to the biology of asthma and allergic inflammation (see Table 2).

Rhinosinusitis

It is well known that rhinitis or rhinosinusitis frequently coexists in patients with asthma, and that the upper airway disease contributes to the expression of lower airway disease. It is now appreciated that cysteinyl-LTs participate in rhinosinusitis

(29). First, these mediators are elevated in nasal lavage fluid of patients with rhinitis and are produced at high levels by nasal tissue from patients with rhinosinusitis. Second, when administered to the nose, cysteinyl-LTs result in rhinorrhea and nasal congestion. Finally, anti-LT agents have clinical utility in rhinosinusitis in patients with and without aspirin-sensitive disease (30). Therefore, cysteinyl-LTs contribute indirectly to the expression of asthma by virtue of their effects on the nose and sinuses.

Eosinophilic Inflammation

Cysteinyl-LTs directly increase the number of inflammatory cells, particularly eosinophils, at sites of inflammation (31,32). This effect involves actions on a variety of the determinants of eosinophil accumulation. First, cysteinyl-LTs promote the generation of eosinophilic precursors in the bone marrow (33), and the reduced numbers of circulating eosinophils consistently observed in patients treated with anti-LT agents (34) likely reflects the abrogation of this systemic effect. Second, these lipids act as potent direct chemoattractants for eosinophils (35). Third, they upregulate endothelial cell expression of adhesion molecules such as P-selectin that are necessary for eosinophil emigration into tissues (36). All of these actions contribute to increased eosinophil recruitment by cysteinyl-LTs. Finally, cysteinyl-LTs are potent inhibitors of eosinophil apoptosis, thereby prolonging the survival of cells that have been recruited (37). These mechanisms explain the ability of anti-LT drugs to reduce eosinophil numbers in the airways under both basal (34) and antigen-challenged (38) conditions.

Interactions Between LTs and Other Mediators

An important advance in our understanding of the biology of the cysteinyl-LTs has been the realization that they interact extensively and bidirectionally with other types of mediators (Fig. 2). Cysteinyl-LTs also activate macrophages, eosinophils, mast cells, and other cells to amplify production of various pro-inflammatory or bronchoconstrictor mediators. These include endothelin, eotaxin, tumor necrosis factor-α, macrophage inflammatory protein-1α, reactive oxygen intermediates, nitric oxide, matrix metalloproteinases, and the T-helper type 2 (Th2) cytokines IL-4 and IL-5.

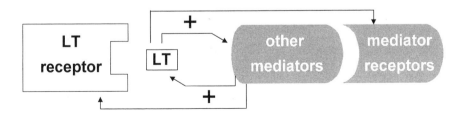

Figure 2 Interactions between LTs and other mediators.

Generation of these same mediators has been shown to be inhibited by anti-LT agents either in vitro or in vivo (39–45). The possible significance of such interactions is apparent from the demonstration that pulmonary eosinophilia induced in animals by the inhalation of LTD_4 could be substantially abrogated by the administration of an anti-IL-5 neutralizing antibody (46). Since some of these mediators also promote eosinophilic inflammation themselves, their inhibition represents an additional indirect mechanism by which anti-LT agents attenuate the inflammatory process. Specificity in the effects of these drugs exists, however, since generation of the Th1 cytokine interferon-γ is not inhibited or is even enhanced by anti-LT agents (43). Consistent with this, lung leukocytes from 5-LO knockout mice produce greater amounts of interferon-γ than do cells from wild-type animals (47). Finally, cysteinyl-LTs not only amplify the generation of other pro-inflammatory mediators, but also have the potential to increase the expression of their cell surface receptors, as has been demonstrated for histamine (48).

Just as cysteinyl-LTs can increase the production of other pro-inflammatory mediators, it is important to note that their own synthesis is likewise enhanced by various other mediators. Substances thought to be involved in various aspects of the airway biology of asthma, including IL-4, IL-5, granulocyte-macrophage colony-stimulating factor (GM-CSF), transforming growth factor-β (TGF-β), and endothelin, have all been shown to upregulate the capacity for cysteinyl-LT production in vitro by a variety of molecular mechanisms (49–53). These mechanisms include increased gene expression as well as alterations in subcellular localization for various enzymes in the LT biosynthetic pathway. Data from animal studies suggest that mediator-induced increases in LT generation are not merely possible, but may be of importance in mediating some of the biological actions of these other mediators. For example, the ability of eotaxin to increase eosinophilic inflammation and BHR in IL-5-transgenic mice was significantly attenuated by inhibitors of cysteinyl-LT synthesis or action (54). In addition, a preliminary report indicated that the ability of the intratracheal administration of IL-13 to induce an asthma-like phenotype was substantially ameliorated in LT-deficient mice with a targeted deletion of 5-LO (55).

Initiation of Immune Responses

Many asthmatics are atopic. Increases in serum IgE also accompany the commonly employed mouse model of asthma in which animals undergo systemic sensitization and then airway challenge with antigen, and this is indicative of a systemic immune response. Mice rendered functionally cysteinyl-LT–deficient, either by treatment with receptor antagonists or by genetic knockout of 5-LO, have been shown to produce decreased levels of serum IgE following antigen sensitization (28,56). These data suggest that cysteinyl-LTs are required for optimal generation of an immune response, and this may reflect the facts that these mediators regulate both the differentiation and the migration to lymph nodes of antigen-presenting dendritic cells (57), processes that are crucial for the initiation of such responses.

β₂-Adrenergic Receptor Desensitization

The β_2-adrenergic bronchodilator, salbutamol, is able to relax human bronchial smooth muscle rings that have been precontracted with carbachol. Moreover, pretreatment of rings with antigen increases the dose of salbutamol required to reverse the carbachol-induced contraction, implying that some type of allergic mechanism results in a form of β_2-adrenergic desensitization. Interestingly, coincubation with a cysteinyl-LT receptor antagonist during the antigen pretreatment period abolishes the desensitization (58). These results suggest that cysteinyl-LTs, likely produced by tissue mast cells, contribute to the β_2-adrenergic desensitization observed in this in vitro model. These data are consistent with the observation that incubation with LTD$_4$ reduced the expression of β_2-adrenergic receptors on peripheral blood lymphocytes (59). It remains to be established whether these interesting findings apply in vivo or whether the LTs might participate more generally in β_2-adrenergic receptor desensitization.

Airway Remodeling

Airway remodeling refers to the structural changes sometimes observed in chronic asthma that may contribute to fixed airflow obstruction and progressive lung function decline. Such structural changes include mucus gland hypertrophy, basement membrane thickening, smooth muscle cell hyperplasia, and subepithelial fibrosis. As will be discussed in detail elsewhere in this volume, these changes are thought to be the result of epithelial injury. It is unclear at the present time whether remodeling is the direct consequence of epithelial injury *per se* or whether it is due in some degree to chronic inflammation, which also occurs in this setting. In the "inflammation begets remodeling" model, the previously described pro-inflammatory actions of cysteinyl-LTs might implicate their participation. However, it is much less well appreciated that cysteinyl-LTs can exert direct actions on smooth muscle cells and fibroblasts, the cells that are responsible for many aspects of the remodeled phenotype. For instance, cysteinyl-LTs augment the mitogenic responses of both smooth muscle cells and fibroblasts to various growth factors in vitro (60,61). In a chronic rodent asthma model involving repeated antigen challenges to the airways over several weeks, increases in airway smooth muscle mass and subepithelial fibrosis are observed. In vivo administration of anti-LT agents during this time period significantly abrogates both of these features (62,63). Further support for a possible role of LTs in airway remodeling derives from observations that these substances are overproduced in other diseases characterized by fibrosis. This has been observed in the lungs of patients with pulmonary parenchymal fibrosis (5) and in patients with hepatic fibrosis (64). In a mouse model of pulmonary fibrosis induced by intratracheal administration of bleomycin, cysteinyl-LT overproduction is observed and fibrosis is abrogated in 5-LO knockout animals (47). This information clearly establishes the *plausibility* that cysteinyl-LTs might participate in airway remodeling. Establishing their actual participation and their contribution will require long-term treatment trials with anti-LT drugs and monitoring of appropriate histopathological and physiological endpoints.

D. Utility of Anti-LT Agents in Asthma Treatment

The accumulated investigational and clinical experience with anti-LT agents indicates a variety of beneficial actions of these drugs (Table 3). As mentioned above,

Table 3 Potential Utility of Anti-LT Agents in Asthma Treatment

Efficacy in rhinosinusitis
Modest acute bronchodilatory action
Protect against bronchoconstriction in response to exercise, antigen, aspirin, pollutants
First-line controller agent in mild-moderate asthma
Add-on controller agent together with ICS in moderate-severe asthma
Steroid-sparing potential
Possible role in acute asthma exacerbation (?)

drugs that inhibit cysteinyl-LT synthesis (zileuton) or action at the $cysLT_1$ receptor (pranlukast, zafirlukast, and montelukast) result in modest acute bronchodilatation, reduce BHR, and protect against bronchoconstrictor challenges including exercise, inhalation of antigen or sulfur dioxide, and ingestion of aspirin. However, it is the efficacy of these agents in longer-term studies in patients with persistent asthma that is of greatest interest. Although no direct comparative studies have been performed among these anti-LT drugs, the data available from individual placebo-controlled trials suggest that the various representatives of this class possess similar activity and are roughly equipotent, and their clinical efficacy will be considered for the class as a whole.

Anti-LT agents have been studied as first-line controller agents in patients with mild-to-moderate persistent asthma. As compared to placebo, these agents have been shown to improve lung function, reduce daytime and nocturnal symptoms, improve asthma-specific quality of life, reduce use of rescue β-agonists, reduce asthma exacerbations necessitating systemic corticosteroid therapy, and reduce health care contacts (reviewed in Ref. 65). No tachyphylaxis has been observed with long-term use. This profile of actions is precisely what is desired in a controller medication and is very similar to that observed with inhaled corticosteroids (ICS). Unlike ICS, however, significant improvements can be detected on the first day of anti-LT therapy (66), which may provide positive reinforcement and encourage compliance. The anti-LTs represent the best genuine alternative to ICS as first-line controller agents with anti-inflammatory activity (67).

At the same time, anti-LT drugs are generally safe and easy to use. Of the agents licensed for use in the United States, zileuton is the least user-friendly of the class: it requires four-times daily dosing and monitoring of liver function tests (because of a ~4% incidence of hepatotoxicity) and can interfere with the metabolism of theophylline. Zafirlukast is dosed twice daily and can interfere with the metabolism of coumadin; there is also some suggestion that optimal efficacy may require doses higher than those approved by the FDA and that some hepatotoxicity exists at such doses. Montelukast is the most user-friendly of these agents: it is dosed once daily, requires no laboratory monitoring, and has no clinically important drug interactions.

Selection of a first-line controller agent for persistent asthma requires a consideration of the relative advantages and disadvantages of ICS vs. anti-LTs. Both classes possess anti-inflammatory activity and a desirable profile of efficacy. In a head-to-head comparison, ICS had an advantage in mean efficacy (68). However, as is true in most such trials, compliance with ICS was ensured at a level (>90%) far exceeding that which is generally achievable in the real world (~50%). During an open extension of that same trial, the advantage of ICS was gradually lost. Although not certain, it is most likely that this decline represents the waning of compliance with ICS to the real-world level. Because ICS use has clearly been limited by suboptimal compliance, oropharyngeal side effects, and persistent concerns about possible systemic side effects, and because patient preference for anti-LTs exceeds that of ICS, it is possible that an efficacy advantage for ICS may be counterbalanced by a compliance advantage for anti-LTs. One final consideration in the selection of a controller agent is its ability to prevent airway remodeling. While some (but not all) clinical studies suggest that ICS may have a modest ability to abrogate remodeling, only preclinical data (discussed above) support the possible utility of anti-LT agents in this regard. Again, appropriate long-term clinical studies of remodeling will be necessary to further inform clinicians' decisions about the use of this new class of medication.

It is apparent from the accumulated experience with anti-LT agents that heterogeneity in responsiveness exists among patients (68). Depending on the therapeutic endpoint examined, it appears that somewhere between 40 and 80% of patients obtain meaningful benefit. The explanation for this heterogeneity remains to be determined. It is logical to envision that the degree of responsiveness is a function of the relative importance of LTs among the myriad of possible candidate mediators in the overall pathophysiology of asthma or of the ability of the drugs to exert their intended effects. These variables, in turn, could reflect individual variations in the amounts of LTs produced, the expression of LT receptors, or the metabolism of anti-LT agents. Such variations could reflect genetic factors, environmental factors, or both. Polymorphisms in certain of the genes encoding LT-forming enzymes or LT receptors have been described. For most of these, the available evidence suggests that they would explain only a small proportion of the observed clinical refractoriness (69). However, preliminary data suggest that a polymorphism in the promoter region of the LTC_4 synthase gene may be quite common and may be an important predictor of the responsiveness to anti-LT agents (70). If this observation is confirmed, genetic testing at this locus *might* provide predictive information about the likelihood of responsiveness to this class of drugs. The application of pharmacogenetic principles to therapy of asthma will be considered in detail in another chapter in this volume. At the present time, there are no clinical markers that predict therapeutic responsiveness in the general population of asthmatics; for example, neither severity of asthma, atopy, nor demographic factors has proven useful. It does appear, however, that the subset of aspirin-sensitive asthmatics exhibits a very high level of LT generation (71), and these patients may in particular benefit from anti-LT drugs (72). Nevertheless, an empiric clinical trial is currently the only practicable approach to determine an individual patient's response to these medications. It seems quite likely that heterogeneity of responsiveness is not unique to anti-LT agents, but, rather, will be observed with all classes of asthma medications, including ICS, if the distribution of responses instead of merely mean responses is examined (73). This would be consistent with the emerging view of asthma as a syndrome encompassing multiple individual phenotypes, rather than a single disease entity.

In addition to their utility as first-line controller agents in patients with mild disease, substantial data also support the efficacy of anti-LTs in more severe asthmatics and in combination with other agents, particularly ICS. Significant benefit with anti-LT drug monotherapy has been observed in patients with severe persistent asthma (74). In patients whose asthma is inadequately controlled despite moderate-dose ICS, the addition of an anti-LT agent has been shown to result in additive improvements in symptoms, lung function, rescue β-agonist use, exacerbations, and eosinophilia (75). Moreover, anti-LT agents possess a steroid-sparing capacity when added to the regimen of patients requiring high-dose ICS (76). The ability of anti-LTs to provide additive benefit in patients already on ICS may be somewhat surprising in view of the common perception that corticosteroids inhibit all aspects of the inflammatory response. This benefit may derive from any of the following: (1) some asthmatics are corticosteroid-resistant; (2) some ICS preparations do not adequately reach the small airways, while a systemically absorbed agent does; (3) corticosteroids inhibit LT generation to a lesser extent and with lesser consistency than they inhibit many other inflammatory mediators (see below); and (4) the broad spectrum of corticosteroid action can be deleterious, since it also extends to inhibition of certain anti-inflammatory molecules such as IL-10 and PGE_2 and to increased expression of receptors for certain cytokines and growth factors.

One further possible application of anti-LT agents is in the treatment of acute asthma exacerbations along with standard systemic corticosteroids. The rationale for this is appealing (77), since systemic corticosteroids may require 12–72 hours to work, since LTs are over-produced during such exacerbations, and since both the bronchodilator and anti-inflammatory actions of anti-LTs occur fairly rapidly. The question is whether inclusion of an anti-LT (administered either with conventional oral dosing or with intravenous preparations currently under investigation) in the regimen administered on presentation to an emergency department will either reduce the need for hospitalization or reduce the length of stay for those patients requiring hospitalization. Preliminary data are encouraging in this regard, but the results of additional ongoing studies are awaited.

VII. Role of Other 5-LO Metabolites and CysLT₂ Receptors in Asthma

Although there is far less information about them than about cysteinyl-LTs, other metabolites derived from the 5-LO pathway may also participate in the pathogenesis of asthma. LTB_4 is not synthesized to an appreciable extent by eosinophils and is only a minor product of mast cells; however, it is the major 5-LO product of human alveolar macrophages and essentially the exclusive LT synthesized by neutrophils. LTB_4 is best known for its ability to serve as a chemoattractant for neutrophils, but is also a potent chemoattractant for eosinophils (78) as well as fibroblasts (79), inhibits neutrophil apoptosis (80), and promotes immune responses (81). 5-HETE has very similar actions as LTB_4 but tends to be less potent. The 5-HETE metabolite 5-oxo-ETE has selective chemoattractant activity against eosinophils (82). Each of these other 5-LO products has been shown to be overproduced either by asthmatics in vivo (83) or by cells derived from them in vitro (84).

In a primate model, a potent LTB_4 antagonist prevented the increased BHR caused by antigen inhalation (85). In a rodent model of antigen-induced asthma, additive effects on airway responses and inflammation were observed by the addition of a BLT antagonist to a $cysLT_1$ antagonist (86). By contrast, no beneficial effect of a BLT antagonist alone was observed in human asthmatics undergoing antigen inhalation challenge (87). However, no trials of a BLT antagonist in chronic asthma have been reported. If 5-LO products other than cysteinyl-LTs were important in asthma, one might expect the 5-LO inhibitor zileuton to possess efficacy that is superior to that of a $cysLT_1$ receptor antagonist. The discovery of a second receptor for cysteiny$_1$-LTs ($cysLT_2$) that is not blocked by the cysteinyl-LT receptor antagonists in clinical use (10) also raises the question of whether it mediates actions relevant to asthma; the fact that $cysLT_2$ is, like $cysLT_1$, expressed on eosinophils suggests that it could. Once again, in the event that this were true, an advantage of a LT synthesis inhibitor (which would block the synthesis of cysteinyl-LTs able to interact with either receptor) over $cysLT_1$ antagonists would be predicted. Although early pilot studies are said to have demonstrated no such advantage of LT synthesis inhibitors, head-to-head comparisons in sufficiently large patient populations have never been conducted. Thus, roles in asthma for 5-LO products other than cysteinyl-LTs and for the $cysLT_2$ receptor remain entirely plausible, but insufficiently studied.

VIII.   Roles of PGD_2 and TxA_2 in Asthma

PGD_2 is the major prostanoid product of mast cells and is also synthesized in smaller quantities by macrophages. Levels of PGD_2 in lung lavage fluid are increased in asthmatics (88). It is a potent bronchoconstrictor in animals and humans and also increases microvascular permeability and BHR. Interestingly, the classically recognized receptor for PGD_2, DP, signals through elevations in cyclic AMP and would therefore be expected to mediate a bronchodilatory effect. Airway obstruction in response to PGD_2 probably reflects some degree of vascular actions resulting in airway edema, mediated by DP, as well as myotropic effects mediated by its ability to also interact with the TxA_2 receptor (89). A second receptor for PGD_2, originally cloned and termed "chemoattractant receptor expressed on Th2 cells" ($CRTH_2$) and now also called DP_2 (90,91), is expressed on eosinophils and basophils as well as Th2 lymphocytes and appears to mediate eosinophilic recruitment by PGD_2. DP receptor knockout mice have been shown to manifest a significant abrogation in BHR, eosinophilic inflammation, and Th2 cytokine expression in the lung in an antigen challenge model of asthma (92); the precise mechanisms for this protection remain to be fully elucidated. In view of the actions of PGD_2 on BHR, airway tone, and eosinophilic inflammation, it must be considered a plausible mediator of asthma.

Selective antagonists for PGD_2 receptors are currently under development, and their efficacy is awaited.

Bioactive lipids, including fatty acids and certain eicosanoids, are regarded as possible endogenous ligands for a PPAR isoform (PPAR-γ), whose activation downregulates transcription of a variety of genes involved in inflammation (7). One of the most potent and best-studied PPAR-γ agonists is a metabolite of PGD_2, 15-deoxy-PGJ_2. When added exogenously to cells, 15-deoxy-PGJ_2 inhibits expression of tumor necrosis factor-α, inducible nitric oxide synthase, and IL-8 in such cells as macrophages, smooth muscle cells, and airway epithelial cells (93,94). While many of these potentially anti-inflammatory and antiasthmatic effects are indeed mediated by PPAR-γ activation, a direct PPAR-γ–independent inhibitory effect of this and structurally related prostanoids on the pro-inflammatory transcription factor, nuclear factor-κB, has also been reported (95). A substantial degree of controversy, however, surrounds the question of whether indeed 15-deoxy-PGJ_2 is produced in vivo and whether it is therefore a plausible endogenous anti-inflammatory mediator (96). Even if it were not, its application as an exogenous agent might be expected to have therapeutic utility.

TxA_2 is synthesized not only by platelets, but also by macrophages, neutrophils, eosinophils, and basophils. As mentioned above, TxA_2 has bronchoconstrictor actions. It also increases microvascular permeability and BHR and impairs mucociliary clearance. Interestingly, a polymorphism in the TxA_2 receptor (TP) gene has been linked with the presence of asthma in Japan (97). Both a TP antagonist (seratrodast) and a TxA_2 synthase inhibitor (ozagrel) are widely prescribed for asthma in Japan. Nevertheless, the reported benefits of these agents have been inconsistent. One study demonstrated no improvement in lung function, but a reduction in symptoms, rescue bronchodilator use, and sputum volume and viscosity (98). Another reported a decrease in BHR but no differences in sputum eosinophils or exhaled NO (99). A comparison of pretreatment with the $cysLT_1$ antagonist pranlukast, ozagrel, or seratrodast showed that the ability of pranlukast to abrogate antigen-induced bronchoconstriction was far superior to that of the TxA_2-directed agents (100). Finally, heterogeneity in responses to seratrodast have also been observed. In one study, 40% of asthmatics were classified as responders on the basis of improvements in symptoms and peak flow rates; interestingly, responders exhibited a significantly higher urinary excretion of a TxA_2 metabolite, suggesting that urinary measurements might be useful in predicting the utility of this agent (101). Larger-scale trials of anti-TxA_2 agents in diverse populations around the world will be necessary to define the potential of this therapeutic approach.

IX. Role of PGE_2 in Asthma

PGE_2 has diverse actions that would tend to be antiasthmatic (Table 4). Inhalation of PGE_2 causes acute bronchodilatation in humans; this is consistent with the recognized ability of this prostanoid to effect smooth muscle relaxation. Pretreatment with inhaled PGE_2 also substantially protects against bronchoconstriction induced by

Table 4 Potential Antiasthmatic Actions of PGE_2

Bronchodilatation
Protect against bronchoconstriction in response to exercise, antigen, aspirin
Reduce BHR
Inhibit leukocyte recruitment
Inhibit lymphocyte proliferation
Inhibit generation of inflammatory mediators
Increase generation of IL-10
Inhibit proliferation of smooth muscle cells and fibroblasts
Inhibit collagen synthesis

exercise, antigen inhalation, and aspirin (in aspirin-sensitive asthmatics) (102). This bronchoprotective effect of PGE_2 likely reflects both a bronchodilatory action as well as its ability to inhibit recruitment of leukocytes and generation of inflammatory mediators. For example, inhaled PGE_2 has been reported to attenuate allergen-induced early and late bronchoconstrictor responses, methacholine hyperresponsiveness, and increases in sputum eosinophils (103). PGE_2 has been reported to inhibit leukocyte chemotaxis, expression of various adhesion molecules and integrins necessary for leukocyte emigration from the vasculature, lymphocyte proliferation, and generation of reactive oxygen intermediates, certain cytokines such as IL-8 and tumor necrosis-α, endothelin, PGD_2, and LTs (104–108). At the same time, it increases the expression of the anti-inflammatory cytokine IL-10 (109). This prostanoid also inhibits the proliferation of smooth muscle cells (110) and fibroblasts (111), inhibits the expression of platelet-derived growth factor-α receptor expression on myofibroblasts (112), and inhibits collagen synthesis by fibroblasts (113). Thus, PGE_2 can exert beneficial effects on bronchial tone, BHR, airway inflammation, and airway remodeling. This broad profile of beneficial actions opposes the pleiotropic asthmagenic actions of LTs. Most of these salutary actions appear to be explained by increases in intracellular cyclic AMP and are assumed to be mediated by the adenyl cyclase-coupled receptors EP2 and EP4. Many of these actions are therefore shared by the prostanoid PGI_2, which also signals via adenyl cyclase. Interestingly, PGE_2 and PGI_2 have also been reported to inhibit activation of the transcription factor nuclear factor-κB (114), and this may also reflect downstream consequences of intracellular cyclic AMP accumulation.

PGE_2 is the major eicosanoid synthesized by airway epithelial cells, and levels of PGE_2 in lung lavage fluid from normal humans are higher than those of other prostanoids (115). PGE_2 is synthesized by airway epithelium in response to various endogenous and exogenous substances known to be bronchoprotective; these include proteases (acting via protease-activated receptors), substance P, and furosemide (102,116). Airway epithelial cells are unusual in that they constitutively express both COX-1 and COX-2 isoforms (117). A growing body of evidence is consistent with the conclusion that endogenously produced PGE_2 is indeed bronchoprotective, just as is exogenously administered PGE_2. For example, administration of COX inhibitors during antigen sensitization and challenge in mice leads to increased BHR, eosinophilia, and expression of cytokines including IL-5 and IL-13 (118). Similar results have been observed in mice who are genetically prostanoid-deficient following COX-1 or COX-2 gene disruption (119). While these results indicate that an endogenously synthesized COX product mediates anti-inflammatory and broncho-protective effects, they do not establish that it is PGE_2. However, considering the airway concentrations and known effects of various prostanoids, PGE_2 is the most likely candidate. Also, COX inhibition or disruption in vivo typically leads to increases in LT production via shunting of AA to the 5-LO pathway; therefore, the consequences of reduced PGE_2 vs. increased LTs can be difficult to distinguish. For both of these reasons, studies of airway responses in mice with disruptions of their EP receptors or with EP-selective antagonists will be necessary to confirm the protective role of endogenous PGE_2 in vivo. In this regard, the ability of substance P to relax airway tone was abrogated in EP2-deficient mice (120).

If indeed PGE_2 is an endogenous bronchoprotective and anti-inflammatory substance, is there any evidence for a deficiency of endogenous PGE_2 in asthma? Very little information on this point is available. However, an inverse relationship between sputum PGE_2 levels and sputum eosinophil numbers was found in subjects with asthma (3). In addition, epithelial strips from horses affected with heaves, a naturally occurring equine variant of asthma, produced less PGE_2 than did strips from unaffected horses, and there was a significant correlation between epithelial PGE_2 production and the time taken for affected animals to develop airway obstruction (121). Expression of COX-1 and COX-2 in bronchial and nasal mucosa of asthmatics has been examined. While no differences from normal subjects have been reported for COX-1, COX-2 expression has been reported to be unchanged (122), increased (123), or decreased (124) in asthmatics and especially aspirin-sensitive asthmatics. It is interesting to note that reduced capacity for synthesis of protective prostanoids has been reported in patients with primary pulmonary hypertension (PGI_2) (125) and idiopathic pulmonary fibrosis (PGE_2) (126), and such reductions have been implicated in the inflammatory and remodeling aspects of these diseases. Further studies will be necessary to determine if this is a component of the pathogenesis or evolution of asthma. In any case, it is clear that administration of exogenous PGE_2 has therapeutic potential in asthma. Cough has been frequently observed in subjects who have received inhaled PGE_2; however, it remains to be determined whether the receptors that mediate cough differ from those that mediate bronchoprotective or anti-inflammatory effects. If cough can be dissociated from these beneficial effects, inhalation of EP receptor-selective PGE_2 agonists may represent an attractive therapeutic approach.

X. Therapeutic Strategies to Alter Eicosanoid Synthesis or Actions

In view of the importance of eicosanoids in airway inflammation and biology, modulation of their tissue concentrations or actions represent appropriate therapeutic targets in asthma. Three generic strategies can be considered. The first is inhibition of the synthesis of a potentially asthmagenic eicosanoid, and the second is antagonism of its receptor. These strategies have been most successfully employed with respect to cysteinyl-LTs and have also been implemented for TxA_2 with more ambiguous results. It is conceivable that other asthmagenic eicosanoids, such as PGD_2, may also be candidates for selective targeting. One unresolved issue involves the relative merits of targeting proximal vs. distal enzymatic steps in eicosanoid synthesis. This has been discussed earlier with regard to inhibition of the 5-LO enzyme (with abrogation of the synthesis of LTB_4, 5-HETE, and metabolites thereof, such as 5-oxo-ETE in addition to the cysteinyl-LTs) vs. selective targeting of cysteinyl-LTs. Here it is unambiguous, at least theoretically, that the broader approach of 5-LO inhibition would be *expected* to be superior to the narrower approach. At other enzymatic steps, the advantages of a more proximal strategy might be less certain. For example, various prostanoids exert either pro- or antiasthmatic actions, as has been discussed. Therefore, inhibition of the COX enzyme(s) might be expected to encompass both deleterious and beneficial effects. The relative importance (i.e., based on relative synthetic rate and receptor expression) of a given prostanoid in any given patient would thus be expected to determine the net outcome of COX inhibition. Examples certainly exist of patients whose asthma is either worsened or improved by treatment with COX inhibitors (nonsteroidal anti-inflammatory drugs). However, most asthmatics can take nonsteroidals without effects on their respiratory status. This is perhaps what might be expected from the symmetrical inhibition of both pro- and antiasthmatic prostanoids of equal importance. The least selective step in the eicosanoid synthetic pathway would be the initial release of AA from membrane phospholipids. This could be accomplished either by the inhibition of PLA_2-mediated deacylation or by reducing the arachidonate content of phospholipids via dietary modifications of fatty acid intake. The latter can be accomplished by supplementation with "fish oil" diets rich in n-3 fatty acids such as eicosapentaenoic acid. The theoretical limitation of a strategy that reduces the levels of available free AA is that synthesis of PGE_2 and PGI_2 (and other potentially protective eicosanoids) would be expected to be reduced along with potentially deleterious eicosanoids. On the other hand, if the production of pro-asthmatic eicosanoids greatly exceeds the production of antiasthmatic eicosanoids, the nonspecificity of inhibiting this most proximal step may not be problematic. Indeed, gene disruption of an important isoform of PLA_2, cytosolic PLA_2, has been demonstrated to protect mice from antigen-induced bronchospasm and BHR (127).

The third and final generic strategy involves administration of or upregulating the synthesis of a potentially beneficial eicosanoid with antiasthmatic actions. The best candidate for such a strategy would be PGE_2. Indeed, inhalation of exogenous PGE_2 has been shown to increase the lung lavage levels of this prostanoid in human subjects (128). As discussed above, selective EP2 and/or EP4 agonists might confer more specificity than would PGE_2 itself. Strategies that result in increased expression of either COX or of PGE_2 synthase could also yield an increase in lung levels of PGE_2 but be more long-lived; these could entail either gene therapy approaches or administration of other agents known to upregulate gene expression of these enzymes. This same strategy could be applied to other eicosanoids with potentially antiasthmatic effects, such as PGI_2 or PPAR-γ agonists. Finally, it is obvious that combination strategies consisting of inhibiting or antagonizing a pro-asthmatic eicosanoid while increasing levels of an antiasthmatic eicosanoid (or its receptor) might have additive benefit.

XI. Effects on Eicosanoid Synthesis of Commonly Used Therapeutic Agents for Asthma

There are a number of pharmacological agents in current use for the treatment of asthma that may modulate the generation of eicosanoids. Nedocramil has been shown to inhibit ex vivo 5-LO metabolism by alveolar macrophages from asthmatics (84), and sodium cromoglycate has been reported to variably inhibit the increase in urinary LTE_4 following allergen challenge of asthmatics (129). Inhibitory effects on LT synthesis in vitro have been reported for theophylline (130) and for β-agonists (131). Inhalation of the long-acting β-agonist salmeterol has been shown to reduce urinary levels of LTE_4 and of a PGD_2 metabolite in parallel with blunted bronchoconstrictor responses following aspirin challenge in aspirin-sensitive asthmatics (131).

The effects of aspirin and other nonsteroidal COX inhibitors have been discussed above. In the minority of asthmatics who develop airway and sometimes systemic reactions to these agents, levels of LTs in urine or lavage fluid have been reported to be extremely high (71). This would not seem to reflect merely shunting of AA from COX to 5-LO pathways, since it is so uncommon and since LT overproduction can be detected in these patients even in the absence of ingestion of nonsteroidals. Aspirin-sensitive asthma has been attributed to increased mast cell expression of LTC_4 synthase (132). However, this does not account for the fact that increased levels of LTB_4 have also been reported in lung lavage fluid following challenge with nonsteroidals (133), nor is it clear that this most distal enzyme in cysteinyl-LT synthesis is ordinarily rate-limiting. One component of the pathogenesis of this syndrome appears to involve the removal of bronchoprotective prostanoids such as PGE_2. While it is unclear whether the relative production of PGE_2 differs between aspirin-sensitive and non–aspirin-sensitive patients, conflicting results regarding COX-2 expression have been reported (123,124). Nevertheless, it has recently been demonstrated that aspirin-sensitive asthmatics can tolerate COX-2-selective inhibitors (134), implying that COX-1 is largely responsible for generating bronchoprotective prostanoids in these patients. It is tempting to speculate that this may reflect the fact that these individuals are deficient in COX-2 expression at baseline.

Corticosteroids (CS) are the mainstay of anti-inflammatory therapy in both chronic asthma (inhaled route) and during asthma exacerbations (systemic route). A large body of literature has addressed the effects of CS on eicosanoid synthesis, but the results have often been conflicting and confusing. To some extent this reflects an array of in vitro and in vivo studies of varying designs carried out in different species. Most studies have focused on LT synthesis, as it is of great interest to determine if this therapeutic mainstay inhibits the production of the best understood asthmagenic eicosanoid. Results of in vitro studies are themselves conflicting. CS failed to inhibit LT synthesis by pulmonary mast cells (135). By contrast, they did have inhibitory effects on alveolar macrophages, but the degree of inhibition in rat cells (136) was far greater than that observed by the same laboratory on human cells (137). In monocytes and monocytic cell lines, CS either had no effect or actually augmented LT production (138) by upregulating the expression of FLAP and/or 5-LO. In vivo administration of CS by either the inhaled or the systemic route has again had inconsistent effects on LT production (139–141). At the very least it seems clear that CS are much less effective and consistent in inhibiting LT synthesis than in inhibiting many other aspects of airway inflammation. The explanation for this inconsistency probably reflects the fact that CS have distinct effects at different enzymatic steps in LT synthesis. Thus, CS inhibit stimulated release of AA from phospholipids, so there is less substrate for the 5-LO pathway. However, this effect is counterbalanced by the fact that they actually increase the expression of 5-LO and/or FLAP in certain cell types. Moreover, CS are potent inhibitors of COX-2 induction and may thereby remove the brake exerted by PGE_2 on LT biosynthesis. At the same time, CS would tend to alter the numbers of LT-generating cells in the airways, reducing the numbers of eosinophils but increasing the numbers of neutrophils. It is likely that in individual patients, the relative importance of each of these enzymatic steps or mechanisms and their susceptibility to inhibition by CS varies, providing an explanation for the inconsistent effects of this class of drug. The failure of CS to adequately inhibit LT synthesis may underlie the observed additive clinical and anti-inflammatory benefits of adding anti-LT agents to CS.

XII. Conclusions

Eicosanoids have long been implicated in the pathogenesis of asthma. The discovery that a mixture of cysteinyl-LTs accounts for SRS bioactivity permitted for the first time the eventual development of a class of pharmacological agents that target a single mediator of asthma. Anti-LT agents represent the first new class of asthma pharmacotherapy in 30 years. The early assumption that involvement of cysteinyl-LTs and other eicosanoids was confined to their effects on bronchial smooth muscle tone has given way to the realization that, instead, eicosanoids are pleiotropic mediators that modulate virtually every aspect of the biology of airway responses. A contemporary perspective conceptualizes eicosanoids as having even broader actions than do the cytokines: they not only affect the "modern" cellular and molecular components of immune responses as well as airway inflammation and remodeling, but also modulate the "old-fashioned" components such as smooth muscle tone, vascular permeability, and mucus secretion and clearance. As is true for cytokines, different eicosanoids possess pro- and antiasthmatic actions. And like bronchoconstrictor responses themselves, immediate and delayed phases of eicosanoid synthesis exist.

The last decade has witnessed a remarkable series of basic advances in our understanding of eicosanoid biology and the roles of these lipid mediators in the pathogenesis and clinical expression of asthma. The first generation of therapeutic modalities capitalizing on these advances has already shown therapeutic utility. Additional basic insights will pave the way for subsequent generations of therapeutic advances over the next decade. These will include not only targeting the inhibition of pro-asthmatic eicosanoids produced in excess, but also efforts to replete antiasthmatic lipids that may be relatively deficient.

Acknowledgments

Research in the author's laboratory supported by NIH grants P50 HL56402 and RO1 HL58897.

References

1. Seeds M, Bass D. Regulation and metabolism of arachidonic acid. Clin Rev Allergy Immunol 1999; 17:5–26.
2. Westcott J. The measurement of leukotrienes in human fluids. Clin Rev Allergy Immunol 1999; 17:153–178.
3. Pavord I, Ward R, Woltmann G, Wardlaw A, Sheller J, Dworski R. Induced sputum eicosanoid concentrations in asthma. Am J Respir Crit Care Med 1999; 160: 1905–1909.
4. Reinhold P, Becher G, Rothe M. Evaluation of the measurement of leukotriene B_4 concentrations in exhaled condensate as a noninvasive method for assessing mediators of inflammation in the lungs of calves. Am J Vet Res 2000; 61:742–749.
5. Wilborn J, Bailie M, Coffey M, Burdick M, Strieter R, Peters-Golden M. Constitutive activation of 5-lipoxygenase in the lungs of patients with idiopathic pulmonary fibrosis. J Clin Invest 1996; 97:1827–1836.
6. Bhattacharya M, Peri K, Almazan G, Ribeiro-da-Silva A, Shichi H, Durocher Y, Abramovitz M, Hou X, Varma D, Chemtob S. Nuclear localization of prostaglandin E_2 receptors. Proc Natl Acad Sci USA 1998; 95:15792–15797.
7. Dussault I, Forman B. Prostaglandins and fatty acids regulate transcriptional signaling via the peroxisome proliferator activated receptor nuclear receptors. Prostaglandins Other Lipid Mediat 2000; 62:1–13.
8. Narumiya S, Sugimoto Y, Ushikubi F. Prostanoid receptors: structures, properties, and functions. Phyisol Rev 1999; 79:1193–1226.
9. Lynch K, O'Neill G, Liu Q, Im D, Sawyer N, Metters K, Coulombe N, Abramovitz M, Figueroa D, Zeng Z, Connolly B, Bai C, Austin C, Chateauneuf A, Stocco R, Greig G, Kargman S, Hooks S, Hosfield E, Williams D, Ford-Hutchinson A, Caskey C, Evans J. Characterization of the human cysteinyl leukotriene $CysLT_1$ receptor. Nature 1999; 399:789–793.
10. Heise C, O'Dowd B, Figueroa D, Sawyer N, Nguyen T, Im D, Stocco R, Bellefeuille J, Abramovitz M, Cheng R, Williams D, Zeng Z, Liu Q, Ma L, Clements M, Coulombe N, Liu Y, Austin C, George S, O'Neill G, Metters K, Lynch K, Evans J. Characterization of the human cysteinyl leukotriene 2 receptor. J Biol Chem 2000; 275: 30531–30536.

11. Yokomizo T, Izumi T, Chang K, Takuwa Y, Shimuzo T. A G-protein-coupled receptor for leukotriene B_4 that mediates chemotaxis. Nature 1997; 387:620–624.

12. Yokomizo T, Kato K, Terawaki K, Izumi T, Shimizu T. A second leukotriene B_4 receptor, BLT_2: a new therapeutic target in inflammation and immunological disorders. J Exp Med 2000; 192:421–431.

13. Kellaway C, Trethewie R. The liberation of a slow reacting smooth muscle stimulating substance of anaphylaxis. Q J Exp Physiol 1940; 30:121–145.

14. Brocklehurst W. The release of histamine and formation of a slow reacting substance (SRS-A) during anaphylactic shock. J Physiol 1960; 151:416–435.

15. Murphy R, Hammarstrom S, Samuelsson B. Leukotriene C: a slow-reacting substance from murine mastocytoma cells. Proc Natl Acad Sci USA 1979; 76:4275–4279.

16. Asano K, Lilly C, O'Donnell W, Israel E, Fischer A, Ransil B, Drazen J. Diurnal variation of urinary leukotriene E_4 and histamine excretion rates in normal subjects and patients with mild-to-moderate asthma. J Allergy Clin Immunol 1995; 96:643–651.

17. Taylor I, Wellings R, Taylor G, Fuller R. Urinary leukotriene E_4 excretion in exercise-induced asthma. J Appl Physiol 1992; 73:743–748.

18. Taylor G, Black P, Turner N, Taylor I, Maltby N, Fuller R, Dollery C. Urinary leukotriene E_4 after antigen challenge and in acute asthma and allergic rhinitis. Lancet 1989; 1:584–588.

19. Knapp H, Sladek K, FitzGerald G. Increased excretion of leukotriene E_4 during aspirin-induced asthma. J Lab Clin Med 1992; 119:48–51.

20. Drazen J, O'Brien J, Sparrow D, Weiss S, Martins M, Israel E. Recovery of leukotriene E_4 from the urine of patients with airway obstruction. Am Rev Respir Dis 1992; 146:104–108.

21. Barnes N, Smith L. Biochemistry and physiology of the leukotrienes. Clin Rev Allergy Immunol 1999; 17:27–42.

22. Israel E, Rubin P, Kemp J, Grossman J, Pierson W, Siegel S, Tinkelman D, Murray J, Busse W, Segal A, Fish J, Kaiser H, Ledford D, Wenzel S, Rosenthal R, Cohn J, Lanni C, Pearlman H, Karahalios P, Drazen J. The effect of inhibition of 5-lipoxygenase by zileuton in mild-to-moderate asthma. Ann Intern Med 1993; 119:1059–1066.

23. Manning P, Watson R, Margolskee D, Williams V, Schwartz J, O'Byrne P. Inhibition of exercise-induced bronchoconstriction by MK-571, a potent LTD_4-receptor antagonist. N Engl J Med 1990; 323:1736–1739.

24. Israel E, Fischer A, Rosenberg M, Lilly C, Callery J, Shapiro J, Cohn J, Rubin P, Drazen J. The pivotal role of 5-lipoxygenase products in the reaction of aspirin-sensitive asthmatics to aspirin. Am Rev Respir Dis 1993; 148:1447–1451.

25. Lazarus S, Wong H, Watts M, Boushey H, Lavins B, Minkwitz M. The leukotriene receptor antagonist zafirlukast inhibits sulfur dioxide-induced bronchoconstriction in patients with asthma. Am J Respir Crit Care Med 1997; 156:1725–1730.

26. O'Hickey S, Hawksworth R, Fong C, Arm J, Spur B, Lee T. Leukotrienes C_4, D_4, and E_4 enhance histamine responsiveness in asthmatic airways. Am Rev Respir Dis 1991; 144:1053–1057.

27. Fischer A, McFadden C, Frantz R, Awni W, Cohn J, Drazen J, Israel E. Effect of chronic 5-lipoxygenase inhibition on airway hyperresponsiveness in asthmatic subjects. Am J Respir Crit Care Med 1995; 152:1203–1207.

28. Irvin C, Tu Y-P, Sheller J, Funk C. 5-Lipoxygenase products are necessary for oval-bumin-induced airway responsiveness in mice. Am J Physiol (Lung Cell Mol Physiol) 1997; 272:L1053–L1058.

29. Simon R. The role of leukotrienes and antileukotriene agents in the pathogenesis and treatment of allergic rhinitis. Clin Rev Allergy Immunol 1999; 17:271–275.

30. Wilson A, Orr L, Sims E, Dempsey O, Lipworth B. Antiasthmatic effects of mediator blockade versus topical corticosteroids in allergic rhinitis and asthma. Am J Respir Crit Care Med 2000; 162:1297–1301.

31. Laitinen L, Laitinen A, Haahtela T, Vilkka V, Spur B, Lee T. Leukotriene E_4 and granulocyte infiltration into asthmatic airways. Lancet 1993; 341:989–990.

32. Diamant Z, Hiltermann J, van Rensen E, Callenbach P, Veselic-Charvat M, van der Veen H, Sont J, Sterk P. The effect of inhaled leukotriene D_4 and methacholine on sputum cell differentials in asthma. Am J Respir Crit Care Med 1997; 155:1247–1253.

33. Cyr M, Denburg J. Systemic aspects of allergic disease: the role of the bone marrow. Curr Opin Immunol 2001; 13:727–732.

34. Pizzichini E, Leff J, Reiss T, Hendeles L, Boulet L, Wei L, Efthimiadis A, Zhang J, Hargreave F. Montelukast reduces airway eosinophilic inflammation in asthma: a randomized, controlled trial. Eur Respir J 1999; 14:12–18.

35. Spada C, Nieves A, Krauss A, Woodward D. Comparison of leukotriene B_4 and D_4 effects on human eosinophil and neutrophil motility in vitro. J Leukoc Biol 1994; 55: 183–191.

36. Pedersen K, Bochner B, Undem B. Cysteinyl leukotrienes induce P-selectin expression in human endothelial cells via a non-cysLT$_1$ receptor-mediated mechanism. J Pharmacol Exp Ther 1997; 281:655–662.

37. Lee E, Robertson T, Smith J, Kilfeather S. Leukotriene receptor antagonists and synthesis inhibitors reverse survival in eosinophils of asthmatic individuals. Am J Respir Crit Care Med 2000; 161:1881–1886.

38. Kane G, Pollice M, Kim C, Cohn J, Dworski R, Murray J, Sheller J, Fish J, Peters S. A controlled trial of the effect of the 5-lipoxygenase inhibitor, zileuton, on lung inflammation produced by segmental antigen challenge in human beings. J Allergy Clin Immunol 1996; 97:646–654.

39. Patrignani P, Modica R, Bertolero F, Patrono C. Differential effects of leukotriene C_4 on endothelin-1 and prostacyclin release by cultured vascular cells. Pharmacol Res 1993; 27:281–285.

40. Menard G, Bissonnette E. Priming of alveolar macrophages by leukotriene D_4: potentiation of inflammation. Am J Respir Cell Mol Biol 2000; 23:572–577.

41. Calhoun W, Lavins B, Minkwitz M, Evans R, Gleich G, Cohn J. Effect of zafirlukast (accolate) on cellular mediators of inflammation. Am J Respir Crit Care Med 1998; 157:1381–1389.

42. Hojo M, Suzuki M, Maghni K, Hamid Q, Powell W, Martin J. Role of cysteinyl leukotrienes in CD4+ T cell-driven late allergic airway responses. J Pharmacol Exp Ther 2000; 293:410–416.

43. Tohda Y, Nakahara H, Kubo H, Haraguchi R, Fukuoka M, Nakajima S. Effects of ONO-1078 (pranlukast) on cytokine production in peripheral blood mononuclear cells of patients with bronchial asthma. Clin Exp Allergy 1999; 29:1532–1536.

44. Rajah R, Nunn S, Herrick D, Grunstein M, Cohen P. Leukotriene D_4 induces MMP-1, which functions as an IGFBP protease in human airway smooth muscle cells. Am J Physiol (Lung Cell Mol Physiol 15) 1996; 271:L1014–L1022.

45. Bisgaard H, Loland L, Anhoj J. NO in exhaled air of asthmatic children is reduced by the leukotriene receptor antagonist montelukast. Am J Respir Crit Care Med 1999; 160:1227–1231.

46. Underwood D, Osborn R, Newsholme S, Torphy T, Hay D. Persistent airway eosinophilia after leukotriene (LT) D_4 administration in the guinea pig: modulation by the LTD_4 receptor antagonist, pranlukast, or an interleukin-5 monoclonal antibody. Am J Respir Crit Care Med 1996; 154:850–857.
47. Peters-Golden M, Bailie M, Marshall T, Wilke C, Phan S, Toews G, Moore B. Protection from pulmonary fibrosis in leukotriene-deficient mice. Am J Respir Crit Care Med 2002; 165:229–235.
48. Pynaert G, Grooten J, van Deventer S, Peppelenbosch M. Cysteinyl leukotrienes mediate histamine hypersensitivity ex vivo by increasing histamine receptor numbers. Molec Med 1999; 5:685–692.
49. Cowburn A, Holgate S, Sampson A. IL-5 increases expression of 5-lipoxygenase-activating protein and translocates 5-lipoxygenase to the nucleus in human blood eosinophils. J Immunol 1999; 163:456–465.
50. Hsieh F, Lam B, Penrose J, Austen K, Boyce J. T helper cell type 2 cytokines coordinately regulate immunoglobulin E-dependent cysteinyl leukotriene production by human cord blood-derived mast cells: profound induction of leukotriene C_4 synthase expression by interleukin 4. J Exp Med 2001; 193:123–133.
51. Brock TG, McNish RW, Coffey MJ, Ojo TC, Phare SM, Peters-Golden M. Effect of granulocyte-macrophage colony-stimulating factor on eicosanoid production by mononuclear phagocytes. J Immunol 1996; 156:2522–2527.
52. Steinhilber D, Radmark O, Samuelsson B. Transforming growth factor β upregulates 5-lipoxygenase activity during myeloid maturation. Proc Natl Acad Sci USA 1993; 90:5984–5988.
53. Yamamura H, Nabe T, Kohno S, Ohata K. Endothelin-1 induces release of histamine and leukotriene C_4 from mouse bone marrow-derived mast cells. Eur J Pharmacol 1994; 257:235–242.
54. Hisada T, Salmon M, Nasuhara Y, Chung K. Cysteinyl-leukotrienes partly mediate eotaxin-induced bronchial hyperresponsiveness and eosinophilia in IL-5 transgenic mice. Am J Respir Crit Care Med 1999; 160:571–575.
55. Rais M, Corry D. IL-13 is required in 5-lipoxygenase mediated allergic inflammation in experimental asthma (abstr). Am J Respir Crit Care Med 2001; 163:A434.
56. Coward S, Marley R, Hill A, Kilfeather S. Cysteinyl leukotriene receptor blockade with SKF 104,353 interrupts antigen-induced sensitisation in BALB/C mice (abstr). Am J Respir Crit Care Med 2000; 161:A20.
57. Robbiani D, Finch R, Jager D, Muller W, Sartorelli A, Randolph G. The leukotriene C_4 transporter MRP_1 regulates CCL19 (MIP-3β, ELC)-dependent mobilization of dendritic cells to lymph nodes. Cell 2000; 103:757–768.
58. Song P, Crimi E, Milanese M, Duan J, Rehder K, Brusasco V. Anti-inflammatory agents and allergen-induced $β_2$-receptor dysfunction in isolated human bronchi. Am J Respir Crit Care Med 1998; 158:1809–1814.
59. Sanz M, de la Cuesta C, Oehling A. Modulation of beta $_2$-adrenoceptors in human lymphocytes by in vitro stimulation with mediators. J Investig Allergol Clin Immunol 1994; 4:116–121.
60. Baud L, Perez J, Denis M, Ardaillou R. Modulation of fibroblast proliferation by sulfidopeptide leukotrienes: effect of indomethacin. J Immunol 1987; 138:1190–1195.
61. Panettieri R, Tan E, Ciocca V, Luttmann M, Leonard T, Hay D. Effects of LTD_4 on human airway smooth muscle cell proliferation, matrix expression, and contraction in vitro: differential sensitivity to cysteinyl leukotriene receptor antagonists. Am J Respir Cell Mol Biol 1998; 19:453–461.

62. Wang C, Du T, Xu L, Martin J. Role of leukotriene D_4 in allergen-induced increases in airway smooth muscle in the rat. Am Rev Respir Dis 1993; 148:413–417.
63. Henderson W, Jr, Tang L-O, Chu S-J, Tsao S-M, Chiang G, Jones F. A role for cysteinyl leukotrienes in airway remodeling in a mouse asthma model. Am J Respir Crit Care Med 2001; 165:108–116.
64. Uemura M, Buchholz U, Kojima H, Keppler A, Hafkemeyer P, Fukui H, Tsujii T, Keppler D. Cysteinyl leukotrienes in the urine of patients with liver diseases. Hepatology 1994; 20:804–812.
65. Drazen J, Israel E, O'Byrne P. Treatment of asthma with drugs modifying the leukotriene pathway. N Engl J Med 1999; 340:197–206.
66. Reiss T, Chervinsky P, Dockhorn R, Shingo S, Seidenberg B, Edwards T. Montelukast, a once-daily leukotriene receptor antagonist, in the treatment of chronic asthma: a multicenter, randomized, double-blind trial. Arch Intern Med 1998; 158:1213–1220.
67. Drazen J, Israel E. Should antileukotriene therapies be used instead of inhaled corticosteroids in asthma? Yes. Am J Respir Crit Care Med 1998; 158:1697–1698.
68. Malmstrom K, Rodriguez-Gomez G, Guerra J, Villaran C, Pineiro A, Wei L, Seidenberg B, Reiss T. Oral montelukast, inhaled beclomethasone, and placebo for chronic asthma. Ann Intern Med 1999; 130:487–495.
69. Drazen J, Yandava C, Dube L, Szczerback N, Hippensteel R, Pillari A, Israel E, Schork N, Silverman E, Katz D, Drajesk J. Pharmacogenetic association between $ALOX_5$ promoter genotype and the response to anti-asthma treatment. Nat Genet 1999; 22:168–170.
70. Sampson A, Siddiqui S, Buchanan D, Howarth P, Holgate S, Holloway J, Sayers I. Variant LTC_4 synthase allele modifies cysteinyl leukotriene synthesis in eosinophils and predicts clinical response to zafirlukast. Thorax 2000; 55(suppl 2):S28–S31.
71. Kumlin M, Dahlen B, Bjork T, Zetterstrom O, Granstrom E, Dahlen S-E. Urinary excretion of leukotriene E_4 and 11-dehydro-thromboxane B_2 in response to bronchial provocations with allergen, aspirin, leukotriene D_4, and histamine in asthmatics. Am Rev Respir Dis 1992; 146:96–103.
72. Dahlen B, Nizankowska E, Szczeklik A, Zetterstrom O, Bochenek G, Kumlin M, Mastalerz L, Pinis G, Swanson L, Boodhoo T, Wright S, Dube L, Dahlen S-E. Benefits from adding the 5-lipoxygenase inhibitor zileuton to conventional therapy in aspirin-intolerant asthmatics. Am J Respir Crit Care Med 1998; 157:1187–1194.
73. Drazen J, Silverman E, Lee T. Heterogeneity of therapeutic responses in asthma. Br Med Bull 2000; 56:1054–1070.
74. Kemp J, Minkwitz M, Bonuccelli C, Warren M. Therapeutic effect of zafirlukast as monotherapy in steroid-naive patients with severe persistent asthma. Chest 1999; 115:336–342.
75. Laviolette M, Malmstrom K, Lu S, Chervinsky P, Pujet J-C, Peszek I, Zhang J, Reiss T. Montelukast added to inhaled beclomethasone in treatment of asthma. Am J Respir Crit Care Med 1999; 160:1862–1868.
76. Tamaoki J, Kondo M, Sakai N, Nakata J, Takemura H, Nagai A, Takizawa T, Konno K. Leukotriene antagonist prevents exacerbation of asthma during reduction of high-dose inhaled corticosteroid. Am J Respir Crit Care Med 1997; 155:1235–1240.
77. Kuitert L, Barnes N. Leukotriene receptor antagonists: useful in acute asthma? Thorax 2000; 55:255–256.
78. Tager A, Dufour J, Goodarzi K, Bercury S, von Andrian U, Luster A. BLTR mediates leukotriene B_4-induced chemotaxis and adhesion and plays a dominant role in eosinophil accumulation in a murine model of peritonitis. J Exp Med 2000; 192:439–446.

79. Mensing H, Czarnetzki B. Leukotriene B$_4$ induces in vitro fibroblast chemotaxis. J Invest Dermatol 1984; 82:9–12.

80. Hebert M-J, Takano T, Holthofer H, Brady H. Sequential morphologic events during apoptosis of human neutrophils. Modulation by lipoxygenase-derived eicosanoids. J Immunol 1996; 157:3105–3115.

81. Yamaoka K, Dugas B, Paul-Eugene N, Mencia-Huerta J, Braquet P, Kolb J-P. Leukotriene B$_4$ enhances IL-4-induced IgE production from normal human lymphocytes. Cell Immunol 1994; 156:124–134.

82. Stamatiou P, Hamid Q, Taha R, Yu W, Issekutz T, Rokach J, Khanapure S, Powell W. 5-Oxo-ETE induces pulmonary eosinophilia in an integrin-dependent manner in Brown Norway rats. J Clin Invest 1998; 102:2165–2172.

83. Wardlaw A, Hay H, Cromwell O, Collins J, Kay A. Leukotrienes, LTC$_4$ and LTB$_4$, in bronchoalveolar lavage in bronchial asthma and other respiratory diseases. J Allergy Clin Immunol 1989; 84:19–26.

84. Damon M, Chavis C, Daures J, Crastes de Paulet A, Michel F, Godard P. Increased generation of the arachidonic metabolites LTB$_4$ and 5-HETE by human alveolar macrophages in patients with asthma: effect in vitro of nedocramil sodium. Eur Respir J 1989; 2:202–209.

85. Turner C, Breslow R, Conklyn M, Andresen C, Patterson D, Lopez-Anaya A, Owens B, Lee P, Watson J, Showell H. In vitro and in vivo effects of leukotriene B$_4$ antagonism in a primate model of asthma. J Clin Invest 1996; 97:381–387.

86. Sakurada T, Abe M, Kodani M, Sakata N, Katsuragi T. Synergistic effects of pranlukast and a leukotriene B$_4$ receptor antagonist on antigen-induced pulmonary reaction. Eur J Pharmacol 1999; 370:153–159.

87. Evans D, Barnes P, Spaethe S, van Alstyne E, Mitchell M, O'Connor B. Effect of a leukotriene B$_4$ receptor antagonist, LY293111, on allergen induced reponses in asthma. Thorax 1996; 51:1178–1184.

88. Liu M, Bleecker E, Lichtenstein L, Kagey-Sobotka A, Niv Y, McLemore T, Permutt S, Proud D, Hubbard W. Evidence for elevated levels of histamine, prostaglandin D$_2$, and other bronchoconstricting prostaglandins in the airways of subjects with mild asthma. Am Rev Respir Dis 1990; 142:121–132.

89. Johnston S, Freezer N, Ritter W, O'Toole S, Howarth P. Prostaglandin D$_2$-induced bronchoconstriction is mediated only in part by the thromboxane prostanoid receptor. Eur Respir J 1995; 8:411–415.

90. Hirai H, Tanaka K, Yoshie O, Ogawa K, Kenmotsu K, Takamori Y, Ichimasa M, Sugamura K, Nakamura M, Takano S, Nagata K. Prostaglandin D$_2$ selectively induces chemotaxis in T helper type 2 cells, eosinophils, and basophils via a seven-transmembrane receptor CRTH2. J Exp Med 2001; 193:255–261.

91. Monneret G, Gravel S, Diamond M, Rokach J, Powell W. Prostaglandin D$_2$ is a potent chemoattractant for human eosinophils that acts via a novel DP receptor. Blood 2001; 98:1942–1948.

92. Matsuoka T, Hirata M, Tanaka H, Takahashi Y, Murata T, Kabashima K, Sugimoto Y, Kobayashi T, Ushikubi F, Aze Y, Eguchi N, Urade Y, Yoshida N, Kimura K, Mizoguchi A, Honda Y, Nagai H, Narumiya S. Prostaglandin D$_2$ as a mediator of allergic asthma. Science 2000; 287:2013–2016.

93. Ricote M, Li A, Willson T, Kelly C, Glass C. The peroxisome proliferator-activated receptor-γ is a negative regulator of macrophage activation. Nature 1998; 391:79–82.

94. Wang A, Dai X, Luu B, Conrad D. Peroxisome proliferator-activated receptor-gamma regulates airway epithelial cell activation. Am J Respir Cell Mol Biol 2001; 24:688–693.

95. Straus D, Pascual G, Welch J, Ricote M, Hsiang C-H, Sengchanthalangsy L, Ghosh G, Glass C. 15-Deoxy-$\delta^{12, 14}$-prostaglandin J_2 inhibits multiple steps in the NF-kB signaling pathway. Proc Natl Acad Sci USA 2000; 97:4844–4849.

96. Narumiya S, FitzGerald G. Genetic and pharmacologic analysis of prostanoid receptor function. J Clin Invest 2001; 108:25–30.

97. Unoki M, Furuta S, Onouchi Y, Watanabe O, Doi S, Fujiwara H, Miyatake A, Fujita K, Tamari M, Nakamura Y. Association studies of 33 single nucleotide polymorphisms (SNPs) in 29 candidate genes for bronchial asthma: positive association with a T924C polymorphism in the thromboxane A_2 receptor gene. Hum Genet 2000; 106:440–446.

98. Tamaoki J, Kondo M, Nakata J, Nagana Y, Isono K, Nagai A. Effect of a thromboxane A_2 antagonist on sputum production and its physicochemical properties in patients with mild to moderate asthma. Chest 2000; 118:73–79.

99. Aizawa H, Inoue H, Nakano H, Matsumoto K, Yoshida M, Fukuyama S, Koto H, Hara N. Effects of a thromboxane A_2 antagonist on airway hyperresponsiveness, exhaled nitric oxide, and induced sputum eosinohils in asthmatics. Prostaglandins Leukot Essent Fatty Acids 1998; 59:185–190.

100. Obase Y, Shimoda T, Matsuo N, Matsuse H, Asai S, Kohno S. Effects of cysteinyl-leukotriene receptor antagonist, thromboxane A_2 receptor antagonist, and thromboxane A_2 synthetase inhibitor on antigen-induced bronchoconstriction in patients with asthma. Chest 1998; 114:1028–1032.

101. Tanaka H, Igarashi T, Saitoh T, Teramota S, Miyazaki N, Kaneko S, Ohmichi M, Abe S. Can urinary eicosanoids be a potential predictive marker of clinical response to thromboxane A_2 receptor antagonist in asthmatic patients? Respir Med 1999; 93: 891–897.

102. Pavord I, Tattersfield A. Bronchoprotective role for endogenous prostaglandin E_2. Lancet 1995; 345:436–438.

103. Gauvreau G, Watson R, O'Byrne P. Protective effects of inhaled PGE_2 on allergen-induced airway responses and airway inflammation. Am J Respir Crit Care Med 1999; 159:31–36.

104. McLeish K, Stelzer G, Wallace J. Regulation of oxygen radical release from murine peritoneal macrophages by pharmacologic doses of PGE_2. Free Radic Biol Med 1987; 3:15–20.

105. Oppenheimer-Marks N, Kavanaugh A, Lipsky P. Inhibition of the transendothelial migration of human T lymphocytes by prostaglandin E_2. J Immunol 1994; 152: 5703–5713.

106. Christman B, Christman J, Dworski R, Blair I, Prakash C. Prostaglandin E_2 limits arachidonic acid availability and inhibits leukotriene B_4 synthesis in rat alveolar macrophages by a nonphospholipase A_2 mechanism. J Immunol 1993; 151:2096–2104.

107. Kunkel S, Spengler M, May M, Spengler R, Larrick J, Remick D. Prostaglandin E_2 regulates macrophage-derived tumor necrosis factor gene expression. J Biol Chem 1988; 263:5380–5384.

108. Prins B, Hu R, Nazario B, Pedram A, Frank H, Weber M, Levin E. Prostaglandin E_2 and prostacyclin inhibit the production and secretion of endothelin from cultured endothelial cells. J Biol Chem 1994; 269:11938–11944.

109. Strassman G, Patil-Koota V, Finkelman F, Fong M, Kambayashi T. Evidence for the involvement of interleukin-10 in the differential deactivation of murine peritoneal macrophages by prostaglandin E_2. J Exp Med 1994; 180:2365–2370.

110. Belvisi M, Saunders M, Yacoub M, Mitchell J. Expression of cyclooxygenase-2 in human airway smooth muscle is associated with profound reductions in cell growth. Br J Pharmacol 1998; 125:1102–1108.

111. Bitterman P, Wewers M, Rennard S, Adelberg S, Crystal R. Modulation of alveolar macrophage-driven fibroblast proliferation by alternative macrophage mediators. J Clin Invest 1986; 77:700–708.

112. Boyle J, Lindroos P, Rice A, Zhang L, Zeldin D, Bonner J. Prostaglandin E_2 counteracts interleukin-1β-stimulated upregulation of platelet-derived growth factor α-receptor on rat pulmonary myofibroblasts. Am J Respir Cell Mol Biol 1999; 20:433–440.

113. Goldstein R, Polgar P. The effect and interaction of bradykinin and prostaglandins on protein and collagen production by lung fibroblasts. J Biol Chem 1982; 257: 8630–8633.

114. D'Acquisto F, Sautebin L, Iuvone T, Di Rosa M, Carnuccio R. Prostaglandins prevent inducible nitric oxide synthase protein expression by inhibiting nuclear factor-κB activation in J_{774} macrophages. FEBS Lett 1998; 440:76–80.

115. Ozaki T, Rennard S, Crystal R. Cyclooxygenase metabolites are compartmentalized in the human lower respiratory tract. J Appl Physiol 1987; 62:219–222.

116. Cocks T, Fong B, Chow J, Anderson G, Frauman A, Goldie R, Henry P, Carr M, Hamilton J, Moffatt J. A protective role for protease-activated receptors in the airways. Nature 1999; 398:156–160.

117. Asano K, Lilly C, Drazen J. Prostaglandin G/H synthase-2 is the constitutive and dominant isoform in cultured human lung epithelial cells. Am J Physiol (Lung Cell Mol Physiol) 1996; 271:L126–L131.

118. Peebles R, Dworski R, Collins R, Jarzecka K, Mitchell D, Graham B, Sheller J. Cyclooxygenase inhibition increases interleukin 5 and interleukin 13 production and airway hyperresponsiveness in allergic mice. Am J Respir Crit Care Med 2000; 162: 676–681.

119. Gavett S, Madison S, Chulada P, Scarborough P, Qu W, Boyle J, Tiano H, Lee C, Langenbach R, Roggli V, Zeldin D. Allergic lung responses are increased in prostaglandin H synthase-deficient mice. J Clin Invest 1999; 104:721–732.

120. Fortner C, Breyer R, Paul R. EP_2 receptors mediate airway relaxation to substance P, ATP, and PGE_2. Am J Physiol (Lung Cell Mol Physiol) 2001; 281:L469–L474.

121. Gray P, Derksen F, Broadstone R, Robinson N, Peters-Golden M. Decreased airway mucosal PGE_2 production during airway obstruction in an animal model of asthma. Am Rev Respir Dis 1992; 146:586–591.

122. Demoly P, Jaffuel D, Lequeux N, Weksler B, Creminon C, Michel F-B, Godard P, Bousquet J. Prostaglandin H synthase 1 and 2 immunoreactivities in the bronchial mucosa of asthmatics. Am J Respir Crit Care Med 1997; 155:670–675.

123. Sousa A, Pfister R, Christie P, Lane S, Nasser S, Schmitz-Schumann M, Lee T. Enhanced expression of cyclooxygenase isoenzyme 2 (COX-2) in asthmatic airways and its cellular distribution in aspirin-sensitive asthma. Thorax 1997; 52:940–945.

124. Picado C, Fernandez-Morata J, Juan M, Roca-Ferrer J, Fuentes M, Xaubet A, Mullol J. Cyclooxygenase-2 mRNA is downexpressed in nasal polyps from aspirin-sensitive asthmatics. Am J Respir Crit Care Med 1999; 160:291–296.

125. Tuder R, Cool C, Geraci M, Wang J, Abman S, Wright L, Badesch D, Voelkel N. Prostacyclin synthase expression is decreased in lungs from patients with severe pulmonary hypertension. Am J Respir Crit Care Med 1999; 159:1925–1932.

126. Wilborn J, Crofford L, Burdick M, Kunkel S, Strieter R, Peters-Golden M. Fibroblasts isolated from patients with idiopathic pulmonary fibrosis have a diminished capacity to synthesize prostaglandin E_2 and to express cyclooxygenase-2. J Clin Invest 1995; 95:1861–1868.

127. Uozumi N, Kume K, Nagase T, Nakatani N, Ishii S, Tashiro F, Komagata Y, Maki K, Ikuta K, Ouchi Y, Miyazaki J, Shimizu T. Role of cytosolic phospholipase A_2 in allergic response and parturition. Nature 1997; 390:618–622.

128. Borok Z, Gillissen A, Buhl R, Hoyt R, Hubbard R, Ozaki T, Rennard S, Crystal R. Augmentation of functional prostaglandin E levels on the respiratory epithelial surface by aerosol administration of prostaglandin E. Am Rev Respir Dis 1991; 144: 1080–1084.

129. Westcott JY, Smith HR, Wenzel SE, Larsen GL, Thomas RB, Felsien D, Voelkel NF. Urinary leukotriene E_4 in patients with asthma: effect of airways reactivity and sodium cromoglycate. Am Rev Respir Dis 1991; 143:1322–1328.

130. Kraft M, Torvik J, Trudeau J, Wenzel S, Martin R. Theophylline: potential antiinflammatory effects in nocturnal asthma. J Allergy Clin Immunol 1996; 97:1242–1246.

131. Szczeklik A, Dworski R, Mastalerz L, Prokop A, Sheller J, Nizankowska E, Cmiel A, Oates J. Salmeterol prevents aspirin-induced attacks of asthma and interferes with eicosanoid metabolism. Am J Respir Crit Care Med 1998; 158:1168–1172.

132. Cowburn A, Sladek K, Soja J, Adamek L, Nizankowska E, Szczeklik A, Lam B, Penrose J, Austen K, Holgate S, Sampson A. Overexpression of leukotriene C_4 synthase in bronchial biopsies from patients with aspirin-intolerant asthma. J Clin Invest 1998; 101:834–846.

133. Langmack E, Wenzel S. Mast cell and eosinophil responses after indomethacin in asthmatics tolerant and intolerant to aspirin. In: Szczellik A, Gryglewski R, Vane J, eds. Eicosanoids, Aspirin, and Asthma. Vol. 114. New York: Marcel Dekker, Inc, 1998:337–350.

134. Stevenson D, Simon R. Lack of cross-reactivity between rofecoxib and aspirin in aspirin-sensitive patients with asthma. J Allergy Clin Immunol 2001; 108:47–51.

135. Cohan V, Undem B, Fox C, Adkinson NJ, Lichtenstein L, Schleimer R. Dexamethasone does not inhibit the release of mediators from human mast cells residing in airway, intestine, or skin. Am Rev Respir Dis 1989; 140:951–954.

136. Peters-Golden M, Thebert P. Inhibition by methylprednisolone of zymosan-induced leukotriene synthesis in alveolar macrophages. Am Rev Respir Dis 1987; 135: 1020–1026.

137. Balter M, Eschenbacher W, Peters-Golden M. Arachidonic acid metabolism in cultured alveolar macrophages from normal, atopic, and asthmatic subjects. Am Rev Respir Dis 1988; 138:1134.

138. Riddick C, Ring W, Baker J, Hodulik C, Bigby T. Dexamethasone increases expression of 5-lipoxygenase and its activating protein in human monocytes and THP-1 cells. Eur J Biochem 1997; 246:112–118.

139. Shindo K, Fukumura M, Miyakawa K. Plasma levels of leukotriene E_4 during clinical course of bronchial asthma and the effect of oral prednisolone. Chest 1994; 105: 1038–1041.

140. O'Shaughnessy K, Wellings R, Gillies B, Fuller R. Differential effects of fluticasone proprionate on allergen-evoked bronchoconstriction and increased urinary leukotriene E_4 excretion. Am Rev Respir Dis 1994; 147:1472–1476.

141. Dworski R, FitzGerald G, Oates J, Sheller J. Effect of oral prednisone on airway inflammatory mediators in atopic asthma. Am J Respir Crit Care Med 1994; 149: 953–959.

30

Nitric Oxide, Reactive Nitrogen Species, and Lipid Mediator Generation in the Lung

JAMES R. COPELAND, MARK T. GLADWIN, and JAMES H. SHELHAMER

Warren G. Magnuson Clinical Center
National Institutes of Health
Bethesda, Maryland, U.S.A.

I. Introduction

The inflammatory process in the airways or the lung parenchyma may be initiated, amplified, and ultimately modulated by a variety of factors. Proteins, such as cytokines, colony-stimulating factors, growth factors, and receptor antagonists; peptides; lipid mediators such as eicosanoids, platelet-activating factors, and lysophospholipids; and signaling molecules, such as nitric oxide (NO) and carbon monoxide, all play roles in this process. How these signaling events are integrated over time is a subject of ongoing interest. This chapter will review mechanisms of NO interactions with lipid mediator generation involved in signaling. Special attention will be paid to potential NO modulation of airway lipid mediator generation.

NO is a free radical diatomic gas molecule generated from the oxidation of L-arginine to citruline by the nitric oxide synthase (NOS) enzymes. All three NOS systems are present in the lung. The predominant NOS isoform present in vascular endothelial cells is the calcium-dependent endothelial NOS (type III or eNOS), while airway epithelial cells contain calcium-independent, inducible NOS (type II or iNOS). Although NO has a potentially short half-life and undergoes unique biochemical interactions, it is capable of reacting with protein heme groups, thiol and tyrosine residues, and protein and lipid radicals to produce physiological effects. Many of these reactions have been explored in detail, such as activation of guanylate cyclase or inactivation of NOS by heme-NO ligation (1,2). However, other mechanisms of signal transduction are currently the subject of intense investigation and sometimes produce contradictory results. Apparent paradoxes reported in the literature may arise from (1) NO reactivity being critically dependent on the oxidation state of the nitrogen (different NO species); (2) the NO concentration present in the reaction conditions (in vivo concentrations < 100 nM); (3) reaction with different NO targets (heme group, thiol, tyrosine); and (4) modification of NO by the microenvironment (alternate reactions competing for NO). Thus, seemingly divergent effects of NO reported in the literature may represent alternate reactions under different conditions. An understanding of the role of NO as a potential modifier of lipid mediator generation requires an understanding of the biochemistry of NO and eicosanoid metabolism. The biochemical mechanisms of NO interactions and pathways for generation of lipid mediators will be reviewed, followed by a discussion of the potential target interactions of NO with lipid-metabolizing enzymes.

II. Biochemistry of Nitric Oxide Protein and Lipid Interactions

The reactions of NO with proteins and lipids can be separated into two major classes of reactions (Fig. 1). The first class involves reactions mediated by low concentrations of NO reacting with high affinity. These include reactions with other radicals (radical-radical coupling) such as superoxide, lipid and tyrosyl radicals, and with heme groups of metalloproteins, such as oxy- and deoxyhemoglobin, guanylate cyclase, and cytochromes. The second class involves reactions mediated by higher concentrations of NO, which reacts slowly with oxygen to form more reactive nitrogen oxide species (RNS). These RNS expand the potential biochemical interactions in addition to those that NO is capable of undergoing. Furthermore, under certain conditions these RNS are longer-lived than NO radical. Thus, generation of RNS allows an expansion of potential NO-mediated effects. Examples of RNS include nitrogen dioxide (NO_2), dinitrogen trioxide (N_2O_3), and peroxynitrite ($ONOO^-$) (3). Determinants of which RNS are generated are concentration of NO, local environment of targeted reaction sites, and concentration of oxygen versus other high-affinity reactants. When multiple reactions are possible, reactants of the faster reaction will compete for NO. This can effectively act to exclude other reactions from occurring, thus modulating the effects of NO signaling (4–7). As will be discussed later, in the lung higher concentrations of oxygen and lower concentrations of heme-containing proteins might favor formation of RNS with subsequent nitration or nitrosation of critical protein amino acids (8).

A. Nitric Oxide Reactions with Protein Heme Groups

NO can react directly with metalloproteins containing heme-iron complexes to form iron-nitrosyl adducts. Examples of such metalloproteins are soluble guanylate cyclase (9,10), producing c-GMP, NOS (1), mediating NO formation, and cytochrome P450 (11,12), which mediates oxidative metabolism of steroids, fatty acids, and

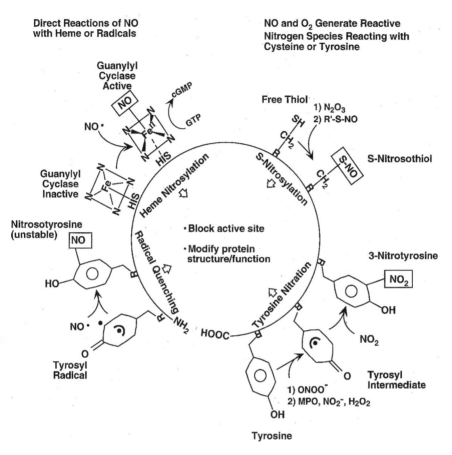

Figure 1 Biochemical interactions of nitric oxide with proteins.

xenobiotics. In the case of soluble guanylate cyclase, NO binds to the iron-heme group similar to oxygen binding to hemoglobin. This results in disruption of the proximal histidine-heme bond in the enzyme protein, allowing the substrates to interact with the catalytic site. Activating the enzyme converts GTP to cGMP, mediating transduction of the NO signal via activation of cGMP-dependent protein kinases, cGMP-gated ion channels, and cGMP-regulated phosphodiesterases (13–16).

NO reacts at diffusion-limited rates with oxyhemoglobin and oxymyoglobin to form nitrate (NO_3^-) and methemoglobin ($HbFe^{III}$). This is the major inactivation pathway for NO, which controls and localizes its bioactivity. For example, studies with the transgenic myoglobin knockout mouse suggest that myoglobin serves to contain NO within the vasculature during sepsis, preventing NO-mediated oxidative inactivation of mitochondrial cytochrome *c* (17). Thus, heme-NO interactions can transduce or terminate signal.

B. Nitric Oxide Reactions with Radicals

Additional direct effects of NO are interactions with other radicals. Tyrosyl radical scavenging by NO has been shown to inhibit ribonucleotide reductase activity (18). Furthermore, NO reacts with lipid peroxides at diffusion-limited rates (19). This can result in NO being a potent antioxidant through termination of lipid radical chain propagation. Another important radical-radical coupling reaction is with superoxide anion to form peroxynitrite ($ONOO^-$) (20). Peroxynitrite is a potent oxidizing agent and is produced rapidly by interaction with superoxide radical. Generation of peroxynitrite during the oxidative burst by activated macrophages and neutrophils has bacteriocidal activity (21). Thus, radical-radical coupling by NO is an important, rapid mechanism for quenching of protein or lipid radicals as well as promotion of oxidation via formation of RNS such as peroxynitrite.

C. Tyrosine Nitration

Protein tyrosine nitration occurs in a wide range of inflammatory pulmonary diseases such as acute respiratory distress syndrome (ARDS), asthma, and cystic fibrosis (8) and serves as a footprint of RNS production. Tyrosine nitration may occur via single electron oxidation by nitrating species ($ONOO^-$, NO_2Cl, $NO_2{}^{\cdot}$) to form a tyrosyl free radical intermediate. This tyrosyl free radical can react with $NO_2{}^{\cdot}$ to form 3-nitro-tyrosine or dimerize to form dityrosine (Fig. 1). Recent studies suggest that neutrophil or eosinophil myeloperoxidases directly nitrate tyrosine residues, using H_2O_2 and nitrite (22,23). While it is clear that tyrosine nitration is widespread in inflammatory diseases and can be used as a marker of inflammation or generation of RNS, a specific role in modification of protein function in vivo is being actively investigated. For example, nitration of surfactant protein A reduces its ability to aggregate lipids. Recently, nitrated surfactant has been found in bronchoalveolar lavage fluid from patients with ARDS (24,25). Several enzymes possess critical tyrosine residues that can be nitrated including ribonucleotide reductase, prostaglandin H synthase, and cytochrome c peroxidase. Whether or not these critical tyrosine residues are oxidized to directly transduce signal, inhibit tyrosine phosphorylation, inactivate proteins, or merely represent markers of inflammation is not yet clear.

D. Thiol Nitrosation

In aerobic aqueous solutions, the primary reaction of NO is with oxygen, ultimately forming nitrite. The reaction of NO with oxygen displays relatively slow, third-order kinetics. This reaction becomes important in conditions where the concentrations of reactants are high and other, high-affinity ligands such as ferrous-heme proteins or radicals are absent. NO and oxygen have greater solubility in hydrophobic environments such as lipid membranes (26). Thus, autooxidation of NO producing RNS, such as N_2O_3, would be expected to be greater in the lipid membrane of a cell. This implies that membrane-associated proteins would be susceptible to nitrosation reactions by NO indirectly via RNS. The reactions proceed as follows:

$$NO + O_2 \rightarrow \cdot ONOO$$
$$NO + \cdot ONOO \rightarrow ONOONO \rightarrow 2NO_2$$
$$NO_2 + NO \rightarrow N_2O_3$$

N_2O_3 can hydrolyze to form nitrite or can react with free thiols to form a covalent thiol-NO bond called an S-nitrosothiol. Although both amines and thiols are capable of being nitrosated, nitrosation of thiols is the preferred reaction under physiological conditions (27). Nitrosothiols are more stable than NO and may serve as a physiological reservoir for NO signaling (28). Intense recent study has focused on the potential role of S-nitrosothiols as vasodilators and on S-nitrosylation as a signal transduction event on par with O-phosphorylation (29). Indeed, S-nitrosothiols circulate in mammalian plasma in low nM concentrations as S-nitrosoalbumin and S-nitrosohemoglobin (30–35) and are capable of *trans*-nitrosation reactions with other proteins. S-nitrosylation of proteins such as caspase (36), p21^{ras} (37), and cardiac calcium release channels (38) have been demonstrated to modify protein activity. It is therefore possible that critical thiol oxidation, S-nitrosylation, or S-thiolation contributes to signal regulation as well.

III. Pathways for Lipid Mediator Generation

Eicosanoids involved in mammalian cell signaling arise from the sequential release and oxidation of arachidonic acid (AA) (Fig. 2). Membrane phospholipids contain a glycerol backbone typically with a saturated fatty acid in the sn-1 position, an unsaturated fatty acid in the sn-2 position, and a base bound via a phosphodiester

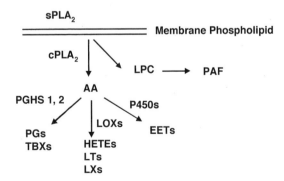

Figure 2 Metabolic pathways in lipid mediator generation. AA, arachidonic acid; CYP450, cytochrome P450; cPLA$_2$, cytosolic phospholipase A$_2$; EETs, epoxyeicosatrienoic acids; HETEs, hydroxyeicosatetraenoic acids; LOXs, lipoxygenases; LPC, lysophosphotidylcholine; LTs, leukotrienes; LXs, lipoxins; PAF, platelet-activating factor; PGs, prostaglandins; PGHS 1, 2, prostaglandin H synthase-1 and prostaglandin H synthase-2; sPLA$_2$, secretory phospholipase A$_2$; TBXs, thromboxanes.

Table 1   Pulmonary Effects of Eicosanoid Mediators

Mediator	Effect	Ref.
PGE_2	Bronchodilation	39–43
	Anti-inflammatory	
PGI_2	Vasodilation	44,45
	Bronchodilation	
	Antiplatelet aggregation	
$PGF_{2\alpha}$	Bronchoconstriction	39,45
	Vasoconstriction	
	Platelet aggregation	
TXA_2	Bronchoconstriction	45,46
	Vasoconstriction	
	Platelet aggregation	
LTC_4, LTD_4	Bronchoconstriction	47,48
	Mucus secretion	
	Vasodilation	
LTB_4	Neutrophil chemotaxis	49–51
HETEs	Vasodilation	52,53
EET (DHET)	Vasodilation	54–58
	Bronchodilation	
	Anti-inflammatory	

bond to the sn-3 position. AA is preferentially bound at the sn-2 position and is released from membrane phospholipids by phospholipase A_2 (PLA$_2$), with the concurrent production of 2-lysophospholipid. Once liberated, AA undergoes oxidation by one of three major enzymatic pathways involving prostaglandin H synthase (PGHS), lipoxygenase (LOX), or cytochrome P450. These three major pathways result in, respectively, the production of (1) prostaglandins, thromboxanes, and prostacyclin; (2) leukotrienes, hydroxyeicosatetraenoic acids (HETEs), and lipoxins; and (3) HETEs and epoxyeicosatrienoic acids (EETs). These products may then interact with specific cellular and nuclear membrane receptors, as second messengers, or autocrine and paracrine factors to produce their biological effects (Table 1).

A. Phospholipase A_2

Three major families of PLA$_2$ enzymes exist in mammalian cells: calcium-independent, or iPLA$_2$, and two families of calcium-dependent PLA$_2$s, cytosolic PLA$_2$ (cPLA$_2$) and secreted PLA$_2$ (sPLA$_2$). Stimulus-initiated liberation of AA involved in cellular signaling pathways occurs via cPLA$_2$ and sPLA$_2$. Little support exists for a role of iPLA$_2$ in stimulus-initiated AA release (59–61).

cPLA$_2$ (e.g., Type IV, cPLA$_2\alpha$) is a high molecular weight ($\sim$85 kDa) enzyme present constitutively in most cells, though its expression can be induced by cytokines and mitogens (62,63). cPLA$_2$ appears to be integrally involved in regulating stimulus-induced early and delayed AA release (61,64,65). Enzymatic release of AA by cPLA$_2$ is calcium dependent, occurring at submicromolar concentrations of intracellular calcium. The calcium dependence for activity appears to be mediated by an N-terminal calcium-binding domain that is required for intracellular translocation of the enzyme to endoplasmic and nuclear membranes where phospholipid substrates reside (66). Serine phosphorylation by mitogen-activated protein kinase (MAPK) has also been shown to regulate enzymatic activity (67,68). Thus, stimulus-induced increases in intracellular calcium may result in translocation of cPLA$_2$ from cytosol to membrane and allow AA to be released in proximity of downstream eicosanoid metabolizing enzymes such as PGHS and LOX, which co-reside with cPLA$_2$ at the membrane (69–71).

The sPLA$_2$s are a diverse group of low molecular weight (~14 kDa) enzymes. Several have been implicated in stimulus-induced AA release (Type IIA, V, X). The sPLA$_2$s require mM concentrations of calcium for activity and have less specificity for AA at the sn-2 position of phospholipids than cPLA$_2$, in vitro (72). sPLA$_2$ contains a signal sequence for transport extracellularly, and its structure consists of several disulfide bonds essential for enzyme activity. Type IIA and V sPLA$_2$s bind cell surface heparan sulfate proteoglycan (HSPG), via C-terminal cationic residues, which appears necessary for catalytic activity and stimulated AA release (61,73). The contribution of sPLA$_2$ to cellular AA metabolism may vary depending upon its expression, which is inducible. There is speculation that cell membrane-bound sPLA$_2$-mediated AA release follows agonist-stimulated perturbation of the cell membrane that facilitates sPLA$_2$ interaction with membrane phospholipid substrate (73,74).

B. Prostaglandin H Synthase

Two isoforms of PGHS have been described. These are heme-containing enzymes catalyzing the committed step in eicosanoid synthesis. PGHS-1 is present in most, but not all, cells and is constitutively expressed. PGHS-2 is undetectable in most cells, but its expression can be transiently induced by a number of cytokines and mitogens and is commonly expressed in inflammatory cells. Both isoforms of PGHS localize to endoplasmic and nuclear membranes (75–77). PGHS catalyzes two reactions at different sites of the enzyme: a cyclooxygenase (bisoxygenase) and a peroxidase reaction. The cyclooxygenase (COX) activity, occurring in a hydrophobic substrate-binding channel of the enzyme, involves a tyrosine radical and mediates the addition of two oxygen molecules to convert AA to 15-hydroperoxy-prostaglandin-9,11-endoperoxide (PGG$_2$). COX activity is inhibited by nonsteroidal anti-inflammatory drugs (NSAIDs). The second enzymatic activity is a peroxidase reaction involving heme-mediated two-electron reduction of PGG$_2$ to 15-hydroxy-prostaglandin-9, 11-endoperoxide (PGH$_2$). The peroxidase heme group requires oxidation in order to initiate the COX reaction located nearby within the protein enzyme. Thus, both activities are absolutely dependent upon the heme iron. The oxidized heme subsequently oxidizes a tyrosine residue forming tyrosyl radical located near the COX activity, which in turn abstracts a hydrogen from AA producing a lipid radical that then interacts with O_2 to produce PGG_2. While peroxidase activity can occur independently of COX, the COX activity is dependent upon oxidation of heme iron by the peroxidase.

Once formed, the endoperoxide PGH_2 is further rearranged to the biologically active eicosanoids PGD_2, PGE_2, $PGF_{2\alpha}$, PGI_2, or TXA_2. Specific synthase enzymes exist for production of these products from PGH_2 (78–81). Which eicosanoid is produced depends on the differential expression of these enzymes within cells (Table 2).

Selective signaling by either of the two isoforms of PGHS can occur based upon differential expression or coordinate expression of PGHS, phospholipases, and specific prostaglandin synthases. In some cells the PGHS-2 levels do not reach more than 20–30% of the level of PGHS-1 (103). The affinity of PGHS peroxidase activity

Table 2   Cellular Eicosanoid Products

Cell type	Eicosanoid	Ref.
Epithelial	PGE_2	82,83
	$PGF_{2\alpha}$	
	12-HETE	
	15-HETE	
Endothelial	PGI_2	84–87
	$PGF_{2\alpha}$	
	PGE_2	
	TXA_2	
Smooth muscle	PGE_2	88–90
	20-HETE	
Fibroblast	PGE_2	91,92
Alveolar macrophage	PGE_2	82,93,94
	TXA_2	
	LTB_4	
	5-HETE	
	15-HETE	
	LTC_4	
Neutrophil	PGE_2	95–98
	TXA_2	
	5-HETE	
	LTB_4	
Eosinophil	15-HETE	82,99
	LTC_4	
Mast cell	PGD_2	100–102
	TXA_2	
	LTB_4	
	LTC_4	
	PAF	

for hydroperoxides such as PGG_2 differs by 10-fold, allowing selective activation of the PGHS-2 isoform at low concentrations of AA (104,105). Lipid peroxides as well as peroxynitrite are capable of oxidizing the heme group thus promoting the COX activity in vitro (106). Of the three types of PLA_2 primarily involved in AA release there are no reports of physical coupling to selective PGHS isozymes. However, $cPLA_2$ appears to have an integral role in eicosanoid synthesis (61,64,65) and may produce AA, which subsequently is involved in coordinate expression of $sPLA_2$ and PGHS-2, thus giving the appearance of a functional coupling between these enzymes under certain conditions (73,107–109). For example, stimulation with IL-1 results in the coexpression of PGHS-2 with PGE_2 and PGI_2 synthases in peritoneal macrophages (110,111) and of PGHS-2 and PGE_2 synthase in A549 cells (79).

C. Lipoxygenase

LOXs are lipid-peroxidating enzymes mediating the stereospecific oxidation of AA to produce hydroperoxyeicosatetraenoic acid (HPETE) intermediates that are subsequently reduced to hydroxyeicosatetraenoic acids (HETE). Three forms of LOX enzyme are recognized based on their positional specificity for oxygenation of AA: 5-, 12-, and 15-LOX (112–114). These enzymes are nonheme iron–containing intracellular enzymes that translocate from soluble cytosolic or intranuclear sites to the nuclear membrane by a calcium-dependent process for activation (115). LOX activity requires activation by hydroperoxy fatty acids (112). Peroxide activation appears to involve oxidizing the resting enzyme ferrous iron to an activated, ferric, form, which subsequently allows lipid hydrogen abstraction leading to lipid radical formation and oxygen insertion. Phosphorylation sites for modulation of 5-LOX activity have also been shown (116,117). 5-LOX is dependent upon an integral nuclear membrane protein, 5-lipoxygenase–activating protein (FLAP), in both resting and activated cells, which binds released AA for presentation to and activation of 5-LOX (118,119).

Leukotriene A_4 is the major product of 5-LOX. LTA_4 may be further metabolized by two major pathways producing either leukotriene B_4 (LTB_4) or the glutathione conjugate leukotriene C_4 (LTC_4). Leukotriene A_4 hydrolase is a 69 kDa zinc-containing cytosolic enzyme mediating epoxide hydrolysis of LTA_4 to form LTB_4. The other major pathway involves an 18 kDa membrane-bound glutathione-S-transferase, leukotriene C_4 synthase. Leukotriene C_4 synthase mediates conjugation of reduced glutathione to LTA_4, producing the cysteinyl leukotriene LTC_4. Once formed, LTC_4 is transported to the extracellular space by an ATP-dependent transporter (120,121). LTC_4 can be further metabolized to biologically active LTD_4 and subsequently LTE_4 by γ-glutamyl transpeptidase and dipeptidases, respectively (122,123).

A third pathway for metabolism of 5-LOX metabolites is coupled to either 12-LOX or 15-LOX to produce lipoxins (LX). Lipoxins are trihydroxytetraenes formed by the coordinate metabolism of AA by either 15-LOX to 15-HPETE followed by 5-LOX, or 5-LOX to LTA_4 followed by 15-LOX to the stereoisomeres lipoxin A_4 (LXA$_4$) or B_4 (LXB$_4$) (124). Lipoxins are unique LOX products in that they have been found to have anti-inflammatory properties (125).

D. Cytochrome P450

Cytochrome P450 enzymes are a family of heme iron–containing, membrane-bound mixed functional oxygenase enzymes which mediate NADPH-dependent oxidation of xenobiotics as well as endogenous lipids. Three types of monooxygenase reactions involving AA are recognized: epoxygenation, midchain hydroxylation, and ω or ω-1 hydroxylation. First, epoxygenation of the four double bonds of AA leads to formation of 5,6-, 8,9-, 11,12-, or 14,15-epoxyeicosatrienoic acids (EET), which can be further hydrolyzed to their corresponding dihydroxyeicosatrienoic acids (DHETE). The second type of reaction consists of oxidation to 5-, 8-, 9-, 11-, 12-, or 15-hydroxyeicosatetraenoic acids (HETE). These products lack the stereospecificity of HETE produced by LOX. The third monooxygenase reaction is ω or ω-1 hydroxylation resulting in 19- or 20-HETE. 20-HETE is further metabolized by PGHS to ω-hydroxy-PGH$_2$ and ω-hydroxy-prostaglandins (126).

Although liberation of AA is considered the committed step in eicosanoid production, as shown above there are extensive enzymatic steps that may be targeted by intracellular signaling mechanisms in the ultimate modulation of final product. The role of NO in this process may result from modification of enzyme activity at the transcription, translation, or posttranslational levels. The following is a discussion of the direct actions of NO, or RNS, on the enzymatic conversion of AA to biologically active eicosanoids.

IV. Interactions of Nitric Oxide and Lipid Mediator Generation

The multiple pathways in eicosanoid mediator generation provide numerous steps for potential direct modulation by NO or RNS. While indirect actions via cGMP-dependent kinases or actions at the gene transcription level can affect the ultimate production of eicosanoids by NO, there are also potential posttranslational effects. Posttranslational modification can occur at several target sites on an enzyme and at several steps in the metabolic process. These targets include heme iron, nonheme iron, free thiols, tyrosine residues, or radical intermediates formed during the catalytic process. The following section and accompanying table (Table 3) attempt to review known and potential sites of interaction by NO and RNS on the eicosanoid mediator pathways.

A. Nitric Oxide Effects on Prostaglandin H Synthase Pathways

Reports in the literature of the effects of NO or RNS on enzymatic activity leading to prostaglandin synthesis are varied and contradictory. Multiple studies have reported inhibition of PGHS function by NO, following induction of endogenous NOS activity or addition of exogenous NO donor agents (127–136). This is in contrast to reports

Table 3 Potential Sites and Mechanism of NO Interaction with Eicosanoid Metabolic Pathways

Enzyme	Mechanism	Ref.
cPLA$_2$	Thiol nitrosation	176,177
PGHS	Heme iron nitrosylation	130,150
	Thiol nitrosation	158,178
	Tyrosine nitration	127,141
	Tyrosyl radical quenching	155,157,179
PGIS	Heme iron nitrosylation	159,161
	Tyrosine nitration	161
TXAS	Heme iron nitrosylation	159,161
LOX	Nonheme iron nitrosylation	130,180
	Lipid radical quenching	6,7
Cytochrome P450	Heme iron nitrosylation	181,182

showing activation of PGHS and increased prostaglandin production under seemingly similar conditions (106,137–147). Still other reports fail to find any significant effect of NO on PGHS activity (148–150). These results imply multiple effects of NO on cellular PGHS activity leading to prostaglandin production. As discussed earlier, such divergent effects can be attributed to differences in NO concentration, duration of exposure, local milieu, or production of RNS producing differing effects.

Investigation of NO-induced modulation of PGHS activity and prostaglandin production using cell culture may yield variable results based on the extent of PGHS isozyme expression. Quiescent cells express primarily PGHS-1 and have low amounts of prostaglandin production, as measured in the extracellular media. Stimulation of cells in culture with inflammatory mediators such as interleukin-1 (IL-1), tumor necrosis factor (TNF), or lipopolysaccharide (LPS) produces increased prostaglandin and NO production as a result of increased expression of PGHS-2 and inducible NOS (iNOS), respectively (106,128,144,149,151). Thus, quiescent and stimulated cells produce prostaglandins under different cellular conditions. This may indicate that divergent results of NO on prostaglandin production may result from differing effects on PGHS-1 and PGHS-2 activity. However, studies comparing purified PGHS-1 and PGHS-2 show no differences in response to NO donors (106,144).

Review of the studies reporting NO-induced inhibition of prostaglandin production in whole cells reveals these studies were performed in cytokine-stimulated cells using prolonged treatment (exceeding 2 hours) with NO donors (128,131,133,136,152). These studies showed that NO-induced decreases in prostaglandin production were associated with downregulation of PGHS-2, without changes in PGHS-1, when compared to stimulated control cells. This suggests that NO-induced reduction of prostaglandin production may occur secondary to decreased expression of PGHS-2 rather than a direct effect on PGHS enzyme function.

However, one study using LPS-stimulated endothelial cells did show decreased prostaglandin production without a reduction of PGHS-2 protein expression following short-term exposure to the NO donor NOC-7 (134). A similar result using the same NO donor was found in vitro using purified enzyme (146). Another study found that prolonged NO donor treatment resulted in increased prostaglandin synthesis in cells stimulated with IL-1β, which did not result in up regulation of NOS activity (153). Although levels of PGHS protein expression were not assessed in this latter report, the increased prostaglandin production appeared to be cGMP dependent. Altogether, these findings suggest that NO may inhibit PGHS activity and prostaglandin production in multiple ways. Whether long-term exposure to NO inhibits PGHS activity directly or primarily occurs through downregulation of enzyme is not clear from the majority of these works.

Reports showing activation of PGHS and prostaglandin synthesis were performed in quiescent cells using short-term treatment with NO donors (139,143,146). Cells used in these experiments expressed primarily PGHS-1. When the level of PGHS protein was measured in these latter studies, no change in PGHS-1 or PGHS-2 was found following NO treatment. However, one study found decreased prostaglandin production in quiescent smooth muscle cells after short-term exposure to an NO donor agent, but this particular response was cGMP dependent (132). Another study using quiescent endothelial cells has shown an increase in PGHS-2 expression following prolonged exposure to the NO donor SIN-1, which liberates peroxynitrite (149). Interestingly, the increased PGHS-2 expression found in this study was not associated with an increase in prostaglandin production, possibly related to altered heme utilization after SIN-1 exposure. In summary, it appears that short-term exposure of cells expressing primarily PGHS-1 to NO results in activation of PGHS and increased prostaglandin production without altering enzyme protein expression. NO can interact with PGHS at multiple sites to potentially modulate its activity, and investigations using purified enzyme are needed to clarify these interactions and their effects.

Binding of NO to ferrous heme occurs with high affinity, and early studies speculated that this may be a mechanism of modification of PGHS activity by NO (2,150). However, heme iron in resting PGHS exists in the ferric state, which has a much lower affinity for NO, which explains why several investigations have failed to detect NO binding to heme iron of PGHS (5,141). Furthermore, reconstitution of PGHS-1 apoprotein with nitrosylated heme produces inactive enzyme (141). Together, these studies indicate that NO binding to heme iron would inhibit PGHS enzyme function, although binding to PGHS heme may not occur at physiological levels of NO.

Tyrosine radical formation is an essential component of the cyclooxygenase catalytic function of PGHS. Nitration of PGHS tyrosine-385 has been reported when treated with NO (154,155). Any formation of nitrotyrosine adducts at this site on PGHS would be expected to produce overall inhibition of PGHS COX activity (141,156,157). However, AA may effectively compete with NO for interaction with the tyrosine radical intermediate and effectively prevent modification at this site as a mechanism for NO modification of PGHS activity (127).

PGHS contains several conserved cysteine residues. Nitrosation of any of these free thiols may be potential sites for enzyme modification. Indirect evidence supporting activation of PGHS by NO may involve S-nitrosation of free thiols (141). Site-directed mutagenesis of these free thiols decreases PGHS activity (158). It remains to be determined if modification of free thiols by NO has any modulating effect on PGHS activity.

While studies of NO acting at specific targets on PGHS predict inactivation of COX function, these studies cannot explain observations of enzyme activation. Peroxynitrite has been shown to act as a reducing substrate for PGHS peroxidase, substituting for hydroperoxides, resulting in activation of PGHS COX function (106,146). Peroxynitrite may be the RNS mediating PGHS activation, rather than NO, in inflammatory models as scavenging of superoxide anion inhibits activation of PGHS (and peroxynitrite formation). Similar studies have shown increased prostaglandin production by addition of peroxynitrite to platelets (127).

Other steps of prostaglandin synthesis downstream from PGHS are also sites of interaction by NO for modulation of prostanoid generation. Prostacyclin synthase (PGIS) and thromboxane synthase (TXS) are heme-containing enzymes mediating the conversion of the endoperoxide PGH_2 to prostacyclin (PGI_2) and thromboxane (TXA_2), respectively. These enzymes contain heme-thiolate bonds, similar to cytochrome P450 enzymes (159), which are potential target sites for oxidation by RNS. It is not known if disruption of these iron-sulfur bonds would produce inhibition of enzymatic activity. Studies using NO have shown partial activation of PGIS at low concentrations and inhibition at higher concentrations of NO (160). Peroxynitrite inhibits PGIS activity but has no effect on TXS. The mechanism by which peroxynitrite inhibits PGIS does not appear to involve disruption of the iron-sulfur bond but correlates with tyrosine nitration (161).

B. Nitric Oxide Effects on Lipoxygenase Pathways

NO donor agents are reported to inhibit LOX activity in intact cells and preparations of purified enzyme (130,147,162,163). LOX is a nonheme iron–containing enzyme that requires oxidation of the resting ferrous to the active ferric form for enzyme activation. Initial studies speculated that NO bound directly to ferrous iron to form an iron-nitrosyl complex, thus blocking enzyme activation. Surprisingly, concentrations of NO required for iron-nitrosyl complex formation are far in excess of that required for inhibition of enzyme activity or what is found in vivo (7,26,164,165). When studied under anaerobic conditions, where only the peroxidase function of LOX enzyme occurs, NO had no effect on enzyme activity despite cycling of the iron through ferrous and ferric oxidation states (6). Inhibition of LOX by NO may occur by binding of the lipid peroxyl radical produced during dioxygenase cycling resulting in lipid peroxynitrite and inactive enzyme (reduced iron state). The reduced enzyme remains in the resting state until activated by peroxide. If the rate of enzyme activation is slower than the rate of dioxygenase activity, a net inhibition of LOX enzyme activity can be achieved by NO scavenging of lipid peroxyl radical. In addition, these studies and others show that peroxide activation of LOX enzyme results in net consumption of two moles of NO per mole of enzyme (6,7). In this model NO is consumed during enzyme activation. Furthermore, any remaining NO would provide a continuous source of resting enzyme as a result of scavenging the lipid radical during enzyme substrate cycling. Thus, in the presence of excess substrate for activation LOX activity would continuously consume NO. Consistent with this model LOX activation in intact platelets resulted in decreased guanylate cyclase activation by NO. This effectively shows that the physiological activity of NO can be altered by competing reactions. A net scavenging effect of NO by LOX activation results in decreased physiological effects of NO.

C. Nitric Oxide Effects on Cytochrome P450 Pathways

NO is thought to cause inhibition of cytochrome P450 activity by binding to heme iron, analogous to that reported for NOS and catalase (1,166,167). Indeed, several investigations have shown inhibition of cellular cytochrome P450 activity by NO (11,168,169), and iron-nitrosyl complexes have been detected following induction of endogenous NOS in smooth muscle cells (170). Sodium nitroprusside (SNP) inhibits formation of the cytochrome P450 product 20-HETE in renal arteries (171). Reduction in 20-HETE contributes to the mechanism of SNP dilation of these vessels.

Inhibition of cytochrome P450 may involve disruption of heme-protein binding, resulting in free heme and inactive apoprotein. NO binding to the heme iron and subsequent axial cysteine bond displacement may allow release of the heme iron (12,172). Release of heme from cytochrome P450 may be a regulatory function for this enzyme by NO (173,174). Several studies have shown NO-dependent inhibition of cytochrome P450 activity in hepatocytes following induction of NOS with endotoxin or cytokines (11,169,175) resulting in decreased cytochrome P450 enzyme levels.

V. Conclusions

NO can affect lipid mediator generation at the transcriptional, translational, and posttranslational levels. Posttranslational regulation can occur via direct reactions with NO or indirectly via RNS. The direct reactions include iron binding and radical quenching. Indirect reactions via autooxidation products of NO include S-nitrosation of cysteine or nitration of tyrosine residues. Given the limited biochemical interactions of NO directly, RNS allow a temporal, spatial, and biochemical expansion of NO reactions and effects. Potential interactions of NO with lipid mediator generation can occur at several steps during eicosanoid metabolism. Limiting cellular sources of AA, altering lipid substrates, and inhibition or stimulation of the various enzymes involved in AA metabolism (PGHS, PG isomerase, LOX, cytochrome P450) are all potential target steps for modification by NO. Unfortunately, understanding the interactions of NO species with eicosanoid metabolic enzymes is complex, as shown by seemingly conflicting studies using purified enzyme protein, whole cell or cell fraction preparations. This may result from involvement of different NO species or different enzyme activities being observed.

Studies using purified enzyme preparations support a role for activation of prostaglandin formation by RNS such as peroxynitrite. Whole cell preparations expressing mainly PGHS-1 also support activation of prostaglandin formation by NO. However, inhibition of prostaglandin formation is also reported and is associated with downregulation of PGHS-2 protein expression following prolonged exposure to NO. Ultimately, downregulation of prostaglandin synthesis pathways may be the major effect, especially in inflammatory cells expressing high levels of PGHS-2 with stimulation. Studies support overall inhibition of LOX and cytochrome P450 pathways by NO or RNS. However, reactivity of NO or of RNS as well as competing reactions for NO or RNS in the target microenvironment can effectively determine the reaction process. The relevant questions are whether the direct or indirect reactions by NO occur under physiological, pathological, or pharmacological conditions and if these reactions result in signal transduction or termination. A clear understanding of the interactions at a biochemical level are necessary to fully understand the physiological and pathological potential for modification of lipid mediator generation by NO or RNS.

References

1. Griscavage JM, Hobbs AJ, Ignarro LJ. Negative modulation of nitric oxide synthase by nitric oxide and nitroso compounds. Adv Pharmacol 1995; 34:215–234.
2. Tsai A. How does NO activate hemeproteins? FEBS Lett 1994; 341(2–3):141–145.
3. Wink DA, Mitchell JB. Chemical biology of nitric oxide: insights into regulatory, cytotoxic, and cytoprotective mechanisms of nitric oxide. Free Radic Biol Med 1998; 25(4–5):434–456.
4. Abu-Soud HM, Hazen SL. Interrogation of heme pocket environment of mammalian peroxidases with diatomic ligands. Biochemistry 2001; 40(36):10747–10755.
5. O'Donnell VB, et al. Catalytic consumption of nitric oxide by prostaglandin H synthase-1 regulates platelet function. J Biol Chem 2000; 275(49):38239–38244.
6. O'Donnell VB, et al. 15-Lipoxygenase catalytically consumes nitric oxide and impairs activation of guanylate cyclase. J Biol Chem 1999; 274(29):20083–20091.
7. Rubbo H, et al. Nitric oxide inhibition of lipoxygenase-dependent liposome and low-density lipoprotein oxidation: termination of radical chain propagation reactions and formation of nitrogen-containing oxidized lipid derivatives. Arch Biochem Biophys 1995; 324(1):15–25.
8. van der Vilet A, et al. Reactive nitrogen species and tyrosine nitration in the respiratory tract: epiphenomena or a pathobiologic mechanism of disease? Am J Respir Crit Care Med 1999; 160(1):1–9.
9. Moncada S, Palmer RM, Higgs EA. Nitric oxide: physiology, pathophysiology, and pharmacology. Pharmacol Rev 1991; 43(2):109–142.
10. Stone JR, Marletta MA. Soluble guanylate cyclase from bovine lung: activation with nitric oxide and carbon monoxide and spectral characterization of the ferrous and ferric states. Biochemistry 1994; 33(18):5636–5640.

11. Khatsenko OG, et al. Nitric oxide is a mediator of the decrease in cytochrome P450-dependent metabolism caused by immunostimulants. Proc Natl Acad Sci USA 1993; 90(23):11147–11151.

12. Wink DA, et al. Inhibition of cytochromes P450 by nitric oxide and a nitric oxide-releasing agent. Arch Biochem Biophys 1993; 300(1):115–123.

13. Ignarro LJ, et al. Endothelium-derived relaxing factor produced and released from artery and vein is nitric oxide. Proc Natl Acad Sci USA 1987; 84(24):9265–9926.

14. Ignarro LJ, et al. Activation of purified guanylate cyclase by nitric oxide requires heme. Comparison of heme-deficient, heme-reconstituted and heme-containing forms of soluble enzyme from bovine lung. Biochim Biophys Acta 1982; 718(1):49–59.

15. Ignarro LJ, Wood KS, Wolin MS. Activation of purified soluble guanylate cyclase by protoporphyrin IX. Proc Natl Acad Sci USA 1982; 79(9):2870–2873.

16. Ignarro LJ, Wood KS, Wolin MS. Regulation of purified soluble guanylate cyclase by porphyrins and metalloporphyrins: a unifying concept. Adv Cyclic Nucleotide Protein Phosphorylation Res 1984; 17:267–274.

17. Flogel U, et al. Myoglobin: a scavenger of bioactive NO. Proc Natl Acad Sci USA 2001; 98(2):735–740.

18. Lepoivre M, Flaman JM, Henry Y. Early loss of the tyrosyl radical in ribonucleotide reductase of adenocarcinoma cells producing nitric oxide. J Biol Chem 1992; 267(32): 22994–23000.

19. O'Donnell VB, Freeman BA. Interactions between nitric oxide and lipid oxidation pathways: implications for vascular disease. Circ Res 2001; 88(1):12–21.

20. Crow JP, Beckman JS. The importance of superoxide in nitric oxide-dependent toxicity: evidence for peroxynitrite-mediated injury. Adv Exp Med Biol 1996; 387:147–161.

21. Ischiropoulos H, Zhu L, Beckman JS. Peroxynitrite formation from macrophage-derived nitric oxide. Arch Biochem Biophys 1992; 298(2):446–451.

22. Baldus S, et al. Endothelial transcytosis of myeloperoxidase confers specificity to vascular ECM proteins as targets of tyrosine nitration. J Clin Invest 2001; 108(12): 1759–1770.

23. Ford PC, Wink DA, Stanbury DM. Autoxidation kinetics of aqueous nitric oxide. FEBS Lett 1993; 326(1–3):1–3.

24. Haddad IY, et al. Nitration of surfactant protein A results in decreased ability to aggregate lipids. Am J Physiol 1996; 270(2 Pt 1):L281–288.

25. Zhu S, et al. Increased levels of nitrate and surfactant protein a nitration in the pulmonary edema fluid of patients with acute lung injury. Am J Respir Crit Care Med 2001; 163(1):166–172.

26. Liu X, et al. Accelerated reaction of nitric oxide with O_2 within the hydrophobic interior of biological membranes. Proc Natl Acad Sci USA 1998; 95(5):2175–2179.

27. Stamler JS, Singel DJ, Loscalzo J. Biochemistry of nitric oxide and its redox-activated forms. Science 1992; 258(5090):1898–1902.

28. Gaston B. Nitric oxide and thiol groups. Biochim Biophys Acta 1999; 1411(2–3): 323–333.

29. Lane P, Hao G, Gross SS. S-Nitrosylation is emerging as a specific and fundamental posttranslational protein modification: head-to-head comparison with O- phosphorylation. Sci STKE 2001; (86): p. RE1.

30. Cannon RO, 3rd, et al. Effects of inhaled nitric oxide on regional blood flow are consistent with intravascular nitric oxide delivery. J Clin Invest 2001; 108(2):279–287.

31. Gladwin MT, et al. Relative role of heme nitrosylation and beta-cysteine 93 nitrosation in the transport and metabolism of nitric oxide by hemoglobin in the human circulation. Proc Natl Acad Sci USA 2000; 97(18):9943–9948.

32. Gladwin MT, et al. Role of circulating nitrite and S-nitrosohemoglobin in the regulation of regional blood flow in humans. Proc Natl Acad Sci USA 2000; 97(21):11482–11487.

33. Jia L, et al. S-nitrosohaemoglobin: a dynamic activity of blood involved in vascular control. Nature 1996; 380(6571):221–226.

34. Marley R, et al. A chemiluminescense-based assay for S-nitrosoalbumin and other plasma S-nitrosothiols. Free Radic Res 2000; 32(1):1–9.

35. Stamler JS, et al. Nitric oxide circulates in mammalian plasma primarily as an S-nitroso adduct of serum albumin. Proc Natl Acad Sci USA 1992; 89(16):7674–7677.

36. Mannick JB, et al. Fas-induced caspase denitrosylation. Science 1999; 284(5414):651–654.

37. Lander HM, et al. A molecular redox switch on p21(ras). Structural basis for the nitric oxide-p21(ras) interaction. J Biol Chem 1997; 272(7):4323–4326.

38. Xu L, et al. Activation of the cardiac calcium release channel (ryanodine receptor) by poly-S-nitrosylation. Science 1998; 279(5348):234–237.

39. Mathe AA, Hedqvist P. Effect of prostaglandins F_2 alpha and E_2 on airway conductance in healthy subjects and asthmatic patients. Am Rev Respir Dis 1975; 111(3):313–320.

40. Bonta IL, Parnham MJ. Immunomodulatory-antiinflammatory functions of E-type prostaglandins. Minireview with emphasis on macrophage-mediated effects. Int J Immunopharmacol 1982; 4(2):103–109.

41. Pavord ID, et al. Effect of inhaled prostaglandin E_2 on allergen-induced asthma. Am Rev Respir Dis 1993; 148(1):87–90.

42. Hartert TV, et al. Prostaglandin E(2) decreases allergen-stimulated release of prostaglandin D(2) in airways of subjects with asthma. Am J Respir Crit Care Med 2000; 162(2 Pt 1):637–640.

43. Klockmann MT, et al. Interaction of human neutrophils with airway epithelial cells: reduction of leukotriene B_4 generation by epithelial cell derived prostaglandin E_2. J Cell Physiol 1998; 175(3):268–275.

44. Hardy CC, et al. Bronchoconstrictor and antibronchoconstrictor properties of inhaled prostacyclin in asthma. J Appl Physiol 1988; 64(4):1567–1574.

45. Hyman AL, et al. Prostaglandins and the lung. Med Clin North Am 1981; 65(4):789–808.

46. Ermert M, et al. Endotoxin priming of the cyclooxygenase-2-thromboxane axis in isolated rat lungs. Am J Physiol Lung Cell Mol Physiol 2000; 278(6):L1195–1203.

47. Adelroth E, et al. Airway responsiveness to leukotrienes C4 and D4 and to methacholine in patients with asthma and normal controls. N Engl J Med 1986; 315(8):480–484.

48. Drazen JM, Austen KF. Leukotrienes and airway responses. Am Rev Respir Dis 1987; 136(4):985–998.

49. Smith MJ, Ford-Hutchinson AW, Bray MA. Leukotriene B: a potential mediator of inflammation. J Pharm Pharmacol 1980; 32(7):517–518.

50. Ford-Hutchinson AW, et al. Leukotriene B, a potent chemokinetic and aggregating substance released from polymorphonuclear leukocytes. Nature 1980; 286(5770):264–265.

51. Gimbrone MA, Jr., Brock AF, Schafer AI. Leukotriene B_4 stimulates polymorphonuclear leukocyte adhesion to cultured vascular endothelial cells. J Clin Invest 1984; 74(4):1552–1555.

52. Zhu D, et al. Hypoxic pulmonary vasoconstriction is modified by P-450 metabolites. Am J Physiol Heart Circ Physiol 2000; 279(4):H1526–1533.

53. Jacobs ER, et al. Airway synthesis of 20-hydroxyeicosatetraenoic acid: metabolism by cyclooxygenase to a bronchodilator. Am J Physiol 1999; 276(2 Pt 1):L280–288.

54. Tan JZ, Kaley G, Gurtner GH. Nitric oxide and prostaglandins mediate vasodilation to 5,6-EET in rabbit lung. Adv Exp Med Biol 1997; 407:561–566.

55. Stephenson AH, Sprague RS, Lonigro AJ. 5,6-Epoxyeicosatrienoic acid reduces increases in pulmonary vascular resistance in the dog. Am J Physiol 1998; 275(1 Pt 2): H100–109.

56. Stephenson AH, et al. Inhibition of cytochrome P-450 attenuates hypoxemia of acute lung injury in dogs. Am J Physiol 1996; 270(4 Pt 2):H1355–1362.

57. Dumoulin M, et al. Epoxyeicosatrienoic acids relax airway smooth muscles and directly activate reconstituted KCa channels. Am J Physiol 1998; 275(3 Pt 1):L423–431.

58. Node K, et al. Anti-inflammatory properties of cytochrome P450 epoxygenase-derived eicosanoids. Science 1999; 285(5431):1276–1279.

59. Balsinde J, Balboa MA, Dennis EA. Antisense inhibition of group VI Ca^{2+}-independent phospholipase A_2 blocks phospholipid fatty acid remodeling in murine P388D1 macrophages. J Biol Chem 1997; 272(46):29317–29321.

60. Balsinde J, Dennis EA. Function and inhibition of intracellular calcium-independent phospholipase A_2. J Biol Chem 1997; 272(26):16069–16072.

61. Murakami M, et al. The functions of five distinct mammalian phospholipase A2S in regulating arachidonic acid release. Type IIa and type V secretory phospholipase A2S are functionally redundant and act in concert with cytosolic phospholipase A_2. J Biol Chem 1998; 273(23):14411–14423.

62. Clark JD, et al. Cytosolic phospholipase A_2. J Lipid Mediat Cell Signal 1995; 12(2–3): 83–117.

63. Leslie CC. Properties and regulation of cytosolic phospholipase A_2. J Biol Chem 1997; 272(27):16709–16712.

64. Bonventre JV, et al. Reduced fertility and postischaemic brain injury in mice deficient in cytosolic phospholipase A_2. Nature 1997; 390(6660):622–625.

65. Uozumi N, et al. Role of cytosolic phospholipase A_2 in allergic response and parturition. Nature 1997; 390(6660):618–622.

66. Schievella AR, et al. Calcium-mediated translocation of cytosolic phospholipase A_2 to the nuclear envelope and endoplasmic reticulum. J Biol Chem 1995; 270(51): 30749–30754.

67. de Carvalho MG, et al. Identification of phosphorylation sites of human 85-kDa cytosolic phospholipase A_2 expressed in insect cells and present in human monocytes. J Biol Chem 1996; 271(12):6987–6997.

68. Lin LL, Lin AY, Knopf JL. Cytosolic phospholipase A_2 is coupled to hormonally regulated release of arachidonic acid. Proc Natl Acad Sci USA 1992; 89(13): 6147–6151.

69. Glover S, et al. Translocation of the 85-kDa phospholipase A_2 from cytosol to the nuclear envelope in rat basophilic leukemia cells stimulated with calcium ionophore or IgE/antigen. J Biol Chem 1995; 270(25):15359–15367.

70. Peters-Golden M, et al. Translocation of cytosolic phospholipase A_2 to the nuclear envelope elicits topographically localized phospholipid hydrolysis. Biochem J 1996; 318(Pt 3):797–803.

71. Serhan CN, Haeggstrom JZ, Leslie CC. Lipid mediator networks in cell signaling: update and impact of cytokines. Faseb J 1996; 10(10):1147–1158.

72. Dennis EA. The growing phospholipase A_2 superfamily of signal transduction enzymes. Trends Biochem Sci 1997; 22(1):1–2.

73. Murakami M, et al. Different functional aspects of the group II subfamily (Types IIA and V) and type X secretory phospholipase A(2)s in regulating arachidonic acid release

and prostaglandin generation. Implications of cyclooxygenase-2 induction and phospholipid scramblase-mediated cellular membrane perturbation. J Biol Chem 1999; 274(44):31435–31444.

74. Zhou Q, et al. Molecular cloning of human plasma membrane phospholipid scramblase. A protein mediating transbilayer movement of plasma membrane phospholipids. J Biol Chem 1997; 272(29):18240–18244.

75. Morita I, et al. Different intracellular locations for prostaglandin endoperoxide H synthase-1 and -2. J Biol Chem 1995; 270(18):10902–10908.

76. Rollins TE, Smith WL. Subcellular localization of prostaglandin-forming cyclooxygenase in Swiss mouse 3T3 fibroblasts by electron microscopic immunocytochemistry. J Biol Chem 1980; 255(10):4872–4875.

77. Spencer AG, et al. Subcellular localization of prostaglandin endoperoxide H synthases-1 and -2 by immunoelectron microscopy. J Biol Chem 1998; 273(16):9886–9893.

78. Hara S, et al. Isolation and molecular cloning of prostacyclin synthase from bovine endothelial cells. J Biol Chem 1994; 269(31):19897–19903.

79. Jakobsson PJ, et al. Identification of human prostaglandin E synthase: a microsomal, glutathione-dependent, inducible enzyme, constituting a potential novel drug target. Proc Natl Acad Sci USA 1999; 96(13):7220–7225.

80. Kuwamoto S, et al. Inverse gene expression of prostacyclin and thromboxane synthases in resident and activated peritoneal macrophages. FEBS Lett 1997; 409(2):242–246.

81. Suzuki T, et al. Induction of hematopoietic prostaglandin D synthase in human megakaryocytic cells by phorbol ester. Biochem Biophys Res Commun 1997; 241(2): 288–293.

82. Conrad DJ. The arachidonate 12/15 lipoxygenases. A review of tissue expression and biologic function. Clin Rev Allergy Immunol 1999; 17(1–2):71–89.

83. Salvail D, Dumoulin M, Rousseau E. Direct modulation of tracheal Cl-channel activity by 5,6- and 11,12- EET. Am J Physiol 1998; 275(3 Pt 1):L432–441.

84. Davidge ST, et al. Biphasic stimulation of prostacyclin by endogenous nitric oxide (NO) in endothelial cells transfected with inducible NO synthase. Gen Pharmacol 1999; 33(5):383–387.

85. Hume R, et al. Prostaglandins PGE_2 and PGF_2 alpha in human fetal lung: immunohistochemistry and release from organ culture. Exp Lung Res 1992; 18(2):259–273.

86. Carley WW, Niedbala MJ, Gerritsen ME. Isolation, cultivation, and partial characterization of microvascular endothelium derived from human lung. Am J Respir Cell Mol Biol 1992; 7(6):620–630.

87. Toivanen JL. Effects of selenium, vitamin E and vitamin C on human prostacyclin and thromboxane synthesis in vitro. Prostaglandins Leukot Med 1987; 26(3):265–280.

88. Vigano T, et al. Cyclooxygenase-2 and synthesis of PGE_2 in human bronchial smooth-muscle cells. Am J Respir Crit Care Med 1997; 155(3):864–868.

89. Bonazzi A, et al. Effect of endogenous and exogenous prostaglandin E(2) on interleukin-1 beta-induced cyclooxygenase-2 expression in human airway smooth-muscle cells. Am J Respir Crit Care Med 2000; 162(6):2272–2277.

90. Frisbee JC, et al. Role of prostanoids and 20-HETE in mediating oxygen-induced constriction of skeletal muscle resistance arteries. Microvasc Res 2001; 62(3):271–283.

91. Zhu YK, et al. Cytokine inhibition of fibroblast-induced gel contraction is mediated by PGE(2) and NO acting through separate parallel pathways. Am J Respir Cell Mol Biol 2001; 25(2):245–253.

92. Vancheri C, et al. Different expression of TNF-alpha receptors and prostaglandin E(2) Production in normal and fibrotic lung fibroblasts: potential implications for the evolution of the inflammatory process. Am J Respir Cell Mol Biol 2000; 22(5):628–634.

93. Beck-Speier I, et al. Agglomerates of ultrafine particles of elemental carbon and TiO_2 induce generation of lipid mediators in alveolar macrophages. Environ Health Perspect 2001; 109(suppl 4):613–618.

94. Coffey MJ, et al. Regulation of 5-lipoxygenase metabolism in mononuclear phagocytes by CD_4 T lymphocytes. Exp Lung Res 1999; 25(7):617–629.

95. Crooks SW, Stockley RA. Leukotriene B_4. Int J Biochem Cell Biol 1998; 30(2): 173–178.

96. Fasano MB, Wells JD, McCall CE. Human neutrophils express the prostaglandin G/ H synthase 2 gene when stimulated with bacterial lipopolysaccharide. Clin Immunol Immunopathol 1998; 87(3):304–308.

97. Feuerstein G, Hallenbeck JM. Leukotrienes in health and disease. FASEB J 1987; 1(3):186–192.

98. Niiro H, et al. Regulation by interleukin-10 and interleukin-4 of cyclooxygenase-2 expression in human neutrophils. Blood 1997; 89(5):1621–1628.

99. Calabrese C, et al. Arachidonic acid metabolism in inflammatory cells of patients with bronchial asthma. Allergy 2000; 55(suppl 61):27–30.

100. Mita H, Ishii T, Akiyama K. Generation of thromboxane A_2 from highly purified human sinus mast cells after immunological stimulation. Prostaglandins Leukot Essent Fatty Acids 1999; 60(3):175–180.

101. Hart PH. Regulation of the inflammatory response in asthma by mast cell products. Immunol Cell Biol 2001; 79(2):149–153.

102. Nishimura H, et al. Acute effects of prostaglandin D_2 to induce airflow obstruction and airway microvascular leakage in guinea pigs: role of thromboxane A_2 receptors. Prostaglandins Other Lipid Mediat 2001; 66(1):1–15.

103. Wilborn J, DeWitt DL, Peters-Golden M. Expression and role of cyclooxygenase iso-forms in alveolar and peritoneal macrophages. Am J Physiol 1995; 268(2 Pt 1): L294–301.

104. Chen W, Pawelek TR, Kulmacz RJ. Hydroperoxide dependence and cooperative cyclooxygenase kinetics in prostaglandin H synthase-1 and -2. J Biol Chem 1999; 274(29):20301–20306.

105. Kulmacz RJ. Cellular regulation of prostaglandin H synthase catalysis. FEBS Lett 1998; 430(3):154–157.

106. Landino LM, et al. Peroxynitrite, the coupling product of nitric oxide and superoxide, activates prostaglandin biosynthesis. Proc Natl Acad Sci USA 1996; 93(26): 15069–15074.

107. Bingham CO, 3rd, et al. A heparin-sensitive phospholipase A_2 and prostaglandin endo-peroxide synthase-2 are functionally linked in the delayed phase of prostaglandin D_2 generation in mouse bone marrow-derived mast cells. J Biol Chem 1996; 271(42): 25936–25944.

108. Kuwata H, et al. Cytosolic phospholipase A_2 is required for cytokine-induced expres-sion of type IIA secretory phospholipase A_2 that mediates optimal cyclooxygenase-2-dependent delayed prostaglandin E_2 generation in rat 3Y1 fibroblasts. J Biol Chem 1998; 273(3):1733–1740.

109. Tada K, et al. Induction of cyclooxygenase-2 by secretory phospholipases A_2 in nerve growth factor-stimulated rat serosal mast cells is facilitated by interaction with fibro-blasts and mediated by a mechanism independent of their enzymatic functions. J Immu-nol 1998; 161(9):5008–5015.

110. Brock TG, McNish RW, Peters-Golden M. Arachidonic acid is preferentially metabo-lized by cyclooxygenase-2 to prostacyclin and prostaglandin E_2. J Biol Chem 1999; 274(17):11660–11666.

111. Matsumoto H, et al. Concordant induction of prostaglandin E_2 synthase with cyclooxygenase-2 leads to preferred production of prostaglandin E_2 over thromboxane and prostaglandin D_2 in lipopolysaccharide-stimulated rat peritoneal macrophages. Biochem Biophys Res Commun 1997; 230(1):110–114.

112. Kuhn H, Borngraber S. Mammalian 15-lipoxygenases. Enzymatic properties and biological implications. Adv Exp Med Biol 1999; 447:5–28.

113. Radmark OP. The molecular biology and regulation of 5-lipoxygenase. Am J Respir Crit Care Med 2000; 161(2 Pt 2):S11–15.

114. Yamamoto S, et al. Arachidonate 12-lipoxygenase isozymes. Adv Exp Med Biol 1999; 447:37–44.

115. Peters-Golden M, Brock TG. Intracellular compartmentalization of leukotriene biosynthesis. Am J Respir Crit Care Med 2000; 161(2 Pt 2):S36–40.

116. Lepley RA, Fitzpatrick FA. Inhibition of mitogen-activated protein kinase kinase blocks activation and redistribution of 5-lipoxygenase in HL-60 cells. Arch Biochem Biophys 1996; 331(1):141–144.

117. Lepley RA, Muskardin DT, Fitzpatrick FA. Tyrosine kinase activity modulates catalysis and translocation of cellular 5-lipoxygenase. J Biol Chem 1996; 271(11): 6179–6184.

118. Abramovitz M, et al. 5-Lipoxygenase-activating protein stimulates the utilization of arachidonic acid by 5-lipoxygenase. Eur J Biochem 1993; 215(1):105–111.

119. Mancini JA, et al. 5-lipoxygenase-activating protein is an arachidonate binding protein. FEBS Lett 1993; 318(3):277–281.

120. Lam BK, et al. The identification of a distinct export step following the biosynthesis of leukotriene C_4 by human eosinophils. J Biol Chem 1989; 264(22):12885–12889.

121. Schaub T, Ishikawa T, Keppler D. ATP-dependent leukotriene export from mastocytoma cells. FEBS Lett 1991; 279(1):83–86.

122. Lee CW, et al. Conversion of leukotriene D_4 to leukotriene E_4 by a dipeptidase released from the specific granule of human polymorphonuclear leucocytes. Immunology 1983; 48(1):27–35.

123. Tate SS, Meister A. Gamma-glutamyl transpeptidase: catalytic, structural and functional aspects. Mol Cell Biochem 1981; 39:357–368.

124. Serhan CN. Lipoxins and novel aspirin-triggered 15-epi-lipoxins (ATL): a jungle of cell-cell interactions or a therapeutic opportunity? Prostaglandins 1997; 53(2): 107–137.

125. McMahon B, et al. Lipoxins: revelations on resolution. Trends Pharmacol Sci 2001; 22(8):391–395.

126. Schwartzman ML, et al. Metabolism of 20-hydroxyeicosatetraenoic acid by cyclooxygenase. Formation and identification of novel endothelium-dependent vasoconstrictor metabolites. J Biol Chem 1989; 264(20):11658–11662.

127. Boulos C, Jiang H, Balazy M. Diffusion of peroxynitrite into the human platelet inhibits cyclooxygenase via nitration of tyrosine residues. J Pharmacol Exp Ther 2000; 293(1): 222–229.

128. Chen JX, et al. NO regulates LPS-stimulated cyclooxygenase gene expression and activity in pulmonary artery endothelium. Am J Physiol Lung Cell Mol Physiol 2001; 280(3):L450–457.

129. Fujimoto Y, et al. Comparison of the effects of nitric oxide and peroxynitrite on the 12-lipoxygenase and cyclooxygenase metabolism of arachidonic acid in rabbit platelets. Prostaglandins Leukot Essent Fatty Acids 1998; 59(2):95–100.

130. Kanner J, Harel S, Granit R. Nitric oxide, an inhibitor of lipid oxidation by lipoxygenase, cyclooxygenase and hemoglobin. Lipids 1992; 27(1):46–49.

131. Kosonen O, et al. Inhibition by nitric oxide-releasing compounds of prostacyclin production in human endothelial cells. Br J Pharmacol 1998; 125(2):247–254.

132. Marcelin-Jimenez G, Escalante B. Functional and cellular interactions between nitric oxide and prostacyclin. Comp Biochem Physiol C Toxicol Pharmacol 2001; 129(4): 349–359.

133. Minghetti L, et al. Interferon-gamma and nitric oxide down-regulate lipopolysaccharide-induced prostanoid production in cultured rat microglial cells by inhibiting cyclooxygenase-2 expression. J Neurochem 1996; 66(5):1963–1970.

134. Onodera M, et al. Differential effects of nitric oxide on the activity of prostaglandin endoperoxide H synthase-1 and -2 in vascular endothelial cells. Prostaglandins Leukot Essent Fatty Acids 2000; 62(3):161–167.

135. Perez Martinez S, et al. Nitric oxide inhibits prostanoid synthesis in the rat oviduct. Prostaglandins Leukot Essent Fatty Acids 2000; 62(4):239–242.

136. Tanaka Y, Igimi S, Amano F. Inhibition of prostaglandin synthesis by nitric oxide in RAW 264.7 macrophages. Arch Biochem Biophys 2001; 391(2):207–217.

137. Bakker EN, Sipkema P. Permissive effect of nitric oxide in arachidonic acid induced dilation in isolated rat arterioles. Cardiovasc Res 1998; 38(3):782–787.

138. Corbett JA, et al. IL-1 beta induces the coexpression of both nitric oxide synthase and cyclooxygenase by islets of Langerhans: activation of cyclooxygenase by nitric oxide. Biochemistry 1993; 32(50):13767–13770.

139. Davidge ST, et al. Nitric oxide produced by endothelial cells increases production of eicosanoids through activation of prostaglandin H synthase. Circ Res 1995; 77(2): 274–83.

140. Farina M, et al. IL1 alpha augments prostaglandin synthesis in pregnant rat uteri by a nitric oxide mediated mechanism. Prostaglandins Leukot Essent Fatty Acids 2000; 62(4):243–247.

141. Hajjar DP, et al. Nitric oxide enhances prostaglandin-H synthase-1 activity by a heme-independent mechanism: evidence implicating nitrosothiols. J Am Chem Soc 1995; 117:3340–3346.

142. Mollace V, et al. The effect of nitric oxide on cytokine-induced release of PGE_2 by human cultured astroglial cells. Br J Pharmacol 1998; 124(4):742–746.

143. Salvemini D, Currie MG, Mollace V. Nitric oxide-mediated cyclooxygenase activation. A key event in the antiplatelet effects of nitrovasodilators. J Clin Invest 1996; 97(11): 2562–2568.

144. Salvemini D, et al. Nitric oxide activates cyclooxygenase enzymes. Proc Natl Acad Sci USA 1993; 90(15):7240–7244.

145. Sautebin L, et al. Modulation by nitric oxide of prostaglandin biosynthesis in the rat. Br J Pharmacol 1995; 114(2):323–328.

146. Upmacis RK, Deeb RS, Hajjar DP. Regulation of prostaglandin H_2 synthase activity by nitrogen oxides. Biochemistry 1999; 38(38):12505–12513.

147. Velardez MO, et al. Role of nitric oxide in the metabolism of arachidonic acid in the rat anterior pituitary gland. Mol Cell Endocrinol 2001; 172(1–2):7–12.

148. Curtis JF, et al. Nitric oxide: a prostaglandin H synthase 1 and 2 reducing cosubstrate that does not stimulate cyclooxygenase activity or prostaglandin H synthase expression in murine macrophages. Arch Biochem Biophys 1996; 335(2):369–376.

149. Eligini S, et al. Induction of cyclo-oxygenase-2 in human endothelial cells by SIN-1 in the absence of prostaglandin production. Br J Pharmacol 2001; 133(7):1163–1171.

150. Tsai AL, Wei C, Kulmacz RJ. Interaction between nitric oxide and prostaglandin H synthase. Arch Biochem Biophys 1994; 313(2):367–372.
151. Knowles RG, Moncada S. Nitric oxide synthases in mammals. Biochem J 1994; 298(Pt 2):249–258.
152. Habib A, et al. Regulation of the expression of cyclooxygenase-2 by nitric oxide in rat peritoneal macrophages. J Immunol 1997; 158(8):3845–3851.
153. Watkins DN, Garlepp MJ, Thompson PJ. Regulation of the inducible cyclo-oxygenase pathway in human cultured airway epithelial (A549) cells by nitric oxide. Br J Pharmacol 1997; 121(7):1482–1488.
154. Goodwin DC, et al. Nitric oxide trapping of tyrosyl radicals generated during prostaglandin endoperoxide synthase turnover. Detection of the radical derivative of tyrosine 385. J Biol Chem 1998; 273(15):8903–8909.
155. Gunther MR, et al. Nitric oxide trapping of the tyrosyl radical of prostaglandin H synthase-2 leads to tyrosine iminoxyl radical and nitrotyrosine formation. J Biol Chem 1997; 272(27):17086–17090.
156. Kulmacz RJ, et al. Prostaglandin H synthase: spectroscopic studies of the interaction with hydroperoxides and with indomethacin. Biochemistry 1990; 29(37):8760–8771.
157. Shimokawa T, et al. Tyrosine 385 of prostaglandin endoperoxide synthase is required for cyclooxygenase catalysis. J Biol Chem 1990; 265(33):20073–20076.
158. Kennedy TA, Smith CJ, Marnett LJ. Investigation of the role of cysteines in catalysis by prostaglandin endoperoxide synthase. J Biol Chem 1994; 269(44):27357–27364.
159. Tanabe T, Ullrich V. Prostacyclin and thromboxane synthases. J Lipid Mediat Cell Signal 1995; 12(2–3):243–255.
160. Wade ML, Fitzpatrick FA. Nitric oxide modulates the activity of the hemoproteins prostaglandin I2 synthase and thromboxane A$_2$ synthase. Arch Biochem Biophys 1997; 347(2):174–180.
161. Zou M, Martin C, Ullrich V. Tyrosine nitration as a mechanism of selective inactivation of prostacyclin synthase by peroxynitrite. Biol Chem 1997; 378(7):707–713.
162. Maccarrone M, et al. Nitric oxide-donor compounds inhibit lipoxygenase activity. Biochem Biophys Res Commun 1996; 219(1):128–133.
163. Nakatsuka M, Osawa Y. Selective inhibition of the 12-lipoxygenase pathway of arachidonic acid metabolism by L-arginine or sodium nitroprusside in intact human platelets. Biochem Biophys Res Commun 1994; 200(3):1630–1634.
164. Brovkovych V, et al. Direct electrochemical measurement of nitric oxide in vascular endothelium. J Pharm Biomed Anal 1999; 19(1–2):135–143.
165. Salerno JC, Siedow JN. The nature of the nitric oxide complexes of lipoxygenase. Biochim Biophys Acta 1979; 579(1):246–251.
166. Brown GC. Reversible binding and inhibition of catalase by nitric oxide. Eur J Biochem 1995; 232(1):188–191.
167. Hurshman AR, Marletta MA. Nitric oxide complexes of inducible nitric oxide synthase: spectral characterization and effect on catalytic activity. Biochemistry 1995; 34(16): 5627–34.
168. Raiford DS, Thigpen MC. Kupffer cell stimulation with *Corynebacterium parvum* reduces some cytochrome P450-dependent activities and diminishes acetaminophen and carbon tetrachloride-induced liver injury in the rat. Toxicol Appl Pharmacol 1994; 129(1):36–45.
169. Stadler J, et al. Inhibition of cytochromes P4501A by nitric oxide. Proc Natl Acad Sci USA 1994; 91(9):3559–3563.

170. Geng YJ, et al. Cytokine-induced expression of nitric oxide synthase results in nitrosy-
      lation of heme and nonheme iron proteins in vascular smooth muscle cells. Exp Cell
      Res 1994; 214(1):418–428.
171. Alonso-Galicia M, et al. Contribution of 20-HETE to the vasodilator actions of nitric
      oxide in renal arteries. Am J Physiol 1998; 275(3 Pt 2):F370–378.
172. Kim YM, et al. Loss and degradation of enzyme-bound heme induced by cellular nitric
      oxide synthesis. J Biol Chem 1995; 270(11):5710–5713.
173. Juckett M, et al. Heme and the endothelium. Effects of nitric oxide on catalytic iron
      and heme degradation by heme oxygenase. J Biol Chem 1998; 273(36):23388–23397.
174. Kim YM, et al. Nitric oxide and intracellular heme. Adv Pharmacol 1995; 34:277–291.
175. Muller CM, et al. Nitric oxide mediates hepatic cytochrome P450 dysfunction induced
      by endotoxin. Anesthesiology 1996; 84(6):1435–1442.
176. Li B, et al. Inactivation of a cytosolic phospholipase A_2 by thiol-modifying reagents:
      cysteine residues as potential targets of phospholipase A_2. Biochemistry 1994; 33(28):
      8594–8603.
177. Li B, et al. Site-directed mutagenesis of Cys324 and Cys331 in human cytosolic phos-
      pholipase A_2: locus of action of thiol modification reagents leading to inactiviation of
      $cPLA_2$. Biochemistry 1996; 35(10):3156–3161.
178. Picot D, Loll PJ, Garavito RM. The X-ray crystal structure of the membrane protein
      prostaglandin H2 synthase-1. Nature 1994; 367(6460):243–249.
179. Guittet O, Roy B, Lepoivre M. Nitric oxide: a radical molecule in quest of free radicals
      in proteins. Cell Mol Life Sci 1999; 55(8–9):1054–1067.
180. Nelson MJ. The nitric oxide complex of ferrous soybean lipoxygenase-1. Substrate, pH,
      and ethanol effects on the active-site iron. J Biol Chem 1987; 262(25):12137–12142.
181. Daiber A, et al. Nitration and inactivation of cytochrome P450BM-3 by peroxynitrite.
      Stopped-flow measurements prove ferryl intermediates. Eur J Biochem 2000; 267(23):
      6729–6739.
182. Mehl M, et al. Peroxynitrite reaction with heme proteins. Nitric Oxide 1999; 3(2):
      142–152.

31

Adenosine Signaling and Lung Inflammation

SUMAN K. BANERJEE and MICHAEL R. BLACKBURN

University of Texas–Houston Medical School
Houston, Texas, U.S.A.

I. Introduction

Inflammatory lung diseases such as asthma and chronic obstructive pulmonary disease (COPD) are associated with cellular damage and airway remodeling that result in the loss of lung function. Adenosine is a signaling nucleoside that is generated during cellular stress and damage and has been implicated to play a role in lung diseases such as asthma and COPD (1,2). Adenosine may therefore serve as an important mediator of the chronic inflammation and ensuing airway remodeling associated with these diseases. There is substantial clinical and experimental evidence that suggests that adenosine and its signaling pathway play an important role in asthma and COPD. In this chapter we will provide an overview of the adenosine signaling pathway and examine the evidence linking adenosine signaling to asthma and COPD. Attention will be given to the description of murine animal models that exhibited severe lung inflammation and damage in association with elevations in lung adenosine levels. In addition, novel adenosine-based therapeutics for the treatment of lung inflammation and damage will be discussed.

II. Adenosine Metabolism and Signaling

Adenosine is a ubiquitous signaling nucleoside that is rapidly generated as a net result of ATP catabolism that occurs in situations of cellular stress or damage.

Intracellularly, adenosine can be derived from the dephosphorylation of adenosine 5′-monophospate (AMP) by a cytosolic form of 5′-nucleotidase (Fig. 1). The majority of intracellular AMP is formed by cleavage of the high-energy phosphate bonds of adenosine diphosphate (ADP) and adenosine triphosphate (ATP) during energy generation. Under normal conditions most of this AMP is reconverted to ADP and ATP, but under conditions of high energy demand and hypoxia AMP can be metabolized to adenosine by cytosolic 5′-nucleotidase. Intracellular adenosine can also be formed from the hydrolysis of S-adenosylhomocysteine, a product of cellular transmethylation reactions that utilize S-adenosylmethionine as a methyl donor (Fig. 1). Intracellular concentrations of adenosine are usually kept low by its rephosphorylation to AMP by the enzyme adenosine kinase (3) or its deamination to inosine by adenosine deaminase (ADA) (4). When intracellular concentrations exceed the capacity of these enzyme systems, adenosine is transported out of the cell through facilitated nucleoside transport systems. Mast cells activated by antigen have been shown to release adenosine (5), which may represent a source of increased adenosine release in the lungs of asthmatics.

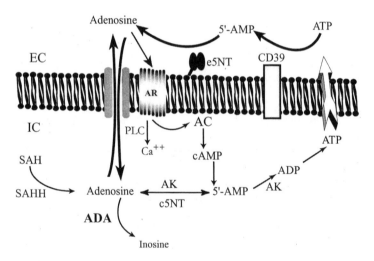

Figure 1 Pathways of adenosine production, metabolism, and transport. Extracellular (EC) adenosine can be generated from the dephosphorylation of 5′AMP by the enzyme ecto-5′-nucleotidase (e5NT). 5′AMP is generated from the dephosphorylation of ADP/ATP by the enzyme NTPDase 1 (CD39). Extracellular adenosine can bind adenosine receptors (AR) that are coupled to effector systems such as adenylate cyclase (AC) and phospholipase C (PLC). These in turn regulate intracellular cAMP and Ca^{2+}, respectively, and can influence cellular physiology in several ways. Extracellular adenosine can also be transported in and out of the cell by facilitated nucleoside transporters. Intracellular (IC) adenosine is can be generated from the dephosphorylation of 5′-AMP by a cytosolic for of 5′-nucleotidase (c5NT) or by the hydrolysis of SAH (S-adenosylhomocysteine) by SAHH (S-adenosylhomecysteine hydrolase). Intracellular adenosine can be phosphorylated to AMP by adenosine kinase (AK) or deaminated to inosine by adenosine deaminase (ADA).

Adenosine can be formed extracellularly from adenine nucleotides released from many cell types by mechanisms that are not yet clearly understood (6). The breakdown of adenine nucleotides by a family of ecto-ATP/ADPases, including CD39 (NTPDase 1), and ecto-5′ nucleotidases, including CD73 (AMPase) (7), can subsequently generate large amounts of adenosine at the cell surface (Fig. 1). Inflammatory cells that have been shown to release nucleotides include neutrophils (8) and eosinophils (9) and likely mast cells. In addition, airway epithelial cells release ATP (10) and possess the ectoenzymes for its conversion to adenosine (10). Hence, there is evidence to suggest that adenosine can be generated in the inflamed lung, but experimental evidence confirming the mechanisms involved is lacking.

Once generated, extracellular adenosine can influence a diverse array of cellular functions by engaging cell surface adenosine receptors (11). Adenosine receptors are seven transmembrane spanning receptors that couple to effector systems through heterotrimeric G-proteins (Fig. 1) (11). Mammals possess four adenosine receptors, termed A_1, A_{2A}, A_{2B}, and A_3 adenosine receptors (12). Each receptor has a unique affinity for adenosine and adenosine receptor analogs, and they have distinct cellular and tissue distributions that can vary among species. Most evidence suggests that the A_1 and A_3 adenosine receptors are coupled to adenylate cyclase by inhibitory G-proteins (α_i), and hence serve to lower the intracellular levels of the second messenger cAMP (13,14). The A_{2A} and A_{2B} adenosine receptors are commonly coupled to adenylate cyclase by the stimulatory G-protein (α_s) and serve to increase intracellular cAMP (13,14). Although most studies demonstrate coupling of the adenosine receptors to adenylate cyclase, evidence exists to suggest that these receptors couple to other effector molecules such as phospholipase C (Fig. 1) (11,14). Therefore, signaling through adenosine receptors plays important roles in the regulation of both intracellular cAMP and Ca^{2+} and can hence influence cellular physiology in a number of ways. The expression of these receptors is widely distributed among tissues, and this signaling pathway has been implicated to exert important physiological effects in the cardiovascular (15), neurological (16), renal (17), and immune systems (18), as well as on aspects of inflammation and tissue damage (19).

III. Adenosine Signaling in Asthma

Asthma is an inflammatory disease that is typified by the infiltration of immune cells into the lung followed by structural changes to the airways that lead to the loss of airway function (20). Adenosine has been implicated to play a role in asthma and other inflammatory lung diseases such as COPD (1). Clinical evidence linking this signaling pathway to asthma includes the observation that lavage fluid collected form asthmatics contains elevated adenosine concentrations (21), asthmatics and individuals with COPD show increased sensitivity to airway challenges with adenosine or its precursor AMP (22,24), and, dipyridamole, a drug that increases extracellular adenosine by blocking adenosine transport, can induce bronchoconstriction in asthmatics (25). In addition, the expression of adenosine receptors is altered in the lungs of individuals suffering from lung inflammation (26), and the nonselective adenosine receptor antagonist theophylline has been shown to have clinical benefit in the treatment of this disease (27,28). These clinical observations not only ascribe a functional role for adenosine signaling in asthma, but have also led to the use of adenosine as a diagnostic tool for this disease.

The underlying mechanism of the acute bronchoconstrictor response to adenosine in asthmatics is reasonably well understood (29). Most studies agree that mast cell activation is central to the asthmatic's response to adenosine. Evidence to support this includes the ability of adenosine- or AMP-induced bronchoconstriction to be inhibited by mast cell stabilizers (30). In addition, adenosine- or AMP-induced bronchoconstriction is attenuated by treatment with receptor antagonists to mediators released from mast cells such as histamine (30) and leukotrienes (31). There is evidence that the A_{2B} adenosine receptor on human mast cells plays an important role in mediating the release of mediators that play a role in acute bronchoconstriction as well as in the release of cytokines (32–34) that may be involved in the more chronic inflammation seen in asthma. These data suggest that adenosine-mediated mast cell activation plays an important role in asthma, but it is less clear why asthmatics exhibit such a heightened response to adenosine. In addition, the effects of adenosine on other cell types that are known to play important roles in asthma have not been adequately examined in asthmatics.

Additional information into possible mechanisms of adenosine-induced bronchoconstriction has come from experimental models of asthma in species such as guinea pigs, rabbits, and rats (reviewed in Ref. 35). Although adenosine has demonstrated effects on bronchoconstriction in most experimental models of asthma, the dependence on mast cell degranulation and the specific receptors involved can vary greatly among models. In most models, occupation of the A_{2A} receptor does not cause bronchospasm (36), and some models have actually suggested A_{2A} receptor–mediated bronchial relaxation (37–39). In conscious guinea pigs sensitized with ovalbumin, adenosine induces a potent bronchoconstrictor response (40), which is not enhanced following ovalbumin challenge. These effects were not inhibited by A_1 antagonists and were mimicked by A_3 agonists, suggesting the A_3 adenosine receptor plays an important role in this model (41). In contrast, adenosine-induced bronchoconstriction in nonsensitized guinea pigs indicate mediation by A_1 receptors (38,39). Adenosine-mediated bronchospasm studies in the allergic rabbit model typify A_1 receptor–mediated effects that are likely a result of direct effects on smooth muscle cells (42–44). The interactions of adenosine with the rat airway in vivo is markedly strain dependent. Brown Norway (BN) and Fisher 344 strains are poorly responsive to adenosine receptor agonists (45). However, BN rats can be sensitized to antigen and also manifest early and late bronchoconstrictor responses to allergen challenge with specific adenosine receptor engagement (46–48). These studies suggest that the response in BN rats occurs against a background of mild pulmonary inflammation, is a consequence of A_{2B} receptor activation, is mast cell dependent, and can be blocked selectively by theophylline. In contrast, BDE rats show reactivity to adenosine agonists in the absence of allergen sensitization as evidenced by bronchoconstriction and spontaneous eosinophilic inflammation (36,45,49). In this model, A_3 receptor activation was associated with mast cell degranulation and release of histamine and 5-HT into the plasma, while the A_1-receptor-mediated component was capable of inducing bronchoconstriction independent of mast cell activation (36). When considering these findings, it appears that the BN rat model exhibits features of adenosine-induced bronchoconstriction that are most consistent with those seen in humans. This model will likely prove useful in the analysis of specific mechanisms involved in adenosine-induced bronchoconstriction and examining the efficacy of adenosine-based therapeutics on this process.

IV. The Role of Adenosine Receptors on Inflammatory Cells

As mentioned above, the mast cell is an inflammatory cell that plays a key role in asthmatic and allergic states. These cells release mediators that have both immediate and chronic effects on airway constriction and inflammation (50). Upon stimulation, mast cells rapidly release preformed mediators such as histamine and tryptase, which are stored inside secretory granules. Lipid mediators and a variety of cytokines are produced and secreted over a more prolonged period. Increasing evidence suggests that adenosine can modulate mast cell degranulation (51). Adenosine, and adenosine analogs in vitro, have been shown to enhance mediator release from mast cells in response to challenge with a variety of stimuli (52–57). While adenosine alone seems to have no effect on mediator release from mast cells in the absence of antigen stimulation in vitro (52,58), a number of studies suggest that adenosine can initiate mast cell degranulation in the absence of additional stimuli in vivo (46,59–61).

Human mast cells have been found to express the A_{2A} and A_{2B} adenosine receptors (62). Stimulation of A_{2B} receptors activate human mast cells and promote IL-8 secretion (34), and there is accumulating evidence that A_{2B} is the predominant receptor that mediates adenosine-induced bronchoconstriction in man (32,34). The A_{2B} receptor appears to promote and A_{2A} receptor inhibits mast cell degranulation. At high adenosine concentrations the mast cell is activated because the low-affinity A_{2B} receptor is occupied, but at low concentrations only the off-signal provided by occupation of the higher A_{2A} receptor predominates. In view of this, the blockade of adenosine-induced bronchoconstriction by theophylline (28) or enprophylline (32) supports the role of the A_{2B} receptor since it is the only relevant purinoceptor blocked at therapeutic blood concentrations of these drugs (2).

Whereas human mast cells appear to only express the A_{2A} and A_{2B} adenosine receptors, rodent mast cells express A_{2A}, A_{2B}, and A_3 adenosine receptors (57,61,63,64). Despite these apparent species differences, the mouse has provided the opportunity to examine the role of adenosine signaling in mast cell degranulation on backgrounds where these receptors have been genetically deleted. Recent studies using genetically modified mice have begun to shed light on the role of the A_3 adenosine receptor in murine mast cells (64). Tilley et al. (61) demonstrated that adenosine, as well as its metabolite inosine, was able to activate cutaneous mast cells and in turn increase vasopermeability. These effects were not seen in mice deficient in the A_3 adenosine receptor, nor were bone marrow–derived mast cells from A_3-deficient mice able to respond to adenosine even in the presence of antigen (64). These studies suggest that the A_3 adenosine receptor is the sole receptor responsible for adenosine-mediated mast cell degranulation in murine bone marrow–derived mast cells and cutaneous mast cells. However, the role of the A_3 adenosine receptor in murine lung mast cell degranulation has not been examined.

In summary, the mechanisms through which adenosine mediates mast cell degranulation are not completely understood. Variabilities in adenosine-mediated mast cell degranulation may be due to differences in receptor expression in various cells, the tissue source of mast cells, species differences, and whether mast cells are primed immunologically prior to degranulation measurements. Most studies suggest that the A_{2B} and A_3 adenosine receptors are predominantly involved in mediating adenosine's effects on mast cells (34,57,65,66), but experimental evidence in animal models and humans is needed to clarify these issues.

Like mast cells, eosinophils have emerged as a major inflammatory cell type in asthma, and increases in eosinophils are often observed in the lungs of asthmatics (67). These cells can release mediators that contribute to the airway damage often associated with asthma, such as bronchial epithelial cell damage and the stimulation of mucus production (68,69). The involvement of adenosine signaling in eosinophil biology has been demonstrated via the anti-inflammatory actions of theophylline in the management of asthma (70–73). The A_3 adenosine receptor has been shown to be expressed on human eosinophils that accumulate in the lung (26). Furthermore, engagement of this receptor on eosinophils is thought to mediate the release of Ca^{2+} from intracellular stores (74) and can inhibit eosinophil degranulation (75,76) and chemotaxis (26,77). A_3 receptor activation also induces apoptosis of eosinophils (74) and may play an important role in the resolution of eosinophilic lung inflammation. These studies indicate A_3 receptor activation as a possible mechanism of anti-inflammatory action of theophylline in vivo and specific A_3 receptor ligands may be useful in the treatment of asthma. However, additional knowledge about the specific role of A_3 receptor engagement within the context of an inflamed lung is needed before such adenosine-based therapeutics can be pursued.

Macrophages constitute another cell population that may be involved at numerous steps in the pathogenesis of asthma by their ability to secrete mediators that enhance inflammatory cell proliferation and survival (78). Adenosine has been known to modulate different functional activities in macrophages. Murine bone marrow–derived macrophages express A_{2B} and A_3 receptor subtypes (79,80), and macrophage A_{2B} receptor expression is upregulated by IFN-γ (79). The engagement of adenosine receptors on macrophages elicits both pro- and anti-inflammatory events including the inhibition of tumor necrosis factor-α expression (80,81) and nitric oxide production (81), increased production of IL-10 (81), increased differentiation of monocytes into macrophages (82–84), and the promotion of multinucleated giant cells (85). The A_3 receptor has been implicated in the inhibition of TNF-α release from human monocytes by LPS (80,86) and from murine macrophage cell lines (87), while A_{2A} receptor activation has been implicated in the in vivo inhibition of TNF-α production in BALB/c mice (81). These studies demonstrate that adenosine can elicit both pro- and anti-inflammatory influences on macrophages. The exact action of adenosine is likely dictated by the state of macrophage activation, the immunological environment in which the macrophage is found, and the concentration of adenosine present. Further investigation into the influence of adenosine signaling on macrophages is warranted by the observation that adenosine levels are elevated in the lungs of asthmatics where these cells likely carry out important functions.

V. The Use of Genetically Modified Mice to Study the Role of Adenosine in Lung Inflammation

A. Importance of Genetically Modified Mice in the Study of Lung Disease

In addition to actions on mast cells, eosinophils, and macrophages, adenosine impacts other cellular processes that contribute to the asthmatic phenotype. These include neuronal signaling (88), smooth muscle contractility (43), and mucus production and/or secretion from airway epithelial cells (89). Significant information can be gathered from examining the influence of adenosine on these processes in vitro. However, a comprehensive understanding of how adenosine influences lung inflammation and damage will only emerge from studies in the whole animal where the complex cellular interactions that dictate lung inflammation and damage are intact. Advances in mouse molecular genetics have provided the opportunity to examine the role of specific gene products in the whole animal. Numerous studies have examined gene products hypothesized to play important roles in asthma by either deleting or over expressing these genes in mice. These include components of numerous cytokine (90,91), chemokine (92), and growth factor (93) signaling pathways. Results from these studies have yielded valuable information as to how these signaling molecules contribute to lung disease. There are numerous approaches one could consider to examine the role of adenosine signaling in lung disease using genetically modified mice, including the targeted deletion or overexpression of the enzymes involved in adenosine metabolism or the adenosine receptors. Mice with targeted deletions in the A_{2A} (94), A_1 (95), and A_3 (64) adenosine receptors have been made and characterized. Deletion of these receptors does not result in any apparent lung phenotype. As mentioned above, A_3-deficient mice have been used to demonstrate the importance of A_3 receptor signaling in mast cell degranulation (61,64). However, studies are still underway to examine the impact of these receptor deficiencies in experimental models of asthma.

A caveat to examining phenotypes in adenosine receptor–deficient mice is the potential for compensating redundancies among the various receptors. Our laboratory has taken an alternative approach to examine the role of adenosine signaling in lung inflammation and damage in the mouse. We generated mice deficient in the purine catabolic enzyme adenosine deaminase (ADA), which catalyzes the deamination of adenosine and 2′-deoxyadenosine to inosine and 2′-deoxyinosine (96). ADA is responsible for controlling the levels of these substrates in tissues and cells, and it was hypothesized that deletion of this enzyme would result in pronounced elevations in adenosine and 2′-deoxyadenosine. It was rationalized that such animals may in turn serve as useful models for studying diseases in which elevations of these substrates is thought to play a role, such as asthma and immunodeficiencies. Deletion of ADA led to pronounced accumulations of adenosine in many tissues including the lung (96). The ADA-deficient mice developed a combined immunodeficiency that appeared to result from the metabolic consequences associated with the accumulation of 2'-deoxyadenosine (96,97). In addition, ADA-deficient mice developed a severe pulmonary phenotype that included defects in alveogenesis and severe lung inflammation and damage that resembled that seen in an asthmatic lung (98). The lung damage in these animals was severe and led to death by 3 weeks of age. Adenosine accumulated to high levels in the lungs of these mice, and many of the phenotypes observed could be attributed to elevations in lung adenosine in that lowering lung adenosine using ADA enzyme therapy either prevented or reversed many of these phenotypes (98,99). Below is a description of the findings in these animals that suggest that adenosine signaling may play an important role in regulating lung inflammation and damage.

B. Pulmonary Phenotypes in ADA-Deficient Mice

Abnormal Lung Development in ADA-Deficient Mice

ADA-deficient newborn mice were visually undistinguishable from ADA-positive control littermates. However, between 10 and 12 days of postnatal life, ADA-deficient mice began to show signs of respiratory distress characterized by rapid breathing and failure to thrive. This respiratory distress was progressive, and the mice died by 3 weeks of age (96). At birth, ADA-deficient lungs were normal, but by postnatal day 5 there was an increase in alveolar airway size. Secondary septation of the alveoli occurs between days 5 and 10 in normal mice; however, alveolar size remained enlarged in ADA-deficient lungs at day 10, suggesting that there was a defect in secondary septation. Adenosine concentrations in the lungs of ADA-deficient mice were normal at birth but were significantly elevated at days 5 and 10 (100), suggesting that elevated adenosine and perhaps abnormal adenosine signaling likely contributed to the abnormal alveogenesis seen. This hypothesis was supported by the observation that treatment of ADA-deficient mice with ADA enzyme therapy from birth to prevent adenosine accumulation resulted in normal secondary septation in the lungs of these animals (99). Nothing is known concerning the expression of adenosine receptors during lung development, and examining the expression of adenosine receptors in normal and ADA-deficient lungs will help clarify the role of adenosine signaling during normal and abnormal lung development.

Adenosine-Dependent Changes in Lung Inflammation and Damage in ADA-Deficient Mice

As mentioned earlier, elevated adenosine levels are found in the lungs of asthmatics (21), and adenosine has been implicated to play a role in the regulation of inflammatory cell types that are central to this disease (1). The status of inflammatory cells was examined in the lungs of ADA-deficient mice to determine if there were similarities between these animals and asthmatics (98). Beginning around postnatal day 15, there was a diffuse increase in activated alveolar macrophages in the alveolar spaces and a pronounced infiltration of eosinophils throughout the lungs. In addition to this severe lung inflammation, the bronchial epithelium in ADA-deficient lungs exhibited a progressive increase in mucus production and an accumulation of mucus and cellular debris in the bronchial airways (98). Hence, ADA-deficient mice develop lung inflammation and damage similar to that seen in the asthmatic lung.

Adenosine levels were greatly elevated in lungs of ADA-deficient mice (98), suggesting that the severe inflammation and mucus metaplasia seen may be a result of perturbations in adenosine signaling. Again, the use of ADA enzyme therapy was able to provide information into the dependence of these cellular changes on elevations in lung adenosine concentrations. A single treatment of ADA-deficient mice with ADA enzyme replacement therapy was able to reverse the lung eosinophilia and mucus metaplasia within 72 hours in association with lowering lung adenosine levels (98). These striking findings demonstrated that merely elevating lung adenosine levels could cause severe lung inflammation and damage that is reminiscent of that seen in asthmatics. The cellular targets and adenosine receptors involved in these processes have yet to be determined, but this model will provide a unique opportunity to examine the influence of endogenously elevated adenosine on cellular processes involved in lung inflammation and damage.

Evidence for Mast Cell Degranulation in ADA-Deficient Lungs

Mast cells release mediators that influence lung inflammation (50). ADA-deficient mice show extensive lung mast cell degranulation in association with elevated adenosine levels (100). Mast cell degranulation was evident at postnatal day 5, and mast cells were completely degranulated by day 10. Interestingly, lung inflammation is not detected in the lungs of ADA-deficient mice until day 15 (98), suggesting that the mast cell degranulation seen was not secondary to adenosine's effects on other inflammatory cells, but rather associated with precipitous increases in lung adenosine levels. This was supported further by the observation that ADA enzyme therapy prevented the accumulation of lung adenosine as well as mast cell degranulation (100). Moreover, treatment of ADA-deficient mice with broad-based adenosine receptor antagonists prevented 30–40% of the mast cell degranulation seen, suggesting the involvement of adenosine receptor signaling (100). These studies demonstrated the ability of endogenously generated adenosine to influence lung mast cell degranulation in a receptor-mediated manner and established ADA-deficient mice as a model system to investigate the specific adenosine receptor responses involved in the degranulation of lung mast cells. The relative contribution of A_3 and A_{2B} in lung mast cell degranulation in ADA-deficient mice is still not clear. Determining which of these receptors are expressed specifically on lung mast cells and associating mast cell degranulation with the levels of adenosine that accumulate in the lungs of humans and mice will be important for understanding this issue.

Gene Expression in ADA-Deficient Lungs

Comparing the expression patterns of several thousand genes in both normal and ADA-deficient mice has considerably enhanced the ability to identify and characterize biological roles for adenosine-regulated genes in mediating pulmonary insufficiency. Mouse cDNA expression arrays were used for high throughput monitoring of gene expression in normal and ADA-deficient lungs. This study allowed us to distinguish genes involved in several biological pathways in the lung and also identify genes that may be regulated by adenosine (101). Changes in gene expression were highly reproducible and represented changes in the expression of a variety of molecular markers, including transcription factors, cell surface antigens, cell cycle regulators, cell adhesion receptors, etc. These findings demonstrated that gene expression patterns in ADA-deficient lungs, which have characteristically elevated adenosine levels, differ from expression patterns in normal lungs.

Lowering adenosine levels using ADA enzyme therapy has striking effects on gene expression that may be associated with resolution of pulmonary eosinophilia (101). Monocyte chemotactic protein (MCP-3), CD32, urokinase plasminogen activator (UPA), osteopontin, VEGF, and P selectin are known genes that can mediate eosinophil trafficking (102–105). The expressions of these genes were elevated in ADA-deficient lungs, and ADA enzyme therapy decreased their expression in conjunction with decreased lung eosinophilia. The expression of several airway-relevant cysteine proteases (cathepsins A, B, D, H, and L) and antiproteases (cystatins) was also affected by ADA enzyme therapy, suggesting that regulating adenosine levels may also help regulate the expression of these genes that have been implicated to play a critical role in maintaining alveolar morphology. Thus, microarray analysis has identified many genes that may be involved in mediating adenosine-related changes in inflamed ADA-deficient lungs. Such primary findings provide important clues to the communications among genes and contribute to exploration of potential target genes for possible molecular diagnosis and therapy.

Airway Hyperresponsiveness in Partially ADA-Deficient Mice

We have recently characterized the impact of endogenously elevated lung adenosine on airway inflammation and physiology in a mouse model of partial ADA deficiency (106). *Partially* ADA-deficient mice were generated by the ectopic expression of an ADA minigene in the gastrointestinal tract of otherwise ADA-deficient mice. These mice do not exhibit the defects in alveogenesis seen in the *completely* ADA-deficient mice described above. *Partially* ADA-deficient mice developed lung inflammation and damage, but at a much later stage than that seen in *completely* ADA-deficient mice (98), and died from respiratory distress at 4–5 months of age instead of 3 weeks of age. Examination of airway physiology at 6 weeks of age revealed an increase in airway responsiveness in association with elevated lung adenosine (106). This airway hyperresponsiveness was reversed following the lowering of lung adenosine levels using ADA enzyme therapy, suggesting a dependence of this feature on elevated adenosine. Furthermore, treatment with the broad-spectrum adenosine receptor antagonist theophylline prevented airway hyperresponsiveness (106), implicating the involvement of adenosine receptors. Whether the effect of receptor engagement in this model is a direct effect on airway smooth muscle or a secondary effect due to activation of other mediator cells (mast cells, nerves, airway epithelium, macrophages) could not be determined from these studies. However, this model will prove useful in deciphering the effects of endogenously elevated adenosine on airway physiology.

VI. Proposed Model for Adenosine Signaling in the Inflamed Lung

Adenosine is a ubiquitous signaling molecule in that most cells in the body generate adenosine and possess adenosine receptors. The challenge in understanding this signaling pathway in health and disease comes from our relative lack of knowledge about the factors that govern the regulation of this signaling pathway and dictate whether it serves to maintain homeostasis, protect tissues from injury, or trigger the promotion of inflammation or tissue damage. In the case of lung inflammation and damage, such as is seen in asthma and COPD, adenosine likely serves both pro- and anti-inflammatory roles that may be dictated by the levels of adenosine found in the lung. A working model addressing this issue is shown in Figure 2. Sensitization and challenge with any number of allergens is known to lead to a Th2-mediated immunological response that can set up the underlying inflammation and airway damage seen in the asthmatic lung. The resultant inflammation and associated hypoxia may then lead to the release of ATP and the local generation of adenosine in

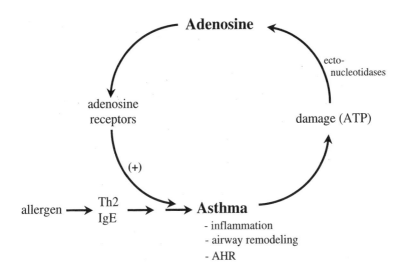

Figure 2 Model of adenosine potentiation of lung inflammation and damage. Inflammation and hypoxia that occurs in the asthmatic lung can result in the release of ATP, which is converted to adenosine by ecto-nucleotidases. Elevations in extracellular adenosine can lead to increased signaling through adenosine receptors that may potentiate the inflammation and damage seen in the asthmatic lung.

the lung. The accumulation of adenosine may then access signaling pathways by engaging specific adenosine receptors on various cell types found in the inflamed lung. As seen in this review, adenosine can influence a number of different cellular processes that are found in the asthmatic lung. It is therefore likely that enhanced signaling resulting from elevated adenosine levels can perpetuate or potentiate inflammation and damage in the asthmatic lung. Evidence to support this hypothesis comes from our work in ADA-deficient mice that shows that chronically elevating adenosine, in the absence of antigen exposure, can lead to lung inflammation and damage. Furthermore, lowering the levels of adenosine in the lung using ADA enzyme therapy is able to reverse certain aspects of lung inflammation and damage. Examination of the specific adenosine receptors involved in these processes must be elucidated to help define the mechanisms involved. In addition, examination of this signaling pathway in other experimental models of asthma, and in the asthmatic lung, is needed so that the full potential of adenosine-based therapeutics can be determined. Finally, if the hypothesis that enhanced adenosine generation and signaling perpetuates lung inflammation and damage holds true, it is likely that this signaling pathway also plays an important role in more chronic forms of lung disease such as pulmonary fibrosis, cystic fibrosis, emphysema, and acute respiratory distress syndrome.

VII. Adenosine-Based Therapeutics

There is an outstanding literature base to suggest that adenosine serves a role in the regulation of inflammatory lung diseases such as asthma and COPD. As the specific expression patterns for the various adenosine receptors are elucidated and their functions determined, they will represent excellent targets for drug development and the treatment of adenosine-dependent features in the asthmatic lung. Given that there are likely species differences in receptor usage, care must be taken in developing receptor agonists and antagonists that are selective for the human forms of these receptors. Another potential approach towards adenosine-based therapeutics for lung disease has arisen from our work in ADA-deficient mice. In this animal model, ADA enzyme therapy can effectively remove adenosine that accumulates in the lungs of these mice, and doing so leads to the reversal of key features of experimental asthma including mast cell degranulation (100), lung eosinophilia (98), mucus metaplasia (98), airway hyperresponsiveness (106), and the expression of proinflammatory molecules (101). Given that adenosine levels are elevated in the lungs of asthmatics, it stands to reason that there may be therapeutic benefit to lowering lung adenosine levels in these patients using ADA enzyme therapy. This may represent a novel and important means of regulating the degree of inflammation and damage seen in asthma. Before such treatments can be considered, experiments must be conducted to examine the efficacy of ADA enzyme therapy in established animal models of asthma.

References

1. Jacobson MA, Bai TR. The role of adenosine in asthma. In: Jacobson KA, Jarvis MF, eds. Purinergic Approaches in Experimental Therapeutics. Danvers, MA: Wiley-Liss, Inc., 1997:315–331.

2. Fozard JR, Hannon JP. Adenosine receptor ligands: potential as therapeutic agents in asthma and COPD. Pulm Pharmacol Ther 1999; 12:111–114.

3. Arch JR, Newsholme EA. The control of the metabolism and the hormonal role of adenosine. Essays Biochem 1978; 14:82–123.

4. Trams EG, Lauter CJ. On the sidedness of plasma membrane enzymes. Biochim Biophys Acta 1974; 345:180–197.

5. Marquardt DL, Gruber HE, Wasserman SI. Adenosine release from stimulated mast cells. Proc Natl Acad Sci USA 1984; 81:6192–6196.

6. Harden TK, Lazarowski ER. Release of ATP and UTP from astrocytoma cells. Prog Brain Res 1999; 120:135–143.

7. Zimmermann H. Extracellular metabolism of ATP and other nucleotides. Naunyn Schmiedebergs Arch Pharmacol 2000; 362:299–309.

8. Madara JL, Patapoff TW, Gillece-Castro B, et al. 5′-Adenosine monophosphate is the neutrophil-derived paracrine factor that elicits chloride secretion from T84 intestinal epithelial cell monolayers. J Clin Invest 1993; 91:2320–2325.

9. Resnick MB, Colgan SP, Patapoff TW, et al. Activated eosinophils evoke chloride secretion in model intestinal epithelia primarily via regulated release of 5′-AMP. J Immunol 1993; 151:5716–5723.

10. Donaldson SH, Lazarowski ER, Picher M, Knowles MR, Stutts MJ, Boucher RC. Basal nucleotide levels, release, and metabolism in normal and cystic fibrosis airways. Mol Med 2000; 6:969–982.

11. Olah ME, Stiles GL. Adenosine receptor subtypes: characterization and therapeutic regulation. Annu Rev Pharmacol Toxicol 1995; 35:581–606.

12. Ralevic V, Burnstock G. Receptors for purines and pyrimidines. Pharmacol Rev 1998; 50:413–492.

13. Londos C, Cooper DM, Wolff J. Subclasses of external adenosine receptors. Proc Natl Acad Sci USA 1980; 77:2551–2554.

14. Stiles G. Adenosine receptor subtypes: new insights from cloning and functional studies. In: Jacobson KA, Jarvis MF, eds. Purinergic Approaches in Experimental Therapeutics. New York: Wiley-Liss, Inc., 1997:29–37.

15. Belardinelli L, Linden J, Berne RM. The cardiac effects of adenosine. Prog Cardiovasc Dis 1989; 32:73–97.

16. Fredholm BB, Dunwiddie TV. How does adenosine inhibit transmitter release? Trends Pharmacol Sci 1988; 9:130–134.

17. Churchill PC. Renal effects of 2-chloroadenosine and their antagonism by aminophylline in anesthetized rats. J Pharmacol Exp Ther 1982; 222:319–323.

18. Huang S, Apasov S, Koshiba M, Sitkovsky M. Role of A2a extracellular adenosine receptor-mediated signaling in adenosine-mediated inhibition of T-cell activation and expansion. Blood 1997; 90:1600–1610.

19. Cronstein BN. Adenosine regulation of neutrophil function and inhibition of inflammation via adenosine receptors. In: Jacobson KA, Jarvis MF, eds. Purinergic approaches in experimental therapeutics. New York: Wiley-Liss, 1997:285–299.

20. Elias JA, Zhu Z, Chupp G, Homer RJ. Airway remodeling in asthma. J Clin Invest 1999; 104:1001–1006.

21. Driver AG, Kukoly CA, Ali S, Mustafa SJ. Adenosine in bronchoalveolar lavage fluid in asthma. Am Rev Respir Dis 1993; 148:91–97.

22. Cushley MJ, Tattersfield AE, Holgate ST. Inhaled adenosine and guanosine on airway resistance in normal and asthmatic subjects. Br J Clin Pharmacol 1983; 15:161–165.

23. Mann JS, Holgate ST, Renwick AG, Cushley MJ. Airway effects of purine nucleosides and nucleotides and release with bronchial provocation in asthma. J Appl Physiol 1986; 61:1667–1676.

24. Oosterhoff Y, de Jong JW, Jansen MA, Koeter GH, Postma DS. Airway responsiveness to adenosine 5′-monophosphate in chronic obstructive pulmonary disease is determined by smoking. Am Rev Respir Dis 1993; 147:553–558.

25. Eagle KA, Boucher CA. Intravenous dipyridamole infusion causes severe bronchospasm in asthmatic patients. Chest 1989; 95:258–259.

26. Walker BA, Jacobson MA, Knight DA, et al. Adenosine A_3 receptor expression and function in eosinophils. Am J Respir Cell Mol Biol 1997; 16:531–537.

27. Mann JS, Cushley MJ, Holgate ST. Adenosine-induced bronchoconstriction in asthma. Role of parasympathetic stimulation and adrenergic inhibition. Am Rev Respir Dis 1985; 132:1–6.

28. Cushley MJ, Tattersfield AE, Holgate ST. Adenosine-induced bronchoconstriction in asthma. Antagonism by inhaled theophylline. Am Rev Respir Dis 1984; 129:380–384.

29. Meade CJ, Dumont I, Worrall L. Why do asthmatic subjects respond so strongly to inhaled adenosine? Life Sci 2001; 69:1225–1240.

30. Phillips GD, Polosa R, Holgate ST. The effect of histamine-H1 receptor antagonism with terfenadine on concentration-related AMP-induced bronchoconstriction in asthma. Clin Exp Allergy 1989; 19:405–409.

31. Van Schoor J, Joos GF, Kips JC, Drajesk JF, Carpentier PJ, Pauwels RA. The effect of ABT-761, a novel 5-lipoxygenase inhibitor, on exercise- and adenosine-induced bronchoconstriction in asthmatic subjects. Am J Respir Crit Care Med 1997; 155: 875–880.

32. Linden J, Thai T, Figler H, Jin X, Robeva AS. Characterization of human A(2B) adenosine receptors: radioligand binding, Western blotting, and coupling to G(q) in human embryonic kidney 293 cells and HMC-1 mast cells. Mol Pharmacol 1999; 56: 705–713.

33. Feoktistov I, Polosa R, Holgate ST, Biaggioni I. Adenosine A_{2B} receptors: a novel therapeutic target in asthma? Trends Pharmacol Sci 1998; 19:148–153.

34. Feoktistov I, Biaggioni I. Adenosine A_{2b} receptors evoke interleukin-8 secretion in human mast cells. An enprofylline-sensitive mechanism with implications for asthma. J Clin Invest 1995; 96:1979–1986.

35. Fozard JR, Hannon JP. Species differences in adenosine receptor-mediated bronchoconstrictor responses. Clin Exp Allergy 2000; 30:1213–1220.

36. Meade CJ, Mierau J, Leon I, Ensinger HA. In vivo role of the adenosine A_3 receptor: N6-2-(4- aminophenyl)ethyladenosine induces bronchospasm in BDE rats by a neurally mediated mechanism involving cells resembling mast cells. J Pharmacol Exp Ther 1996; 279:1148–1156.

37. Ali S, Metzger WJ, Olanrewaju HA, Mustafa SJ. Adenosine receptor-mediated relaxation of rabbit airway smooth muscle: a role for nitric oxide. Am J Physiol 1997; 273: L581–587.

38. Farmer SG, Canning BJ, Wilkins DE. Adenosine receptor-mediated contraction and relaxation of guinea-pig isolated tracheal smooth muscle: effects of adenosine antagonists. Br J Pharmacol 1988; 95:371–378.

39. Ghai G, Zimmerman MB, Hopkins MF. Evidence for A_1 and A_2 adenosine receptors in guinea pig trachea. Life Sci 1987; 41:1215–1224.

40. Thorne JR, Broadley KJ. Adenosine-induced bronchoconstriction in conscious hyperresponsive and sensitized guinea pigs. Am J Respir Crit Care Med 1994; 149:392–399.

41. Thorne JR, Danahay H, Broadley KJ. Analysis of the bronchoconstrictor responses to adenosine receptor agonists in sensitized guinea-pig lungs and trachea. Eur J Pharmacol 1996; 316:263–271.

42. Ali S, Mustafa SJ, Metzger WJ. Adenosine receptor-mediated bronchoconstriction and bronchial hyperresponsiveness in allergic rabbit model. Am J Physiol 1994; 266: L271–277.

43. Ali S, Mustafa SJ, Metzger WJ. Adenosine-induced bronchoconstriction and contraction of airway smooth muscle from allergic rabbits with late-phase airway obstruction: evidence for an inducible adenosine A1 receptor. J Pharmacol Exp Ther 1994; 268: 1328–1334.

44. Nyce JW, Metzger WJ. DNA antisense therapy for asthma in an animal model. Nature 1997; 385:721–725.

45. Pauwels RA, Van der Straeten ME. An animal model for adenosine-induced bronchoconstriction. Am Rev Respir Dis 1987; 136:374–378.

46. Tigani B, Hannon JP, Mazzoni L, Fozard JR. Effects of wortmannin on bronchoconstrictor responses to adenosine in actively sensitised brown norway rats. Eur J Pharmacol 2000; 406:469–476.

47. Hannon JP, Tigani B, Williams I, Mazzoni L, Fozard JR. Mechanism of airway hyperresponsiveness to adenosine induced by allergen challenge in actively sensitized Brown Norway rats. Br J Pharmacol 2001; 132:1509–1523.

48. Elwood W, Lotvall JO, Barnes PJ, Chung KF. Characterization of allergen-induced bronchial hyperresponsiveness and airway inflammation in actively sensitized brown Norway rats. J Allergy Clin Immunol 1991; 88:951–960.

49. Pauwels RA, Joos GF. Characterization of the adenosine receptors in the airways. Arch Int Pharmacodyn Ther 1995; 329:151–160.

50. Shimizu Y, Schwartz LB. Mast cell involvement in asthma. In: Barnes PJ, Leff AR, Grunstein MM, Woolcock AJ, eds. Asthma. Vol. 1. Philadelphia: Lippincott-Raven, 1997:353–365.

51. Forsythe P, Ennis M. Adenosine, mast cells and asthma. Inflamm Res 1999; 48: 301–307.

52. Marquardt DL, Parker CW, Sullivan TJ. Potentiation of mast cell mediator release by adenosine. J Immunol 1978; 120:871–878.

53. Church MK, Holgate ST, Hughes PJ. Adenosine inhibits and potentiates IgE-dependent histamine release from human basophils by an A2-receptor mediated mechanism. Br J Pharmacol 1983; 80:719–726.

54. Hughes PJ, Holgate ST, Church MK. Adenosine inhibits and potentiates IgE-dependent histamine release from human lung mast cells by an A2-purinoceptor mediated mechanism. Biochem Pharmacol 1984; 33:3847–3852.

55. Marquardt DL, Walker LL, Wasserman SI. Adenosine receptors on mouse bone marrow-derived mast cells: functional significance and regulation by aminophylline. J Immunol 1984; 133:932–937.

56. Peachell PT, Lichtenstein LM, Schleimer RP. Differential regulation of human basophil and lung mast cell function by adenosine. J Pharmacol Exp Ther 1991; 256:717–726.

57. Ramkumar V, Stiles GL, Beaven MA, Ali H. The A_3 adenosine receptor is the unique adenosine receptor which facilitates release of allergic mediators in mast cells. J Biol Chem 1993; 268:16887–16890.

58. Marquardt DL, Gruber HE, Wasserman SI. Adenosine release from stimulated mast cells. Proc Natl Acad Sci USA 1984; 81:6192–6196.
59. Doyle MP, Linden J, Duling BR. Nucleoside-induced arteriolar constriction: a mast cell-dependent response. Am J Physiol 1994; 266:H2042–2050.
60. Hannon JP, Pfannkuche HJ, Fozard JR. A role for mast cells in adenosine A_3 receptor-mediated hypotension in the rat. Br J Pharmacol 1995; 115:945–952.
61. Tilley SL, Wagoner VA, Salvatore CA, Jacobson MA, Koller BH. Adenosine and inosine increase cutaneous vasopermeability by activating A(3) receptors on mast cells. J Clin Invest 2000; 105:361–367.
62. Feoktistov I, Biaggioni I. Pharmacological characterization of adenosine A_{2B} receptors: studies in human mast cells co-expressing A_{2A} and A_{2B} adenosine receptor subtypes. Biochem Pharmacol 1998; 55:627–633.
63. Marquardt DL, Walker LL, Heinemann S. Cloning of two adenosine receptor subtypes from mouse bone marrow-derived mast cells. J Immunol 1994; 152:4508–4515.
64. Salvatore CA, Tilley SL, Latour AM, Fletcher DS, Koller BH, Jacobson MA. Disruption of the A(3) adenosine receptor gene in mice and its effect on stimulated inflammatory cells. J Biol Chem 2000; 275:4429–4434.
65. Auchampach JA, Jin X, Wan TC, Caughey GH, Linden J. Canine mast cell adenosine receptors: cloning and expression of the A_3 receptor and evidence that degranulation is mediated by the A_{2B} receptor. Mol Pharmacol 1997; 52:846–860.
66. Gao Z, Li BS, Day YJ, Linden J. A(3) adenosine receptor activation triggers phosphorylation of protein kinase B and protects rat basophilic leukemia 2H3 mast cells from apoptosis. Mol Pharmacol 2001; 59:76–82.
67. Strek MK, Leff AR. Eosinophils. In: Barnes PJ, Leff AR, Grunstein MM, Woolcock AJ, eds. Asthma. Vol. 1. Philadelphia: Lippincott-Raven, 1997:353–365.
68. Leff AR. Inflammatory mediation of airway hyperresponsiveness by peripheral blood granulocytes. The case for the eosinophil. Chest 1994; 106:1202–1208.
69. Gleich GJ. The eosinophil and bronchial asthma: current understanding. J Allergy Clin Immunol 1990; 85:422–436.
70. Pauwels RA. New aspects of the therapeutic potential of theophylline in asthma. J Allergy Clin Immunol 1989; 83:548–553.
71. Kips JC, Peleman RA, Pauwels RA. The role of theophylline in asthma management. Curr Opin Pulm Med 1999; 5:88–92.
72. Pauwels R. The effects of theophylline on airway inflammation. Chest 1987; 92:32S–37S.
73. Barnes PJ, Pauwels RA. Theophylline in the management of asthma: time for reappraisal? Eur Respir J 1994; 7:579–591.
74. Kohno Y, Ji X, Mawhorter SD, Koshiba M, Jacobson KA. Activation of A_3 adenosine receptors on human eosinophils elevates intracellular calcium. Blood 1996; 88:3569–3574.
75. Ezeamuzie CI, Philips E. Adenosine A_3 receptors on human eosinophils mediate inhibition of degranulation and superoxide anion release. Br J Pharmacol 1999; 127:188–194.
76. Ezeamuzie CI. Involvement of A(3) receptors in the potentiation by adenosine of the inhibitory effect of theophylline on human eosinophil degranulation: possible novel mechanism of the anti-inflammatory action of theophylline. Biochem Pharmacol 2001; 61:1551–1559.
77. Knight D, Zheng X, Rocchini C, Jacobson M, Bai T, Walker B. Adenosine A_3 receptor stimulation inhibits migration of human eosinophils. J Leukoc Biol 1997; 62:465–468.

78. Toews GB. Macrophages. In: Barnes PJ, Leff AR, Grunstein MM, Woolcock AJ, eds. Asthma. Vol. 1. Philadelphia: Lippincott-Raven, 1997:381–398.
79. Xaus J, Mirabet M, Lloberas J, et al. IFN-gamma up-regulates the A_{2B} adenosine receptor expression in macrophages: a mechanism of macrophage deactivation. J Immunol 1999; 162:3607–3614.
80. Sajjadi FG, Takabayashi K, Foster AC, Domingo RC, Firestein GS. Inhibition of TNF-alpha expression by adenosine: role of A_3 adenosine receptors. J Immunol 1996; 156: 3435–3442.
81. Hasko G, Szabo C, Nemeth ZH, Kvetan V, Pastores SM, Vizi ES. Adenosine receptor agonists differentially regulate IL-10, TNF-alpha, and nitric oxide production in RAW 264.7 macrophages and in endotoxemic mice. J Immunol 1996; 157:4634–4640.
82. Eppell BA, Newell AM, Brown EJ. Adenosine receptors are expressed during differentiation of monocytes to macrophages in vitro. Implications for regulation of phagocytosis. J Immunol 1989; 143:4141–4145.
83. Najar HM, Ruhl S, Bru-Capdeville AC, Peters JH. Adenosine and its derivatives control human monocyte differentiation into highly accessory cells versus macrophages. J Leukoc Biol 1990; 47:429–439.
84. Salmon JE, Brogle N, Brownlie C, et al. Human mononuclear phagocytes express adenosine A1 receptors. A novel mechanism for differential regulation of Fc gamma receptor function. J Immunol 1993; 151:2775–2785.
85. Merrill JT, Shen C, Schreibman D, et al. Adenosine A_1 receptor promotion of multinucleated giant cell formation by human monocytes: a mechanism for methotrexate-induced nodulosis in rheumatoid arthritis. Arthritis Rheum 1997; 40:1308–1315.
86. Le Vraux V, Chen YL, Masson I, et al. Inhibition of human monocyte TNF production by adenosine receptor agonists. Life Sci 1993; 52:1917–1924.
87. Bowlin TL, Borcherding DR, Edwards CK, 3rd, McWhinney CD. Adenosine A_3 receptor agonists inhibit murine macrophage tumor necrosis factor-alpha production in vitro and in vivo. Cell Mol Biol 1997; 43:345–349.
88. Polosa R, Rajakulasingam K, Church MK, Holgate ST. Repeated inhalation of bradykinin attenuates adenosine 5′-monophosphate (AMP) induced bronchoconstriction in asthmatic airways. Eur Respir J 1992; 5:700–706.
89. Johnson HG, McNee ML. Adenosine-induced secretion in the canine trachea: modification by methylxanthines and adenosine derivatives. Br J Pharmacol 1985; 86:63–67.
90. Zhu Z, Homer RJ, Wang Z, et al. Pulmonary expression of interleukin-13 causes inflammation, mucus hypersecretion, subepithelial fibrosis, physiologic abnormalities, and eotaxin production. J Clin Invest 1999; 103:779–788.
91. McKenzie GJ, Fallon PG, Emson CL, Grencis RK, McKenzie AN. Simultaneous disruption of interleukin (IL)-4 and IL-13 defines individual roles in T helper cell type 2-mediated responses. J Exp Med 1999; 189:1565–1572.
92. Kim Y, Sung S, Kuziel WA, Feldman S, Fu SM, Rose CE, Jr. Enhanced airway Th2 response after allergen challenge in mice deficient in CC chemokine receptor-2 (CCR2). J Immunol 2001; 166:5183–5192.
93. Munger JS, Huang X, Kawakatsu H, et al. The integrin alpha v beta 6 binds and activates latent TGF beta 1: a mechanism for regulating pulmonary inflammation and fibrosis. Cell 1999; 96:319–328.
94. Ledent C, Vaugeois JM, Schiffmann SN, et al. Aggressiveness, hypoalgesia and high blood pressure in mice lacking the adenosine A_{2a} receptor. Nature 1997; 388:674–678.
95. Sun D, Samuelson LC, Yang T, et al. Mediation of tubuloglomerular feedback by adenosine: evidence from mice lacking adenosine 1 receptors. Proc Natl Acad Sci USA 2001; 98:9983–9988.

96. Blackburn MR, Datta SK, Kellems RE. Adenosine deaminase-deficient mice generated using a two-stage genetic engineering strategy exhibit a combined immunodeficiency. J Biol Chem 1998; 273:5093–5100.

97. Blackburn MR, Datta SK, Wakamiya M, Vartabedian BS, Kellems RE. Metabolic and immunologic consequences of limited adenosine deaminase expression in mice. J Biol Chem 1996; 271:15203–15210.

98. Blackburn MR, Volmer JB, Thrasher JL, et al. Metabolic consequences of adenosine deaminase deficiency in mice are associated with defects in alveogenesis, pulmonary inflammation and airway obstruction. J Exp Med 2000; 129:159–170.

99. Blackburn MR, Aldrich M, Volmer JB, et al. The use of enzyme therapy to regulate the metabolic and phenotypic consequences of adenosine deaminase deficiency in mice: differential impact on pulmonary and immunologic abnormalities. J Biol Chem 2000; 275:32114–32121.

100. Zhong H, Chunn JL, Volmer JB, Fozard JR, Blackburn MR. Adenosine-mediated mast cell degranulation in adenosine deaminase- deficient mice. J Pharmacol Exp Ther 2001; 298:433–440.

101. Banerjee S, Young H, Volmer J, Blackburn M. Gene expression profiling in inflammatory airway disease associated with elevated adenosine. Am J Physiol Lung Cell Mol Physiol 2002; in press.

102. Broide DH, Sullivan S, Gifford T, Sriramarao P. Inhibition of pulmonary eosinophilia in P-selectin- and ICAM-1-deficient mice. Am J Respir Cell Mol Biol 1998; 18:218–225.

103. Giachelli CM, Lombardi D, Johnson RJ, Murry CE, Almeida M. Evidence for a role of osteopontin in macrophage infiltration in response to pathological stimuli in vivo. Am J Pathol 1998; 152:353–358.

104. Mabilat-Pragnon C, Janin A, Michel L, et al. Urokinase localization and activity in isolated eosinophils. Thromb Res 1997; 88:373–379.

105. Ying S, Meng Q, Zeibecoglou K, et al. Eosinophil chemotactic chemokines (eotaxin, eotaxin-2, RANTES, monocyte chemoattractant protein-3 (MCP-3), and MCP-4), and C-C chemokine receptor 3 expression in bronchial biopsies from atopic and nonatopic (intrinsic) asthmatics. J Immunol 1999; 163:6321–6329.

106. Chunn JL, Young HW, Banerjee SK, Colasurdo GN, Blackburn MR. Adenosine-dependent airway inflammation and hyperresponsiveness in partially adenosine deaminase-deficient mice. J Immunol 2001; 167:4676–4685.

32

Complement Factor 5 in Asthma

MARSHA WILLS-KARP, JÖRG KÖHL, and CHRISTOPHER L. KARP

Cincinnati Children's Hospital Medical Center
Cincinnati, Ohio, U.S.A.

I. Introduction

The worldwide prevalence and severity of allergic asthma have increased dramatically in recent decades. Therapeutic advances have unfortunately not kept pace, and asthma morbidity and mortality continue to rise. The cardinal features of allergic asthma include airway hyperresponsiveness (AHR) to a variety of specific and non-specific stimuli, excessive airway mucus production, pulmonary eosinophilia, and elevated concentrations of serum immunoglobulin E (IgE). Although asthma is multifactorial in origin, it is generally accepted that it arises as a result of inappropriate immunological responses to common environmental antigens in genetically susceptible individuals (1). Specifically, a multitude of evidence suggests that CD4+ T cells producing Th2 cytokines (IL-4, IL-5, IL-13) play a pivotal role in disease pathogenesis. Although extensive research is ongoing into the processes underlying the development of deleterious immune responses to the ubiquitous, otherwise harmless, antigens that drive the expression of allergic asthma, these mechanisms remain a mystery.

Recent years have brought growing mechanistic awareness of the profound influence of the innate immune system on adaptive immune responses. The complement system, a phylogenetically ancient part of the innate immune system, is no exception. In addition to its long-recognized role as a lytic effector system that protects against microbial pathogens, it is clear that the complement system regulates adaptive immunity at many levels. First, the complement system is an important regulator of B-cell activation, providing an important mechanism for pathogen (or "danger") recognition by B lymphocytes. Second, the engagement of complement receptors on antigen-presenting cells (APC) leads to potent effects on the production of immunoregulatory cytokines such as IL-12. Third, while the anaphylatoxins (the complement activation products C3a and C5a) have long been appreciated for their effects on myeloid cell migration, activation, and effector functions, it has recently become clear these these molecules also regulate the functions of dendritic cells and activated T and B cells.

The complement system had been distinguished, until quite recently, by a relative lack of attention from those engaged in research into asthma pathogenesis. Such neglect took place despite knowledge of the fact that the anaphylatoxins can induce critical parts of the phenotype of type I hypersensitivity reactions (of presumed relevance to allergic asthma) such as smooth muscle contraction, activation of mast cells, and increased vascular permeability. Recent awareness of the key immunoregulatory role of complement in other infectious and inflammatory disease models has fueled new interest in the role of complement in asthma and allergic disease. In this chapter we will discuss our current understanding of the role of complement in the pathogenesis of allergic asthma and highlight the potential of targeting complement pathways for therapeutic drug development.

II. Complement Activation Pathways

The complement system is made up of more than 30 soluble and membrane-bound proteins, about half of which are involved in keeping complement activation under tight control by a variety of redundant mechanisms. Most soluble complement components are synthesized principally in the liver. Not surprisingly, their production is regulated as part of the acute-phase response. Plasma complement components are synthesized elsewhere as well, however. Monocyte/macrophages make essentially the entire complement cascade, and, of particular note for present purposes, airway epithelial cells are capable of synthesizing complement components as well. Three pathways of complement activation are recognized: the alternative pathway, the classical pathways, and the MBLectin pathway (Fig. 1) (reviewed in Refs. 2,3). All involve a initial proteolytic cascade carried out by serine proteases. All lead to the activation of C3 by cleavage to C3b, exposing a cryptic, highly reactive thioester bond that binds covalently with surrounding nucleophiles, such as NH_2 or OH groups on nearby molecules.

A. Alternative Pathway

Phylogenetically the oldest pathway, the alternative pathway provides for a unique mode of pathogen recognition. Nonself is recognized not by the presence of pathogen-associated molecular patterns, but by the absence of host-associated molecular patterns. Low-level activation of the pathway occurs constitutively, both in plasma

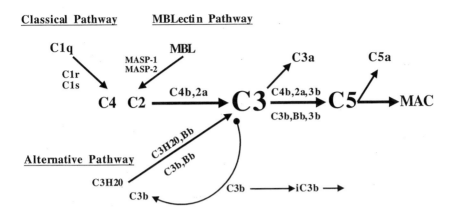

Figure 1 Schematic overview of complement activation and degradation.

and on surfaces. Massive pathway amplification (leading to physiologically relevant activation of complement) results when the C3b so generated attaches to an "activator" surface: one not protected by host sialic acid molecules or host complement-regulatory molecules.

The details are worth sketching. Reaction of the internal thioester bond of C3 with H_2O, leading to the generation of a molecule with a C3b-like conformation (iC3 or $C3H_2O$), occurs continuously at very low levels, a phenomenon referred to as "C3-tickover." $C3H_2O$ can, in turn, associate with factor B, rendering the latter susceptible to cleavage by factor D. The resulting complex ($C3H_2O,Bb$) is an active C3 convertase, leading to the generation of C3b. This initial alternative pathway C3 convertase has a short half-life: factor H binds $C3H_2O$, displacing Bb and allowing factor I–mediated degradation of $C3H_2O$, which prevents it from becoming part of a new C3 convertase. The C3b thereby generated, however, is available for covalent binding to nearby molecules, either in the fluid phase or on cell surfaces. Like $C3H_2O$, C3b can associate with factor B, rendering the latter susceptible to cleavage by factor D and leading to the formation of the C3 convertase C3b,Bb. In fluids and on nonactivator surfaces (e.g., host cell membranes), this convertase is rapidly dissociated by factor H, with C3b being degraded by factor I. The lack of complement amplification on such surfaces is largely a function of the affinity of factor H for negatively charged sialic acid residues on host cell surface glycoproteins. The lower affinity of factor H for surfaces not thereby protected (activator surfaces), however, allows for massive upregulation of the alternative pathway—deposited C3b forming new C3 convertases in a feed-forward loop of amplification. The presence of membrane-bound proteins from the regulators of complement activation (RCA) family (see below) provides a second level of control of alternative pathway activation on host cell surfaces.

B. Classical Pathway

The classical pathway is driven by antigen-antibody interactions. Self/nonself (or danger/nondanger) discrimination by this pathway is thus not direct, depending as it largely does on prior signals from the innate immune system to the adaptive immune system during initial presentation of the antigen involved.

Activation of the pathway begins with the activation of C1, a complex, consisting of a C1q molecule in association with two C1r and two C1s molecules. C1q is itself made up of six identical subunits, each with a C-terminal globular domain tethered to a collagen-like domain. The globular domains of C1q bind to the conformationally altered Fc portions of antibodies that have engaged their cognate antigens. One IgM or at least 2 IgG antibodies in close proximity (of the proper isotype: IgG_3 or IgG_1 in human, IgG_{2a}, IgG_{2b}, or IgG_3 in mice) are required for C1q activation. Such activation involves reciprocal cleavage and activation of C1r, followed by C1r-mediated cleavage and activation of C1s. C1s, in turn, cleaves C4 and C2, leading to generation of the classical pathway C3 convertase. Cleavage of C4 generates C4a, a molecule with minor anaphylatoxin activity in guinea pigs, but not in mice or humans (4). It also leads to the exposing of an internal thioester bond in the other molecule so generated, C4b. A minor amount of the C4b thereby generated undergoes covalent attachment to surfaces (as opposed to H_2O) contiguous with the antigen/antibody/activated C1 complex. C2 subsequently forms a complex with C4b, rendering it accessible for cleavage-mediated activation by C1s. In turn, C4b,2a, the classical pathway C3 convertase, activates C3.

It has recently become clear that there is constitutive low-level activation of the classical pathway in vivo, like that seen with alternative pathway (5). Analogous to C3-tickover in the alternative pathway, C1-tickover occurs in a process that is immunoglobulin-dependent (low levels of circulating immune complexes; spontaneous formation of immunoglobulin aggregates) and upregulated by blood stasis.

C. MBLectin Pathway

Mannan (or mannose)–binding lectin (MBL) is a soluble pattern recognition receptor in the collectin family. A C-type lectin, MBL engages highly repetitive carbohydrate ligands on pathogens. The structure of MBL is reminiscent of C1q, with multiple C-terminal globular domains tethered to a central collagen-like domain, and, in fact, MBL leads to C1-independent activation of the classical pathway. The globular domains of MBL are carbohydrate recognition domains. The iterative engagement of several such domains leads to the activation of MBL-associated homologues of C1r and C1s, MASP-1 and MASP-2. In turn, MASP-2 cleaves C4 and C2, leading to the generation of the classical pathway C3 convertase.

D. C3 Activation by Other Means

Other proteases, both endogenous (e.g., plasmin) and exogenous (e.g., cobra venom factor), are capable of activating C3, although physiological relevance for endogenous C3 activators apart from the C3 convertases described above is doubtful. Additionally, immunoglobulin-independent activation of C1 can occur through both en-dogenous (e.g., C-reactive protein) and exogenous (e.g., HIV gp41) means. It is perhaps notable, as discussed below, that many human allergens are themselves serine proteases.

III. C3 and Downstream

All three pathways lead to C3 activation, with liberation of the anaphylatoxin C3a and generation of C3b. In turn, C3b forms part of the classical (C4b,2a,3b) and alternative (C3b,Bb,3b) pathway C5 convertases. C5 convertase activity leads to cleavage of C5, with liberation of the anaphylatoxin C5a and generation of C5b. In turn, C5b nucleates the (nonenzymatic) formation of the membrane attack complex. As with C3, C5 can be cleaved by endogenous, non–complement-related enzymes (e.g., trypsin, thrombin, elastase), although the (patho)physiological relevance of this fact remains unclear.

Not surprisingly, C3 also forms a principal point of control for the complement system (3). In addition to factor H, described above, other members of the RCA family play critical roles in such regulation. Members with decay acceleration activity lead to dissociation of C3 convertases. These include CR1 and DAF (CD55) on cell membranes (active on both convertases), along with the soluble members C4bp and factor H, which have activity on classical and alternative pathway convertases, respectively. Members with membrane cofactor activity render C3b and C4b cleavable by factor I from plasma. These include CR1 and MCP (CD46) on cell membranes (active on both C3b and C4b), along with the soluble members C4bp and factor H, which have activity on C4b and C3b, respectively.

A variety of biological outcomes are downstream of C3 activation. In addition to microbial lysis by membrane attack complexes, these include: (1) activation of granulocytes and endothelia by sublytic quantities of attack complexes; (2) deposition of C3 fragments on membranes and/or particles (e.g., antigen-antibody complexes, microbes) leading to phagocytosis; immune complex clearance; clearance of apoptotic bodies; B-cell activation; and alterations in immune cell signal transduction, adhesion, activation, and cytokine production; and (3) anaphylatoxin-mediated effects (detailed below). Most such activities depend upon the engagement of specific complement receptors. These include RCA family members, the β-integrins CR3 and CR4, the anaphylatoxin receptors C3aR and C5aR, and receptors for C1q and factor H. All provide potential therapeutic targets.

IV. Complement Fragments and Immunoregulation: Effects on Cytokine Production by Antigen-Presenting Cells

C3b and iC3b were the first complement activation fragments to be shown to affect immunoregulatory cytokine production by APC. IL-12 is a heterodimeric cytokine that is central to the orchestration of both innate and acquired cellular immune responses. Among its activities, IL-12 is: (1) a potent inducer of IFNγ from T and natural killer (NK) cells, (2) critical for the development of Th1 responses in most systems (leading to secondary increases in IFNγ and TNF production, macrophage activation, and the production of complement-fixing antibodies), and (3) an enhancer of cytotoxicity by CD8+ cytolytic T cells and NK cells (6). Working in a measles virus system, it was initially discovered that cross-linking (with measles virus, monoclonal antibodies, or dimerized C3b) of the RCA member CD46 led to potent inhibition of the production of IL-12 by human monocytes (7). This was subsequently shown to be but a particular instance of a more general phenomenon: engagement of the ß-integrin CR3 (CD11b/CD18, Mac-1) with antibody or certain particulate ligands (including particles coated with iC3b) also inhibited IL-12 production by both murine and human monocyte/macrophages (8,9). In all of these systems, the cytokine phenotype was one of a profound suppression of IL-12 with little if any downregulation of the production of other proinflammatory cytokines or chemokines. The ability of complement receptor ligation to specifically inhibit IL-12 production suggested that complement activation products could directly regulate the class of immune response (inhibiting Th1 responses, augmenting Th2 responses) through interaction with antigen-presenting cells.

An analogous linkage between complement and acquired immunity was already known. CD19 is part of a signal transduction complex on B cells, the ligand-binding subunit of which is the RCA member CR2. Cross-linking of membrane immunoglobulin (mIg) to CD19, effected by the binding of a complement-opsonized immunogen to CR2 and mIg, dramatically lowers the threshold for B-cell activation (10). The ability of monocytic receptors for C3 degradation products to specifically inhibit IL-12 suggested that the complement system not only augments humoral immune responses (through CR2-mediated upregulation of B cell activation), but inhibits cellular immune responses (through CD46- and CR3-mediated inhibition of IL-12 production). Genetic approaches to asthma led to the realization that the anaphylatoxin C5a also has effects on immunoregulation.

V. C3a and C5a

Complement activation by any pathway results in formation of C3a and C5a. These anaphylatoxins are peptides that were initially defined functionally by their activities on small blood vessels, smooth muscle, mast cells, and peripheral blood leukocytes. C3a and C5a have a plethora of proinflammatory actions, including (1) promotion of leukocyte chemotaxis; (2) enhancement of neutrophil-endothelial cell adhesion; (3) upregulation of vascular permeability; (4) induction of granule secretion by phagocytes; and (5) induction of the production and release of a variety of proinflammatory cytokines and chemokines (e.g., IL-1, IL-6, TNF-α, and IL-8) (Fig. 2). The potent effects of the anaphylatoxins on the trafficking and activation of effector cells of the allergic response are of particular relevance to asthma. Notably, C5a is chemotactic for macrophages, neutrophils, activated B and T lymphocytes, and basophils; and both C3a and C5a are chemotactic for eosinophils and mast cells. In

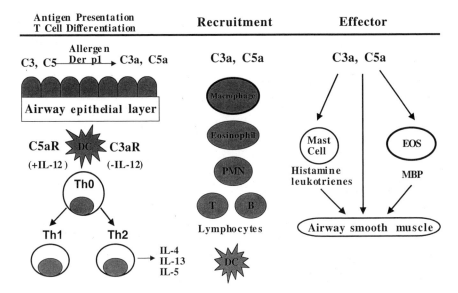

Figure 2 Proposed functions of anaphylatoxins in allergic asthma. C3 and C5 are produced at the airway surface by epithelial cells and/or via leakage from the vascular compartment. These precursor molecules can be cleaved by allergens themselves or proteases released as a result of the inflammatory process. Once produced, C3a and C5a may bind their respective receptors on a variety of cells. It has recently been hypothesized that through binding receptors on macrophages/dendritic cells, these mediators can direct the nature of the immune response to inhaled antigens. Specifically, C5a may enhance IL-12 production and drive a Th1-mediated immune response, while C3a may inhibit direct Th2 immune responses. In addition, these potent mediators are chemotactic for a variety of cells important in the allergic response, including eosinophils, neutrophils, dendritic cells, macrophages, and lymphocytes. In turn, C3a and C5a activate the major effector cells of the allergic response, mast cells and eosinophils, resulting in release of bronchoactive substances such as histamine, leukotrienes, and MBP, respectively. Through these combined actions, the anaphylatoxins play a major role in the development of allergic airway responses.

addition to recruiting granulocytes into the airways, the anaphylatoxins also stimulate their effector mechanisms, leading to rapid release of histamine from basophils and mast cells and to upregulation of the synthesis of eosinophil cationic protein. C3a and C5a are also able to induce smooth muscle contraction. The contractile actions of anaphylatoxins are thought to be mediated via the induction of leukotrienes, prostanoids, and platelet-activating factor by mast cells and eosinophils, although direct effects on smooth muscle have not been ruled out (11).

C3a and C5a exert their effects by interacting with their receptors, C3aR and C5aR respectively (12,13). Both of these receptors belong to the large family of seven-transmembrane-domain G-protein-coupled receptors. In addition to being present on myeloid cells, dendritic cells, and and activated lymphocytes (14–19),

C3aR and C5aR are present on a variety of cell types in the lung, including bronchial smooth muscle cells and vascular endothelial cells. Of note, the expression of these receptors on bronchial smooth muscle appears to be regulated by exposure to various environmental agents such as allergens and endotoxin (20). Specifically, C3aR is upregulated on bronchial smooth muscle cells by both allergen challenge and LPS exposure in mice, whereas C5aR expression is only elevated following LPS. C5aR expression has been noted on bronchial and alveolar epithelial cells in some studies (20,21), but not others (22,23).

VI. Role of Complement Fragments in Experimental Models of Asthma

In addition to its well-recognized proinflammatory actions, an immunoregulatory role for C5a has recently been proposed. Through combined genetic and genomic approaches, Karp et al. identified C5 as a susceptibility gene for allergen-induced AHR (24). Susceptibility to the development of allergen-induced AHR is associated with a Th2 dominant cytokine pattern, whereas resistance is associated with Th1 cytokine production. As might therefore be expected, allergen-induced AHR is prevented or ablated by exogenous IL-12 in susceptible strains (25), whereas neutralization of IL-12 renders resistant strains susceptible (26). In this model, A/J mice are susceptible, exhibiting AHR along with mucous metaplasia and an inflammatory response characterized by marked pulmonary eosinophilia and elevated IgE levels after antigen challenge. C3H/HeJ mice are resistant and do not develop AHR or elevations in IgE production and exhibit a reduced eosinophilic inflammatory response (26). A/J mice have a 2-base-pair deletion in a 5′ exon of the C5 gene, which renders them deficient in C5 mRNA and protein production (and devoid of functional C5); C3H/HeJ mice are C5 sufficient (27). Abnormal C5 gene expression was found to be associated with susceptibility to Th2-driven immune responses.

Given the facts noted above that (1) C3 fragments (C3b, C3b1)inhibit APC production of IL-12 and (2) C5a promotes monocyte/macrophage production of TNF-α, IL-1, and IL-6, Karp et al. (24) examined the effects of ablating C5a-mediated signaling in monocytic cells in a mechanistic search for the link between C5 and susceptibility to allergen-induced AHR. To model the in vivo lack of access to C5a in the macrophages of susceptible mice, ablation of C5a-mediated signaling was studied in human monocyte/macrophages cultured in the absence of serum. C5aR signaling was ablated with a C5aR antagonist (28). Of note, blockade of the C5aR caused marked dose-dependent inhibition of the IL-12 productive capacity of primary human monocytes. Such blockade also inhibited the secretion of TNFα, albeit less potently. Interestingly, while inhibition of C5aR signaling had no overall effect on bacterially driven IL-10 production, IFNγ-mediated suppression of IL-10 production was reversed (24).

This finding that ablation of C5aR signaling compromises monocytic cell production of IL-12 appeared, superficially, to be in conflict with other published data demonstrating that C5a can itself lead to IL-12 inhibition (9,29). Suppression of IL-12 production induced by C5a is mechanistically separable from that resulting from ablation of C5aR signaling, however. The C5aR is coupled to a pertussis toxin–sensitive G protein (12). C5a-mediated IL-12 suppression is pertussis toxin–sensitive and only occurs in the presence of serum. C5aR antagonist–mediated suppression is neither pertussis toxin–sensitive nor dependent upon the presence of serum (24). Modulation of IL-12 production by both a C5aR antagonist and C5a suggests a model in which some C5aR signaling is needed to render monocyte/macrophages competent for IL-12 production, while further exposure to C5a leads to inhibition of the production of this potentially toxic cytokine.

The stimulated production of IL-12 was subsequently compared in A/J and C3H/HeJ mice: peritoneal macrophages from C5-deficient A/J mice produce significantly less IL-12 than those obtained from C5-sufficient C3H/HeJ mice (24). Similar, biologically relevant, differences in IL-12 production by C5 deficient (A/J) and C5 sufficient (C57BL/6) strains have also been found in a model of malaria infection (30). Taken together, these studies suggested that C5 deficiency may lead to impaired IL-12 production, thereby predisposing to the mounting deleterious Th2 immune responses upon allergen exposure.

Other data in the literature are consistent with this hypothesis. Skamene and colleagues have shown that the susceptibility of A/J mice to *Listeria* infection is due to the aberrant C5 gene (31). Successful resolution of *Listeria* infection has clearly been shown to be dependent on IL-12. Similarly, Tsuji et al. (32,33) have shown that C5 (in particular, C5a) is essential for the development of Th1-directed contact sensitivity (CS) responses. Specifically, they demonstrated that (1) mice deficient in C5 or the C5aR had impaired CS responses and (2) blockade of C5a with a specific C5a antiserum resulted in impaired CS responses in C5 sufficient mice. Consistent with the importance of C5 in Th1-mediated immune responses, C5 appears to be important in development of collagen-induced arthritis (34) and endotoxic shock (35). Taken together these studies suggest that C5a normally serves to facilitate IL-12 production by APCs and that a deficiency in C5a may skew the immune response towards a Th2 cytokine pattern due to the lack of production of IL-12 by antigen-presenting cells.

Interestingly, recent studies in several animal models have implicated C3 and C3a in asthma pathogenesis. Specifically, Humbles and colleagues (36) demonstrated that C3aR-deficient mice (Balb/c × 129) do not develop allergen-driven AHR following allergen sensitization and challenge. Of note, the pattern and magnitude of infiltration of inflammatory cells into the lung was similar in allergen-exposed C3aR wild-type and Knockout (KO) mice, suggesting that, in contrast to current dogma, C3 plays a major role in the allergic response that is independent of its chemoattractant properties. Similarly, Walters et al. (37) showed that AHR induced in mice by airway exposure to a nonantigenic environmental stimulus, urban ambient air–derived particulate matter, is also dependent on C3: C3-deficient mice failed to develop AHR. The particulate matter–induced inflammatory response was unchanged in the knockouts in this model as well. Airway challenge with particulate matter was associated with marked deposition of C3 along the airway epithelium and subepithelial smooth muscle in wild-type mice. Guinea pigs with a naturally occurring deficiency in the C3aR exhibited a significant decrease in late-phase bronchoconstriction as compared to control strains (38). Early-phase bronchoconstriction was demonstrated to depend on activation of the C3aR pathway as well. Furthermore, using C3 knockout mice, Drouin and colleagues (39) demonstrated that C3-deficient mice have dramatically lower numbers of IL-4–producing cells in their lungs following allergen exposure, along with a reduction in Th2-driven IgE and IgG1 antibody levels and an increase in Th1-driven IgG2a levels. In contrast to the above studies, this study linked C3 deficiency to alterations in the inflammatory response, with reduced eosinophil and enhanced neutrophil recruitment into the lung compartment. Altogether, these studies suggest that C3 is important in the development of AHR induced by a variety of stimuli. Although the exact mechanism(s) remain unclear, the data are consistent with an upstream immunoregulatory role for C3 ad C3a (promotion of T-cell polarization towards a Th2 phenotype) rather than activity solely as a chemoattractant.

Collectively, studies in animal models strongly support a role for complement components in the development of allergic asthma. In contrast to the well-recognized role of C3a and C5a as chemoattractants, these studies highlight a likely role in directing the class of the specific immune response. Specifically, a predominance of C3a production may predispose to a Th2 immune response, while a dominant C5a response may mediate protection from Th2-driven allergic responses. Although the exact mechanisms by which these complement fragments reciprocally regulate the allergic response are unknown, such mechanisms are likely to involve regulation of IL-12 production by antigen-presenting cells.

VII. Role of Complement in Human Asthma

The importance of complement pathways in allergic disorders in humans is supported by numerous reports of exaggerated anaphylatoxin production in asthma (36,40,41) Van de Graaf et al. (40) showed that C3a is increased in BAL fluid of stable asthmatics compared to healthy controls. Humbles and colleagues (36) demonstrated that segmental allergen challenge induced elevations in BAL C3a-C3a des-arginine levels from asthmatic individuals, but not in normal controls. Interestingly, Krug et al. (41) demonstrated elevations in BAL levels of both C3a and C5a 24 hours following segmental allergen challenge of asthmatic individuals, whereas no elevations were observed following such challenge in normal individuals.

Consistent with the accumulating biological evidence of the importance of complement in the pathogenesis of asthma, recent studies suggest that asthma-related traits are linked to chromosomal regions containing the C5 and C5aR genes. Specifically, two genome-wide screens for asthma susceptibility loci have found linkage to the C5 chromosomal region (9q34) (42,43). Furthermore, the human C5aR gene is located at 19q13.3, a susceptibility locus for asthma in several different cohorts (43,44). People with homozygous defects in the C5 gene, like others with deficiencies in late complement components, suffer a high incidence of disseminated neisserial infection. They are protected, however, from the fulminant shock that often accompanies such disease in the face of complement sufficiency, a phenomenon that may be due to the effects of a lack of C5a on TNF-α and IL-12 production (35). It is not known whether C5 null individuals are prone to development of asthma. However, in preliminary experiments, we have identified a T-to-C change at position -245 of the promoter of the C5aR gene (M. Wills-Karp and K. B. Barnes, unpublished results). Preliminary results suggest that the promoter polymorphism in the C5aR gene is moderately associated with atopic asthma in a Caucasian population in Cincinnati, Ohio (M. Wills-Karp, unpublished results), but additional studies are necessary to confirm an association with increased susceptibility to asthma in other populations.

VIII. Mechanisms of Complement Activation in Asthma

The mechanisms underlying the generation of anaphylatoxins in allergic asthma remain unclear. There are multiple possibilities. First, complement is likely to be activated through the classical pathway as a result of allergen-antibody complex formation. However, (1) this would be an event downstream of antigen-presentation events, the time when effects on immunoregulatory cytokine production would seem to be most pertinent to Th2 polarization, and (2) the antibody classes and isotypes upregulated by Th2 cytokines are poor at complement fixation. Second, C5 and C3 could be cleaved by proteases released from mast cells and other inflammatory cells (e.g., trypsin, thrombin, elastase) in the airway wall as a secondary consequence of IgE-mediated processes. Such a scenario suffers from the same kinetic considerations. Third, pattern recognition of carbohydrate structures on allergens might lead to activation of the MBLectin pathway. Fourth, alternative pathway activation may occur on allergen-related surfaces, or proteases derived from allergens may themselves may cleave the C3 and C5 that is constitutively produced at the airway surface by airway epithelial cells. Indeed, several investigators have reported the generation of anaphylatoxins during in vitro incubation of serum with extracts from different allergens (45,46). Interestingly, Castro et al. (46) demonstrated that house dust mite extract induced potent complement activation in the serum of both asthmatic and healthy subjects. Mauro and colleagues (47) subsequently formally demonstrated that proteases derived from *Dermatophagoides* species (*Der p 3* and *Der f 3*) cleave both C3 and C5 into their active fragments in vitro. Thus, the biochemical properties of allergens themselves may play an important role in generation of anaphylatoxins at the airway interface with the environment, a place where they would be uniquely positioned to direct the immune response. Although this is an intriguing hypothesis, it does not explain why complement levels are preferentially elevated in the lungs of asthmatic individuals, as both normals and asthmatics are exposed to similar levels of these allergens. Clearly much remains to be learned about the exact mechanisms of complement activation in the asthmatic lung.

IX. Conclusion

Substantial evidence suggests that complement activation plays an important role in the development of allergic airway responses. Traditionally, C3a and C5a have been thought to contribute to the allergic response via their potent proinflammatory and chemotactic activity. New insights into the biology of complement suggest a much more complex role for complement in asthma. Collectively, studies in animal models of asthma support the imputation of an important immunoregulatory role for these anaphylatoxins. Specifically, a dominance of C3a production may predispose to a Th2 immune response, while a dominance of C5a production may mediate protection from Th2-driven allergic responses. If the murine data can be extrapolated to human disease, we would predict that the Th2-polarized immune responses associated with asthma may arise as either a result of impaired generation of C5a (or C5aR activation) or enhanced generation of C3a (or C3aR activation). Support for a causal role for altered anaphylatoxin production in human disease comes from reports of exaggerated complement production in the lungs of asthmatics as well as the putative genetic linkages to chromosomal regions containing the C5a and C5aR genes. Although much remains to be learned about the complex role played by anaphylatoxins in asthma, identification of a role for complement in the development of allergic asthma provides a focus for the development of novel therapeutic strategies for an increasingly important disease. Direct modulation of the C3aR or C5aR G-protein coupled receptors may provide tractable targets for therapeutic development.

Acknowledgments

The authors acknowledge the support of NIH grants HL58527, HL67736, HL66623 to MWK, and AI40507 to CLK.

References

1. Wills-Karp M. Immunologic basis of antigen-induced airway hyperresponsiveness. Annu Rev Immunol 1999; 17:255–281.
2. Prodinger WM, Würzner R, Erdei A, Dierich MP. Complement. In: Paul W, ed. Fundamental Immunology, 4th ed. Philadelphia: Lippincott-Raven Press, 1998:967–996.
3. Liszewski MK, Farries TC, Lublin DM, Rooney IA, Atkinson JP. Control of the complement system. Adv Immunol 1996; 61:201–283.
4. Lienenklaus S, Ames RS, Tornett MA, Sarau HM, Foley JJ, Crass T, Sohns B, Raffetseder U, Grove M, Hölzer Am Klos A, Köhl J, Bautsch W. Cutting edge: human anaphylatoxin C4a is a potent agonist of the guinea pig but not the human C3a receptor. J Immunol 1998; 161:2089–2093.
5. Manderson AP, Pickering MC, Botto M, Walport MJ, Parish CR. Continual low-level activation of the classical complement pathway. J Exp Med 2001; 194:747–756.
6. Trinchieri G. Interleukin-12: a cytokine at the interface of inflammation and immunity. Adv Immunol 1998; 70:83–243.
7. Karp CL, Wysocka M, Wahl LM, Ahearn JM, Cuomo PJ, Sherry B, Trinchieri G, Griffin DE, et al. Mechanism of suppression of cell-mediated immunity by measles virus. Science 1996; 273:228–231.
8. Marth T, Kelsall BL. Regulation of interleukin-12 by complement receptor 3 signaling. J Exp Med 1997; 185:1987–1995.

9. Sutterwala FS, Noel GJ, Clynes R, Mosser DM. Selective suppression of interleukin-12 induction after macrophage receptor ligation. J Exp Med 1997; 185:1977–1985.

10. Fearon DT, Carter RH. The CD19/CR2/TAPA-1 complex of B lymphocytes: linking natural to acquired immunity. Annu Rev Immunol 1995; 13:127–149.

11. Stimler-Gerard NP. Immunopharmacology of anaphylatoxin-induced bronchoconstrictor responses. Complement 1986; 3:137–151.

12. Gerard C, Gerard NP. C5A anaphylatoxin and its seven transmembrane-segment receptor. Annu Rev Immunol 1994; 12:775–808.

13. Crass T, Raffetseder U, Martin U, Grove M, Klos A, Kohl J, Bautsch W. Expression cloning of the human C3a anaphylatoxin receptor (C3aR) from differentiated U-937 cells. Eur J Immunol 1996; 26:1944–1950.

14. Ames RS, Li Y, Sarau HM, Nuthulaganti P, Foley JJ, Ellis C, Zeng Z, Su K, Jurewicz AJ, Hertzberg RP, Bergsma DJ, Kumar C. Molecular cloning and characterization of the human anaphylatoxin C3a receptor. J Biol Chem 1996; 271:20231–20234.

15. Fischer WH, Hugli TE. Regulation of B cell functions by C3a and C3a(desArg): suppression of TNF-alpha, IL-6, and the polyclonal immune response. J Immunol 1997; 159: 4279–4286.

16. Ottonello L, Corcione A, Tortolina G, Airoldi I, Albesiano E, Favre A, D'Agostino R, Malavasi F, Pistoia V, Dallegri F. rC5a directs the in vitro migration of human memory and naive tonsillar B lymphocytes: implications for B cell trafficking in secondary lymphoid tissues. J Immunol 1999; 62:6510–6517.

17. Nataf S, Davoust N, Ames RS, Barnum SR. Human T cells express the C5a receptor and are chemoattracted to C5a. J Immunol 1999; 62:4018–4023.

18. Werfel T, Kirchhoff K, Wittmann M, Begemann G, Kapp A, Heidenreich F, Gotze O, Zwirner J. Activated human T lymphocytes express a functional C3a receptor. J Immunol 2000; 165:6599–6605.

19. Martin U, Bock D, Arseniev L, Tornetta MA, Ames RS, Bautsch W, Kohl J, Ganser A, Klos A. The human C3a receptor is expressed on neutrophils and monocytes, but not on B or T lymphocytes. J Exp Med 1997; 186:199–207.

20. Drouin SM, Kildsgaard J, Haviland J, Zabner J, Jia HP, McCray PB Jr, Tack BF, Wetsel RA. Expression of the complement anaphylatoxin C3a and C5a receptors on bronchial epithelial and smooth muscle cells in models of sepsis and asthma. J Immunol 2001; 166:2025–2032.

21. Haviland DL, McCoy RL, Whitehead WT, Akama H, Molmenti EP, Brown A, Haviland JC, Parks WC, Perlmutter DH, Wetsel RA. Cellular expression of the C5a anaphylatoxin receptor (C5aR): demonstration of C5aR on nonmyeloid cells of the liver and lung. J Immunol 1995; 154:1861–1869.

22. Fayyazi A, Sandau R, Duong LQ, Gotze O, Radzun HJ, Schweyer S, Soruri A, Jorg Zwirner.C5a receptor and interleukin 6 are expressed in tissue macrophages and stimulated keratinocytes but not in pulmonary and intestinal epithelial cells. Am J Pathol 1999; 154:495–501.

23. Zwirner J, Fayyazi A, Goetz O. Expression of the anaphylatoxin C5a receptor in nonmyeloid cells. Mol Immunol 1999; 36:877–884.

24. Karp CL, Grupe A, Schadt E, Ewart SL, Keane-Moore M, Cuomo PJ, Kohl J, Wahl L, Kuperman D, Germer S, Aud D, Peltz G, Wills-Karp M. Identification of complement factor 5 as a susceptibility locus for experimental allergic asthma. Nat Immunol 2000; 1:221–226.

25. Gavett SH, O'Hearn DJ, Li X, Huang S, Finkelman FD, Wills-Karp M. Interleukin 12 inhibits antigen-induced airway hyperresponsiveness, inflammation, and Th2 cytokine expression in mice. J Exp Med 1995; 182:1527–1536.

26. Keane-Myers A, Wysocka M, Trinchieri G, Wills-Karp M. Resistance to antigen-induced airway hyperresponsiveness requires endogenous production of IL-12. J Immunol 1998; 161:919–926.

27. Wetsel RA, Fleischer DT, Haviland DL. Deficiency of the murine fifth complement component (C5). A 2-base pair gene deletion in a 5'-exon. J Biol Chem 1990; 265: 2435–2440.

28. Heller T, Hennecke M, Baumann U, Gessner JE, Vilsendorf AM, Baensch M, Boulay F, Kola A, Klos A, Bautsch W, Kohl J. Selection of a C5a receptor antagonist from phage libraries attenuating the inflammatory response in immune complex disease and ischemia/reperfusion injury. J Immunol 1999; 163:985–994.

29. Wittman M, Zwirner J, Larsson VA, Kirchhoff K, Begemann G, Kapp A, Gotze O, Werfel T. C5a suppresses the production of IL-12 by IFN-gamma-primed and lipopolysaccharide-challenged human monocytes. J Immunol 1999; 162:6763–6769.

30. Sam H, Stevenson MM. Early IL-12 p70, but not p40, production by splenic macrophages correlates with host resistance to blood-stage *Plasmodium chabaudi* AS malaria. Clin Exp Immunol 1999; 117:343–349.

31. Gervais F, Stevenson M, Skamene, E. Genetic control of resistance to Listeria monocytogenes: regulation of leukocyte inflammatory responses by the Hc locus. J Immunol 1984; 132:2078–2083.

32. Tsuji RF, Geba GP, Wang Y, Kawamoto K, Matis LA, Askenase PW. Required early complement activation in contact sensitivity with generation of local C5-dependent chemotactic activity, and late T cell interferon gamma: a possible initiating role of B cells. J Exp Med 1997; 186:1015–1026.

33. Tsuji RF, Kawikova I, Ramabhadran R, Akahira-Azuma M, Taub D, Hugli TE, Gerard C, Askenase PW. Early local generation of C5a initiates the elicitation of contact sensitivity by leading to early T cell recruitment. J Immunol 2000; 165:1588–1598.

34. Wang Y, Rollins SA, Madri JA, Matis LA. Anti-C5 monoclonal antibody therapy prevents collagen-induced arthritis and ameliorates established disease. Proc Natl Acad Sci USA 1995; 92:8955–8959.

35. Barton PA, Warren JS. Complement component C5 modulates the systemic tumor necrosis factor response in murine endotoxic shock. Infect Immun 1993; 61:1474–1481.

36. Humbles AA, Lu B, Nilsson CA, Lilly C, Israel E, Fujiwara Y, Gerard NP, Gerard C. A role for C3a anaphylatoxin receptor in the effector phase of asthma. Nature 2000; 406:998–1001.

37. Walters DM, Breyesse PN, Schofield B, Wills-Karp M. Complement factor 3 mediates particulate matter-induced airway hyperresponsiveness. Am J Respir Cell Mol Biol. In press.

38. Bautsch W, Hoymann HG, Zhang Q, Meier-Wiedenbach I, Raschke U, Ames RS, Sohns B, Flemme N, Meyer zu Vilsendorf A, Grove M, Klos A, Kohl J. Cutting edge: guinea pigs with a natural C3a-receptor defect exhibit decreased bronchoconstriction in allergic airway disease: evidence for an involvement of the C3a anaphylatoxin in the pathogenesis of asthma. J Immunol 2000; 165:5401–5405.

39. Drouin SM, Corry DB, Kildsgaard, Wetsel RA. Cutting edge: the absence of C3 demonstrates a role for complement in Th2 effector functions in a murine model of pulmonary allergy. J Immunol 2001; 167:4141–4145.

40. Van de Graaf EA, Jansen HM, Bakker MM, Alberts C, Schattenkerk JKE, Out TA. ELISA of complement C3a in bronchoalveolar lavage fluid. J Immunol Methods 1992; 147:241.

41. Krug N, Tschernig T, Erpenbeck VJ, Hohlfeld JM, Kohl J. Complement factors C3a and C5a are increased in bronchoalveolar lavage fluid after segmental allergen provocation in subjects with asthma. Am J Respir Crit Care Med 2001; 164:1841–1843.

42. Ober C, Cox NJ, Abney M, Di Rienzo A, Lander ES, Changyaleket B, Gidley H, Kurtz B, Lee J, Nance M, Pettersson A, Prescott J, Richardson A, Schlenker E, Summerhill E, Willadsen S, Parry R. Genome-wide search for asthma susceptibility loci in a founder population. The Collaborative Study on the Genetics of Asthma. Hum Mol Genet 1998; 7:1393–1398.

43. Wjst M, Fischer G, Immervoll T, Jung M, Saar K. et al. A genome-wide search for linkage to asthma. German Asthma Genetics Group. Genomics 1999; 58:1–8.

44. A genome-wide search for asthma susceptibility loci in ethnically diverse populations. The Collaborative Study on the Genetics of Asthma (CSGA). Nat Genet 1997; 15: 389–392.

45. Nagata S, Glovsky MM. Activation of human serum complement with allergens. I. Generation of C3a, C4a, C5a and induction of human neutrophil aggregation. J Allergy Clin Immunol 1987; 80:24–32.

46. Castro FFM, Schmitz-Schumann M, Rother U, Kirschfink M. Complement activation by house dust: reduced reactivity of serum complement in patients with bronchial asthma. Int Arch Allergy Appl Immunol 1991; 96:305–310.

47. Mauro K, Akaike T, Ono T, Okamoto T, Maeda H. Generation of anaphylatoxins through proteolytic processing of C3 and C5 by house dust mite protease. J Allergy Clin Immunol 1997; 100:253–260.

33

Complement Anaphylatoxin Receptors in Asthma

NORMA P. GERARD and CRAIG GERARD

Harvard Medical School
Boston, Massachusetts, U.S.A.

A recent series of investigations using animal models of allergic airways disease as well as correlative studies in human asthmatics have suggested that C3a and C5a anaphylatoxins are significant mediators of inflammation in the airways. Receptors for the anaphylatoxins are present in airway epithelium and upregulated in the presence of inflammation. The C3a receptor is also present on airway smooth muscle. In this chapter we will briefly review the pathways leading to complement activation, the animal models implicating a role for C3a and C5a in asthma, and the clinical studies that correlate asthma with complement activation. The development of small molecule antagonists for the C3a and C5a receptors, which has finally been achieved, may soon allow for a proof-of-concept trial in human disease.

I. Introduction

The complement system, composed of some 30 proteins, has evolved as a major bulwark of the innate immune system, and is a bridge to the acquired immune system (1). Three individual pathways lead to complement activation, known as the classical, alternative, and mannan-binding lectin pathways. In all three, the anaphylatoxins C3a and C5a are liberated from the N-termini of the complement components C3 and C5, respectively, by proteolysis, and an oligomeric membrane attack complex is produced by association of C5b, C6, C7, C8, and C9 (2). The classical pathway is activated by immune complexes consisting of antigen and IgA, IgM, IgG2, or IgG4. The alternative pathway is activated by interaction of factor B and properdin with xenobiotic surfaces. Finally, the mannan-binding lectin pathway is activated by recognition of patterns of carbohydrates on foreign surfaces. Mannan-binding protein is a serum protein associated with several serine proteases called mannan-associated serine proteases (MASPs). Thus, recognition of nonself substances leads to activation of a proteolytic cascade that aims to (1) lyse the foreign cell membrane, (2) opsonize the substance with C3 fragments leading to phagocytosis and clearance, (3) participate in the development of acquired immune responses via C3 receptors on B cells, (4) recruit bone marrow–derived cells to perform host defense functions, and (5) regulate local vascular permeability. Although this list is far from complete, it does provide a broad sense of the complex functions of the complement system.

The anaphylatoxins have long been known as mediators of host defense and inflammation (3). C3a and C5a function by binding to G protein–coupled receptors expressed on a wide variety of cells, including myeloid cells, lymphoid cells, mast cells and basophils, endothelial and epithelial cells, neurons, microglial cells, and smooth muscle cells (4). The most easily studied signaling properties of these receptors include chemotaxis, exocytosis of granule-bound enzymes or mediators, and activation of NADPH oxidase. Less clear are the functions of anaphylatoxin receptors on nonmotile cells, such as lung epithelium. Linkage of anaphylatoxin to various inflammatory diseases is well known, but it is only recently that a number of groups have identified a potential pathological role for C3a and C5a in asthma. This chapter will review these data.

II. C3a in Asthma

There has been considerable speculation as to the role of complement activation in asthma for some time (5). However, a number of recent studies using mice and guinea pigs have provided evidence for a significant role for C3a and its receptor in antigen-induced airways hyperresponsiveness (AHR) (6–8).

Humbles et al. (6) attempted to use mice deficient in the C3a receptor as controls for mice deficient in the eotaxin receptor CCR3. The rationale behind this experiment was that CCR3 was thought to be the major eosinophil chemoattractant in antigen-induced airways hyperresponsiveness and that this cell type was responsible for the physiological changes. Since the C3a receptor is also highly expressed on eosinophils (9), but was not expected to play a role in this model, we felt it was a good control for mouse strains and eosinphil targeting. Surprisingly, we found the results to be exactly the opposite of what we expected; mice deficient in CCR3 displayed excessive AHR to methacholine compared to wild-type animals, while C3a receptor deficient mice were protected from antigen-induced AHR (6,10). In the case of the C3a receptor–deleted animals, we observed no apparent differences in the inflammatory response or cytokine profile. Thus, aside from the observation that the C3a receptor is present and upregulated directly on smooth muscle in human

Table 1 C3a/C3a des-Arg Levels in Human BAL Fluid

		Asthmatics ($n = 8$)		
	Normals ($n = 5$)	Preallergen	Sham	Allergen
Median	59	64	69	123*
IQR	58–107	42–79	46–91	55–357

C3a/C3a des Arg levels (ng/mL) were assessed in BAL fluid by radioimmunoassay. Results are the medians and interquartile ranges (IQR) for 5 normal and 8 asthmatic subjects that underwent segmental sham or allergen challenge.
*$p < 0.01$, significant difference between sham and allergen groups (Wilcoxin signed-ranks test).

and mouse models of asthma (8), we are at a loss to explain these findings. Further, because the C3a receptor has been detected on human activated T cells (both CD4 + and CD8 +), there are a number of mechanistic details to be determined.

Because of the surprising result, we assessed airway bronchoalveolar lavage (BAL) fluid for C3a in samples from asthmatics and controls who received subsegmental antigen challenge. We observed a significant increase in C3a in several patients, which correlated with the presence of BAL neutrophils (Table 1). These data have been independently replicated in a larger study performed recently by Krug and colleagues (11), who demonstrated significant elevations of C3a and C5a in mild asthmatics after antigen challenge, with essentially no change in normal controls. Further, as we had suggested previously, these investigators also found that the levels of C3a and C5a correlated with the number of eosinophils and neutrophils in the BAL fluid. Subsequent to the report by Humbles and colleagues (6), both mice and guinea pigs deficient in C3 or the C3a receptor, respectively, also showed reduced AHR after antigen challenge in vivo, as did mice treated with a C3a receptor antagonist (7). Table 2 summarizes these findings.

Mechanistically, several potential pathways could lead to complement activation in these models. First, it is possible that immune complexes activate complement through the classical pathway (1). Second, recognition of carbohydrate structures by the mannan-binding lectin pathway could participate. Finally, direct cleavage of

Table 2 Studies Indicating Role for Complement Activation in the Pathogenesis of Asthma

	Mouse	Rat	Guinea pig	Human
C3a	Humbles et al. (6) Drouin et al. (8)		Kohl (3) Regal and Klos (14)	Humbles et al. (6) Krug et al. (11)
C5a	Humbles et al. (10) Karp et al. (12)	Abe et al. (13)		Humbles et al. (6) Krug et al. (11)

C3 and C5 by mast cell proteases released via IgE-induced degranulation could also generate the anaphylatoxins. Thus, at present we have only correlative data in humans in an antigen-challenge setting. However, given the preliminary studies with C3a receptor–deficient mice and guinea pigs, this receptor seems to be an excellent target for asthma therapy.

Given that no change in the inflammatory milieu was observed in the animal studies, where protection from airway hyperresponsiveness correlated with lack of the C3a receptor or ligand precursor C3, what might the mechanism be for the protective effect? Our leading hypothesis is that activation of the C3a receptor, like the cysteinyl leukotriene receptors, may represent a direct action mediated at the level of airway smooth muscle. We demonstrated some time ago that human lung tissues in organ bath underwent spasmogenic contraction when treated with C3a or C5a (15). Drouin and colleagues (8) demonstrated the presence of C3a receptors on smooth muscle of mouse and human lung, which were upregulated in protein expression after mice were sensitized to ovalbumin. Clinical studies with human asthmatic tissues must attempt now to confirm the presence and possible overexpression of C3aR in smooth muscle.

III. C5 in Asthma

As mentioned above, a number of reports provide evidence for detectable levels of the complement fragment C5a in the BAL fluid of allergic asthmatics, as well as in the nasal lavage of patients with atopic rhinitis subsequent to specific antigen challenge (9,16–19). C5a is a very powerful mediator, affecting virtually all cells of the myeloid lineage, mast cells, as well as parenchymal cells (8). Additionally, C5b-9, which forms the lytic membrane attack complex of complement, has also been demonstrated to exhibit signaling functions, eliciting calcium flux, PKC, and MAP kinase activation (20–23). Thus, there are at least two potential pathways by which C5 may be implicated in asthma, one via C5a receptor activation, and the other by sublytic membranolysis by C5b-9.

In the past year, two studies have appeared in animal models with diametrically opposite results. Karp and colleagues (12) in an elegant genomic/proteomic approach, noted that mouse strains at the extreme of airways hyperresponsiveness to methacholine following ovalbumin sensitization were naturally deficient in complement component C5. Based on this observation, a quantitative trait locus analysis was performed, which also implicated the C5 region. Independently, differential expression of genes in the lung of susceptible and resistant backcross mice further linked the expression of C5 with the level of airways hyperresponsiveness. In order to approach this phenomenon mechanistically, the authors measured the level of IL-12 released from the monocytes of animals sufficient or deficient in C5 (24), or treated with a phage display–derived peptide antagonist (25). The data presented indicate that C5a, acting through the C5a receptor, is anti-inflammatory, resulting in decreased secretion of type 1 cytokines and increased secretion of type 2 cytokines in monocytes treated with lipopolysaccharide (LPS) and *Staphylococcus aureus*

Cowen strain. The authors, however, did not present data from the in vivo setting relating to the degree of inflammation or cytokine levels. Also unclear from the presentation is the mechanism for the effect of the C5a antagonist, which suppressed IL-12 production. Were the cells presumed to be making C5a in an autocrine fashion, activity of which was presumably blocked by the antagonist? In sum, the conclusion of these authors was that C5, acting through C5a, is a locus that confers decreased susceptibility to experimental asthma in the mouse.

The second recent study examined a similar model in the rat. Abe and colleagues (13) used Brown Norway rats, which were sensitized with ovalbumin and then examined after one, two, or three aerosol antigen challenges. In this model, an early phase component is observed, consisting of changes in resistance following antigen challenge, and after three challenges a late phase component occurs ~6 hours following challenge. Notably, there is no late phase response after one or two challenges, and unlike the mouse, where airways hyperresponsiveness occurs after 24 hours, the late phase in the rat occurs after 6 hours.

The investigators employed three methods to inhibit complement activation; soluble CR1, futhan (a nonspecific protease inhibitor that blocks coagulation as well as complement cascades), and the oligopeptide (Nme-Phe-Lys-Pro-dCha-Trp-dArg) identified by phage-display, which is described as a nanomolar antagonist of the C5a receptor. Using these reagents, the authors showed that (1) all three complement inhibitors blocked the early phase, but more significantly the late phase in sensitized rats; (2) this was associated with a decrease in histological evidence of inflammation; (3) there was a decrease in measured BAL cytokines IL-12, IL-4, IL-5, and IFNγ (but not eotaxin); (4) responses could be restored in complement blocked animals by addition of rat C5adesArg, but not C3adesArg. The authors concluded that blockade of C5a receptor is associated with decreased airways hyperresponsiveness—exactly the opposite result to Karp and colleagues.

It is difficult to reconcile these results, but the following should be considered. First, the Karp manuscript describing linkage to C5 may actually reflect a linkage disequilibrium with another gene. Second, the Abe work was done with rat, and, although unlikely, the effects may be species specific. Third, using C5a receptor-deficient mice on a Balb/c background, we see a small protection in AHR following sensitization and challenge (similar but smaller in magnitude than the Abe result), but this paled in comparison to our reported results with C3a receptor-deficient mice (6). Fourth, we have recently cloned a second serpentine receptor for C5a anaphylatoxin, present in both mouse and human, that is not coupled to G proteins by virtue of a mutation in a critical G protein interaction site on the receptor (26). Thus, in the absence of C5, both receptors would go without ligand, which may influence the result in a complex way.

IV. Conclusions

Several recent reports using novel genetically engineered animals have provided evidence for a critical role for C3a/C3a receptor interactions in allergen-induced airways hyperresponsiveness, and two groups have independently provided evidence for anaphylatoxins specifically in the antigen-challenged human lung. Armed with these data, it is now feasible to perform a clinical test of efficacy in humans using complement inhibitors. Several inhibitors are available for such a clinical trial, including soluble CR1, anti-C5 monoclonal antibody, and small molecule antagonists for both the C3a and C5a receptors.

References

1. Medzhitov R, Janeway C Jr. Innate immunity. N Engl J Med 2000; 343:338–344.
2. Lambris JD, Reid KB, Volanakis JE. The evolution, structure, biology and pathophysiology of complement. Immunol Today 1999; 20:207–211.
3. Kohl J. Anaphylatoxins and infectious and non-infectious inflammatory diseases. Mol Immunol 2001; 38:175–187.
4. Gerard C, Gerard NP. C5a anaphylatoxin and its seven transmembrane-segment receptor. Annu Rev Immunol 1994; 12:775–808.
5. Gerard NP. Complement fragments. In: Barnes PJ, Grunstein M, Leff A, Woolcock AJ, eds. New York: Raven Press, 1997:639–652.
6. Humbles AA, Lu B, Nilsson CA, Lilly C, Israel E, Fujiwara Y, Gerard NP, Gerard C. A role for the C3a anaphylatoxin receptor in the effector phase of asthma. Nature 2000; 406:998–1001.
7. Bautsch W, Hoymann HG, Zhang Q, Meier-Wiedenbach I, Raschke U, Ames RS, Sohns B, Flemme N, Meyer zu Vilsendorf A, Grove M, Klos A, Kohl J. Cutting edge: guinea pigs with a natural C3a-receptor defect exhibit decreased bronchoconstriction in allergic airway disease: evidence for an involvement of the C3a anaphylatoxin in the pathogenesis of asthma. J Immunol 2000; 165:5401–5405.
8. Drouin SM, Kildsgaard J, Haviland J, Zabner J, Jia HP, McCray PB Jr, Tack BF, Wetsel RA. Expression of the complement anaphylatoxin C3a and C5a receptors on bronchial epithelial and smooth muscle cells in models of sepsis and asthma. J Immunol 2001; 166:2025–2032.
9. Daffern PJ, Pfeifer PH, Ember JA, Hugli TE. C3a is a chemotaxin for human eosinophils but not for neutrophils. I. C3a stimulation of neutrophils is secondary to eosinophil activation. J Exp Med 1995; 181:2119–2127.
10. Humbles AA, Lu B, Friend DS, Okinaga S, Lora J, Algarawi A, Martin TR, Gerard NP, Gerard C. The murine CCR3 receptor regulates both the role of eosinophils and mast cells in allergen-induced airway inflammation and hyperresponsiveness. Proc Natl Acad Sci USA 2002; 99:1479–1484.
11. Krug N, Tschernig T, Erpenbeck VJ, Hohlfeld JM, Kohl J. Complement factors C3a and C5a are increased in bronchoalveolar lavage fluid after segmental allergen provocation in subjects with asthma. Am J Respir Crit Care Med 2001; 164:1841–1843.
12. Karp CL, Grupe A, Schadt E, Ewart SL, Keane-Moore M, Cuomo PJ, Kohl J, Wahl L, Kuperman D, Germer S, Aud D, Peltz G, Wills-Karp M. Identification of complement factor 5 as a susceptibility locus for experimental allergic asthma. Nat Immunol 2000; 1:221–226.
13. Abe M, Shibata K, Akatsu H, Shimizu N, Sakata N, Katsuragi T, Okada H. Contribution of anaphylatoxin C5a to late airway responses after repeated exposure of antigen to allergic rats. J Immunol 2001; 167:4651–4660.

14. Regal JF, Klos A. Minor role of the C3a receptor in systemic anaphylaxis in the guinea pig. Immunopharmacology 2000; 46(1):15–28.

15. Stimler NP, Gerard C, O'Flaherty JT. Platelet-activating factor (AAGPC) contracts human lung tissues in vitro. In: Benveniste J, et al., eds. Proc. 1st Intl. Symp. on Platelet-Activating Factor, Inserm Symp. Vol. 23. Amsterdam: Elsevier 1983:195–204.

16. Lukacs NW, Glovsky MM, Ward PA. Complement-dependent immune complex-induced bronchial inflammation and hyperreactivity. Am J Physiol Lung Cell Mol Physiol 2001; 280:L512–518.

17. Andersson M, Michel L, Llull JB, Pipkorn U. Complement activation on the nasal mucosal surface—a feature of the immediate allergic reaction in the nose. Allergy 1994; 49:242–245.

18. Teran LM, Campos MG, Begishvilli BT, Schroder JM, Djukanovic R, Shute JK, Church MK, Holgate ST, Davies DE. Identification of neutrophil chemotactic factors in bronchoalveolar lavage fluid of asthmatic patients. Clin Exp Allergy 1997; 27:396–405.

19. Castro FF, Schmitz-Schumann M, Rother U, Kirschfink M. Complement activation by house dust: reduced reactivity of serum complement in patients with bronchial asthma. Int Arch Allergy Appl Immunol 1991; 96:305–310.

20. Nicholson-Weller A, Halperin JA. Membrane signaling by complement C5b-9, the membrane attack complex. Immunol Res 1993; 12:244–257.

21. Benzaquen LR, Nicholson-Weller A, Halperin JA. Terminal complement proteins C5b-9 release basic fibroblast growth factor and platelet-derived growth factor from endothelial cells. J Exp Med 1994; 179:985–992.

22. Wang C, Gerard NP, Nicholson-Weller A. Signalling by hemolytically inactive C5b67 (iC5b67), an agonist of polymorphonuclear leukocytes. J Immunol 1996; 156:786–792.

23. Dobrina A, Pausa M, Fischetti F, Bulla R, Vecile E, Ferrero E, Mantovani A, Tedesco F. Cytolytically inactive terminal complement complex causes transendothelial migration of polymorphonuclear leukocytes in vitro and in vivo. Blood 2002; 99:185–192.

24. Karp CL, Wills-Karp M. Complement and IL-12: yin and yang. Microbes Infect 2001; 2:109–119.

25. Heller T, Hennecke M, Baumann U, Gessner JE, zu Vilsendorf AM, Baensch M, Boulay F, Kola A, Klos A, Bautsch W, Kohl J. Selection of a C5a receptor antagonist from phage libraries attenuatingthe inflammatory response in immune complex disease and ischemia/reperfusion injury. J Immunol 1999; 163:985–994.

26. Slattery D, Okinaga S, Humbles A, Zsengeller Z, Morteau O, Kincade MB, Brodbeck RM, Krause JE, Choe H-R, Gerard NP, Gerard C. A second serpentine receptor for C5a anaphylatoxins.

34

Inflammatory and Structural Changes in Airway Remodeling of Asthma

ANTHONY E. REDINGTON

University of Hull
Hull, England

STEPHEN T. HOLGATE

University of Southampton
Southampton, England

I. Pathology of Airway Remodeling

A. Airway Thickening

Thickening of the airway wall was first recognized as a feature of asthma in several necropsy studies (1–4). In their classic study published in 1922, for example, Huber and Koessler (1) measured airway dimensions in postmortem tissue from six subjects with fatal asthma and seven nonasthmatic subjects. In bronchi of external diameter greater than 2 mm, the thickness of the airway wall was increased in those with asthma. These early reports relied on qualitative descriptions or on relatively imprecise methods of quantitation. The later recognition that the internal perimeter of an airway remains relatively constant at different lung volumes and with different degrees of airway smooth muscle shortening allowed internal perimeter to be used as a marker of airway size in comparative studies (5–7). Using this approach, James et al. (8) examined postmortem lung tissue from 18 subjects with asthma, the majority of whom had died during a severe episode, and 23 nonasthmatic control subjects. These authors confirmed an increase in total wall area in cartilaginous and membranous airways of all sizes, including small airways defined on the basis of an internal perimeter of <2 mm.

Other investigators have measured airway dimensions in tissue from subjects with fatal asthma and from subjects with a history of asthma who have died of other causes. Comparing study subjects with nonasthmatic controls, Carroll et al. (9) reported that the thickening in fatal asthma was most marked in large and small cartilaginous airways, although it was also evident in small membranous bronchioles. In nonfatal asthma, in contrast, airway thickening was confined to the small peripheral airways. In another study of similar design, Kuwano et al. (10) reported a stepwise increase in total wall area of membranous airways in nonasthmatic control subjects, subjects with nonfatal asthma, and subjects with fatal asthma.

B. Airway Smooth Muscle Hypertrophy and Hyperplasia

Thickening of the airway smooth muscle layer in asthma was described in many of the early postmortem reports (1,3,4,11–14), and in most (8–10), but not all (15), of the more recent morphometric studies. Carroll et al. (9), for example, found that in fatal asthma the area of this layer was more than doubled in cartilaginous airways of all sizes compared with nonasthmatic control cases. In nonfatal asthma, the increase was restricted to the larger membranous airways. Kuwano et al. (10) similarly reported that in fatal asthma the smooth muscle layer was two- to threefold thicker in all but the smallest airways.

In an early study confined to large airways, Heard and Hossain (13) suggested that hyperplasia rather than hypertrophy was the principal cellular pathology accounting for the increased airway smooth muscle mass. Detailed morphometric analyses later suggested two distinct types of smooth muscle thickening (16,17). In some cases, the process was restricted to large central airways and was associated exclusively with hyperplasia. In others, thickening was evident throughout the bronchial tree, with hypertrophy from the segmental bronchi to the terminal bronchioles and mild hyperplasia only in the larger bronchi. The significance of these two patterns is uncertain.

C. Subepithelial Fibrosis and Myofibroblast Hyperplasia

One of the most characteristic pathological features in asthmatic airways is the deposition of a layer of excess connective tissue beneath the airway epithelium (Fig. 1). This was first described in postmortem reports (1–4,18,19) and in studies using rigid bronchoscopy (20,21). Many bronchoscopy-based studies later confirmed the presence of subepithelial fibrosis in allergic asthma (22–31) and in other forms of the disease including intrinsic asthma (32), occupational asthma (33), and cough-variant asthma (34). Most reports have suggested that the depth of this layer is increased by a factor of 1.5- to 2.5-fold. Electron microscopy has demonstrated that it is the lamina reticularis that becomes thickened, whereas the lamina rara and lamina densa appear normal at the ultrastructural level (24,30,32,35,36). Because it can be measured fairly easily, depth of subepithelial fibrosis is frequently used as an index of airway remodeling. No detailed studies, however, have examined how closely this reflects other aspects of the remodeling response.

Immunohistochemical analysis has provided information regarding the molecular immunopathology of the subepithelial region. Roche et al. (23) described deposition of fibronectin and the interstitial collagens types III and V in the thickened

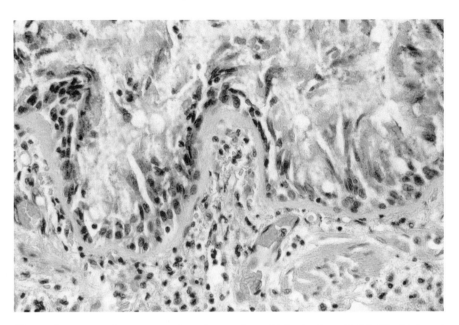

Figure 1 Section of postmortem tissue from patient with fatal asthma (H&E). The thickened layer of connective tissue beneath the airway epithelium is clearly visible. (Courtesy of Dr. A. Campbell, Hull Royal Infirmary.)

subepithelial band. Other investigators have confirmed an excess of interstitial collagens (33,37) and also of the adhesive glycoprotein tenascin-C (38). It was initially suggested that the pattern of immunostaining for laminin and collagen IV—molecules localized to the lamina rara and the lamina densa—was unaltered in asthma (23). In a detailed study using a range of laminin chain–specific antibodies, however, Altraja et al. (39) showed that chronic asthma is associated with the presence of laminin α2 and β2 chains in the subepithelial basement membrane, variants that normally are expressed only during fetal development.

Immediately below the lamina reticularis is a population of subepithelial mesenchymal cells that have the ultrastructural features of myofibroblasts (24,37). These cells appear to correspond to the "attenuated fibroblast sheath" described in the basement membrane zone in rat trachea (40) and to similar cell populations that exist in small airways (41) and in the pulmonary interstitium (42). Although myofibroblasts are morphologically intermediate between fibroblasts and smooth muscle cells (43), they are not functional intermediates. In particular, their ability to synthesize collagen, especially types I and III, is greater than that of fibroblasts in vitro (44,45), and they are the cells principally responsible for increased lung collagen gene expression in an animal model of pulmonary fibrosis (46). Brewster et al. (24) reported increased numbers of subepithelial myofibroblasts in bronchoscopic biopsy specimens from asthmatics. Moreover, there was a correlation between cell number and depth of the lamina reticularis, suggesting that these cells are responsible for connective tissue deposition in the region. More recently, Gizycki et al. (47) showed that acute exposure to allergen resulted in a marked increase in the numbers of these cells in bronchial biopsy specimens from sensitized asthmatic subjects.

The fibrotic process in asthma may extend to the deeper layers of the airway wall, but there have been some conflicting reports. Minshall et al. (48) reported a stepwise increase in fibrosis in the lamina propria in biopsy specimens from patients with mild, moderate, and severe asthma. Increased immunostaining for collagen types III and V at this site has also been reported (29). On the other hand, Chu et al. (31) could detect no difference in total collagen, detected by Sirius red staining, or in collagen types I and III evaluated immunohistochemically in asthmatics with disease of varying grades of severity compared to nonasthmatic control subjects. In another study, Godfrey et al. (49) found no alteration in the proportion of subepithelial area occupied by collagen fibers in either mild or more severe asthma.

D. Vascularity

Dilatation of capillary blood vessels in the bronchial mucosa was described as a striking feature in a report of 20 cases of fatal asthma (4). Several recent studies have quantitated changes in vessel numbers and vascular volume in the airway wall in asthma. In a study confined to peripheral airways, Kuwano et al. (10) found that the proportion of submucosal area occupied by vessels was increased from 0.6% in nonasthmatic individuals to 3.3% in those with asthma. Carroll et al. (50) reported that the number and area of large blood vessels were increased in large cartilaginous airways in cases of fatal asthma, although the total number of vessels and area occupied were similar in fatal asthma, nonfatal asthma, and control tissue. Several bronchoscopy-based studies have now confirmed increases in submucosal vascularity in biopsy specimens from subjects with mild asthma (51–54) and with more severe disease (55).

E. Glandular Changes

Prominence of mucus-secreting submucosal glands was described in most (3,11,12,18), although not all (20), of the early fatal asthma autopsy reports. Several subsequent morphometric studies have found increases in the proportion of the bronchial wall occupied by mucous glands in fatal and severe asthma (9,56,57). In the study of Carroll et al. (9), the mucous gland area was increased in fatal asthma compared to nonasthmatic control subjects in cartilaginous airways of all sizes. Measurements in nonfatal asthma were intermediate between those in fatal asthma and in control subjects. The relative proportions of mucous and serous acini appear to be preserved in asthma (20).

An increase in the area of the airway epithelium occupied by goblet cells has also been described by several investigators (56–58). Ordoñez et al. (58), for example, used the approach of "design-based stereology" to measure goblet cell size and numbers in bronchial biopsy specimens. These authors reported that the number of goblet cells was 2.5-fold greater in specimens from individuals with mild and moderate asthma, but that their size was not altered. There was an accompanying increase in stored mucin. Increased goblet cell numbers might result from either hyperplasia or metaplasia.

F. Elastic Tissue

Godfrey et al. (49) used electron-microscopy-based morphometric methods to determine the relative area of the subepithelial zone in bronchial biopsy specimens that was occupied by elastic fibers. No significant differences were apparent between subjects with mild asthma, asthmatic subjects receiving short-term or long-term treatment with inhaled corticosteroids, subjects with fatal asthma, and nonasthmatic control subjects. On the other hand, Bousquet et al. (59) described histochemical and ultrastructural evidence of elastolysis in asthmatic airways. Carroll et al. (60) studied the network of elastic fibers that form longitudinal bundles, in association with collagen and myofibroblasts, in the airway submucosa. In fatal asthma, the area of these bundles was increased in large and small airways, but their elastin content was reduced.

G. Cartilage

Early studies found no alterations in the proportional area of the airway wall occupied by cartilage in asthma (11,12). Carroll et al. (9), however, reported that the area of cartilage was increased in segmental and subsegmental airways in subjects with fatal asthma. In another morphometric study, Haraguchi et al. (61) described degenerative change in cartilage and perichondrial fibrosis in airways 3–8 mm in diameter in three subjects with fatal asthma.

II. Imaging of Airway Remodeling

In many cases of uncomplicated asthma, the plain chest radiograph may be normal or simply show evidence of hyperinflation (62). Bronchial wall thickening is also a frequent finding, however, with prevalence figures of 46% (63) and 71% (64) reported in two surveys. This feature appears most common in those subjects with the most severe disease (63).

High-resolution computed tomographic (HRCT) scanning provides more detailed information about the airways and lung parenchyma. Qualitative surveys of HRCT images of the lungs have demonstrated a number of abnormalities in asthma, especially bronchial wall thickening, cylindric bronchiectasis, and emphysema (63–68). In particular, the reported prevalence of bronchial wall thickening has been over 80% in several of these studies (64,66,68). This feature has been interpreted as the radiographic correlate of airway remodeling, although additional factors such as edema and inflammatory cell infiltration may contribute to bronchial wall thickening.

Several investigators have examined the relationship between airway dimensions on HRCT scans and indexes of disease severity. Boulet et al. (69) determined the wall thickness: outer diameter ratio of a large airway, the intermediate bronchus, in asthmatic subjects with and without fixed airflow obstruction and in nonasthmatic control subjects. In their initial report, measurements did not differ significantly between the three groups, although in asthmatic subjects with fixed airflow obstruction there was a negative correlation between this ratio and the methacholine PC_{20} (69). In a subsequent study of a larger number of subjects with incomplete reversibility of airflow obstruction, however, Hudon et al. (70) found that the wall thickness: diameter ratio of the intermediate bronchus was increased. Okazawa et al. (71) studied small airway dimensions and found a significant increase in wall thickness in subjects with mild to moderate asthma. Finally, Awadh et al. (72) measured airway dimensions in 40 asthmatics with disease of varying severity. There was a small increase in wall thickness and area in patients with mild asthma compared to healthy control subjects, but more marked increases in subjects with moderate asthma and with near-fatal asthma. The pattern of changes observed was similar in both large and small airways.

Ethical considerations regarding the radiation dose associated with HRCT mean that it is probably unsuitable for use in epidemiological studies requiring repeated measurements in large numbers of subjects. There is, therefore, a need for alternative strategies to image the airways. The technique of optical coherence tomography, which has been used to define upper respiratory tract anatomy in patients with suspected obstructive sleep apnea (73), holds some promise in this regard.

III. Mechanisms of Airway Remodeling

A. Epithelial Dysfunction

The airway epithelial layer forms a physical barrier between the external environment and the internal milieu of the lung and is subject to repeated contact with allergens, viruses, air pollutants, and other potentially injurious stimuli. Many investigators have suggested that damage to or fragility of the airway epithelium is a characteristic pathological feature of asthma. For example, epithelial desquamation in asthma has been described in autopsy tissue (1,2,4,18) and in bronchial biopsy specimens obtained by rigid (21,74) or fiberoptic (22,75) bronchoscopy. Increased numbers of epithelial cells in bronchoalveolar lavage (BAL) fluid have been reported in several studies (76–78). Finally, clusters of columnar epithelial cells (Creola bodies) are frequently present in sputum of patients with asthma (79). The principal site of disruption appears to lie at the plane between the basal and suprabasal cell layers (80).

Not all studies have confirmed these findings (9,27,81), and some investigators have expressed concern that the changes described might be artifactual (82). Lackie et al. (83), however, reported that expression of the cell-surface proteoglycan CD44 was strongly increased in areas of asthmatic epithelium where basal cells had lost their columnar cell attachments, but not in comparable areas of nonasthmatic epithelium (Fig. 2). Increased CD44 expression is also associated with bronchial epithelial repair in vitro (84), supporting the view that the in vivo damage is intrinsic rather than a consequence of the biopsy procedure or of tissue processing. Similar findings have been reported in relation to the epidermal growth factor receptor (EGFR) (85,86). In nonasthmatic tissue, immunostaining for this molecule was largely confined to basal cells, whereas in asthmatic airways it was seen throughout the epithelial layer, and the proportion of the epithelial area immunostained was positively correlated with the extent of subepithelial fibrosis. Furthermore, intense EGFR immunostaining was seen in areas of epithelial damage in bronchial biopsy specimens from asthmatic subjects, but not in similar areas from control subjects.

Expression of the EGFR is also associated with a repair phenotype in vitro. Using a model of epithelial wounding and repair in 16HBE 14o- human bronchial epithelial cell monolayers, Puddicombe et al. (85) showed that injury by mechanical scraping resulted in a localized increase in EGFR immunostaining at the wound edge and rapid phosphorylation/activation of the receptor. Increased EGFR expression appears not to be paralleled by a hyperproliferative response, however, as basal cell expression of proliferating cell nuclear antigen (PCNA) is unaltered in asthma despite extensive epithelial shedding (87). This may be due to high local levels of antiproliferative growth factors such as transforming growth factor (TGF)-β1 and TGF-β2, which are released and activated in response to injury (85,88) and elevated in BAL fluid from asthmatic subjects in vivo (89). These observations have led to the hypothesis that the airway epithelium in asthma has an increased susceptibility

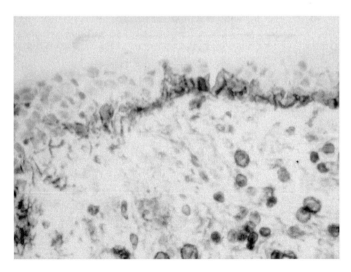

Figure 2   Immunohistochemical staining for CD44 in bronchial biopsy specimen from patient with asthma. Increased immunostaining of basal cells can be seen at the site of epithelial disruption. Positively staining cells are also evident in the subepithelial region. (Courtesy of J. E. Baker, Southampton General Hospital.)

to injury and an impaired ability to repair itself, resulting from an imbalance in signaling by members of the EGF and TGF-β families. Structurally intact epithelium may therefore be "locked" into a repair phenotype in which it sustains airway inflammation and remodeling by continued release of proinflammatory and profibrotic mediators.

The likely functional impact of epithelial injury on the underlying mesenchymal cells has been explored using three-dimensional in vitro coculture systems. Zhang et al. (90) embedded myofibroblasts derived from human bronchial wall in a collagen gel and cultured 16HBE 14o- cells on the surface of the gel. Chemical injury to the epithelial cell layer by poly-L-arginine, a surrogate for eosinophil granule cationic proteins, stimulated a myofibroblast proliferative response. Conditioned medium from mechanically damaged epithelial cells also increased myofibroblast proliferation. Levels of TGF-β2, platelet-derived growth factor (PDGF), fibroblast growth factor (FGF)-2, and endothelin (ET)-1 in the culture supernatants increased after epithelial injury, and the proliferative response could be reduced by 76% by blocking these growth factors.

Another system involves guinea pig tracheal epithelial cells cultured on an amniotic membrane with tracheal fibroblasts cultured beneath (91). The epithelial cells differentiate into a pseudostratified layer that closely resembles the tracheal epithelium in vivo. Morishima et al. (92) used this model to examine the consequences of epithelial injury induced by mechanical scraping. In parallel with reepithelialization and epithelial redifferentiation, fibroblasts were induced to adopt a transient myofibroblastic phenotype, as determined by α-smooth muscle actin (SMA) expression and ultrastructural features, and expression of collagen type I and III precursors was increased. These processes were associated with the release of extracellular matrix–bound TGF-β1, and the critical role of TGF-β1 in myofibroblast induction in this model was confirmed by neutralizing experiments.

Bronchoscopy-based studies have reported overexpression of several epithelium-derived growth factors in asthma, including TGF-β1 (89,93), FGF-2 (53,94), and ET-1 (95–97). Considered together with the in vitro findings, these studies point to an important role for airway epithelial cells in initiating and maintaining the remodeling process through their interactions with subepithelial mesenchymal cells. In this respect, the airway epithelium and the underlying mesenchyme may be considered together as an anatomical and functional configuration that has been termed the epithelial-mesenchymal trophic unit (EMTU). The recently described pores in the basement membrane may act to facilitate communication between the two compartments (98).

B. Airway Inflammation

Most forms of asthma are characterized by a chronic inflammatory process, in which infiltration and activation of mast cells and eosinophils are prominent features. Both these cell types are capable of synthesizing and releasing mediators that may contribute directly to airway remodeling. Several studies have identified eosinophils as an important source of TGF-β1 gene expression in asthmatic airways, particularly in patients with severe disease (48,93,99). Furthermore, Minshall et al. (48) reported a direct correlation between the number of TGF-β1 mRNA+ cells and depth of subepithelial fibrosis. Similarly, eosinophils have been shown to represent a major cellular source of PDGF in bronchial biopsy specimens from patients with severe asthma (100). Mast cells also express several growth factors including TGF-β1 (101) and FGF-2 (102). In addition the mast cell enzyme tryptase, a major product released upon degranulation, is able to stimulate fibroblasts to proliferate (103) and to synthesize collagen type I (104).

The airway inflammatory response in asthma is believed to be orchestrated by a population of T lymphocytes that are polarized towards a Th2 phenotype (105). These cells secrete a specific profile of cytokines including interleukin (IL)-3, -4, -5, -9, and -13, and granulocyte-macrophage colony-stimulating factor (GM-CSF), all of which are encoded in a gene cluster on chromosome 5q31–33 (106). Although these Th2 cytokines have been characterized as proinflammatory mediators in asthmatic airways, many are also able to reproduce one or more components of the remodeling response. For example, overexpression of cytokines such as IL-1β (107), IL-6 (108), IL-9 (109), IL-11 (110), IL-13 (111), tumor necrosis factor (TNF)-α (112), and GM-CSF (113,114) in rodent lungs—achieved using either adenovirus vectors or genetically transgenic animals—leads to a fibrotic response and in some cases also to myofibroblast hyperplasia.

The mechanism of this response has been explored in detail in the case of IL-13. Targeted overexpression of an IL-13 transgene in murine lungs using the CC10 promoter reproduces many of the features of the remodeling response in asthmatic airways, including subepithelial fibrosis, mucus hypersecretion, and airway hyperresponsiveness to methacholine (111). The profibrotic properties of IL-13 in vitro are relatively weak: it dose have some mitogenic activity for human bronchial fibroblasts, but does not induce myofibroblastic transformation or activate collagen synthesis (115). IL-13 does, however, induce release of TGF-β2 by cultured airway epithelial cells (115), suggesting that its profibrotic effect may be mainly secondary to epithelial activation. The dependence of IL-13–induced fibrosis on stimulation and activation of TGF-β has also been demonstrated in vivo using a soluble antagonist (116).

These findings illustrate how the Th2 airway inflammatory response may functionally interact with the EMTU to cause airway remodeling. In this respect, the EMTU may be seen as an integrated unit that coordinates the airway responses both to injury and to Th2 cytokines through the release and activation of TGF-β.

C. Mechanical Stress

A recent hypothesis has proposed that airway remodeling may be instigated by the sustained mechanical stresses associated with bronchoconstriction and buckling of the epithelial layer. Using a system of cocultured human bronchial epithelial cells and human lung fibroblasts, Swartz et al. (117) showed that a hydrostatic pressure difference across the epithelial layer resulted in increased synthesis of collagens, particularly type III, by the fibroblasts. The mechanisms involved in this response are not yet fully understood. Epithelial fibronectin expression was increased, but conditioned medium from epithelial cells exposed to mechanical stress failed to reproduce the fibroblast response. Nevertheless, in the presence of a susceptible epithelium this novel mechanism provides a potential route for airway remodeling to occur in the absence of any inflammatory stimulus.

IV. Pathophysiological Consequences of Airway Remodeling

A. Airway Hyperresponsiveness

Several studies have examined the functional consequences of airway remodeling mathematically by calculating its potential effects on the mechanics of the airway and its ability to conduct airflow (118–120). These models are based on a consideration of the geometric effects of airway thickening and on simulated computational dose-response curves. They predict that small increases in the thickness of the peripheral airway walls that do not reduce baseline resistance to airflow can amplify the effect of smooth muscle shortening on airway caliber. On this basis, Wiggs et al. (120) predicted that the magnitude of airway thickening observed in morphometric studies could contribute substantially to airway hyperresponsiveness in asthma. This is consistent with the inverse correlation demonstrated between methacholine responsiveness and bronchial wall thickness on HRCT (69). In a later modification of the mathematical model, Lambert et al. (121) suggested that the increase in the airway smooth muscle layer was the most important feature accounting for hyperresponsiveness.

Mathematical models also provide information about how airway remodeling can alter the pattern of mucosal folding, or buckling, that occurs with smooth muscle shortening. These studies have suggested that differences in mucosal folding patterns can have important effects on airway narrowing (122,123). In particular, thickening or stiffening of the thin inner structural layer may lead to a reduced number of mucosal folds and an enhancement of luminal narrowing (124). The mechanical properties of the thickened subepithelial collagen layer in asthma may therefore contribute to airway hyperresponsiveness. In support of this, there are now many reports of inverse correlations between the depth of this layer and methacholine or histamine responsiveness measurement as the PC_{20} in asthma (26–28,30,125).

B. Decline of Lung Function

Many investigators have reported that subjects with asthma have an accelerated decline of lung function in adult life compared with the general population (126–130). In a longitudinal community-based study in Copenhagen, Denmark, for example, Lange et al. (130) found that unadjusted FEV_1 declined by an average of 38 mL per year among adults with self-reported asthma and 22 mL per year in nonasthmatic control subjects (130) The negative influence of asthma on FEV_1 was seen in both smokers and nonsmokers. Some patients experience very steep rates of decline in lung function, leading to poorly reversible or irreversible airflow obstruction (70,131,132). Cross-sectional studies have also shown that lung function measurements are lower than predicted in adults with asthma (133–136). The degree of impairment appears related to both the duration and severity of disease.

There has been speculation that loss of lung function in asthma is a consequence of longstanding airway inflammation leading to the chronic and irreversible structural changes of remodeling. There is, however, little experimental evidence for this at present. In part, this no doubt reflects the inherent difficulty in studying the question, and in particular the lack of a validated noninvasive marker of remodeling that can be used in longitudinal studies. Some support derives from the HRCT studies discussed above, demonstrating increased airway wall thickening in those subjects with irreversible airflow obstruction (70) and those with the most severe disease (72). Furthermore, a recent study of airway morphometry in fatal asthma showed that the degree of airway thickening was greatest in those older individuals with the longest duration of disease (137). On the other hand, bronchoscopy-based (23,26–28,30,31,125) and postmortem (137) studies have repeatedly failed to demonstrate a correlation between depth of subepithelial fibrosis and disease duration, and reports of inverse correlations between subepithelial fibrosis and FEV_1 have been inconsistent.

C. Airway Distensibility

Two studies have shown that the airways of subjects with asthma are less distensible than normal airways (138,139). Stiffer airways, lacking the ability to passively dilate normally, may contribute to nonreversible airflow limitation. There has been speculation that this phenomenon is caused by airway remodeling, but this has not been examined directly.

V. Antiasthma Therapies and Airway Remodeling

A. Inhaled Corticosteroids

The first study to investigate treatment with an inhaled corticosteroid and airway remodeling failed to demonstrate an effect. Jeffery et al. (25) measured subepithelial basement membrane thickness in 11 subjects with mild atopic asthma before and after regular inhaled treatment for 4 weeks with either budesonide (400 µg daily) or terbutaline. Pretreatment values were higher than in nonasthmatic control subjects, but there was no significant change after the inhaled corticosteroid. The small sample size and the low dose and short duration of treatment may all have limited the ability of this study to detect a significant change. Measurements were also very similar, however, in a separate group of 10 subjects with severe asthma who had taken inhaled corticosteroid treatment for at least 6 months.

More recent bronchoscopic studies, in contrast, have reported treatment-related improvements in indexes of remodeling in subjects receiving inhaled corticosteroids. In a placebo-controlled parallel group study, Olivieri et al. (140) found that treatment with fluticasone propionate 500 µg daily for 6 weeks significantly reduced the depth of the subepithelial reticular layer. Unfortunately, interpretation of this report is limited by the fact that the two groups were poorly matched for pretreatment baseline values. Sont et al. (141) studied 75 adults with mild-to-moderate asthma whose dose of inhaled corticosteroid (budesonide or beclometasone dipropionate) was adjusted using either a reference strategy, based on symptoms, PEF variability, and FEV_1, or an airway hyperresponsiveness strategy aimed additionally at improving methacholine PC_{20}. Over the 2-year study period, the median dose of inhaled corticosteroid was 400 μg daily higher in the airway hyperresponsiveness group. In those patients who underwent bronchoscopy before and after treatment, the thickness of the subepithelial layer was significantly reduced in the airway hyperresponsiveness strategy group, but not in the reference-strategy group.

Other investigators have used immunohistochemical methods to study the effects of inhaled corticosteroids on specific molecular components. In a placebo-controlled study, Trigg et al. (142) described reduced subepithelial expression of collagen type III after 4 months of treatment with inhaled beclometasone dipropionate 1000 μg daily. However, despite randomization, the subjects receiving placebo in that study had higher pretreatment measurements than those receiving active treatment. There was therefore no significant difference between the two groups in posttreatment values. In patients with birch-pollen sensitive asthma, Laitinen et al. (38) reported that immunoreactive tenascin-C expression was decreased after treatment with inhaled budesonide 800 μg daily.

B. Short-Acting β₂-Agonists

Few reports have specifically addressed the effects of short-acting β_2-agonists on airway remodeling. Jeffery et al. (25) studied five subjects with mild asthma who had previously been taking a short-acting β_2-agonist less than once daily and found no effect of regular treatment with terbutaline 500 μg four times daily on the thickness of the lamina reticularis. Altraja et al. (143), however, reported that albuterol (salbuterol) 200 μg four times daily significantly reduced subepithelial expression of tenascin-C. This is a surprising result that, until replicated, should perhaps be treated with caution.

C. Long-Acting β₂-Agonists

Roberts et al. (144) reported a study of treatment for 6 weeks with the long-acting β_2-agonist salmeterol 50 μg twice daily in subjects with mild asthma. No effect was identified on the depth of the sub-basement membrane collagen layer measured in electron micrographs. This is consistent with the reported failure of salmeterol to exert a demonstrable airway anti-inflammatory effect in this (144) and in other (145,146) bronchoscopy-based studies. There is some evidence that formoterol may exert a weak anti-inflammatory effect in the airways (147,148), but its possible effect on remodeling has not been reported.

D. Cromones

Nedocromil sodium inhibits the activation of many inflammatory cells in vitro (149–152), but two bronchoscopy-based studies have suggested that its airway anti-inflammatory properties in vivo are at best weak (143,153). Consistent with this, Altraja et al. (143) reported that treatment with nedocromil sodium 4 mg four times daily for 12 weeks did not result in significant changes in subepithelial expression of collagen types III, IV, or VII, or of tenascin-C. The possible influence of sodium cromoglycate on airway remodeling has not been reported.

E. Leukotriene Receptor Antagonists

The cysteinyl leukotriene LTD_4 can augment mitogen-induced proliferation of airway smooth muscle cells (154), and leukotriene pathways have recently been implicated in a murine model of airway remodeling (155). Although there is evidence that the leukotriene receptor antagonists montelukast (156), zafirlukast (157), and pranlukast (158) exert anti-inflammatory effect in the airways, the ability of these agents to influence airway remodeling has not been reported in human asthma.

F. Theophylline

Several bronchoscopic studies have suggested that theophylline has anti-inflammatory properties in asthma (159–161). Furthermore, theophylline and other phosphodiesterase inhibitors can modulate the proliferative and synthetic properties of fibroblasts and airway smooth muscle cells in vitro (162,163). The possible influence of these agents on remodeling in vivo has not been reported.

VI. Prevention of Airway Remodeling

A potentially important question is whether some form of intervention strategy, for example with drug treatment or allergen avoidance, might prevent airway remodeling from occurring.

There is no direct information about this at present, but some indirect evidence derives from several studies suggesting that early introduction of inhaled corticosteroids in asthma is associated with the greatest potential for improvement. Haahtela et al. (164,165) studied more than 100 asthmatic patients with recently diagnosed asthma who had not previously taken any form of anti-inflammatory therapy. They were randomly assigned to receive regular treatment with either an inhaled corticosteroid (budesonide 1200 μg daily) or an inhaled short-acting β_2-agonist (terbutaline). Treatment with budesonide led to a reduction in symptoms, improvements in PEF and FEV_1, and a decrease in airway hyperresponsiveness. In the terbutaline-treated subjects, by contrast, there were no significant changes in symptoms or lung function. The study then continued into a third year, during which 37 subjects who had received terbutaline during the initial 2-year period were crossed over in an open manner to treatment with budesonide. Although improvements in lung function did occur in patients starting budesonide treatment more than 2 years after diagnosis, these responses were significantly smaller than those in subjects who had commenced treatment soon after diagnosis.

This is consistent with information about the relation between duration of disease and response to inhaled corticosteroids. Selroos et al. (166) retrospectively studied changes in lung function after starting budesonide therapy in a group of over 100 adult patients with mild or moderate asthma. Patients were stratified according to the duration of their pretreatment symptoms, which ranged from 6 months to more than 10 years. The authors found an inverse relationship between duration of asthma symptoms and maximum improvements in FEV_1 and PEF, suggesting that a delay in treatment may lead to irreversible airways obstruction. Agertoft et al. (167) made similar observations in asthmatic children starting budesonide therapy: the annual increase in FEV_1 was greatest in those children whose asthma was shortest in duration.

There is also evidence that inhaled corticosteroids may modify the accelerated loss of lung function in asthma. Dompeling et al. (168) studied 56 patients with obstructive lung disease—about half of whom had asthma—who had been shown to have a rate of decline of FEV_1 of at least 80 mL per year. These subjects, all previously treated with bronchodilators alone, then received treatment with beclometasone dipropionate 800 μg daily for 2 years. In the asthmatic group, there was a marked improvement in FEV_1 over the first 6 months, followed by a progressive decline during months 7–24. However, the rate of decline in prebronchodilator FEV_1 (100 mL/yr) was significantly less than in the preceding period of treatment with bronchodilators alone (173 mL/yr).

Considered together, these studies suggest that some capacity for functional reversibility is lost when treatment with inhaled corticosteroids is delayed, and that these agents may modify the unfavorable disease course seen with bronchodilators alone, at least in those subjects with the steepest rates of decline. Although these observations are intriguing, the studies are nonrandomized and are open to other methodological criticisms. Additionally, it must be emphasized that remodeling has not been examined directly. The relation between airway remodeling and both lung-function parameters and clinical indexes of disease severity is uncertain.

The natural history of remodeling also needs to be considered in this context. At least in the case of subepithelial fibrosis, it is clear that this develops very early in the course of disease. For example, it is already established in adult asthmatics with early and mild disease (169), i.e., appears soon after exposure to occupational sensitizers (33), and has been described in postmortem tissue (36,170), resected lung tissue (36), and bronchoscopic biopsy specimens (171) from children with asthma. Indeed, there is evidence that subepithelial fibrosis may be present in the airways of children up to 2 years before the onset of clinical symptoms of asthma (172). There may therefore be difficulties if a "window of opportunity" exists, after which intervention is less effective or ineffective.

VII. Conclusions and Future Directions

The pathological changes in airway remodeling are now reasonably clear, and rapid progress is being made to unravel the cellular and molecular mechanisms that underlie them. When viewing remodeling as a therapeutic target in asthma, however, there are a number of issues that must be considered. At present, the physiological significance of airway remodeling and its relationship to the natural history of the disease are still poorly understood, relying to a large extent on inference and on mathematical modeling. A biomarker that would predict remodeling would be extremely valuable to define these issues more clearly. It may be that some asthmatic patients are at risk of developing clinically significant remodeling, while others are not. Identification of those who are at risk, perhaps on the basis of particular polymorphisms that determine differences in host response, might allow antiremodeling therapies to be targeted appropriately. Novel therapies will likely be developed, and animal models of airway remodeling, based on overexpression of candidate mediators or on chronic antigen exposure, will no doubt be informative in identifying appropriate targets. However, it seems unlikely that any single mediator will be sufficient to account for the complexity of the remodeling response seen in vivo.

References

1. Huber HL, Koessler KK. The pathology of bronchial asthma. Arch Intern Med 1922; 30:689–760.
2. Houston JC, de Navasquez S, Trounce JR. A clinical and pathological study of fatal cases of status asthmaticus. Thorax 1953; 8:207–213.
3. Messer JW, Peters GA, Bennett WA. Causes of death and pathologic findings in 304 cases of bronchial asthma. Dis Chest 1960; 38:616–624.
4. Dunnill MS. The pathology of asthma, with special reference to changes in the bronchial mucosa. J Clin Pathol 1960; 13:27–33.
5. James AL, Paré PD, Moreno RH, Hogg JC. Quantitative measurement of smooth muscle shortening in isolated pig trachea. J Appl Physiol 1987; 63:1360–1365.
6. James AL, Hogg JC, Dunn LA, Paré PD. The use of the internal perimeter to compare airway size and to calculate smooth muscle shortening. Am Rev Respir Dis 1988; 138: 136–139.
7. James AL, Paré PD, Hogg JC. Effects of lung volume, bronchoconstriction, and cigarette smoke on morphometric airway dimensions. J Appl Physiol 1988; 64:913–919.
8. James AL, Paré PD, Hogg JC. The mechanics of airway narrowing in asthma. Am Rev Respir Dis 1989; 139:242–246.
9. Carroll N, Elliot J, Morton A, James A. The structure of large and small airways in nonfatal and fatal asthma. Am Rev Respir Dis 1993; 147:405–410.
10. Kuwano K, Bosken CH, Paré PD, Bai TR, Wiggs BR, Hogg JC. Small airways dimensions in asthma and in chronic obstructive pulmonary disease. Am Rev Respir Dis 1993; 148:1220–1225.
11. Dunnill MS, Massarella GR, Anderson JA. A comparison of the quantitative anatomy of the bronchi in normal subjects, in status asthmaticus, in chronic bronchitis, and in emphysema. Thorax 1969; 24:176–179.
12. Takizawa T, Thurlbeck WM. Muscle and mucous gland size in the major bronchi of patients with chronic bronchitis, asthma, and asthmatic bronchitis. Am Rev Respir Dis 1971; 104:331–336.
13. Heard BE, Hossain S. Hyperplasia of bronchial muscle in asthma. J Pathol 1972; 110: 319–331.

14. Hossain S. Quantitative measurement of bronchial muscle in men with asthma. Am Rev Respir Dis 1973; 107:99–109.
15. Thomson RJ, Bramley AM, Schellenberg RR. Airway muscle stereology: implications for increased shortening in asthma. Am J Respir Crit Care Med 1996; 154:749–757.
16. Ebina M, Yaegashi H, Chiba R, Takahashi T, Motomiya M, Tanemura M. Hyperreactive site in the airway tree of asthmatic patients revealed by thickening of bronchial muscles: a morphometric study. Am Rev Respir Dis 1990; 141:1327–1332.
17. Ebina M, Takahashi T, Chiba T, Motomiya M. Cellular hypertrophy and hyperplasia of airway smooth muscles underlying bronchial asthma: a 3-D morphometric study. Am Rev Respir Dis 1993; 148:720–726.
18. Cardell BS, Pearson RSB. Death in asthmatics. Thorax 1959; 14:341–352.
19. Sobonya RE. Quantitative structural alterations in long-standing allergic asthma. Am Rev Respir Dis 1984; 130:289–292.
20. Glynn AA, Michaels L. Bronchial biopsy in chronic bronchitis and asthma. Thorax 1960; 15:142–153.
21. Salvato G. Some histological changes in chronic bronchitis and asthma. Thorax 1968; 23:168–172.
22. Jeffery PK, Wardlaw AJ, Nelson FC, Collins JV, Kay AB. Bronchial biopsies in asthma: an ultrastructural, quantitative study and correlation with hyperreactivity. Am Rev Respir Dis 1989; 140:1745–1753.
23. Roche WR, Beasley R, Williams JH, Holgate ST. Subepithelial fibrosis in the bronchi of asthmatics. Lancet 1989; i:520–524.
24. Brewster CEP, Howarth PH, Djukanovic R, Wilson J, Holgate ST, Roche WR. Myofibroblasts and subepithelial fibrosis in bronchial asthma. Am J Respir Cell Mol Biol 1990; 3:507–511.
25. Jeffery PK, Godfrey RW, Ädelroth E, Nelson F, Rogers A, Johansson S-A. Effects of treatment on airway inflammation and thickening of basement membrane reticular collagen in asthma: a quantitative light and electron microscopic study. Am Rev Respir Dis 1992; 145:890–899.
26. Cho SH, Seo JY, Choi DC, Yoon HJ, Cho YJ, Min KU, Lee GK, Seo JW, Kim YY. Pathological changes according to the severity of asthma. Clin Exp Allergy 1996; 26: 1210–1219.
27. Boulet L-P, Laviolette M, Turcotte H, Cartier A, Dugas M, Malo J-L, Boutet M. Bronchial subepithelial fibrosis correlates with airway responsiveness to methacholine. Chest 1997; 112:45–52.
28. Chetta A, Foresi A, Del Donno M, Bertorelli G, Pesci A, Olivieri D. Airways remodeling is a distinctive feature of asthma and is related to severity of disease. Chest 1997; 111:852–857.
29. Wilson JW, Li X. The measurement of reticular basement membrane and submucosal collagen in the asthmatic airway. Clin Exp Allergy 1997; 27:363–371.
30. Hoshino M, Nakamura Y, Sim JJ. Expression of growth factors and remodelling of the airway wall in bronchial asthma. Thorax 1998; 53:21–27.
31. Chu HW, Halliday JL, Martin RJ, Leung DYM, Szefler SJ, Wenzel SE. Collagen deposition in large airways may not differentiate severe asthma from milder forms of the disease. Am J Respir Crit Care Med 1998; 158:1936–1944.
32. Molina C, Brun J, Coulet M, Betail G, Delage J. Immunopathology of the bronchial mucosa in "late-onset" asthma. Clin Allergy 1977; 7:137–145.
33. Saetta M, Di Stefano A, Maestrelli P, De Marzo N, Milani GF, Pivirotto F, Mapp CE, Fabbri LM. Airway mucosal inflammation in occupational asthma induced by toluene diisocyanate. Am Rev Respir Dis 1992; 145:160–168.

34. Niimi A, Matsumoto H, Minakuchi M, Kitaichi M, Amitani R. Airway remodelling in cough-variant asthma. Lancet 2000; 356:564–565.

35. McCarter JH, Vazquez JJ. The bronchial basement membrane in asthma: immunohisto-chemical and ultrastructural observations. Arch Path 1966; 82:328–335.

36. Cutz E, Levison H, Cooper DM. Ultrastructure of airways in children with asthma. Histopathology 1978; 2:407–421.

37. Chakir J, Laviolette M, Boutet M, Laliberté R, Dubé J, Boulet L-P. Lower airways remodeling in nonasthmatic subjects with allergic rhinitis. Lab Invest 1996; 75: 735–744.

38. Laitinen A, Altraja A, Kämpe M, Linden M, Virtanen I, Laitinen LA. Tenascin is increased in airway basement membrane of asthmatics and decreased by an inhaled steroid. Am J Respir Crit Care Med 1997; 156:951–958.

39. Altraja A, Laitinen A, Virtanen I, Kämpe M, Simonsson BG, Karlsson S-E, Håkansson L, Venge P, Sillastu H, Laitinen LA. Expression of laminins in the airways in various types of asthmatic patients: a morphometric survey. Am J Respir Cell Mol Biol 1996; 15:482–488.

40. Evans MJ, Guha SC, Cox RA, Moller PC. Attenuated fibroblast sheath around the basement membrane zone in the trachea. Am J Respir Cell Mol Biol 1993; 8:188–192.

41. Plopper CA, Mariassy AT, Hill LH. Ultrastructure of the nonciliated bronchiolar epithe-lial (Clara) cell of mammalian lung: I. A comparison of rabbit, guinea pig, rat, hamster, and mouse. Exp Lung Res 1980; 1:139–154.

42. Kapanci Y, Assimacopoulos A, Irle C, Zwahlen A, Gabbiani G. "Contractile interstitial cells" in pulmonary alveolar septa: a possible regulator of ventilation-perfusion ratio? Ultrastructural, immunofluorescence, and in vitro studies. J Cell Biol 1974; 60: 375–392.

43. Gabbiani G, Ryan GB, Majno G. Presence of modified fibroblasts in granulation tissue and their possible role in wound contraction. Experientia 1971; 27:549–550.

44. Oda D, Gown AM, Vande Berg JS, Stern R. Instability of the myofibroblast phenotype in culture. Exp Mol Pathol 1990; 52:221–234.

45. Darby I, Skalli O, Gabbiani G. α-smooth muscle actin is transiently expressed by myofibroblasts during experimental wound healing. Lab Invest 1990; 63:21–29.

46. Zhang K, Rekhter MD, Gordon D, Phan SH. Myofibroblasts and their role in lung collagen gene expression during pulmonary fibrosis: a combined immunohistochemical and in situ hybridization study. Am J Pathol 1994; 145:114–125.

47. Gizycki MJ, Ädelroth E, Rogeres AV, O'Byrne PM, Jeffery PK. Myofibroblast in-volvement in the allergen-induced late response in mild atopic asthma. Am J Respir Cell Mol Biol 1997; 16:664–673.

48. Minshall EM, Leung DYM, Martin RJ, Song YL, Cameron L, Ernst P, Hamid Q. Eosinophil-associated TGF-β1 mRNA expression and airways fibrosis in bronchial asthma. Am J Respir Cell Mol Biol 1997; 17:326–333.

49. Godfrey RWA, Lorimer S, Majumdar S, Adelroth E, Johnston PW, Rogers AV, Johans-son S-A, Jeffery PK. Airway and lung elastic fibre is not reduced in asthma nor in asthmatics following corticosteroid treatment. Eur Respir J 1995; 8:922–927.

50. Carroll NG, Cooke C, James AL. Bronchial blood vessel dimensions in asthma. Am J Respir Crit Care Med 1997; 155:689–695.

51. Li X, Wilson JW. Increased vascularity of the bronchial mucosa in mild asthma. Am J Respir Crit Care Med 1997; 156:229–233.

52. Orsida BE, Li X, Hickey B, Thien F, Wilson JW, Walters EH. Vascularity in asthmatic airways: relation to inhaled steroid dose. Thorax 1999; 54:289–295.

53. Hoshino M, Takahsahi M, Aoike N. Expression of vascular endothelial growth factor, basic fibroblast growth factor, and angiogenin immunoreactivity in asthmatic airways and its relationship to angiogenesis. J Allergy Clin Immunol 2001; 107:295–301.

54. Salvato G. Quantitative and morphological analysis of the vascular bed in bronchial biopsy specimens from asthmatic and non-asthmatic subjects. Thorax 2001; 56: 902–906.

55. Vrugt B, Wilson S, Bron A, Holgate ST, Djukanovic R, Aalbers R. Bronchial angiogenesis in severe glucocorticoid-dependent asthma. Eur Respir J 2000; 15:1014–1021.

56. Aikawa T, Shimura S, Sasaki H, Ebina M, Takishima T. Marked goblet cell hyperplasia with mucus accumulation in the airways of patients who died of severe acute asthma attack. Chest 1992; 101:916–921.

57. Shimura S, Andoh Y, Haraguchi M, Shirato K. Continuity of airway goblet cells and intraluminal mucus in the airways of patients with bronchial asthma. Eur Respir J 1996; 9:1395–1401.

58. Ordoñez CL, Khashayar R, Wong HH, Ferrando R, Wu R, Hyde DM, Hotchkiss JA, Zhang Y, Novikov A, Dolganov G, Fahy JV. Mild and moderate asthma is associated with airway goblet cell hyperplasia and abnormalities in mucin gene expression. Am J Respir Crit Care Med 2001; 163:517–523.

59. Bousquet J, Lacoste J-Y, Chanez P, Vic P, Godard P, Michel F-B. Bronchial elastic fibers in normal subjects and asthmatic patients. Am J Respir Crit Care Med 1996; 153:1648–1654.

60. Carroll NG, Perry S, Karkhanis A, Harji S, Butt J, James AL, Green FHY. The airway longitudinal elastic fiber network and mucosal folding in patients with asthma. Am J Respir Crit Care Med 2000; 161:244–248.

61. Haraguchi M, Shimura S, Shirato K. Morphometric analysis of bronchial cartilage in chronic obstructive pulmonary disease and bronchial asthma. Am J Respir Crit Care Med 1999; 159:1005–1013.

62. Kinsella M, Müller NL, Staples C, Vedal S, Chan-Yeung M. Hyperinflation in asthma and emphysema: assessment by pulmonary function testing and computed tomography. Chest 1988; 94:286–289.

63. Paganin F, Trussard V, Seneterre E, Chanez P, Giron J, Godard P, Sénac JP, Michel FB, Bousquet J. Chest radiography and high resolution computed tomography of the lungs in asthma. Am Rev Respir Dis 1992; 146:1084–1087.

64. Lynch DA, Newell JD, Tschomper BA, Cink TM, Newman LS, Bethel R. Uncomplicated asthma in adults: comparison of CT appearance of the lungs in asthmatic and healthy subjects. Radiology 1993; 188:829–833.

65. Neeld DA, Goodman LR, Gurney JW, Greenberger PA, Fink JN. Computerized tomography in the evaluation of allergic bronchopulmonary aspergillosis. Am Rev Respir Dis 1990; 142:1200–1205.

66. Angus RM, Davies M-L, Cowan MD, McSharry C, Thomson NC. Computed tomographic scanning of the lung in patients with allergic bronchopulmonary aspergillosis and in asthmatic patients with a positive skin test to *Aspergillus fumigatus*. Thorax 1994; 49:586–589.

67. Paganin F, Séneterre E, Chanez P, Daurés JP, Bruel JM, Michel FB, Bousquet J. Computed tomography of the lungs in asthma: influence of disease severity and etiology. Am J Respir Crit Care Med 1996; 153:110–114.

68. Grenier P, Mourey-Gerosa I, Benali K, Brauner MW, Leung AN, Lenoir S, Cordeau MP, Mazoyer B. Abnormalities of the airways and lung parenchyma in asthmatics:

CT observations in 50 patients and inter- and intraobserver variability. Eur Radiol 1996; 6:199–206.

69. Boulet L-P, Bélanger M, Carrier G. Airway responsiveness and bronchial-wall thickness in asthma with or without fixed airflow obstruction. Am J Respir Crit Care Med 1995; 152:865–871.

70. Hudon C, Turcotte H, Laviolette M, Carrier G, Boulet L-P. Characteristics of bronchial asthma with incomplete reversibility of airflow obstruction. Ann Allergy Asthma Immunol 1997; 78:195–202.

71. Okazawa M, Müller N, McNamara AE, Child S, Verburgt L, Paré PD. Human airway narrowing measured using high resolution computed tomography. Am J Respir Crit Care Med 1996; 154:1557–1562.

72. Awadh N, Müller NL, Park CS, Abboud RT, FitzGerald JM. Airway wall thickness in patients with near fatal asthma and control groups: assessment with high resolution computed tomographic scanning. Thorax 1998; 53:248–253.

73. Pitris C, Brezinski ME, Bouma B, Tearney GJ, Southern JF, Fujimoto JG. High resolution imaging of the upper respiratory tract with optical coherence tomography: a feasibility study. Am J Respir Crit Care Med 1998; 157:1640–1644.

74. Laitinen LA, Heino M, Laitinen A, Kava T, Haahtela T. Damage of the airway epithelium and bronchial reactivity in patients with asthma. Am Rev Respir Dis 1985; 131: 599–606.

75. Ohashi Y, Motojima S, Fukuda T, Makino S. Airway hyperresponsiveness, increased intracellular spaces of bronchial epithelium, and increased infiltration of eosinophils and lymphocytes in bronchial mucosa in asthma. Am Rev Respir Dis 1992; 1450: 1469–1476.

76. Wardlaw AJ, Dunnette S, Gleich GJ, Collins JV, Kay AB. Eosinophils and mast cells in bronchoalveolar lavage in subjects with mild asthma: relationship to bronchial hyperreactivity. Am Rev Respir Dis 1988; 137:62–69.

77. Beasley R, Roche WR, Roberts JA, Holgate ST. Cellular events in the bronchi in mild asthma and after bronchial provocation. Am Rev Respir Dis 1989; 139:806–817.

78. Chanez P, Vignola AM, Vic P, Guddo F, Bonsignore G, Godard P, Bousquet J. Comparison between nasal and bronchial inflammation in asthmatic and control subjects. Am J Respir Crit Care Med 1999; 159:588–595.

79. Naylor B. The shedding of the mucosa in the bronchial tree in asthma. Thorax 1962; 17:69–72.

80. Montefort S, Roberts JA, Beasley R, Holgate ST, Roche WR. The site of disruption of the bronchial epithelium in asthmatic and non-asthmatic subjects. Thorax 1992; 47: 499–503.

81. Lozewicz S, Wells C, Gomez E, Ferguson H, Richman P, Devalia J, Davies RJ. Morphological integrity of the bronchial epithelium in mild asthma. Thorax 1990; 45: 12–15.

82. Ordóñez C, Ferrando R, Hyde DM, Wong HH, Fahy JV. Epithelial desquamation in asthma: artifact or pathology? Am J Respir Crit Care Med 2000; 162:2324–2329.

83. Lackie PM, Baker JE, Günthert U, Holgate ST. Expression of CD44 isoforms is increased in the airway epithelium of asthmatic subjects. Am J Respir Cell Mol Biol 1997; 16:14–22.

84. Leir S-H, Baker JE, Holgate ST, Lackie PM. Increased CD44 expression in human bronchial epithelial cell repair after damage or plating at low cell densities. Am J Physiol 2000; 278:L1129–L1137.

85. Puddicombe SM, Polosa R, Richter A, Krishna MT, Howarth PH, Holgate ST, Davies DE. Involvement of the epidermal growth factor receptor in epithelial repair in asthma. FASEB J 2000; 14:1362–1374.

86. Polosa R, Puddicombe SM, Krishna MT, Tuck AB, Howarth PH, Holgate ST, Davies DE. Expression of c-erbB receptors and ligands in the bronchial epithelium of asthmatic subjects. J Allergy Clin Immunol 2002; 109:75–81.

87. Demoly P, Simony-Lafontaine J, Chanez P, Pujol J-L, Lequeux N, Michel F-B, Bousquet J. Cell proliferation in the bronchial mucosa of asthmatics and chronic bronchitics. Am J Respir Crit Care Med 1994; 150:214–217.

88. Howat WJ, Holgate ST, Lackie PM. TGF-β isoform release and activation during in vitro bronchial epithelial wound repair. Am J Physiol 2002; 282:L115–L123.

89. Redington AE, Madden J, Frew AJ, Djukanovic R, Roche WR, Holgate ST, Howarth PH. Transforming growth factor-beta 1 in asthma: measurement in bronchoalveolar lavage fluid. Am J Respir Crit Care Med 1997; 156:642–647.

90. Zhang S, Smart H, Holgate ST, Roche WR. Growth factors secreted by bronchial epithelial cells control myofibroblast proliferation: an in vitro co-culture model of airway remodeling in asthma. Lab Invest 1999; 79:395–405.

91. Goto Y, Noguchi Y, Nomura A, Sakamoto T, Ishii Y, Bitoh S, Picton C, Fujita Y, Watanabe T, Hasegawa S, Uchida Y. In vitro reconstitution of the tracheal epithelium. Am J Respir Cell Mol Biol 1999; 20:312–318.

92. Morishima Y, Nomura A, Uchida Y, Noguchi Y, Sakamoto T, Ishii Y, Goto Y, Masuyama K, Zhang MJ, Hirano K, Mochizuki M, Ohtsuka M, Sekizawa K. Triggering the induction of myofibroblast and fibrogenesis by airway epithelial shedding. Am J Respir Cell Mol Biol 2001; 24:1–11.

93. Vignola AM, Chanez P, Chiappara G, Merendino A, Pace E, Rizzo A, la Rocca AM, Bellia V, Bonsignore G, Bousquet J. Transforming growth factor-β expression in mucosal biopsies in asthma and chronic bronchitis. Am J Respir Crit Care Med 1997; 156:591–599.

94. Redington AE, Roche WR, Madden J, Frew AJ, Djukanovic R, Holgate ST, Howarth PH. Basic fibroblast growth factor in asthma: measurement in bronchoalveolar lavage fluid basally and following allergen challenge. J Allergy Clin Immunol 2001; 107:384–387.

95. Springall DR, Howarth PH, Counihan H, Djukanovic R, Holgate ST, Polak JM. Endothelin immunoreactivity of airway epithelium in asthmatic patients. Lancet 1991; 337:697–701.

96. Redington AE, Springall DR, Ghatei MA, Lau LCK, Holgate ST, Polak JM, Howarth PH. Endothelin in bronchoalveolar lavage fluid and its relation to airflow obstruction in asthma. Am J Respir Crit Care Med 1995; 151:1034–1039.

97. Redington AE, Springall DR, Meng Q-H, Tuck AB, Holgate ST, Polak JM, Howarth PH. Immunoreactive endothelin in bronchial biopsy specimens: increased expression in asthma and modulation by corticosteroid therapy. J Allergy Clin Immunol 1997; 100:544–552.

98. Howat WJ, Holmes JA, Holgate ST, Lackie PM. Basement membrane pores in human bronchial epithelium: a conduit for infiltrating cells? Am J Pathol 2001; 158:673–680.

99. Ohno I, Nitta Y, Yamauchi K, Hoshi H, Honma M, Woolley K, O'Byrne P, Tamura G, Jordana M, Shirato K. Transforming growth factor β1 (TGFβ1) gene expression by eosinophils in asthmatic airway inflammation. Am J Respir Cell Mol Biol 1996; 15:404–409.

100. Ohno I, Nitta Y, Yamauchi K, Hoshi H, Honma M, Wooley K, O'Byrne P, Dolovich J, Jordana M, Tamura G, Tanno Y, Shirato K. Eosinophils as a potential source of platelet-derived growth factor B-chain (PDGF-B) in nasal polyposis and bronchial asthma. Am J Respir Cell Mol Biol 1995; 13:639–647.

101. Gordon JR, Galli SJ. Promotion of mouse fibroblast collagen gene expression by mast cells stimulated via the FcεRI: role for mast cell-derived transforming growth factor β and tumor necrosis factor α. J Exp Med 1994; 180:2027–2037.

102. Inoue Y, King Jr. TE, Tinkle SS, Dockstader K, Newman LS. Human mast cell basic fibroblast growth factor in pulmonary fibrotic disorders. Am J Pathol 1996; 149: 2037–2054.

103. Ruoss SJ, Hartmann T, Caughey GH. Mast cell tryptase is a mitogen for cultured fibroblasts. J Clin Invest 1991; 88:493–499.

104. Cairns JA, Walls AF. Mast cell tryptase stimulates the synthesis of type I collagen in human lung fibroblasts. J Clin Invest 1997; 99:1313–1321.

105. Robinson DS, Hamid Q, Ying S, Tsicopoulos A, Barkans J, Bentley AM, Corrigan C, Durham SR, Kay AB. Predominant T_{H2}-like bronchoalveolar T-lymphocyte population in atopic asthma. N Engl J Med 1992; 326:298–304.

106. Boulay J-L, Paul WE. The interleukin-4 family of lymphokines. Curr Opin Immunol 1992; 4:294–298.

107. Kolb M, Margetts PJ, Anthony DC, Pitossi F, Gauldie J. Transient expression of IL-1β induces acute lung injury and chronic repair leading to pulmonary fibrosis. J Clin Invest 2001; 107:1529–1536.

108. DiCosmo BF, Geba GP, Picarella D, Elias JA, Rankin JA, Stripp BR, Whitsett JA, Flavell RA. Airway epithelial cell expression of interleukin-6 in transgenic mice: uncoupling of airway inflammation and bronchial hyperreactivity. J Clin Invest 1994; 94:2028–2035.

109. Temann U-A, Geba GP, Rankin JA, Flavell RA. Expression of interleukin 9 in the lungs of transgenic mice causes airway inflammation, mast cell hyperplasia, and bronchial hyperresponsiveness. J Exp Med 1998; 188:1307–1320.

110. Tang W, Geba GP, Zheng T, Ray P, Homer RJ, Kuhn III C, Flavell RA, Elias JA. Targeted expression of IL-11 in the murine airway causes lymphocytic inflammation, bronchial remodeling, and airways obstruction. J Clin Invest 1996; 98:2845–2853.

111. Zhu Z, Homer RJ, Wang Z, Chen Q, Geba GP, Wang J, Zhang Y, Elias JA. Pulmonary expression of interleukin-13 causes inflammation, mucus hypersecretion, subepithelial fibrosis, physiologic abnormalities, and eotaxin production. J Clin Invest 1999; 103: 779–788.

112. Sime PJ, Marr RA, Gauldie D, Xing Z, Hewlett BR, Graham FL, Gauldie J. Transfer of tumor necrosis factor-α to rat lung induces severe pulmonary inflammation and patchy interstitial fibrogenesis with induction of transforming growth factor-β1 and myofibroblasts. Am J Pathol 1998; 153:825–832.

113. Xing Z, Ohkawara Y, Jordana M, Graham FL, Gauldie J. Transfer of granulocyte-macrophage colony-stimulating factor gene to rat lung induces eosinophilia, monocytosis, and fibrotic reactions. J Clin Invest 1996; 97:1102–1110.

114. Xing Z, Tremblay GM, Sime PJ, Gauldie J. Overexpression of granulocyte-macrophage colony-stimulating factor induces pulmonary granulation tissue formation and fibrosis by induction of transforming growth factor-β1 and myofibroblast accumulation. Am J Pathol 1997; 150:59–66.

115. Richter A, Puddicombe SM, Lordan JL, Bucchieri F, Wilson SJ, Djukanovic R, Dent G, Holgate ST, Davies DE. The contribution of interleukin (IL)-4 and IL-13 to the

epithelial-mesenchymal trophic unit in asthma. Am J Respir Cell Mol Biol 2001; 25: 385–391.

116. Lee CG, Homer RJ, Zhu Z, Lanone S, Wang X, Koteliansky V, Shipley JM, Gotwals P, Noble P, Chen Q, Senior RM, Elias JA. Interleukin-13 induces tissue fibrosis by selectively stimulating and activating transforming growth factor β_1. J Exp Med 2001; 194:809–821.

117. Swartz MA, Tschumperlin DJ, Drazen JM. Mechanical stress is communicated between different cell types to elicit matrix remodeling. Proc Natl Acad Sci USA 2001; 98: 6180–6185.

118. Moreno RH, Hogg JC, Paré PD. Mechanics of airway narrowing. Am Rev Respir Dis 1986; 133:1171–1180.

119. Wiggs BR, Moreno R, Hogg JC, Hilliam C, Paré PD. A model of the mechanics of airway narrowing. J Appl Physiol 1990; 69:849–860.

120. Wiggs BR, Bosken C, Paré PD, James A, Hogg JC. A model of airway narrowing in asthma and in chronic obstructive pulmonary disease. Am Rev Respir Dis 1992; 145: 1251–1258.

121. Lambert RK, Wiggs BR, Kuwano K, Hogg JC, Paré PD. Functional significance of increased airway smooth muscle in asthma and COPD. J Appl Physiol 1993; 74: 2771–2881.

122. Lambert RK. Role of bronchial basement membrane in airway collapse. J Appl Physiol 1991; 71:666–673.

123. Lambert RK, Codd SL, Alley MR, Pack RJ. Physical determinants of bronchial mucosal folding. J Appl Physiol 1994; 77:1206–1216.

124. Wiggs BR, Hrousis CA, Drazen JM, Kamm RD. On the mechanism of mucosal folding in normal and asthmatic airways. J Appl Physiol 1997; 83:1814–1821.

125. Chetta A, Foresi A, Del Donno M, Consigli GF, Bertorelli G, Pesci A, Barbee RA, Olivieri D. Bronchial responsiveness to distilled water and methacholine and its relationship to inflammation and remodeling of the airways in asthma. Am J Respir Crit Care Med 1996; 153:910–917.

126. Schachter EN, Doyle CA, Beck GJ. A prospective study of asthma in a rural community. Chest 1984; 85:623–630.

127. Peat JK, Woolcock AJ, Cullen K. Rate of decline of lung function in subjects with asthma. Eur J Respir Dis 1987; 70:171–179.

128. Ulrik CS, Backer V, Dirksen A. A 10 year follow up of 180 adults with bronchial asthma: factors important for the decline in lung function. Thorax 1992; 47:14–18.

129. Ulrik CS, Lange P. Decline of lung function in adults with bronchial asthma. Am J Respir Crit Care Med 1994; 150:629–634.

130. Lange P, Parner J, Vestbo J, Schnohr P, Jensen G. A 15-year follow-up study of ventilatory function in adults with asthma. N Engl J Med 1998; 339:1194–1200.

131. Backman KS, Greenberger PA, Patterson R. Airways obstruction in patients with long-term asthma consistent with "irreversible asthma." Chest 1997; 112:1234–1240.

132. Ulrik CS, Backer V. Nonreversible airflow obstruction in life-long nonsmokers with moderate to severe asthma. Eur Respir J 1999; 14:892–896.

133. Brown PJ, Greville HW, Finucane KE. Asthma and irreversible airflow obstruction. Thorax 1984; 39:131–136.

134. Finucane KE, Greville HW, Brown PJE. Irreversible airflow obstruction: evolution in asthma. Med J Aust 1985; 142:602–604.

135. Connolly CK, Chan NS, Prescott RJ. The relationship between age and duration of asthma and the presence of persistent airflow obstruction in asthma. Postgrad Med J 1988; 64:422–425.

136. Braman SS, Kaemmerlen JT, Davis SM. Asthma in the elderly: a comparison between patients with recently acquired and long-standing disease. Am Rev Respir Dis 1991; 143:336–340.
137. Bai TR, Cooper J, Koelmeyer T, Paré PD, Weir TD. The effect of age and duration of disease on airway structure in fatal asthma. Am J Respir Crit Care Med 2000; 162: 663–669.
138. Wilson JW, Li X, Pain MCF. The lack of distensibility of asthmatic airways. Am Rev Respir Dis 1993; 148:806–809.
139. Johns DP, Wilson J, Harding R, Walters EH. Airway distensibility in healthy and asthmatic subjects: effect of lung volume history. J Appl Physiol 2000; 88:1413–1420.
140. Olivieri D, Chetta A, Del Donno M, Bertorelli G, Casalini A, Pesci A, Testi R, Foresi A. Effect of short-term treatment with low-dose inhaled fluticasone propionate on airway inflammation and remodeling in mild asthma: a placebo-controlled study. Am J Respir Crit Care Med 1997; 155:1864–1871.
141. Sont JK, Willems LNA, Bel EH, van Krieken JHJM, Vandenbroucke JP, Sterk PJ, AMPUL study group. Clinical control and histopathologic outcome of asthma when using airway hyperresponsiveness as an additional guide to long-term treatment. Am J Respir Crit Care Med 1999; 159:1043–1051.
142. Trigg CJ, Manolitsas ND, Wang J, Calderón M, McAulay A, Jordan SE, Herdman MJ, Jhalli N, Duddle JM, Hamilton SA, Devalia JL, Davies RJ. Placebo-controlled immunopathologic study of four months of inhaled corticosteroids in asthma. Am J Respir Crit Care Med 1994; 150:17–22.
143. Altraja A, Laitinen A, Meriste S, Marran S, Märtson T, Sillastu H, Laitinen LA. Regular albuterol or nedocromil sodium—effects on airway subepithelial tenascin in asthma. Respir Med 1999; 93:445–453.
144. Roberts JA, Bradding P, Britten KM, Walls AF, Wilson S, Gratziou C, Holgate ST, Howarth PH. The long-acting β_2-agonist salmeterol xinafoate: effects on airway inflammation in asthma. Eur Respir J 1999; 14:275–282.
145. Gardiner PV, Ward C, Booth H, Allison A, Hendrick DJ, Walters EH. Effect of eight weeks of treatment with salmeterol on bronchoalveolar lavage inflammatory indices in asthmatics. Am J Respir Crit Care Med 1994; 150:1006–1011.
146. Kraft M, Wenzel SE, Bettinger CM, Martin RJ. The effect of salmeterol on nocturnal symptoms, airway function, and inflammation in asthma. Chest 1997; 111:1249–1254.
147. Wallin A, Sandström T, Söderberg M, Howarth P, Lundbäck B, Della-Cioppa G, Wilson S, Judd M, Djukanovic R, Holgate S, Lindberg A, Larssen L. The effects of regular inhaled formoterol, budesonide, and placebo on mucosal inflammation and clinical indices in mild asthma. Am J Respir Crit Care Med 1998; 158:79–86.
148. Wilson SJ, Wallin A, Della-Cioppa G, Sandström T, Holgate ST. Effects of budesonide and formoterol on NF-κB, adhesion molecules, and cytokines in asthma. Am J Respir Crit Care Med 2001; 164:1047–1052.
149. Leung KBP, Flint KC, Brostoff J, Hudspith BN, Johnson NM, Lau HYA, Liu WL, Pearce FL. Effects of sodium cromoglycate and nedocromil sodium on histamine secretion from human lung mast cells. Thorax 1988; 43:756–761.
150. Mekori YA, Baram D, Goldberg A, Hershkoviz R, Reshef T, Sredni D. Nedocromil sodium inhibits T-cell function in vitro and in vivo. J Allergy Clin Immunol 1993; 91:817–824.
151. Bruijnzeel PLB, Hamelink ML, Kok PMT, Kreukniet JK. Nedocromil sodium inhibits the A23187- and opsonized zymosan-induced leukotriene formation by human eosinophils but not by human neutrophils. Br J Pharmacol 1989; 96:631–636.

152. Bruijnzeel PLB, Warringa RAJ, Kok PTM, Kreukniet J. Inhibition of neutrophil and eosinophil induced chemotaxis by nedocromil sodium and disodium cromoglycate. Br J Pharmacol 1990; 99:798–802.

153. Manolitsas ND, Wang J, Devalia JL, Trigg CJ, McAulay AE, Davies RJ. Regular albuterol, nedocromil sodium, and bronchial inflammation in asthma. Am J Respir Crit Care Med 1995; 151:1925–1930.

154. Panettieri Jr. RA, Tan EML, Ciocca V, Luttmann MA, Leonard TB, Hay DWP. Effects of LTD$_4$ on human airway smooth muscle proliferation, matrix expression, and contraction in vitro: differential sensitivity to cysteinyl leukotriene receptor antagonists. Am J Respir Cell Mol Biol 1998; 19:453–461.

155. Henderson Jr. WR, Tang LO, Chu SJ, Tsao SM, Chiang GK, Jones F, Jonas M, Pae C, Wang H, Chi EY. A role for cysteinyl leukotrienes in airway remodeling in a mouse asthma model. Am J Respir Crit Care Med 2002; 165:108–116.

156. Pizzichini E, Leff JA, Reiss TF, Hendele L, Boulet L-P, Wei LX, Efthimiadis AE, Zhang J, Hargreave FE. Montelukast reduces airway eosinophilic inflammation in asthma: a randomized, controlled trial. Eur Respir J 1999; 14:12–18.

157. Calhoun WJ, Lavins BJ, Minkwitz MC, Evans R, Gleich GJ, Cohn J. Effect of zafirlukast (Accolate) on cellular mediators of inflammation: bronchoalveolar lavage findings after segmental antigen challenge. Am J Respir Crit Care Med 1998; 157:1381–1389.

158. Nakamura Y, Hoshino M, Sim JJ, Ishii K, Hosaka K, Sakamoto T. Effect of the leukotriene receptor antagonist pranlukast on cellular infiltration in the bronchial mucosa of patients with asthma. Thorax 1998; 53:835–841.

159. Sullivan P, Bekir S, Jaffar Z, Page C, Jeffery P, Costello J. Anti-inflammatory effects of low-dose oral theophylline in atopic asthma. Lancet 1994; 343:1006–1008.

160. Kidney J, Dominguez M, Taylor PM, Rose M, Chung KF, Barnes PJ. Immunomodulation by theophylline in asthma: demonstration by withdrawal of therapy. Am J Respir Crit Care Med 1995; 151:1907–1914.

161. Finnerty JP, Lee C, Wilson S, Madden J, Djukanovic R, Holgate ST. Effects of theophylline on inflammatory cells and cytokines in asthmatic subjects: a placebo-controlled parallel group study. Eur Respir J 1996; 9:1672–1677.

162. Levi-Schaffer F, Touitou E. Xanthines inhibit 3T3 fibroblast proliferation. Skin Pharmacol 1991; 4:286–290.

163. Billington CK, Joseph SK, Swan C, Scott MG, Jobson TM, Hall IP. Modulation of human airway smooth muscle proliferation by type 3 phosphodiesterase inhibition. Am J Physiol 1999; 276:L412–L419.

164. Haahtela T, Järvinen M, Kava T, Kiviranta K, Koskinen S, Lehtonen K, Nikander K, Persson T, Reinikainen K, Selroos O, Sovijärvi A, Stenius-Aarniala B, Svahn T, Tammivaara R, Laitinen LA. Comparison of a β2-agonist, terbutaline, with an inhaled corticosteroid, budesonide, in newly detected asthma. N Engl J Med 1991; 325: 388–392.

165. Haahtela T, Järvinen M, Kava T, Kiviranta K, Koskinen S, Lehtonen K, Nikander K, Persson T, Selroos O, Sovijärvi A, Stenius-Aarniala B, Svahn T, Tammivaara R, Laitinen LA. Effects of reducing or discontinuing inhaled budesonide in patients with mild asthma. N Engl J Med 1994; 331:700–705.

166. Selroos O, Pietinalho A, Löfroos A-B, Riska H. Effect of early vs late intervention with inhaled corticosteroids in asthma. Chest 1995; 108:1228–1234.

167. Agertoft L, Pedersen S. Effects of long-term treatment with an inhaled corticosteroid on growth and pulmonary function in asthmatic children. Respir Med 1994; 88:373–381.

168. Dompeling E, van Schayck CP, van Grunsven PM, van Herwaardeen CLA, Akkermans R, Molema J, Folgering H, van Weel C. Slowing the deterioration of asthma and chronic obstructive pulmonary disease observed during bronchodilator therapy by adding inhaled corticosteroids: a 4-year prospective study. Ann Intern Med 1993; 118: 770–778.

169. Vignola AM, Chanez P, Campbell AM, Souques F, Lebel B, Enander I, Bousquet J. Airway inflammation in mild intermittent and in persistent asthma. Am J Respir Crit Care Med 1998; 157:403–409.

170. Richards W, Patrick JR. Death from asthma in children. Am J Dis Child 1965; 110: 4–21.

171. Çokugras H, Akçakaya N, Seçkin I, YC, Sarimurat N, Aksoy F. Ultrastructural examination of bronchial biopsy specimens from children with moderate asthma. Thorax 2001; 56:25–29.

172. Pohunek P, Roche WR, Turzikova J, Kudrmann J, Warner JO. Eosinophilic inflammation in the bronchial mucosa of children with bronchial asthma (abstr). Eur Respir J 1997; 10(suppl 25):160s.

35

The Role of Proteases in Airway Remodeling

FARRAH KHERADMAND and KIRTEE RISHI

Baylor College of Medicine
Houston, Texas, U.S.A.

I. Introduction

Immune cells and their bioactive products are mediators of allergic lung disease and the physiological consequences of this inflammation. These same inflammatory cells and molecules also dictate formation of peribronchovascular granulation tissue, which we will refer to here as provisional matrix or reactive stroma, and activate various proteolytic enzymes (1–4). These enzymes are capable of degrading various connective tissue, or matrix proteins but also many other biologically active proteins. As reviewed here, the functional consequences of inflammatory proteolysis are complex and highly relevant to the expression and regulation of diseases such as asthma and thus demand equally complex regulatory pathways.

Inflammatory cells themselves secrete various types of degrading enzymes, and inflammatory cytokines can induce connective tissue, or mesenchymal cells to express extracellular matrix (ECM)–degrading enzymes (5–8). Regardless of the source, it appears that members of several classes of proteases are strongly expressed at sites of acute and chronic inflammation. Besides their historic role as basement membrane–degrading enzymes, many new functions have been described for proteases in the reactive stroma. The description of the cross talk between inflammatory cells and the stromal tissue that manifests as expression and activation of ECM-degrading enzymes in response to proinflammatory cytokines is a concept that seemed unlikely only a few years ago.

In this chapter we will review recent advances that elucidate the role of proteases in a provisional matrix or reactive stroma and how they may alter airway remodeling in allergic diseases. In particular we will focus on experimental studies examining the spatio-temporal regulation of the matrix metalloprotease (MMP) family of enzymes in acute and chronic inflammatory conditions. We will discuss the emerging views that shed light on the function of proteases beyond their historical roles as extracellular protein–cleaving molecules. Targeted mutations in mice, combined with animal models of allergic inflammation, are also beginning to reveal functions of many members of the MMP family in vivo. Complicating our attempts to fully understand how MMPs function in vivo is the fact that new members of this already sizable family are still being discovered. In addition, the enormous degrading capability of MMPs demands a multitude of regulatory processes at pre- and posttranscriptional stages that are still only vaguely understood (9). Can we use MMP inhibitors to alter pathological outcomes during inflammation? As we will develop below, our knowledge base is currently insufficient to allow the safe targeting of these molecules with the goal of treating inflammatory conditions such as asthma and chronic obstructive pulmonary disease (COPD). However, the importance of this expanding family of regulatory molecules suggests that their manipulation will eventually become an important means for treating these highly morbid conditions.

II. ECM Proteases in the Lung

The ECM proteases that cleave internal peptide bonds (the endopeptidases) are grouped into four major classes—the serine, cysteine, aspartic, and metalloproteases—based on their essential catalytic group (10–12). Proteases are also classified based on their sensitivity to class-specific endogenous or nonendogenous inhibitors, such as phenylmethylsufonyl fluoride, soybean trypsin inhibitor, α_1-antiprotease (α_1-antitrypsin) for serine proteases; E-64 for cysteine proteases; pepstatin A for aspartic proteases; and EDTA, tissue inhibitor of metalloproteases (TIMPs), and 1,10-phenanthroline for metalloproteases (13,14). A considerable body of literature indicates that proteases, in particular serine and MMP, together with their endogenous inhibitors, take part in inflammation, wound repair, and fibrosis (15–17). However, details of how such diverse roles can be attributed to individual proteolytic enzymes are lacking.

The family of MMPs consists of over 26 secreted or membrane-bound zinc-dependent endopeptidases that have been reported in organisms ranging from protozoa to mammals (9,11). MMPs are characterized for their ability to cleave extracellular and transmembrane proteins, as well as factors that are embedded within the matrix, e.g., growth factors, chemokines, and cytokines (9). Several members of the MMP gene family are upregulated during allergic inflammation (18,19) and may participate in the pathogenesis of several lung diseases, especially COPD and asthma

(18,20–24). MMPs also facilitate inflammatory cell recruitment across the endothelial basement membrane (25–27).

As part of the essential regulatory processes in the development of embryonic lung, timely expression and regulation of extracellular proteases of the MMP family are required for release of many transmembrane growth and differentiation factors, e.g., epidermal growth factors, as well as for proteolysis of ECM molecules (28,29). Such regulatory processes can be complex. For instance, MMP2, which is critical for alveogenesis, requires epidermal growth factor–dependent expression of MMP14 (MT1-MMP) in the epithelium and mesenchyme during lung development (30). MMP14 proteolytically activates the latent MMP2, without affecting mRNA synthesis.

While proteolysis is critical in lung development, the resurgence of proteolytic activity within the reactive stroma during chronic inflammatory processes of the mature lung is viewed as part of the irreversible tissue remodeling that can favor fibrosis (16,31,32). Thus, in order to understand lung remodeling, it is critical to understand why mediators of inflammation result in programs of gene activation that favor degradation and paradoxically fibrotic reactions.

Degrading structural proteins within the ECM, the main function of MMPs, appears quite simple, and yet the mechanisms by which proteolysis alters immune cell function is decisively complex (9,33). For instance, elastin, a complex structural ECM in the lung that provides elasticity and resilience, when degraded by gelatinase A (MMP2) or gelatinase B (MMP9), forms fragments that are potent chemoattractant factors for inflammatory cells (34,35). Similarly, MMPs mediate cleavage of other ECM molecules, growth factors, chemokines, or cytokines in inflamed tissue, which can render these factors inactive (36–39). However, the cleaved products from these molecules can in turn exert opposing functions (37). Thus, as we learn more about substrate and enzyme interaction in vivo, new and diverse functions of the MMP multigene family emerge that can affect all aspects of tissue remodeling. In the case of inflammation, there may be dual pro- and anti-inflammatory functions (37).

Most studies to date provide evidence that MMPs are present at the site of inflammation, although insight into their possible function during inflammation has proved difficult to show (40). Several interesting questions remain unanswered: What is the role of proteases in lung inflammation? What are the key proteases implicated in the pathogenesis of lung reactive stroma? Where are proteases expressed and how would we decipher their role in inflammatory reactions in the lung? The most challenging question, however, is how MMPs could alter remodeling in chronic allergic disease when there is not yet a unified understanding of spatio-temporal regulation of MMPs under normal or pathological conditions. Specifically, several studies have detected MMPs in the epithelium of peribronchial glands and conducting airways under a variety of conditions (41–45). Others have reported expression of MMP7 (Matrilysin), but not MMP1 (collagenase-1), MMP2 (gelatinase A), MMP3 (stromelysin-1), or MMP9 (gelatinase B) in the same cells (30,46,47). Furthermore, even following inflammation or acute injury, only MMP7 and none of MMP1, MMP2, MMP3, or MMP9 was upregulated in the more proximal and distal epithelial lining cell in the lung (47). Thus, we await further research that may help to clarify some of these basic unanswered questions regarding the spatio-temporal regulation of MMPs during allergic airway inflammation.

III. Airway Remodeling and Reactive Stroma Formation in Asthma

The term "airway remodeling" is often applied to describe the constellation of ana-tomical changes observed in the lungs during acute and chronic allergic inflammation (3,48,49). Although variously defined, airway remodeling may conservatively in-clude changes such as goblet cell metaplasia and mucus gland hyperplasia, subepi-thelial collagen deposition, smooth muscle hyperplasia and/or hypertrophy, airway mucus plugging, and other changes that are believed to contribute to the airway obstruction of asthma (50).

Autopsy series of patients dying of severe asthma have demonstrated a more potent degree of airway inflammation compared to biopsy specimens from mild to moderate asthmatics and also demonstrate occlusive airway impaction due to inflammatory cells and mucus (51–53). The major clinical endpoints in asthma, death, dyspnea, and cough, are strongly related to, and likely caused by, airway obstruction. Indeed, mortality from asthma appears to be due to asphyxiation (54). Airway obstruction in asthma consists of at least three components: airway hyperre-sponsiveness (AHR), physical obstruction, and fibrosis. AHR is defined as an en-hanced constrictive response to provocative challenges with cholinergic agonists, and physical obstruction due to mucus and other debris develops in early stages of disease. There is widespread agreement that these acute components of airway obstruction are mediated, either directly or indirectly by T cells, particularly CD4 + T cells (termed Th2 cells), which secrete a restricted repertoire of cytokines, namely interleukin 4 (IL-4), IL-5, IL-9, and IL-13 (3,4,48,55,56).

A third component of airway obstruction, airway remodeling due to fibrosis, is less well described but likely contributes to chronic, irreversible airway dysfunction. Several studies have identified asthmatic inflammation alone as the cause for irrever-sible airflow obstruction, independent of compounding factors such as cigarette smoking (57–59). Fiberoptic bronchoscopy specimens obtained from lungs of pa-tients with mild, moderate, or severe asthma show excess deposition of collagen beneath the bronchial epithelial basement membrane (60–62). Although in some studies subepithelial collagen deposition does not determine the severity of asthma (62), others have shown a positive correlation between the degree of collagen accu-mulation in the airway and the severity of asthma symptoms (63,64). While this debate remains unresolved, permanent reorganization of the airway due to deposition of collagen may explain why asthmatics have residual airway obstruction during asymptomatic phases and why in children, AHR predisposes them to lower values for forced expiratory volume in one second (FEV_1) (65). Indeed, the natural history of lung function in adult patients with asthma reveals a substantially greater decline in FEV_1 over time than in nonasthmatics (58,66). This finding is in keeping with an earlier report linking poorly controlled asthma to chronic mucus hypersecretion, also a marker of a greater decline in FEV_1 in asthmatics, and increased mortality in asthmatics through substantial compromise in ventilatory function (53,67). However, in pathological states such as asthma, where active matrix remodeling is observed, the presence of chronic inflammatory cells and their secretory products, especially proteases, is presumed responsible for much of the irreversible architectural reorganization (61). However, what remains unresolved is the contribution of MMPs in the pathogenesis of subepithelial fibrosis and perhaps other aspects of airway remodeling (16,50).

IV. Matrix Proteases and Their Inhibitors

The theory of protease/antiprotease imbalance in the pathogenesis of subepithelial fibrosis remains quite controversial (9,15,68). In favor of this hypothesis, several studies have shown a strong association between increases in the bronchoalveolar lavage (BAL) fluid (18,61,69) and tissue (70) levels for MMP9 and disease activity in asthma. Furthermore, treatment with inhaled corticosteroids was shown to increase TIMP1 and decrease MMP9 immunoreactivities in the bronchial tissue, with a concomitant decrease in subepithelial collagen type III deposition (71). From these data it was concluded that corticosteroid treatment of asthma can reduce subepithelial collagen deposition by downregulation of MMP9 expression and upregulation of TIMP1 (71). While these findings point to the well-established role of steroids in resolving the underlying inflammatory cell infiltrates in asthma, the correlation with decreases in MMP9 and collagen III does not imply a causal relation because both findings may be unrelated. Thus, decreases in MMP9 and collagen III may both be a consequence of steroid therapy. Furthermore, at the transcriptional level, both MMP9 and TIMP1 are coregulated, such that activators and repressors will generally affect both genes in the same direction (11). It is therefore not surprising that dexamethasone decreased both MMP9 and TIMP1 in human alveolar macrophages (72,73).

Although TIMPs have been more classically described as inhibitors of MMPs, by far the most abundant inhibitors of MMPs in vivo are circulating α_2-macroglobulins and α_1-proteinase inhibitor (9,74). In contrast, the principal function of locally produced TIMPs is to finely orchestrate MMP activation. Furthermore, several regulatory pathways beyond TIMPs play key roles in localizing the pericellular proteolytic activity of MMPs (9,75). Specifically, mechanisms for localizing MMPs to the cell surface membrane include binding of MMP2 via the C-terminal domain to $\alpha v \beta 3$ integrin; expression of transmembrane MMPs, e.g., membrane-bound MT-MMPs; and activation of many cell surface serine class proteases that require MMPs for activation, e.g., thrombin and plasminogen (13,76–79). Concentration of MMP activity within localized pockets of the target cell–ECM neighborhood limit the extent of proteolysis and the need for endogenous MMP inhibitors (75). In addition, MMPs can undergo proteolytic inactivation by binding to their natural inhibitors, such as α_1-macroglobulin or thrombospondin 2, which can result in removal of the protease-antiprotease complex by endocytosis (74). Thus, the popular method of elucidating

MMP regulation through immunohistochemical analysis of MMP and TIMP expression is simplistic and fails to account for the full diversity and function of MMPs and their regulators expressed as part of any inflammatory process (12,80).

V. Extracellular Matrix Composition and Function in Normal and Inflamed Lung

Proteolysis of structural matrix molecules was first discovered as an integral part of cell-cell and cell-matrix interaction. The ECM proteins that are expressed in the adult lung include collagen I, III, and IV (Fig. 1); elastin; laminins; fibronectin; entactin/nidogen; proteoglycans; and dystroglycans (81–84). Various methods used to analyze and quantify collagen in the human lung parenchyma have estimated that collagen I, III, and IV constitute 69, 21, and 8% of the total collagen, respectively (85,86). Although a minor component of total collagen measured in the lung, collagen IV in the basement membrane accounts for most of the strength of the blood-

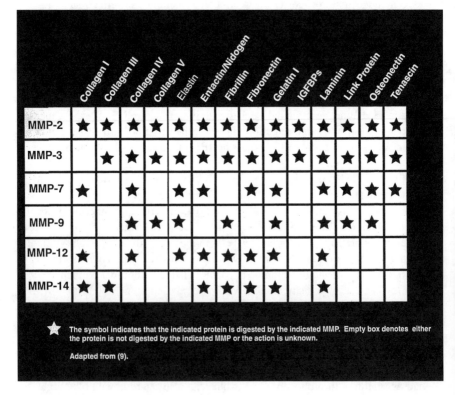

Figure 1 Lung ECM degradation and MMPs.

gas barrier separating the thin capillaries from the alveolar epithelium (87). Indeed, MMP2 and MMP9 were first identified as 72 and 92 kDa type IV collagenases, and it is not surprising that the same enzymes have been implicated in the pathogenesis of chronic inflammatory conditions such as COPD and asthma (88).

The newly synthesized matrix within the reactive stroma of the inflamed lung, also known as the provisional matrix, is quite fluid, with its exact composition not fully understood (89). It is important to note that the provisional matrix is synthesized only as a reaction to injury and differs from what is normally present in the lung. Many newly synthesized matrix molecules, such as collagen V, entactin, fibronectin, and tenascin, are only transiently expressed (90). A plausible role for expression of these matrix molecules may mirror the role of these molecules during lung development (91,92). Our current understanding of the composition and biological roles of molecules in the basement membrane is therefore partly driven from embryonic lung studies, where some of the basement membrane proteins are transiently expressed and thought to act as morphogens. In the case of tenascin and entactin, minor constituents of the basement membrane of the adult lung, mRNA and protein are highly expressed during lung development and again during lung injury and repair (91,93,94). Similarly, collagen XVIII expression, localized to the epithelial tip at the initiation of lung organogenesis, is induced by instructive signals from the primordial lung mesenchyme (95). The function of the known components of the provisional matrix is only partially described (82,89), but what is certain is that in order to reestablish normal lung architecture, the provisional matrix must eventually reorganize into the permanent matrix of the lung. As such, proteases play a crucial role in reestablishing the original matrix composition by degrading the newly formed provisional matrix (29).

VI. ECM and Other Regulatory Molecules as MMP Substrates

The discrete expression and multiplicity of MMP member profiles suggests that different MMPs have unique functions, even though their similar substrate specificities may suggest otherwise. This overlapping substrate specificity also means that less is known about the function of individual MMP family members in vivo. Before we can understand the role of matrix metalloproteinases in lung matrix remodeling, we need to examine where MMPs are expressed and how are they regulated in inflammation In vitro studies have identified numerous candidates as substrates for MMPs, although in the majority of cases, solid in vivo correlative data are lacking (9).

In vitro studies show that several MMPs cleave many of the ECM proteins in the lung. In the case of interstitial collagen, the cleavage sites identified in breakdown products from the tissue agree with those that are generated in vitro (9,96). This type of information is of limited value, since several members of the MMP family can produce the same cleavage fragments (9,97). Although the list of potential MMP substrates is lengthy, the number of proven in vivo substrates is rather short (11).

ECM degradation results in disruption and remodeling of structural barriers, which can allow inflammatory cell movement along the inflamed tissue (11,98). Although this role for ECM degradation is not disputed, alternative outcomes from the proteolysis of extracellular matrix are now being entertained (33,99). Specifically, the instructive information embedded within the extracellular matrices is the target of MMP cleavage, such that release of sequestered bioactive molecules such as cytokines and chemokines, or shedding of the surface molecules such as L-selectins can alter immune cell function (12,27). MMP2, for instance, cleaves fibroblast growth factor receptor 1, a tyrosine kinase receptor, rendering it inaccessible for fibroblast growth factor binding and releasing a soluble receptor fragment of unknown direct biological function (100). On the other hand, MMP9 was shown to cleave the IL-2 receptor α chain on T cells, which results in downregulation of IL-2–dependent autocrine proliferation (101). The cleavage of laminin-5 by MMP2 generates new fragments that expose a normally inaccessible site to the epithelial cells, resulting in their enhanced motility (36). Availability of transforming growth factor-β to carry out its biological function was also shown to depend on degradation of decorin, a small collagen-associated proteoglycan that binds and sequesters its activity (102).

Generation and inactivation of bioactive molecules during inflammation can also alter cellular function. For instance, MMPs can cleave many serine class proteases, such as plasminogen and urokinase-type plasminogen activators that are potent mitogenic factors for lung fibroblasts (103). Similarly, MMP2 MMP7, and MMP9 can cleave α_1-proteinase inhibitor, the major endogenous serine class protease inhibitor (11). This cleavage inactivates the α_1-proteinase inhibitor and also generates a new biologically active fragment that is a powerful neutrophil chemoattractant factor (104). Since α_1-proteinase inhibitor is a potent endogenous inhibitor of neutrophil elastase, its degradation by MMP9 may indirectly activate neutrophil elastase by removing its natural inhibitor, which results in the elastin degradation seen in inflammatory lung disease (90,105). Thus, interfering with inhibitory molecules may be a plausible mechanism by which the prominent presence of MMP9 may participate in tissue remodeling (97).

Recent screening methods have identified potential physiological substrates for MMPs. For instance, using the MMP2 C-terminal domain as bait in a yeast two-hybrid screen, monocyte chemoattractant protein-3 was identified as an MMP2 substrate (37). Furthermore, searching the protein databases for specific peptide sequences identified the prodomain of transforming growth factor β as a potential target for MMP cleavage (106).

VII. Regulation of MMPs by Th2 Cytokines

As discussed earlier, recent studies show activated CD4 + T cells producing Th2 cytokines, including IL-4, IL-5, IL-10, and IL-13, in asthmatic lung (107). Despite the role of Th2 cytokines in mediating the acute asthma phenotype, the literature remains divided on their role in orchestrating a microenvironment that allows formation of a reactive stroma and progression of the subepithelial fibrosis that is believed to underlie chronic airway dysfunction. In contrast to the stimulation of macrophages by IL-4, IL-5, or IL-10, it has been shown that fibroblasts and chondrocytes downregulate MMPs in vitro (108–111). Bronchoalveolar lavage (BAL) fluid from asthma patients expressing the same cytokines shows upregulated production of MMPs (61,112). IFN-γ acts as an antifibrotic agent by downregulating collagen synthesis from human lung fibroblasts (113). Interestingly, clinical studies have shown an increase in IFN-γ expression following steroid treatment that corresponds with disease amelioration, although the effect on collagen synthesis was not examined (114). While only correlative, these studies nonetheless demonstrate a consistent relationship between airway inflammation and airway dysfunction and suggest that cytokine manipulation may influence disease expression. However, a clear understanding of the role of MMPs and reactive stroma formation in AHR and lung remodeling is lacking.

VIII. New and Old Functional Roles of MMPs in Allergic Lung Disease

The diversity in the role of proteases stems from their action as part of a complex interplay between cytokines, cell surface, transmembrane, and extracellular molecules that can influence local composition of bioactive molecules (Fig. 2). A significant advance in our understanding of how MMPs interact with ECM in the reactive

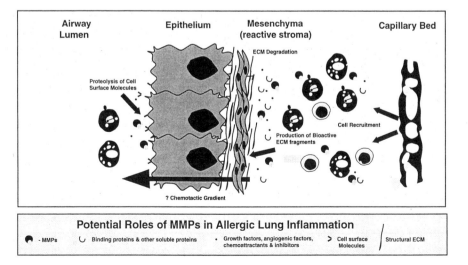

Figure 2 Potential roles of MMPs in allergic lung inflammation.

stroma has come from genetic analysis of mutational deletion of MMPs in mice. In particular, mice deficient in MMP2 when sensitized with allergens exhibited a robust allergic phenotype. Histopathology of lungs revealed that compared to the wild type, numerous eosinophils accumulated abnormally in the lungs of MMP2-/- mice concomitant with marked overexpression of mRNA for Th2 cytokines. Although excess eosinophils might account for this aberrant cytokine expression, lymphocytes produce the majority of Th2 cytokine mRNA in murine lungs following antigen challenge and are therefore a more likely source (4). Thus, both activated Th2 cells and eosinophils accumulate excessively in the absence of active MMP2. MMP2-dependent cell egression may therefore be a general mechanism required for the elimination of recruited inflammatory cells. Th2 cells and eosinophils especially are strongly implicated in the pathogenesis of allergic diseases such as asthma (115), and their accumulation, together with their excess cytokine products, would be expected to correlate with more severe disease.

The clearance of leukocytes in lung is not clearly understood, but it may proceed through one of three known routes: apoptosis and phagocytosis, lymphatic recirculation, and cell egression into the lumen (116). Recent studies show that in vitro clearance of apoptotic neutrophils is mediated through phagocytosis by macrophages (117). In acute allergic airway inflammation, however, eosinophils and macrophages constitute over 80% of total recovered leukocytes (118–120).

Although allergic inflammation may be deleterious to any organ, the host is particularly susceptible to lung involvement because of the potentially lethal effects of the inflammatory exudate on gas exchange (121). In this regard, luminal clearance of inflammatory cells is a potentially important means of inflammatory cell clearance. The lung epithelial basement membrane, rather than an insurmountable barrier, is readily degraded by members of the MMP clan (29). Further, transmigration of IL-5–activated eosinophils through an artificial basement membrane was partially blocked by synthetic MMP inhibitors (122). Surprisingly, recent studies have demonstrated that extravasation of inflammatory cells across the endothelial basement membrane occurs independently of the MMPs required for luminal clearance. Thus, the processes of extravasation and luminal clearance, while obviously related, rely on distinct mechanisms with MMP2 participating significantly only in the latter.

IX. Immune-Mesenchymal Cross-Talk: Role of MMPs in Inflammation

To understand the immune-mesenchymal cross-talk that must underlie the repair phase of allergic inflammation, the role of MMP2 and its regulation in allergic airway disease has been investigated. MMP2 expression in the lung is upregulated in the presence of Th2 cells and it requires the IL-4/IL-13-receptor–specific signaling chain IL-4Rα (124). Furthermore, lung mesenchymal cells secrete MMP2 directly in response to stimulation by IL-13 (20,123). Mice deficient in MMP2 or treated with MMP inhibitor develop allergic lung disease and a grossly abnormal phenotype marked by the massive accumulation in the lung of inflammatory cells, concomitant reduction in bronchoalveolar lavage cellularity, and extreme susceptibility to lethal asphyxiation (124). Thus, while IL-13 and IL-4Rα are required to initiate the asthma phenotype and associated inflammation, they also function to resolve allergic inflammation by directly eliciting MMP2 secretion from mesenchymal cells. In promoting the clearance of inflammatory cells through the airway lumen, MMP2 therefore serves a novel, beneficial role and represents an essential link in an IL-13/IL-4Rα–dependent regulatory loop that dampens inflammation.

X. Conclusions

The ongoing search for potential targets of ECM-degrading enzymes promises a better understanding of how MMPs may alter cell function. Although many MMPs share similar substrate profiles, differential expression and mechanisms that control activation of these enzymes provide clues as to their specific roles in lung inflammation and repair. Specifically, regulatory steps that ensure proteolytic activity against components of the basement membrane will also potentiate ECM remodeling by generating several different biologically active molecules, such as chemokines and fibronectin fragments that will alter immune cell function.

Among the major tasks that lie ahead is to determine the transcriptional regulation of the cytokines and chemokines that is needed as part of the inflammatory regulatory loop required for clearance of the recruited inflammatory cells. While excess production of proteases during inflammation may indeed be a necessary phase of repair process, identification of novel, functional genetic variants in the human MMP gene family may be a plausible explanation for genetic predisposition to over- or underproduction of MMPs (9). Knowledge gained from studies of especially animal models of allergic inflammation will provide the insight into MMP function that is required to determine the utility of proteases and protease inhibitors in the clinical management of diseases such as asthma.

References

1. Kumar RK, Foster PS. Murine model of chronic human asthma. Immunol Cell Biol 2001; 79:141–144.
2. Busse WW, Banks-Schlegel S, Wenzel SE. Pathophysiology of severe asthma. J Allergy Clin Immunol 2000; 106:1033–1042.
3. Fahy JV, Corry DB, Boushey HA. Airway inflammation and remodeling in asthma. Curr Opin Pulm Med 2000; 6:15–20.
4. Corry DB. IL-13 in allergy: home at last. Curr Opin Immunol 1999; 11:610–614.
5. Baram D, et al. Human mast cells release metalloproteinase-9 on contact with activated T cells: juxtacrine regulation by tnf-alpha. J Immunol 2001; 167:4008–4016.
6. Sempowski GD, Derdak S, Phipps RP. Interleukin-4 and interferon-gamma discordantly regulate collagen biosynthesis by functionally distinct lung fibroblast subsets. J Cell Physiol 1996; 167:290–296.
7. Doucet C, et al. Interleukin (IL) 4 and IL-13 act on human lung fibroblasts. Implication in asthma. J Clin Invest 1998; 101:2129–2139.

8. Renauld JC. New insights into the role of cytokines in asthma. J Clin Pathol 2001; 54:577–589.

9. Sternlicht MD, Werb Z. How matrix metalloproteinases regulate cell behavior. Annu Rev Cell Dev Biol 2001; 17:463–516.

10. Birkedal-Hansen, H. Matrix metalloproteinases. Adv Dent Res 1995; 9:16.

11. Sternlicht MD, Werb Z. ECM Proteinases. In: Kreis T, Vale R. Guidebook to the Extracellular Matrix and Adhesion Proteins. New York: Oxford University Press, 1999: 503–562.

12. Murray GI. Matrix metalloproteinases: a multifunctional group of molecules. J Pathol 2001; 195:135–137.

13. Birkedal-Hansen, H. Proteolytic remodeling of extracellular matrix. Curr Opin Cell Biol 1995; 7:728–735.

14. Stocker W, et al. The metzincins—topological and sequential relations between the astacins, adamalysins, serralysins, and matrixins (collagenases) define a superfamily of zinc-peptidases. Protein Sci 1995; 4:823–840.

15. Strieter RM. Mechanisms of pulmonary fibrosis: conference summary. Chest 2001; 120:77S–85S.

16. Mautino G, Capony F, Bousquet J, Vignola AM. Balance in asthma between matrix metalloproteinases and their inhibitors. J Allergy Clin Immunol 1999; 104:530–533.

17. Parks WC. Matrix metalloproteinases in repair. Wound Repair Regen 1999; 7:423–432.

18. Becky Kelly EA, Busse WW, Jarjour NN. Increased matrix metalloproteinase-9 in the airway after allergen challenge. Am J Respir Crit Care Med 2000; 162:1157–1161.

19. Vignola AM, et al. Sputum metalloproteinase-9/tissue inhibitor of metalloproteinase-1 ratio correlates with airflow obstruction in asthma and chronic bronchitis. Am J Respir Crit Care Med 1998; 158:1945–1950.

20. Zheng T, et al. Inducible targeting of IL-13 to the adult lung causes matrix metalloproteinase- and cathepsin-dependent emphysema. J Clin Invest 2000; 106:1081–1093.

21. Kumagai K, et al. Inhibition of matrix metalloproteinases prevents allergen-induced airway inflammation in a murine model of asthma. Journal of Immunology 1999; 162: 4212–4219.

22. Boushey H. Targets for asthma therapy. Allergie Immunol 2000; 32:336–341.

23. Holla LI, Vasku A, Stejskalova A, Znojil V. Functional polymorphism in the gelatinase B gene and asthma. Allergy 2000; 55:900–901.

24. Cataldo D, et al. MMP-2- and MMP-9-linked gelatinolytic activity in the sputum from patients with asthma and chronic obstructive pulmonary disease. Int Arch Allergy Immunol 2000; 123:259–267.

25. Haas TL, Madri JA. Extracellular matrix-driven matrix metalloproteinase production in endothelial cells: implications for angiogenesis. Trends Cardiovasc Med 1999; 9: 70–77.

26. Madri JA, Graesser D, Haas T. The roles of adhesion molecules and proteinases in lymphocyte transendothelial migration. Biochem Cell Biol 1996; 74:749–757.

27. Faveeuw C, Preece G, Ager A. Transendothelial migration of lymphocytes across high endothelial venules into lymph nodes is affected by metalloproteinases. Blood 2001; 98:688–695.

28. Kheradmand F, Werb Z. Shedding light on shedasses: role in growth and development. BioEssays 2002; 24:8–12.

29. Vu TH, Werb Z. Matrix metalloproteinases: effectors of development and normal physiology. Genes Dev 2000; 14:2123–2133.

30. Kheradmand P, Rishi K, Werb Z. Signaling through the EGF receptor controls lung morphogenesis in part by regulating MT1-MMP-mediated activation of gelatinase A/ MMP2. J Cell Sci 2002; 115:839–848.

31. Jeffery PK, Laitinen A, Venge P. Biopsy markers of airway inflammation and remodelling. Respir Med 2000; 94(suppl F):S9–15.

32. Bousquet J, Jeffery PK, Busse WW, Johnson M, Vignola AM. Asthma. From broncho-constriction to airways inflammation and remodeling. Am J Respir Crit Care Med 2000; 161:1720–1745.

33. McCawley LJ, Matrisian LM. Matrix metalloproteinases: they're not just for matrix anymore! Curr Opin Cell Biol 2001; 13:534–540.

34. Senior RM, Connolly NL, Cury JD, Welgus HG, Campbell EJ. Elastin degradation by human alveolar macrophages. A prominent role of metalloproteinase activity. Am Rev Respir Dis 1989; 139:1251–1256.

35. Senior RM, et al. Val-Gly-Val-Ala-Pro-Gly, a repeating peptide in elastin, is chemotactic for fibroblasts and monocytes. J Cell Biol 1984; 99:870–874.

36. Giannelli G, Falk-Marzillier J, Schiraldi O, Stetler-Stevenson WG, Quaranta V. Induction of cell migration by matrix metalloprotease-2 cleavage of laminin-5. Science 1997; 277:225–228.

37. McQuibban GA, et al. Inflammation dampened by gelatinase A cleavage of monocyte chemoattractant protein-3. Science 2000; 289:1202–1206.

38. Kang T, et al. Subcellular distribution and cytokine- and chemokine-regulated secretion of leukolysin/MT6-MMP/MMP-25 in neutrophils. J Biol Chem 2001; 276:21960–21968.

39. Overall CM. Matrix metalloproteinase substrate binding domains, modules and exosites. Overview and experimental strategies. Methods Mol Biol 2001; 151:79–120.

40. Corbel M, et al. Modulation of airway remodeling-associated mediators by the antifibrotic compound, pirfenidone, and the matrix metalloproteinase inhibitor, batimastat, during acute lung injury in mice. Eur J Pharmacol 2001; 426:113–121.

41. Yao PM et al. Cell-matrix interactions modulate 92-kD gelatinase expression by human bronchial epithelial cells. Am J Respir Cell Mol Biol 1998; 18:813–822.

42. d'Ortho MP, et al. Alveolar epithelial cells in vitro produce gelatinases and tissue inhibitor of matrix metalloproteinase-2. Am J Physiol 1997; 273:L663–675.

43. Yao PM, et al. Expression of matrix metalloproteinase gelatinases A and B by cultured epithelial cells from human bronchial explants. J Biol Chem 1996; 271:15580–15589.

44. Buisson AC, et al. Wound repair-induced expression of a stromelysins is associated with the acquisition of a mesenchymal phenotype in human respiratory epithelial cells. Lab Invest 1996; 74:658–669.

45. Pardo A, Ridge K, Uhal B, Sznajder JI, Selman M. Lung alveolar epithelial cells synthesize interstitial collagenase and gelatinases A and B in vitro. Int J Biochem Cell Biol 1997; 29:901–910.

46. Reponen P, et al. Molecular cloning of murine 72-kDa type IV collagenase and its expression during mouse development. J Biol Chem 1992; 267:7856–7862.

47. Dunsmore SE, et al. Matrilysin expression and function in airway epithelium. J Clin Invest 1998; 102:1321–1331.

48. Barnes PJ. Pathophysiology of asthma. Br J Clin Pharmacol 1996; 42:3–10.

49. Sears MR. Consequences of long-term inflammation. The natural history of asthma. Clin Chest Med 2000; 21:315–329.

50. Fish JE, Peters SP. Airway remodeling and persistent airway obstruction in asthma. J Allergy Clin Immunol 1999; 104:509–516.

51. Weitzman JB, Kanarek NF, Smialek JE. Medical examiner asthma death autopsies: a distinct subgroup of asthma deaths with implications for public health preventive strategies. Arch Pathol Lab Med 1998; 122:691–699.

52. Aikawa T, Shimura S, Sasaki H, Ebina M, Takishima T. Marked goblet cell hyperplasia with mucus accumulation in the airways of patients who died of severe acute asthma attack. Chest 1992; 101:916–921.

53. Openshaw PJ, Turner-Warwick M. Observations on sputum production in patients with variable airflow obstruction; implications for the diagnosis of asthma and chronic bronchitis. Respir Med 1989; 83:25–31.

54. Molfino NA, Nannini LJ, Martelli AN, Slutsky AS. Respiratory arrest in near-fatal asthma. N Engl J Med 1991; 324:285–288.

55. Abbas AK, Murphy KM, Sher A. Functional diversity of helper T lymphocytes. Nature 1996; 383:787–793.

56. Coffman RL, Mocci S, O'Garra A. The stability and reversibility of Th1 and Th2 populations. Curr Topics Microbiol Immunol 1999; 238:1–12.

57. Anthonisen NR, et al. Effects of smoking intervention and the use of an inhaled anticholinergic bronchodilator on the rate of decline of FEV_1. The Lung Health Study. JAMA 1994; 272:1497–1505.

58. Lange P, Parner J, Vestbo J, Schnohr P, Jensen G. A 15-year follow-up study of ventilatory function in adults with asthma. N Engl J Med 1998; 339:1194–1200.

59. Ollerenshaw SL, Woolcock AJ. Characteristics of the inflammation in biopsies from large airways of subjects with asthma and subjects with chronic airflow limitation. Am Rev Respir Dis 1992; 145:922–927.

60. Roche WR, Beasley R, Williams JH, Holgate ST. Subepithelial fibrosis in the bronchi of asthmatics. Lancet 1989; 1:520–524.

61. Hoshino M, Nakamura Y, Sim J, Shimojo J, Isogai S. Bronchial subepithelial fibrosis and expression of matrix metalloproteinase-9 in asthmatic airway inflammation. J Allergy Clin Immunol 1998; 102:783–788.

62. Chu HW, et al. Collagen deposition in large airways may not differentiate severe asthma from milder forms of the disease. Am J Respir Crit Care Med 1998; 158: 1936–1944.

63. Boulet LP, et al. Bronchial subepithelial fibrosis correlates with airway responsiveness to methacholine. Chest 1997; 112:45–52.

64. Wenzel SE, et al. Evidence that severe asthma can be divided pathologically into two inflammatory subtypes with distinct physiologic and clinical characteristics. Am J Respir Crit Care Med 1999; 160:1001–1008.

65. Weiss ST, et al. Effects of asthma on pulmonary function in children. A longitudinal population-based study. Am Rev Respir Dis 1992; 145:58–64.

66. Vestbo J, Prescott E, Lange P. Association of chronic mucus hypersecretion with FEV1 decline and chronic obstructive pulmonary disease morbidity. Copenhagen City Heart Study Group. Am J Respir Crit Care Med 1996; 153:1530–1535.

67. Connolly CK, Murthy NK, Alcock SM, Prescott RJ. Sputum and pulmonary function in asthma. Chest 1997; 112:994–999.

68. Vaillant B, Chiaramonte MG, Cheever AW, Soloway PD, Wynn TA. Regulation of hepatic fibrosis and extracellular matrix genes by the Th response: new insight into the role of tissue inhibitors of matrix metalloproteinases. J Immunol 2001; 167:7017–7026.

69. Mautino G, Oliver N, Chanez P, Bousquet J, Capony F. Increased release of matrix metalloproteinase-9 in bronchoalveolar lavage fluid and by alveolar macrophages of asthmatics. Am J Respir Cell Mol Biol 1997; 17:583–591.

70. Lemjabbar H, et al. Contribution of 92 kDa gelatinase/type IV collagenase in bronchial inflammation during status asthmaticus. Am J Respir Crit Care Med 1999; 159: 1298–1307.

71. Hoshino M, Takahashi M, Takai Y, Sim J. Inhaled corticosteroids decrease subepithelial collagen deposition by modulation of the balance between matrix metalloproteinase-9 and tissue inhibitor of metalloproteinase-1 expression in asthma (see comments). J Allergy Clin Immunol 1999; 104:356–363.

72. Shapiro SD, Campbell EJ, Kobayashi DK, Welgus HG. Dexamethasone selectively modulates basal and lipopolysaccharide-induced metalloproteinase and tissue inhibitor of metalloproteinase production by human alveolar macrophages. J Immunol 1991; 146:2724–2729.

73. Shapiro SD, Kobayashi DK, Welgus HG. Identification of TIMP-2 in human alveolar macrophages. Regulation of biosynthesis is opposite to that of metalloproteinases and TIMP-1. J Biol Chem 1992; 267:13890–13894.

74. Sottrup-Jensen L, Birkedal-Hansen H. Human fibroblast collagenase-alpha-macroglobulin interactions. Localization of cleavage sites in the bait regions of five mammalian alpha-macroglobulins. J Biol Chem 1989; 264:393–401.

75. Werb Z. ECM and cell surface proteolysis: regulating cellular ecology. Cell 1997; 91: 439–442.

76. Boger DL, Goldberg J, Silletti S, Kessler T, Cheresh DA. Identification of a novel class of small-molecule antiangiogenic agents through the screening of combinatorial libraries which function by inhibiting the binding and localization of proteinase MMP2 to integrin alpha(V)beta(3). J Am Chem Soc 2001; 123:1280–1288.

77. Brooks PC, et al. Localization of matrix metalloproteinase MMP-2 to the surface of invasive cells by interaction with integrin alpha v beta 3. Cell 1996; 85:683–693.

78. Deryugina EI, et al. MT1-MMP initiates activation of pro-MMP-2 and integrin alphavbeta3 promotes maturation of MMP-2 in breast carcinoma cells. Exp Cell Res 2001; 263:209–223.

79. Caterina JJ, et al. Inactivating mutation of the mouse tissue inhibitor of metalloproteinases-2(Timp-2) gene alters proMMP-2 activation. J Biol Chem 2000; 275: 26416–26422.

80. Kotra LP, et al. Insight into the complex and dynamic process of activation of matrix metalloproteinases. J Am Chem Soc 2001; 123:3108–3113.

81. Wright C, Strauss S, Toole K, Burt AD, Robson SC. Composition of the pulmonary interstitium during normal development of the human fetus. Pediatr Dev Pathol 1999; 2:424–431.

82. Starcher BC, Lung elastin and matrix. Chest 2000; 117:229S–234S.

83. Cantor JO, Cerreta JM, Armand G, Osman M, Turino GM. The pulmonary matrix, glycosaminoglycans and pulmonary emphysema. Connect Tissue Res 1999; 40: 97–104.

84. O'Donnell MD, et al. Ultrastructure of lung elastin and collagen in mouse models of spontaneous emphysema. Matrix Biol 1999; 18:357–360.

85. Takubo Y, et al. Age-associated changes in elastin and collagen content and the proportion of types I and III collagen in the lungs of mice. Exp Gerontol 1999; 34:353–364.

86. van Kuppevelt TH, Veerkamp JH, Timmermans JA. Immunoquantification of type I, III, IV and V collagen in small samples of human lung parenchyma. Int J Biochem Cell Biol 1995; 27:775–782.

87. Berg JT, Breen EC, Fu Z, Mathieu-Costello O, West JB. Alveolar hypoxia increases gene expression of extracellular matrix proteins and platelet-derived growth factor-B in lung parenchyma. Am J Respir Crit Care Med 1998; 158:1920–1928.

88. Senior RM, et al. Human 92- and 72-kilodalton type IV collagenases are elastases. J Biol Chem 1991; 266:7870–7875.

89. Roman J. Extracellular matrix and lung inflammation. Immunol Res 1996; 15:163–178.

90. Jeffery P. Remodeling in asthma and chronic obstructive lung disease. Am J Respir Crit Care Med 2001; 164:S28–S38.

91. Warburton D, et al. The molecular basis of lung morphogenesis. Mech Dev 2000; 92: 55–81.

92. Warburton D, et al. Do lung remodeling, repair, and regeneration recapitulate respiratory ontogeny. Am J Respir Crit Care Med 2001; 164:S59–62.

93. Laitinen A, et al. Tenascin is increased in airway basement membrane of asthmatics and decreased by an inhaled steroid. Am J Respir Crit Care Med 1997; 156:951–958.

94. Senior RM, et al. Entactin expression by rat lung and rat alveolar epithelial cells. Am J Respir Cell Mol Biol 1996; 14:239–247.

95. Lin Y, et al. Induced repatterning of type XVIII collagen expression in ureter bud from kidney to lung type: association with sonic hedgehog and ectopic surfactant protein C. Development 2001; 128(suppl):1573–1585.

96. Woessner JF, Jr. MMPs and TIMPs. An historical perspective. Methods Mol Biol 2001; 151:1–23.

97. Ashworth JL, et al. Fibrillin degradation by matrix metalloproteinases: implications for connective tissue remodelling. Biochem J 1999; 340:171–181.

98. Stetler-Stevenson WG, Yu AE. Proteases in invasion: matrix metalloproteinases. Semin Cancer Biol 2001; 11:143–152.

99. Xu J, et al. Proteolytic exposure of a cryptic site within collagen type IV is required for angiogenesis and tumor growth in vivo. J Cell Biol 2001; 154:1069–1079.

100. Levi E, et al. Matrix metalloproteinase 2 releases active soluble ectodomain of fibroblast growth factor receptor 1. Proc Natl Acad Sci USA 1996; 93:7069–7074.

101. Sheu BC, et al. A novel role of metalloproteinase in cancer-mediated immunosuppression. Cancer Res 2001; 61:237–242.

102. Imai K, Hiramatsu A, Fukushima D, Pierschbacher MD, Okada Y. Degradation of decorin by matrix metalloproteinases: identification of the cleavage sites, kinetic analyses and transforming growth factor-betal release. Biochem J 1997; 322:809–814.

103. Brown JK, et al. Tryptase, the dominant secretory granular protein in human mast cells, is a potent mitogen for cultured dog tracheal smooth muscle cells. Am J Respir Cell Mol Biol 1995; 13:227–236.

104. Banda MJ, Rice AG, Griffin GL, Senior RM. The inhibitory complex of human alpha 1-proteinase inhibitor and human leukocyte elastase is a neutrophil chemoattractant. J Exp Med 1988; 167:1608–1615.

105. Debelle L, Alix AJ. The structures of elastins and their function. Biochimie 1999; 81: 981–994.

106. Yu Q, Stamenkovic I. Cell surface-localized matrix metalloproteinase-9 proteolytically activates TGF-beta and promotes tumor invasion and angiogenesis. Genes Dev 2000; 14:163–176.

107. McKenzie GJ, et al. Impaired development of Th2 cells in IL-13-deficient mice. Immunity 1998; 9:423–432.

108. Lacraz S, Nicod LP, Chicheportiche R, Welgus HG, Dayer JM. IL-10 inhibits metalloproteinase and stimulates TIMP-1 production in human mononuclear phagocytes. J Clin Invest 1995; 96:2304–2310.

109. Nemoto O, et al. Suppression of matrix metalloproteinase-3 synthesis by interleukin-4 in human articular chondrocytes. J Rheumatol 1997; 24:1774–1779.

110. Prontera C, Crescenzi G, Rotilio D. Inhibition by interleukin-4 of stromelysin expression in human skin fibroblasts: role of PKC. Exp Cell Res 1996; 224:183–188.

111. Corcoran ML, Stetler-Stevenson WG, Brown PD, Wahl LM. Interleukin 4 inhibition of prostaglandin E2 synthesis blocks interstitial collagenase and 92-kDa type IV collagenase/gelatinase production by human monocytes. J Biol Chem 1992; 267:515–519.

112. Ohno I, et al. Eosinophils as a source of matrix metalloproteinase-9 in asthmatic airway inflammation. Am J Respir Cell Mol Biol 1997; 16:212–219.

113. Clark JG, Dedon TF, Wayner EA, Carter WG. Effects of interferon-gamma on expression of cell surface receptors for collagen and deposition of newly synthesized collagen by cultured human lung fibroblasts. J Clin Invest 1989; 83:1505–1511.

114. Leung DY, et al. Dysregulation of interleukin 4, interleukin 5, and interferon gamma gene expression in steroid-resistant asthma. J Exp Med 1995; 181:33–40.

115. Foster PS, et al. Elemental signals regulating eosinophil accumulation in the lung. Immunol Rev 2001; 179:173–181.

116. Savill J. Apoptosis in resolution of inflammation. Kidney Blood Pressure Res 2000; 23:173–174.

117. Savill J, Fadok V. Corpse clearance defines the meaning of cell death. Nature 2000; 407:784–788.

118. Corry DB, et al. Interleukin 4, but not interleukin 5 or eosinophils, is required in a murine model of acute airway hyperreactivity. J Exp Med 1996; 183:109–117.

119. Corry DB, et al. Requirements for allergen-induced airway hyperreactivity in T and B cell-deficient mice. Mol Med 1998; 4:344–355.

120. Grunig G, et al. Requirement for IL-13 independently of IL-4 in experimental asthma. Science 1998; 282:2261–2263.

121. Azzawi M, Johnston PW, Majumdar S, Kay AB, Jeffery PK. T lymphocytes and activated eosinophils in airway mucosa in fatal asthma and cystic fibrosis. Am Rev Respir Dis 1992; 145:1477–1482.

122. Okada S, Kita H, George TJ, Gleich GJ, Leiferman KM. Migration of eosinophils through basement membrane components in vitro: role of matrix metalloproteinase-9. Am J Respir Cell Mol Biol 1997; 17:519–528.

123. Zhu Z, et al. of Pulmonary expression interleukin-13 causes inflammation, mucus hypersecretion, subepithelial fibrosis, physiologic abnormalities, and eotaxin production. J Clin Invest 1999; 103:779–788.

124. Corry D, Rishi K, Kanelis J, Kiss A, Song L, Xu J, Feng L, Werb Z, Kheradmand F. Decreased allergic lung inflammatory cell egression and increased susceptibility to asphyxiation in MMP-2-deficiency. Nature Immunol 2002; 3:347–353.

36

Airway Smooth Muscle
An Immunomodulatory Cell?

AILI L. LAZAAR and REYNOLD A. PANETTIERI, Jr.

University of Pennsylvania Medical Center
Philadelphia, Pennsylvania, U.S.A.

I. Introduction

Asthma, a chronic disease with a prevalence of 3–5% in the United States, is characterized by reversible airway obstruction, airway inflammation, and airway smooth muscle (ASM) cell hyperplasia. The traditional view of airway smooth muscle in asthma, that of a purely contractile tissue, is rapidly changing. New evidence suggests that ASM cells play an important role, not only in regulating bronchomotor tone, but also in the perpetuation of airway inflammation and in the remodeling of the airways. In this chapter we will review the synthetic function of ASM cells, defined as the ability to secrete immune modulatory cytokines and chemokines and to express surface receptors that are important for cell adhesion and leukocyte activation. We will examine pharmacological approaches to modifying the synthetic function of ASM cells and discuss how altered synthetic function may contribute to airway remodeling.

II. Chemokine and Cytokine Release by Airway Smooth Muscle Cells

Following antigen exposure, eosinophils, macrophages, and lymphocytes are activated and/or recruited into the airways, where they initiate and perpetuate airway inflammation. The production of pro-inflammatory mediators by these cells has a profound influence on ASM cells. Evidence suggests that exposure of ASM to cytokines or growth factors alters contractility and calcium homeostasis (1) and induces SMC hypertrophy and hyperplasia (reviewed in Ref. 2). Recent data, however, convincingly demonstrate that ASM cells themselves can secrete a number of cytokines and chemoattractants, as shown in Figure 1. Studies of bronchial biopsies in mild asthmatics reveal constitutive staining of ASM for RANTES, a C-C chemokine that is involved in lymphocyte recruitment (3); in vitro, RANTES secretion is induced by TNFα and IFNγ (4–6). Similarly, the C-X-C chemokine IL-8, a neutrophil chemoattractant, is also secreted by ASM in response to TNFα, IL-1β, and bradykinin, a contractile agonist (7–9). Eotaxin is present in vivo in smooth muscle in asthmatics and is released by cultured ASM upon stimulation with TNFα, IL-1β, IL-4, or IL-13 (10–12). Eotaxin is critically important for eosinophil recruitment in asthma and other allergic conditions. Other chemokines that are secreted by ASM cells in vivo

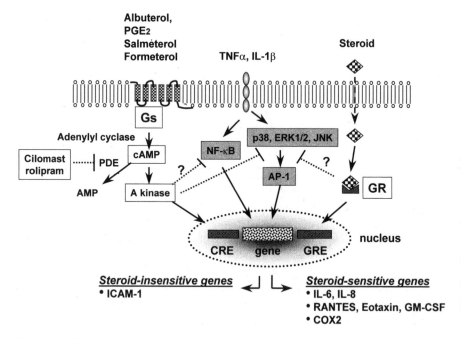

Figure 1   Putative signaling pathways that regulate cytokine-induced synthetic responses in airway smooth muscle cells. [cAMP]$_i$-mobilizing agents inhibit cytokine-induced chemokine and cell adhesion molecule expression. Il-6 secretion, however, is augmented by agents that increase [cAMP]$_i$. Cytokine-induced NF-κB activation in human airway smooth muscle is corticosteroid-insensitive. A kinase, cAMP-dependent protein kinase A; NF-κB, nuclear factor κB; CRE, cAMP response element; GRE, glucocorticoid response element; GR, glucocorticoid receptor; Gs, guanine-nucleotide binding protein; PDE, phosphodiesterase; JNK, jun kinase; ERK, extracellular signal-regulated kinase. (From Ref. 85.)

and in vitro include the family of monocyte chemotactic proteins MCP-1, MCP-2, and MCP-3 (5,13).

IL-6, a pleiotropic cytokine, induces smooth muscle cell hyperplasia (14), but also modulates B- and T-cell proliferation and immunoglobulin secretion. IL-6 secretion by ASM cells is inducible by multiple stimuli, including IL-1β, TNFα, TGF-β, and sphingosine-1-phosphate, a recently described mediator in asthma (6,9,15–17). Engagement of CD40 also induces IL-6 secretion by ASM cells (18). This has implications for clinical asthma where activated T lymphocytes, which express CD40L, are abundant and found in apposition to smooth muscle cell bundles. Interestingly, transgenic expression of IL-6 in the murine lung evokes a peribronchiolar inflammatory infiltrate but the animals are relatively *hypo*responsive to challenge with acetylcholine (19,20). Collectively, these studies suggest an intriguing role for IL-6 in controlling local inflammation and regulating airway reactivity and is consistent with the known ability of IL-6 to inhibit TNFα and IL-1β secretion.

ASM cells may also play a role in promoting both the recruitment and survival of eosinophils by secretion of GM-CSF and IL-5 (21–23). IL-5 and other Th2 cytokines may also play a role in sensitizing ASM cells to the effects of contractile agonists, independent of their effects on airway eosinophilia (23–25). Finally, additional cytokines that are secreted by human ASM cells include IL-1β, IFNβ, and other IL-6 family cytokines, such as leukemia inhibitory factor and IL-11, which are secreted following exposure of ASM cells to viral particles (9,15,26–28). IL-11 transgenic mice also exhibit submucosal thickening, but, in contrast to IL-6 transgenic mice, these animals display airway hyperreactivity (29). The differing effects of IL-6 and IL-11 on airway hyperreactivity are likely mediated through their unique receptor subunits and differences in downstream signaling pathways (30).

III. Receptors Involved in Cell Adhesion and Lymphocyte Activation

Cell adhesion molecules (CAMs) mediate leukocyte–endothelial cell interactions during the process of cell recruitment and homing (31). The expression and activation of a cascade of CAMs that include selectins, integrins, and members of the immunoglobulin superfamily, as well as the local production of chemoattractants, leads to leukocyte adhesion and transmigration into lymph nodes and sites of inflammation involving nonlymphoid tissues. The mechanisms that regulate extravasation of leukocytes from the circulation during the establishment of a local inflammatory response are rapidly being delineated. Less defined are the subsequent interactions of the infiltrating leukocytes with other cell types in the bronchial submucosa or with the extracellular matrix, which may be important for sustaining the inflammatory response.

In addition to mediating leukocyte extravasation and transendothelial migration, CAMs promote submucosal or subendothelial contact with cellular and extracellular matrix components and serve as co-stimulatory molecules in the activation of leukocytes. Evidence suggests that CAMs mediate inflammatory cell-stromal cell interactions that may contribute to airway inflammation. ASM cells express ICAM-1 and VCAM-1, which are inducible by a wide range of inflammatory mediators (32). In contrast, contractile agonists such as bradykinin and histamine have little effect on ASM CAM expression. ASM cells also constitutively express CD44, the primary receptor of the matrix protein hyaluronan (32). Recent data suggest that ASM cells express variable levels of integrin subunits, with the α_v, α_5, and β_1 subunits predominating (33). Activated T lymphocytes adhere via LFA-1 and VLA-4 to cytokine-induced ICAM-1 and VCAM-1 on cultured human airway smooth muscle cells. Moreover, an integrin-independent component of lymphocyte-smooth muscle cell adhesion appears to be mediated by CD44-hyaluronan interactions (32).

CAMs can function as accessory molecules for leukocyte activation (31,34,35). Whether CAMs expressed on smooth muscle serve this function, however, remains controversial. ASM cells do express MHC class II and CD40 following stimulation with IFNγ (18,36). Recent studies also suggest that human ASM cells express low levels of CD80 (B7.1) and CD86 (B7.2) (37). The physiological relevance of these findings remains unknown since ASM cells cannot present alloantigen to CD4 T cells, despite the expression of MHC class II and co-stimulatory molecules (36).

Functionally, however, adhesion of stimulated CD4 T cells can induce smooth muscle cell DNA synthesis (32). This appears to require direct cell-cell contact and is not mimicked by treatment of the cells with T-cell–conditioned medium. Adhesion of activated T cells also appears to alter smooth muscle cell contractility in a contact-dependent manner (37). Ligation of CD40, a co-stimulatory molecule upregulated by IFNγ, increases intracellular calcium as well as IL-6 secretion, while engagement of VCAM-1 activates phosphatidylinositol 3-kinase and augments growth factor–induced ASM cell proliferation (18,38). In addition, investigators have demonstrated that ASM cells express Fas in vivo. In vitro, expression of Fas is upregulated by TNFα, and, importantly, crosslinking of Fas induces smooth muscle cell apoptosis (39). These studies highlight the concept that direct interactions between leukocytes and smooth muscle cells via immune receptors such as CD40 and Fas or adhesion receptors such as ICAM-1 and VCAM-1 contribute to the modulation of the local milieu resulting in smooth muscle cell activation and growth.

IV. Other Immunomodulatory Proteins

Increased amounts of exhaled nitric oxide (NO) have been detected in patients with asthma (reviewed in Ref. 40). Nitric oxide appears to have a selective suppressive effect on the Th1 subset of helper T cells, suggesting that increased levels of nitric oxide may therefore lead to the predominantly Th2 type response associated with asthma. Nitric oxide synthase has been demonstrated in airway smooth muscle cells in vitro, where it results in an inhibition of ASM cell proliferation (41,42). In contrast, there is only indirect evidence that ASM cells produce nitric oxide in situ (43). ASM cells also produce large amounts of PGE_2 and, to a lesser extent, other prostanoids, following stimulation with pro-inflammatory cytokines (44). Although PGE_2 is a potent bronchodilator, it also has significant immunological effects. For example,

PGE_2 can decrease expression of CD23 (FcγRII), which has been shown to be expressed on human ASM cells (45) and may have a role as a negative regulator of airway inflammation and hyperresponsiveness (46–48). PGE_2 inhibits cytokine-induced secretion of GM-CSF and RANTES in vitro (6,49) and allergen-induced release of PGD_2 in patients with asthma (50). In contrast, PGE_2 also primes dendritic cells towards a Th2-promoting capacity and synergizes with IL-4 to induce IgE synthesis (51,52). Thus the roles of ASM-derived NO and PGE_2 need to be further defined, as they may have both beneficial and deleterious effects in the airway.

Leukotrienes are potent bronchoconstrictors in normal and asthmatic subjects and ASM cells express both receptors for the cysteinyl leukotrienes, LTC_4, LTD_4, and LTE_4 (53,54). Expression of the CysLT1 receptor is increased by exposure to IFNγ and results in an increase in LTD_4-mediated force generation in cultured ASM cells (55). The association between CysLT1 receptor expression and contractility may explain the increase in airway hyperresponsiveness following viral infection, a Th1-predominant environment. It also suggests that leukotriene receptor antagonists may have a therapeutic role in this clinical setting. Finally, receptors for the complement-derived anaphylatoxin peptides C3a and C5a have also been described on ASM cells. These peptides may play an important role in the pathogenesis of asthma by altering airway hyperresponsiveness, rather than airway inflammation (56,57).

V. Airway Smooth Muscle Cells and Extracellular Matrix

The importance of airway remodeling in chronic severe asthma has only recently been appreciated. ASM cells, by production of extracellular matrix (ECM) components, as well as matrix-modifying enzymes, may contribute to this process. ASM cell hypertrophy and hyperplasia is a hallmark of asthma. While ASM cells respond to exogenous growth factor stimulation by activating a complex array of signaling pathways that result in cell proliferation and growth, ASM cells may also produce endogenous growth factors that contribute to this process. Early reports demonstrated that IL-1β acts as a smooth muscle cell mitogen due to autocrine secretion of PDGF (58). More recently, it has been shown that TGF-β is secreted from ASM cells and, in turn, induces smooth muscle cell synthesis of hyaluronan and collagen (59–61). Recent studies have demonstrated that ASM cells secrete VEGF, a potent endothelial mitogen (62). While increased VEGF in bronchoalveolar lavage fluid of asthmatics appears to correlate with airway hyperreactivity (63), the effects of VEGF on ASM cell proliferation and synthetic function are currently unknown.

ASM cells secrete a wide variety of matrix proteoglycans, including fibronectin, collagen, hyaluronan, laminin, and versican, which are critical for maintaining the structure and function of the airways. The composition of the ECM is tightly controlled and involves a dynamic process of matrix deposition and degradation. Inflammatory processes such as asthma disturb this balance, resulting not only in an abnormal amount of matrix deposition, but also in an altered composition of matrix components. In asthma, there is an increase in hyaluronan, fibronectin, tenascin, versican, laminin, and collagen types I, III, and V (64,65). In vitro, serum from asthmatic patients increases smooth muscle cell release of fibronectin, laminin, perlecan, and chondroitin sulfate (66). Treatment of cells with corticosteroids, however, had no effect on the production of matrix proteins by ASM cells (66). This has been borne out in human studies where inhaled corticosteroids had minimal effect on altering ECM composition in asthmatics (67). These data support the finding that while corticosteroids are effective at inhibiting inflammation, newer therapies are needed to prevent and/or reverse airway fibrosis seen in asthma.

The derangement in matrix components seen in asthma likely is multifactorial. Not only is there increased matrix deposition, there is also an imbalance between matrix-degrading enzymes and inhibitors of these proteases. One class of proteins that has been intensively studied is the matrix metalloproteinase (MMP) family. MMP-1 expression is elevated in the smooth muscle cells of asthmatics, and studies have shown that LTD_4 increases expression of MMP-1, which acts to degrade insulin-like growth factor binding protein, a growth inhibitor (68). $TNF\alpha$ induces the release of MMP-9, which can degrade matrix but also plays a critical role in cleaving latent $TGF-\beta$ to its active form (69). Progelatinase A (MMP-2) is constitutively released by ASM cells, but remains inactive because of high levels of tissue inhibitor of metalloproteinases (TIMP)-2 on the cell membrane (70). In contrast, TIMP-1 is secreted in large amounts into the conditioned media of ASM cells (70). Membrane type 1 MMP is also found on ASM (70); this proteinase can activate MMP-2 and has been shown to cleave CD44 from the cell surface and promote cell migration (71). Clearly, ASM cells play an active role in modifying their environment. Further studies will be necessary to understand the interaction between ECM, MMPs, and TIMPs in the development of airway remodeling.

Thus, ASM cells provide a rich source of cytokines and chemokines and under certain conditions can express a wide variety of adhesion receptors, co-stimulatory molecules, and other immunomodulatory proteins (Table 1). Taken together, these

Table 1 Immunomodulatory Proteins Expressed by Human ASM Cells

Cytokines	Chemokines	CAMs	Other
IL-1β	IL-8	ICAM-1	CD40
IL-5	RANTES	VCAM-1	Fas
IL-6	MCP-1,-2,-3	CD44	HLA-DR
IL-8	Eotaxin	LFA-1	FcγRII
IL-11	GM-CSF	$\alpha_9\beta_1$	FcγRIII
LIF		$\alpha_5\beta_1$	NO
IFNβ		α_v, α_6 subunits	PGE$_2$
			CysLT receptors
			C3a/C5a receptors
			MMP/TIMP
			VEGF

data provide support for the potential role of ASM cells not only in perpetuating airway inflammation but also in leukocyte activation.

VI. Airway Smooth Muscle as a Target for Anti-Inflammatory Therapy

To date, the most effective therapeutic approaches in asthma are corticosteroids and β-adrenergic receptor agonists, which abrogate airway inflammation and reverse bronchoconstriction, respectively. Given the new evidence that ASM cells secrete and express immunomodulatory proteins, investigators are now studying the cellular and molecular processes that regulate ASM synthetic function and examining the role of dexamethasone and β agonists in modulating cytokine-induced synthetic responses.

A. Effects of [cAMP]$_i$-Mobilizing Agents on Cytokine-Induced Synthetic Responses

In asthma, β-agonists such as isoproterenol, albuterol, salmeterol, and formoterol are therapeutic agents that promote bronchodilation by stimulating receptors coupled to Gs, which in turn activates adenylyl cyclase, increases [cAMP]$_i$, and stimulates cAMP-dependent protein kinase (A-kinase) in ASM. In a similar manner, PGE$_2$, which is produced in large quantities at sites of inflammation, also increases [cAMP]$_i$ in human ASM cells and is a potent and effective bronchodilator (72). New evidence suggests that [cAMP]$_i$-mobilizing agents in ASM cells also modulate cytokine-induced synthetic function. In TNFα-stimulated ASM cells, both eotaxin and RANTES expression are effectively inhibited by isoproterenol, PGE$_2$, dibutyl-[cAMP]$_i$, or the phosphodiesterase inhibitors rolipram and cilomast (6,73,74). TNFα-induced IL-8 secretion was also inhibited by the combination of [cAMP]$_i$ mobilizing agents and corticosteroids (75). Similarly, sphingosine-1-phosphate, which activates a Gs protein–coupled receptor and increases [cAMP]$_i$, abrogated TNFα-induced RANTES secretion in ASM cells (17).

In contrast to the effects of [cAMP]$_i$ on chemokine secretion, pharmacological agents that increase [cAMP]$_i$ markedly stimulate secretion of IL-6 in human ASM cells (6). This appears to be due to effects on basal IL-6 promoter activity (76). Whether the secreted IL-6 modulates ASM cell function in an autocrine manner or alters leukocyte function in the submucosa remains unknown. Since studies show that overexpression of IL-6 decreases acetylcholine responsiveness in transgenic mice (19), the role of IL-6 in asthma may be that of an anti-inflammatory signal. More recently, it has been shown that cAMP decreases secretion of GM-CSF by ASM cells. Cyclooxygenase inhibitors reduce PGE$_2$ and enhance cytokine-induced secretion of GM-CSF (49,77), while PDE type IV inhibitors reduce GM-CSF secretion in vitro and antigen-induced airway hyperresponsiveness in an animal model (49,78). Taken together, current evidence suggests that some but not all pro-inflammatory functions in ASM cells are inhibited by [cAMP]$_i$-mobilizing agents.

Conflicting reports exist, however, concerning effects of increased $[cAMP]_i$ on lymphocyte adhesion and migration through cytokine-activated endothelial cells (79,80). The controversy regarding the role of $[cAMP]_i$ in modulating cell adhesion likely reflects differences in the cytokines used to stimulate endothelial cells or the temporal differences in the addition of the agonists used to increase $[cAMP]_i$. Far less is known concerning $[cAMP]_i$ effects on smooth muscle-leukocyte adhesion. In human ASM cells, activation of $[cAMP]_i$-dependent pathways inhibited, in part, both TNFα-mediated induction of ICAM-1 and VCAM-1 expression and adhesion of activated T cells to ASM cells. Interestingly, the basal expression of ICAM-1 and VCAM-1, as well as the binding of activated T cells to unstimulated ASM, was resistant to increases in $[cAMP]_i$ (81). Together these studies show that cytokine-induced expression of cell adhesion molecules and T-cell adhesion to ASM cells are modulated by changes in $[cAMP]_i$.

B. Corticosteroids Alter Cytokine-Induced Synthetic Responses

One of the most effective medications to date for controlling airway inflammation in asthma has been inhaled corticosteroids. Despite their use for over 25 years, the precise mechanisms by which steroids improve lung function in asthma remain unclear. Current evidence suggests that chemokine and cytokine secretion induced by inflammatory mediators is inhibited by dexamethasone in human ASM cells. Cytokine-induced secretion of RANTES (4–6), MCP (5), eotaxin (73), GM-CSF (21), and IL-6 (16) is abrogated by corticosteroids. In most of these studies, corticosteroid and $[cAMP]_i$-mobilizing agents also act additively to inhibit chemokine and cytokine secretion. Recent data suggest that the effects of dexamethasone on RANTES expression are mediated through inhibition of the transcription factor AP-1 (76).

NF-κB is another transcriptional factor mediating chronic inflammatory responses in asthma, rheumatoid arthritis, psoriasis, and inflammatory bowel disease (82). Interestingly, dexamethasone had no effect on TNFα- or IL-1 β–induced NF-κB activation in human ASM cells (83). Furthermore, cytokine-induced ICAM-1 expression in ASM cells, which is completely dependent on NF-κB activation, was modestly affected by dexamethasone, and IL-6 secretion is only partially inhibited (76). In contrast, IL-1β–induced cyclooxygenase-2 expression was abrogated (44,83,84). Collectively these data support the notion that anti-inflammatory effects of steroids in asthma may not be due solely to modulation of cytokine-induced NF-κB activation and are likely regulated by pathways such as AP-1 or other transcription factors.

VII. Summary

The biology of ASM is complex and fascinating. The myriad pathways regulating cell growth and proliferation, combined with the emerging role of ASM as a modulator of inflammation, provide a rich area of investigation (see Fig. 1). Future studies will focus on mechanisms regulating both acute inflammation and the chronic repair processes leading to airway remodeling in the hopes of expanding the repertoire of useful therapeutic agents in the treatment of asthma.

References

1. Amrani Y, Panettieri RA, Jr. Cytokines induce airway smooth muscle cell hyperresponsiveness to contractile agonists. Thorax 1998; 53:713–716.
2. Lazaar AL, Amrani Y, Panettieri RA, Jr. The role of inflammation in the regulation of airway smooth muscle cell function and growth. In: Busse W, Holgate S, eds. Asthma and Rhinitis. Oxford, UK: Blackwell Science, Ltd., 2000:1402–1413.
3. Berkman N, Krishnan VL, Gilbey T, Newton R, O'Connor B, Barnes PJ, Chung KF. Expression of RANTES mRNA and protein in airways of patients with mild asthma. Am J Respir Crit Care Med 1996; 154:1804–1811.
4. John M, Hirst SJ, Jose PJ, Robichaud A, Berkman N, Witt C, Twort CHC, Barnes PJ, Chung KF. Human airway smooth muscle cells express and release RANTES in response to T helper 1 cytokines. Regulation by T helper 2 cytokines and corticosteroids. J Immunol 1997; 158:1841–1847.
5. Pype JL, Dupont LJ, Menten P, Van Coillie E, Opdenakker G, Van Damme J, Chung KF, Demedts MG, Verleden GM. Expression of monocyte chemotactic protein (MCP)-1, MCP-2, and MCP-3 by human airway smooth-muscle cells. Modulation by corticosteroids and T-helper 2 cytokines. Am J Respir Cell Mol Biol 1999; 21:528–536.
6. Ammit AJ, Hoffman RK, Amrani Y, Lazaar AL, Hay DWP, Torphy TJ, Penn RB, Panettieri RA, Jr. TNFα-induced secretion of RANTES and IL-6 from human airway smooth muscle cells: modulation by cAMP. Am J Respir Cell Mol Biol 2000; 23:794–802.
7. John M, Au B-T, Jose PJ, Lim S, Saunders M, Barnes PJ, Mitchell JA, Belvisi MG, Chung KF. Expression and release of interleukin-8 by human airway smooth muscle cells: Inhibition by Th-2 cytokines and corticosteroids. Am J Respir Cell Mol Biol 1998; 18:84–90.
8. Pang L, Knox AJ. Bradykinin stimulates IL-8 production in cultured human airway smooth muscle cells: role of cyclooxygenase products. J Immunol 1998; 161:2509–2515.
9. Hedges JC, Singer CA, Gerthoffer WT. Mitogen-activated protein kinases regulate cytokine gene expression in human airway myocytes. Am J Respir Cell Mol Biol 2000; 23:86–94.
10. Ghaffar O, Hamid Q, Renzi PM, Allahkverdi Z, Molet S, Hogg JC, Shore SA, Luster AD, Lamkhioued B. Constitutive and cytokine-stimulated expression of eotaxin by human airway smooth muscle cells. Am J Respir Crit Care Med 1999; 159:1933–1942.
11. Chung KF, Patel HJ, Fadlon EJ, Rousell J, Haddad E-B, Jose PJ, Mitchell J, Belvisi M. Induction of eotaxin expression and release from human airway smooth muscle cells by IL-1β and TNFα: effects of IL-10 and corticosteroids. Br J Pharmacol 1999; 127:1145–1150.
12. Moore PE, Church TL, Chism DD, Panettieri RA, Jr., Shore SA. IL-13 and IL-4 cause eotaxin release in human airway smooth muscle cells: a role for ERK. Am J Physiol (Lung Cell Mol Physiol) 2002; 282:L847–853.

13. Sousa AR, Lane SJ, Nakhosteen JA, Yoshimura T, Lee TH, Poston RN. Increased expression of the monocyte chemoattractant protein-1 in bronchial tissue from asthmatic subjects. Am J Respir Cell Mol Biol 1994; 10:142–147.

14. De S, Zelazny ET, Souhrada JF, Souhrada M. IL-1β and IL-6 induce hyperplasia and hypertrophy of cultured guinea pig airway smooth muscle cells. J Appl Physiol 1995; 78:1555–1563.

15. Elias JA, Wu Y, Zheng T, Panettieri RA, Jr. Cytokine- and virus-stimulated airway smooth muscle cells produce IL-11 and other IL-6-type cytokines. Am J Physiol (Lung Cell Mol Physiol) 1997; 273/17:L648–L655.

16. McKay S, Hirst SJ, Bertrand-de Haas M, de Jonste JC, Hoogsteden HC, Saxena PR, Sharma HS. Tumor necrosis factor-α enhances mRNA expression and secretion of interleukin-6 in cultured human airway smooth muscle cells. Am J Respir Cell Mol Biol 2000; 23:103–111.

17. Ammit AJ, Hastie AT, Edsall LC, Hoffman RK, Amrani Y, Krymskaya VP, Kane SA, Peters SP, Penn RB, Spiegel S, Panettieri RA, Jr. Sphingosine 1-phosphate modulates human airway smooth muscle cell functions that promote inflammation and airway remodeling in asthma. FASEB J 2001; 15:1212–1214.

18. Lazaar AL, Amrani Y, Hsu J, Panettieri RA, Jr., Fanslow WC, Albelda SM, Puré E. CD40-mediated signal transduction in human airway smooth muscle. J Immunol 1998; 161:3120–3127.

19. DiCosmo BF, Geba GP, Picarella D, Elias JA, Rankin JA, Stripp BR, Whitsett JA, Flavell RA. Airway epithelial cell expression of interleukin-6 in transgenic mice. Uncoupling of airway inflammation and bronchial hyperreactivity. J Clin Invest 1994; 94:2028–2035.

20. Wang J, Homer RJ, Chen Q, Elias JA. Endogenous and exogenous IL-6 inhibit aeroallergen-induced Th2 inflammation. J Immunol 2000; 165:4051–4061.

21. Saunders MA, Mitchell JA, Seldon PM, Yacoub MH, Barnes PJ, Giembycz MA, Belvisi MG. Release of granulocyte-macrophage colony stimulating factor by human cultured airway smooth muscle cells: suppression by dexamethasone. Br J Pharmacol 1997; 120:545–546.

22. Hallsworth MP, Soh CPC, Twort CHC, Lee TH, Hirst SJ. Cultured human airway smooth muscle cells stimulated by interleukin-1β enhance eosinophil survival. Am J Respir Cell Mol Biol 1998; 19:910–919.

23. Hakonarson H, Maskeri N, Carter C, Chuang S, Grunstein MM. Autocrine interaction between IL-5 and IL-1β mediates altered responsiveness of atopic asthmatic sensitized airway smooth muscle. J Clin Invest 1999; 104:657–667.

24. Rizzo CA, Yang R, Greenfeder S, Egan RW, Pauwels RA, Hey JA. The IL-5 receptor on human bronchus selectively primes for hyperresponsiveness. J Allergy Clin Immunol 2002; 109:404–409.

25. Venkayya R, Lam M, Willkom M, Grunig G, Corry DB, Erle DJ. The Th2 lymphocyte products IL-4 and IL-13 rapidly induce airway hyperresponsiveness through direct effects on resident airway cells. Am J Respir Cell Mol Biol 2002; 26:202–208.

26. Knight DA, Lydell CP, Zhou D, Weir TD, Schellenberg RR, Bai TR. Leukemia inhibitory factor (LIF) and LIF receptor in human lung: distribution and regulation of LIF release. Am J Respir Cell Mol Biol 1999; 20:834–841.

27. Hakonarson H, Carter C, Maskeri N, Hodinka R, Grunstein MM. Rhinovirus-mediated changes in airway smooth muscle responsiveness: induced autocrine role of interleukin-1β. Am J Physiol (Lung Cell Mol Physiol) 1999; 277/21:L13–L21.

28. Rodel J, Assefa S, Prochnau D, Woytas M, Hartmann M, Groh A, Straube E. Interferon-β induction by *Chlamydia pneumoniae* in human smooth muscle cells. FEMS Immunol Med Microbiol 2001; 32:9–15.

29. Kuhn C, Homer RJ, Zhu Z, Ward N, Elias JA. Morphometry explains variation in airway responsiveness in transgenic mice overexpressing interleukin-6 and interleukin-11 in the lung. Chest 2000; 117:260S–262S.

30. Lahiri T, Laporte JD, Moore PE, Panettieri RA, Jr., Shore SA. Interleukin-6 family cytokines: signaling and effects in human airway smooth muscle cells. Am J Physiol (Lung Cell Mol Physiol) 2001; 280:L1225–L1232.

31. Springer TA. Adhesion receptors of the immune system. Nature 1990; 346:425–434.

32. Lazaar AL, Albelda SM, Pilewski JM, Brennan B, Puré E, Panettieri RA, Jr. T lympho-cytes adhere to airway smooth muscle cells via integrins and CD44 and induce smooth muscle cell DNA synthesis. J Exp Med 1994; 180:807–816.

33. Freyer AM, Johnson SR, Hall IP. Effects of growth factors and extracellular matrix on survival of human airway smooth muscle cells. Am J Respir Cell Mol Biol 2001; 25:569–576.

34. Dustin ML, Springer TA. Role of lymphocyte adhesion receptors in transient interactions and cell locomotion. Annu Rev Immunol 1991; 9:27–66.

35. van Seventer GA, Newman W, Shimuzu Y, Nutman TB, Tanaka Y, Horgan KJ, Gopal TV, Ennis E, O'Sullivan D, Grey H. Analysis of T cell stimulation by superantigen plus major histocompatibility complex class II molecules or by CD3 monoclonal antibody: costimulation by purified adhesion ligands VCAM-1, ICAM-1, but not ELAM-1. J Exp Med 1991; 174:901–913.

36. Lazaar AL, Reitz HE, Panettieri RA, Jr., Peters SP, Puré E. Antigen receptor-stimulated peripheral blood and bronchoalveolar lavage-derived T cells induce MHC class II and ICAM-1 expression on human airway smooth muscle. Am J Respir Cell Mol Biol 1997; 16:38–45.

37. Hakonarson H, Kim C, Whelan R, Campbell D, Grunstein MM. Bi-directional activation between human airway smooth muscle cells and T lymphocytes: role in induction of altered airway responsiveness. J Immunol 2001; 166:293–303.

38. Lazaar AL, Krymskaya VP, Das SK. VCAM-1 activates phosphatidylinositol 3-kinase and induces p120(Cb1) phosphorylation in human airway smooth muscle cells. J Immunol 2001; 166:155–161.

39. Hamann KJ, Vieira JE, Halayko AJ, Dorscheid D, White SR, Forsythe SM, Camoretti-Mercado B, Rabe KF, Solway J. Fas cross-linking induces apoptosis in human airway smooth muscle cells. Am J Physiol (Lung Cell Mol Physiol) 2000; 278:L618.

40. Gaston B, Drazen JM, Loscalzo J, Stamler JS. The biology of nitrogen oxides in the airways. Am J Respir Crit Care Med 1994; 149:538–551.

41. Hamad AM, Johnson SR, Knox AJ. Antiproliferative effects of NO and ANP in cultured human airway smooth muscle. Am J Physiol 1999; 277:L910–L918.

42. Patel HJ, Belvisi MG, Donnelly LE, Yacoub MH, Chung KF, Mitchell JA. Constitutive expressions of type I NOS in human airway smooth muscle cells: evidence for an antiproliferative role. FASEB J 1999; 13:1810–1816.

43. Gow AJ, Chen Q, Hess DT, Day BJ, Ischiropoulos H, Stamler JS. Basal and stimulated protein S-nitrosylation in multiple cell types and tissues. J Biol Chem 2002; 277:9637–9640.

44. Belvisi MG, Saunders MA, Haddad E-B, Hirst SJ, Yacoub MH, Barnes PJ, Mitchell JA. Induction of cyclo-oxygenase-2 by cytokines in human cultured airway smooth muscle cells: novel inflammatory role of this cell type. Br J Pharmacol 1997; 120:910–916.

45. Hakonarson H, Grunstein MM. Autologously up-regulated Fc receptor expression and action in airway smooth muscle mediates its altered responsiveness in the atopic asthmatic sensitized state. Proc Natl Acad Sci USA 1998; 95:5257–5262.

46. Cernadas M, De Sanctis GT, Krinzman SJ, Mark DA, Donovan CE, Listman JA, Kobzik L, H. Kikutani, Christiani DC, Perkins DL, Finn PW. CD23 and allergic pulmonary inflammation: potential role as an inhibitor. Am J Respir Cell Mol Biol 1999; 20:1.

47. Dasic G, Juillard P, Graber P, Herren S, Angell T, Knowles R, Bonnefoy JY, Kosco-Vilbois MH, Chvatchko Y. Critical role of CD23 in allergen-induced bronchoconstriction in a murine model of allergic asthma. Eur J Immunol 1999; 29:2957.

48. Haczku A, Takeda K, Hamelmann E, Loader J, Joetham A, Redai I, Irvin CG, Lee JJ, Kikutani H, Conrad D, Gelfand EW. CD23 exhibits negative regulatory effects on allergic sensitization and airway hyperresponsiveness. Am J Respir Crit Care Med 2000; 161:952–960.

49. Lazzeri N, Belvisi MG, Patel HJ, Yacoub MH, Fan Chung K, Mitchell JA. Effects of prostaglandin E(2) and cAMP elevating drugs on GM-CSF release by cultured human airway smooth muscle cells. Relevance to asthma therapy. Am J Respir Cell Mol Biol 2001; 24:44–48.

50. Hartert TV, Dworski RT, Mellen BG, Oates JA, Murray JJ, Sheller JR. Prostaglandin E_2 decreases allergen-stimulated release of prostaglandin D_2 in airways of subjects with asthma. Am J Respir Crit Care Med 2000; 162:637.

51. Kapsenberg ML, Hilkens CM, Wierenga EA, Kalinski P. The paradigm of type 1 and type 2 antigen-presenting cells. Implications for atopic allergy. Clin Exp Allergy 1999; 29 (suppl 2):33–36.

52. Roper RL, Conrad DH, Brown DM, Warner GL, Phipps RP. Prostaglandin E2 promotes IL-4-induced IgE and IgG1 synthesis. J Immunol 1990; 145:2644–2651.

53. Lynch KR, O'Neill GP, Liu Q, Im DS, Sawyer N, Metters KM, Coulombe N, Abramovitz M, Figueroa DJ, Zeng Z, Connolly BM, Bai C, Austin CP, Chateauneuf A, Stocco R, Greig GM, Kargman S, Hooks SB, Hosfield E, Williams DL, Jr., Ford-Hutchinson AW, Caskey CT, Evans JF. Characterization of the human cysteinyl leukotriene CysLT1 receptor. Nature 1999; 399:789.

54. Heise CE, O'Dowd BF, Figueroa DJ, Sawyer N, Nguyen T, Im D-S, Stocco R, Bellefeu-ille JN, Abramovitz M, Cheng R, Williams DL, Jr., Zeng Z, Liu Q, Ma L, Clements MK, Coulombe N, Liu Y, Austin CP, George SR, O'Neill GP, Metters KM, Lynch KR, Evans JF. Characterization of the human cysteinyl leukotriene 2 receptor. J Biol Chem 2000; 275:30531–30536.

55. Amrani Y, Moore PE, Hoffman R, Shore SA, Panettieri RA, Jr. Interferon-γ modulates cysteinyl leukotriene receptor-1 expression and function in human airway myocytes. Am J Respir Crit Care Med 2001; 164:2098–2101.

56. Humbles AA, Lu B, Nilsson CA, Lilly C, Israel E, Fujiwara Y, Gerard NP, Gerard C. A role for the C3a anaphylatoxin receptor in the effector phase of asthma. Nature 2000; 406:998.

57. Karp CL, Grupe A, Schadt E, Ewart SL, Keane-Moore M, Cuomo PJ, Kohl J, Wahl L, Kuperman D, Germer S, Aud D, Peltz G, Wills-Karp M. Identification of complement factor 5 as a susceptibility locus for experimental allergic asthma. Nature Immunol 2000; 1:221.

58. De S, Zelazny ET, Souhrada JF, Souhrada M. Interleukin-1β stimulates the proliferation of cultured airway smooth muscle cells via platelet-derived growth factor. Am J Respir Cell Mol Biol 1993; 9:645–651.

59. Black PN, Young PG, Skinner SJ. Response of airway smooth muscle cells to TGF-beta 1: effects on growth and synthesis of glycosaminoglycans. Am J Physiol (Lung Cell Mol Physiol) 1996; 271:L910.

60. McKay S, de Jongste JC, Saxena PR, Sharma HS. Angiotensin II induces hypertrophy of human airway smooth muscle cells: expression of transcription factors and transforming growth factor-β_1. Am J Respir Cell Mol Biol 1998; 18:823.

61. Coutts A, Chen G, Stephens N, Hirst S, Douglas D, Eichholtz T, Khalil N. Release of biologically active TGF-β from airway smooth muscle cells induces autocrine synthesis of collagen. Am J Physiol (Lung Cell Mol Physiol) 2001; 280:L999.

62. Knox AJ, Corbett L, Stocks J, Holland E, Zhu YM, Pang L. Human airway smooth muscle cells secrete vascular endothelial growth factor: up-regulation by bradykinin via a protein kinase C and prostanoid-dependent mechanism. FASEB J 2001; 15:2480–2488.

63. Hoshino M, Nakamura Y, Hamid QA. Gene expression of vascular endothelial growth factor and its receptors and angiogenesis in bronchial asthma. J Allergy Clin Immunol 2001; 107:1034–1038.

64. Roberts CR, Burke A. Remodelling of the extracellular matrix in asthma: proteoglycan synthesis and degradation. Can Respir J 1998; 5:48–50.

65. Laitinen A, Altraja A, Kampe M, Linden M, Virtanen I, Laitinen LA. Tenascin is increased in airway basement membrane of asthmatics and decreased by an inhaled steroid. Am J Respir Crit Care Med 1997; 156:951–958.

66. Johnson PRA, Black JL, Cralin S, Ge Q, Underwood PA. The production of extracellular matrix proteins by human passively sensitized airway smooth-muscle cells in culture: The effect of beclomethasone. Am J Respir Crit Care Med 2000; 162:2145–2151.

67. Laitinen LA, Laitinen A. Inhaled corticosteroid treatment and extracellular matrix in the airways in asthma. Int Arch Allergy Immunol 1995; 107:215–216.

68. Rajah R, Nunn S, Herrick D, Grunstein MM, Cohen P. LTD-4 induces matrix metalloproteinase-1 which functions as an IGFBP protease in airway smooth muscle cells. Am J Physiol (Lung Cell Mol Physiol) 1996; 271:L1014–L1022.

69. Yu A, Stamenkovic I. Cell surface-localized matrix metalloproteinase-9 proteolytically activates TGF-β and promotes tumor invasion and angiogenesis. Genes Develop 2000; 14:163.

70. Foda HD, George S, Rollo E, Drews M, Conner C, Cao J, Panettieri RA, Jr., Zucker S. Regulation of gelatinases in human airway smooth muscle cells: mechanism of progelatinase A activation. Am J Physiol (Lung Cell Mol Physiol) 1999; 277/21:L174–L182.

71. Kajita M, Itoh Y, Chiba T, Mori H, Okada A, Kinoh H, Seiki M. Membrane-type 1 matrix metalloproteinase cleaves CD44 and promotes cell migration. J Cell Biol 2001; 153:893.

72. Hall IP, Widdop S, Townsend P, Daykin K. Control of cyclic AMP levels in primary cultures of human tracheal smooth muscle cells. Br J Pharmacol 1992; 107:422–428.

73. Pang L, Knox AJ. Regulation of TNF-α-induced eotaxin release from cultured human airway smooth muscle cells by β_2-agonists and corticosteroids. FASEB J 2001; 115:261–269.

74. Hallsworth MP, Twort CH, Lee TH, Hirst SJ. β_2-adrenoceptor agonists inhibit release of eosinophil-activating cytokines from human airway smooth muscle cells. Br J Pharmacol 2001; 132:729.

75. Pang L, Knox AJ. Synergistic inhibition by β_2-agonists and corticosteroids on tumor necrosis factor-α-induced interleukin-8 release from cultured human airway smooth-muscle cells. Am J Respir Cell Mol Biol 2000; 23:79–85.

76. Ammit AJ, Lazaar AL, Irani C, O'Neill GM, Gordon ND, Amrani Y, Penn RB, Panettieri RA, Jr. Tumor necrosis factor-α-induced secretion of RANTES and interleukin-6 from human airway smooth muscle cells: modulation by glucocorticoids and β-agonists. Am J Respir Cell Mol Biol 2002; 26:465–474.

77. Bonazzi A, Bolla M, Buccellati C, Hernandez A, Zarini S, Vigano T, Fumagalli F, Viappiani S, Ravasi S, Zannini P, Chiesa G, Folco G, Sala A. Effect of endogenous and exogenous prostaglandin E_2 on interleukin-1β-induced cyclooxygenase-2 expression in human airway smooth-muscle cells. Am J Respir Crit Care Med 2000; 162:2272.

78. Kanehiro A, Ikemura T, Makela MJ, Lahn M, Joetham A, Dakhama A, Gelfand EW. Inhibition of phosphodiesterase 4 attenuates airway hyperresponsiveness and airway inflammation in a model of secondary allergen challenge. Am J Respir Crit Care Med 2001; 163:173.

79. Oppenheimer-Marks N, Kavanaugh AF, Lipsky PE. Inhibition of the transendothelial migration of human T lymphocytes by prostaglandin E2. J Immunol 1994; 152: 5703–5713.

80. To SS, Schreiber L. Effect of leukotriene B4 and prostaglandin E2 on the adhesion of lymphocytes to endothelial cells. Clin Exp Immunol 1990; 81:160–165.

81. Panettieri RA, Jr., Lazaar AL, Puré E, Albelda SM. Activation of cAMP-dependent pathways in human airway smooth muscle cells inhibits TNF-α-induced ICAM-1 and VCAM-1 expression and T lymphocyte adhesion. J Immunol 1995; 154:2358–2365.

82. Barnes PJ, Karin M. Nuclear factor-κB—a pivotal transcription factor in chronic inflammatory diseases. N Engl J Med 1997; 336:1066–1071.

83. Amrani Y, Lazaar AL, Panettieri RA, Jr. Up-regulation of ICAM-1 by cytokines in human tracheal smooth muscle cells involves an NF-κB-dependent signaling pathway that is only partially sensitive to dexamethasone. J Immunol 1999; 163:2128–2134.

84. Pang L, Knox AJ. Effect of interleukin-1β, tumour necrosis factor-α and interferon-γ on the induction of cyclo-oxygenase-2 in cultured human airway smooth muscle cells. Br J Pharmacol 1997; 121:579–587.

85. Lazaar AL, Panettieri RA, Jr. Airway smooth muscle as an immunomodulatory cell: a new target for pharmacotherapy? Curr Opin Pharmacol 2001; 1:259–264.

37

Cellular Trafficking of β₂-Adrenergic Receptors

ROBERT H. MOORE

Baylor College of Medicine
Houston, Texas, U.S.A.

BRIAN J. KNOLL

University of Houston
Houston, Texas, U.S.A.

I. Introduction

The β_2-adrenergic receptor (β_2AR) is a member of the G protein–coupled receptor (GPCR) family and is an important target for catecholamine hormones in physiological actions such as the relaxation of vascular and airway smooth muscle. Agonist-bound β_2ARs work principally by activating adenylyl cyclase through a coupled stimulatory heterotrimeric G protein (G_s), consisting of α, β, and γ subunits (1). Upon receptor activation, the G protein α subunit binds guanosine triphosphate (GTP) and dissociates into G_α and $G_{\beta\gamma}$. G_α activates adenylyl cyclase, causing a rise in the intracellular levels of cyclic AMP, a second messenger that eventually mediates most downstream physiological effects. Signaling via G_α terminates when its intrinsic GTP hydrolysis stimulates the reassociation of the α, β, and γ subunits and recoupling to receptors (1).

In the lung, β_2ARs are expressed on the surface of a variety of cell types including airway and vascular smooth muscle cells, epithelial and endothelial cells, sensory neurons, and multiple inflammatory cell types (2). Although the major clinical effect of activating pulmonary β_2ARs with β-agonists is airway smooth muscle relaxation and the bronchodilation of constricted airways, in vitro studies suggest that β-agonists may also have anti-inflammatory effects (2). In cellular and animal studies, β-agonists have been shown to inhibit the release of mediators by inflammatory cells such as mast cells and neutrophils, reduce substance P release by neurons, and decrease vascular permeability and airway mucosa edema (2–6). Despite these findings, anti-inflammatory effects of β-agonists have been difficult to demonstrate in clinical trials, and many studies indicate that clinically relevant anti-inflammatory effects of β-agonists are at best marginal. In fact, the chronic use of β_2-agonists in patients with asthma may increase mediator release from mast cells and heighten airway inflammation and hyperresponsiveness in response to inhaled allergen (7–9). The reasons for this apparent discrepancy between preclinical and clinical data may relate in part to the lower number and increased desensitization of β_2ARs expressed on inflammatory cells as compared with airway smooth muscle cells (10–14).

II. Mechanisms of β_2AR Desensitization

Desensitization of the β_2AR proceeds by at least three distinct mechanisms. Following activation by agonists, receptors are rapidly phosphorylated, which functionally uncouples them from transductional G proteins (1). Homologous desensitization, induced specifically by receptor activation, is mediated by G protein–coupled receptor kinases (GRKs). Phosphorylation by protein kinase A (PKA) and protein kinase C (PKC) mediate heterologous desensitization, which can be induced by processes distinct from receptor activation (15). After a short exposure to agonist (5 min), a large fraction of receptors move into endocytic vesicles by clathrin/dynamin-mediated endocytosis where they undergo dephosphorylation, which is probably mediated by a membrane-associated protein phosphatase (16), and then rapidly recycle back to the cell surface (17). These steps are likely prerequisite for receptor recoupling to G protein/cyclase (18,19). With prolonged exposures to agonist, there is a decrease in the total number of receptors within the cell, a process termed downregulation. It recently has been shown that downregulation proceeds by at least two mechanisms: (1) a high-affinity process that occurs at very low agonist concentrations and does not require receptor internalization and (2) a low-affinity process that occurs at higher concentrations of agonist and which is associated with receptor endocytosis (20). Following endocytosis, a fraction of receptors are sorted to lysosomes, where they are downregulated, and to the pericentriolar recycling endosome, from which they slowly recycle (21). Decreased receptor synthesis may also contribute to downregulation, probably as a result of increased mRNA degradation (22).

III. β_2AR Desensitization and Inflammatory Cell Function

On mast cells, the activation of β_2ARs reduces the degranulation of secretory vesicles containing spasmogens and proinflammatory mediators (2). Chronic desensitization of mast cell β_2ARs may be of clinical relevance since the bronchoprotective effects of β_2-agonists against agents that induce mast cell degranulation, such as adenosine monophosphate (AMP), decrease significantly with prolonged β_2-agonist use (23).

In addition, regular β_2-agonist administration causes an increase in airway reactivity to allergen (a process that is probably mediated, at least in part, through mast cell degranulation) and increases in both early and late asthmatic responses (8,9).

Mast cells express much higher levels of GRK2 than airway smooth muscle cells, and this may promote greater acute and chronic desensitization of mast cell β_2ARs (12,24). Several in vivo and in vitro studies have shown that β_2ARs on mast cells are profoundly downregulated and desensitized following the prolonged use of β_2-agonists (14,25–27). The administration to human subjects of the short-acting β_2-agonist albuterol for only 24 hours causes a substantial downregulation ($\sim$70%) and functional desensitization of β_2ARs on airway epithelial cells, indicating that receptor function can be significantly modified in vivo using standard β-agonist therapy (26).

IV. β_2AR Phosphorylation and Endocytosis

A. Overview of Clathrin-Mediated Endocytosis

Endocytosis is a basic and crucial process utilized by all cells for the uptake of material from the extracellular milieu and the plasma membrane (28). While there are several distinct mechanisms by which endocytosis may proceed, endocytosis via clathrin-coated pits is of particular importance in the regulation of a variety of cell surface receptors, including GPCRs (29,30). Therefore, a discussion of the basic mechanisms governing clathrin-mediated endocytosis is essential to understanding the cellular trafficking of β_2ARs.

The major structural component of the coated pit is clathrin, consisting of three light chains and three heavy chains that form three-legged trimers called triskelions (28,31). Interlocking triskelions form a polygonal lattice on the cytoplasmic surface of the plasma membrane at the site of an envaginating endocytic pit (28,31). A second major component of the coated pit is the heterotetrameric adaptor protein, AP-2 (28,32). AP-2 is crucial for clathrin-coat assembly and for the recruitment of other proteins, such as amphiphysin, epsin, AP180, and eps15, to the clathrin-coated vesicle (32). In many cases, AP-2 also recruits cell surface receptors to coated pits via a direct interaction between the μ2 subunit of AP-2 and an internalization signal within the cytoplasmic domain of the receptor (33,34). However, for GPCRs such as the β_2AR, the interaction of receptor and AP-2 apparently is indirect and requires the presence of β-arrestin complexed with receptor (35).

The mechanism by which coated pits pinch off from the plasma membrane to become coated vesicles is not completely understood, other than that this process requires dynamin (28,36). Dynamin is a cytoplasmic 100 kDa GTPase that undergoes polymerization at high concentrations and localizes to the necks of elongated coated pits (37). GTP hydrolysis by dynamin is required for scission of coated pits to form coated vesicles and is the rate-limiting step in clathrin-mediated endocytosis (38). However, it is unclear if the dynamin GTPase directly induces constriction of the coated pit neck or if it activates other effectors that mediate scission (28,39–41). Whatever the mechanisms, it is established that the expression of a dominant negative mutant dynamin-1 inhibits clathrin-mediated endocytosis, including that of β_2ARs (42,43).

B. Role of GRKs and β-Arrestins in β₂AR Endocytosis

Agonist-induced (homologous) desensitization of the β_2AR begins when the intracellular carboxyl-terminal (C-terminal) domain of agonist-occupied receptor is phosphorylated by a GRK, primarily the GRK2 isoform, which is recruited to the cell surface via an interaction with $G_{\beta\gamma}$ and agonist-occupied receptors. Receptors are then bound by nonvisual arrestins (β-arrestin 1 and β-arrestin 2), causing the uncoupling of receptors from G_s (44–46). GRK2 also may mediate β_2AR endocytosis by recruiting phosphoinositide 3-kinase to the plasma membrane, resulting in the generation of phosphoinositides (47). The exact receptor serine/threonine residues that serve as substrates for GRK phosphorylation are still unclear. In vitro studies reveal five serine/threonine residues as phosphorylation sites for GRK2 and these five plus two additional sites for GRK5 (48). However, when β_2ARs mutated at the GRK2 or GRK5 sites are expressed in vivo, no alterations in either agonist-induced receptor desensitization or endocytosis are observed (49). More recent data reveal a serine cluster at positions 355, 356, and 364 in the C-terminal tail of the β_2AR that may be critical for rapid receptor desensitization (50). β_2ARs mutated at these sites and expressed in vivo are markedly impaired in their ability to undergo agonist-induced phosphorylation, desensitization, and endocytosis, suggesting that these residues serve as in vivo substrates for GRK phosphorylation (50). Further, partial agonists that promote lower levels of rapid β_2AR phosphorylation are also less efficient at targeting receptors to the endocytic pathway (17,51).

Numerous studies indicate a central role for β-arrestins in the dynamin-mediated endocytosis of a variety of GPRCs via clathrin-coated vesicles (52–58). Live-cell imaging studies using β-arrestin green fluorescent protein (GFP) chimeras have shown that following the binding of agonists to GPCRs, β-arrestin translocates from the cytosol to the plasma membrane, where they interact with GRK-phosphorylated receptors (56,58–60). β-Arrestins are known to interact directly with two key structural components of clathrin-coated pits: clathrin, via a step that requires the dephosphorylation of β-arrestin and allows β-arrestin to function as a clathrin adaptor (52,61), and AP-2 (35). These interactions greatly promote the endocytosis of β_2ARs into early endosomes via clathrin-coated vesicles, and β-arrestin mutants lacking the AP-2 interactive domain are deficient in their ability to recruit receptors into coated pits (62). Studies in genetically engineered mice lacking β-arrestin 1, β-arrestin 2, or both, suggest that β-arrestin 2 is the predominant arrestin that mediates β_2AR endocytosis, although both β-arrestins can promote receptor desensitization and downregulation (63).

The intracellular complement of both GRK2 and β-arrestin has marked effects on the kinetics of β_2AR internalization (64,65). The overexpression of dominant negative mutants of either GRK2 or β-arrestin 1 markedly impairs agonist-induced β_2AR internalization (66,67), while overexpressing wild-type GRK2 or β-arrestin 1 can rescue an internalization defective mutant (Y326A) β_2AR (68). Although the overexpression of β-arrestin 1 does not increase β₂AR internalization in HEK293 cells (69), the downmodulation of β-arrestins using antisense mRNAs results in a significant impairment in β₂AR internalization (70).

Some evidence indicates a function for β-arrestins as scaffolds to promote the recruitment of signaling proteins and regulators of endocytic traffic into a receptor-arrestin complex. Among the signaling proteins recruited to this complex is Src tyrosine kinase, which links β₂AR signaling to the mitogen-activated protein (MAP) kinase cascade (71). In addition, two endocytic regulatory proteins, the small GTPase ARF6 and its nucleotide exchange factor ARNO, have recently been shown to interact with β-arrestin (72). ARNO is found in a complex with β-arrestin and upon agonist stimulation, β-arrestin then interacts with GDP-bound ARF6. The formation of this complex promotes the ARNO-mediated loading of ARF6 with GTP, resulting in ARF6 activation (72). Thus, the interaction of ARNO and ARF6 with β-arrestin provides a mechanism by which activated ARF6 can function in close proximity to the β₂AR and promote receptor internalization.

C. Ubiquitination and β₂AR Endocytosis

A role for ubiquitination in the endocytosis of membrane receptors such as the GPCRs yeast α-phermone receptor and human CXCR4 and the receptor tyrosine kinase human growth hormone receptor has been well-documented (73–75). Recently, such a regulatory role for ubiquitination in β₂AR endocytosis and degradation has been suggested (76). Agonist treatment leads to the rapid ubiquitination of both the β₂AR and β-arrestin 2. The ubiquitination of β-arrestin 2 by the E3 ubiquitin ligase Mdm2 is required for β₂AR endocytosis, and ubiquitinated β-arrestin may serve to recruit other E3 ligases that then ubiquitinate β₂ARs. Although ubiquitination of the β₂AR is not necessary for its internalization, receptor ubiquitination may be necessary for its degradation in lysosomes (76).

V. Dynamics of β₂AR Endocytosis and Recycling

Using both radioligand binding and immunological assays, the rates of β₂AR endocytosis and recycling have been carefully measured and the dynamic nature of these processes defined. Upon exposure to full agonists such as epinephrine and isoproterenol, approximately 60–70% of β₂ARs are removed from the plasma membrane into a vesicular pool defined morphologically as early endosomes (77,78), where they localize with internalized transferrin (see Fig. 1A,B). The half-time for this endocytic step after stimulation with a full agonist is approximately 3 minutes. Both the rate and extent of β₂AR endocytosis are reduced following treatment with partial agonists to a degree reflected by their ability to trigger receptor signaling (17,51). Once in the early endosome, β₂ARs are dephosphorylated by protein phosphatases and most receptors recycle back to the plasma membrane and recouple to G_s-adenylyl cyclase (16,17). Endocytosis and recycling is required for receptor resensitization and manipulations that disrupt either of these steps also alter β₂AR resensitization (18,79). Further, β₂ARs undergo continuous rounds of endocytosis and recycling as long as

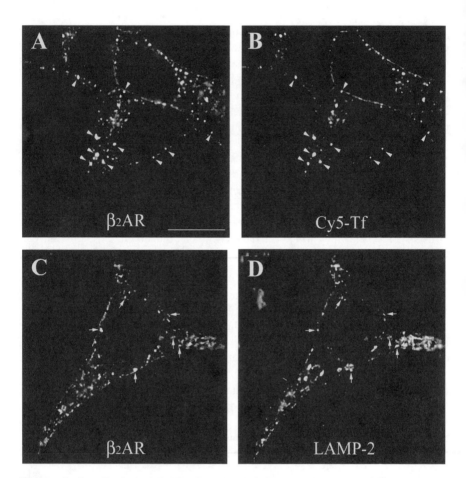

Figure 1 Localization of β₂ARs following brief and prolonged exposures to agonist. HEK293 cells expressing epitope-tagged human β₂ARs were treated with isoproterenol (ISO, 5 μM) for 15 minutes (A, B) or 6 hours (C, D). Cells in panels A and B were fed fluorescently tagged transferrin (Cy5-Tf) for 30 minutes to label endosomes, while those in panels C and D were treated with the protease inhibitor leupeptin (100 μM) to allow the accumulation of β₂ARs in lysosomes. Cells were labeled with antibodies against β₂AR alone (A, B) or against receptors and the late endosome/lysosome marker lysosome–associated membrane protein-2 (LAMP-2, panels C and D), followed by species-appropriate fluorescently conjugated secondary antibodies. Images were collected at an optical section depth of 150 nm using a Zeiss epifluorescence microscope equipped with a 100× lens (NA 1.4) and optimized using Deltavision deconvolution software. Scale bar = 10 μm. (A, B) Following a brief exposure to agonist, β₂ARs appear in punctate vesicles in a distribution that almost completely overlaps with that of Cy5-transferrin (arrowheads), indicating the endocytosis of receptors into early endosomes. (C, D) Following a prolonged exposure to agonist, β₂ARs also localize to vesicles that are positive for LAMP-2 (arrows), indicating the trafficking of some receptors to late endosomes and lysosomes.

agonist remains present (17,80). However, both the rate and extent of β_2AR recycling diminish with prolonged exposures to agonist, a phenomenon associated with the shunting of some receptors into protease-containing late endosomes and lysosomes (see Fig. 1C,D) and possibly into the pericentriolar recycling endosome (21,43,81,82).

VI. Intracellular Sorting of β_2ARs

While it is well established that the main destination for internalized β_2ARs is the rapid recycling pathway from early endosomes directly to the plasma membrane, it is now recognized that with prolonged exposures to agonists, some receptors are diverted to other intracellular compartments including late endosomes and lysosomes, where they are degraded, and perhaps to the pericentriolar recycling endosome, from which they slowly recycle (21,43,81,82) (see Fig. 2 for model). The mechanisms by which the β_2ARs are properly directed to these cellular destinations are not fully understood, although several recent studies have indicated that a variety of trafficking proteins may directly or indirectly regulate the endosome sorting of receptors. Further, it is known that endosome sorting of β_2ARs is pH dependent, as treatment with the proton pump inhibitor bafilomycin A1, which raises endosome pH, blocks receptor traffic to lysosomes and induces their accumulation within the pericentriolar recycling endosome (21).

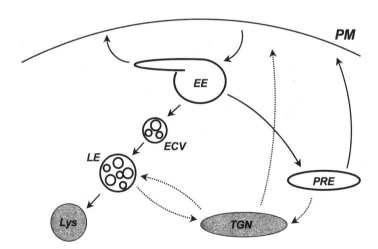

Figure 2 Intracellular trafficking of β_2ARs. The solid arrows indicate trafficking steps known to be utilized by β_2ARs, while the dashed arrows show steps in the endosome/lysosome system not known to involve β_2ARs. PM, plasma membrane; EE, early endosome; LE, late endosome; ECV, endocytic carrier vesicles; TGN, *trans*-Golgi network; PRE, perinuclear recycling endosome.

A. Rab GTPases and β₂AR Trafficking

Rab proteins are members of the small GTPase superfamily, and as with all GTPases, they shuttle between two activity states that are determined by the phosphorylation status of a bound guanine nucleotide, with rab-GTP conferring an active state and rab-GDP being inactive (83,84). Every rab protein has a characteristic subcellular distribution where it functions as an essential regulator of vectorial traffic (85–88). On the endocytic pathway, rab7 is localized to late endosomes and lysosomes and rab11 to the pericentriolar recycling endosome, while rab4 and rab5 are present on early endosomes (89–93). Rab5 plays a role in the fusion of uncoated endocytic vesicles to form early endosomes and regulates endocytosis in vivo (91,94), while rab4 may participate in the recycling of receptors from the early endosome directly to the cell surface (95).

    While no direct evidence has been published that identifies either rab7 or rab11 as regulators of β₂AR trafficking or function, recent data have shown that rab4 and rab5 do participate in the regulation of β₂AR endocytosis, recycling, and function (96,97). The overexpression of a constitutively activated rab5 mutant (rab5Q79L) induces the internalization of β₂ARs into dilated endosomes without altering receptor dephosphorylation or recycling (96). Conversely, expressing the dominant-negative rab5S34N mutant impairs receptor internalization and redistributes receptors to peripheral vesicles at or near the plasma membrane (96). Further, expressing a dominant-negative rab4 mutant (rab4N121I) slows β₂AR recycling from early endosomes to the plasma membrane, thereby disrupting receptor resensitization (96). These data also indicate that β₂AR dephosphorylation occurs as receptors traffic from rab5- to rab4-positive compartments (96).

B. β₂AR Sorting Signals and Interacting Proteins

Many plasma membrane proteins contain signals within their cytoplasmic domains that regulate their internalization, intracellular sorting, or both (34,98–100). For the β₂AR, two potential C-terminal tail signals have been identified: a dileucine motif at positions 339 and 340, which is required for efficient internalization but is not known to regulate intracellular trafficking (101), and a protein interaction domain comprised of the receptor's three or four terminal amino acids (DSLL) that appears to mediate β₂AR recycling (102–104). Transplantation of this four-amino-acid domain to the C-terminal tail of the nonrecycling δ opioid receptor creates a receptor chimera that is efficiently recycled (104).

    Recent evidence suggests that two proteins, EBP50 [ezrin-radixin-moesin (ERM)-binding phosphoprotein-50] and NSF (*N*-ethylmaleimide-sensitive factor), interact with the β₂AR and regulate receptor recycling (102,103). EBP50 contains two protein-binding domains: a PDZ domain that binds the β₂AR via an interaction with the DSLL sequence of the receptor C-terminal tail and an ERM-binding domain that binds the cortical actin cytoskeleton (102,105). Interruption of the β₂AR/EBP50 interaction by the addition of a single alanine to the receptor's cytoplasmic tail, by replacing the serine in the DSLL domain (serine 411) with aspartic acid or alanine, or by overexpressing GRK5, which phosphorylates serine 411 in vitro, inhibits β₂AR recycling, and leads to the apparent missorting of receptors to lysosomes. Similarly, β₂ARs are missorted to lysosomes and degraded in cells expressing mutant EBP50 lacking the ERM-binding domain (102). Further, depolymerization of the actin cytoskeleton with latrunculin B also appears to disrupt β₂AR recycling, causing internalized receptors to be diverted to a perinuclear compartment (102). Together, these data suggest that the interaction of β₂ARs with the actin cytoskeleton via EBP50 is critical to the proper sorting of receptors to the recycling pathway (102).

However, two other studies raise questions about the role of EBP50 as a regulator of β₂AR traffic. First, the addition of a 6-histidine tag to the receptor C-terminal tail, a maneuver that should disrupt receptor interaction with EBP50, does not affect the steady-state pool of internalized receptors (a balance between receptor endocytosis and recycling), nor does it alter the rate of receptor recycling to the plasma membrane when directly quantified (50). In addition, a β₂AR mutated at leucine 412 within the DS<u>L</u>L domain maintains its ability to interact with EBP50 but is recycling deficient, suggesting that other proteins may be more important in the regulation of β₂AR recycling (103).

Using a yeast two-hybrid screen, NSF was identified as a protein that interacts with the C-terminal tail of the β₂AR (103). NSF participates in a 20S protein complex that is critical in the fusion of intracellular membranes along the endocytic and exocytic pathways (106,107). Mutation of any of the terminal three amino acids (SLL) of the β₂AR significantly reduces NSF binding, an interaction that is required for efficient receptor endocytosis and recycling (103). Further, the overexpression of NSF increases the rates of endocytosis and recycling of wild-type β₂ARs but not mutant receptors deficient in NSF binding (103). Together, these data suggest a role for NSF in the regulation of both β₂AR endocytosis and recycling via a direct protein-protein interaction.

VII. Conclusions

Considerable evidence exists that β₂ARs are expressed on multiple inflammatory cells within the airway and that activation of these receptors in vitro decreases the release of inflammatory mediators (2–6). Unfortunately, due to a series of complex acute and chronic events that induce receptor desensitization, significant in vivo anti-inflammatory effects for β₂-agonists are limited at best (2,7,14,27). These cellular processes provide targets for potential therapeutics, based on the interruption of receptor desensitization, that may enhance the anti-inflammatory effects of β₂-agonists in vivo. Potential therapeutic targets include the disruption of β₂AR phosphorylation by GRKs, the enhancement of receptor resensitization by altering the rates of endocytosis or recycling, and the limiting of chronic desensitization and downregulation by decreasing the targeting of β₂ARs to the degradative pathway. Thus, understanding the cellular mechanisms underlying the acute and chronic desensitization of β₂ARs, particularly those expressed on inflammatory cells, is critical given the central role of β₂-agonists in the treatment of respiratory diseases such as asthma.

Acknowledgments

This work was supported by grants from the National Institutes of Health RO-1 HL64934 (RHM) and HL50047 (BJK).

References

1. Liggett SB. Molecular basis of G protein-coupled receptor signaling. In: Crystal RG, West JB, Barnes PJ, Weibel ER, eds. The Lung: Scientific Foundations. Philadelphia: Lippincott-Raven, 1997:19–36.
2. Barnes PJ. Effect of beta-agonists on inflammatory cells. J Allergy Clin Immunol 1999; 104:S10–17.
3. Lau HY, Wong PL, Lai CK, Ho JK. Effects of long-acting beta 2-adrenoceptor agonists on mast cells of rat, guinea pig, and human. Int Arch Allergy Immunol 1994; 105: 177–180.
4. Lau HYA, Wong PL, Lai CKW. Effects of β_2-adrenergic agonists on isolated guinea pig lung mast cells. Agents Actions 1994; 42:92–94.
5. Chong LK, Cooper E, Vardey CJ, Peachell PT. Salmeterol inhibition of mediator release from human lung mast cells by beta-adrenoceptor-dependent and independent mechanisms. Br J Pharmacol 1998; 123:1009–1015.
6. Shichijo M, Inagaki N, Nakai N, Kimata M, Nakahata T, Serizawa I, Iikura Y, Saito H, Nagai H. The effects of anti-asthma drugs on mediator release from cultured human mast cells. Clin Exp Allergy 1998; 28:1228–1236.
7. Swystun VA, Gordon JR, Davis EB, Zhang X, Cockcroft DW. Mast cell tryptase release and asthmatic responses to allergen increase with regular use of salbutamol. J Allergy Clin Immunol 2000; 106:57–64.
8. Cockcroft DW, McParland CP, Britto SA, Swystun VA, Rutherford BC. Regular inhaled salbutamol and airway responsiveness to allergen. Lancet 1993; 342:833–837.
9. Cockcroft DW, O'Byrne PM, Swystun VA, Bhagat R. Regular use of inhaled albuterol and the allergen-induced late asthmatic response. J Allergy Clin Immunol 1995; 96: 44–49.
10. Chong LK, Peachell PT. Beta-adrenoceptor reserve in human lung: a comparison between airway smooth muscle and mast cells. Eur J Pharmacol 1999; 378:115–122.
11. Drury DE, Chong LK, Ghahramani P, Peachell PT. Influence of receptor reserve on β-adrenoceptor-mediated responses in human lung mast cells. Br J Pharmacol 1998; 124:711–718.
12. McGraw DW, Liggett SB. Heterogeneity in β-adrenergic receptor kinase expression in the lung accounts for cell-specific desensitization of the β_2-adrenergic receptor. J Biol Chem 1997; 272:7338–7344.
13. McGraw DW, Donnelly ET, Eason MG, Green SA, Liggett SB. Role of βARK in long-term agonist-promoted desensitisation of the β_2-adrenergic receptor. Cell Signal 1998; 10:197–204.
14. Chong LK, Morice AH, Yeo WW, Schleimer RP, Peachell PT. Functional desensitization of β agonist responses in human lung mast cells. Am J Respir Cell Mol Biol 1995; 13:540–546.
15. Pitcher J, Lohse MJ, Codina J, Caron MG, Lefkowitz RJ. Desensitization of the isolated β_2-adrenergic receptor by β-adrenergic receptor kinase, cAMP-dependent protein ki-

nase, and protein kinase-C occurs via distinct molecular mechanisms. Biochemistry 1992; 31:3193–3197.

16. Krueger KM, Daaka Y, Pitcher JA, Lefkowitz RJ. The role of sequestration in G protein-coupled receptor resensitization. Regulation of β₂-adrenergic dephosphorylation by vesicular acidification. J Biol Chem 1997; 272:5–8.

17. Morrison KJ, Moore RH, Carsrud NDV, Millman EE, Trial J, Clark RB, Barber R, Tuvim M, Dickey BF, Knoll BJ. Repetitive endocytosis and recycling of the β₂-adrenergic receptor during agonist-induced steady-state redistribution. Mol Pharmacol 1996; 50:692–699.

18. Yu SS, Lefkowitz RJ, Hausdorff WP. β-adrenergic receptor sequestration—a potential mechanism of receptor resensitization. J Biol Chem 1993; 268:337–341.

19. Pippig S, Andexinger S, Lohse MJ. Sequestration and recycling of β₂-adrenergic receptors permit receptor resensitization. Mol Pharmacol 1995; 47:666–676.

20. Williams BR, Barber R, Clark RB. Kinetic analysis of agonist-induced down-regulation of the beta(2)-adrenergic receptor in BEAS-2B cells reveals high- and low-affinity components. Mol Pharmacol 2000; 58:421–430.

21. Moore RH, Tuffaha A, Millman EE, Hall HS, Dai W, Dickey BF, Knoll BJ. Agonist-induced sorting of human β₂-adrenergic receptors to lysosomes during downregulation. J Cell Sci 1999; 112:329–338.

22. Bouvier M, Collins S, O'Dowd BF, Campbell PT, de Blasi A, Kobilka BK, MacGregor C, Irons GP, Caron MG, Lefkowitz RJ. Two distinct pathways for cAMP-mediated down-regulation of the β₂-adrenergic receptor. Phosphorylation of the receptor and regulation of its mRNA level. J Biol Chem 1989; 264:16786–16792.

23. O'Connor BJ, Aikman SL, Barnes PJ. Tolerance to the nonbronchodilator effects of inhaled β₂ agonists in asthma. N Engl J Med 1992; 327:1204–1208.

24. McGraw DW, Donnelly ET, Eason MG, Green SA, Liggett SB. Role of βARK in long-term agonist-promoted desensitization of the β-adrenergic receptor. Cell Signal 1998; 10:197–204.

25. Nishikawa M, Mak JCW, Barnes PJ. Effect of short- and long-acting β₂-adrenoceptor agonists on pulmonary β₂-adrenoceptor expression in human lung. Eur J Pharmacol 1996; 318:123–129.

26. Turki J, Green SA, Newman KB, Meyers MA, Liggett SB. Human lung cell β₂-adrenergic receptors desensitize in response to in vivo administered β-agonist. Am J Physiol Lung Cell Mol Physiol 1995; 13:709–714.

27. Yates DH, Worsdell M, Barnes PJ. Effect of an inhaled glucocorticosteroid on mast cell and smooth muscle β₂ adrenergic tolerance in mild asthma. Thorax 1998; 53:110–113.

28. Marsh M, McMahon HT. The structural era of endocytosis. Science 1999; 285:215–220.

29. Takei K, Haucke V. Clathrin-mediated endocytosis: membrane factors pull the trigger. Trends Cell Biol 2001; 11:385–391.

30. Ferguson SS. Evolving concepts in G protein-coupled receptor endocytosis: the role in receptor desensitization and signaling. Pharmacol Rev 2001; 53:1–24.

31. Kirchhausen T. Clathrin. Annu Rev Biochem 2000; 69:699–727.

32. Traub LM, Downs MA, Westrich JL, Fremont DH. Crystal structure of the alpha appendage of AP-2 reveals a recruitment platform for clathrin-coat assembly. Proc Natl Acad Sci USA 1999; 96:8907–8912.

33. Boll W, Ohno H, Zhou SY, Rapoport I, Cantley LC, Bonifacino JS, Kirchhausen T. Sequence requirements for the recognition of tyrosine-based endocytic signals by clathrin AP-2 complexes. EMBO J 1996; 15:5789–5795.

34. Kirchhausen T, Bonifacino JS, Riezman H. Linking cargo to vesicle formation: receptor tail interactions with coat proteins. Curr Op Cell Biol 1997; 9:488–495.

35. Laporte SA, Oakley RH, Zhang J, Holt JA, Ferguson SS, Caron MG, Barak LS. The beta2-adrenergic receptor/beta arrestin complex recruits the clathrin adaptor AP-2 during endocytosis. Proc Natl Acad Sci USA 1999; 96:3712–3717.

36. De Camilli P, Takei K, McPherson PS. The function of dynamin in endocytosis. Curr Opin Neurobiol 1995; 5:559–565.

37. Schmid SL, McNiven MA, De Camilli P. Dynamin and its partners: a progress report. Curr Op Cell Biol 1998; 10:504–512.

38. Sever S, Damke H, Schmid SL. Dynamin: GTP controls the formation of constricted coated pits, the rate limiting step in clathrin-mediated endocytosis. J Cell Biol 2000; 150:1137–1148.

39. Stowell MH, Marks B, Wigge P, McMahon HT. Nucleotide-dependent conformational changes in dynamin: evidence for a mechanochemical molecular spring. Nat Cell Biol 1999; 1:27–32.

40. Marks B, Stowell MH, Vallis Y, Mills IG, Gibson A, Hopkins CR, McMahon HT. GTPase activity of dynamin and resulting conformation change are essential for endocytosis. Nature 2001; 410:231–235.

41. Sever S, Muhlberg AB, Schmid SL. Impairment of dynamin's GAP domain stimulates receptor-mediated endocytosis. Nature 1999; 398:481–486.

42. Damke H, Baba T, Warnock DE, Schmid SL. Induction of mutant dynamin specifically blocks endocytic coated vesicle formation. J Cell Biol 1994; 127:915–934.

43. Gagnon AW, Kallal L, Benovic JL. Role of clathrin-mediated endocytosis in agonist-induced downregulation of the β_2-adrenergic receptor. J Biol Chem 1998; 273: 6976–6981.

44. Lefkowitz RJ. G protein-coupled receptors III. New roles for receptor kinases and β-arrestins in receptor signaling and desensitization. J Biol Chem 1998; 273: 18677–18680.

45. Lefkowitz RJ. G protein-coupled receptor kinases. Cell 1993; 74:409–412.

46. Krupnick JG, Benovic JL. The role of receptor kinases and arrestins in G protein-coupled receptor regulation. Annu Rev Pharmacol Toxicol 1998; 38:289–319.

47. Naga Prasad SV, Barak LS, Rapacciuolo A, Caron MG, Rockman HA. Agonist-dependent recruitment of phosphoinositide 3-kinase to the membrane by beta-adrenergic receptor kinase 1. A role in receptor sequestration. J Biol Chem 2001; 276: 18953–18959.

48. Fredericks ZL, Pitcher JA, Lefkowitz RJ. Identification of the G protein-coupled receptor kinase phosphorylation sites in the human β_2-adrenergic receptor. J Biol Chem 1996; 271:13796–13803.

49. Seibold A, January BG, Friedman J, Hipkin RW, Clark RB. Desensitization of β_2-adrenergic receptors with mutations of the proposed G protein coupled receptor kinase phosphorylation sites. J Biol Chem 1998; 273:7637–7642.

50. Seibold A, Williams B, Huang ZF, Friedman J, Moore RH, Knoll BJ, Clark RB. Localization of the sites mediating desensitization of the beta(2)-adrenergic receptor by the GRK pathway. Mol Pharmacol 2000; 58:1162–1173.

51. January B, Seibold A, Whaley BS, Hipkin RW, Lin D, Schonbrunn A, Barber R, Clark RB. β_2-Adrenergic receptor desensitization, internalization, and phosphorylation in response to full and partial agonists. J Biol Chem 1997; 272:23871–23879.

52. Goodman OB, Jr., Krupnick JG, Santini F, Gurevich VV, Penn RB, Gagnon AW, Keen JH, Benovic JL. β-arrestin acts as a clathrin adaptor in endocytosis of the β_2-adrenergic receptor. Nature 1996; 383:447–450.

53. Mukherjee S, Palczewski K, Gurevich V, Benovic JL, Banga JP, Hunzicker-Dunn M. A direct role for arrestins in desensitization of the luteinizing hormone/choriogonadotropin receptor in porcine ovarian follicular membranes. Proc Natl Acad Sci USA 1999; 96:493–498.

54. Pals-Rylaarsdam R, Gurevich VV, Lee KB, Ptasienski JA, Benovic JL, Hosey MM. Internalization of the m2 muscarinic acetylcholine receptor—arrestin-independent and -dependent pathways. J Biol Chem 1997; 272:23682–23689.

55. Ferguson SSG, Downey WE, III, Colapietro A-M, Barak LS, Ménard L, Caron MG. Role of β-arrestin in mediating agonist-promoted G protein- coupled receptor internalization. Science 1996; 271:363–366.

56. Zhang J, Barak LS, Anborgh PH, Laporte SA, Caron MG, Ferguson SSG. Cellular trafficking of G protein-coupled receptor/β-arrestin endocytic complexes. J Biol Chem 1999; 274:10999–11006.

57. Barak LS, Warabi K, Feng X, Caron MG, Kwatra MM. Real-time visualization of the cellular redistribution of G protein-coupled receptor kinase 2 and β-arrestin 2 during homologous desensitization of the substance P receptor. J Biol Chem 1999; 274: 7565–7569.

58. Groarke DA, Wilson S, Krasel C, Milligan G. Visualization of agonist-induced association and trafficking of green fluorescent protein-tagged forms of both beta-arrestin-1 and the thyrotropin-releasing hormone receptor-1. J Biol Chem 1999; 274: 23263–23269.

59. Mundell SJ, Benovic JL. Selective regulation of endogenous G protein-coupled receptors by arrestin in HEK293 cells. J Biol Chem 1999; 275:12900–12908.

60. Oakley RH, Laporte SA, Holt JA, Barak LS, Caron MG. Association of β-arrestin with G protein-coupled receptors during clathrin-mediated endocytosis dictates the profile of receptor resensitization. J Biol Chem 1999; 274:32248–32257.

61. Lin F-T, Krueger KM, Kendall HE, Daaka Y, Fredericks ZL, Pitcher JA, Lefkowitz RJ. Clathrin-mediated endocytosis of the β₂-adrenergic receptor is regulated by phosphorylation/dephosphorylation of β-arrestin 1. J Biol Chem 1998; 272:31051–31057.

62. Laporte SA, Oakley RH, Holt JA, Barak LS, Caron MG. The interaction of beta-arrestin with the AP-2 adaptor is required for the clustering of beta 2-adrenergic receptor into clathrin-coated pits. J Biol Chem 2000; 275:23120–23126.

63. Kohout TA, Lin FS, Perry SJ, Conner DA, Lefkowitz RJ. Beta-arrestin 1 and 2 differentially regulate heptahelical receptor signaling and trafficking. Proc Natl Acad Sci USA 2001; 98:1601–1606.

64. Ménard L, Ferguson SSG, Zhang J, Lin F-T, Lefkowitz RJ, Caron MG, Barak LS. Synergistic regulation of β₂-adrenergic receptor sequestration: Intracellular complement of β-adrenergic receptor kinase and β-arrestin determine kinetics of internalization. Mol Pharmacol 1997; 51:800–808.

65. Ménard L, Ferguson SS, Zhang J, Lin FT, Lefkowitz RJ, Caron MG, Barak LS. Synergistic regulation of beta2-adrenergic receptor sequestration: intracellular complement of beta-adrenergic receptor kinase and beta-arrestin determine kinetics of internalization. Mol Pharmacol 1997; 51:800–808.

66. Kong G, Penn R, Benovic JL. A β-adrenergic receptor kinase dominant negative mutant attenuates desensitization of the β₂-adrenergic receptor. J Biol Chem 1994; 269: 13084–13087.

67. Orsini MJ, Benovic JL. Characterization of dominant-negative arrestins that inhibit β₂-adrenergic receptor internalization by distinct mechanisms. J Biol Chem 1998; 273: 34616–34622.

68. Ferguson SSG, Ménard L, Barak LS, Koch WJ, Colapietro A-M, Caron MG. Role of phosphorylation in agonist-promoted β_2-adrenergic receptor sequestration—Rescue of a sequestration-defective mutant receptor by βARK1. J Biol Chem 1995; 270: 24782–24789.

69. Marullo S, Faundez V, Kelly RB. Beta 2-adrenergic receptor endocytic pathway is controlled by a saturable mechanism distinct from that of transferrin receptor. Receptors Channels 1999; 6:255–269.

70. Mundell SJ, Loudon RP, Benovic JL. Characterization of G protein-coupled receptor regulation in antisense mRNA-expressing cells with reduced arrestin levels. Biochemistry 1999; 38:8723–8732.

71. Luttrell LM, Ferguson SS, Daaka Y, Miller WE, Maudsley S, Della Rocca GJ, Lin F, Kawakatsu H, Owada K, Luttrell DK, Caron MG, Lefkowitz RJ. Beta-arrestin-dependent formation of beta2 adrenergic receptor-Src protein kinase complexes. Science 1999; 283:655–661.

72. Claing A, Chen W, Miller WE, Vitale N, Moss J, Premont RT, Lefkowitz RJ. Beta-arrestin-mediated ADP-ribosylation factor 6 activation and beta 2-adrenergic receptor endocytosis. J Biol Chem 2001; 276:42509–42513.

73. Hicke L, Riezman H. Ubiquitination of a yeast plasma membrane receptor signals its ligand-stimulated endocytosis. Cell 1996; 84:277–287.

74. Strous GJ, Van Kerkhof P, Govers R, Ciechanover A, Schwartz AL. The ubiquitin conjugation system is required for ligand-induced endocytosis and degradation of the growth hormone receptor. EMBO J 1996; 15:3806–3812.

75. Marchese A, Benovic JL. Agonist-promoted ubiquitination of the G protein-coupled receptor CXCR4 mediates lysosomal sorting. J Biol Chem 2001; 276:45509–45512.

76. Shenoy SK, McDonald PH, Kohout TA, Lefkowitz RJ. Regulation of receptor fate by ubiquitination of activated beta 2-adrenergic receptor and beta -arrestin. Science 2001; 294:1307–1313.

77. von Zastrow M, Kobilka BK. Ligand-regulated internalization and recycling of human β_2-adrenergic receptors between the plasma membrane and endosomes containing transferrin receptors. J Biol Chem 1992; 267:3530–3538.

78. Moore RH, Sadovnikoff N, Hoffenberg S, Liu S, Woodford P, Angelides K, Trial J, Carsrud NDV, Dickey BF, Knoll BJ. Ligand-stimulated β_2-adrenergic receptor internalization via the constitutive endocytic pathway into rab5-containing endosomes. J Cell Sci 1995; 108:2983–2991.

79. Zhang J, Barak LS, Winkler KE, Caron MG, Ferguson SSG. A central role for β-arrestins and clathrin-coated vesicle-mediated endocytosis in β_2-adrenergic receptor resensitization. Differential regulation of receptor resensitization in two distinct cell types. J Biol Chem 1997; 272:27005–27014.

80. von Zastrow M, Kobilka BK. Antagonist-dependent and -independent steps in the mechanism of adrenergic receptor internalization. J Biol Chem 1994; 269: 18448–18452.

81. Moore RH, Hall HS, Rosenfeld JL, Dai W, Knoll BJ. Specific changes in β_2-adrenoceptor trafficking kinetics and intracellular sorting during downregulation. Eur J Pharm 1999; 369:113–123.

82. Kallal L, Gagnon AW, Penn RB, Benovic JL. Visualization of agonist-induced sequestration and down-regulation of a green fluorescent protein-tagged β_2-adrenergic receptor. J Biol Chem 1998; 273:322–328.

83. Bourne HR. GTPases: a turn-on and a surprise. Nature 1993; 366:628–629.

84. Schimmöller F, Simon I, Pfeffer SR. Rab GTPases, directors of vesicle docking. J Biol Chem 1998; 273:22161–22164.
85. Somsel RJ, Wandinger-Ness A. Rab GTPases coordinate endocytosis. J Cell Sci 2000; 113(pt2):183–192.
86. Pfeffer SR. Rab GTPases: specifying and deciphering organelle identity and function. Trends Cell Biol 2001; 11:487–491.
87. Zerial M, McBride H. Rab proteins as membrane organizers. Nat Rev Mol Cell Biol 2001; 2:107–117.
88. Segev N. Ypt/rab gtpases: regulators of protein trafficking. Sci STKE 2001; 2001: RE11.
89. Chavrier P, Parton RG, Hauri HP, Simons K, Zerial M. Localization of low molecular weight GTP binding proteins to exocytic and endocytic compartments. Cell 1990; 62: 317–329.
90. van der Sluijs P, Hull M, Zahraoui A, Tavitian A, Goud B, Mellman IS. The small GTP-binding protein rab4 is associated with early endosomes. Proc Natl Acad Sci USA 1991; 88:6313–6317.
91. Gorvel J-P, Chavrier P, Zerial M, Gruenberg J. Rab5 controls early endosome fusion in vitro. Cell 1991; 64:915–925.
92. Méresse S, Gorvel JP, Chavrier P. The rab7 GTPase resides on a vesicular compartment connected to lysosomes. J Cell Sci 1995; 108:3349–3358.
93. Ullrich O, Reinsch S, Urbe S, Zerial M, Parton RG. Rab11 regulates recycling through the pericentriolar recycling endosome. J Cell Biol 1996; 135:913–924.
94. Bucci C, Parton RG, Mather IH, Stunnenberg H, Simons K, Hoflack B, Zerial M. The small GTPase rab5 functions as a regulatory factor in the early endocytic pathway. Cell 1992; 70:715–728.
95. van der Sluijs P, Hull M, Webster P, Male P, Goud B, Mellman IS. The small GTP-binding protein rab4 controls an early sorting event on the endocytic pathway. Cell 1992; 70:729–740.
96. Seachrist JL, Anborgh PH, Ferguson SS. Beta 2-adrenergic receptor internalization, endosomal sorting, and plasma membrane recycling are regulated by rab GTPases. J Biol Chem 2000; 275:27221–27228.
97. Rosenfeld JL, Moore RH, Zimmer K-P, Alpizar-Foster E, Dai W, Zarka MN, Knoll BJ. Lysosome proteins are redistributed during expression of a GTP-hydrolysis defective rab5a. J Cell Sci 2001; 114:4499–4508.
98. Trowbridge IS, Collawn JF, Hopkins CR. Signal-dependent membrane protein trafficking in the endocytic pathway. Annu Rev Cell Biol 1993; 9:129–161.
99. Gruenberg J, Maxfield FR. Membrane transport in the endocytic pathway. Curr Op Cell Biol 1995; 7:552–563.
100. Bonifacino JS, Marks MS, Ohno H, Kirchhausen T. Mechanisms of signal-mediated protein sorting in the endocytic and secretory pathways. Proc Assoc Am Physicians 1996; 108:285–295.
101. Gabilondo AM, Hegler J, Krasel C, Boivin-Jahns V, Hein L, Lohse MJ. A dileucine motif in the C terminus of the β₂-adrenergic receptor is involved in receptor internalization. Proc Natl Acad Sci USA 1997; 94:12285–12290.
102. Cao TT, Deacon HW, Reczek D, Bretscher A, von Zastrow M. A kinase-regulated PDZ-domain interaction controls endocytic sorting of the β2-adrenergic receptor. Nature 1999; 401:286–289.
103. Cong M, Perry SJ, Hu LA, Hanson PI, Claing A, Lefkowitz RJ. Binding of the beta 2 adrenergic receptor to N-ethylmaleimide-sensitive factor regulates receptor recycling. J Biol Chem 2001; 276:45145–45152.

104. Gage RM, Kim KA, Cao TT, von Zastrow M. A transplantable sorting signal that is sufficient to mediate rapid recycling of G protein-coupled receptors. J Biol Chem 2001; 276:44712–44720.

105. Reczek D, Berryman M, Brestscher A. Identification of EBP50: a PDZ-containing phosphoprotein that associates with members of the ezrin-radixin-moesin family. J Cell Biol 1997; 139:169–179.

106. Rothman JE. The protein machinery of vesicle budding and fusion. Protein Sci 1996; 5:185–194.

107. Hay JC, Scheller RH. SNAREs and NSF in targeted membrane fusion. Curr Opin Cell Biol 1997; 9:505–512.

38

Genetic Targets in Asthma

**ARJUN B. CHATTERJEE, TIMOTHY D. HOWARD, and
EUGENE R. BLEECKER**

Wake Forest University School of Medicine
Winston-Salem, North Carolina, U.S.A.

I. Introduction

The purpose of this chapter is to review overall methodology and perspectives on the identification of potential genetic targets in allergy and asthma. Three examples of these approaches will be described in detail. Genetic studies have already led to advances in our understanding of basic disease processes, disease expression, and characterization of the asthmatic and allergic phenotypes (1,2). Multiple genes influence susceptibility to asthma, and disease expression is affected by these genetic factors. Complex genetic disorders are common in the population and are more prevalent than single-gene disorders, which are relatively rare (Table 1). Understanding the specific phenotype, as well as understanding relevant intermediate phenotypes, is important in dissecting the genetic components of these disorders (3). Genetic studies of allergy, bronchial hyperresponsiveness (BHR), and asthma require comprehensive scientific approaches since these conditions are characterized by heterogeneous phenotypic expression related to the complex interaction of environmental factors with multiple susceptibility genes. In addition, clinical disease, progression, and severity may be further influenced by different genes that influence disease expression as well as by viral respiratory infections, bacterial respiratory infections (endotoxin exposure), frequency of exposure to allergens, as well as other diverse environmental factors (4,5) (Fig. 1). Thus, delineating the role of genetic

Table 1   Characteristics of Complex Genetic Diseases

Multifactorial traits are influenced by multiple genes and environmental factors
Often common disorders
Mode of inheritance not fitting a monogenic gene model
Other confounding variables include genetic heterogeneity (2 or more genes acting independ-
    ently) and sporadic or nongenetic causes

susceptibility in the expression and development of complex disorders and understanding the interaction between genes and the environment are of major public
health significance.

Several genome-wide screens have improved our understanding of genetic
contributions to the development of asthma. Analyses of these genome screens have
detected several chromosomes with linkage to various phenotypes of atopy, IgE
levels, BHR and asthma (6). Positional cloning and sequencing of specific chromosomal regions have led to novel gene detection and candidate gene studies in multiple
population samples. Candidate gene studies and novel genes have been examined
for the presence of polymorphisms that may be associated with various phenotypic
factors (7–11). Linkage in some chromosomes has been reproduced across many
populations, while others have only been found in specific ethnic populations. To
interpret the biological significance of genetic associations with asthma and allergy,
investigators are performing gene expression and function studies to complement
these genetic approaches. These studies will delineate the functional relationship
between sequence variants in candidate genes and disease phenotype.

Genetic approaches will provide further insight into the pathophysiology of
these diseases and should ultimately lead to new and more effective therapeutic

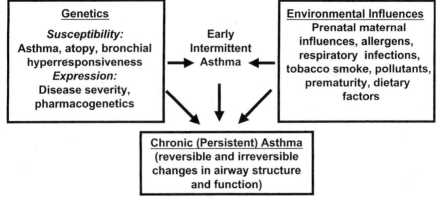

Figure 1   Interplay between genetics, environment, and disease.

interventions. In addition, identification of susceptibility genes for asthma and allergy may lead to new diagnostic methods for presymptomatic diagnosis, development of strategies for disease prevention in susceptible individuals, and delineation of the interaction between genotype and response to specific treatments (pharmacogenetics) (2). Genetic studies of complex disorders such as asthma require the collaborative efforts of investigators involved in phenotype definition, molecular and statistical genetics, and functional biological studies.

II. Definition of Asthma/Diagnostic Criteria

Asthma is characterized by BHR and variable airway obstructions. Atopic traits such as elevated total serum immunoglobulin E (IgE) levels and positive skin responses are closely associated with asthma and bronchial hyperresponsiveness and may predispose to the development of symptomatic allergy and asthma (12–15). Atopic diseases, such as asthma, allergic rhinitis, and eczema, are characterized by an elevated and prolonged immunoglobulin E (IgE) antibody response after allergen exposures. Atopy is generally considered to be caused by the interaction of genetic and environmental factors (16). Changes in environmental factors, such as lifestyle, diet, air pollution, allergen exposure, microbial environment (endotoxins), and viral respiratory infections, are likely to play an important role in the increasing worldwide rise of atopic diseases (17–19). Genetic studies have identified several chromosomal regions that may contain genes that contribute to asthma, atopy, or closely associated phenotypes (16,20).

The diagnosis of asthma is based on the recurrence of a characteristic set of clinical symptoms (wheezing, intermittent dyspnea, cough, nocturnal cough, exercise-induced asthma, and dyspnea) and physiological manifestations of the disease (variable airflow obstruction and BHR) (21). Since asthma is a chronic inflammatory disease of the airways and reliable noninvasive biomarkers of bronchial inflammation are not readily available, this definition does not provide criteria that reflect the extent and severity of bronchial inflammation. There is heterogeneity in the clinical presentation of asthma, with some individuals having a milder form of asthma while others have a much more severe and often progressive disease characterized by morphological changes in the airways (22). In some patients asthma is characterized by recurrent acute episodes presumably triggered by inflammatory events, while other patients display more persistent asthma. These differences are felt to be caused by chronic inflammation associated with structural changes in the bronchi (airways remodeling). It is also possible that differences in disease severity may be influenced by polymorphisms or sequence variants in genes that effect disease expression (severity) (10,23).

Bronchial hyperresponsiveness, which is defined as an increased bronchoconstrictor response to a variety of physical or chemical stimuli, can be measured using pharmacological, physical, or allergen-challenge methods (24). BHR, a phenotypic trait that is present in almost every patient with asthma, may reflect inflammatory events in the airway and can be studied in all members of a family or population sample (25). BHR can be found in family members without asthma symptoms (asymptomatic bronchial hyperresponsiveness), making this phenotypic trait not specifically definitive for asthma. Other individuals without asthma may display bronchial hyperresponsiveness, including individuals with early or established chronic obstructive pulmonary disease (COPD), chronic cigarette smokers, and nonasthmatic subjects with allergic rhinitis (26–29). However, despite these other etiologies that cause BHR, assessment of airways responsiveness in genetic studies remains an important approach in characterizing the asthma phenotype. There is no other single physiological test for asthma with sufficient sensitivity and specificity; in addition, there are no convenient or validated noninvasive measures of airways inflammation that can be used reproducibly in large population samples to diagnose asthma. Thus, it is appears necessary to rely on both the presence of symptoms and objective measures of pulmonary function and BHR in characterizing asthma phenotype (30,31).

III. Asthma and Obstructive Lung Disease

There is also an overlap between asthma and other obstructive lung diseases. In childhood, diseases that may resemble asthma, e.g., cystic fibrosis and bronchiectasis, can be excluded using clinical criteria and diagnostic tests. In adults, the principal disease that can resemble asthma in some of its clinical manifestations is COPD. COPD is a chronic disease of the airways that is characterized by progressive airflow obstruction that primarily occurs in individuals with a long history of cigarette smoking and chronic bronchitis. This disease occurs almost exclusively in middle-aged or older individuals with at least a 20-year history of smoking one or more packages of cigarettes each day. The cardinal clinical feature is dyspnea, which results from impairment of ventilatory function due to airflow obstruction. Many patients also develop emphysema, a destructive process in the lung parenchyma in which there is both a reduction in lung elasticity as well as dilation and loss of the alveolar-capillary surface for exchange of O_2 in the lungs (32,33).

Symptoms and the presence of reversible airways disease in smokers may lead to a clinical picture consistent with asthma. Often this is referred to as chronic obstructive bronchitis or chronic asthmatic bronchitis (34). Some individuals with smoking-related lung disease may have a history of asthma earlier in life. This overlap between asthma and chronic progressive obstructive airways disease has been named the "Dutch hypothesis." This hypothesis proposes that different obstructive airways diseases are interrelated and require host susceptibility (genes) as well as environmental exposures for their expression (35). Interestingly, only a relatively small proportion of chronic cigarette smokers (~20%) develop COPD and/or emphysema; this suggests that there is genetic susceptibility to the pulmonary responses to the toxic effects of tobacco smoke in the lungs.

IV. Phenotype Definition in Genetic Studies

Disease definition in asthma and allergy needs to be specific and reproducible so that results from different genetic studies may be compared. It is often useful to evaluate associated phenotypes, especially those that represent objective or quantitative measures that can be assessed in all family members in studies of common polygenic disorders. Clinical diagnosis of asthma, historical information, and questionnaires are often used, but criteria must be clearly defined a priori and not open to variable interpretations to prevent the introduction of heterogeneity into study design and interpretation. In performing family studies, individuals who are difficult to classify because of the presence of confounding factors such as smoking and individuals who have minimal symptoms of the disease will be present. Thus, family units may be ascertained through a proband who meets both objective and subjective criteria for asthma, but other family members may be more difficult to classify. These individuals, who only meet some of the disease criteria, are important to follow over time, especially if they have the same genotype as their affected family members, to determine if they develop the disorder over time after additional environmental exposures. Family members with intermediate phenotypes represent a target population for studies on early disease identification and disease prevention.

When all individuals in families or extended pedigrees are studied clinically, it is useful to classify the phenotypes into one of a limited number of categories such as asthma, possible asthma, uncertain airways disease, COPD, or unaffected, using a defined set or algorithm (21). Family members who meet only some of the criteria for asthma may be classified as having possible or probable asthma, and this group may be given less weight than the groups with definite asthma during genetic analysis. The *"uncertain"* category is needed for individuals who are difficult to classify due to confounding factors. For example, an individual with a significant history of tobacco smoking who has airways hyperresponsiveness and no airway obstruction will be difficult to classify because of the known relationship between smoking, airways obstruction, and BHR (26). Another group will be individuals with asymptomatic bronchial hyperresponsiveness who have evidence of abnormal airway function but do not have asthma symptoms.

While assessment of bronchial inflammation should be considered in genetic studies of asthma, the usual methods include the use of investigative bronchoscopy with bronchial biopsies and examination of respiratory fluids and cells obtained using bronchoalveolar lavage. These are invasive techniques that cannot be performed in a large number of individuals (36–38). Measures that may be more appropriate for family studies should be considered such as serum IgE level, analysis of induced sputum, and total blood eosinophil counts (39,40). In specific instances other bronchial challenge techniques (histamine, adenosine or AMP, exercise, allergen) may be considered. Additional biomarkers and related measures of inflammation need to be developed to provide a sensitive and specific assessment of bronchial inflammation and airways remodeling in asthma that can be routinely used in large sample studies.

V. Evidence for a Genetic Component in Asthma and Allergy

Asthma is an excellent example of a complex genetic disease that is caused by the interaction of multiple genes and environmental exposures in susceptible and at-risk individuals. It is possible that the level of genetic susceptibility may vary in different ethnic groups. Different combinations of susceptibility genes accompanied by variations in environmental exposures may determine whether an individual at risk develops mild asthma or more progressive disease (25,41). Children may develop wheezing from viral infections of the lower respiratory tract, which are frequent in childhood (30). However, not all children who wheeze will develop asthma or long-term bronchial hyperresponsiveness (42). Thus, understanding genetic factors that determine susceptibility and progression of asthma will result in the ability to predict future disease development and institute early interventions.

A. Twin Studies

There is an increased frequency of asthma and related phenotypes in monozygotic (MZ) twins as compared with dizygotic (DZ) twins (concordance). Twin studies are helpful in assessing the heritable component of a disease because MZ twins are genetically identical and DZ twins are related as nontwin siblings. Within a twin pair, other environmental variables are usually similar if the twins are raised in the same environment. In a large twin study of 7000 same-sex twins born between 1886 and 1925, the concordance rate for self-reported asthma in MZ pairs was 19%, while it was 4.8% in DZ twins (43). In a large Australian study, the MZ concordance rate was 30% while the DZ concordance rate was only 12%. Similar results were noted when BHR was used as a marker instead of self-reported asthma (44,45).

B. Familial Aggregation and Genetic Epidemiology in Asthma and Allergy (Segregation Studies)

Another method of demonstrating that there is a genetic component to disease is to use genetic epidemiological approaches to evaluate familial aggregation. This approach is confounded by the inability to completely evaluate multiple genes and control for all gene-environment interactions. However, the use of segregation analytical techniques may be an appropriate method to evaluate a population before embarking on more complicated genetic studies that include genome screening and linkage analysis. Asthma, BHR, total serum IgE, and other associated phenotypes have been found to have familial aggregation (45–50).

Some of these approaches will be illustrated by describing an ongoing Dutch study of the genetics of allergy and asthma. In this study, families were ascertained through a single proband, an individual with asthma who was originally studied at a referral hospital in northern Holland between 1962 and 1975. The probands were restudied between 1990 and 1999 for several phenotypes, including asthma and allergy, along with their spouse, children, and grandchildren. The only criteria for evaluation were that the proband initially had an asthma phenotype and a living spouse with at least two offspring. In addition to a standardized clinical characterization, all the subjects had DNA isolated for genotyping. This study was designed for segregation analysis (since families were chosen by the presence of only one affected individual or proband), association studies, familial aggregation studies, and genome-wide screen with fine mapping studies. First-degree relatives of asthmatics had an increased frequency of asthma and atopy when compared to control subjects and their families (20,21). In the initial analysis, 18% of the offspring of probands had asthma, 8% had probable asthma, 21% had unclassified airways disease (asymptomatic BHR, smokers with mild asthmatic symptoms), 4% had COPD, and 49% were unaffected. Approximately one-quarter of the offspring were found to have an asthmatic phenotype (21). When atopy was defined as a positive specific IgE to aeroallergens (Phadiatop assay), 29% of children with nonatopic parents were atopic, 47% of children with one atopic parent were atopic, and 62% of children with two atopic parents were atopic (20). These studies support a genetic component, but they do not identify the specific mode of inheritance.

Segregation analysis is an analytical technique that uses family data to identify a likely mode of inheritance. Modeling software helps to differentiate between dominant, recessive, co-dominant, and polygenic modes of inheritance. This type of analysis may not be sufficient for most complex diseases because it is currently limited to evaluating one or two genetic modes of inheritance. In some populations it has yielded evidence of polygenic inheritance and has shown evidence for a two-locus inheritance model for total serum IgE in the Dutch (51–53). In the Dutch study, a one-locus model segregation analysis was performed for IgE, a quantitative trait showing evidence for a mixed recessive model with a residual genetic effect. However, a mixed two-major-gene model with a residual genetic effect fit the data significantly better than the one-locus model. Using the two-locus model, there was evidence that the second gene modified the effect of the first recessive gene, and individuals homozygous for the first risk gene with one risk allele from the second dominant gene had the highest serum IgE levels (Fig. 2). The results of this segregation analysis can be used for subsequent linkage analyses and aid in fine mapping studies for gene localization (41,54).

C. Linkage Studies/Genome-Wide Screens

Linkage can be defined as the co-inheritance of two or more loci because of close proximity on the same chromosome so that after meiosis they remain associated more often than the 50% expected for independent assortment (Table 2). These linked loci can be associated with different phenotypes for genome-wide screens within any given population. In a genome screen, polymorphic genetic markers (Fig. 3) are used that span each chromosome at regular intervals (e.g., for a density map of approximately 10 cm, 350–400 markers would be necessary in order to cover the 22 chromosomes).

Several genome-wide screens have been performed in different ethnic populations: Amish (55), French (56,57), Australian, English (58), Afro-Caribbean (59), Tristan da Cunha, Canadian (60), heterogeneous United States (61), Hutterites (CSGA) (62,63), Italian (64), German (65), Dutch (41), Japanese (66), and Finnish (67). We will focus on two populations in whom genome-wide screens have been performed: the Dutch (20,41) and a heterogeneous U.S. population (54,61).

Since serum immunoglobulin E is closely related to atopy, a genome-wide screen for total serum IgE in the Dutch was performed and analyzed using variance

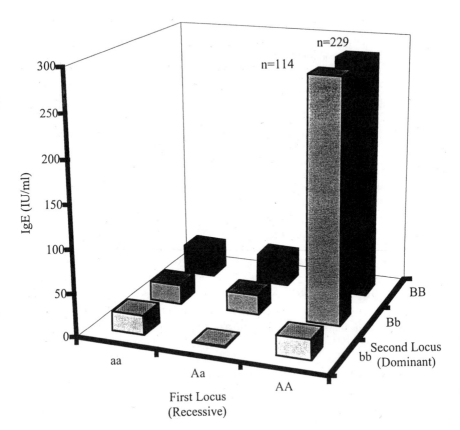

Figure 2 Segregation analysis of total serum IgE under the two-locus model (200 Dutch families). (Modified from Ref. 41.)

component analysis. Evidence for linkage was found on chromosomes 1p, 2q, 3q, 5q, 6p, 7q, 12q, and 13q (41). The highest LOD score of 3.65 was obtained on chromosome 7q with the addition of fine mapping markers while LOD scores of 2.73 and 2.46 were found on chromosomes 5q and 12q using genome screen markers (41). A subsequent genome-wide screen was performed in the Dutch using several different markers of atopy. These markers included specific IgE to *Der p 1*, specific

Table 2 Characteristics of Linkage Analysis

Families with disease or trait
Use of polymorphic genetic markers
Statistical association of disease with chromosomal region (*p*-value or LOD score)

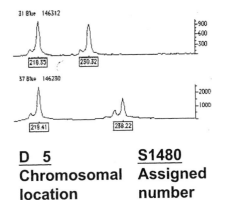

PCR product that amplifies a single unique chromosomal region whose physical location is known

D 5 **Chromosomal location**   **S1480** **Assigned number**   **Usually characterized by a number of different alleles**

Figure 3 Example of a polymorphic genetic marker.

IgE to a group of common aeroallergens (Phadiatop assay), peripheral blood eosinophils, and skin test responsiveness to 16 common aeroallergens. For specific IgE to *Der p 1*, linkage was found on 3q, 18p, and 22q, with the highest LOD score of 1.53 on 3q. For the phadiatop assay, linkage was found on 7q, 11q, 17q, 22q, with the highest LOD score of 1.38 on 17q. For skin test responsiveness to house dust mite, linkage was found on 5p, 8p, 10q, 11q, 12p, 13q, 17q, and 22q, with the highest LOD score of 1.71 on 8p. For peripheral blood eosinophils, linkage was found on 2q, 6p, 15q, and 17q with the highest LOD score of 2.19 on 15q (20).

In the United States Collaborative Study for the Genetics of Asthma (CSGA), a heterogeneous group of families from three ethnic groups was studied for asthma. Families were ascertained through two affected sibling probands. Other family members, including parents, siblings, and offspring, were also phenotyped, and DNA was collected for further genotypic analysis. A genome-wide screen was performed with 323 polymorphic DNA markers evenly spaced across the genome in 266 families. Evidence for linkage with asthma susceptibility was found in several different ethnic subpopulations and on several different chromosomes, including 14q, 12q, and 5q (54). Ethnically specific analyses showed evidence of linkage for 1p in the Hispanic population, 11q in the African American population, and 6p in the European American population.

Conditional analyses were performed on each of four chromosomal regions: the region showing the highest LOD score for the entire group (14q) and the regions with the highest LOD in each ethnic subgroup. This analysis was performed using a positive (gene-gene interaction) and negative (heterogeneity gene-gene interaction) weighting scheme. Significant evidence for a positive gene-gene interaction was found (Fig. 4). This supported the idea that multiple genes regulate susceptibility to asthma (Fig. 5). Several of these chromosomal regions identified using conditional analysis have been observed in other genome-wide screens indicating their importance for further study and gene identification.

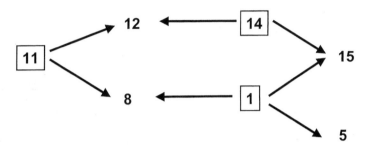

Figure 4 Summary of the conditional analysis performed in the CSGA. Linkage region on chromosome 11 interacts with linkage regions on chromosomes 8 and 12. Chromosome 6 showed no conditional effect and is not included in the figure. (Adapted from Ref. 54.)

The CSGA was an ethnically and genetically heterogeneous group. The Dutch population from Gröningen, a provence in northeastern Holland, is a relatively isolated population with little immigration to other regions of the country that provides a more homogeneous population. Other important populations to evaluate in genetic studies would be more isolated populations with a founder effect. The Hutterite population in South Dakota has been studied for asthma and allergy. A genome-wide screen was performed using 563 markers in 693 Hutterites. Evidence for linkage to multiple genes was found on chromosomes 1, 2, 3, 5, 8, 9, 11, 13, 14, 16, 18, 19, and 20 (63).

The linkage areas identified in these studies provide insight into the biology and pathogenesis of asthma. Genes within these chromosomal regions may identify specific genes that may prove to represent biological or therapeutic targets important in the pathogenesis and treatment of asthma. Some of these potential gene targets will be considered below.

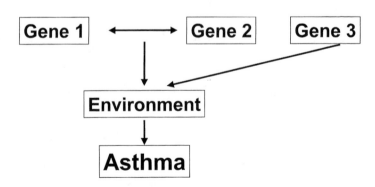

Figure 5 Multilocus interactions of multiple genes and the environment.

VI. Genetically Identified Biological Targets in Asthma

In-depth discussions reviewing the biological targets for inflammatory airways diseases can be found elsewhere in this volume as well as in the literature and will not be discussed in this chapter.

Investigators have delineated potential biological targets using molecular techniques, cell biology, and animal models of disease, as well as human studies in normals and patients with allergic disorders and asthma. The findings from genetic studies in humans represent another approach to define biological targets that complement previous biological approaches. Candidate genes that have been identified using biological studies can be evaluated using association studies that are variations on case-control study designs. In addition, investigators of biological candidate genes that are located on chromosomal regions that are linked to either primary or associated asthma phenotypes represent an important approach during mapping studies (Table 3). The overall approach is to evaluate sequence variants or single nucleotide polymorphisms (SNPs) in a specific gene (Fig. 6).

Specific information about SNPs within a candidate gene can be ascertained using informatic approaches or by direct sequencing of the gene in a smaller popula-

Table 3 Positional Candidate Genes for Asthma or Atopy in Selected Regions of Linkage

Location	Candidate gene	Function
1p31	IL-12 receptor	Cytokine receptor
2q33	CTLA4	T-cell proliferation
	CD28	T-cell proliferation
	ICOS	T-cell antigen-specific immune response
3q	IL-12A	Cytokine
5q23–q31	Il-3,-4,-5,-9, -13	B-cell switching, mast cell proliferation
	β2AR	G-protein–coupled receptor in lung
	GRL	Glucocorticoid receptor
	CD14	High-affinity LPS receptor
6p21–p22	HLA region	Antigen presentation
	TNF	Mediates inflammatory response
7q	IPLA2γ	Arachidonic acid release in airway epithelium
8p	Defensin α	Increases IL-8 in airway epithelium
11q13	FcεRiβ	High-affinity IgE receptor
12q23	NOS-1	Pro-inflammatory/bronchodilator
	IFNγ	Inhibits IL-4 activity
14q	TRAF-3	TNF-receptor associated protein
15q	GABA Receptor	Neural control of respiration
16p	IL-4R	Induction of IgE with IL4
17q	ICAM2	Intercellular adhesion molecule
	CCR7	Chemokine CC receptor 7
	RANTES	Eosinophil chemoattractant

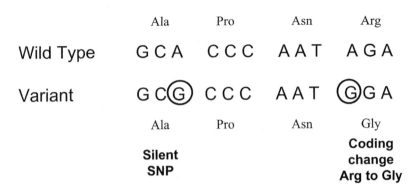

Figure 6 Examples of two different types of single nucleotide polymorphisms (SNPs).

tion sample to identify SNPs for genotyping in a larger population sample. Usually a combination of these SNPs preferably located in the promoter or coding regions can be genotyped in larger population samples to evaluate potential associations with allergy or asthma. One does not need to limit evaluation to SNPs that cause an amino acid change or splice variant because a specific SNP may be in linkage disequilibrium or represent a component of a haplotypes with the gene. To illustrate this approach, we will describe studies using three different candidate genes that are located in regions of linkage.

A. IL-4/IL-13/IL-4R, Th$_2$ Differentiation and IgE Production

Interleukin-4 (IL-4, chromosome 5q) mediates important pro-inflammatory functions in asthma including induction of the IgE isotype switch, expression of vascular cell adhesion molecule-1 (VCAM-1, chromosome 1p), promotion of eosinophil transmigration across endothelium, mucus secretion, and differentiation of T helper type 2 (Th$_2$) lymphocytes leading to cytokine release (68). A further role that IL-4 plays in the pathogenesis of asthma has been indicated from actively sensitized IL-4 knockout mice. Neither specific IgE induction nor BHR was detected in these mice (69,70), suggesting a critical role for the IL-4/IL-4R pathway in these phenotypes. Interleukin-13 (IL-13, chromosome 5q) contributes to the maintenance of the Th$_2$ lymphocyte profile that leads to elevated baseline IgE levels, and murine models have demonstrated the critical nature of IL-13 independent of IL-4 (71). The pleiotropic effects of IL-13 and IL-4 are mediated through the IL-4 receptor (IL-4R, chromosome 16p), which is composed of the high-affinity α subunit and either the common γ subunit or the IL-13 receptor α subunit (IL-13R, chromosome Xq) (Fig. 7). The complete IL-4R is composed of the α and γ subunits. The IL-13R is composed of the IL-4Rα subunit and either a low-affinity IL-13Rα1 (72) or a high-affinity IL-13Rα2 subunit (73). Soluble recombinant IL-4R lacks transmembrane and cytoplasmic activating domains and therefore, can sequester IL-4 without mediating cellular activation (68). Therefore, it is possible that different polymorphisms in

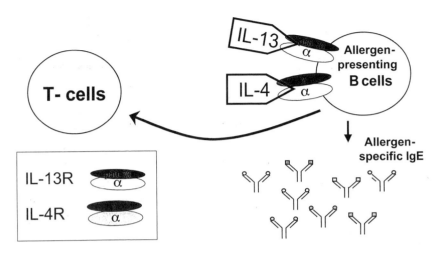

Figure 7 Role of IL-13 and IL-4 in inflammation.

these receptors, as well as in the IL-13 and IL-4 cytokines, contribute to the complex regulation of atopy or asthma phenotypes.

At least 16 SNPs in the large (~51 kb) IL-4Rα gene have been reported (9,74–78) (Fig. 8). The 150V, S478P, and Q551R variants have been associated with a greater risk for atopy (75,79), a greater risk for atopic asthma (76), and

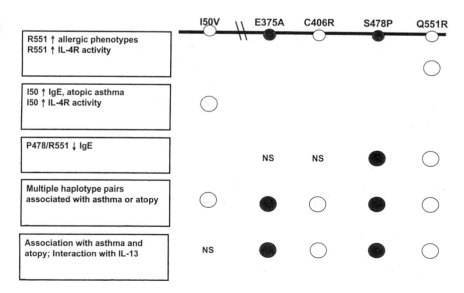

Figure 8 Polymorphisms in the IL-4Rα gene.

variation in IgE levels (77). In addition, specific variants were shown to modulate the activity of IL-4Rα (75,80) and the levels of soluble IL-4Rα (78). Eight polymorphisms in IL-4Rα (7 in exon 12) were studied in inbred and ethnically diverse outbred populations, and significant evidence for an association between several of these variants, as well as the resulting haplotypes, and asthma and atopy was observed (9).

Howard and coworkers evaluated five polymorphisms in IL-4Rα in the Dutch population to determine the importance of these variants in regard to susceptibility to and expression of asthma and atopy in this population. The hypothesis was to test for differences in total serum IgE levels between IL-4Rα genotypes and then to investigate associated phenotypes (8).

Table 4 summarizes the allele frequencies and the associations of the various SNPs in IL-4Rα with IgE level, skin response, and BHR. These data show associations with total serum IgE and skin test responses to allelic variation in the IL4R gene, suggesting that this gene may be important in regulating allergic responses and the development of inflammation in allergic asthma. Since IL-13 interacts with the IL-4α receptor (Fig. 7) and is located on chromosome 5q, a region that has been linked to allergy (IgE) and asthma (BHR) (47,55,81), this gene has been resequenced and evaluated for associations with allergic and asthmatic phenotypes (Fig. 9) (77,82). Since IL-13 and IL-4R have a biological interaction, possible gene-gene interaction between the two genes was also studied. The hypothesis was that individuals with risk alleles for both genes would have either more severe or a greater risk for asthma.

Howard and colleagues analyzed individuals with the highest-risk genotype for interaction with the previously reported high-risk IL-13 SNP (-1111 C/T) (7,8). Each SNP was individually associated with the asthma phenotype. The interaction effect observed was most notable in IL-4Rα S478 homozygotes when combined with the IL-13 SNP in a dominant fashion (CT and TT polymorphisms). The odds ratio was 4.87 ($p = 0.0004$) (Fig. 10). This analysis was repeated using the IgE level and was also found to be significant; however, the effect was similar to the effect of s478 alone.

The IL-13 promoter polymorphism most likely affects transcriptional regulation of the gene, whereas it has been suggested that the S478P variation of IL-4Rα

Table 4 SNP Allele Frequencies in IL-4Rα in a Dutch Population

SNP	Allele frequency	IgE level	Skin response	BHR
V50	0.47	$p = 0.07$	$p = 0.16$	$p = 0.79$
A375	0.12	$p = 0.02$	$p = 0.09$	$p = 0.16$
R406	0.12	$p = 0.01$	$p = 0.05$	$p = 0.09$
P478	0.16	$p = 0.0007$	$p = 0.03$	$p = 0.04$
R551	0.20	$p = 0.06$	$p = 0.2$	$p = 0.64$

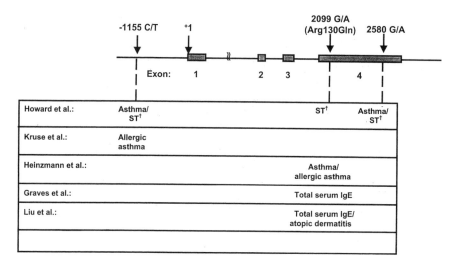

Figure 9 Selected association studies with IL-13 in allergy and asthma. †Skin test sensitivity. (Modified from Ref. 8.)

alters the conformation of the receptor protein and possibly modifies downstream signaling (77). Increased amounts of IL-13 cytokine may enhance the effect of the altered IL-4R complex, intensifying the downstream response.

Criteria have been suggested to assess the validity of biological candidate genes in complex disease. These are (1) a consistent association of the gene with the disease; (2) the gene should be located in a region with linkage to the phenotype in

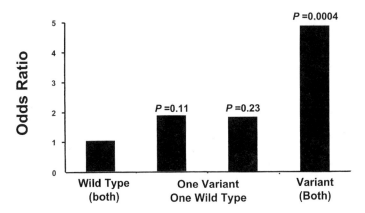

Figure 10 Interaction of IL-4R and IL-13 genes on asthma susceptibility in the Dutch. (Modified from Ref. 7.)

question; (3) the polymorphism should result in a functional change in transcription, translation, or activity of the gene product; and (4) the gene in question should have a plausible biological role (51). Applying these criteria, we find that the IL-13/IL-4/IL-4R pathways appear to fulfill these criteria. IL-4R has been associated with atopy and asthma in several populations, as noted above. The genes are located on 5q and 16p, where linkage has already been shown to the various asthma phenotypes. Some of the SNPs discussed above cause a measurable biological effect [decreased IgE levels for P478/R551 haplotype (77)]. However, since the many SNPs in exon 12 are in such high linkage disequilibrium with each other, we will not know which known SNP or which as-yet-undiscovered SNP actually causes a functional or conformational change without functional expression studies to determine effect. The IL-13/IL-4R pathway is important in the immune response and hence has a plausible biological role in the pathogenesis of asthma.

These observations add support to the hypothesis that asthma is a complex disease whose risk, pathogenesis, and severity are modified though a complex interplay of gene-gene and gene-environment interactions.

B. CD28/CTLA-4 and IgE Synthesis and Regulation

A key control point for IgE synthesis and regulation is the necessity for co-stimulation and activation of T cells. T cells recognize antigen-presenting cells by the antigen bound to MHC class II molecules, but this binding alone is insufficient to activate T cells. Co-stimulation by other receptor-ligand complexes facilitates efficient and appropriate activation of T cells. Two of the main co-stimulation complexes are the B7-1 (CD80) and B7-2 (CD86) ligands with CD28 (chromosome 2q33) and cytotoxic T-lymphocyte–associated 4 (CTLA-4, chromosome 2q33) receptors. CD28 is constitutively expressed on T cells and acts as a positive co-stimulator of T-cell activation. CTLA-4 is only expressed on activated T cells and acts as a negative feedback regulator of T-cell activation. CTLA-4–deficient mice have elevated immunoglobulin levels (83). Since CTLA-4 and CD28 are intricately associated with regulation of T-cell activation and T cells have a critical role in asthma, both CD28 and CTLA-4 would be reasonable targets for further genetic investigation.

Both CTLA-4 and CD28 have been examined in asthma and allergy phenotypes. No association was observed in a group of German individuals ascertained randomly or through an individual with atopy (84) or in a Japanese group of atopic asthma subjects (85). In the CSGA population, chromosome 2q33 has been linked to the "asthma" phenotype in the Hispanic subpopulation (54,61). In the Hutterites, a founder population in the United States that originated in the Tyrolean Alps in the 1500s, evidence for linkage to 2q (peak marker D2S2944) was observed with positive skin test response to cockroach and house dust mite (63). This region was also noted to have linkage with total serum IgE levels in a primarily German population (65). Linkage has also been shown in the French population (EGEA) to 2q33 with total serum IgE levels (57). Xu and colleagues reported linkage with total serum IgE levels to 2q33 in the Dutch population mentioned previously (4). CTLA-4 is within the candidate region (86).

Three polymorphisms have been examined for their relationship with immune diseases: a C/T polymorphism at position −318 in the promoter (87), an A/G change at position +49 of exon 1 (codes for an amino acid change of Thr to Ala) (88), and a microsatellite AT repeat in the 3′ UTR (89). One or more of these polymorphisms have been shown to be associated with type 1 diabetes, autoimmune thyroid disease, celiac disease, Graves' disease, and multiple sclerosis (90–97). Additional data suggests that the +49 A/G and the 3′ UTR microsatellite may have functional significance (98,99).

In a study comparing patients with asthma to healthy controls, the CTLA-4 polymorphisms were more associated with elevated total serum IgE levels in patients with asthma (100). Also, this group noted a multiplicative interaction between polymorphisms in the promoter of CTLA-4 (−318 C/T) and $F_C\varepsilon R1_\beta$ (−109 C/T) and total serum IgE levels (100). In data presented in abstract form, Howard and colleagues (101) reported that they detected novel SNPs in CTLA-4 and in CD28. These polymorphisms in CTLA-4 were examined in the Dutch population described earlier. Using the probands and their spouses in a case-control study design, they observed a significant association between the CTLA-4 polymorphisms and atopy and asthma. These results are suggestive that the co-stimulation pathway, especially CTLA-4, is important in the development of atopy and asthma-related phenotypes (101).

C. CD14/LPS

Recent studies have suggested that bacterial infections in infancy may protect against the development of allergy (102). In 1997 Holt and coworkers (103) hypothesized that bacterial signals play a functional role in the maturation of the Th1-type immune response, thereby suppressing the Th2-type response, which may produce an atopic phenotype. Microbial products, such as lipopolysaccharides (LPS), may provide activation signals for Th1-maturation.

One pathway through which LPS exerts its function includes high- and low-affinity LPS receptors. An important high-affinity receptor for LPS and other bacterial wall components is CD14 (chromosome 5q), a 55 kDa glycosylphosphatidylinositol-anchored protein localized on monocytes, macrophages, and polymorphonuclear cells. Binding of LPS to CD14 is facilitated by lipopolysaccharide-binding protein. CD14 is also present as soluble CD14 (sCD14) in serum, where it acts like membrane-bound CD14 in cells that do not express CD14 (104).

The gene encoding CD14 is a positional candidate gene for atopy, as it is localized on chromosome 5q31.1 (105), a region that has been linked to asthma and atopic responses (47,53,55,106–108). Baldini and coworkers (109) reported the association of a polymorphism in the CD14 gene and atopy. In the promoter region of the CD14 gene, a C-to-T transition was identified at position −159 upstream from the major transcription site (CD14/−159). In a Caucasian subset ($n = 5314$) of a general population sample of 11-year-old children from the United States, children homozygous for TT alleles had higher serum levels of sCD14 than those homozygous for the CC alleles. In addition, skin test–positive children with the TT genotype had

Table 5 Genotype Frequencies of the CD14 Promoter Polymorphism in
the Dutch Population

Group	CC	CT	TT
Probands	32.1%	47.8%	20.1%
Spouse controls	19.6%	53.8%	26.6%

lower levels of serum total IgE and a lower number of positive skin prick tests when compared with the pooled group of subjects carrying CC and CT (109).

Koppelman and coworkers (110) performed a study in the Dutch population previously described to assess whether the C allele was associated with serum IgE, skin test positivity, allergic rhinitis, or asthma phenotypes. In this case-control study, single gene polymorphisms were evaluated in 159 probands (as cases) and 158 spouses (as controls) (Table 5).

In subjects with a positive skin test, serum IgE levels were significantly higher in the CC homozygotes than CT heterozygotes or TT homozygotes. In individuals with positive skin prick tests, the number of allergens that were positive was significantly higher in the subjects with the CC genotype (5 positive allergens) than the CT or TT genotypes (4 and 3, respectively). The odds ratio that a CC genotype individual would have hay fever was 2.15 more likely than CT or TT. Interestingly, specific asthma phenotypes such as BHR, FEV_1, reversibility, and peripheral blood eosinophil count were not associated with the CD14 gene at all. This study suggests that the CD14 polymorphism is associated with expression of asthma rather than with susceptibility.

Association with CD14 appears important since there have been several reports showing association of the gene with disease (109,111). The gene is located on 5q, an area with chromosomal linkage to a variety of asthma phenotypes. The sequence variation in question results in a functional change as evidenced by the reduced level of sCD14 in the CC homozygous individuals (109), and CD14 has a plausible biological role in asthma and atopy.

VII. Conclusion

Genetic approaches have provided and will continue to provide insight into the pathophysiology and development of these allergic diseases and asthma. With the developing understanding of the complex mechanisms involved in allergy and asthma, additional candidate genes will be identified and novel genes will be discovered that may lead to new therapeutic targets and presymptomatic identification and prevention.

References

1. Daser A, Daheshia M, De Sanctis GT. Genetics of allergen-induced asthma. J Allergy Clin Immunol 2001; 108(2):167–174.

2. Bleecker ER, Postma DS, Meyers DA. Genetic susceptibility to asthma in a changing environment. Ciba Found Symp 1997; 206:90–99.

3. Xu J, Wiesch DG, Meyers DA. Genetics of complex human diseases: genome screening, association studies and fine mapping. Clin Exp Allergy 1998; 28(suppl 5):1–5; discussion 26–28.

4. Peat JK, Gray EJ, Mellis CM, Leeder SR, Woolcock AJ. Differences in airway responsiveness between children and adults living in the same environment: an epidemiological study in two regions of New South Wales. Eur Respir J 1994; 7(10):1805–1813.

5. Roorda RJ, Gerritsen J, van Aalderen WM, Schouten JP, Veltman JC, Weiss ST, Knol K. Follow-up of asthma from childhood to adulthood: influence of potential childhood risk factors on the outcome of pulmonary function and bronchial responsiveness in adulthood. J Allergy Clin Immunol 1994; 93(3):575–584.

6. Bleecker ER, Postma DS, Meyers DA. Evidence for multiple genetic susceptibility loci for asthma. Am J Respir Crit Care Med 1997; 156(4 pt 2):S113–116.

7. Howard TD, Koppelman GH, Xu J, Zheng SL, Postma DS, Meyers DA, Bleecker ER. Gene-gene interaction in asthma: IL4RA and IL13 in a Dutch population with asthma. Am J Hum Genet 2002; 70(1):230–236.

8. Howard TD, Whittaker PA, Zaiman AL, Koppelman GH, Xu J, Hanley MT, Meyers DA, Postma DS, Bleecker ER. Identification and association of polymorphisms in the interleukin-13 gene with asthma and atopy in a Dutch population. Am J Respir Cell Mol Biol 2001; 25(3):377–384.

9. Ober C, Leavitt SA, Tsalenko A, Howard TD, Hoki DM, Daniel R, Newman DL, Wu X, Parry R, Lester LA, Solway J, Blumenthal M, King RA, Xu J, Meyers DA, Bleecker ER, Cox NJ. Variation in the interleukin 4-receptor alpha gene confers susceptibility to asthma and atopy in ethnically diverse populations. Am J Hum Genet 2000; 66(2): 517–526.

10. Li Kam Wa TC, Mansur AH, Britton J, Williams G, Pavord I, Richards K, Campbell DA, Morton N, Holgate ST, Morrison JF. Association between −308 tumour necrosis factor promoter polymorphism and bronchial hyperreactivity in asthma. Clin Exp Allergy 1999; 29(9):1204–1208.

11. Albuquerque RV, Hayden CM, Palmer LJ, Laing IA, Rye PJ, Gibson NA, Burton PR, Goldblatt J, Lesouef PN. Association of polymorphisms within the tumour necrosis factor (TNF) genes and childhood asthma. Clin Exp Allergy 1998; 28(5):578–584.

12. Burrows B, Martinez FD, Halonen M, Barbee RA, Cline MG. Association of asthma with serum IgE levels and skin-test reactivity to allergens. N Engl J Med 1989; 320(5): 271–277.

13. Burrows B. Allergy and the development of asthma and bronchial hyperresponsiveness. Clin Exp Allergy 1995; 25(suppl 2):15–18.

14. Sears MR, Burrows B, Flannery EM, Herbison GP, Hewitt CJ, Holdaway MD. Relation between airway responsiveness and serum IgE in children with asthma and in apparently normal children. N Engl J Med 1991; 325(15):1067–1071.

15. Halonen M, Stern D, Taussig LM, Wright A, Ray CG, Martinez FD. The predictive relationship between serum IgE levels at birth and subsequent incidences of lower respiratory illnesses and eczema in infants. Am Rev Respir Dis 1992; 146(4):866–870.

16. Postma DS, Bleecker ER. Genetics of asthma. In: Barnes PJ, Grunstein MM, Lett AR, Woolcock AJ, eds. Asthma. Philadelphia: Lippincott-Raven, 1997:145–154.

17. Burney PGJ. Epidemiologic trends. In: Barnes PJ, Grunstem MM, Lett AR, Woolcock AJ, eds. Asthma. Philadelphia: Lippincott-Raven, 1997:35–47.

18. Strachan DP. Lifestyle and atopy. Lancet 1999; 353(9163):1457–1458.

19. Hopkin JM. Mechanisms of enhanced prevalence of asthma and atopy in developed countries. Curr Opin Immunol 1997; 9(6):788–792.
20. Koppelman GH, Stine OC, Xu J, Howard TD, Zheng SL, Kauffman HF, Bleecker ER, Meyers DA, Postma DS. Genome-wide search for atopy susceptibility genes in Dutch families with asthma. J Allergy Clin Immunol 2002; 109(3):498–506.
21. Panhuysen CI, Bleecker ER, Koeter GH, Meyers DA, Postma DS. Characterization of obstructive airway disease in family members of probands with asthma. An algorithm for the diagnosis of asthma. Am J Respir Crit Care Med 1998; 157(6 pt 1):1734–1742.
22. Busse WW, Banks-Schlegel S, Wenzel SE. Pathophysiology of severe asthma. J Allergy Clin Immunol 2000; 106(6):1033–1042.
23. Drazen JM, Weiss ST, Cooper D. Beta 2 adrenoceptor polymorphisms. Thorax 1996; 51(11):1168.
24. Crapo RO, Casaburi R, Coates AL, Enright PL, Hankinson JL, Irvin CG, MacIntyre NR, McKay RT, Wanger JS, Anderson SD, Cockcroft DW, Fish JE, Sterk PJ. Guidelines for methacholine and exercise challenge testing—1999. This official statement of the American Thoracic Society was adopted by the ATS Board of Directors, July 1999. Am J Respir Crit Care Med 2000; 161(1):309–329.
25. Lester LA, Rich SS, Blumenthal MN, Togias A, Murphy S, Malveaux F, Miller ME, Dunston GM, Solway J, Wolf RL, Samet JM, Marsh DG, Meyers DA, Ober C, Bleecker ER. Ethnic differences in asthma and associated phenotypes: collaborative study on the genetics of asthma. J Allergy Clin Immunol 2001; 108(3):357–362.
26. Tashkin DP, Altose MD, Bleecker ER, Connett JE, Kanner RE, Lee WW, Wise R. The lung health study: airway responsiveness to inhaled methacholine in smokers with mild to moderate airflow limitation. The Lung Health Study Research Group. Am Rev Respir Dis 1992; 145(2 pt 1):301–310.
27. Sparrow D, O'Connor GT, Basner RC, Rosner B, Weiss ST. Predictors of the new onset of wheezing among middle-aged and older men. The Normative Aging Study. Am Rev Respir Dis 1993; 147(2):367–371.
28. Sporik R, Holgate ST, Platts-Mills TA, Cogswell JJ. Exposure to house-dust mite allergen (Der p I) and the development of asthma in childhood. A prospective study. N Engl J Med 1990; 323(8):502–507.
29. Woolcock AJ, Anderson SD, Peat JK, Du Toit JI, Zhang YG, Smith CM, Salome CM. Characteristics of bronchial hyperresponsiveness in chronic obstructive pulmonary disease and in asthma. Am Rev Respir Dis 1991; 143(6):1438–1443.
30. Busse WW, Lemanske Jr. RF, Dick EC. The relationship of viral respiratory infections and asthma. Chest 1992; 101(6 suppl):385S–388S.
31. Schwartz J, Weiss ST. Relationship of skin test reactivity to decrements in pulmonary function in children with asthma or frequent wheezing. Am J Resp Crit Care Med 1995; 152(6 pt 1):2176–2180.
32. Pauwels RA, Buist AS, Calverley PM, Jenkins CR, Hurd SS. Global strategy for the diagnosis, management, and prevention of chronic obstructive pulmonary disease. NHLBI/WHO Global Initiative for Chronic Obstructive Lung Disease (GOLD) Workshop summary. Am J Respir Crit Care Med 2000; 163(5):1256–1276.
33. Gross NJ. The GOLD standard for chronic obstructive pulmonary disease. Am J Respir Crit Care Med 2001; 163(5):1047–1048.
34. ATS. Standards for the diagnosis and care of patients with chronic obstructive pulmonary disease. American Thoracic Society. Am J Respir Crit Care Med 1995; 152(5 pt 2):S77–121.

35. Orie NG, de Vries K, Sluiter HJ, Tammeling GJ, Booy-Noord H, Grobler NJ, von der Lende R. [Chronic bronchitis and cancer from the standpoint of the clinician]. Hefte Unfallheilkd 1966; 87:25–33.

36. Bleecker ER, McFadden Jr. ER, Hurd SS, Goldstein RA, Ram JS. Investigative bronchoscopy in subjects with asthma and other obstructive pulmonary diseases. Whether and when. Chest 1992; 101(2):297–298.

37. Wenzel SE, Szefler SJ, Leung DY, Sloan SI, Rex MD, Martin RJ. Bronchoscopic evaluation of severe asthma. Persistent inflammation associated with high dose glucocorticoids. Am J Respir Crit Care Med 1997; 156(3 pt 1):737–743.

38. Moore WC, Hasday JD, Meltzer SS, Wisnewski PL, White B, Bleecker ER. Subjects with mild and moderate asthma respond to segmental allergen challenge with similar, reproducible, allergen-specific inflammation. J Allergy Clin Immunol 2001; 108(6): 908–914.

39. Fahy JV, Wong H, Liu J, Boushey HA. Comparison of samples collected by sputum induction and bronchoscopy from asthmatic and healthy subjects. Am J Respir Crit Care Med 1995; 152(1):53–58.

40. Maestrelli P, Saetta M, Di Stefano A, Calcagni PG, Turato G, Ruggieri MP, Roggeri A, Mapp CE, Fabbri LM. Comparison of leukocyte counts in sputum, bronchial biopsies, and bronchoalveolar lavage. Am J Resp Crit Care Med 1995; 152(6 pt 1): 1926–1931.

41. Xu J, Postma DS, Howard TD, Koppelman GH, Zheng SL, Stine OC, Bleecker ER, Meyers DA. Major genes regulating total serum immunoglobulin E levels in families with asthma. Am J Hum Genet 2000; 67(5):1163–1173.

42. Martinez FD. Recognizing early asthma. Allergy 1999; 54(suppl 49):24–28.

43. Edfors-Lubs ML. Allergy in 7000 twin pairs. Acta Allergol 1971; 26(4):249–285.

44. Duffy DL, Martin NG, Battistutta D, Hopper JL, Mathews JD. Genetics of asthma and hay fever in Australian twins. Am Rev Respir Dis 1990; 142(6 pt 1):1351–1358.

45. Hopp RJ, Bewtra AK, Biven R, Nair NM, Townley RG. Bronchial reactivity pattern in nonasthmatic parents of asthmatics. Ann Allergy 1988; 61(3):184–186.

46. Holberg CJ, Elston RC, Halonen M, Wright AL, Taussig LM, Morgan WJ, Martinez FD. Segregation analysis of physician-diagnosed asthma in Hispanic and non-Hispanic white families. A recessive component? Am J Respir Crit Care Med 1996; 154(1): 144–150.

47. Postma DS, Bleecker ER, Amelung PJ, Holroyd KJ, Xu J, Panhuysen CI, Meyers DA, Levitt RC. Genetic susceptibility to asthma—bronchial hyperresponsiveness coinherited with a major gene for atopy. N Engl J Med 1995; 333(14):894–900.

48. Meyers DA, Beaty TH, Freidhoff LR, Marsh DG. Inheritance of total serum IgE (basal levels) in man. Am J Hum Genet 1987; 41(1):51–62.

49. Meyers DA, Hasstedt SJ, Marsh DG, Skolnick M, King MC, Bias WB, Amos DB. The inheritance of immunoglobulin E: genetic linkage analysis. Am J Med Genet 1983; 16(4):575–581.

50. Marsh DG, Meyers DA, Bias WB. The epidemiology and genetics of atopic allergy. N Engl J Med 1981; 305(26):1551–1559.

51. Lander E, Kruglyak L. Genetic dissection of complex traits: guidelines for interpreting and reporting linkage results. Nat Genet 1995; 11(3):241–247.

52. Martinez FD, Holberg CJ. Segregation analysis of physician-diagnosed asthma in Hispanic and non-Hispanic white families. Clin Exp Allergy 1995; 25(suppl 2):68–70.

53. Xu J, Levitt RC, Panhuysen CI, Postma DS, Taylor EW, Amelung PJ, Holroyd KJ, Bleecker ER, Meyers DA. Evidence for two unlinked loci regulating total serum IgE levels. Am J Hum Genet 1995; 57(2):425–430.

54. Xu J, Meyers DA, Ober C, Blumenthal MN, Mellen B, Barnes KC, King RA, Lester LA, Howard TD, Solway J, Langefeld CD, Beaty TH, Rich SS, Bleecker ER, Cox NJ. Genomewide screen and identification of gene-gene interactions for asthma-susceptibility loci in three U.S. populations: collaborative study on the genetics of asthma. Am J Hum Genet 2001; 68(6):1437–1446.

55. Marsh DG, Neely JD, Breazeale DR, Ghosh B, Freidhoff LR, Ehrlich-Kautzky E, Schou C, Krishnaswamy G, Beaty TH. Linkage analysis of IL4 and other chromosome 5q31.1 markers and total serum immunoglobulin E concentrations. Science 1994; 264(5162):1152–1156.

56. Kauffmann F, Dizier MH. EGEA (Epidemiological study on the Genetics and Environment of Asthma, bronchial hyperresponsiveness and atopy)—design issues. EGEA Co-operative Group. Clin Exp Allergy 1995; 25(suppl 2):19–22.

57. Dizier MH, Besse-Schmittler C, Guilloud-Bataille M, Annesi-Maesano I, Boussaha M, Bousquet J, Charpin D, Degioanni A, Gormand F, Grimfeld A, Hochez J, Hyne G, Lockhart A, Luillier-Lacombe M, Matran R, Meunier F, Neukirch F, Pacheco Y, Parent V, Paty E, Pin I, Pison C, Scheinmann P, Thobie N, Vervloet D, Kauffmann F, Feingold J, Lathrop M, Demenais F. Genome screen for asthma and related phenotypes in the French EGEA study. Am J Respir Crit Care Med 2000; 162(5):1812–1818.

58. Daniels SE, Bhattacharrya S, James A, Leaves NI, Young A, Hill MR, Faux JA, Ryan GF, Le Souef PN, Lathrop GM, Musk AW, Cookson WO. A genome-wide search for quantitative trait loci underlying asthma. Nature 1994; 383(6597):247–250.

59. Barnes KC, Neely JD, Duffy DL, Freidhoff LR, Breazeale DR, Schou C, Naidu RP, Levett PN, Renault B, Kucherlapati R, Iozzino S, Ehrlich E, Beaty TH, Marsh DG. Linkage of asthma and total serum IgE concentration to markers on chromosome 12q: evidence from Afro-Caribbean and Caucasian populations. Genomics 1996; 37(1): 41–50.

60. Slutsky AS, Zamel N. Genetics of asthma: the University of Toronto Program. University of Toronto Genetics of Asthma Research Group. Am J Respir Crit Care Med 1997; 156(4 Pt 2):S130–132.

61. A genome-wide search for asthma susceptibility loci in ethnically diverse populations. The Collaborative Study on the Genetics of Asthma (CSGA). Nat Genet 1997; 15(4): 389–392.

62. Ober C, Cox NJ, Abney M, Di Rienzo A, Lander ES, Changyaleket B, Gidley H, Kurtz B, Lee J, Nance M, Pettersson A, Prescott J, Richardson A, Schlenker E, Summerhill E, Willadsen S, Parry R. Genome-wide search for asthma susceptibility loci in a founder population. The Collaborative Study on the Genetics of Asthma. Hum Mol Genet 1998; 7(9):1393–1398.

63. Ober C, Tsalenko A, Parry R, Cox NJ, 2000. A second-generation genomewide screen for asthma-susceptibility alleles in a founder population. Am J Hum Genet 2000; 67(5): 1154–1162.

64. Malerba G, Trabetti E, Patuzzo C, Lauciello MC, Galavotti R, Pescollderungg L, Boner AL, Pignatti PF. Candidate genes and a genome-wide search in Italian families with atopic asthmatic children. Clin Exp Allergy 1999; 29(suppl 4):27–30.

65. Wjst M, Fischer G, Immervoll T, Jung M, Saar K, Rueschendorf F, Reis A, Ulbrecht M, Gomolka M, Weiss EH, Jaeger L, Nickel R, Richter K, Kjellman NI, Griese M,

von Berg A, Gappa M, Riedel F, Boehle M, van Koningsbruggen S, Schoberth R, Szczepanski R, Dorsch W, Silbermann M, Wichmann HE, et al. A genome-wide search for linkage to asthma. German Asthma Genetics Group. Genomics 1999; 58(1): 1–8.

66. Yokouchi Y, Nukaga Y, Shibasaki M, Noguchi E, Kimura K, Ito S, Nishihara M, Yamakawa-Kobayashi K, Takeda K, Imoto N, Ichikawa K, Matsui A, Hamaguchi H, Arinami T. Significant evidence for linkage of mite-sensitive childhood asthma to chromosome 5q31-q33 near the interleukin 12 B locus by a genome-wide search in Japanese families. Genomics 2000; 66(2):152–160.

67. Laitinen T, Daly MJ, Rioux JD, Kauppi P, Laprise C, Petays T, Green T, Cargill M, Haahtela T, Lander ES, Laitinen LA, Hudson TJ, Kere J. A susceptibility locus for asthma-related traits on chromosome 7 revealed by genome-wide scan in a founder population. Nat Genet 2001; 28(1):87–91.

68. Steinke JW, Borish L. Th2 cytokines and asthma. Interleukin-4: its role in the pathogenesis of asthma, and targeting it for asthma treatment with interleukin-4 receptor antagonists. *Respir Res* 2001; 2(2):66–70.

69. Brusselle GG, Kips JC, Tavernier JH, van der Heyden JG, Cuvelier CA, Pauwels RA, Bluethmann H. Attenuation of allergic airway inflammation in IL-4 deficient mice. Clin Exp Allergy 1994; 24(1):73–80.

70. Brusselle G, Kips J, Joos G, Bluethmann H, Pauwels R. Allergen-induced airway inflammation and bronchial responsiveness in wild-type and interleukin-4-deficient mice. Am J Respir Cell Mol Biol 1995; 12(3):254–259.

71. Grunig G, Warnock M, Wakil AE, Venkayya R, Brombacher F, Rennick DM, Sheppard D, Mohrs M, Donaldson DD, Locksley RM, Corry DB. Requirement for IL-13 independently of IL-4 in experimental asthma. Science 1998; 282(5397):2261–2263.

72. Aman MJ, Tayebi N, Obiri NI, Puri RK, Modi WS, Leonard WJ. cDNA cloning and characterization of the human interleukin 13 receptor alpha chain. J Biol Chem 1996; 271(46):29265–29270.

73. Gauchat JF, Schlagenhauf E, Feng NP, Moser R, Yamage M, Jeannin P, Alouani S, Elson G, Notarangelo LD, Wells T, Eugster HP, Bonnefoy JY. A novel 4-kb interleukin-13 receptor alpha mRNA expressed in human B, T, and endothelial cells encoding an alternate type-II interleukin-4/interleukin-13 receptor. Eur J Immunol 1997; 27(4): 971–978.

74. Deichmann K, Bardutzky J, Forster J, Heinzmann A, Kuehr J. Common polymorphisms in the coding part of the IL4-receptor gene. Biochem Biophys Res Commun 1997; 231(3):696–697.

75. Hershey GK, Friedrich MF, Esswein LA, Thomas ML, Chatila TA. The association of atopy with a gain-of-function mutation in the alpha subunit of the interleukin-4 receptor. N Engl J Med 1997; 337(24):1720–1725.

76. Mitsuyasu H, Izuhara K, Mao XQ, Gao PS, Arinobu Y, Enomoto T, Kawai M, Sasaki S, Dake Y, Hamasaki N, Shirakawa T, Hopkin JM. Ile50Val variant of IL4R alpha upregulates IgE synthesis and associates with atopic asthma. Nat Genet 1998; 19(2): 119–120.

77. Kruse S, Japha T, Tedner M, Sparholt SH, Forster J, Kuehr J, Deichmann KA. The polymorphisms S503P and Q576R in the interleukin-4 receptor alpha gene are associated with atopy and influence the signal transduction. Immunology 1999; 96(3): 365–371.

78. Hackstein H, Hecker M, Kruse S, Bohnert A, Ober C, Deichmann KA, Bein G. A novel polymorphism in the 5′ promoter region of the human interleukin-4 receptor

alpha-chain gene is associated with decreased soluble interleukin-4 receptor protein levels. Immunogenetics 2001; 53(4):264–269.

79. Kruse S, Forster J, Kuehr J, Deichmann KA. Characterization of the membrane-bound and a soluble form of human IL-4 receptor alpha produced by alternative splicing. Int Immunol 1999; 11(12):1965–1970.

80. Deichmann KA, Heinzmann A, Forster J, Dischinger S, Mehl C, Brueggenolte E, Hildebrandt F, Moseler M, Kuehr J. Linkage and allelic association of atopy and markers flanking the IL4-receptor gene. Clin Exp Allergy 1998; 28(2):151–155.

81. Meyers DA, Postma DS, Panhuysen CI, Xu J, Amelung PJ, Levitt RC, Bleecker ER. Evidence for a locus regulating total serum IgE levels mapping to chromosome 5. Genomics 1994; 23(2):464–470.

82. Liu X, Nickel R, Beyer K, Wahn U, Ehrlich E, Freidhoff LR, Bjorksten B, Beaty TH, Huang SK. An IL13 coding region variant is associated with a high total serum IgE level and atopic dermatitis in the German multicenter atopy study (MAS-90). J Allergy Clin Immunol 2000; 106(1 pt 1):167–170.

83. Waterhouse P, Penninger JM, Timms E, Wakeham A, Shahinian A, Lee KP, Thompson CB, Griesser H, Mak TW. Lymphoproliferative disorders with early lethality in mice deficient in Ctla-4. Science 1995; 270(5238):985–988.

84. Heinzmann A, Plesnar C, Kuehr J, Forster J, Deichmann KA. Common polymorphisms in the CTLA-4 and CD28 genes at 2q33 are not associated with asthma or atopy. Eur J Immunogenet 2000; 27(2):57–61.

85. Nakao F, Ihara K, Ahmed S, Sasaki Y, Kusuhara K, Takabayashi A, Nishima S, Hara T. Lack of association between CD28/CTLA-4 gene polymorphisms and atopic asthma in the Japanese population. Exp Clin Immunogenet 2000; 17(4):179–184.

86. Dariavach P, Mattei MG, Golstein P, Lefranc MP. Human Ig superfamily CTLA-4 gene: chromosomal localization and identity of protein sequence between murine and human CTLA-4 cytoplasmic domains. Eur J Immunol 1988; 18(12):1901–1905.

87. Deichmann K, Heinzmann A, Bruggenolte E, Forster J, Kuehr J. An Mse I RFLP in the human CTLA4 promotor. Biochem Biophys Res Commun 1996; 225(3):817–818.

88. Nistico L, Buzzetti R, Pritchard LE, Van der Auwera B, Giovannini C, Bosi E, Larrad MT, Rios MS, Chow CC, Cockram CS, Jacobs K, Mijovic C, Bain SC, Barnett AH, Vandewalle CL, Schuit F, Gorus FK, Tosi R, Pozzilli P, Todd JA. The CTLA-4 gene region of chromosome 2q33 is linked to, and associated with, type 1 diabetes. Belgian Diabetes Registry. Hum Mol Genet 1996; 5(7):1075–1080.

89. Polymeropoulos MH, Xiao H, Rath DS, Merril CR. Dinucleotide repeat polymorphism at the human CTLA4 gene. Nucleic Acids Res 1991; 19(14):4018.

90. Abe T, Takino H, Yamasaki H, Ozaki M, Sera Y, Kondo H, Sakamaki H, Kawasaki E, Awata T, Yamaguchi Y, Eguchi K. CTLA4 gene polymorphism correlates with the mode of onset and presence of ICA512 Ab in Japanese type 1 diabetes. Diabetes Res Clin Pract 1999; 46(2):169–175.

91. Lee YJ, Huang FY, Lo FS, Wang WC, Hsu CH, Kao HA, Yang TY, Chang JG. Association of CTLA4 gene A-G polymorphism with type 1 diabetes in Chinese children. Clin Endocrinol (Oxf) 2000; 52(2):153–157.

92. Naluai AT, Nilsson S, Samuelsson L, Gudjonsdottir AH, Ascher H, Ek J, Hallberg B, Kristiansson B, Martinsson T, Nerman O, Sollid LM, Wahlstrom J. The CTLA4/CD28 gene region on chromosome 2q33 confers susceptibility to celiac disease in a way possibly distinct from that of type 1 diabetes and other chronic inflammatory disorders. Tissue Antigens 2000; 56(4):350–355.

93. Marron MP, Raffel LJ, Garchon HJ, Jacob CO, Serrano-Rios M, Martinez Larrad MT, Teng WP, Park Y, Zhang ZX, Goldstein DR, Tao YW, Beaurain G, Bach JF, Huang HS, Luo DF, Zeidler A, Rotter JI, Yang MC, Modilevsky T, Maclaren NK, She JX. Insulin-dependent diabetes mellitus (IDDM) is associated with CTLA4 polymorphisms in multiple ethnic groups. Hum Mol Genet 1997; 6(8):1275–1282.

94. Badenhoop K. CTLA4 variants in type 1 diabetes: some stirrups serve better backing endocrine autoimmunity. Clin Endocrinol (Oxf) 2000; 52(2):139–140.

95. Donner H, Braun J, Seidl C, Rau H, Finke R, Ventz M, Walfish PG, Usadel KH, Badenhoop K. Codon 17 polymorphism of the cytotoxic T lymphocyte antigen 4 gene in Hashimoto's thyroiditis and Addison's disease. J Clin Endocrinol Metab 1997; 82(12):4130–4132.

96. Ligers A, Xu C, Saarinen S, Hillert J, Olerup O. The CTLA-4 gene is associated with multiple sclerosis. J Neuroimmunol 1999; 97(1–2):182–190.

97. Harbo HF, Celius EG, Vartdal F, Spurkland A. CTLA4 promoter and exon 1 dimorphisms in multiple sclerosis. Tissue Antigens 1999; 53(1):106–110.

98. Kouki T, Sawai Y, Gardine CA, Fisfalen ME, Alegre ML, DeGroot LJ. CTLA-4 gene polymorphism at position 49 in exon 1 reduces the inhibitory function of CTLA-4 and contributes to the pathogenesis of Graves' disease. J Immunol 2000; 165(11): 6606–6611.

99. Huang D, Giscombe R, Zhou Y, Pirskanen R, Lefvert AK. Dinucleotide repeat expansion in the CTLA-4 gene leads to T cell hyper-reactivity via the CD28 pathway in myasthenia gravis. J Neuroimmunol 2000; 105(1):69–77.

100. Hizawa N, Yamaguchi E, Jinushi E, Konno S, Kawakami Y, Nishimura M. Increased total serum IgE levels in patients with asthma and promoter polymorphisms at CTLA4 and FCER1B. J Allergy Clin Immunol 2001; 108(1):74–79.

101. Howard TD, Postma D, Hawkins GA, Koppelman GH, Zheng SL, Xu J, Meyers DA, Bleecker ER. Fine-Mapping of an Increased Total IgE Susceptibility Gene on Chromosome 2q: Analysis of CTLA-4 and CD28. New York: American Academy of Asthma, Allergy, and Immunology, 2002.

102. Martinez FD, Holt PG. Role of microbial burden in aetiology of allergy and asthma. Lancet 1999; 354(suppl 2):SII121–125.

103. Holt PG, Sly PD, Bjorksten B. Atopic versus infectious diseases in childhood: a question of balance? Pediatr Allergy Immunol 1997; 8(2):53–58.

104. Wright SD. Innate recognition of microbial lipids. In: Inflammation: Basic Principles and Clinical Correlates, 3rd ed. Philadelphia: Lippincott Williams & Wilkins, 1999: 525–535.

105. Haziot A, Chen S, Ferrero E, Low MG, Silber R, Goyert SM. The monocyte differentiation antigen, CD14, is anchored to the cell membrane by a phosphatidylinositol linkage. J Immunol 1988; 141(2):547–552.

106. Hizawa N, Freidhoff LR, Ehrlich E, Chiu YF, Duffy DL, Schou C, Dunston GM, Beaty TH, Marsh DG, Barnes KC, Huang SK. Genetic influences of chromosomes 5q31-q33 and 11q13 on specific IgE responsiveness to common inhaled allergens among African American families. Collaborative Study on the Genetics of Asthma (CSGA). J Allergy Clin Immunol 1998; 102(3):449–453.

107. Noguchi E, Shibasaki M, Arinami T, Takeda K, Maki T, Miyamoto T, Kawashima T, Kobayashi K, Hamaguchi H. Evidence for linkage between asthma/atopy in childhood and chromosome 5q31-q33 in a Japanese population. Am J Respir Crit Care Med 1997; 156(5):1390–1393.

108. Martinez FD, Solomon S, Holberg CJ, Graves PE, Baldini M, Erickson RP. Linkage of circulating eosinophils to markers on chromosome 5q. Am J Respir Crit Care Med 1998; 158(6):1739–1744.

109. Baldini M, Lohman IC, Halonen M, Erickson RP, Holt PG, Martinez FD. A polymorphism in the 5′ flanking region of the CD14 gene is associated with circulating soluble CD14 levels and with total serum immunoglobulin E. Am J Respir Cell Mol Biol 1999; 20(5):976–983.

110. Koppelman GH, Reijmerink NE, Colin Stine O, Howard TD, Whittaker PA, Meyers DA, Postma DS, Bleecker ER. Association of a promoter polymorphism of the CD14 gene and atopy. Am J Respir Crit Care Med 2001; 163(4):965–969.

111. Gao PS, Mao XQ, Baldini M, Roberts MH, Adra CN, Shirakawa T, Holt PG, Martinez FD, Hopkin JM. Serum total IgE levels and CD14 on chromosome 5q31. Clin Genet 1999; 56(2):164–165.

39

Application of Pharmacogenetics to the Therapeutics of Asthma

ERIC S. SILVERMAN

Brigham and Women's Hospital
Harvard Medical School
Harvard School of Public Health
Boston, Massachusetts, U.S.A.

**JOSEPHINE HJOBERG,
LYLE J. PALMER, KELAN TANTISIRA,
SCOTT T. WEISS, and
JEFFREY M. DRAZEN**

Brigham and Women's Hospital
Harvard Medical School
Boston, Massachusetts, U.S.A.

I. Introduction

There is great heterogeneity in the way asthmatics respond to medications, and a substantial portion of this heterogeneity is genetic in origin. This therapeutic heterogeneity, or variable drug response, may take a variety of forms, such as interindividual differences in absolute drug efficacy, differences in the amount or duration of drug required for effect, or predisposition to adverse drug reactions. Pharmacogenomics is a rapidly evolving discipline and approach to patient care that uses genetic information and genomic technologies to identify the genetic loci and underlying mechanisms responsible for variable therapeutic outcomes. Once pharmacogenetic* loci are identified, they can be used to prospectively tailor an individual's therapeutic regimen to optimize efficacy and avoid adverse reactions. Ideally, this approach would allow physicians to bypass therapeutic trials, during which a patient is placed on sequential drugs to see which particular class of drug or individual preparation is best suited for that patient. This approach to patient care has obvious benefits and is applicable to all diseases.

---

* The term pharmacogenetics is generally used in a more restrictive manner to refer to specific examples of genetic variants that impact response to drugs.

In this chapter we describe pharmacogenomic principles in the context of asthma with an emphasis on research methodology, specific examples, and "functional pharmacogenomics" (i.e., the molecular mechanisms by which these genetic variants alter drug response). Although the principles and applicability of pharmacogenomics are likely to be relevant to all asthma drugs and therapeutic targets of airway inflammation, there are currently only three genes with polymorphisms known to impact asthma treatment: the β_2-adrenergic receptor, the 5-lipoxygenase gene, and the LTC_4 synthase gene. This chapter will emphasize polymorphisms of the leukotriene pathway as examples of asthma pharmacogenetics.

II. Asthma and Its Treatment

Asthma is a common syndrome of the airways affecting approximately 5–10% of the population in industrialized countries (1). Of great concern is the 30% increase in the worldwide prevalence of asthma over the past 20 years (2). In the United States, the cost of direct health care attributed to asthma was approximately $8.1 billion per annum in 2000, and almost 40% of this expenditure was for medications alone (3). Although many asthma medications are available, they have modest therapeutic efficacy, in part because of the highly variable response of individual patients. These data underscore the need for more uniformly effective asthma therapeutic agents and new algorithms for their prescription.

Asthma is a heterogeneous and genetically complex syndrome characterized by reversible airflow obstruction, airway hyperresponsiveness, and inflammation of the airways. Asthma is not a single disease but a syndrome with a variety of phenotypes that share these three cardinal features. The phenotypic variability of asthma between patients reflects the multiple genetic and environmental determinants among different patients. Individual differences in responses to drugs and in predisposition to adverse reactions are just other examples of these phenotypic differences.

Despite these individual differences, today's therapies make asthma a highly manageable disease. The two main types of asthma drugs are the so-called reliever or rescue drugs that target the acute bronchconstriction and the so-called controller treatments that are used to reduce the severity of airway inflammation and the severity and frequency of obstruction (4). The main reliever drugs are rapid-acting β_2-agonists (e.g., albuterol, terbutaline, isoetharine), which relax the bronchial smooth muscle by activation of β_2-adrenergic receptors. This is the treatment of choice for mild intermittent asthma. For mild, moderate, and severe persistent asthma, the reliever treatment is usually combined with controller treatment. The two commonly used classes of controller agents are the inhaled corticosteroids and the leukotriene modifiers. The inhaled corticosteroids (e.g., budesonide, beclomethasone, and fluticasone) and the leukotriene modifiers (e.g., zileuton, montelukast, zafirlukast) modify the inflammatory micro-environment of the airway to reduce airway obstruction and hyperresponsiveness. It has been estimated that as many as one half of asthmatic patients do not respond to treatment with β_2-agonists, leukotriene antagonists, or an inhaled corticosteroid (5,6). How much of this variability is due to genetic factors is currently unknown but can be estimated.

III. Heterogeneity of the Asthma Therapeutic Response

In asthma, the variability in therapeutic response among different individuals is greater than the variation seen in the same individual on two different occasions (5). The variability between subjects can be of genetic or environmental origin or due to differences in examination technique or other measurement errors. One obvious nongenetic factor that may influence the efficacy of a treatment is age. The reactions of infants, children, adolescents, and the elderly to a drug may be different from that of adults because of developmental effects on the pharmacokinetics or pharmacodynamic pathways of the drug (7). Another obvious nongenetic factor is drug compliance; most individuals prefer pills over metered-dose inhalers and may not be taking the most commonly prescribed asthma drugs as directed.

The genetic factors are much less obvious. There are four general paradigms by which sequence variants may lead to heterogeneity in therapeutic response for all diseases. The simplest and best-described paradigm in pharmacogenomics is that of sequence variants that alter the metabolism, distribution, or excretion of a drug and thereby enhancing or inhibiting drug effects (pharmacokinetic paradigm). This phenomenon was first observed in the 1950s when patients with inherited deficiency of plasma cholinesterase had a prolonged paralytic response to suxamethonium (8). The second paradigm involves sequence variants that result in an unintended consequence of a drug outside of its therapeutic target (idiosyncratic paradigm). This paradigm was also appreciated early on, when it was discovered that inherited differences in the ability of an individual to acetylate isoniazide was associated with predisposition to the development of peripheral neuropathy (9). A third paradigm consists of sequence variants in the drug target or the drug target pathway that leads to altered drug efficacy (pharmacodynamic). The β_2-adrenergic receptor LTC_4 synthase and 5-lipoxygenase gene polymorphisms are good examples of this paradigm. A fourth possible paradigm involves the genetic heterogeneity leading to the development of the disease itself or differences in disease severity that may indirectly impact drug response (asthma genesis or severity factors). In other words, asthma may be caused by abnormalities in multiple pathways, or combinations of pathways, modulating the inflammatory response to allergen and, thus, be more or less responsive to a class of drugs depending on the inflammatory pathway targeted by that class of drugs. Table 1 lists common genetic and nongenetic "environmental" causes of variable drug response in asthma. Although all known examples of asthma pharmacogenetics follow the pharmacodynamic paradigm, we believe that examples representative of each pathway will be found in the near future.

To better illustrate the heterogeneity of asthma therapeutic response, we provide a specific example using data from a large clinical trial of the β_2-agonist albuterol for mild asthma (10). Figure 1 shows the number of patients as a function of percent change in the forced expiratory volume in one second (FEV_1) after treatment

Table 1   Causes of Heterogeneity of Asthma Therapeutic Response

Genetic factors	Environmental factors
Pharmacokinetic	Allergen exposure
Idiosyncratic reaction	Infectious complications
Pharmacodynamic	Toxic exposure
Disease severity	Compliance
	Inhaler technique
	Concomitant illness
	Drug–drug interactions
	Age, size of patient
	Measurement error

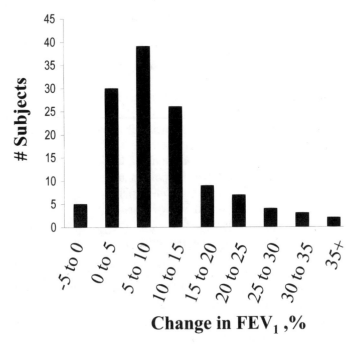

Figure 1   Variable response to the β_2-agonist albuterol: patients with mild-to-moderate asthma are treated with a standard dose of inhaled albuterol. Numbers of patients are shown as a function of change in FEV_1 as a percent of baseline. Note wide range of response among asthmatics given the same treatment. (Unpublished data courtesy of Dr. Jeffrey M. Drazen.)

with albuterol. Some patients had a dramatic response, with a >35% improvement in FEV$_1$, but, many patients had little or no response. Moreover, some patients seemed to deteriorate after β-agonist administration with a fall in baseline FEV$_1$. In the study illustrated in Figure 1, patients were carefully selected and closely followed to minimize confounding factors such as poor compliance and poor MDI technique; nevertheless, the genetic and nongenetic factors are still difficult to separate. Since variance is additive, one approach to estimating the fraction of variance that has a genetic origin is to estimate the intraindividual variance in treatment response (nongenetic) and compare this to the interindividual variance (nongenetic + genetic). The repeatability (*r*) of the treatment response reflects the upper limit of heritability and is defined by the equation

$$r = \frac{(V_G + V_{Eg})}{V_P}$$

where V_G is the genetic variance, V_{Eg} is the overall environmental variance from known or unknown sources, and V_P is the total variance. With the use of this approach, the repeatability of response to various asthma treatments has been estimated to be approximately 60–85% of the total population variance (5). However, this is an upper limit estimate; only by identifying pharmacogenetic loci and prospectively randomizing patients by genotype can the genetic variance be determined precisely.

IV. SNPs and Other Genetic Polymorphisms

The human genome is not a static entity but is shaped continuously by heritable mutations passed down from parent to progeny. If more than one allele is present at a given locus and the alleles differ by a single base pair, such a mutation is called a single nucleotide polymorphism (SNP, pronounced snip). The term haplotype refers to the ordered arrangement of alleles at different loci on a chromosome. SNPs have received more attention than other sequence variants (i.e., tandem repeats, insertion, deletions) because these variants are probably responsible for the majority of phenotypic differences between individuals with common diseases. Moreover, these variants are particularly suited for genetic studies designed to find loci responsible for complex disease traits because they are more frequent, dense, and stable and are more amenable to high-throughput genotyping strategies than other sequence variants. More than 2 million SNPs have already been found in the human genome, and the number is increasing exponentially as a result of large-scale sequencing efforts (11). However, as demonstrated by the 5-lipoxygenase promoter polymorphisms (a tandem repeat) and discussed in detail below, sequence variants other than SNPs may have important pharmacogenetic consequences.

Although SNPs are likely to be the variants responsible for phenotypic differences among individuals, most of these variants are functionally silent. Many SNPs are common, occurring in the human genome at a frequency of 10% or higher (12). They may be located in coding regions (cSNPs), noncoding regions such as upstream regulatory elements (promoters) or 3′, 5′ untranslated regions (perigenic SNPs), introns (intronic SNPs), or between genes (intergenic SNPs). A SNP in a coding region that changes the amino acid sequence is called a nonsynonymous SNP. One that does not change an amino acid sequence is called a synonymous SNP. Although the distribution of SNPs varies greatly across the genome, the average is approximately 1 SNP per 1000 bases (12). The estimated number of cSNPs in the human genome resulting in alterations in amino acid sequence is around 50,000–100,000 (13), however, the relative importance of SNPs in altering regulatory regions (e.g., promoter elements, slice sites) is difficult to predict and should not be underestimated. Regardless of mechanism by which a genetic variant causes a phenotypic change, the major challenge for investigators is finding a functionally significant polymorphism in the approximately 3 billion base pairs that constitute the human genome and associating the polymorphism with a specific phenotype.

V. Dissecting Complex Traits: The Association Study

Most genetic studies used to map disease susceptibility or disease modifier genes can be categorized into two fundamental types: genome scans based on linkage analysis and candidate gene studies based on case-control association. Genome scans make no assumption about the location of the variant in the genome, rather use genetic markers (i.e., microsatellites) to follow regions of the genome as they cosegregate with a phenotype in a study pedigree, usually consisting of a family or inbred population. Once a chromosomal region has been identified and narrowed, positional cloning techniques can be used to isolate the gene and its functionally relevant variant. While this design is well suited for simple Mendelian traits caused by variants in one or a few genes and has been successfully used to identify the disease genes and specific variants involved in many such diseases, the utility of genome scans for genetically complex diseases has been limited and somewhat disappointing.

In contrast, association studies are intrinsically more powerful than linkage analysis in detecting multiple weak effects found in genetic complex diseases and are generally the only study designs suitable for pharmacogenetic investigation (14). Although genome-wide association studies on outbred populations using large numbers of genetic markers (>50,000 SNPs) may be possible, most association studies focus on a few polymorphisms in candidate genes thought to be biologically relevant to the phenotype of interest. These studies are usually based on a case-control design and, in the case of asthma pharmacogenetics, involve the collection of asthmatics "cases" with enhanced response to a drug and a group of asthmatics consisting of poor responders to serve as a "control" for comparison. If side effects were the major outcome of interest, the cases would consist of asthmatics with frequent or severe reactions to treatment and the control group would consist of asthmatics without adverse reactions to the treatment. By genotyping case individuals and comparing the frequency of an allele or haplotype with controls, it may be possible to establish an association. A positive association does not necessarily establish causality, because a SNP may be in linkage disequilibrium with the functionally relevant SNP. Thus, providing additional evidence of a functional genomic nature is essential to establish the precise location of a biologically relevant polymorphism. While

Table 2   Issues to Consider when Designing Association Studies

Issue	Key question	Possible solution
Selection of cases and controls	a. Selected without bias? b. Meet phenotype criteria? c. Free of confounding factors? d. Matched regarding demographic factors? e. Matched regarding environmental factors?	a. Population-based selection b. Family-based association design
Sample size	Are there enough subjects?	a. Power calculations b. Large studies
Population stratification	Are cases and controls matched?	a. Match ethnicity b. Family-based design c. Genotype at unlinked markers
Selection of candidate gene	a. Biologically feasible? b. All variants identified?	a. Demonstrate functional effect b. Completely sequence gene
Linkage disequilibrium	a. Other genes? b. Other polymorphisms?	a. Haplotype analysis b. Completely sequence gene
Multiple comparisons	a. How many alleles tested? b. How many phenotypes tested?	a. Bonferroni correction b. Estimate empirical *p*-values

association studies are intuitively obvious, there are many theoretical and technical pitfalls that have tainted reported association studies (15). These are listed in Table 2 and briefly discussed in the next section.

VI. Problems with Association Studies: Statistical Power, Linkage Disequilibrium, and Population Stratification

The association of a polymorphism with an altered therapeutic response may have no functional explanation because it is caused by a type I error, i.e., an association is accepted as real when it is in fact false. Experience suggests that many published studies are confounded by this problem (15). In the setting of multiple testing, with many loci in a candidate gene, or a few loci in many genes, erroneous associations are likely to be made because of statistical artefacts. By correcting for multiple comparisons and using relatively conservative thresholds of significance, type 1 errors can be avoided. One approach, called the Bonferroni correction, sets the threshold of significance at $p = 0.05/n$, where n equals the number of independent associations performed, not at the conventional 0.05 level of significance. However, this may be too stringent and lead to excess type II error—failure to detect true associations. These power issues and other essential features of a sound association study are detailed by Silverman and Palmer (15).

A SNP may also be associated with a particular phenotype in the absence of an obvious functional effect because of linkage disequilibrium, i.e., two or more alleles at different loci occur together more often than expected by chance because of their close proximity in the genome and infrequent recombinations. In the case of pharmacogenomics, the nonfunctional SNP is associated with altered drug response because it is in linkage disequilibrium with a functional SNP that is the true pharmacogenetic locus. Alternatively, a pharmacogenetic phenotype may require the interaction of two or more SNPs within a gene or among several genes. These issues are further complicated by the inheritance of families of SNPs together in a given narrow chromosomal region; the group of linked SNPs is known as a SNP haplotype. Moreover, the complex patterns of linkage disequilibrium resulting in the formation of haplotypes are extremely variable across the human genome, even over relatively short sequence stretches, and cannot be reliably predicted based on proximity alone (16). Experience with the SNP haplotypes suggests that they are more useful than single SNPs for predicting drug response (6); however, large study populations are necessary to identify all the common haplotypes and to achieve adequate statistical power.

Another common cause of an erroneous association is the use of poorly chosen populations that contain undetected stratification, usually due to recent admixture of populations. For example, there may be an ethnic or racial imbalance between drug responders and nonresponders such that a SNP that is more frequent in one group reflects the ethnic or racial differences and not the genetic basis of the altered drug response. Such confounding factors can be avoided by choosing cases and controls carefully; however, stratification is not always obvious, especially in the ethnically and racially diverse populations in the United States. Methods developed to detect population stratification include the genotyping of random panels of SNPs unrelated to the phenotype of interest (17). The absence of an association in this panel can provide reassurance that cases and controls are appropriately matched. With improved high-throughput genotyping methods, these new approaches will be easier to apply and will help avoid erroneous associations.

VII. Pharmacogenetics of Antileukotriene Therapy

Identifying candidate genes to screen for sequence variants and to test for association can be a great challenge because the molecular pathways through which asthma therapeutics mediate their effects are manifold and extremely complicated. All pathways contain multiple receptors, signal transduction components, transcription factors, metabolizing enzymes, regulatory cytokines, and chemokines that may contain modifying genetic variants. In short, there are many good candidate genes that must be screened for polymorphisms and tested for association. Furthermore, because of the inevitable weaknesses of association studies discussed above, it is necessary to verify positive associations with follow-up studies using other populations and statistical techniques. It is also essential to bolster a positive association studies with functional data, i.e., identify a realistic molecular mechanism by which a polymorphism mediates a pharmacogenetic effect. Of the three examples of asthma pharmacogenetics (β_2-agonist receptor polymorphisms, 5-lipoxygenase polymorphisms, and the LTC_4 synthase polymorphism) identified to date, only the β_2-agonist receptor polymorphisms have been firmly established as pharmacogenetic loci. These pharmacogenetic polymorphisms have been identified by association studies, verified in several follow-up studies, and shown to have effects on receptor function in vitro and in vivo. Although the significance of the 5-lipoxygenase and LTC_4 synthase polymorphisms have not yet been replicated in multiple association studies, data are emerging to support their role in altered response to antileukotriene drugs and are now discussed in depth.

A. Pharmacology of the Leukotriene Pathway

Leukotrienes are a family of eicosatetraenoic acids with profound effects on airway biology (18). The major source of leukotrienes derives from the release of arachidonic acid from the cell membrane by a number of potential phospholipase A2s (PLA_2) (Fig. 2). The arachidonic acid is converted to LTA_4 by 5-lipoxygenase (5-LO or ALOX5). The 5-LO–activating protein (FLAP) serves as an essential cofactor along with Ca^{2+} and ATP (19). LTA_4 hydrolase catalyses the production of LTB_4

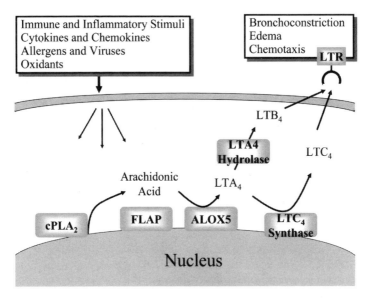

Figure 2 Simplified view of the leukotriene pathway: multiple enzymes and cofactors interact to form leukotrienes. cPLA$_2$, cytoplasmic phospholipase A$_2$; FLAP; 5-lipoxygenase–activating protein; ALOX5, 5-lipoxygenase; LTR, leukotriene receptors.

from LTA$_4$ (20), and the cysteinyl-leukotriene LTC$_4$ is formed from LTA$_4$ by the action of LTC$_4$ synthase (21). LTC$_4$ exits the cell by a specific carrier-mediated membrane transporter (22) and is further converted via LTD$_4$ to LTE$_4$ by enzymes in the extracellular space (23). The cysteinyl-leukotrienes (LTC$_4$, LTD$_4$, LTE$_4$) are among the most potent bronchoconstrictors ever identified (23), and these effects are mediated by binding to the Cys-LT$_1$ receptor (24). LTB$_4$ is not a bronchoconstrictor but a chemotactic agent that attracts neutrophils, eosinophils, and monocytes (25). Asthmatics have increased levels of LTB$_4$ and cysteinyl-leukotrienes in their airways (26), and antileukotriene therapy has been associated with improvement in various types of asthma (27). Currently, two classes of antileukotriene drugs have been approved for asthma treatment: the leukotriene Cys-LT$_1$ receptor antagonists (e.g., pranlukast, zafirlukast, and montelukast) and the 5-lipoxygenase inhibitor (zileuton).

B. Variable Therapeutic Responses to Antileukotriene Therapy

As with all asthma medications, individuals vary greatly in their response to antileukotriene drugs. In a study by Malmstrom et al., 644 patients were randomized to receive montelukast (10 mg/day) or placebo over a 12-week period (28). The subjects receiving montelukast had a mean increase in FEV$_1$ of 7.4%, whereas the placebo group had an increase of 0.7%, indicating that montelukast is an effective asthma drug (Fig. 3). However, when the data are analyzed on an individual basis,

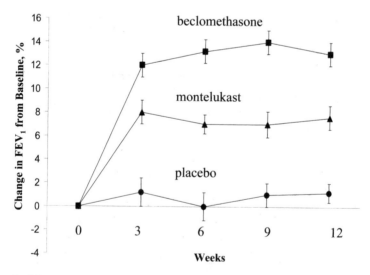

Figure 3   Mean percentage change from baseline ($\pm$ SE) in FEV$_1$ over the 12-week treatment period: black squares represent patients receiving inhaled beclomethasone, 200 µg twice daily; black triangles represent patients receiving montelukast, 10 mg once daily; black circles represent patients receiving placebo. Beclomethasone increased mean FEV$_1$ approximately 13.1% at 12 weeks, whereas montelukast increased mean FEV$_1$ approximately 7.4%. (Modified from Ref. 28.)

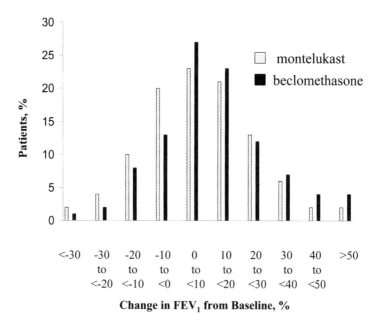

Figure 4 Distribution of treatment responses for FEV$_1$: response distributions (% of patients) are shown as histograms for predefined intervals of % change in FEV$_1$. Note wide variation in therapeutic response among patients. (Modified from Ref. 28.)

it becomes clear that there was tremendous variability in response, similar to the response to beclomethasone (Fig. 4). The mean values are skewed by a small number of individuals with a dramatic improvement in FEV$_1$. Many patients had no significant improvement, and the condition of some patients even deteriorated. On the basis of these data and other studies with similar results, it has been hypothesized that genetic factors might be responsible for some of this heterogeneity (5).

C. 5-Lipoxygenase and LTC$_4$ Synthase Gene Promoter Polymorphisms

Several of the genes controlling leukotriene synthesis have been screened for sequence variants and subjected to association studies as part of an effort to identify the genetic basis for variable response to antileukotriene drugs. Polymorphisms with pharmacogenetic significance have been found in two of these genes, 5-LO and LTC4 synthase, although others genes are likely to exist.

Expression of 5-LO protein is regulated at a number of levels (29). At the transcriptional level, binding of different transcription factors to specific consensus binding sites in the 5-LO gene promoter region has been shown to be important for expression in vitro. Two transcription factors, Sp1 and early growth response factor-1 (Egr-1), bind to the promoter in a series of tandem consensus sites located in a

G + C-rich core promoter region between − 179 to − 56 bp relative to the transcriptional start site (30). The SP1-binding sites are adjacent to the Egr-1–binding sites, and Egr-1 can displace Sp1 from this promoter region and increase transcription above basal levels by recruiting the transcriptional coactivator CREB-binding protein (CBP) (31). A family of polymorphisms has been identified in this region that consists of a deletion of one or two Egr-1 -GGGCGG- consensus binding sites or the addition of one of these sites (Fig. 5) (32). Approximately 94% of subjects have one wild-type allele at this locus. The pharmacogenetic significance of this polymorphism was investigated in a clinical drug trial of the zileuton-like 5-LO inhibitor, ABT-761, in asthmatics (33). Overall, ABT-761 resulted in a significant improvement of FEV_1 above baseline. As in the Malmstrom et al. study (28), there was marked variability in individual responses. When the patients (114 with high-dose ABT-761 and 107 with placebo) were stratified for genotype at the 5-LO promoter, it became apparent that subjects with at least one wild-type allele had an improvement in FEV_1 of approximately 19%, whereas patients with no wild-type allele had a decrease in FEV_1 of 1% (Fig. 6). This locus represents a pharmacogenetic pattern suggesting that the 6% of patients with asthma who do not carry a wild-type allele at this locus are less likely to respond to this type of antileukotriene treatment.

A transversion SNP (A to C) at − 444 bp in the LTC_4 synthase gene promoter represents a second pharmacogenetic locus of relevance to the leukotriene pathway. The C allele creates an activator protein-2 consensus binding site that may increase the expression of the gene and be associated with enhanced production of cysteinyl-leukotriene (34). Sampson and colleagues found that among asthmatic subjects treated with zafirlukast (20 mg bid), those homozygous for the A allele ($n = 10$ subjects) at the − 444 locus had a diminished FEV_1 response compared with those with the C/C or C/A ($n = 13$) genotype (34). A similar relationship has been found between this polymorphism and response to pranlukast. It is also of interest that Sanak et al. have shown that this polymorphism may be associated with the diagnosis of aspirin-induced asthma and may represent the first example of the idiosyncratic paradigm of asthma pharmacogenetics (35). As additional loci are detected, it will

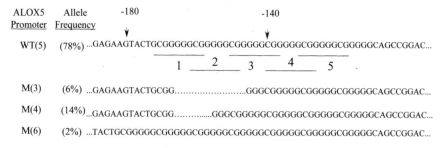

Figure 5 Location and characteristics of ALOX5 polymorphisms: WT allele has 5 Sp1/ Egr-1 transcription factor consensus binding sites. Alleles M(3), M(4), and M(5) have 3, 4, and 5 binding sites, respectively. Allele frequencies are noted.

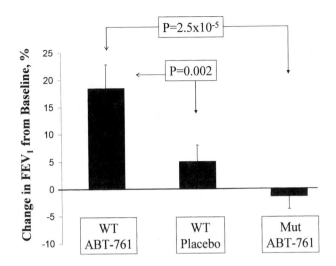

Figure 6 ALOX5 genotype predicts antileukotriene response: improvement in FEV_1 at 84 days of treatment was significantly greater for WT subjects treated with ABT-761 (300 mg/ day) compared with subjects possessing any ALOX5 mutant allele. ABT-761 is an ALOX5 inhibitor similar to zileuton. (Modified from Ref. 33.)

be interesting to determine if there are additive or synergistic effects of multiple variant alleles in the genes of the leukotriene pathway.

VIII. Conclusions: The Future of Asthma Pharmacogenetics

The use of pharmacogenetics and pharmacogenomics will most certainly be crucial for the development of safer, more effective, and less expensive therapy for asthma and other genetically complex diseases. In this post–Human Genome Project era, the extensive genomic information that is rapidly accumulating and is readily available over the Internet will make it easier to detect pharmacogenetic phenomena and to establish causal associations with loci in candidate genes. The use of emerging high-throughput microarray technology will make it possible to genotype patients at many loci simultaneously to create detailed profiles of their likely responses to drugs. In the near future it may be possible to obtain a small buccal brush sample in the clinic from a person with asthma and send it to the laboratory for an "asthma pharmacogenetic panel." There the DNA would be extracted and genotyped at the established pharmacogenetic loci so that therapeutic recommendations could be made (i.e., which drugs would be more or less likely to work and will be more or less likely to have adverse effects).

We have outlined some of the formidable obstacles that remain, including the large number of candidate genes that must be considered and the pressing need for properly designed genetic studies to elucidate complex and subtle pharmacogenetic association and to eliminate erroneous conclusions. Finding these SNPs will require pooling of patient samples and data from many clinical trials and great technical resources to screen the many candidate genes for SNPs and to genotype individuals at many loci in each candidate gene. Despite these difficulties, it seems likely that many of these SNPs will soon be used routinely in clinical practice for optimizing drug therapy for asthma and other genetically complex diseases. We and others speculate that by the year 2010 personalized medicine based on pharmacogenetics will be a reality (6).

Acknowledgments

This work was funded National Institutes of Health HLBI HL70573 and UO1 HL65899.

References

1. Barnes PJ, Thomson NC, Rodger IW. Preface. In: Barnes PJ, Rodger IW, Thomson NC, eds. Asthma: Basic Mechanisms and Clinical Management, 3rd ed. San Diego, CA: Academic Press, 1998.
2. Sullivan SD, Weiss KB. Pharmacoeconomics of asthma treatments. In: Barnes PJ, Rodger IW, Thomson NC, eds. Asthma: Basic Mechanisms and Clinical Management, 3rd ed. San Diego, CA: Academic Press, 1998:903–916.
3. American Lung Association's Epidemiology and Statistics Unit. Trends in asthma morbidity and mortality. Vol. 2001: American Lung Association, 2001. Accessed online at www.lungusa.org.
4. NHLBI/WHO Workshop. Global initiative from asthma management and prevention. National Institutes of Health, National Heart, Lung, and Blood Institute and the World Health Organization, 1998. Accessed online at www.ginasthma.com.
5. Drazen JM, Silverman EK, Lee TH. Heterogeneity of therapeutic responses in asthma. Br Med Bull 2000; 56:1054–1070.
6. Liggett SB. Pharmacogenetic applications of the Human Genome Project. Nat Med 2001; 7:281–283.
7. Leeder JS. Pharmacogenetics and pharmacogenomics. Pediatr Clin North Am 2001; 48: 765–781.
8. Kalow W. Familial incidence of low pseudocholinesterase level. Lancet 1956; 271:576.
9. Hughes HB, Biehl JP, Jones AP, Schmidt LH. Metabolish of isoniazid in man as related to the occurrence of peripheral neuritis. Am Rev Tuberc 1954; 70:266–273.
10. Drazen JM, Israel E, Boushey HA, Chinchilli VM, Fahy JV, Fish JE, Lazarus SC, Lemanske RF, Martin RJ, Peters SP, Sorkness C, Szefler SJ. Comparison of regularly scheduled with as-needed use of albuterol in mild asthma. Asthma Clinical Research Network. N Engl J Med 1996; 335:841–847.
11. The International SNP Map Working Group. A map of human genome sequence variation containing 1.42 million single nucleotide polymorphisms. Nature 2001; 409: 928–933.

12. Brookes AJ. The essence of SNPs. Gene 1999; 234:177–186.
13. Ingelman-Sundberg M. Pharmacogenetics: an opportunity for a safer and more efficient pharmacotherapy. J Intern Med 2001; 250:186–200.
14. Elston RC. The genetic dissection of multifactorial traits. Clin Exp Allergy 1995; 25(suppl 2): 103–106.
15. Silverman EK, Palmer LJ. Case-control association studies for the genetics of complex respiratory diseases. Am J Respir Cell Mol Biol 2000; 22:645–648.
16. Clark DA, Weiss KM, Nickerson DA, Taylor SL, Buchanan A, Stengard J, Salomaa V, Vartiainen E, Perola M, Boerwinkle E, Sing CF. Haplotype structure and population genetic inferences from nucleotide-sequence variation in human lipoprotein lipase. Am J Human Genet 1998; 63:595–612.
17. Pritchard JK, Rosenberg NA. Use of unlinked genetic markers to detect population stratification in association studies. Am J Hum Genet 1999; 65:220–228.
18. Samuelson B. leukotrienes: mediators of immediate hypersensitivity reactions and inflammation. Science 1983; 220:568–575.
19. Dixon RA, Diehl RE, Opas E, Rands E, Vickers PJ, Evans JF, Gillard JW, Miller DK. Requirement of a 5-lipoxygenase-activating protein for leukotriene synthesis. Nature 1990; 343:282–284.
20. Samuelsson B, Funk CD. Enzymes involved in the biosynthesis of leukotriene B4. J Biol Chem 1989; 264:19469–19472.
21. Yoshimoto T, Soberman RJ, Lewis RA, Austen KF. Isolation and characterization of leukotriene C4 synthetase of rat basophilic leukemia cells. Proc Natl Acad Sci USA 1985; 82:8399–8403.
22. Lam BK, Owen WF, Jr., Austen KF, Soberman RJ. The identification of a distinct export step following the biosynthesis of leukotriene C4 by human eosinophils. J Biol Chem 1989; 264:12885–12889.
23. Drazen JM. Cysteinyl leukotrienes. In: Barnes PJ, Rodger IW, Thomson NC, eds. Asthma: Basic Mechanisms and Clinical Management, 3rd ed. San Diego, CA: Academic Press, 1998:281–295.
24. Lynch KR, O'Neill GP, Liu Q, Im DS, Sawyer N, Metters KM, Coulombe N, Abramovitz M, Figueroa DJ, Zeng Z, Connoly BM, Bai C. Austin CP, Chateauneuf A, Stocco R, Greig GM, Kargman S, Hooks SB, Hosfield E, Williams DR, Ford-Hutchinson AW, Caskey CT, Evans JF. Characterization of the human cysteinyl leukotriene CysLT1 receptor. Nature 399:789–793.
25. Lewis RA, Austen KF, Soberman RJ. Leukotrienes and other products of the 5-lipoxygenase pathway. Biochemistry and relation to pathobiology in human diseases. N Engl J Med 1990; 323:645–655.
26. Holgate ST, Bradding P, Sampson AP. Leukotriene antagonists and synthesis inhibitors: new directions in asthma therapy. J Allergy Clin Immunol 1996; 98:1–13.
27. Drazen JM, Israel E, O'Byrne PM. Treatment of asthma with drugs modifying the leukotriene pathway. N Engl J Med 1999; 340:197–206.
28. Malmstrom K, Rodriguez-Gomez G, Guerra J, et al. Oral montelukast, inhaled beclomethasone, and placebo for chronic asthma. A randomized, controlled trial. Montelukast/Beclomethasone Study Group. Ann Intern Med 1999; 130:487–495.
29. Silverman ES, Drazen JM. The biology of 5-lipoxygenase: function, structure, and regulatory mechanisms. Proc Assoc Am Physicians 1999; 111:525–536.
30. Silverman ES, Du J, De Sanctis GT, Radmark O, Samuelsson B, Drazen JM, Collins T. Egr-1 and Sp1 interact functionally with the 5-lipoxygenase promoter and its naturally occurring mutants. Am J Respir Cell Mol Biol 1998; 19:316–323.

31. Silverman ES, Du J, Williams AJ, Wadgaonkar R, Drazen JM, Collins T. cAMP-response-element-binding-protein-binding protein (CBP) and p300 are transcriptional coactivators of early growth response factor-1 (Egr-1). Biochem J 1998; 336:183–189.

32. In KH, Asano K, Beier D, Grobholz J, Finn PW, Silverman EK, Silverman ES, Collins T, Fischer AR, Keith TP, Serino K, Kim SW, De Sanctis GT, Yandava C, Pillari A, Rubin P, Kemp J, Israel E, Busse W, Ledford D, Murray JJ, Segal A, Tinkleman D, Drazen JM. Naturally occurring mutations in the human 5-lipoxygenase gene promoter that modify transcription factor binding and reporter gene transcription. J Clin Invest 1997; 99:1130–1137.

33. Drazen JM, Yandava CN, Dube L, Szczerback N, Hippensteel R, Pillari A, Israel E, Schork N, Silverman ES, Katz DA, Drajesk J. Pharmacogenetic association between ALOX5 promoter genotype and the response to anti-asthma treatment. Nat Genet 1999; 22:168–170.

34. Sampson AP, Siddiqui S, Buchanan D, Howarth PH, Holgate ST, Holloway JW, Sayers I. Variant LTC(4) synthase allele modifies cysteinyl leukotriene synthesis in eosinophils and predicts clinical response to zafirlukast. Thorax 55(suppl 2):28–31.

35. Sanak M, Pierzchalska M, Bazan-Socha S, Szczeklik A. Enhanced expression of the leukotriene C(4) synthase due to overactive transcription of an allelic variant associated with aspirin-intolerant asthma. Am J Respir Cell Mol Biol 2000; 23:290–296.

40

DNA-Based Immunotherapy for Asthma

DAVID H. BROIDE and EYAL RAZ

University of California, San Diego
La Jolla, California, U.S.A.

I. Introduction

Our improved understanding of the cellular and molecular mechanisms mediating the pathogenesis of allergen-induced asthma has led to attempts to downregulate the Th2-mediated inflammatory response in the airway using DNA-based therapies. A variety of DNA-based therapies are currently being investigated in animal models as well as human clinical trials. The different DNA-based therapies being evaluated in allergen-induced asthma include immunostimulatory DNA sequences (ISS, or CpG DNA motif), allergen protein–ISS conjugate, DNA vaccines encoding allergens (plasmid DNA or pDNA), and antisense oligonucleotides. In this chapter we discuss the theory and mechanism of action of each of these DNA-based therapeutics and review results of therapeutic efficacy and toxicity in animal models of asthma and human disease.

II. Immunostimulatory DNA

A. Immunostimulatory DNA and the Hygiene Hypothesis

The prevalence of allergic asthma has increased over the last two decades in industrialized countries especially in young children (1). Allergic diseases affect as many as 30% of individuals in some populations. The U.S. Centers for Disease Control (CDC) reports that more than 17 million people in the United States currently suffer from asthma, about 7% of the population (2). The increasing prevalence of allergic diseases is occurring despite the availability of effective therapies (e.g., inhaled corticosteroids). The reasons for these trends are poorly understood and could be related to the "hygiene hypothesis," which argues that reduced exposure to microbial stimuli as a consequence of modern hygiene practices plays a major role in the rising prevalence of allergic diseases (3). Thus, in industrialized countries higher hygiene standards such as frequent vaccinations, the overuse of antibiotics, the consumption of pasteurized or "sterilized" foods and cleaner water, all contribute to the modification of the microbial environment in which we live. As a consequence of this reduction in microbial exposures, genetically predisposed children are hypothesized to be biased toward the development Th2 immune deviation (4).

The hygiene hypothesis offers a provocative rationale for consideration of bacterial DNA-based therapeutics for the treatment of allergic diseases. The immunological activities of DNA-based immunotherapeutics are dependent on immunostimulatory DNA sequences (ISS), which are abundant in many microbial genomes but are rare in mammalian DNA. Therefore, DNA-based therapeutics are likely to elicit immunity, in part by mimicry of natural infectious exposures. If the sterilization of the environment we live in proves to be a contributing factor in the rising prevalence of allergic diseases, as the hygiene hypothesis proposes, then DNA-based immunotherapeutics represent novel and rational approaches for their treatment (5).

B. Immune Response to Immunostimulatory DNA

Immunostimulatory DNA sequences (ISS or CpG motif) which are derived from bacterial DNA are strong inducers of Th1 responses to antigen and have therefore been investigated in the treatment of Th2-mediated diseases such as asthma (6). Immunostimulatory DNA sequences contain unmethylated CpG dinucleotides within a given hexamer that follows the formula: 5′-purine-purine-CG-pyrimidine-pyrimidine-3′ (e.g., 5′-GACGTC-3′) or 5′-purine-TCG-pyrimidine-pyrimidine-3′ (e.g., 5′-GTCGTC-3′) (7). Interestingly, CpG dinucleotides generally occur at near the expected frequency (1 in 16) in many prokaryotic genomes but are much less frequent in eukaryotic DNA. In addition, less than 5% of the cytosines in prokaryotic CpG dinucleotides are methylated, whereas 70–90% of the CpG dinucleotides in eukaryotic genomes contain an inactivating methylated cytosine (8). These observations have led to the proposal that the vertebrate innate immune system has evolved the ability to detect these CpG motifs found in bacterial genomes, as is the case with other microbial products such as lipopolysaccharide (LPS) or dsRNA. This hypothesis is further supported by recent work establishing that ISS binds to Toll-like receptor (TLR) 9 to activate similar intracellular signaling pathways, which are activated by other microbial ligands that interact with other members of the TLR family (9,10). The cloning and characterization of the mouse and human TLR-9 receptor may explain differences in ISS sequences which optimally bind to mouse or human TLR-9. Because only approximately 75% of the amino acids in the mouse TLR-9 are present in human TLR-9, differences in the TLR-9 amino acid sequences could contribute to the specificity of recognition of ISS sequences (9).

Functionally, ISS activate cells of the innate immune system, including dendritic cells, macrophages, and natural killer (NK) cells, and induce B-cell proliferation and IgM antibody production (6,11–16). The antigen/allergen-independent (innate) immune response induced by ISS is characterized by the production of interleukin (IL)-12, IL-18, interferons (IFNs), IL-6, and IL-10 (6,11–16). In addition, ISS induces the expression of a number of co-stimulatory molecules on the surface of B cells and antigen-presenting cells (APCs) (17). ISS has also recently been shown to increase expression of the IFN-γ receptor (CD119) and reduce expression of the IL-4 receptor (CD124) on human B cells (11). ISS induces cytokines (IL-12, IFN-γ, and IL-10), which inhibit IL-4–dependent IgE synthesis in human B cells (11). In contrast to ISS, vertebrate DNA, methylated bacterial DNA, and methylated ISS do not elicit an immune response.

Studies with ISS as a vaccine adjuvant have shown that it elicits a robust and multifaceted adaptive immune response to co-administered proteins, analogous to the immune response elicited by gene vaccines (6,18,19). Furthermore, ISS has a long-lasting Th1-biasing adjuvant effect on antigens (and potentially allergens) encountered at the site of delivery. In fact, ISS delivery 1–7 days before antigen (prepriming) leads to immune responses of greater magnitude than those seen with antigen/ISS co-delivery (18). This is likely to be due to ISS-induced APC activation, which has been shown to last for up to 2 weeks in mice (17,18). The robust and persistent immune activation and Th1 adjuvant activity elicited by ISS has prompted its study as an antiallergic vaccine adjuvant and immunomodulator for the prevention and reversal of Th2-biased (allergic) immune deviation and the immediate hypersensitivity responses that characterize asthma (20–23), allergic conjunctivitis (24), and anaphylaxis (25) (Fig. 1).

C. Bacterial DNA and TLR-9

The TLRs expressed predominantly on a variety of innate immune cells including monocytes and dendritic cells belong to a family of pattern recognition receptors that allow the innate immune system to sense different classes of microbial products (26,27). Currently there are 10 known TLRs. Peptidoglycan is known to activate innate immune cells via TLR-2, dsRNA via TLR-3, LPS via TLR-4, flagellin via TLR-5 while bacterial DNA, i.e., ISS-DNA, via TLR-9 (26,27). Bacterial DNA, as do other ligands of the TLR family, initiates a signaling cascade, which is mediated via MyD88, IRAK, and TRAF6 to activate MAPK and NF-κB pathways (26,27). Activation of immune cells by ISS has also been shown to require cellular uptake of the DNA by DNA sequence–independent endocytosis and, later, by endosomal acidification (28). The required acidification in mediating signaling by ISS is unique and necessary for TLR-9 signaling (29). This finding supports the assumption that certain TLRs (e.g., TLR-9) are recruited into the phagosome where they are activated by their ligands released from the lysed pathogen (30) and further suggests that different microbial TLR ligands induce cell activation at various stages of endosomal

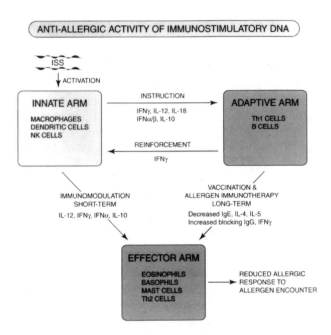

Figure 1   Simplified schema for the anti-allergic activities of immunostimulatory DNA sequences (ISS). Cryptic immunostimulatory DNA contained in allergen-gene vaccination plasmids and synthetic ISS directly activate cells of the innate arm of the immune system to produce a number of antiallergic and Th1-promoting cytokines. This acute burst of cytokines directly inhibits the effector arm of the allergic hypersensitivity response, including the response of precommitted Th2 cells. In addition, ISS-induced innate immune activation promotes the development of Th1- and inhibits Th2-biased adaptive responses to allergens. This Th1-biased adaptive response reinforces the activities of innate immune response, while mediating long-lasting inhibition of the effector arm of the allergic immediate hypersensitivity response. Thus, ISS activation of two separate but complementary arms of the immune response (innate and adaptive) has the potential to provide both rapid and long-lasting inhibition of the allergic response. (From Ref. 5.)

maturation. Activation of signaling cascades mediated by ISS (MAPK and NF-κB) is impaired in TLR9-deficient dendritic cells and is restored by genetic complementation using hTLR9 cDNA transfection (31,32). In addition, TLR9-deficient mice are resistant to ISS-mediated lethal shock and do not mount a Th1-like immune response to antigen mixed with ISS (9).

D.   Bacterial DNA and DNA-PK

Once ISS are taken up into cells, they are thought to signal via intracellular molecules. One such molecule is the DNA-dependent protein kinase (DNA-PK) (10). DNA-PK is a member of phosphatidylinositol 3 (PI3) kinase–like family that also includes ATM, FRAP, and FRP1 (33). DNA-PK can be detected in both the nucleus and cytoplasm. In the nucleus, DNA-PK plays a pivotal role in the repair of DNA double-stranded breaks created by environmental insults, such as ionizing radiation, or by intrinsic nuclear processes, such as programmed DNA rearrangements during lymphocyte differentiation (e.g., VDJ recombination) (33). In contrast, the cytoplasmic functions of DNA-PK are unclear. At physiological salt concentrations, DNA-PK requires two components for activity: a DNA-binding protein, Ku, and a catalytic subunit, DNA-PKcs. Ku is a heterodimer of 70 and 86 kDa polypeptides that binds to double-stranded DNA ends, nicks, single-stranded DNA or transitions between double- and single-strand DNA. DNA-PKcs has double- and single-strand DNA-binding domains and are activated by both double- and single-stranded DNA ends (34).

In vivo administration of bacterial-DNA or ISS to mice lacking the catalytic subunit of DNA-PK (DNA-PKcs) and in vitro ISS stimulation of bone marrow–derived macrophages from these mice results in defective induction of IL-6 and IL-12. Further analysis using bone marrow–derived macrophages from IKKβ-/- mice revealed that both DNA-PKcs and IKKβ are essential for normal cytokine production in response to ISS or bacterial DNA. ISS and bacterial DNA both activate DNA-PK, which in turn contributes to the activation of IKK of NF-κB (10). The relationship between TLR-9 and DNA-PKcs in mediating ISS-induced cell activation is still unclear (10,29). However, a potential explanation for such an interaction was recently described. TIRAP, a MyD88 analog, was shown to interact with PKR (protein kinase of dsRNA) to mediate LPS signaling (35). The dependence of ISS-mediated signaling on MyD88 (but not on TIRAP) suggests that MyD88 may interact with DNA-PK in an analogous fashion to mediate ISS signaling.

E. ISS in Mouse Models of the Prevention of Allergy and Asthma

Several studies have demonstrated that ISS can inhibit Th2 cytokine responses, as well as eosinophilic inflammation and airway hyperreactivity to methacholine in mouse models of asthma (Fig. 2) (20–23). In addition to inhibiting eosinophilia of the airway and lung parenchyma, ISS also significantly inhibits blood eosinophilia, suggesting that ISS exerts a significant effect on the bone marrow production and/ or release of eosinophils (20). The inhibition of the bone marrow production of eosinophils is associated with a significant inhibition of T-cell–derived cytokine production (IL-5, GM-CSF, and IL-3). As IL-5 is an important lineage-specific eosinophil growth factor as well as an inducer of the bone marrow release of eosinophils, the inhibitory effect of ISS on the generation of IL-5 plays an important role in mediating the effect of ISS on bone marrow production and/or release of eosinophils. The onset of the ISS effect on reducing the number of tissue eosinophils is both immediate (within 1 day of administration) and not due to ISS directly inducing eosinophil apoptosis (20). ISS is effective in inhibiting eosinophilic airway inflammation when administered either systemically or mucosally (i.e., intranasally or intratracheally) (20). Interestingly, a single dose of ISS has been shown to reduce

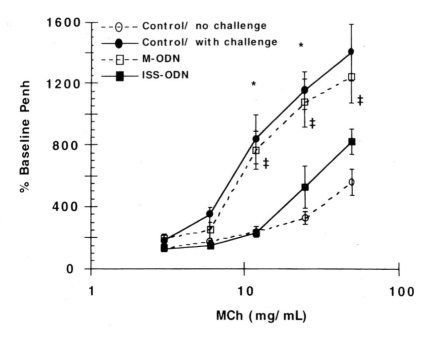

Figure 2 The effect of ISS on methacholine (MCh) responsiveness. OVA-sensitized BALB/c mice received ISS-ODN (50 μg) or M-ODN (50 μg) i.p. 24 hours before OVA inhalation challenges, and MCh responsiveness was measured 48 hours after the last OVA challenge. Airway responsiveness to increasing concentrations of MCh (0–50 mg/mL) was assessed by barometric whole-body plethysmography, and Penh values were calculated. The mean ± SEM for 12 mice in three experiments is expressed as a percentage of baseline Penh values observed after PBS exposure. Administration of ISS-ODN significantly reduced the increase in MCh responsiveness by 69 ± 9.9% compared with M-ODN–treated mice ($p < 0.05$ by Turkey-Kramer HSD test). (From Ref. 20.)

airway eosinophilia as effectively as daily injections of corticosteroids for 7 days (20) (Fig. 3). Furthermore, while both ISS and corticosteroids inhibited IL-5 production, only ISS was able to induce allergen-specific IFN-γ production and redirect the immune system toward a Th1 response (20) (Fig. 4).

The cellular mechanism of action of ISS in vivo may be more complex than that initially hypothesized based on results from in vitro studies. While ISS induces a strong Th1 response, the antiallergic effect of ISS may not be mediated by this mechanism in vivo. In support of this hypothesis are studies demonstrating that adoptive transfer of antigen specific Th1 cells do not protect against eosinophilic airway inflammation in a mouse model of asthma (36,37) and studies demonstrating that ISS can mediate its antiallergic effect in vivo independent of the Th1 cytokines IFN-γ and IL-12 (38). ISS can also inhibit eosinophilic inflammation and airway hyperreactivity in mice depleted of NK cells, a major source of IFN-γ induced by

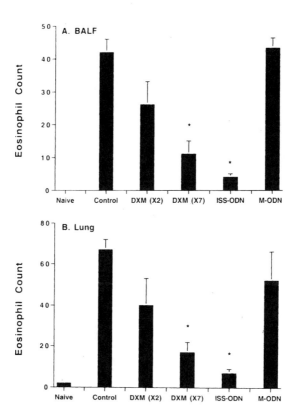

Figure 3 The effect of ISS or corticosteroids on eosinophilic inflammation of the lungs. OVA-sensitized BALB/c mice received either ISS-ODN (100 μg), M-ODN (100 μg), twice-daily doses of dexamethasone (5 mg/kg), or 7 daily doses of dexamethasone (5 mg/kg), i.p., prior to OVA inhalation challenges. The number of BAL fluid eosinophils (A) or lung eosinophils (B) were quantitated. Both ISS-ODN and 7 days of dexamethasone significantly inhibited BAL and lung eosinophilia. (From Ref. 20.)

ISS (39) (Fig. 5). Thus, the ability of ISS to induce a Th1 response and IFN-γ expression may not be essential to its inhibitory effect on allergic inflammation in vivo. However, some studies suggest that the induction of IFN-γ and a Th1 response is essential to the antiallergic effect of ISS (22).

While a single systemic dose of ISS is very effective in inhibiting IL-5, eosinophilic airway inflammation, and bronchial hyperresponsiveness, the duration of inhibition of Th2 responses is not permanently sustained (40). The reversible inhibition of Th2 responses at 4 weeks suggests that it may be necessary to administer ISS repeatedly at monthly intervals to maintain inhibition of airway inflammation and airway hyperreactivity (40). However, studies with mucosal delivery of two doses of ISS have demonstrated a prolonged inhibition of eosinophilic airway inflammation for 2 months (22).

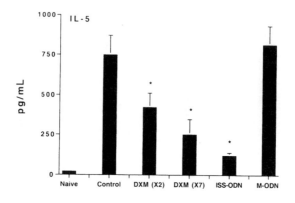

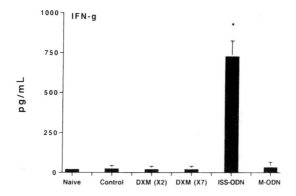

Figure 4 The effect of ISS or corticosteroids on Th1 and Th2 cytokine responses. OVA-sensitized BALB/c mice received either ISS-ODN (100 μg), M-ODN (100 μg), twice-daily doses of dexamethasone (5 mg/kg), or 7 daily doses of dexamethasone (5 mg/kg), i.p., prior to OVA inhalation challenges. The cytokine profile of CD4 + splenocyte supernatants were assayed by ELISA from cells incubated for 72 hours with 100 μg/mL of OVA. Both ISS-ODN and dexamethasone (2 or 7 daily doses) significantly inhibited IL-5 (A), whereas only ISS-ODN induced IFN-γ (B). (From Ref. 20.)

F. ISS in Mouse Models: Therapy of Established Asthma

When ISS is administered as acute therapy for established allergic airway inflammation such as might occur during an acute episode of asthma (as opposed to as preventive therapy as discussed above), ISS decreases airway hyperreactivity as effectively as dexamethasone and the combination of ISS and dexamethasone therapy is more effective than monotherapy with either agent alone in reducing airway hyperreactivity. The mechanism by which either ISS or corticosteroids inhibit airway hyperreactivity is likely to be mediated by distinct and shared cellular pathways. Both ISS and corticosteroids inhibit the bone marrow generation of eosinophils and the result-

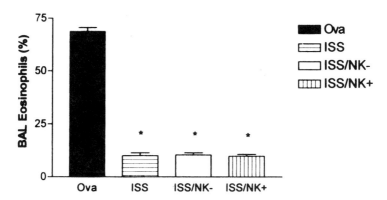

Figure 5 Effect of ISS and NK-cell depletion on BAL eosinophilis. There was a significant inhibition in the number of BAL eosinophilis in OVA-challenged mice that received ISS, as well as OVA-challenged mice that received ISS plus NK-depleting (ISS/NK−) or control (ISS/NK+) antibody ($n = 12$). *$p < 0.001$ versus OVA-challenged mice. (From Ref. 39.)

ant influx of eosinophils into the lung. Distinct anti-inflammatory pathways are suggested by the fact that ISS and corticosteroids differ in their mechanism of eosinophil clearance to regional lymph nodes, induction of apoptosis in peribronchial regions, and induction of the Th1 cytokine IFN-γ, which has antieosinophilic effects (41). Corticosteroids, but not ISS, increase apoptosis and clearance of airway eosinophils, whereas ISS and not corticoseroids induce IFN-γ. Shared anti-inflammatory pathways are suggested by the fact that ISS and corticosteroids both inhibit Th2 cytokine responses (IL-5) and mucus production to a similar degree. The combination of the shared and distinct anti-inflammatory pathways (some of which have been identified) may account for the additive effect of ISS and corticosteroids on inhibiting airway hyperreactivity.

G. ISS and Mouse Models of RSV-Induced Asthma

ISS activate the innate immune system to generate antiviral cytokines such as IFN-γ (42). In a mouse model of respiratory syncytial virus (RSV)–induced airway inflammation, mice pretreated with ISS expressed the antiviral cytokine IFN-γ in the lung, and this was associated with significantly reduced RSV viral titers (Fig. 6), peribronchial inflammation (Fig. 7), and mucus secretion (Fig. 8) (43). Although ISS significantly reduced the RSV viral titer, peribronchial inflammation, and mucus cells in the airway, ISS reduced, but did not significantly inhibit, RSV-induced airway hyperreactivity to methacholine. The mechanism(s) by which ISS induces these effects is not known but may involve the induction by ISS of antiviral cytokines such as IFN-γ, IFN-α/β, and the activation by ISS of other innate immune system cells (i.e., macrophages, dendritic cells, NK cells, B cells) whose functions may be important in viral clearance (6,12).

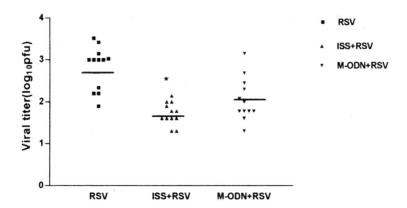

Figure 6 ISS inhibits RSV replication in the lung. ISS inhibits the number of RSV plaque-forming units (log 10 scale) in the lungs of mice infected with RSV and treated with ISS compared with that seen in mice infected with RSV and treated with M-ODN ($n = 12$; *$p < 0.001$). (From Ref. 43.)

The potential importance of IFN-γ in host defense against RSV is suggested from in vitro and in vivo studies. The ability of IFN-γ to inhibit RSV replication in vivo is suggested from studies of IFN-γ DNA gene delivery and RSV/IFN-γ gene vaccines administered prior to RSV infection in mice (44). As these IFN-γ–expressing vectors inhibited RSV replication early following RSV infection in

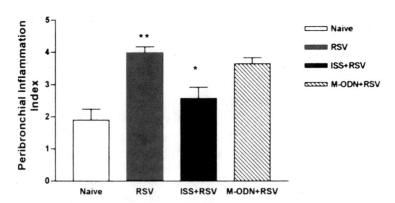

Figure 7 Effect of ISS on RSV-induced peribronchial inflammation. RSV infection induced significant numbers of peribronchial inflammatory cells compared with that seen in uninfected mice ($n = 12$ mice; **$p < 0.05$). ISS significantly inhibited the number of peribronchial inflammatory cells in the airways of RSV-infected mice treated with ISS compared with in RSV-infected mice that had not received ISS ($n = 12$ mice; *$p < 0.05$). (From Ref. 43.)

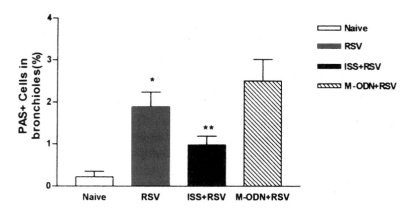

Figure 8 ISS inhibit RSV-induced mucus expression. RSV infection induced the expression of a significant percentage of PAS-positive cells in the airway compared with that seen in uninfected naïve mice ($n = 12$; *$p < 0.01$). ISS significantly inhibited the number of PAS-positive cells in the airways of RSV-infected mice treated with ISS compared with that seen in RSV-infected mice that had not received ISS ($n = 12$; **$p < 0.05$). (From Ref. 43.)

vivo, it seems likely that IFN-γ effects on innate immunity such as activation of macrophages rather than IFN-γ effects on adaptive immunity such as induction of a Th1 response mediate its antiviral effect. In contrast to gene vaccines containing IFN-γ cDNA, ISS stimulates NK cells to generate IFN-γ (14). The effect of ISS on NK cells is predominantly indirect and is mediated by macrophage generation of IL-12 stimulating NK cells to generate IFN-γ (45). Like IFN-γ gene delivery, administration of ISS inhibits RSV replication within days of RSV infection in vivo, suggesting that its effect is primarily due to activation of innate immunity as opposed to adaptive immunity.

In contrast to gene delivery of IFN-γ, ISS also induces the expression of IFN-α and IFN-β, which have additional antiviral effects (6,12). The importance of IFNs to the control of viral infections is suggested from studies of viral infections in mice deficient in IFN-α receptors or IFNs (46,47). In addition, studies have demonstrated that IFNs-α/β inhibit RSV replication in vitro and that ISS induces IFNs-α/β (6,12). The potent activity of IFN against viral infections is based on the expression of IFN-inducible protective genes (e.g., 2′,5′-oligoadenylate synthetase, double-stranded RNA-activated protein kinase, guanylate-binding protein, and MxA protein) that inhibit viral replication, impede viral dissemination, and confer cellular resistance (48,49). The 2′,5′-oligoadenylate synthetase gene is induced by viral infection and IFN and plays a major role in the antiviral activity of host cells by activating RNase L to cleave viral RNA and thereby inhibit viral protein synthesis (48,49). However, ISS influences a broad range of innate immune system functions, making it possible that effects independent of generating IFNs could also mediate its effect on inhibiting RSV replication and mucus secretion in vivo.

If ISS were used as a therapy to prevent allergen-induced asthma, the development of an intercurrent respiratory infection with RSV may be cleared more efficiently with less mucus production. Thus, ISS therapy administered to prevent allergen-induced inflammation and airway hyperreactivity would have additional potential benefits in reducing the severity of RSV infections.

H. Allergen Protein: ISS Conjugates

Recently, interest has developed in the use of allergen protein conjugated to ISS DNA (allergen-ISS conjugate, or AIC) for the treatment of allergic diseases, as this approach has certain theoretical advantages compared to unconjugated ISS. The primary advantage of AIC that physically linking ISS to allergens would increase the likelihood of their delivery to the same APC, resulting in an amplified, antigen-specific Th1 immune response (50,51), which is much less likely to occur when ISS and allergen are administered separately. The same APC would therefore process the antigen and present the antigen to Th cells, while ISS would induce the APC to release IL-12, thus biasing the well-targeted Th cell to differentiate toward a Th1 phenotype. Furthermore, theoretically AIC might be less allergenic than the ISS allergen protein mixture as steric hindrance or electrostatic blockade of IgE binding epitopes could occur with ISS coating the allergen (50).

I. Immune Response to Allergen Protein–ISS Conjugate

The immune response to Amb a 1, the major short ragweed allergen, conjugated to ISS has been investigated in mice, rabbits, and monkeys (50). In mice, injection of Amb a 1 alone generated a Th2 response characterized by high IL-5 production and low levels of IFN-γ, whereas injection of the Amb a 1–ISS conjugate induced a Th1 response characterized by high levels of IFN-γ production and low levels of IL-5. Injection of a mixture of Amb a 1 and ISS was much less effective than the Amb a 1–ISS conjugate in generating a Th1 immune response. Furthermore, in mice primed for a Th2 response with injections of Amb a 1 in alum, the Amb a 1–ISS conjugate induced a Th1 immune response and reversed the preexisting Th2-biased immune deviation (50). The Amb a 1–ISS conjugate also prevented an increase in IgE antibody formation after challenge with Amb a 1 and inhibited the release of histamine from human basophils in patients with ragweed allergy in vitro by 30-fold, whereas a mixture of Amb a 1 and ISS did not suppress histamine release (50). These results demonstrate that allergen conjugated to ISS can enhance the Th1 immune response, reverse a preexisting Th2 immune bias, and potentially reduce the allergenicity of allergen protein immunotherapy.

J. Allergen Protein–ISS Conjugate Therapy and Mouse Models of Allergy and Asthma

In a mouse model of asthma, concomitant administration of AIC intratracheally prior to allergen challenge reduced airway eosinophilia and airway hyperreactivity to methacholine, downregulated the Th2 immune response, and enhanced Th1 cytokine expression (52). The OVA-conjugated ISS was found to be 100-fold more efficient than the unconjugated mixture in reducing airway eosinophilia and bronchial hyper-reactivity, with this inhibitory effect observed for at least 2 months (52). AIC therefore offer significant promise as therapy for asthma and other allergic disorders, although investigation of its immune modulating properties in humans requires further study.

III. Gene Vaccination

A. Method of Administration

The surprising finding that a gene encoded on a plasmid (pDNA) injected intramuscularly could be expressed in vivo (53) opened an entirely new approach to vaccine development. Since that discovery, investigators have embarked upon a number of applications of direct plasmid injection including prevention of infectious disease and treatment of cancer and allergic diseases (5,54). The T-cell–mediated responses to gene vaccination can be attributed to the in vivo expression of the encoded antigen as well as ISS in the vector. A number of terms (e.g., genetic vaccination, genetic immunization, pDNA immunization or vaccination, and DNA or gene vaccination) have been used to describe the injecting of pDNA encoding a protein antigen. The pDNA is circular, with several functional elements, which include an origin of replication, along with an antibiotic resistance gene, which allows the plasmid to be replicated and produced in high quantities in *E. coli* under selective pressure. Expression of the gene encoding the antigen is usually under the control of a strong viral or eukaryotic promoter, such as the human cytomegalovirus (HCMV) E1 promoter. The appropriate termination and polyadenylation sequences follow the antigen gene sequence so that any mammalian cell that takes up the plasmid can express the protein.

Delivery of the pDNA can be performed in a variety of ways. While most studies have used intramuscular and intradermal routes of immunization, other routes of injection such as intravenous, intranasal, subcutaneous, and intraperitoneal methods have also been tested (55). The pDNA may simply be dissolved in normal saline and injected intradermally (56) or intramuscularly (53). Alternatively, a "gene gun" can be used to transduce skin cells with gold microprojectiles coated with pDNA encoding the antigen (also known as particle-mediated gene-delivery technology) (57,58). The delivery of pDNA has also been enhanced by encapsulation with liposomes (59,60). These different methods of injection elicit slightly different immune responses and will be discussed further below.

B. The Immune Response Induced by Gene Vaccination

Immunization with pDNA results in both humoral and cellular immune responses that are specific to the expressed antigen. Not only is the adaptive immune system responsive to plasmid expression, but the innate immune system is activated by the presence of unmethylated CpG or ISS found in the plasmid vector. There is thus an interplay between the innate and the adaptive immune responses, whereby the innate response augments the adaptive response through cytokine secretion and activation of antigen-presenting cells.

An important advantage of gene vaccination is the type of immune response induced in CD4 + T helper (Th) cells. Th cells differentiate from Th0 precursors into two readily discernible populations, Th1 and Th2, based on the types of cytokines they produce (61). Th1 cells produce IL-2, IFN-γ, and tumor necrosis factor (TNF-α), while Th2 cells produce IL-4, IL-5, IL-6, and IL-13 (62). Such differentiation is determined by the cytokines present during the priming period (63). Th1 cells mediate delayed-type hypersensitivity (DTH) reactions, increase IgG2a and IgG3 isotype synthesis via IFN-γ secretion (in the mouse) (64), and are associated with a strong cytotoxic T-lymphocyte (CTL) response. In contrast, Th2 cells activate B cells to produce IgG1 and IgE subclasses and also stimulate eosinophils via IL-5 (65). These two polarized responses are cross-regulated by the cytokines they secrete in vivo.

Plasmid DNA immunization by direct intradermal, injection induces Th cell differentiation to the Th1 type. Subsequently, antigen-specific T cells secrete high levels of IFN-γ, which leads to the production of IgG2a antibodies as well as the activation of strong MHC class I–restricted CTL responses (66). Not only can an ongoing antigen-specific Th2 response induced by protein in alum be "switched" to an antigen-specific Th1 response by "naked" pDNA immunization, but the Th1 response induced by pDNA immunization also prevails over a later attempt to induce a Th2 response by protein in alum immunization (67).

The bias in the T-cell cytokine profile and the potent response relative to the quantitatively small amount of protein produced by pDNA injection suggested that the same DNA was acting as an adjuvant to enhance the response. The elements that augment the immune response have been localized to the noncoding region in the backbone of the plasmid vector and shown to consist of ISS. The immunogenicity of the pDNA vaccine is significantly reduced by methylating its CpG motifs and increased by co-administering exogenous ISS (68). Altering the number of ISS within the pDNA can change the magnitude of the Th1 response (69). In addition, co-injection of protein and ISS (6), or antigen combined with incomplete Freund's adjuvant and ISS (70), can similarly elicit an antigen-specific Th1 response. Oligonucleotides covalently linked to protein antigens (i.e., AIC) are more potent in raising a Th1 response than immunization with mixtures of antigen- and ISS-containing oligonucleotides (71,72).

However, despite the suggestive in vitro evidence of a role for cytokines from antigen-presenting cells such as monocytes/macrophages in the promotion of Th1 differentiation in gene vaccination, the mechanism by which gene vaccines induce an antigen-specific Th1 response in vivo is still not precisely defined. Antigen is expressed at the site of injection by myocytes (53), keratinocytes, fibroblasts, and cells with the morphological appearance of dendritic cells (56). Additional antigen-expressing dendritic cells have been detected in the draining lymph nodes of mice immunized with pDNA (73–76). If the APCs are directly transfected by pDNA, they may be stimulated by ISS in the pDNA backbone to induce Th1 cytokines (like IL-12) and prime naive antigen-specific Th precursor cells to become Th1 cells.

However, Th-cell priming may occur by a professional APC, which takes up exogenous protein synthesized by other transfected cells. APCs such as monocytes/macrophages do make several Th1-inducing cytokines and upregulate several co-stimulators in response to the ISS present on the pDNA (17). Perhaps ISSs affect the APC in its ability to process extracellular antigens in a more efficient manner to present on MHC class I and II, or the ISS may change the overall environment of injected tissues to promote Th1 differentiation.

C. Gene Vaccination: Immunization with Antigen and Co-Stimulatory Molecules or Cytokines

Gene vaccination is being widely investigated as a potential prophylactic or therapeutic intervention for a variety of applications including asthma and allergy. The ease with which plasmid constructs can be manipulated allows the generation of different forms of an antigen (e.g., secreted, membrane-bound, or even antigen with deleted sequences to avoid the expression of unwanted antigenic epitopes). Furthermore, gene vaccination gives the added advantage of ectopically expressing membrane-bound molecules such as potential antigen-presenting molecules or co-stimulatory ligands, which may alter the overall immune response. Gene vaccination with combinations of plasmids expressing antigen and co-stimulators has proved to be effective in enhancing different arms of the immune system. For example, expression of B7.1 is useful for cytotoxic T-cell priming and B7.2 to enhance antibody responses (77–79). Other studies have also shown enhanced immune responses using co-linear expression of co-stimulatory molecules (80). The expression of the co-stimulator ligand appears to act locally and is dependent on the presence of the plasmid expressing the co-stimulator molecule at the same site as the antigen-encoding plasmid (77). In addition, plasmid encoding CD40 ligand, a co-stimulatory molecule upregulated on activated T cells to stimulate APCs, enhances antibody and CTL activity when co-immunized with plasmid encoding antigen (81,82).

The immune response may also be modulated by simply mixing different plasmids co-expressing soluble cytokines to skew toward a desired immune response. For example, pDNA expressing granulocyte-macrophage colony-stimulating factor (GM-CSF) (which may affect antigen presentation) has been shown to stimulate both Th and B-cell responses in a number of systems (83–85). Chow and colleagues (86) demonstrated that co-immunization of the hepatitis B virus (HBV) DNA vaccine with IL-12 or IFN-γ gene exhibited a significant enhancement of Th1 responses while maintaining inhibition of Th2 responses. On the other hand, co-injection of HBV DNA vaccine with the IL-4 gene significantly enhanced the development of specific Th2 cells while Th1 differentiation was suppressed. IL-2 or GM-CSF enhanced the development of Th1 cells without affecting the development of Th2 cells (86). The co-delivery of antigen with cytokine can also be achieved by expressing the antigen and the cytokine as a fusion product (87). Variations of these immunization strategies show promise in a number of areas including allergy, infectious diseases, and cancer immunotherapies.

D.　Gene Vaccines and Mouse Models of Allergy and Asthma

Gene vaccines encoding an allergen are able to inhibit IgE and Th2 immune responses as well as airway hyperreactivity in animal models of asthma (67,88,89). Both humoral and cellular immune responses to encoded allergens can be generated following intramuscular or intradermal injection of pDNA encoding a specific antigen (67). ISS sequences in the noncoding plasmid backbone of the pDNA vaccinated mice acts as a Th1 adjuvant and explains why the same antigen when delivered as pDNA induces a Th1 response but when delivered as protein induces a Th2 response. Since asthma is characterized by a Th2 response to antigen, these findings suggested the potential use of pDNA encoding allergens to downregulate the Th2 immune response to allergens by generating a Th1 response. Gene vaccination with pDNA encoding β-gal inhibited both IgE and IL-5 cytokine response to β-gal protein in alum (67). In a mouse model of asthma, mice sensitized to develop a Th2 response to ova protein and pretreated with intradermal injections of pDNA encoding ova protein developed significantly less bronchoalveolar lavage fluid eosinophils, lung eosinophils, and bone marrow eosinophils after inhalation of OVA protein compared to mice injected with a control pDNA construct (88). Studies using a rat model of asthma have demonstrated that the IgE response, histamine release into bronchoalveolar lavage fluid, and bronchial hyperreactivity following challenge with aerosolized dust mite allergen Der p5 were inhibited in rats immunized with a pDNA encoding the Der p 5 allergen (89). The response to the gene vaccine was antigen specific, as the rats immunized with pDNA encoding the Der p 5 allergen were protected against Der p 5 allergen challenge, but not against a different allergen, i.e., ovalbumin challenge (89). Gene vaccines also prevent anaphylactic reactions in mouse models of anaphylaxis (90,91) as well as allergic responses to birch pollen (92,93) and latex allergens (94).

IV.　Antisense

A.　Mechanism of Action of Antisense Therapy

The goal of antisense therapy is to selectively inhibit the expression of a specific gene product by preventing the translation of mRNA into protein (95). Antisense ODN therapy acts by sequence specific hybridization to mRNA, inhibiting the expression of that specific gene product while not affecting the expression of other genes. In order for antisense ODNs to be synthesized, the coding sequence of the gene to be inhibited must be known. Antisense compounds are generally about 20 base pairs of deoxynucleotides that have a sequence that is complementary to a portion of the targeted mRNA.

B.　Antisense and Animal Models of Allergy and Asthma

Several gene products important to asthma and allergic inflammation have been targeted with antisense ODN in animal models of asthma. These include cell surface receptors (adenosine A1, IL-5 receptor) (96–98), cytokines (IL-4, IL-5) (99,100), intracellular signaling molecules (Syk protein tyrosine kinases) (101), and transcription factors (GATA-3) (102).

The feasibility of using antisense therapy in asthma was first suggested in studies using antisense targeted to the adenosine A1 receptor in a rabbit model of asthma (96,97). Pretreatment of rabbits with inhaled adenosine A1 receptor antisense resulted in at least an order of magnitude increase in the dose of aerosolized adenosine required to reduce dynamic compliance of the lung (a measure of bronchoconstriction) by 50% (96). Airway smooth muscle derived from rabbits treated with inhaled adenosine A1 receptor antisense demonstrated an approximately 75% decrease in the adenosine A1 receptor density but did not affect the adenosine A2 receptor density indicating the specificity of the targeted antisense therapy (96).

GATA-3 is a transcription factor that is preferentially expressed in Th2 cells and regulates the expression of Th2 cytokine genes important to allergic inflammation. Studies with antisense targeted to GATA-3 in mouse models of asthma have demonstrated that GATA-3 antisense inhibits eosinophilic airway inflammation, airway hyperreactivity, and cytokine expression including IL-4 and IL-5 (104). The advantages of targeting a transcription factor that regulates the expression of several Th2 cytokine genes includes the fact that one is selectively targeting Th2 as opposed to Th1 cytokine genes, as well as the fact that more than one gene is being inhibited by targeting a single transcription factor. However, not all Th2 cytokine genes are inhibited by the GATA-3 antisense as cytokines such as IL-9 continue to be expressed. Antisense has also been delivered directly to the airway to inhibit stem cell factor, a mast cell growth factor. Inhibition of stem cell factor by antisense therapy suppresses airway inflammation and IL-4 production (103).

V. Potential for DNA-Based Therapy in Human Allergy and Asthma

A. ISS

Evidence that ISS can activate human cells is derived from several in vitro studies demonstrating that human monocytes, dendritic cells, B cells, and NK cells are activated by ISS (15,16,104–107). Human mononuclear cells secrete IFN-γ, IL-6, IL-12, and TNF-α in response to ISS stimulation (105). ISS directly activates human dendritic cells to express increased levels of co-stimulatory molecules, which results in the dendritic cells becoming more effective inducers of allogeneic T-cell proliferative responses (16). In studies of mononuclear cells from dust mite–allergic individuals ISS inhibits Der p 1–induced IL-4 production and induces Der p 1 IFN-γ production (108).

At present there are no published studies investigating the safety and efficacy of ISS in vivo in human allergy and asthma. However, clinical studies with antisense phosphorothioate oligodeoxynucleotide sequences have been used in doses up to 10 mg/kg with little related toxicity (109,110). This dose is 3–30 times the 10–100 μg dose of ISS used in studies demonstrating ISS efficacy in mouse models of asthma.

B. Allergen Protein: ISS Conjugate

In human studies a ragweed protein (i.e., Amb a 1)–ISS conjugate induces significantly less basophil histamine release compared to ragweed alone (50). In studies
of human mononuclear cells, an Amb a 1–ISS conjugate was more effective at
enhancing IFN-γ production and inhibiting IL-4 production compared to ISS alone
(111). Preliminary studies suggest that an Amb a 1–ISS conjugate is less allergenic
than the allergen protein based on skin test reactivity (112). However, further studies
are needed to demonstrate whether this approach is safe and effective in the therapy
of human allergy and asthma.

C. Gene Vaccines

Studies of gene vaccines in humans have best been evaluated in the field of infectious
disease and oncology where no serious adverse events related to injection of pDNA
have been reported (54). Gene vaccines for the prevention of HIV, malaria, and
hepatitis B are currently undergoing clinical evaluation. Although gene vaccines
alone can elicit humoral and cellular immune responses to many antigens, the immune response may be suboptimal for protection against infectious disease (54).
Strategies to increase gene vaccine immunogenicity by modifying the plasmids and/
or their method of delivery to improve the immune and clinical response are currently
in development. At present there are no published studies of the human immune
response to gene vaccines encoding allergens.

D. Antisense

The potential for antisense to be utilized in human disease has best been applied to
cytomegalavirus (CMV) infection in subjects with AIDS. Vitravene, an antisense
therapy that inhibits CMV replication, is FDA approved for local therapy of CMV
retinitis in patients with AIDS and provides conceptual proof of principal that antisense therapy can be used to treat human disease (113). At present there is no
published information on the use of antisense therapy in the treatment of human
allergic disease or asthma.

VI. Safety Issues Related to the Use of DNA-Based Therapies

Several potential safety concerns regarding gene vaccines have been addressed in
animal models and will need to be addressed in all human studies (114). These
include the theoretic potential for integration of the injected pDNA into the host
genome (with the theoretic risk of increasing the risk for malignancy) as well as the
potential for triggering autoimmune responses to injected DNA (114).

   Available evidence suggests that gene vaccines currently being tested clinically
rarely integrate into the host genome (114). Integration of DNA fragments from the
injected gene vaccine into the host genome have been investigated using sizing gels
to obtain host DNA from various tissues injected with pDNA (pDNA is separated

from host genome DNA as it is much smaller in size) (115). The genomic DNA is then assayed for integrated pDNA using a sensitive PCR-based assay. Studies of influenza hemagglutinin and HIV gag gene vaccines injected into the quadriceps have found no evidence of genome integration above the spontaneous mutation rate (114). Preclinical studies in mice and rabbits suggest that the vast majority of pDNA is detected in the muscle and skin near the injection site, with lower levels also detected in the draining lymph nodes (116,117). Much lower levels of intramuscularly injected pDNA also reach all highly vascularized organs including the gonads. Plasmid DNA reaching the gonads rapidly dissipates and was extrachromosomal, indicating a low risk of germline transmission. Long-term persistence of pDNA has only been detected at the site of injection and not at distant sites. Modifications of gene vaccines that increase cellular uptake will need to be monitored to ensure that increased uptake of the gene vaccine is not associated with an increased risk of genomic integration.

The potential of gene vaccination to trigger autoimmunity is another potential concern (114). Gene vaccines might stimulate the production of autoantibodies against the injected DNA (i.e., anti-DNA antibodies), potentially inducing or aggravating autoimmune diseases such as systemic lupus erythematosus. Preclinical studies in mice suggest that the low levels of autoantibodies that can be induced by repeated gene vaccination are insufficient to cause disease in normal or SLE-prone mice (118,119).

Studies with ISS, which induce a Th1 immune response, will also carefully need to monitor that Th1 immune–mediated diseases are not exacerbated by this form of DNA-based therapy (120,121).

VII. Conclusion

A variety of DNA-based therapeutic strategies have shown significant promise in animal models of asthma. Studies currently being conducted in human subjects should determine whether DNA-based therapeutics are safe and effective therapies in patients with allergic rhinitis and asthma.

Acknowledgments

Supported by NIH grants AI 33977 and AI38425 to DHB. ER was supported by NIH grant AI 40682 and a grant from Dynavax incorporation.

References

1. Holgate ST. The epidemic of allergy and asthma. Nature 1999; 402:B2–4.
2. Forecasted state-specific estimates of self-reported asthma prevalence—United States, 1998. MMWR 1998; 47:1022–1025.

3. Anderson WJ, Watson L. Asthma and the hygiene hypothesis. N Engl J Med 2001; 344:1643–1644.

4. Diaz-Sanchez D. Pollution and the immune response: atopic diseases—are we too dirty or too clean? Immunology 2000; 101:11–18.

5. Horner AA, Van Uden JH, Zubeldia JM, Broide D, Raz E. DNA-based immunotherapeutics for the treatment of allergic disease. Immunol Rev 2001; 179:102–118.

6. Roman M, Martin-Orozco E, Goodman JS, Nguyen MD, Sato Y, Ronaghy A, Kornbluth RS, Richman DD, Carson DA, Raz E. Immunostimulatory DNA sequences function as T helper-1-promoting adjuvants. Nat Med 1997; 3:849–854.

7. Yamamoto S, Yamamoto T, Tokunaga T. The discovery of immunostimulatory DNA sequence. In: Raz E, ed. Immunostimulatory DNA Sequences. Berlin: Springer-Verlag, 2000:11–20.

8. Bird AP. DNA methylation and the frequency of CpG in animal DNA. Nucleic Acids Res 1980; 8:1499–1504.

9. Hemmi H, Takeuchi O, Kawai T, Kalsho T, Sato S, Snajo H, Matsumato M, Hoshino K, Wagner H, Takeda K and Akira S. A Toll like receptor recognizes bacterial DNA. Nature 2000; 408:740–745.

10. Chu W-M, Gong X, Li Z-W, Takabaysahi K, Ouyang H-H, Chen Y, Lois A, Chen DJ, Li GC, Karin M, Raz E. DNA-PKcs is required for activation of innate immunity by immunostimulatory DNA. Cell 2000; 103:909–918.

11. Horner AA, Widhopf GF, Burger J, Takabayashi K, Cinman N, Ronaghy A, Spiegelberg H, Raz E. Immunostimulatory DNA mediated inhibition of IL-4 dependent IgE synthesis from human B cells. J Allergy Clin Immunol 2001; 108:417–423.

12. Klinman DM, Yi AK, Beaucage SL, Conover J, Krieg AM. CpG motifs present in bacteria DNA rapidly induce lymphocytes to secrete interleukin 6, interleukin 12, and interferon gamma. Proc Natl Acad Sci USA 1996; 93:2879–2883.

13. Krieg AM, Yi AK, Matson S, Waldschmidt TJ, Bishop GA, Teasdale R, Koretzky GA, Klinman DM. CpG motifs in bacterial DNA trigger direct B-cell activation. Nature 1995; 374:546–549.

14. Ballas ZK, Rasmussen WL, Krieg AM. Induction of natural killer activity in murine and human cells by CpG motifs in oligodeoxynucleotides and bacterial DNA. J Immunol 1996; 157:1840–1845.

15. Liang H, Nishioka Y, Reich CF, Pisetsky DS, Lipsky, PE. Activation of human B cells by phosphorothioate oligodeoxynucleotides. J Clin Invest 1996; 98:1119–1129.

16. Hartmann G, Weiner GJ, Krieg AM. CpG DNA: a potent signal for growth, activation, and maturation of human dendritic cells. Proc Natl Acad Sci USA 1999; 96:9305–9310.

17. Martin-Orozco E, Kobayashi H, Van Uden J, Nguyen M-D, Kornbluth RS, Raz E. Enhancement of antigen-presenting cell surface molecules involved in cognate interactions by immunostimulatory DNA sequences. Int Immunol 1999; 11:1111–1118.

18. Kobayashi H, Horner AA, Takabayashi K, Nguyen MD, Huang E, Cinman N, Raz E. Immunostimulatory DNA pre-priming: a novel approach for prolonged Th1-biased immunity. Cell Immunol 1999; 198:69–75.

19. Horner AA, Datta S, Takabayashi K, Belikov I, Hayashi T, Cinman N, Nguyen MD, Van Uden JH, Berzofsky JA, Richman DD, Raz E. Immunostimulatory DNA-based vaccines elicit multifaceted immune responses against HIV at systemic and mucosal sites. J Immunol 2001; 167:1584–1591.

20. Broide D, Schwarze J, Tighe H, Gifford T, Nguyen MD, Malek S, Van Uden J, Martin-Orozco E, Gelfand EW, Raz E. Immunostimulatory DNA sequences inhibit IL-5,

eosinophilic inflammation, and airway hyperresponsiveness in mice. J Immunol 1998; 161:7054–7062.

21. Kline JN, Waldschmidt TJ, Businga TR, Lemish JE, Weinstock JV, Thorne PS, Krieg AM. Modulation of airway inflammation by CpG oligodeoxynucleotides in a murine model of asthma. J Immunol 1998; 160:2555–2559.

22. Sur S, Wild JS, Choudhury BK, Sur N, Alam R, Klinman DM. Long-term prevention of allergic lung inflammation in a mouse model of asthma by CpG oligodeoxynucleotides. J Immunol 1999; 162:6284–6293.

23. Serebrisky D, Teper AA, Huang CK, Lee SY, Zhang TF, Schofield BH, Kattan M, Sampson HA, Li XM. CpG oligonucleotides can reverse Th2 associated allergic airway responses and alter the B7.1/B7.2 expression in a murine model of asthma. J Immunol 2000; 165:5906–5912.

24. Magone MT, Chan CC, Beck L, Whitcup SM, Raz E. Systemic or mucosal administration of immunostimulatory DNA inhibits early and late phases of murine allergic conjunctivitis. Eur J Immunol 2000; 30:1841–1850.

25. Horner AA, Nguyen MD, Ronaghy A, Cinman N, Verbeek S, Raz E. DNA-based vaccination reduces the risk of lethal anaphylactic hypersensitivity in mice. J Allergy Clin Immunol 2000; 106:349–356.

26. Ozinsky A, Underhill DM, Fontenot JD, Hajjar AM, Smith KD, Wilson CB, Schroeder L, Aderem A. The repertoire for pattern recognition of pathogens by the innate immune system is defined by cooperation between toll-like receptors. Proc Natl Acad Sci USA 2000; 97:13766–13771.

27. Aderem A, Ulevitch RJ. Toll like receptors in the induction of the innate immune response. Nature 2000; 406:782–787.

28. Yi AK, Tuetken R, Redford T, Waldschmidt M, Kirsch J, Krieg AM. CpG motifs in bacterial DNA activate leukocytes through the pH-dependent generation of reactive oxygen species. J Immunol 1998; 160:4755–4761.

29. Akira S, Takeda K, Kaisho T. Toll-like receptors: critical proteins linking innate and acquired immunity. Nat Immunol 2001; 2:675–680.

30. Ozinsky A, Underhill DM, Fontenot JD, Hajjar AM, Smith KD, Wilson CB, Schroeder L, Aderem A. The repertoire for pattern recognition of pathogens by the innate immune system is defined by cooperation between toll-like receptors. Proc Natl Acad Sci USA 2000; 97:13766–13771.

31. Bauer S, Kirschning CJ, Hacker H, Redecke V, Hausmann S, Akira S, Wagner H, Lipford GB. Human TLR-9 confers responsiveness to bacterial DNA via species-specific CpG motif recognition. Proc Natl Acad Sci USA 2001; 98:9237–9242.

32. Takeshiata F, Leifar CA, Gursel I, Ishii KJ, Takeshita S, Gursel M, Klinman DM. Role of TLR-9 in CpG DNA-induced activation of human cells. J Immunol 2001; 167: 3555–3558.

33. Durocher D, Jackson SP. DNA-PK, ATM and ATR as sensors of DNA damage: variations on a theme? Curr Opinion Cell Biol 2001; 13:225–231.

34. Smith GC, Jackson SP. The DNA-dependent protein kinase. Genes Dev 1999; 13: 916–13934.

35. Horng T, Barton GM, Medzhitov R. TIRAP: an adapter molecule in the Toll signaling pathway. Nat Immunol 2001; 2:835–841.

36. Hansen G, Berry G, DeKruyff RH, Umetsu DT. Allergen-specific Th1 cells fail to counterbalance Th2 cell-induced airway hyperreactivity but cause severe airway inflammation. J Clin Invest 1999;103:175–183.

37. Randolph DA, Stephens R, Carruthers CJ, Chaplin DD. Cooperation between Th1 and Th2 cells in a murine model of eosinophilic airway inflammation. J Clin Invest 1999; 104:1021–1029.

38. Kline JN, Krieg AM, Waldschmidt TJ, Ballas, ZK, Jain, V, Businga TR. CpG oligode-oxynucleotides do not require Th1 cytokines to prevent eosinophilic airway inflammation in a murine model of asthma. J Allergy Clin Immunol 1999; 104:1258–1264.

39. Broide DH, Stachnick G, Castaneda D, Nayar J, Miller M, Cho JY, Rodriguez M, Roman M, Raz E. Immunostimulatory DNA mediates inhibition of eosinophilic inflammation and airway hyperreactivity independent of natural killer cells in vivo. J Allergy Clin Immunol 2001; 108:759–763.

40. Broide D, Stachnick G, Castaneda D, Nayar J, Miller M, Cho JY, Roman M, Zubeldia J, Hayashi T, Raz E. Systemic administration of immunostimulatory DNA sequences mediate reversible inhibition of Th2 responses in a mouse model of asthma J Clin Immunol 2001; 21:163–170.

41. Ikeda RK, Nayar J, Broide DH. Effect of ISS on the resolution of ongoing eosinophilic airway inflammation. Am J Respir Crit Care Med 2001; 107:A321.

42. Yamamoto S, Yamamoto T, Kataoka T, Kuramoto E, Yano O, Tokunaga T. Unique palindromic sequence in synthetic oligonucleotides are required to induce IFN and augment IFN-mediated natural killer activity. J Immunol 1992; 148:4072–4076.

43. Cho J, Miller M, Baek K, Castaneda D, Nayar J, Roman M, Raz E, Broide D. Immuno-stimulatory DNA sequences inhibit respiratory syncytial viral load, airway inflammation, and mucus secretion. J Allergy Clin Immunol 2001; 108:697–702.

44. Bukreyev A, Whitehead SS, Bukreyeva N, Murphy BR, Collins PL. Interferon-γ expressed by a recombinant respiratory syncytial virus attenuates virus replication in mice without compromising immunogenicity. Proc Natl Acad Sci USA 1999; 96: 2367–2372.

45. Chace JH, Hooker NA, Mildenstein KL, Krieg AM, Cowdery JS. Bacterial DNA-induced NK cell IFN-γ production is dependent on macrophage secretion of IL-12. Clin Immunol Immunopathol 1997; 84:185–193.

46. van den Broek MF, Muller U, Huang S, Zinkernagel RM, Aguet M. Immune defence in mice lacking type I and/or type II interferon receptors. Immunol Review 1995; 148: 5–18.

47. Bogdan C. The function of type I interferons in antimicrobial immunity. Curr Opin Immunol 2000; 12:419–424.

48. Hovanessian AG. Interferon-induced and double RNA-activated enzymes: a specific protein kinase and $2'$, $5'$-oligoadenylate synthetases. J Interferon Res 1991; 11: 199–205.

49. Will A, Hemmann U, Horn F, Rollinghoff M, Gessner A. Intracellular murine IFN-γ mediates virus resistance, expression of oligoadenylate synthetase and activation of STAT transcription factors. J Immunol 1996; 157:4576–4583.

50. Tighe H, Takabayashi K, Schwartz D, Van Nest G, Tuck S, Eiden JJ, Kagey-Sobotka A, Creticos PS, Lichtenstein LM, Spiegelberg HL, Raz E. Conjugation of immunostim-ulatory DNA to the short ragweed allergen amb a 1 enhances its immunogenicity and reduces its allergenicity. J Allergy Clin Immunol 2000; 106:124–134.

51. Shirota H, Sano K, Hirasawa K, Terui T, Ohuchi K, Hattori T, Shirato K, Tamura, G. Novel roles of CpG oligodeoxynucleotides as a leader for the sampling and presentation of CpG tagged antigen by dendritic cells. J Immunol 2001; 167:66–74.

52. Shirota H, Sano K, Kikuchi T, Tamura G, Shirato K. Regulation of murine airway eosinophilia and Th2 cells by antigen-conjugated CpG oligodeoxynucleotides as a novel antigen specific modulator J Immunol 2000; 164:5575–5582.

53. Wolff JA, Malone RW, Williams P, Chong W, Acsadi G, Jani A, Felgner PL. Direct gene transfer into mouse muscle in vivo. Science 1990; 247:1465–1468.

54. Gurunathan S, Klinman DM, Seder RA. DNA vaccines: immunology, application, and optimization. Annu Rev Immunol 2000; 18:927–974.

55. Fynan EF, Webster RG, Fuller DH, Haynes JR, Santoro JC, Robinson HL. DNA vaccines: protective immunizations by parenteral, mucosal, and gene-gun inoculations. Proc Natl Acad Sci USA 1993; 90:11478–11482.

56. Raz E, Carson DA, Parker SE, Parr TB, Abai AM, Aichinger G, Gromkowski SH, Singh M, Lew D, Yankauckas MA, Baird SM, Rhodes GH. Intradermal gene immunization: the possible role of DNA uptake in the induction of cellular immunity to viruses. Proc Natl Acad Sci USA 1994; 91:9519–9523.

57. Tang DC, DeVit M, Johnston SA. Genetic immunization is a simple method for eliciting an immune response. Nature 1992; 356:152–154.

58. Johnston SA, Tang DC. Gene gun transfection of animal cells and genetic immunization. Methods Cell Biol 1994; 43:353–365.

59. Wheeler CJ, Felgner PL, Tsai YJ, Marshall J, Sukhu L, Doh SG, Hartikka J, Nietupski J, Manthorpe M, Nichols M, Plewe M, Liang X, Norman J, Smith A, Cheng SH. A novel cationic lipid greatly enhances plasmid DNA delivery and expression in mouse lung. Proc Natl Acad Sci USA 1996; 93:11454–11459.

60. Okada E, Sasaki S, Ishii N, Aoki I, Yasuda T, Nishioka K, Fukushima J, Miyazaki J, Wahren B, Okuda K. Intranasal immunization of a DNA vaccine with IL-12- and granulocyte-macrophage colony-stimulating factor (GM-CSF)-expressing plasmids in liposomes induces strong mucosal and cell-mediated immune responses against HIV-1 antigens. J Immunol 1997; 159:3638–3647.

61. Mosmann TR, Cherwinski H, Bond MW, Giedlin MA, Coffman RL. Two types of murine helper T cell clone. I. Definition according to profiles of lymphokine activities and secreted proteins. J Immunol 1986; 136:2348–2357.

62. Abbas AK, Murphy KM, Sher A. Functional diversity of helper T lymphocytes. Nature 1996; 383:787–793.

63. Seder RA, Paul WE. Acquisition of lymphokine-producing phenotype by CD4+ T cells. Annu Rev Immunol 1994; 12:635–673.

64. Street NE, Mosmann TR. Functional diversity of T lymphocytes due to secretion of different cytokine patterns. FASEB J 1991; 5:171–177.

65. Drazen JM, Arm JP, Austen KF. Sorting out the cytokines of asthma [comment]. J Exp Med 1996; 183:1–5.

66. Ulmer JB, Donnelly JJ, Parker SE, Rhodes GH, Felgner PL, Dwarki VJ, Gromkowski SH, Deck RR, DeWitt CM, Friedman A. Heterologous protection against influenza by injection of DNA encoding a viral protein. Science 1993; 259:1745–1749.

67. Raz E, Tighe H, Sato Y, Corr M, Dudler JA, Roman M, Swain SL, Spiegelberg HL, Carson DA. Preferential induction of a Th1 immune response and inhibition of specific IgE antibody formation by plasmid DNA immunization. Proc Natl Acad Sci USA 1996; 93:5141–5145.

68. Klinman DM, Yamshchikov G, Ishigatsubo Y. Contribution of CpG motifs to the immunogenicity of DNA vaccines. J Immunol 1997; 158:3635–3639.

69. Sato Y, Roman M, Tighe H, Lee D, Corr M, Nguyen MD, Silverman GJ, Lotz M, Carson DA, Raz E. Immunostimulatory DNA sequences necessary for effective intradermal gene immunization. Science 1996; 273:352–354.

70. Chu RS, Targoni OS, Krieg AM, Lehmann PV, Harding CV. CpG oligodeoxynucleo-tides act as adjuvants that switch on T helper 1 (Th1) immunity. J Exp Med 1997; 186:1623–1631.

71. Tighe H, Takabayashi K, Schwartz D, Marsden R, Beck L, Corbeil J, Richman DD, Eiden JJ Jr, Spiegelberg HL, Raz E. Conjugation of protein to immunostimulatory DNA results in a rapid, long-lasting and potent induction of cell-mediated and humoral immunity. Eur J Immunol 2000; 30:1939–1947.

72. Cho HJ, Takabayashi K, Cheng PM, Nguyen MD, Corr M, Tuck S, Raz E. Immunostim-ulatory DNA-based vaccines induce cytotoxic lymphocyte activity by a T-helper cell-independent mechanism. Nat Biotechnol 2000; 18:509–514.

73. Condon C, Watkins SC, Celluzzi CM, Thompson K, Falo LD Jr. DNA-based immuni-zation by in vivo transfection of dendritic cells. Nat Med 1996; 2:1122–1128.

74. Porgador A, Irvine KR, Iwasaki A, Barber BH, Restifo NP, Germain RN. Predominant role for directly transfected dendritic cells in antigen presentation to CD8+ T cells after gene gun immunization. J Exp Med 1998; 188:1075–1082.

75. Casares S, Inaba K, Brumeanu TD, Steinman RM, Bona CA. Antigen presentation by dendritic cells after immunization with DNA encoding a major histocompatibility complex class II-restricted viral epitope. J Exp Med 1997; 186:1481–1486.

76. Akbari O, Panjwani N, Garcia S, Tascon R, Lowrie D, Stockinger B. DNA vaccination: transfection and activation of dendritic cells as key events for immunity. J Exp Med 1999; 189:169–178.

77. Corr M, Tighe H, Lee D, Dudler J, Trieu M, Brinson DC, Carson DA. Costimulation provided by DNA immunization enhances antitumor immunity. J Immunol 1997; 159: 4999–5004.

78. Iwasaki A, Torres CA, Ohashi PS, Robinson HL, Barber BH. The dominant role of bone marrow-derived cells in CTL induction following plasmid DNA immunization at different sites. J Immunology 1997; 159:11–14.

79. Kim JJ, Bagarazzi ML, Trivedi N, Hu Y, Kazahaya K, Wilson DM, Ciccarelli R, Chattergoon MA, Dang K, Mahalingam S, Chalian AA, Agadjanyan MG, Boyer JD, Wang B, Weiner DB. Engineering of in vivo immune responses to DNA immunization via codelivery of costimulatory molecule genes. Nat Biotechnol 1997; 15:641–646.

80. Iwasaki A, Stiernholm BJ, Chan AK, Berinstein NL, Barber BH. Enhanced CTL re-sponses mediated by plasmid DNA immunogens encoding costimulatory molecules and cytokines. J Immunol 1997; 158:4591–4601.

81. Mendoza RB, Cantwell MJ, Kipps TJ. Immunostimulatory effects of a plasmid express-ing CD40 ligand (CD154) on gene immunization. J Immunol 1997; 159:5777–5781.

82. Gurunathan S, Irvine KR, Wu CY, Cohen JI, Thomas E, Prussin C, Restifo NP, Seder RA. CD40 ligand/trimer DNA enhances both humoral and cellular immune responses and induces protective immunity to infectious and tumor challenge. J Immunol 1998; 161:4563–4571.

83. Xiang Z, Ertl HC. Manipulation of the immune response to a plasmid-encoded viral antigen by coinoculation with plasmids expressing cytokines. Immunity 1995; 2: 129–135.

84. Pasquini S, Xiang Z, Wang Y, He Z, Deng H, Blaszczyk-Thurin M, Ertl HC. Cytokines and costimulatory molecules as genetic adjuvants. Immunol Cell Biol 1997; 75: 397–401.

85. Svanholm C, Lowenadler B, Wigzell H. Amplification of T-cell and antibody responses in DNA-based immunization with HIV-1 Nef by co-injection with a GM-CSF expres-sion vector. Scand J Immunol 1997; 46:298–303.

86. Chow YH, Chiang BL, Lee YL, Chi WK, Lin WC, Chen YT, Tao MH. Development of Th1 and Th2 populations and the nature of immune responses to hepatitis B virus DNA vaccines can be modulated by codelivery of various cytokine genes. J Immunol 1998; 160:1320–1329.

87. Maecker HT, Umetsu DT, DeKruyff RH, Levy S. DNA vaccination with cytokine fusion constructs biases the immune response to ovalbumin. Vaccine 1997; 15: 1687–1696.

88. Broide D, Orozco EM, Roman M, Carson DA, Raz E. Intradermal gene vaccination down-regulates both arms of the allergic response. J Allergy Clin Immunol 1997; 99: S129.

89. Hsu CH, Chua KY, Tao MH, Lai YL, Wu HD, Huang SK, Hsieh KH. Immunoprophylaxis of allergen-induced immunoglobulin E synthesis and airway hyperresponsiveness in vivo by genetic immunization. Nat Med 1996; 2:540–544.

90. Roy K, Mao HQ, Huang SK, Leong KW. Oral gene delivery with chitosan—DNA nanoparticles generate immunologic protection in a murine model of peanut allergy. Nat Med 1999; 5:387–391.

91. Horner AA, Nguyen MD, Ronaghy A, Cinman N, Verbeek S, Raz E. DNA-based vaccination reduces the risk of lethal anaphylactic hypersensitivity in mice. J Allergy Clin Immunol 2000; 106:349–356.

92. Hartl A, Kiesslich J, Weiss R, Bernhaupt A, Mostböck S, Scheiblhofer S, Flöckner H, Sippl M, Ebner C, Ferreira F, Thalhamer J. Isoforms of the major allergen of birch pollen induce different immune responses after genetic immunization. Int Arch Allergy Immunol 1999; 120:17–29.

93. Hartl A, Kiesslich J, Weiss R, Bernhaupt A, Mostböck S, Scheiblhofer S, Ebner C, Ferreira F, Thalhamer J. Immune response after immunization with plasmid DNA encoding Bet v 1, the major allergen of birch pollen. J Allergy Clin Immunol 1999; 103:107–113.

94. Slater JE, Paupore E, Zhang YT, Colberg-Poley AM. The latex allergen Hev b 5 transcript is widely distributed after subcutaneous injection in BALB/c mice of its DNA vaccine. J Allergy Clin Immunol 1998; 102:469–475.

95. Metzger W, Nyce J. Oligonucleotide therapy of allergic asthma. J Allergy Clin Immunol 1999; 104:260–266.

96. Richardson PJ. Asthma. Blocking adenosine with antisense. Nature 1997; 385: 684–685.

97. Nyce JW, Metzger W. DNA antisense therapy in an animal model. Nature 1997; 385: 721–725.

98. Lach-Trifilieff E, McKay RA, Monia BP, Karras JG, Walker C. In vitro and in vivo inhibition of interleukin (IL)-5-mediated eosinopoiesis by murine IL-5R alpha antisense oligonucleotide. Am J Respir Cell Mol Biol 2001; 24:116–122.

99. Karras JG, McGraw K, McKay RA, Cooper SR, Lerner D, Lu T, Walker C, Dean NM, Monia BP. Inhibition of antigen-induced eosinophilia and late phase airway hyperresponsiveness by an IL-5 antisense oligonucleotide in mouse models of asthma. J Immunol 2000; 164:5409–5415.

100. Molet S, Ramos-Barbon D, Martin JG, Hamid Q. Adoptively transferred late allergic response is inhibited by IL-4, but not IL-5, antisense oligonucleotide. J Allergy Clin Immunol 1999; 104:205–214.

101. Stenton GR, Kim MK, Nohara O, Chen CF, Hirji N, Wills FL, Gilchrist M, Hwang PH, Park JG, Finlay W, Jones RL, Befus AD, Schreiber AD. Aerosolized Syk antisense

        suppresses Syk expression, mediator release from macrophages, and pulmonary inflam-
        mation. J Immunol 2000; 164:3790–3797.
102.   Finotto S, De Sanctis GT, Lehr HA, Herz U, Buerke M, Schipp M, Bartsch B, Atreya
        R, Schmitt E, Galle PR, Renz H, Neurath MF. Treatment of allergic airway inflamma-
        tion and hyperresponsiveness by antisense-induced local blockade of GATA-3 expres-
        sion. J Exp Med 2001; 193:1247–1260.
103.   Finotto S, Buerke M, Lingnau K, Schmitt E, Galle PR, Neurath MF. Local administra-
        tion of antisense phosphorothioate oligonucleotides to the c-kit ligand, stem cell factor,
        suppresses airway inflammation and IL-4 production in a murine model of asthma. J
        Allergy Clin Immunol 2001; 107:279–286.
104.   Hartmann G, Weeratna RD, Ballas ZK, Payette P, Blackwell S, Suparto I, Rasmussen
        WL, Waldschmidt M, Sajuthi D, Purcell RH, Davis HL, Krieg AM. Delineation of a
        CpG phosphorothioate oligodeoxynucleotide for activating primate immune responses
        in vitro and in vivo. J Immunol 2000; 164:1617–1624.
105.   Hartmann G, Krieg AM. CpG DNA and LPS induce distinct patterns of activation in
        human monocytes. Gene Therapy 1999; 6:893–903.
106.   Iho S, Yamamoto T, Takahashi T, Yamamoto S. Oligodeoxynucleotides containing
        palindromic sequences with internal 5'-CpG-3' act directly on human NK and activated
        T cells to induce IFN-gamma production in vitro. J Immunol 1999; 163:3642–3652.
107.   Bauer M, Heeg K, Wagner H, Lipford GB. DNA activates human immune cells through
        a CpG sequence-dependent manner. Immunology 1999; 97:699–705.
108.   Bohle B, Jahn-Schmid B, Maurer D, Kraft D, Ebner C. Oligodeoxynucleotides contain-
        ing CpG motifs induce IL-12, IL-18, and IFN-gamma production in cells from allergic
        individuals and inhibits IgE synthesis in vitro. Eur J Immunol 1999; 29:2344–2353.
109.   Agrawal S. Antisense oligonucleotides: towards clinical trials. Trends Biotechnol 1996;
        14:376–387.
110.   Monteith DK, Geary RS, Leeds JM, Johnston J, Monia BP, Levin AA. Preclinical
        evaluation of the effects of a novel antisense compound targeting C-raf kinase in mice
        and monkeys. Toxicol Sci 1998; 46:365–375.
111.   Marshall JD, Abtahi S, Eiden J, Tuck S, Milley R, Haycock F, Reid MJ, Kagey-
        Sobotka A, Creticos PS, Lichtenstein LM, Van Nest G. Immunostimulatory sequence
        DNA linked to the Amb a 1 allergen promotes Th1 cytokine expression while downreg-
        ulating Th2 cytokine expression in PBMC's from human patients with ragweed allergy.
        J Allergy Clin Immunol 2001; 108:191–197.
112.   Creticos PS, Eiden JJ, Balcer SL, Van Nest G, Kagey-Sobotka A, Tuck SF, Norman
        PS, Lichtenstein LM. Immunostimulatory oligodeoxynucleotides conjugated to Amb
        a 1: safety, skin test reactivity, and basophil histamine release. J Allergy Clin Immunol
        2000; 105:S70.
113.   Galderisi U, Cascino A, Giordano A. Antisense oligonucleotides as therapeutic agents.
        J Cell Physiol 1999; 181:251–257.
114.   Smith HA, Klinman DM. The regulation of DNA vaccines. Curr Opin Biotechnol
        2001; 12:299–303.
115.   Ledwith BJ, Manam S, Troilo PJ, Barnum AB, Pauley CJ, Nichols WW. Plasmid DNA
        vaccines: assay for integration into host genomic DNA. Dev Biol 2000; 104:33–43.
116.   Martin T, Parker SE, Hedstrom R, Le T, Hoffman SL, Norman J, Hobart P, Lew D.
        Plasmid DNA malaria vaccine: the potential for integration after intramuscular injec-
        tion. Hum Gene Ther 1999; 10:759–768.
117.   Parker SE, Borellinin F, Wenk ML, Hobart P, Hoffman SL, Norman JA. Plasmid DNA
        malaria vaccine: tissue distribution and safety studies in mice and rabbits. Hum Gene
        Ther 1999; 10:741–758.

118. Klinman DM, Takeshita F, Kamstrup S, Takeshita S, Ishii K, Ichino M, Yamada H. DNA vaccines: capacity to induce autoimmunity and tolerance. Dev Biol 2000; 104: 45–51.
119. Mor G, Yamshchikov G, Sedagah M, Takeno M, Wang R, Houghten RA, Hoffman S, Klinman DM. Induction of neonatal tolerance by plasmid DNA vaccination of mice. J Clin Invest 1996; 98:2700–2705.
120. Castro M, Chaplin DD, Walter MJ, Holtzman MJ. Could asthma be worsened by stimulating the T-helper type 1 immune response? Am J Respir Cell Mol Biol 2000; 2:143–146.
121. von Hertzen LC, Haahtela T. Could the risk of asthma and atopy be reduced by a vaccine that induces a strong T helper type 1 response? Am J Respir Cell Mol Biol 2000; 22:139–142.

41

Allergen Immunotherapy
Therapeutic Vaccines for Allergic Diseases

JEAN BOUSQUET and
PASCAL DEMOLY

Hôpital Arnaud de Villeneuve
Montpellier, France

ANTONIO M. VIGNOLA

Istituto di Fisiopatologia Respiratoria
Palermo, Italy

I. Introduction

Allergen-specific immunotherapy is the practice of administering gradually increasing quantities of an allergen extract to an allergic subject to ameliorate the symptoms associated with the subsequent exposure to the causative allergen. Allergen immunotherapy was introduced to treat "pollinosis" or allergic rhinitis by Noon and Freeman in 1911 (1). There is good evidence that immunotherapy using inhalant allergens to treat seasonal or perennial allergic rhinitis and asthma is clinically effective. Guidelines and indications for specific immunotherapy with inhalant allergens were published in 1998 by the World Health Organization (WHO) following several other guidelines (2) and updated in the Allergic Rhinitis and its Impact on Asthma (ARIA) document (3).

Vaccines are utilized in medicine as immune modifiers. So, too, is allergen-specific immunotherapy. Knowledge gained from studies of allergic mechanisms, such as the importance of Th1 and Th2 cells, cytokine regulation of the immune responses, and specific inhibition or ablation of pathogenic immune responses by means of tolerance induction, may be applicable to a variety of allergic and other immunological diseases. This is especially true for autoimmune diseases such as juvenile diabetes mellitus and multiple sclerosis. Thus, the concepts utilized and the scientific data that support the use of allergen immunotherapy to treat allergic diseases are now being applied scientifically for other immunological diseases. The recent WHO position paper was therefore entitled "Allergen Immunotherapy, Therapeutic Vaccines for Allergic Diseases" to indicate that vaccines (allergen extracts) that modify or downregulate the immune response for allergic diseases are part of this broad-based category of therapies developed to treat other immunological diseases (2).

The nasal and bronchial mucosa present similarities, and most patients with asthma also have rhinitis (4,5). Dysfunction of the upper and lower airways frequently coexist. Epidemiological (6), pathophysiological, and clinical studies have strongly suggested a relationship between rhinitis and asthma. These data have led to the concept that the upper and lower airways may be considered as a unique entity influenced by a common and probably evolving inflammatory process, which may be sustained and amplified by intertwined mechanisms. Thus, it is important to consider asthma, rhinitis, and conjunctivitis as a single entity when immunotherapy is prescribed.

II. Allergen Standardization

The quality of the allergen vaccine is critical for both diagnosis and treatment. Where possible, standardized vaccines with known potency and shelf life should be used. The most common vaccines used in clinical allergy practice are now available as standardized products or are pending standardization. However, there are many vaccines currently being marketed (many of which are only used occasionally), and it is neither feasible nor economic to standardize all of them.

Both European and U.S. recommendations require measurements of total allergenic potency and biological activity. Allergen vaccines are biologically standardized using skin tests, and the in vitro potency is measured by methods derived from RAST inhibition (7). The rapid development of new technologies for both DNA and protein analysis offers opportunities for improved standardization. Many important allergens from pollen, dust mites, animal danders, insects, and foods have now been cloned and are being expressed as homogeneous recombinant proteins, which, in several cases, have allergenic activity comparable to the that of the natural protein allergen. With these new technologies, an allergen extract can be defined by major allergen content in mass units, and the consistency of each lot can be accurately monitored. When possible, the use of standardized allergen vaccines is favored (8). The application of new technologies to allergen standardization, particularly measurement of well-defined allergens and the use of recombinant allergens, will greatly facilitate objective comparisons of allergen extracts. Measuring specific allergens (or marker proteins) allows quantitative comparison of the allergen composition of different extracts in absolute units (ng or μg). The measurement of major allergens for standardization is now a realistic and desirable goal, which should be encouraged (9).

Several allergen units are used, including:

IU (international unit)
AU (allergy unit)

BAU (biological allergy unit)
BU (biological unit)
IR (index of reactivity)
TU (therapeutic unit)

In the European Pharmacopeia, allergen preparations for specific immunotherapy include (9):

Unmodified vaccines
Vaccines modified chemically (e.g., formaldehyde allergoids)
Vaccines modified by adsorption onto different carriers (so-called depot vaccines)
Modified and depot vaccines have been developed to make specific immunotherapy more effective and reduce the risks of side effects.

Allergen vaccines should be distributed, provided their potency, composition, and stability have been documented as one of the following:

Vaccines from a single source material
Mixtures of related, cross-reacting allergen vaccines such as grass pollen vaccines, deciduous tree pollen vaccines, related ragweed pollen vaccines, and related mite vaccines
Mixtures of other allergen vaccines provided that stability data (10) and data on clinical efficacy are available (where mixtures are marketed, the relative amounts of each component of the mixture should be indicated.)

III. Mechanisms

Specific immunotherapy (SIT) is specific to the antigen administered (11). The mechanisms of specific immunotherapy are complex (12,13) and may differ depending on the allergen (venoms or inhalant allergens) and the route of immunization.

A. IgE and IgG Antibodies

Early studies focused on immunoglobulin levels (IgE, IgG, and IgG subclasses) (14,15) and, in particular, on the so-called "blocking" IgG (16). Characteristic changes in serum immunoglobulins are found, with an initial increase in IgE followed by a blunting of seasonal increases in IgE in pollen-sensitive patients and a gradual decline in allergen-specific IgE levels over several years. This is accompanied by an increase in allergen-specific IgG (blocking antibodies), although neither appears to correlate closely with the clinical response to immunotherapy (17). It is, however, possible that the binding capacity of immunoglobulins is modified during specific immunotherapy. Data are lacking to confirm this hypothesis. In venom immunotherapy, it was found that early increase in serum specific IgG was correlated with clinical improvement (18), but after some years of treatment, the protection by IgG no longer exists.

However, new compelling data may shed light on the role of IgG antibodies (19). High amounts of allergen administered in SIT preferentially generate Th1 cytokines in T cells and IgG4 antibodies in memory B cells (20). Moreover, blocking antibodies induced by specific allergy vaccination prevent the activation of CD4 + T cells by inhibiting serum IgE–facilitated allergen presentation (21), and T-cell epitope–containing hypoallergenic recombinant fragments of the major birch pollen allergen, Bet v 1, induce blocking antibodies (22).

B. T-Cell Reactivity

Many studies suggest that specific immunotherapy acts by modifying the T-lymphocyte response to subsequent natural allergen exposure (23). Besides anti-IgE therapy, SIT is the only current immunomodulatory treatment of allergic rhinitis and asthma. Studies in blood and within the target organ have demonstrated a shift in the balance of T-cell subsets away from Th2 type (producing particularly IL-4 and IL-5) in favor of a Th1 type T-lymphocyte response (with the preferential production of IFN-γ). Studies of the nasal mucosa before and after immunotherapy have demonstrated suppression of the late nasal response and increases in the numbers of cells expressing mRNA for IFN-γ and IL-12. Immunotherapy may therefore act by modifying T-cell responses by either immune deviation (increase in Th0/Th1) or T-cell anergy (decrease in Th2/Th0) or, more likely, both (24,25). Change in cytokine patterns occurs early in the course of immunotherapy (26). These immunomodulatory effects were correlated with the efficacy of SIT, at least in grass pollen allergy (27). During and after immunotherapy the proliferative response of allergen-specific T lymphocytes in response to the administered antigen are significantly reduced. According to recent publications, this effect is due to the production of the immunosuppressive cytokine IL-10 (28). IL-10 elicits anergy in T cells by selective inhibition of the CD28 co-stimulatory pathway and controls suppression and development of antigen-specific immunity (29). An alternative may be amplification of suppressor CD8 + T cells, which may have a down-regulatory effect.

C. Target Organ Reactivity

Specific immunotherapy may act by reducing inflammatory cell recruitment, activation, or mediator secretions (17). Immunotherapy resulted in a decrease in mast cells in nasal tissues as well as a reduction in histamine and PGD2 levels in nasal secretions following allergen challenge. In pollen-sensitive patients, conventional immunotherapy inhibited immediate release of mast cell mediators (30) and eosinophil numbers in nasal lavage and biopsies in response to allergen provocation (31,32). Moreover, anti-inflammatory effects of SIT were still observed, albeit reduced, one year after SIT cessation (33). Reduction in the size of the allergen-induced late-phase reaction (LPR) is seen as a consequence of successful allergen-specific immunotherapy, which was associated with a reduction of Th2 responses (34). Recently, an interesting observation has been made. Th2 lymphocytes from atopic patients treated with immunotherapy undergo rapid apoptosis after culture with specific allergens (35), suggesting a new role for immunotherapy.

The mechanisms of local immunotherapy are still unclear, but a systemic effect is likely since serum immunoglobulin changes can be seen. The role of this form of treatment in the Th1/Th2 cytokine network needs further study (36).

IV. Immunotherapy Alters the Course of Allergic Diseases

Although drugs are highly effective and usually without important side effects, they only represent a symptomatic treatment, while specific immunotherapy is the only treatment that may alter the natural course of the disease (2). Long-term efficacy of specific immunotherapy after it has been stopped has been shown for subcutaneous specific immunotherapy (33,37,38). Durham et al. (38) conducted a randomized, double-blind, placebo-controlled trial of the discontinuation of immunotherapy for grass pollen allergy in patients in whom 3–4 years of this treatment had previously been shown to be effective. Scores for seasonal symptoms and the use of rescue antiallergic medication remained low after the discontinuation of immunotherapy, and there was no significant difference between patients who continued immunotherapy and those who discontinued it. However, in the study of Naclerio et al. (33), 1 year after discontinuation of ragweed immunotherapy nasal challenges showed partial recrudescence of mediator responses, even though reports during the season appeared to indicate continued suppression of symptoms. Long-term efficacy still has to be documented for local specific immunotherapy.

Specific immunotherapy has been used for the curative treatment of allergic diseases, but there are some suggestions indicating that specific immunotherapy may have a preventive efficacy. Allergic sensitization usually begins early in life, and symptoms often start within the first decade. It has been shown that specific immunotherapy was less effective in older patients than in children and that inflammation and remodeling of the airways in asthma provide poor prognosis for an effective specific immunotherapy. Moreover, if specific immunotherapy is used as a preventive treatment, it should be started as soon as allergy has been diagnosed (39).

To determine whether specific immunotherapy with standardized allergen extracts could prevent the development of new sensitizations over a 3-year follow-up survey, a prospective nonrandomized study was carried out in a population of asthmatic children aged under 6 years whose only allergic sensitivity was to house dust mites (40). In this study, 22 children monosensitized to house dust mites who were receiving specific immunotherapy with standardized allergen extracts were compared with 22 age-matched subjects monosensitized to house dust mites who were taken as controls. Around 45% of children receiving specific immunotherapy did not develop new sensitivities versus none in the control group. This study suggested that specific immunotherapy in children monosensitized to house dust mites alters the natural course of allergy in preventing the development of new sensitizations. Newer studies confirmed the results of Des-Roches (41).

When specific immunotherapy is introduced to patients with only allergic rhino-conjunctivitis, specific immunotherapy may stop the development of asthma.

The early study of Johnstone (42) with several different allergens showed that children receiving specific immunotherapy developed asthma in 28% compared to placebo-treated children, who had asthma in 78%. To answer the question, "Does specific allergen-specific immunotherapy stop the development of asthma?" the Preventive Allergy Treatment (PAT) study was initiated in children 7–13 years of age (43). This multicenter study was conducted in Austria, Denmark, Finland, Germany, and Sweden. After 2 years of specific immunotherapy, a significantly greater number of children in the control group developed asthma compared to the active specific immunotherapy group. More studies are needed to determine how specific immunotherapy may modify the allergic disease or impair progression to asthma (44). It has been proposed that specific immunotherapy should be started early in the disease process in order to modify the spontaneous long-term progress of the allergic inflammation and disease (2,45,46).

V. Subcutaneous Immunotherapy

A. Efficacy

Controlled studies demonstrate that allergen immunotherapy is effective for patients with stinging insect hypersensitivity (for review, see Ref. 47) and allergic rhinitis/conjunctivitis and allergic asthma. The efficacy of subcutaneous specific immunotherapy has been documented in most double-blind, placebo-controlled studies published in the following areas:

Hymenoptera venom (48)
Birch and Betulaceae pollen (49–51)
Grass pollen [a study found that calcium phosphate immunotherapy was effective (52)]
Ragweed pollen
Parietaria pollen (53)
A few other pollen species, including mountain cedar and coco
Pollen-induced asthma (some studies found a significant improvement, whereas fewer found no benefit)
House dust mite (specific immunotherapy was found to be effective in some studies in asthma and rhinitis. Fewer studies found no efficacy in asthma)
Cat (many studies found that bronchial symptoms during cat-specific immunotherapy are usually improved, but nasal symptoms were not recorded clearly Thus, by analogy to asthma, it is proposed that specific immunotherapy in cat-induced rhinitis is effective)
Molds: *Alternaria* and *Cladosporium*
Specific immunotherapy with house dust. *Candida albicans*, bacterial vaccines (54) or other undefined allergens is ineffective and not recommended (for review see Ref. 2)
Studies with immune complexes (allergen-antibody) have been performed and efficacy was demonstrated

In asthma, a large study found no benefit in children sensitized to many allergens (55), but a meta-analysis using the Cochrane collaboration (56) found that immunotherapy was effective. Fifty-four randomized controlled trials were analyzed. There were 25 trials of immunotherapy for house mite allergy: 13 pollen allergy trials, 8 animal dander allergy trials, 2 *Cladosporium* mold allergy, and 6 looking at multiple allergens. Concealment of allocation was assessed as clearly adequate in only 11 of these trials. Significant heterogeneity was present in a number of comparisons. Overall, there was a significant reduction in asthma symptoms and medication following immunotherapy. There was also a significant improvement in asthma symptom scores [standardized mean difference -0.52; 95% confidence interval (CI) -0.70 to -0.35]. People receiving immunotherapy were less likely to report a worsening of asthma symptoms than those randomized to placebo (odds ratio 0.27; 95% CI 0.21–0.35). People randomized to immunotherapy were less likely to require medication than those randomized to placebo (odds ratio 0.28; 95% CI 0.19–0.42). Allergen immunotherapy reduced allergen-specific bronchial hyperreactivity, with some reduction in-specific bronchial hyperreactivity as well. These effects on nonspecific bronchial hyperreactivity were further confirmed in newer studies (57–59). There was no consistent effect on lung function. The reviewer's conclusions were that immunotherapy may reduce asthma symptoms and use of asthma medications, but the size of the benefit compared to other therapies is not known. The possibility of adverse effects (such as anaphylaxis) must be considered.

The level of evidence for the efficacy of subcutaneous specific immunotherapy in asthma, rhinitis, and conjunctivitis is A according to guidelines used by WHO (60) (Tables 1, 2).

Table 1 Classification Schemes of Statements of Evidence

Category of evidence:
Ia: Evidence for meta-analysis of randomized controlled trials
Ib: Evidence from at least one randomized controlled trial
IIa: Evidence from at least one controlled study without randomization
IIb: Evidence from at least one other type of quasi-experimental study
III: Evidence from nonexperimental descriptive studies, such as comparative studies, correlation studies, and case-control studies
IV: Evidence from expert committee reports or opinions or clinical experience of respected authorities, or both
Strength of recommendation:
A: Directly based on category I evidence
B: Directly based on category II evidence or extrapolated recommendation from category I evidence
C: Directly based on category III evidence or extrapolated recommendation from category I or II evidence
D: Directly based on category IV evidence or extrapolated recommendation from category I, II or III evidence

---

Source: Ref. 60.

Table 2 Categories of Evidence for Immunotherapy

Administration		Seasonal, adults	Seasonal, children	Perennial, adults	Perennial, children
Subuctaneous	Asthma	A (Ia)	A (Ia)	A (Ia)	A (Ia)
	Rhinitis + conjunctivitis	A (Ib)	A (Ib)	A (Ib)	A (Ib)
Sublingual	Rhinitis + conjunctivitis	A (Ib)	A (Ib)	A (Ib)	
Intranasal	Rhinitis + conjunctivitis	A (Ib)	A (Ib)	A (Ib)	

Source: Ref. 3.

The use of allergen immunotherapy requires specialist assessment, especially in children, because there are special problems and questions in this age group. Immunotherapy started early in the disease process may modify the spontaneous long-term progress of the allergic inflammation and disease (45,46). Immunotherapy is rarely started before the age of 5 years.

B. Safety

The major risk of allergen immunotherapy is anaphylaxis (61,62). Asthma appears to be a significant risk factor for systemic reactions (63–65). Therefore, allergen immunotherapy should be administered by or under the close supervision of a trained physician who can recognize early symptoms and signs of anaphylaxis and administer emergency treatment (63). It is possible that immunotherapy with grass pollen induces more systemic reactions than that with other allergens (66). There are recommendations to minimize risks of immunotherapy (Table 3).

Premedication with oral H1-antihistamines was proposed to reduce mild systemic reactions (68), and this treatment was even proposed to increase safety of

Table 3 Recommendations to Minimize Risk and Improve Efficacy of Immunotherapy

Specific immunotherapy needs to be prescribed by specialists and administered by physicians trained to manage systemic reactions if anaphylaxis occurs.

Patients with multiple sensitivities may not benefit as much as do patients with a single sensitivity from specific immunotherapy. More data are necessary.

Patients with nonallergic triggers will not benefit from specific immunotherapy

Specific immunotherapy is more effective in children and young adults than later in life.

It is essential for safety reasons that patients be asymptomatic at the time of injections because lethal adverse reactions are more often found in asthma patients with severe airways obstruction.

FEV_1 with pharmacological treatment should reach at least 70% of predicted values for both efficacy and safety reasons.

Source: Ref. 67.

specific immunotherapy in venom-allergic patients (69). It was found in rush immunotherapy with house dust mites and pollens that a combined treatment with oral H1-blockers and corticosteroids reduced the risk of anaphylactic reactions (70,71).

C. Indications

The treatment of allergic diseases is based on allergen avoidance, pharmacotherapy, allergen immunotherapy, and patient education. Physicians should know the local and regional aerobiology and be aware of the potential allergens in the patient's indoor and outdoor environments. Only physicians with a training in allergology can select the clinically relevant allergen vaccines for therapy. Immunotherapy, where appropriate, should be used in combination with other forms of therapy with the hope that the patient will become as symptom-free as medically possible.

Allergen immunotherapy is indicated for patients who have demonstrable evidence of specific IgE antibodies to clinically relevant allergens and whose allergic symptoms warrant the time and risk of allergen immunotherapy. Contraindications for inhalant allergen and venom immunotherapy may be absolute or relative (45). Patient selection is important, and efficacy must always be balanced against the risk of side effects. The necessity for initiating allergen immunotherapy depends on the degree to which symptoms can be reduced by medication, the amount and type of medication required to control symptoms, and whether effective allergen avoidance is possible (Table 4).

The indications for venom immunotherapy are provided in the Position Paper of EAACI (47). An absolute indication is a history of severe allergic systemic reactions with respiratory and/or cardiovascular symptoms and positive diagnostic tests (skin tests and/or serum-specific IgE).

The indications for immunotherapy in asthma and rhinitis have been separated in some guidelines (67,72,73), and this artificial separation has led to unresolved questions (74,75), possibly because the IgE-mediated reaction has not been considered as a multiple organ involvement. It is therefore important to consider immunotherapy based on the allergen sensitization rather than on a particular disease manifestation (44,76) (Fig. 1).

Immunotherapy for treatment of allergic rhinitis conjunctivitis is indicated (1) when antihistamines and topical drugs insufficiently control symptoms (2) in patients who do not wish to be on pharmacotherapy, (3) when pharmacotherapy produces undesirable side effects, (4) when the patient is concerned about long-term pharmacological therapy, and (5) if the season is prolonged or polysensitized patients are exposed to several subsequent pollen seasons (i.e., tree, grass, and weed pollen sensitivity) (2). The risk/benefit ratio should be considered in every case.

Although efficacy of immunotherapy has been shown for treatment of allergic asthma, the increased risk of systemic reactions in patients with asthma has been considered a contraindication in the U.K. guidelines (77), although not in other published national or international guidelines (2,3). Patients allergic to mites are candidates for mite allergen immunotherapy if they have significant symptoms of rhinitis or asthma when they are exposed to domestic mite allergens.

Table 4 Considerations for Initiating Immunotherapy

1. Presence of a demonstrated IgE-mediated disease
   Positive skin tests and/or serum-specific IgE
2. Documentation that specific sensitivity is involved in symptoms
   Exposure to the allergen(s) determined by allergy testing related to appearance of symptoms
   If required allergen challenge with the relevant allergen(s)
3. Characterization of other triggers that may be involved in symptoms
4. Severity and duration of symptoms
   Subjective symptoms
   Objective parameters, e.g., work loss, school absenteeism
   Pulmonary function (*essential*): exclude patients with severe asthma
   Monitoring of the pulmonary function by peak flow
5. Response of symptoms to nonimmunological treatment
   Response to allergen avoidance
   Response to pharmacotherapy
6. Availability of standardized or high-quality vaccines
7. Contraindications
   Treatment with β-blocker
   Other immunological disease
   Inability of patients to comply
8. Sociological factors
   Cost
   Occupation of candidate
   Impaired quality of life despite adequate pharmacological treatment
9. Objective evidence of efficacy of immunotherapy for the selected patient (availability of controlled clinical studies)

Source: Ref. 2.

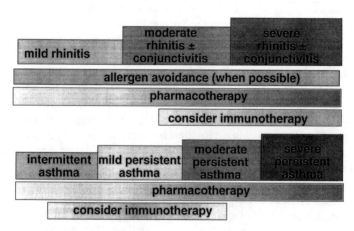

Figure 1 Specific immunotherapy in patients with asthma and rhinitis.

Avoidance is the treatment of choice for animal dander–induced allergic diseases. However, complete avoidance is often impossible due to exposure to animal allergens in environments in which animals are not present (78). Immunotherapy may be prescribed for patients in whom avoidance of animal allergens is not fully effective, as in cases of occupational exposure or refusal to evict an animal from the home.

For mold allergy, avoidance, where possible, of indoor mold allergens is the treatment of choice. Some studies have demonstrated clinical improvement when well-characterized vaccines of *Cladosporium* or *Alternaria* have been used in the treatment of mold-induced allergy. Patients with positive skin tests and symptoms when exposed to other relevant mold allergens may be considered for immunotherapy. Vaccines of undefined allergens such as house dust, bacteria, *Candida albicans*, or *Trichophyton* should not be used for immunotherapy (2).

The duration of immunotherapy required to maintain improvement in clinical symptoms is still unknown. A duration of 3 years has been found to be optimal for grass pollen immunotherapy (38). For patients who respond to treatment, many clinicians advise 3–5 years of therapy. However, the decision as to when to discontinue allergen immunotherapy should be individualized. Several studies suggest that venom immunotherapy may be discontinued after 3–5 years in most patients.

VI. Other Routes of Immunotherapy

New routes of administration of immunotherapy currently being explored include nasal, sublingual-swallow, or oral immunotherapy using high allergen doses.

A. Efficacy

Intranasal Immunotherapy

Efficacy of intranasal specific immunotherapy has been documented in most double-blind, placebo-controlled studies carried out in allergic rhinitis (and often also conjunctivitis) to (for review, see Refs. 2,3):

> Birch and alder pollen
> Grass pollen (79)
> Ragweed pollen
> *Parietaria* pollen (80)
> House dust mite

The level of evidence for the efficacy of intranasal specific immunotherapy in rhinitis and conjunctivitis is A according to WHO guidelines (3,60) (see Table 1, 2).

Sublingual Immunotherapy

Efficacy of high-allergen dose sublingual swallow-specific immunotherapy has been documented in double-blind, placebo-controlled studies carried out in allergic rhinitis to (for review, see Refs. 2,3,81):

Birch pollen (82) [in a small study of 30 patients, sublingual-swallow specific
   immunotherapy was not found to be significantly effective (83)]
Grass pollen (84–86)
Parietaria pollen (80,87,88)
House dust mite (89–94) [in the study of Bousquet et al. (89) results were
   difficult to analyze since the study was a corticosteroid-tapering study,
   which is notoriously difficult to be carried out]

The level of evidence for the efficacy of high-dose sublingual specific immunotherapy in rhinitis and conjunctivitis is A according to WHO guidelines (3,60) (see
Tables 1, 2). However, sublingual immunotherapy is still under investigation since
most studies have used a small number of patients (95,96). Moreover, the efficacy
of low-dose sublingual immunotherapy is still a matter of debate since adequate
trials have not been carried out.

Others

Efficacy of oral specific immunotherapy has been documented in some but not most
double-blind, placebo-controlled studies carried out in allergic rhinitis to (for review,
see Ref. 2). Intrabronchial immunotherapy does not seem to be safe enough to be
recommended (for review, see Ref. 2).

B. Safety

With intranasal specific immunotherapy, the only systemic side effect reported is
asthma (probably caused by incorrect administration of allergen extract).
   With sublingual specific immunotherapy, serious systemic side effects
(asthma, urticaria, and gastrointestinal complaints) were observed in children in one
study (92). However, in all other studies, only mild reactions were observed, even
in children with asthma (82,84,85,87–91,97–101). Postmarketing surveillance studies of sublingual specific immunotherapy showed that this procedure appeared to
be well tolerated in children (102,103).
   Since local specific immunotherapy is self-administered at home, patients
should be informed of the potential risks of a systemic reaction and how to treat
such a reaction should it occur (2).

C. Indications

Local nasal and high dose sublingual specific immunotherapy may be indicated in
(2,104):

Carefully selected patients with rhinitis, conjunctivitis, and/or asthma caused
   by pollen and mite allergy
Patients insufficiently controlled by conventional pharmacotherapy
Patients who have presented with systemic reactions during injection-specific
   immunotherapy
Patients showing poor compliance with or refusing injections

These recommendations do not apply to low-dose sublingual immunotherapy.

VII. Future Vaccines

New technologies and the improvement of our knowledge of the basic mechanisms of allergic diseases may completely alter the way allergen immunotherapy is utilized in the future. These advances should result in new, safer, and substantially more effective methods of manipulating the human immune response. These new approaches will be directed at every disease induced by antigen, such as asthma, as well as autoimmune disease such as type I diabetes and multiple sclerosis.

Many of the important allergens inducing an IgE-mediated immune response have now been cloned, key epitopes have been identified, and modified allergens are available. Recombinant DNA technology allows the large-scale production of highly pure and defined allergens for diagnostic and therapeutic purposes (105). Specific approaches for immunotherapy of allergy are currently being tested (106). Several approaches may be used (for review, see Ref. 107).

The knowledge of the molecular and crystal structure of allergens will clearly improve immunotherapy (108,109). Recombinant allergen molecules represent tools to study effector cell activation (110), but they can also be used for therapeutic purposes. Engineering of allergens has been started (111–114). It may be of great importance for food allergens in order to reduce systemic reactions during immunotherapy (115). Patient-tailored cocktails of recombinant venom allergens or isoforms may be of interest (116).

Pollen allergen mimotopes identified by phage display peptide library inhibit allergen-human IgE antibody interaction (117,118). Monovalent fusion proteins of IgE mimotopes were found to be safe for immunotherapy (119).

T-cell–targeted strategies used have involved the development of nonanaphylactic allergens, allergen fragments, or peptides for active immunotherapy (106). T-cell peptides were used for immunotherapy (120), but due to side effects they were discontinued. This form of treatment has been reassessed (121) and phase 2 trials are ongoing (122–124), but the results of the study in cat-allergic patients are not yet conclusive (125). In venom allergy, recent studies with T-cell epitope peptides from the major bee venom allergen phospholipase A_2 look promising (116,126).

IgE-binding haptens of major allergens have been for passive saturation of effector cells and induction of blocking antibodies. Allergen-specific antibodies and antibody fragments for passive therapy in the allergic effector organs may be more difficult to use.

Plasmid DNA immunization (127–129) has been widely studied. The mechanism of the pDNA-induced Th1 immune response was shown to be the result of stimulation by distinct noncoding immunostimulatory DNA sequences (ISS) containing CpG motifs in the backbone of the pDNA. The ISS induced antigen-presenting cells to secrete cytokines that cause naive T cells to differentiate into Th1 cells (e.g., IFN-α, IL-12) as well as eosinophilic inflammation when ISS was administered before or coadministered with inhaled allergen challenge. The data indicate that gene vaccination induces a Th1 immune response that is capable of downregulating a preexisting Th2 response and IgE antibody formation. Thus, immunization with pDNA encoding for allergens may provide a novel type of immunotherapy for allergic diseases. Conjugation of immunostimulatory DNA to allergen may be used as a Th1 adjuvant (130), and it has been shown that conjugation with the short ragweed allergen amb a 1 enhances its immunogenicity and reduces its allergenicity (131) Phase 1 and 2 studies are ongoing in allergic patients.

Many vaccines currently under development are composed of synthetic, recombinant, or highly purified subunit antigens. Vaccines composed of these subunit antigens may be safer than current allergen vaccination, but they may be less immunogenic. Immunological adjuvants are agents that enhance specific immune responses to vaccines (for review, see Refs. 107,132). Adjuvants have diverse mechanisms of action and should be selected for use based on the route of administration and the type of immune response (antibody, cell-mediated, or mucosal) desired for a particular vaccine. Through modulation of cytokine responses, adjuvant formulations can be designed that favor the development of Th1 or Th2 immune responses to vaccine antigens. Crystalline cell surface layers (S-layers) from gram-positive eubacteria were investigated as vaccine carriers for treatment of Type I allergy using Bet v 1 (133). Stimulation of human allergen–specific Th2 lymphocytes with S-layer–conjugated Bet v 1 led to a modulation of the cytokine production pattern from Th2 to Th0/Th1. However, these adjuvants may have some toxic potential. Oral administration of a small amount of antigen-conjugated cholera toxin B subunit is known to induce tolerance to the antigen, but cholera toxin is very toxic. A new approach was able to separate toxicity from adjuvanticity by constructing a fusion protein that combines the enzymatically active cholera toxin A1 subunit (CTA1) with targeting to B cells (134). This may be applicable for preventing the development of allergy.

Nonspecific approaches have also been proposed (for review, see Ref. 107). In view of the pivotal role of IgE in the pathogenesis of allergic disease, inhibition of the IgE response at either the level of IgE synthesis or the effector phase through the use of neutralizing anti-IgE antibodies should be of potential therapeutic value.

VIII. Key Concepts

Several guidelines for specific immunotherapy with inhalant allergens have been published. The 1998 WHO document endorsed the conclusions of previous guidelines published with an update using newly published randomized, double-blind and placebo-controlled trials. A new document is pending, with another update and recommendations based on evidence-based medicine.

The standardization of allergen vaccines is essential. They should be labeled in amounts or major allergens.

The mechanisms of immunotherapy are based on a restored balance between Th2 and Th0/Th1 cells inducing a reduction of inflammation of the target organ.

Subcutaneous immunotherapy is effective when the optimal dose of high-quality vaccine is administered. The majority of patients with allergic diseases can tolerate this target dose without difficulty. However, in selected individuals who have experienced reactions during their build-up treatment phase, a lower maintenance dose may be necessary.

The optimal dose of allergen vaccine administered is similar for all allergen species.

Local nasal and sublingual immunotherapy is effective provided high doses of vaccines are administered. Low-dose local immunotherapy is ineffective and cannot be recommended.

The indications for immunotherapy are based on a precise allergy diagnosis.

IX. Therapeutic Principles

Allergen immunotherapy is indicated for patients who have demonstrable evidence of specific IgE antibodies to clinically relevant allergens and whose allergic symptoms warrant the time and risk of allergen immunotherapy. Contraindications for inhalant allergen and venom immunotherapy may be absolute or relative. Patient selection is important, and efficacy must always be balanced against the risk of side effects. The necessity for initiating allergen immunotherapy depends on the degree to which symptoms can be reduced by medication, the amount and type of medication required to control symptoms, and whether effective allergen avoidance is possible.

References

1. Noon L. Prophylactic inoculation against hay fever. Lancet 1911; i:1572–1573.
2. Bousquet J, Lockey R, Malling H. WHO Position Paper. Allergen immunotherapy: therapeutic vaccines for allergic diseases. Allergy 1998; 53(suppl 54).
3. Bousquet J, Van Cauwenberge P, Khaltaev N. Allergic rhinitis and its impact on asthma. J Allergy Clin Immunol 2001; 108(5 suppl):S147–334.
4. Vignola AM, Chanez P, Godad P, Bousquet J. Relationships between rhinitis and asthma. Allergy 1998; 53(9):833–839.
5. Immunobiology of Asthma and Rhinitis. Pathogenic factors and therapeutic options. Am J Respir Crit Care Med 1999; 160(5):1778–1787.
6. Leynaert B, Bousquet J, Neukirch C, Liard R, Neukirch F. Perennial rhinitis: an independent risk factor for asthma in nonatopic subjects: results from the European Community Respiratory Health Survey. J Allergy Clin Immunol 1999; 301–304.
7. Bousquet J, Michel F. Standardization of allergens. In: Spector S, ed. Provocation Testing in Clinical Practice. New York: Marcel Dekker, 1994:15–50.
8. Nelson HS. The use of standardized extracts in allergen immunotherapy. J Allergy Clin Immunol 2000; 106(1 pt 1):41–45.
9. Allergen products (Producta allergenica). Eur Pharmacop 1997; 1063–1068.
10. Nelson HS, Ikle D, Buchmeier A. Studies of allergen extract stability: the effects of dilution and mixing. J Allergy Clin Immunol 1996; 98(2):382–388.
11. Norman PS, Lichtenstein LM. Comparisons of alum-precipitated and unprecipitated aqueous ragweed pollen extracts in the treatment of hay fever. J Allergy Clin Immunol 1978; 61(6):384–389.
12. Durham SR, Till SJ. Immunologic changes associated with allergen immunotherapy. J Allergy Clin Immunol 1998; 102(2):157–164.
13. Akdis CA, Blaser K. Immunologic mechanisms of specific immunotherapy. Allergy 1999; 56:31–32.

14. Gleich GJ, Zimmermann EM, Henderson LL, Yunginger JW. Effect of immunotherapy on immunoglobulin E and immunoglobulin G antibodies to ragweed antigens: a six-year prospective study. J Allergy Clin Immunol 1982; 70(4):261–271.

15. Van-der-Zee JS, Aalberse RC. The role of IgG in immediate-type hypersensitivity. Eur Respir J Suppl 1991; 13:91s–96s.

16. Lichtenstein L, Holtzman N, Burnett L. A quantitative in vitro study of the chromatographic distribution and immunoglobulin characteristics of human blocking antibody. J Immunol 1968; 101:317–324.

17. Bousquet J, Maasch H, Martinot B, Hejjaoui A, Wahl R, Michel FB. Double-blind, placebo-controlled immunotherapy with mixed grass-pollen allergoids. II. Comparison between parameters assessing the efficacy of immunotherapy. J Allergy Clin Immunol 1988; 82(3 pt 1):439–446.

18. Golden DB, Meyers DA, Kagey-Sobotka A, Valentine MD, Lichtenstein LM. Clinical relevance of the venom-specific immunoglobulin G antibody level during immunotherapy. J Allergy Clin Immunol 1982; 69(6):489–493.

19. Platts-Mills T, Vaughan J, Squillace S, Woodfolk J, Sporik R. Sensitisation, asthma, and a modified Th2 response in children exposed to cat allergen: a population-based cross-sectional study. Lancet 2001; 357(9258):752–756.

20. Blaser K, Akdis CA, Faith A. Differential regulation of allergen-specific antibodies in allergy and specific immunotherapy. Arb Paul Ehrlich Inst Bundesamt Sera Impfstoffe Frankf A M 1999; 93:243–251.

21. van Neerven RJ, Wikborg T, Lund G, Jacobsen B, Brinch-Nielsen A, Arnved J, et al. Blocking antibodies induced by specific allergy vaccination prevent the activation of CD4+ T cells by inhibiting serum-IgE-facilitated allergen presentation. J Immunol 1999; 163(5):2944–2952.

22. Vrtala S, Akdis CA, Budak F, Akdis M, Blaser K, Kraft D, et al. T cell epitope-containing hypoallergenic recombinant fragments of the major birch pollen allergen, Bet v 1, induce blocking antibodies. J Immunol 2000; 165(11):6653–6659.

23. Rolland JM, Douglass J, O'Hehir RE. Allergen immunotherapy: current and new therapeutic strategies. Expert Opin Investig Drugs 2000; 9(3):515–527.

24. Varney VA, Hamid QA, Gaga M, Ying S, Jacobson M, Frew AJ, et al. Influence of grass pollen immunotherapy on cellular infiltration and cytokine mRNA expression during allergen-induced late-phase cutaneous responses. J Clin Invest 1993; 92(2):644–651.

25. Ebner C, Siemann U, Bohle B, Willheim M, Wiedermann U, Schenk S, et al. Immunological changes during specific immunotherapy of grass pollen allergy: reduced lymphoproliferative responses to allergen and shift from TH2 to TH1 in T-cell clones specific for Phl p 1, a major grass pollen allergen [see comments]. Clin Exp Allergy 1997; 27(9):1007–1015.

26. Moverare R, Elfman L, Bjornsson E, Stalenheim G. Changes in cytokine production in vitro during the early phase of birch-pollen immunotherapy. Scand J Immunol 2000; 52(2):200–206.

27. Wilson DR, Nouri-Aria KT, Walker SM, Pajno GB, O'Brien F, Jacobson MR, et al. Grass pollen immunotherapy: symptomatic improvement correlates with reductions in eosinophils and IL-5 mRNA expression in the nasal mucosa during the pollen season. J Allergy Clin Immunol 2001; 107(6):971–976.

28. Akdis CA, Blaser K. IL-10-induced anergy in peripheral T cell and reactivation by microenvironmental cytokines: two key steps in specific immunotherapy. FASEB J 1999; 13(6):603–609.

29. Akdis CA, Blaser K. Role of IL-10 in allergen-specific immunotherapy and normal response to allergens. Microbes Infect 2001; 3(11):891–898.

30. Creticos PS, Adkinson N, Jr., Kagey-Sobotka A, Proud D, Meier HL, Naclerio RM, et al. Nasal challenge with ragweed pollen in hay fever patients. Effect of immunotherapy [published erratum appears in J Clin Invest 1986; 78(5):1421]. J Clin Invest 1985; 76(6):2247–2253.

31. Hedlin G, Silber G, Naclerio R, Proud D, Lamas AM, Eggleston P, et al. Comparison of the in-vivo and in-vitro response to ragweed immunotherapy in children and adults with ragweed-induced rhinitis. Clin Exp Allergy 1990; 20(5):491–500.

32. Durham SR, Ying S, Varney VA, Jacobson MR, Sudderick RM, Mackay IS, et al. Grass pollen immunotherapy inhibits allergen-induced infiltration of CD4 + T lymphocytes and eosinophils in the nasal mucosa and increases the number of cells expressing messenger RNA for interferon-gamma. J Allergy Clin Immunol 1996; 97(6): 1356–1365.

33. Naclerio RM, Proud D, Moylan B, Balcer S, Freidhoff L, Kagey-Sobotka A, et al. A double-blind study of the discontinuation of ragweed immunotherapy. J Allergy Clin Immunol 1997; 100(3):293–300.

34. Eberlein-Konig B, Jung C, Rakoski J, Ring J. Immunohistochemical investigation of the cellular infiltrates at the sites of allergoid-induced late-phase cutaneous reactions associated with pollen allergen-specific immunotherapy. Clin Exp Allergy 1999; 29(12):1641–1647.

35. Guerra F, Carracedo J, Solana-Lara R, Sanchez-Guijo P, Ramirez R. TH2 lymphocytes from atopic patients treated with immunotherapy undergo rapid apoptosis after culture with specific allergens. J Allergy Clin Immunol 2001; 107(4):647–653.

36. Fanta C, Bohle B, Hirt W, Siemann U, Horak F, Kraft D, et al. Systemic immunological changes induced by administration of grass pollen allergens via the oral mucosa during sublingual immunotherapy. Int Arch Allergy Immunol 1999; 120(3):218–224.

37. Des-Roches A, paradis L, Knani J, Hejjaoui A, Dhivert H, Chanez P, et al. Immunotherapy with a standardized *Dermatophagoides pteronyssinus* extract. V-Duration of efficacy of immunotherapy after its cessation. Allergy 1996; 51:430–433.

38. Durham SR, Walker SM, Varga EM, Jacobson MR, O'Brien F, Noble W, et al. Long-term clinical efficacy of grass-pollen immunotherapy [see comments]. N Engl J Med 1999; 341(7):468–475.

39. Demoly P, Bousquet J, Michel FB. Immunotherapy in allergic rhinitis: a prevention for asthma? Curr Probl Dermatol 1999; 28:119–123.

40. Des-Roches A, Paradis L, Ménardo J-L, Bouges S, Daurès J-P, Bousquet J. Immunotherapy with a standardized *Dermatophagoides pteronyssinus* extract. VI. Specific immunotherapy prevents the onset of new sensitizations in children. J Allergy Clin Immunol 1997; 99:450–453.

41. Purello-D'Ambrosio F, Gangemi S, Merendino RA, Isola S, Puccinelli P, Parmiani S, et al. Prevention of new sensitizations in monosensitized subjects submitted to specific immunotherapy or not. A retrospective study. Clin Exp Allergy 2001; 31(8): 1295–1302.

42. Johnstone DE. Immunotherapy in children: past, present, and future. (Part I). Ann Allergy 1981; 46(1):1–7.

43. Jacobsen L, Dreborg S, Møller C, Valovirta E, Wahn U, Niggemann B, et al. Immunotherapy as a preventive treatment (abstr). J Allergy Clin Immunol 1996; 97:232.

44. Bousquet J. Pro: immunotherapy is clinically indicated in the management of allergic asthma. Am J Respir Crit Care Med 2001; 164(12):2139–2140.

45. Malling H, Weeke B. Immunotherapy. Position Paper of the European Academy of Allergy and Clinical Immunology. Allergy 1993; 48(suppl 14):9–35.

46. Ownby DR, Adinoff AD. The appropriate use of skin testing and allergen immunotherapy in young children. J Allergy Clin Immunol 1994; 94(4):662–665.

47. Muller U, Mosbech H. Position paper: immunotherapy with Hymenoptera venoms. Allergy 1993; 48(suppl 14):37–46.

48. Muller U, Mosbech H. Position paper: immunotherapy with Hymenoptera venoms. Allergy 1993; 48(suppl 14):37–46.

49. Balda BR, Wolf H, Baumgarten C, Klimek L, Rasp G, Kunkel G, et al. Tree-pollen allergy is efficiently treated by short-term immunotherapy (STI) with seven preseasonal injections of molecular standardized allergens. Allergy 1998; 53(8):740–748.

50. Klimek L, Dormann D, Jarman ER, Cromwell O, Riechelmann H, Reske-Kunz AB. Short-term preseasonal birch pollen allergoid immunotherapy influences symptoms, specific nasal provocation and cytokine levels in nasal secretions, but not peripheral T-cell responses, in patients with allergic rhinitis. Clin Exp Allergy 1999; 29(10): 1326–1335.

51. Winther L, Malling HJ, Moseholm L, Mosbech H. Allergen-specific immunotherapy in birch- and grass-pollen-allergic rhinitis. I. Efficacy estimated by a model reducing the bias of annual differences in pollen counts. Allergy 2000; 55(9):818–826.

52. Leynadier F, Banoun L, Dollois B, Terrier P, Epstein M, Guinnepain MT, et al. Immunotherapy with a calcium phosphate-adsorbed five-grass-pollen extract in seasonal rhinoconjunctivitis: a double-blind, placebo-controlled study. Clin Exp Allergy 2001; 31(7):988–996.

53. Ariano R, Kroon AM, Augeri G, Canonica GW, Passalacqua G. Long-term treatment with allergoid immunotherapy with Parietaria. Clinical and immunologic effects in a randomized, controlled trial. Allergy 1999; 54(4):313–319.

54. Malling HJ. Bacterial vaccines: anything but placebo. Allergy 2000; 55(3):214–218.

55. Adkinson N, Jr., Eggleston PA, Eney D, Goldstein EO, Schuberth KC, Bacon JR, et al. A controlled trial of immunotherapy for asthma in allergic children. N Engl J Med 1997; 336(5):324–331.

56. Abramson M, Puy R, Weiner J. Immunotherapy in asthma: an updated systematic review. Allergy 1999; 54(10):1022–1041.

57. Walker SM, Pajno GB, Lima MT, Wilson DR, Durham SR. Grass pollen immunotherapy for seasonal rhinitis and asthma: a randomized, controlled trial. J Allergy Clin Immunol 2001; 107(1):87–93.

58. Gruber W, Eber E, Mileder P, Modl M, Weinhandl E, Zach MS. Effect of specific immunotherapy with house dust mite extract on the bronchial responsiveness of paediatric asthma patients. Clin Exp Allergy 1999; 29(2):176–181.

59. Pichler CE, Helbling A, Pichler WJ. Three years of specific immunotherapy with house-dust-mite extracts in patients with rhinitis and asthma: significant improvement of allergen-specific parameters and of nonspecific bronchial hyperreactivity. Allergy 2001; 56(4):301–306.

60. Shekelle PG, Woolf SH, Eccles M, Grimshaw J. Clinical guidelines: developing guidelines. Br Med J 1999; 318(7183):593–596.

61. Lockey RF, Benedict LM, Turkcltaub PC, Bukantz SC. Fatalities from immunotherapy (IT) and skin testing (ST). J Allergy Clin Immunol 1987; 79(4):660–677.

62. Stewart Gd, Lockey RF. Systemic reactions from allergen immunotherapy (editorial). J Allergy Clin Immunol 1992; 90(4 pt 1):567–578.

63. Personnel and equipment to treat systemic reactions caused by immunotherapy with allergenic extracts. American Academy of Allergy and Immunology. J Allergy Clin Immunol 1986; 77(2):271–273.

64. Bousquet J, Hejjaoui A, Dhivert H, Clauzel AM, Michel FB. Immunotherapy with a standardized Dermatophagoides pteronyssinus extract. III. Systemic reactions during the rush protocol in patients suffering from asthma. J Allergy Clin Immunol 1989; 83(4):797–802.

65. Bousquet J, Michel FB. Safety considerations in assessing the role of immunotherapy in allergic disorders. Drug Safety 1994; 10(1):5–17.

66. Winther L, Malling HJ, Mosbech H. Allergen-specific immunotherapy in birch- and grass-pollen-allergic rhinitis. II. Side-effects. Allergy 2000; 55(9):827–835.

67. International Consensus Report on Diagnosis and Management of Asthma. International Asthma Management Project. Allergy 1992; 47(13 suppl):1–61.

68. Jarisch R, Gotz M, Aberer W, Sidl R, Stabel A, Zajc J, et al. Reduction of side effects of specific immunotherapy by premedication with antihistaminics and reduction of maximal dosage to 50,000 SQ-U/ml. Arb Paul Ehrlich Inst Bundesamt Sera Impfstoffe Frankf A M 1988; 82:163–175.

69. Muller U, Hari Y, Berchtold E. Premedication with antihistamines may enhance efficacy of specific-allergen immunotherapy. J Allergy Clin Immunol 2001; 107(1):81–86.

70. Hejjaoui A, Dhivert H, Michel FB, Bousquet J. Immunotherapy with a standardized *Dermatophagoides pteronyssinus* extract. IV. Systemic reactions according to the immunotherapy schedule. J Allergy Clin Immunol 1990; 85(2):473–479.

71. Hejjaoui A, Ferrando R, Dhivert H, Michel FB, Bousquet J. Systemic reactions occurring during immunotherapy with standardized pollen extracts. J Allergy Clin Immunol 1992; 89(5):925–933.

72. International Consensus Report on Diagnosis and Management of Rhinitis. International Rhinitis Management Working Group. Allergy 1994; 49(19 suppl):1–34.

73. Global strategy for asthma management and prevention. WHO/NHLBI workshop report: National Institutes of Health, National Heart, Lung and Blood Institute, Publication Number 95–3659, January 1995.

74. Norman P. Is there a role for immunotherapy in the treatment of asthma? Yes. Am J Respir Crit Care Med 1996; 154:1225–1227.

75. Barnes P. Is there a role for immunotherapy in the treatment of asthma? No. Am J Respir Crit Care Med 1996; 154:1227–1228.

76. Bousquet J, Demoly P, Michel FB. Specific immunotherapy in rhinitis and asthma. Ann Allergy Asthma Immunol 2001; 87(1 suppl 1):38–42.

77. Frew AJ. Injection immunotherapy. British Society for Allergy and Clinical Immunology Working Party. Br Med J 1993; 307(6909):919–923.

78. Custovic A, Green R, Taggart SC, Smith A, Pickering CA, Chapman MD, et al. Domestic allergens in public places. II: Dog (Can f 1) and cockroach (Bla g 2) allergens in dust and mite, cat, dog and cockroach allergens in the air in public buildings. Clin Exp Allergy 1996; 26(11):1246–1252.

79. Bertoni M, Cosmi F, Bianchi I, Di Berardino L. Clinical efficacy and tolerability of a steady dosage schedule of local nasal immunotherapy. Results of preseasonal treatment in grass pollen rhinitis. Ann Allergy Asthma Immunol 1999; 82(1):47–51.

80. Purello-D'Ambrosio F, Gangemi S, Isola S, La Motta N, Puccinelli P, Parmiani S, et al. Sublingual immunotherapy: a double-blind, placebo-controlled trial with Parietaria judaica extract standardized in mass units in patients with rhinoconjunctivitis, asthma, or both. Allergy 1999; 54(9):968–973.

81. Passalacqua G, Canonica GW. Allergen-specific sublingual immunotherapy for respiratory allergy. BioDrugs 2001; 15(8):509–519.

82. Horak F, Stubner P, Berger UE, Marks B, Toth J, Jager S. Immunotherapy with sublingual birch pollen extract. A short-term double-blind placebo study. J Invest Allergol Clin Immunol 1998; 8(3):165–171.

83. Voltolini S, Modena P, Minale P, Bignardi D, Troise C, Puccinelli P, et al. Sublingual immunotherapy in tree pollen allergy. Double-blind, placebo-controlled study with a biologically standardised extract of three pollens (alder, birch and hazel) administered by a rush schedule. Allergol Immunopathol (Madr) 2001; 29(4):103–110.

84. Clavel R, Bousquet J, Andre C. Clinical efficacy of sublingual-swallow immunotherapy: a double-blind, placebo-controlled trial of a standardized five-grass-pollen extract in rhinitis. Allergy 1998; 53(5):493–498.

85. Hordijk GJ, Antvelink JB, Luwema RA. Sublingual immunotherapy with a standardised grass pollen extract; a double-blind placebo-controlled study. Allergol Immunopathol 1998; 26(5):234–240.

86. Caffarelli C, Sensi LG, Marcucci F, Cavagni G. Preseasonal local allergoid immunotherapy to grass pollen in children: a double-blind, placebo-controlled, randomized trial. Allergy 2000; 55(12):1142–1147.

87. La Rosa M, Ranno C, Andri C, Carat F, Tosca MA, Canonica GW. Double-blind placebo-controlled evaluation of sublingual-swallow immunotherapy with standardized *Parietaria judaica* extract in children with allergic rhinoconjunctivitis. J Allergy Clin Immunol 1999; 104(2 pt 1):425–432.

88. Passalacqua G, Albano M, Riccio A, Fregonese L, Puccinelli P, Parmiani S, et al. Clinical and immunologic effects of a rush sublingual immunotherapy to parietaria species: a double-blind, placebo-controlled trial. J Allergy Clin Immunol 1999; 104(5): 964–968.

89. Bousquet J, Scheinmann P, Guinnepain MT, Perrin-Fayolle M, Sauvaget J, Tonnel AB, et al. Sublingual-swallow immunotherapy (SLIT) in patients with asthma due to house-dust mites: a double-blind, placebo-controlled study. Allergy 1999; 54(3): 249–260.

90. Mungan D, Misirligil Z, Gurbuz L. Comparison of the efficacy of subcutaneous and sublingual immunotherapy in mite-sensitive patients with rhinitis and asthma—a placebo controlled study. Ann Allergy Asthma Immunol 1999; 82(5):485–490.

91. Passalacqua G, Albano M, Fregonese L, Riccio A, Pronzato C, Mela G, et al. Randomised controlled trial of local allergoid immunotherapy on allergic inflammation in mite-induced rhinoconjunctivitis. Lancet 1998; 351:629–632.

92. Tari MG, Mancino M, Monti G. Efficacy of sublingual immunotherapy in patients with rhinitis and asthma due to house dust mite. A double-blind study. Allergol Immunopathol Madr 1990; 18(5):277–284.

93. Bahceciler NN, Isik U, Barlan IB, Basaran MM. Efficacy of sublingual immunotherapy in children with asthma and rhinitis: a double-blind, placebo-controlled study. Pediatr Pulmonol 2001; 82(1):49–55.

94. Pajno GB, Morabito L, Barberio G, Parmiani S. Clinical and immunologic effects of long-term sublingual immunotherapy in asthmatic children sensitized to mites: a double-blind, placebo-controlled study. Allergy 2000; 55(9):842–849.

95. Brown JL, Frew AJ. The efficacy of oromucosal immunotherapy in respiratory allergy. Clin Exp Allergy 2001; 81(1):8–10.

96. Lockey RF. "ARIA": global guidelines and new forms of allergen immunotherapy. J Allergy Clin Immunol 2001; 108(4):497–499.

97. Sabbah A, Hassoun S, Le-Sellin J, Andre C, Sicard H. A double-blind, placebo-controlled trial by the sublingual route of immunotherapy with a standardized grass pollen extract. Allergy 1994; 49(5):309–313.

98. Feliziani V, Lattuada G, Parmiani S, Dall'Aglio PP. Safety and efficacy of sublingual rush immunotherapy with grass allergen extracts. A double blind study. Allergol Immunopathol Madr 1995; 23(5):224–230.

99. Troise C, Voltolini S, Canessa A, Pecora S, Negrini AC. Sublingual immunotherapy in Parietaria pollen-induced rhinitis: a double-blind study. J Investig Allergol Clin Immunol 1995; 5(1):25–30.

100. Vourdas D, Syrigou E, Potamianou P, Carat F, Batard T, Andre C, et al. Double-blind, placebo-controlled evaluation of sublingual immunotherapy with standardized olive pollen extract in pediatric patients with allergic rhinoconjunctivitis and mild asthma due to olive pollen sensitization. Allergy 1998; 53(7):662–672.

101. Andre C, Vatrinet C, Galvain S, Carat F, Sicard H. Safety of sublingual-swallow immunotherapy in children and adults. Int Arch Allergy Immunol 2000; 121(3): 229–234.

102. Dj Rienzo V, Pagani A, Parmiani S, Passalacqua G, Canonica GW. Post-marketing surveillance study on the safety of sublingual immunotherapy in pediatric patients. Allergy 1999; 54(10):1110–1113.

103. Lombardi C, Gargioni S, Melchiorre A, Tiri A, Falagiani P, Canonica GW, et al. Safety of sublingual immunotherapy with monomeric allergoid in adults: multicenter post-marketing surveillance study. Allergy 2001; 56(10):989–992.

104. Malling HJ, Abreu-Nogueira J, Alvarez-Cuesta E, Bjorksten B, Bousquet J, Caillot D, et al. Local immunotherapy. Allergy 1998; 53(10):933–944.

105. van-Ree R. Analytical aspects of standardization of allergenic extracts. Allergy 1997; (52):795–806.

106. Valenta R, Vrtala S. Recombinant allergens for specific immunotherapy. Allergy 1999; 4(suppl 56):43–44.

107. Bousquet J, Yssel H, Demoly P. Prospects for a vaccine in allergic diseases and asthma. BioDrugs 2000; 13(3):61–75.

108. Chapman MD, Smith AM, Vailes LD, Arruda LK, Dhanaraj V, Pomes A. Recombinant allergens for diagnosis and therapy of allergic disease. J Allergy Clin Immunol 2000; 106(3):409–418.

109. Lascombe MB, Gregoire C, Poncet P, Tavares GA, Rosinski-Chupin I, Rabillon J, et al. Crystal structure of the allergen Equ c 1. A dimeric lipocalin with restricted IgE-reactive epitopes. J Biol Chem 2000; 75(28):21572–21577.

110. Valenta R, Kraft D. Recombinant allergen molecules: tools to study effector cell activation. Immunol Rev 2001; 179:119–127.

111. Thomas WR, Smith W, Hales BJ. House dust mite allergen characterisation: implications for T-cell responses and immunotherapy. Int Arch Allergy Immunol 1998; 115(1): 9–14.

112. Vrtala S, Hirtenlehner K, Susani M, Akdis M, Kussebi F, Akdis CA, et al. Genetic engineering of a hypoallergenic trimer of the major birch pollen allergen Bet v 1. Faseb J 2001; 15(11):2045–2047.

113. Takai T, Mori A, Yuuki T, Okudaira H, Okumura Y. Non-anaphylactic combination of partially deleted fragments of the major house dust mite allergen Der f 2 for allergen-specific immunotherapy. Mol Immunol 1999; 36(15–16):1055–1065.

114. Bonura A, Amoroso S, Locorotondo G, Di Felice G, Tinghino R, Geraci D, et al. Hypoallergenic variants of the Parietaria judaica major allergen Par j 1: a member of

the non-specific lipid transfer protein plant family. Int Arch Allergy Immunol 2001; 126(1):32–40.

115. Burks W, Bannon G, Lehrer SB. Classic specific immunotherapy and new perspectives in specific immunotherapy for food allergy. Allergy 2001; 56(suppl 67):121–124.

116. Muller UR. New developments in the diagnosis and treatment of hymenoptera venom allergy. Int Arch Allergy Immunol 2001; 124(4):447–453.

117. Davies JM, O'Hehir RE, Suphioglu C. Use of phage display technology to investigate allergen-antibody interactions. J Allergy Clin Immunol 2000; 105(6 pt 1):1085–1092.

118. Suphioglu C, Schappi G, Kenrick J, Levy D, Davies JM, O'Hehir RE. A novel grass pollen allergen mimotope identified by phage display peptide library inhibits allergen-human IgE antibody interaction. FEBS Lett 2001; 502(1–2):46–52.

119. Ganglberger E, Barbara S, Scholl I, Wiedermann U, Baumann S, Hafner C, et al. Monovalent fusion proteins of IgE mimotopes are safe for therapy of type I allergy. FASEB J 2001; 15(13):2524–2526.

120. Norman PS, Ohman J, Jr., Long AA, Creticos PS, Gefter MA, Shaked Z, et al. Treatment of cat allergy with T-cell reactive peptides. Am J Respir Crit Care Med 1996; 154(6 pt 1):1623–1628.

121. Hirahara K, Tatsuta T, Takatori T, Ohtsuki M, Kirinaka H, Kawaguchi J, et al. Preclinical evaluation of an immunotherapeutic peptide comprising 7 T-cell determinants of Cry j 1 and Cry j 2, the major Japanese cedar pollen allergens. J Allergy Clin Immunol 2001; 108(1):94–100.

122. Kay AB. T cells in allergy and anergy. Allergy 1999; 4(suppl 56):29–30.

123. Haselden BM, Larche M, Meng Q, Shirley K, Dworski R, Kaplan AP, et al. Late asthmatic reactions provoked by intradermal injection of T-cell peptide epitopes are not associated with bronchial mucosal infiltration of eosinophils or T(H)2-type cells or with elevated concentrations of histamine or eicosanoids in bronchoalveolar fluid. J Allergy Clin Immunol 2001; 108(3):394–401.

124. Haselden BM, Syrigou E, Jones M, Huston D, Ichikawa K, Chapman MD, et al. Proliferation and release of IL-5 and IFN-gamma by peripheral blood mononuclear cells from cat-allergic asthmatics and rhinitics, non-cat-allergic asthmatics, and normal controls to peptides derived from Fel d 1 chain 1. J Allergy Clin Immunol 2001; 108(3):349–356.

125. Oldfield WL, Kay AB, Larche M. Allergen-derived T cell peptide-induced late asthmatic reactions precede the induction of antigen-specific hyporesponsiveness in atopic allergic asthmatic subjects. J Immunol 2001; 167(3):1734–1739.

126. Muller U, Akdis CA, Fricker M, Akdis M, Blesken T, Bettens F, et al. Successful immunotherapy with T-cell epitope peptides of bee venom phospholipase A2 induces specific T-cell anergy in patients allergic to bee venom. J Allergy Clin Immunol 1998; 101(6 pt 1):747–754.

127. Raz E, Spiegelberg HL. Deviation of the allergic IgE to an IgG response by gene immunotherapy. Int Rev Immunol 1999; 18(3):271–289.

128. Broide D, Raz E. DNA-based immunization for asthma. Int Arch Allergy Immunol 1999; 118(2–4):453–456.

129. Horner AA, Van Uden JH, Zubeldia JM, Broide D, Raz E. DNA-based immunotherapeutics for the treatment of allergic disease. Immunol Rev 2001; 179:102–118.

130. Kumar M, Behera AK, Hu J, Lockey RF, Mohapatra SS. IFN-gamma and IL-12 plasmid DNAs as vaccine adjuvant in a murine model of grass allergy. J Allergy Clin Immunol 2001; 108(3):402–408.

131. Tighe H, Takabayashi K, Schwartz D, Van Nest G, Tuck S, Eiden JJ, et al. Conjugation of immunostimulatory DNA to the short ragweed allergen amb a 1 enhances its immunogenicity and reduces its allergenicity. J Allergy Clin Immunol 2000; 106(1 pt 1): 124–134.
132. Campbell D, DeKruyff RH, Umetsu DT. Allergen immunotherapy: novel approaches in the management of allergic diseases and asthma. Clin Immunol 2000; 7(3):193–202.
133. Jahn-Schmid B, Graninger M, Glozik M, Kupcu S, Ebner C, Unger FM, et al. Immunoreactivity of allergen (Bet v 1) conjugated to crystalline bacterial cell surface layers (S-layers). Immunotechnology 1996; 2(2):103–113.
134. Agren LC, Ekman L, Lowenadler B, Nedrud JG, Lycke NY. Adjuvanticity of the cholera toxin A1-based gene fusion protein, CTA1-DD, is critically dependent on the ADP-ribosyltransferase and Ig-binding activity. J Immunol 1999; 62(4):2432–2440.

42

Peptide-Based Therapy for Asthma

A. BARRY KAY, F. RUNA ALI, and MARK LARCHÉ

National Heart and Lung Institute
Imperial College
Royal Brompton Hospital
London, England

I. Introduction

Atopic allergic diseases such as asthma, rhinoconjunctivitis, and eczema are rising in prevalence and are a common cause of chronic morbidity in industrialized nations. Direct and indirect consequences include greater financial burden upon health care systems and wide-ranging socioeconomic effects. A number of palliative pharmacological approaches are available that address symptoms, including antihistamines, topical corticosteroids, and inhaled bronchodilators. However, many patients with moderate to severe disease experience only partial to poor symptom control. Furthermore, they are often unable to adopt standard allergen avoidance techniques, as the aeroallergens responsible for disease are often widespread in the environment and difficult to control.

At present the only immunologically specific treatment for atopic allergic disease is allergen immunotherapy. This has proven efficacy in prevention against allergic rhinitis, insect sting anaphylaxis, and mild allergic asthma. It involves the administration, usually by subcutaneous (s.c.) injection, of increasing doses of allergen extracts (1–3). However, specific immunotherapy (SIT) is associated with a significant risk of IgE-mediated adverse events including systemic anaphylaxis. Furthermore, allergen extracts are difficult to standardize, and uncertainties remain regarding the optimal duration of treatment. Thus, efforts are currently being focused on the development of other strategies to induce immunological unresponsiveness to common allergens.

The role of T lymphocytes in allergic responses has been studied extensively. CD4 + T-helper type 2 (Th2) cells are increased at tissue sites in allergic diseases and asthma (4–6) accumulate at sites of allergen challenge (7–9), and correlate with symptoms (10). Th2 cells are capable of orchestrating the allergic response as cytokines such as IL-4 and IL-5, promote immunoglobulin class switching to IgE, and can initiate and stimulate the differentiation, survival, and chemotaxis of eosinophils and other effector cells that release mediators in target tissues (11). Thus, the ability to downregulate Th2-type cell function represents an important therapeutic strategy.

T-cell peptide immunotherapy is an approach that predominantly targets CD4 + T cells and uses allergen-derived peptides containing short linear T-cell epitopes to induce tolerance. The principle has been established in animal models, and the reduced ability of short peptide epitopes to cross-link surface-bound IgE may provide significant improvements in safety, enabling substantial expansion in numbers of individuals who may benefit from this form of therapy. Although most studies in humans have been of allergic disorders, there have been analogous approaches to autoimmune conditions such as multiple sclerosis (12,13). This chapter will focus on the rationale behind T-cell peptide immunotherapy in allergic disease of the airways.

II. T-Cell Activation In Vitro

T-cell activation occurs in two stages. The initial step is transient ligation of the T-cell receptor (TCR) by an antigen-derived peptide bound in the peptide-binding groove of a major histocompatibility complex (MHC) molecule on the surface of an antigen-presenting cell (APC). The second is a costimulatory signal provided by triggering of cell surface molecules on the APC, such as the B7 (CD80 and CD86) family, which are ligands for the CD28 and CTLA-4 molecules on the T cell (Fig. 1). Subtle alterations to the complex series of events that gives rise to T-cell activation have been shown to affect the outcome of T-cell recognition of their cognate ligand.

In vitro experiments have demonstrated that different concentrations of peptides can induce activation, or hyporesponsiveness, depending on dose. Lamb and colleagues (14) employed high doses (50 μg) of peptide in vitro to render human T cells nonresponsive. Influenza virus hemagglutinin-specific human Th0 T-cell clones were exposed to supraoptimal doses of peptide in the absence of antigen-presenting cells. Subsequent whole antigen challenge was characterized by antigen-specific T-cell hyporesponsiveness (anergy), which could be prevented or reversed by the addition of IL-2 (15). Changes in T-cell phenotype such as downregulation of the TCR/CD3 receptor complex and enhanced expression of CD2 and CD25 were observed after the induction of hyporesponsiveness in common with productive T-cell activation events (16,17). Further studies using supraoptimal doses of peptides in human CD4 + T-cell clones reactive to house dust mite reproduced clonal anergy

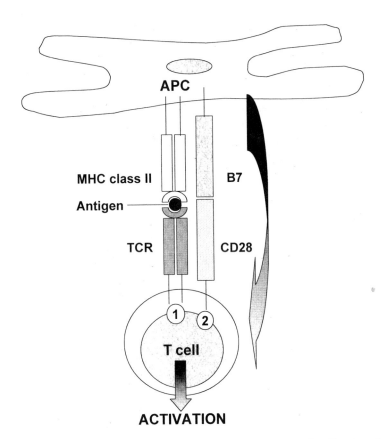

Figure 1 The two-signal model of T-cell activation. Signal 1: transient ligation of the T-cell receptor (TCR) by antigen-derived peptide bound to the peptide-binding groove of a major histocompatibility complex (MHC) class II molecule on the surface of an antigen-presenting cell (APC). Signal 2: full activation requires a further costimulatory signal provided by triggering of cell surface molecules on the same APC, e.g., B7 (CD80 and CD86) family, which are ligands for the CD28 molecule on the T cell.

and showed that this state was accompanied by downregulation of IL-2 and IL-4 and maintenance of IFN-γ secretion (18).

III. Investigation of T-Cell Responses in In Vivo Animal Models

The principle that T-cell peptide epitopes may be used to induce antigen-specific hyporesponsiveness has been extensively investigated in rodent models of autoimmune disease and, more recently, in models of allergic sensitization.

Briner and colleagues established a murine model of cat allergy. Two peptides, IPC-1 and IPC-2, derived from chain 1 of Fel d 1 were administered (19). Soluble IPC-2 was given subcutaneously to naive animals before challenge with peptide in adjuvant. The peptide-specific T-cell response was assessed 10 days after challenge by the culture of mononuclear cells from draining lymph nodes. Decreased IPC-2–specific production of IL-2, IL-4, and IFN-γ was demonstrated. In addition, antigen-specific T-cell proliferation was reduced. The effects of subcutaneous IPC-2 administration on animals already primed with Fel d 1 was also examined. Inhibition of T-cell function was demonstrated by a reduction in IL-2 production and accompanied by reduced levels of IgG antibodies directed against IPC-2. Furthermore, combined administration of IPC-1 and IPC-2 resulted in a decrease in the T-cell response (IL-2 production) to stimulation with the whole Fel d 1 chain 1 protein.

Hoyne and coworkers performed peptide challenge and demonstrated the induction of T-cell tolerance using the mucosal route (20). Thus, intranasal administration of peptides derived from the house dust mite allergen Der p 1 prevented sensitization and also inhibited T-cell responses in primed mice. Transient T-cell activation was shown to precede the induction of hyporesponsiveness (21). Activation of CD4 + T cells from lymph node or splenic tissue was observed, peaking 4 days after peptide treatment. However, at day 14, IL-2 and IFN-γ secretion and proliferative responses were downregulated. Hyporesponsiveness was short-lived in this model, since rechallenge at day 21 elicited a further transient T-cell response, which was subsequently downregulated over time.

Peptide immunotherapy via the mucosal route has been further evaluated in a murine model of bee venom allergy. A mixture of three peptides covering the entire sequence of phospholipase A_2, the major bee venom allergen, was employed. Prophylactic administration led to suppression of the specific IgE response, whereas therapeutic administration to primed presensitised mice induced a greater than 60% decrease in PLA_2-specific IgE and a decline in the IL-4:IFN-γ ratio (22).

IV. Clinical Studies

Early clinical studies of T-cell peptide immunotherapy addressed both perennial and seasonal allergy, specifically cat and ragweed pollinosis. Approximately 95% of individuals with a clinical history of cat allergy have specific IgE directed against Fel d 1 (*Felis domesticus*), a protein found in cat dander and saliva. This allergen is ubiquitous in the environment, present in the homes of cat owners, in public places, and is transported on clothing (23). In initial studies the combination of cloning, sequencing, epitope mapping, and preclinical observations resulted in the selection of two 27-amino-acid sequences, IPC-1 and IPC-2 (both derived from chain 1) and used for subsequent evaluation in clinical trials (24). Thus, the efficacy of Allervax®CAT (IPC-1/IPC-2) was assessed using a double-blind, placebo-controlled trial involving 95 cat-sensitive individuals (25). Following four weekly subcutaneous injections of either placebo, 7.5μg, 75 μg, or 750 μg peptides, clinical efficacy was observed in the highest dose group, 6 weeks after treatment. Clinical outcomes included nasal and lung symptoms during a 60-minute exposure in a room inhabited by live cats. Peptide injections were associated with a significant number of early and late adverse events, including chest tightness, nasal congestion, and flushing. These occurred a few minutes, to several hours after administration of the peptides. Interestingly, in the 750 μg group the incidence and severity of symptoms decreased progressively with each subsequent dose, implying the induction of tolerance to the peptides. In a related study, a decrease in IL-4 production by IPC-1/IPC-2–specific T-cell lines from subjects in the 750 μg group was demonstrated, although there was no alteration in cytokine-production by T-cell lines specific for the whole extract. Furthermore, the proliferative responses to either peptide or whole allergen remained unchanged (26).

Peptide immunotherapy was also evaluated in cat allergic asthmatic subjects using inhaled allergen challenge as an outcome measure (27). Pène and colleagues performed allergen PD_{20} before and after a variable cumulative dose of Allervax® CAT. Subjects received between two and six injections of placebo or peptides (7.5, 75 or 750 μg per injection). Six weeks after the injections, posttreatment $PD_{20}FEV_1$ was not significantly different between the treated and placebo groups. However, in the 75 and 750 μg groups there was a significant improvement between baseline and posttreatment days (within group). In addition, IL-4 release was significantly reduced in the high dose group. No change was observed in IFN-γ production.

In a randomized, double-blind, parallel-group study (28), 40 cat-allergic subjects received s.c. injections of 250 μg peptides or placebo weekly for 4 consecutive weeks. Peptide treatment did not result in reduced early- or late-phase skin reactivity to whole cat extract up to 24 weeks after the last injection. Furthermore, in vitro cell culture assays showed no significant change in cat antigen–specific cytokine production. Frequent adverse events including symptoms of asthma, rhinitis, and pruritus were reported.

Maguire and coworkers performed a multicent, randomized, double-blind, placebo-controlled study of 133 cat-allergic patients who were chronically exposed to cats or had failed previous conventional SIT (29). Subjects received s.c. injections of either 75 or 750μg peptides or placebo twice weekly for 2 weeks in two treatment phases, 4 months apart (a total of eight injections). Pulmonary function was improved in the 750 μg group, but only in those subjects with reduced baseline FEV_1 at a single time point 3 weeks after initial treatment phase. Frequent adverse events were recorded, including three requiring systemic epinephrine. The majority of adverse events were associated with respiratory symptoms, occurred a few hours after injection, and declined with successive doses.

V. Adverse Events in Peptide Immunotherapy

Clinical application of Allervax®CAT peptides were associated with frequent adverse events occurring immediately and up to several hours after peptide injection. Early events may have been due to the length of IPC-1 and IPC-2, since each peptide was 27 residues in length and may have contained conformational determinants (B-cell epitopes) capable of triggering IgE-mediated reactions through the crosslinking of surface-bound IgE upon mast cells and basophils. Late reactions diminished with successive injections and may have been the correlate of the transient T-cell activation and subsequent hyporesponsiveness observed in murine models. The high frequency of adverse events, together with only modest improvement in symptom scores, led to the withdrawal of Allervax ®CAT and a related product (Allervax® RAGWEED) from further clinical studies.

VI. Peptide Therapy for Bee Venom Allergy

In bee venom–sensitized individuals, phospholipase A_2 (PLA_2) is a major allergen. Müller and colleagues used an equimolar mixture of three T-cell epitopes of PLA_2 (each between 11 and 18 residues long) to treat five patients who had experienced IgE-mediated systemic allergic reactions to bee stings (30). Ten patients allergic to bee venom receiving whole allergen SIT served as control subjects. Peptides were administered in an induction phase consisting of an incremental dosing schedule starting at 0.1 μg followed by three maintenance injections of 100 μg each. The total dose received was 397.1 μg over 2 months. The dosing schedule resulted in the delivery of approximately 40 times more PLA_2 than conventional SIT. Allergen challenge in the skin served as the primary outcome measure. Patients received subcutaneous PLA_2 (corresponding approximately to the PLA_2 content of a bee sting) followed 1 week later by a live bee sting. No allergic side effects were reported during peptide therapy. All subjects tolerated the PLA_2 challenge without systemic symptoms. Two peptide-treated patients developed mild systemic allergic symptoms after the bee sting challenge. After peptide immunotherapy, specific proliferative responses by PBMCs to PLA_2 and the peptides were decreased in the three successfully treated patients. The production of Th1 (IL-2, IFN-γ) and Th2 (IL-4, IL-5, IL-13) cytokines was also inhibited, and B cells were unaffected in their capacity to produce specific IgE and IgG4 antibodies. However, after whole allergen challenge, antibody levels increased in favor of IgG4, as often observed in conventional SIT. Further experiments revealed an increase in allergen-specific IL-10 production in these individuals (C. Akdis and K. Blaser, personal communication), findings that support earlier data from whole bee venom–treated patients (31).

VII. Induction of Isolated Late Asthmatic Reactions with Peptides

Peptide challenge has been employed to directly activate allergen-specific T cells resulting in the induction of T-cell–dependent bronchospasm. Haselden and colleagues synthesized three overlapping peptides (designated FC1P) spanning the central region of chain 1 of Fel d 1 and challenged cat-allergic asthmatic subjects by intradermal injection (32). Each peptide was 16/17 residues in length, and in vitro histamine release assays supported the reduced ability of the FC1P preparation to crosslink surface-bound IgE. A dose of 80 μg FC1P was administered as a single

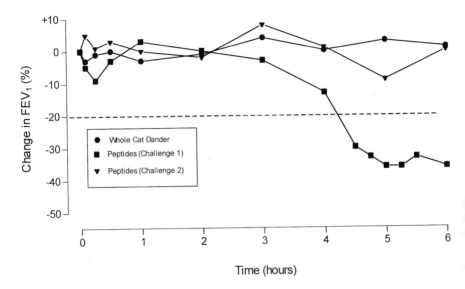

Figure 2 Induction of isolated late asthmatic reaction (LAR) by intradermal injection of Fel d 1–derived peptides and demonstration of attenuation of the reaction at repeat challenge. The percent changes in FEV_1 after intradermal administration of 5 μg multiple overlapping Fel d 1–derived peptides (■), during a control day when intradermal cat dander was administered (●), and at repeat challenge with peptides (▼).

injection to 40 cat-allergic asthmatics. No reaction was observed at the injection site. However, 9 out of the 40 subjects experienced an isolated late asthmatic reaction (LAR), defined as a fall in FEV_1 of 20% or more 2–3 hours after challenge and reaching a plateau at 6 hours. The induction of an isolated LAR without the preceding early phase suggested that peptides bound to MHC molecules could directly activate T cells in the absence of mast cell activation. Rechallenge of subjects with the same dose of FC1P demonstrated the induction of peptide-specific hyporesponsiveness in the lung suggesting the induction of antigen-specific T-cell "tolerance" following transient T-cell activation (Fig. 2).

VIII. Major Histocompatibility Complex in Peptide Therapy

Approximately 25% of subjects experienced LARs (>20% fall in FEV_1) after administration of FC1P. HLA haplotyping identified DR molecules, which appeared to be present at high frequency in the group of subjects developing LARs. Using cat allergen–specific T-cell lines and a panel of fibroblasts transfected with human HLA-DR molecules, out of 9 "reactors" were found to express HLA-DR13 as opposed to 1 out of 31 "nonreactors." DR13-transfected L cells presented the third of the FC1P peptides to autologous T-cell lines. Similarly, DR1 and DR4 bound and presented FC1P peptides. Furthermore "promiscuous" binding of peptides was observed, in that one peptide bound to both DR1 and DR13. Thus, strong support was provided for MHC restriction of two of the three FC1P peptides.

The conclusion of these studies is that successful immunotherapy must take into account the differing HLA haplotypes present in an outbred population. This implies that the number of peptides required to treat all allergic individuals must necessarily be larger than the small number used in studies with inbred animal strains. This may account for the limited clinical benefit seen with IPC1/IPC2 where MHC restriction was not considered and fewer peptides were administered. However, the observation that individual peptides may bind to more than one MHC molecule suggests that only relatively small numbers of peptides may be required to achieve vaccines with broad population activity.

IX. MHC-Based Peptide Vaccines

In further studies, 12 overlapping peptides (16 or 17 residues long each) spanning the majority of chains 1 and 2 of Fel d 1, were synthesized increasing the number of HLA haplotypes able to bind and present peptide (33). Using this preparation of peptides termed multiple overlapping peptides, (MOP), it was demonstrated that the magnitude, as well as the frequency, of isolated LARs in cat-allergic asthmatic subjects was dose dependent, with 50% of individuals developing a LAR when challenged with a single dose of 5 μg of peptides. A second injection of peptides was associated with a marked reduction or absence of the LAR with a return to baseline values over up to 40 weeks (Fig 3). Maximal attenuation occurred 2–4 weeks after the initial peptides challenge, suggesting an active immunological process.

More recently, an open study employing an up-dosing protocol with peptides (0.1, 1.0, 5, 10, 25 μg) injected at 2-weekly intervals demonstrated the ability to induce T-cell hyporesponsiveness in the absence of LARs. These results indicate that incremental dosing protocols, starting at a dose that is too low to induce LARs, may allow peptide immunotherapy to be used safely, without undesirable adverse effects (34).

Following a single peptide injection, cutaneous late phase reactions (LPRs) to intradermal challenge with whole cat dander extract were significantly reduced (33). To confirm these observations in a blinded study, 24 cat-allergic subjects were recruited into a double-blind, placebo-controlled study with 16 subjects randomized to peptides via an incremental dosing protocol, to a total dose of 90 μg (35). After peptide treatment a significant reduction in both the early and late cutaneous reactions to Fel d 1 and also to whole cat dander were observed, indicating peptide-induced modulation of both B-cell (early phase reaction) and T-cell function (late-phase reaction), respectively. Changes in late cutaneous reactions were observed within 3 weeks of completing treatment and persisted for several months. Changes in early cutaneous reactions were only apparent at long-term follow-up (4–12 months). No

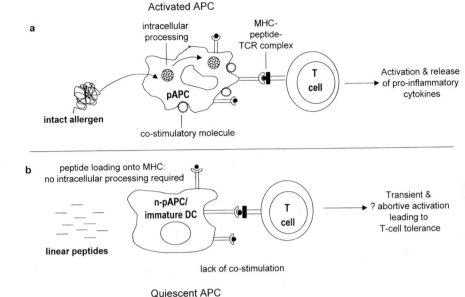

Figure 3 Differing APC responses to intact allergen and short allergen-derived peptides may contribute to differences in T-cell reactivity. (a) The activation of professional APCs (pAPC), e.g., dendritic cells, can be induced by uptake of whole allergen, resulting in upregulation of co-stimulatory molecules on the APC cell surface. Intact allergen is intracellularly processed before peptide loading onto MHC molecules. Subsequent activation of naive T cells occurs by recognition of a peptide-MHC complex accompanied by co-stimulation, leading to pro-inflammatory cytokine production. (b) Short allergen–derived peptides are loaded onto the MHC molecule of immature dendritic cells and nonprofessional APCs (n-pAPC), e.g., lung epithelial and endothelial cells, without the requirement for intracellular processing. Peptide recognition in the absence of APC activation and co-stimulation leads to transient, and possibly abortive, activation resulting in T-cell tolerance.

significant differences were demonstrated in bronchial responsiveness to either methacholine or whole cat dander, although actively treated subjects were better able to tolerate exposure to cats.

In vitro T-cell responses before and after peptide treatment demonstrated a significant decrease in peptide- and whole allergen–induced proliferation of PBMCs and the production of IL-4, IL-13, and IFN-γ in cultures. Similar inhibitory responses to four additional Fel d 1–derived peptides that did not form constituents of the mixture injected were demonstrated, suggesting the induction of linked suppression (33). Furthermore, peptide treatment was associated not only with decreases in whole cat dander–induced pro-inflammatory cytokines by PBMCs, but also with increased IL-10 production (unpublished data). Thus, induction of T-cell hyporesponsiveness in humans may be associated with the induction/expansion of a population of regulatory/suppressor T cells.

X. Potential Mechanisms of T-Cell Peptide Immunotherapy

The nature of T-cell hyporesponsiveness induced by allergen-derived peptides remains incompletely understood. Peripheral T cells may be inactivated by a number of mechanisms including induction of T-cell anergy (unresponsiveness without a decrease in cell numbers), clonal deletion (activation-induced cell death), the induction of active suppression via a regulatory T-cell population, or immune deviation (a shift in phenotype from Th2 to Th1).

XI. T-Cell Anergy

T-cell anergy has been well described in murine studies using allergen-derived peptides (21–23) and in human CD4 + cells in vitro (14–17). The mechanism of inhibition of T-cell responses remains enigmatic. Lack of appropriate co-stimulation has been proposed, although transient CD4 + T-cell activation has been observed in certain studies and is thus difficult to reconcile with suboptimal cell signaling (21,32,33). It now appears that many previous descriptions of T-cell anergy as a functional outcome may have been models in which immunoregulatory, antigen-specific T cells were induced.

XII. Regulatory T Cells

The role of regulatory T cells has been the focus of much recent interest. Elevated levels of IL-10 secondary to peptide treatment supports a mechanism of active suppression (Fig. 4). Animal models of autoimmune diseases have shown that regulatory T-cell populations and cytokines including IL-10 and TGF-β appear to be important factors in the modulation of Th1 and Th2 responses (36,37). Adkis and coworkers, employing either whole bee venom or peptides from PLA_2, have demonstrated that successful immunotherapy in bee venom–sensitive subjects was associated with the production of IL-10 (31). However, T-cell hyporesponsiveness in this model was partially reversed in vitro by the addition of exogenous IL-2 or IL-15 (38), suggesting that further clarification is required to either unify or dissociate the classical anergy model and active suppression by regulatory T cells (38). Recently, Levings and colleagues have demonstrated the ability to expand cultured regulatory T cells in vitro by the addition of exogenous IL-2 (39). Thus, in vitro hyporesponsiveness after venom immunotherapy may have been due to the induction of regulatory T cells. The presence of elevated levels of IL-10 production post-therapy in this model adds further support.

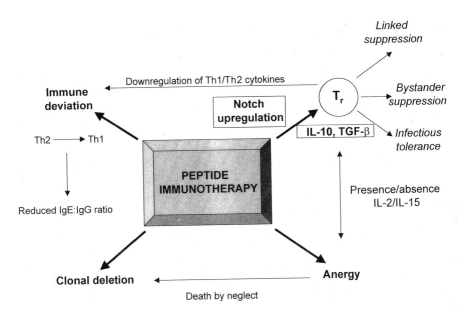

Figure 4 Potential mechanisms of tolerance induced by peptide immunotherapy. Peripheral T cells may be inactivated by a number of routes, including induction of T-cell anergy, clonal deletion, immune deviation (Th2 to Th1/Th0), or the induction of active suppression via a regulatory T-cell population (Tr), acting via the production of immunosuppressive cytokines, such as IL-10 and TGF-β, or upregulation of Notch receptor.

XIII. Intra- and Intermolecular Suppression

A number of studies have described the ability of antigen-specific T cells induced by peptide or whole antigen to modulate the response of distinct populations of T cells specific for other epitopes located within the same or different molecules. These include descriptions of regulatory CD4 + T cells that can confer nonresponsiveness to either other epitopes within the whole molecule (linked or intramolecular epitope suppression) (40), adjacent molecules (bystander tolerance or intermolecular suppression), or the next generation of regulatory T cells (infectious tolerance) (41). Studies using overlapping Fel d 1–derived peptides have shown that T-cell responses to noninjected peptides and to whole allergen were downregulated at the same time as those to injected epitopes (33). Taken together these findings provide evidence of linked suppression in human studies and suggest that in the future, peptide immunotherapy may be successfully based on only a limited number of peptides.

XIV. Cell Contact–Dependent Regulation

Regulatory T cells may induce suppressive effects via cell-to-cell contact. Using a mouse model, Hoyne and colleagues have shown a role for cognate interaction between T cells mediated by Notch/Delta signaling to induce and maintain peripheral T-cell tolerance to Der p 1. Intranasal peptide administered at high doses was found to produce transient expression of Delta1 on inhibitory CD4 + T cells. Ligation of the Notch 1 receptor on adjacent T cells by Delta1 + regulatory cells prevented clonal expansion (42,43).

XV. Clonal Deletion

Clonal deletion is known to play a major role in central tolerance during thymic maturation. In an experimental model of mucosal tolerance employing transgenic mice overexpressing the ovalbumin-specific TCR gene, high-dose treatment with antigen induced clonal deletion via apoptosis. Interestingly, low-dose ovalbumin produced TGF-β–and IL-10–secreting regulatory cells, which inhibited specific T-cell responses (44). However, from the studies available, it appears unlikely that this mechanism plays a major role in the hyporesponsiveness induced by peptides.

XVI. Immune Deviation

Immune deviation from a Th2 to a Th1/Th0 profile has been demonstrated in a large number of studies using conventional SIT and has been associated with a change in the IFN-γ:IL-4 ratio in favor of the former (45). Two studies investigating IPC-1 and IPC-2 in humans found a reduction in Fel d 1-specific IL-4 production by PBMCs or T-cell lines in the high-dose treatment group without a change in IFN-γ (27,28). Immunosuppressive cytokines such as IL-10 and TGF-β were not measured in these studies. Results from our group and also from Müller and coworkers have demonstrated, in peripheral blood mononuclear cells, a generalized reduction in proliferative and Th1/Th2 cytokine responses (30,33) together with an increase in IL-10 production, following peptide treatment. It may be, therefore, that as a result of the way in which soluble peptides are presented to the immune system (perhaps by immature, nonactivated, or nonprofessional antigen-presenting cells), a form of immune deviation is induced. In contrast to that induced by conventional whole allergen immunotherapy, peptide therapy may result in the induction of regulatory T cells that suppress both Th1 and Th2 responses. As a result, peptide immunotherapy may also be of particular interest in autoimmune diseases in which peptide epitopes have been identified.

XVII. Conclusions

An increasing number of studies in both murine and human models suggests that peptide immunotherapy may offer a safe and effective approach for the management of allergic disease. While further work is undertaken to determine the exact mechanism of induction of tolerance, the contributory role of regulatory T cells appears to be a common feature of many studies. The use of short peptides in order to eliminate the likelihood of IgE-mediated side effects may be a prerequisite for success in allergic disease. For maximal efficacy with the minimum number of peptides, the identification of T-cell epitopes which have a broad MHC-binding ability may be considered when designing peptide vaccines. Dose and dose interval selection may also prove critical for the development of optimal hyporesponsiveness in the absence of adverse events. Peptide immunotherapy may be broadly applicable in all areas in which immunopathology is controlled by T lymphocytes. The ability to deliver safe and effective vaccines for allergic conditions that do not require extensive time and resource commitments from patient and physician may substantially expand the market for disease-modifying therapy.

References

1. Varney VA, Gaga M, Frew AJ, Aber VR, Kay AB, Durham SR. Usefulness of immunotherapy in patients with severe summer hayfever uncontrolled by antiallergic drugs. Br Med J 1991; 302:265–269.
2. Varney VA, Edwards J, Tabbah K, Brewster H, Mavroleon G, Frew AJ. Clinical efficacy of specific immunotherapy to cat dander: a double-blind placebo-controlled trial. Clin Exp Allergy 1997; 27:860–867.
3. Durham SR, Walker SM, Varga E-M, Jacobson MR, O'Brien F, Noble W, Till SJ, Hamid QA, Nouri-Aria KT. Long-term clinical efficacy of grass-pollen immunotherapy. N Engl J Med 1999; 341:468–475.
4. Hamid Q, Azzawi M, Ying S, Moqbel R, Wardlaw AJ, Corrigan CJ, Bradley B, Durham SR, Collins JV, Jeffery PK, Quint DJ, Kay AB. Expression of mRNA for interleukin-5 in mucosal bronchial biopsies from asthma. J Clin Invest 1991; 87:1541–1546.
5. Robinson DS, Hamid Q, Ying S, Tsicopoulos A, Barkans J, Bentley AM, Corrigan C, Durham SR, Kay AB. Predominant TH2-like bronchoalveolar T-lymphocyte population in atopic asthma. N Engl J Med 1992; 326:298–304.
6. Ying S, Durham SR, Corrigan CJ, Hamid Q, Kay AB. Phenotype of cells expressing mRNA for TH2-type (interleukin 4 and interleukin 5) and TH1-type (interleukin 2 and interferon gamma) cytokines in bronchoalveolar lavage and bronchial biopsies from atopic asthmatic and normal control subjects. Am J Respir Cell Mol Biol 1995; 12: 477–487.
7. Bentley AM, Meng Q, Robinson DS, Hamid Q, Kay AB, Durham SR. Increases in activated T lymphocytes, eosinophils, and cytokine mRNA expression for interleukin-5 and granulocyte/macrophage colony-stimulating factor in bronchial biopsies after allergen inhalation challenge in atopic asthmatics. Am J Respir Cell Mol Biol 1993; 8: 35–42.
8. Robinson D, Hamid Q, Bentley A, Ying S, Kay AB, Durham SR. Activation of CD4+ T cells, increased TH2-type cytokine mRNA expression, and eosinophil recruitment in bronchoalveolar lavage after allergen inhalation challenge in patients with atopic asthma. J Allergy Clin Immunol 1993; 92:313–324.
9. Huang SK, Xiao HQ, Kleine-Tebbe J, Paciotti G, Marsh DG, Lichtenstein LM, Liu MC. IL-13 expression at the sites of allergen challenge in patients with asthma. J Immunol 1995; 155:2688–2694.

10. Robinson DS, Ying S, Bentley AM, Meng Q, North J, Durham SR, Kay AB, Hamid Q. Relationships among numbers of bronchoalveolar lavage cells expressing messenger ribonucleic acid for cytokines, asthma symptoms, and airway methacholine responsiveness in atopic asthma. J Allergy Clin Immunol 1993; 92:397–403.

11. Kay AB. Allergy and allergic diseases. First of two parts. N Engl J Med 2001; 344: 30–37.

12. Karin N, Binah O, Grabie N, Mitchell DJ, Felzen B, Solomon MD, Conlon P, Gaur A, Ling N, Steinman L. Short peptide-based tolerogens without self-antigenic or pathogenic activity reverse autoimmune disease. J Immunol 1998; 160:5188–5194.

13. Warren KG, Catz I, Wucherpfennig KW. Tolerance induction to myelin basic protein by intravenous synthetic peptides containing epitope P85 VVHFFKNIVTP96 in chronic progressive multiple sclerosis. J Neurol Sci 1997; 152:31–38.

14. Lamb JR, Skidmore BJ, Green N, Chiller JM, Feldmann M. Induction of tolerance in influenza virus-immune T lymphocyte clones with synthetic peptides of influenza haemagglutinin. J Exp MedI 1983; 157:1434–1447.

15. Essery G, Feldmann M, Lamb JR. Interleukin-2 can prevent and reverse antigen-induced unresponsiveness in cloned human T lymphocytes. Immunology 1988; 64:413–417.

16. O'Hehir RE, Lamb JR. Induction of specific clonal anergy in human T lymphocytes by *Staphylococcus aureus* enterotoxins. Proc Natl Acad Sci USA 1990; 87:8884–8888.

17. O'Hehir RE, Aguilar BA, Schmidt TJ, Gollnick SO, Lamb JR. Functional inactivation of *Dermatophagoides* spp. (house dust mite) reactive human T-cell clones. Clin Exp Allergy 1991; 21:209–215.

18. O'Hehir RE, Yssel H, Verma S, de Vries JE, Spits H, Lamb JR. Clonal analysis of differential lymphokine production in peptide and superantigen induced T cell anergy. Int Immunol 1991; 3:819–826.

19. Briner T, Kuo M, Keating K, Rogers B, Greenstein J. Peripheral T-cell tolerance induced in naive and primed mice by subcutaneous injection of peptides from the major cat allergen Fel d 1. Proc Natl Acad Sci USA 1993; 90:7608–12.

20. Hoyne G, O'Hehir RE, Wraith D, Thomas WR, Lamb JR. Inhibition of T-cell and antibody responses to house dust mite allergen by inhalation of the dominant T-cell epitope in naive and sensitised mice. J Exp Med 1993; 178:1783–1788.

21. Hoyne GF, Askonas BA, Hetzel C, Thomas WR, Lamb JR. Regulation of house dust mite responses by intranasally administered peptide: transient activation of CD4+ T cells precedes the development of tolerance in vivo. Int Immunol 1996; 8:335–342.

22. Astori M, von Garnier C, Kettner A, Dufour N, Corradin G, Spertini F. Inducing tolerance by intranasal administration of long peptides in naive and primed CBA/J mice. J Immunol 2000; 165:3497–3505.

23. Custovic A, Fletcher A, Pickering CAC, Francis HC, Green R, Smith A, Chapman M, Woodcock A. Domestic allergens in public places. III. House dust mite, cat, dog, and cockroach allergens in British hospitals. Clin Exp Allergy 1998; 28:53–59.

24. Counsell CM, Bond JF, Ohman JL, Greenstein JL, Garman RD. Definition of the human T-cell epitopes of Fel d 1, the major allergen of the domestic cat. J Allergy Clin Immunol 1996; 98:884–894.

25. Norman PS, Ohman JL, Long AA, Creticos PS, Gefter MA, Shaked Z, Wood RA, Eggleston PA, Hafner KB, Rao P, Lichtenstein LM, Jones NH, Nicodemus CF. Treatment of cat allergy with T-cell reactive peptides. Am J Respir Crit Care Med 1996; 154:1623–1628.

26. Marcotte GV, Braun CM, Norman PS, Nicodemus CF, Kagey-Sobotka A, Lichtenstein LM, Essayan DM. Effects of peptide therapy on ex-vivo T-cell responses. J Allergy Clin Immunol 1998; 101:506–513.

27. Pène J, Desroches A, Paradis L, Lebel B, Farce M, Nicodemus CF, Yssel H, Bousquet J. Immunotherapy with Fel d 1 peptides decreases IL-4 release by peripheral blood T cells of patients allergic to cats. J Allergy Clin Immunol 1998; 102:571–578.

28. Simons F, Imada M, Li Y, Watson W, Hayglass K. Fel d 1 peptides: effect on skin tests and cytokine synthesis in cat-allergic human subjects. Int Immunol 1996; 8:1937–1945.

29. Maguire P, Nicodemus C, Robinson D, Aaronson D, Umetsu DT. The safety and efficacy of ALLERVAX CAT in cat-allergic patients. Clin Immunol 1999; 93:222–231.

30. Müller U, Akdis CA, Fricker M, Akdis M, Blesken T, Bettens F, Blaser K. Successful immunotherapy with T-cell epitope peptides of bee venom phospholipase A2 induces specific T-cell anergy in patients allergic to bee venom. J Allergy Clin Immunol 1998; 101:747–754.

31. Akdis CA, Blesken T, Akdis M, Wuthrich B, Blaser K. Role of interleukin-10 in specific immunotherapy. J Clin Invest 1998; 102:98–106.

32. Haselden BM, Kay AB, Larché M. IgE-independent MHC-restricted T cell peptide epitope-induced late asthmatic reactions. J Exp Med 1999; 189:1885–1894.

33. Oldfield WLG, Kay AB, Larché M. Allergen-derived T-cell peptide-induced late asthmatic reactions precede the induction of antigen-specific hyporesponsiveness in atopic allergic asthmatic subjects. J Immunol 2001; 167:1734–1739.

34. Alexander C, Oldfield WLG, Shirley KE, Larché M, Kay AB. A dosing protocol of allergen-derived T-cell peptide epitopes for the treatment of allergic disease (abstr). J Allergy Clin Immunol 2001; 107:716.

35. Oldfield WLG, Larché M, Kay AB. Effect of T-cell peptides derived from Fel d 1 on allergic reactions and cytokine production in patients sensitive to cats: a randomised controlled trial. Lancet 2002; 360:47–53.

36. Powrie F, Carlino J, Leach MW, Mauze S, Coffman RL. A critical role for transforming growth factor-beta but not interleukin 4 in the suppression of T helper type 1-mediated colitis by CD45RB(low) CD4+ T cells. J Exp Med 1996; 183:2669–2674.

37. Weiner HL, Inobe J, Kuchroo V, Chen Y. Induction and characterisation of TGFβ secreting Th3 cells. FASEB J 1996; 10:A1444.

38. Akdis CA, Akdis M, Blesken T, Wymann D, Alkan SS, Muller U, Blaser K. Epitope-specific T cell tolerance to phospholipase A2 in bee venom immunotherapy and recovery by IL-2 and IL-15 in vitro. J Clin Invest 1996; 98:1676–1683.

39. Levings MK, Sangregorio R, Roncarolo MG. Human CD25(+)CD4(+) t regulatory cells suppress naive and memory T cell proliferation and can be expanded in vitro without loss of function. J Exp Med 2001; 193:1295–1302.

40. Hoyne GF, Jarnicki AG, Thomas WR, Lamb JR. Characterization of the specificity and duration of T cell tolerance to intranasally administered peptides in mice: a role for intramolecular epitope suppression. Int Immunol 1997; 9:1165–1173.

41. Cobbold S, Waldmann H. Infectious tolerance. Curr Opin Immunol 1998; 10:518–524.

42. Hoyne GF, Le Roux I, Corsin-Jimenez M, Tan K, Dunne J, Forsyth LM, Dallman MJ, Owen MJ, Ish-Horowicz D, Lamb JR. Serrate 1-induced notch signalling regulates the decision between immunity and tolerance made by peripheral CD4(+) T cells. Int Immunol 2000; 12:177–185.

43. Hoyne GF, Dallman MJ, Lamb JR. T-cell regulation of peripheral tolerance and immunity: the potential role for Notch signalling. Immunology 2000; 100:281–288.
44. Chen Y, Inobe J, Marks R, Gonnella P, Kuchroo VK, Weiner HL. Peripheral deletion of antigen-reactive T cells in oral tolerance. Nature 1995; 376(6536):177–180.
45. Rolland J, O'Hehir R. Immunotherapy of allergy: anergy, deletion, and immune deviation. Curr Opin Immunol 1998; 10:640–645.

43

Reducing IgE Levels as a Strategy for the Treatment of Asthma

JOHN V. FAHY

University of California, San Francisco
San Francisco, California

I. Introduction

A principal goal of research into mechanisms of disease is to identify mediators that might be targeted as treatments. For example, inhibitors of pro-inflammatory mediators may improve the clinical outcomes of disease. Mediators of disease that do not have also have important functions in maintaining host health are particularly attractive therapeutic targets because their inhibition is unlikely to cause serious side effects.

The story of the development of a therapeutic anti-IgE monoclonal antibody is a good example of how investigations into mechanisms of disease (allergy) identified a key mediator (IgE), which led to the development of a specific inhibitor (anti-IgE) for the purposes of treating human disease (allergic rhinitis and asthma). This review will provide a brief review of this story. I will first address the safety issues that surround the inhibition of IgE in human subjects. Then I will review the three phases of clinical trials of anti-IgE in asthma that have recently been completed. My review will indicate that anti-IgE treatment is well tolerated and effective for the treatment of asthma. The story is not yet finished, however. At the time of writing, anti-IgE was not yet approved as a treatment in the United States or Europe, and the place of anti-IgE in current guidelines for asthma management has not yet been established.

II. Safety of the Anti-IgE Treatment Strategy

IgE is a key mediator of allergy (1). IgE mediates its effects through interactions with high- and low-affinity receptors on a variety of effector cells. The interaction of IgE with its high-affinity receptor (FcεR1) on basophils and mast cells is the key event initiating type 1 hypersensitivity reactions and anaphylaxis. The interaction of IgE and its low-affinity receptor (FcεR2, also known as CD23) is also important, because CD23 expression is found on a wide variety of structural, regulatory, and inflammatory cells in the airway (2,3).

IgE is viewed as a logical target for novel drug development in asthma because several lines of evidence suggest an important role for IgE in asthmatic airway inflammation. First, IgE levels are higher than normal in asthmatic subjects of all ages (4,5). Second, IgE-mediated type 1 hypersensitivity reactions are the likely mechanisms of acute bronchospasm in allergic asthmatic subjects exposed to aeroallergen (1). The approach taken to interfere with the interaction of IgE and its high- and low-affinity receptors has been to develop a monoclonal antibody that reduces IgE levels without causing allergic reactions (6–8). Such therapeutic anti-IgE antibodies are required to have a set of unique binding properties that ensure safety. Research programs at Genentech, Tanox, and Novartis were established to engineer a suitable therapeutic anti-IgE monoclonal antibody, and three candidate antibodies have been tested in humans. The Novartis/Tanox antibodies (CGP 51901 and CGP 56901) and the Genentech antibody (rhuMAb-E25) have undergone clinical testing in human subjects. Based on these data, the companies agreed in 1996 to jointly develop rhuMAb-E25 (omalizumab, "Xolair") as the most promising of these antibodies for further clinical development.

Reducing IgE levels in human subjects using a monoclonal antibody raises at least three possible safety issues: anti-IgE treatment may cause anaphylaxis, may predispose to parasitic infections, or may provoke immune responses, including complement fixation or antibody formation.

A. Anti-IgE Treatment and the Risk of Anaphylaxis

IgE molecules on the surface of effector cells such as basophils or mast cells represent a challenging target for a therapeutic antibody, because anti-IgE antibody binding to cell bound IgE will cross-link adjacent IgE molecules and trigger cell activation, degranulation, and anaphylaxis. Therefore, a characteristic of all therapeutic anti-IgE antibodies is that they have been selected because they bind circulating or "free" IgE but do not bind IgE on the surface of effector cells such as mast cells. This binding specificity occurs because therapeutic anti-IgE binds IgE in the CH3 domain of the IgE heavy chain, i.e., in the same Fc region containing the binding sites for the high- and low-affinity IgE receptors (7,9). Overlap in the binding regions for anti-IgE, FcεR1, and FcεR2 in the CH3 region means that IgE binding to anti-IgE prevents simultaneous binding of IgE to FcεR1 or FcεR2 (10).

The Fc of an IgE molecule is composed of two ε-heavy chains, and therefore each IgE molecule has two identical binding epitopes for anti-IgE, FcεR1, and

FcεR2. Fortunately, another important characteristic of therapeutic anti-IgE antibodies such as omalizumab is that they cannot bind to the vacant or "contralateral" CH3 domain in cell-bound IgE, presumably because of conformational changes in Fc of IgE induced by interaction of IgE with its native receptors. This fact means that anti-IgE will not interact with the free CH3 domain of cell bound IgE and results in a nonanaphylactogenic antibody that can be used for therapeutic purposes (Fig. 1).

Treatment with therapeutic anti-IgE antibody such as omalizumab reduces circulating IgE levels, because omalizumab binds free IgE in the circulation, and the complexes are eliminated by the reticulo-endothelial system. In addition, omalizumab in tissue compartments actively binds any IgE dissociating from FcεR1 and FcεR2 receptors on effector cells. In this way IgE effector cells are "disarmed" of IgE, and IgE-dependent allergic reactions should be prevented. The antiallergic effect of anti-IgE cannot be expected to be immediate, because disarming effector cells of IgE will not be immediate. The kinetics of IgE binding to high-affinity receptors on mast cells and basophils in vivo is unknown, but available data suggest that disarming high-affinity receptors on these cells is likely to take weeks rather than hours or days.

Circulating levels of IgE have important effects in regulating IgE receptor expression on IgE effector cells. This fact was discovered in human experiments using omalizumab. The expression of IgE and FcεR1 on human basophils was mea-

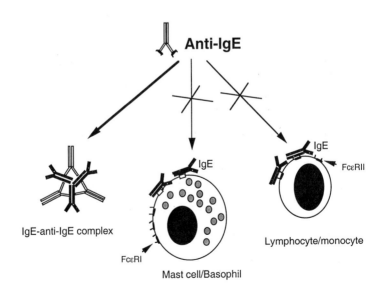

Figure 1 Mechanism of action of nonanaphylactogenic anti-IgE antibodies. Anti-IgE binds free IgE and small complexes can form. These are removed via the reticuloendothelial system. Anti-IgE does not bind IgE already bound to high- or low-affinity IgE receptors, and IgE effector cells are not activated (i.e., it is nonanaphylactogenic). (Modified with permission from Ref. 7.)

sured in 15 subjects receiving omalizumab intravenously. Treatment with omalizumab decreased free IgE levels to 1% of pretreatment levels and also resulted in a marked downregulation of FcεR1 on basophils; median receptor densities were approximately 220,000 receptors per basophil at baseline and fell to approximately 8300 receptors per basophil after 3 months of treatment (26). These data have important consequences for treatment with anti-IgE, because a reduction in IgE receptor density levels will magnify the functional consequences of a reduction in free IgE levels (Fig. 2).

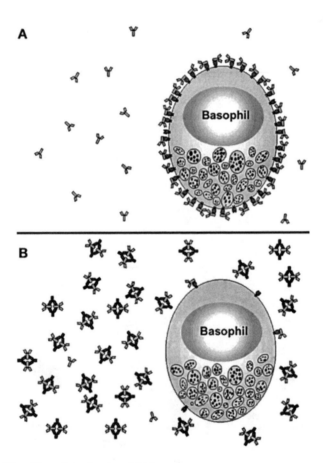

Figure 2 The effect of continual anti-IgE treatment on accumulation of IgE–anti-IgE immune complexes and the downregulation of FcεR1. (A) Normal relationships between free IgE, cell-bound IgE, and IgE receptor density. (B) The effect of anti-IgE treatment. Free IgE is complexed to anti IgE, IgE receptors on effector cells become "disarmed," and IgE receptor density on effector cells decreases. (From Ref. 7.)

B. Anti-IgE Treatment and the Risk of Parasitic Infections

IgE antibody has long been considered an important part of humoral immune defense against parasites (11). Recently, however, the role of IgE in host defense against parasitic infections such as *Schistosoma mansoni* has been debated, and some authors have suggested that the IgE plays a detrimental, rather than beneficial role for the host in parasitic diseases such as schistosomiasis (12–14). Support for this opinion comes from experiments in which mice pretreated with anti-IgE and then infected with *S. mansoni* show *a* reduction in the IgE response to the worm burden but improvement in clinical indicators of infection severity (e.g., a decrease in the number of hepatic granulomas) (13). Interestingly, however, the consequences of parasitic infection are worse if IgE is reduced by gene deletion rather than by antibody inhibition. For example, mice with a null mutation of the Cε gene, and thus incapable of making IgE, are significantly more susceptible to primary infection with *S. mansoni* and develop worm burdens twofold greater than those of wild-type mice (14). Taken together, these data suggest that the method of IgE reduction is important in determining the consequences in terms of risk of parasitic infections. The fact that parasitic infection is better tolerated by animals whose IgE is reduced by antibody treatment than by gene deletion suggest that IgE–anti-IgE complexes may be beneficial. This concept has been raised by Chang (7), who notes that IgE–anti-IgE complexes are not large, are cleared more slowly from the circulation than IgE, and may retain their capacity to interact with antigen. Therefore, these complexes may serve as a reservoir of IgE antibody capable of neutralizing parasitic antigens (Fig. 1).

To date, the safety data from patients treated with omalizumab have not suggested any increased liklihood of parasitic infection, but it will be prudent to maintain vigilance about this possible side effect until larger numbers of patients in more diverse settings are treated.

C. Anti-IgE and the Risk of an Autoimmune Response

The concern that anti-IgE may provoke an immune response is generic to all protein therapeutics, but is considerably reduced by the "humanization step" in the engineering of anti-IgE molecules (15,16). Precursor antibodies to omalizumab were generated in mice, and "humanization" of these murine antibodies involves selective removal of murine residues not essential for binding of the antibody to IgE (15). Omalizumab contains less than 5% murine residues and is thus rendered nonimmunogenic. In addition, although omalizumab has an IgG1 kappa structural framework, it does not fix complement. Clinical studies of omalizumab have been vigilant in testing for antibody responses to omalizumab. However, such antibodies against omalizumab have not been detected in studies of over 1500 patients where the drug has been administered parenterally (17–22). Interestingly, the aerosol route of administration may be more immunogenic than the intravenous or subcutaneous route, because aerosolized omalizumab treatment in 20 patients was associated with development of an antibody to rhuMAb-E25 in one patient (23).

As mentioned above, omalizumab does not bind to the vacant CH3 domain cell bound IgE, but omalizumab can bind to the vacant CH3 domain on IgE bound to omalizumab (7) (Fig. 1). The result is that each IgE molecule can be bound by two omalizumab molecules, and IgE–anti-IgE complexes can form (Fig. 1). Fortunately, omalizumab-IgE complexes are of limited size (1 million MW or smaller) (24,25), and studies in cynomolgous monkeys indicate that these relatively small complexes do not accumulate in any body organs, including the kidney (25). To date, immune complex–mediated complications from omalizumab treatment have not been reported in human studies and seem unlikely to occur based on the in vitro and animal data described above.

III. Dose Selection of Anti-IgE

To achieve therapeutic efficacy with nonanaphylactogenic anti-IgE antibodies, it is necessary to use a dose that greatly decreases IgE levels. The experiments of MacGlashan and colleagues (26) help explain this feature of the anti-IgE treatment strategy. First, FcεR1 densities on basophils from allergic and nonallergic persons range from 10^4 to 10^6 per cell, and several hundred thousand IgE receptors are usually occupied with IgE (26). Second, only about 2000 IgE molecules are required for a half-maximal release of histamine from basophils exposed to specific allergen (27). This explains why anything less than near complete suppression of IgE levels will allow sufficient IgE binding to FcεR1 for full basophil activation. Thus, a little IgE goes a long way, and anti-IgE dosing for therapeutic efficacy will need to reduce IgE levels below a threshold value low enough to prevent IgE effector cell activation. From a practical therapeutic standpoint, this means that anti-IgE dosing needs to be individualized to a patient's total IgE level, and IgE levels on treatment need to undetectable, or nearly so.

The important variables in determining the dose of anti-IgE necessary to reduce IgE to below the level of detection are: antibody affinity for IgE, patient weight (volume of distribution), and patient baseline IgE level. The dosing formula was refined several times during the course of the early phase testing of omalizumab as additional data from clinical trials became available. These data indicate that consistent suppression of IgE to levels below detectable requires omalizumab concentrations significantly in excess of IgE levels (initial omalizumab:IgE ratio of 10:1–15:1) (20). These data also indicate that omalizumab is just as effective when administered subcutaneously as intravenously (20). Therefore, omalizumab is now administered subcutaneously and the dose required per 4-week interval is calculated according to the following formula: 0.016 mg × weight (kg) × IgE level (IU/mL). If the calculated dose per 4-week interval is greater than 300 mg, then the dosing is divided so that subjects receive 225, 300, or 375 mg every 2 weeks (21).

IV. Clinical Studies of Omalizumab in Asthma

A. Phase 1 Studies of Efficacy

The effects of omalizumab treatment on the lower airway responses to aerosolized allergen challenge in asthmatic subjects was studied in two clinical trials (28,29).

In both studies a baseline allergen challenge was followed by intravenous omalizumab or placebo for approximately 9 weeks, and the response to treatment was assessed by the effects on the early or late phase response to allergen or both. In both of these studies omalizumab treatment was associated with a significant attenuation of the early phase response. The change in the allergen PC15 was nearly three doubling doses, with evidence for a slightly greater effect 77 days after treatment initiation than 27 days after treatment initiation (28). Omalizumab treatment was also associated with a 60% attenuation of the late phase response (Fig. 3), which was statistically significant (29).

These clinical studies of the effects of omalizumab on lower airway response to allergen confirmed a suspected role for IgE in mediating the early phase response

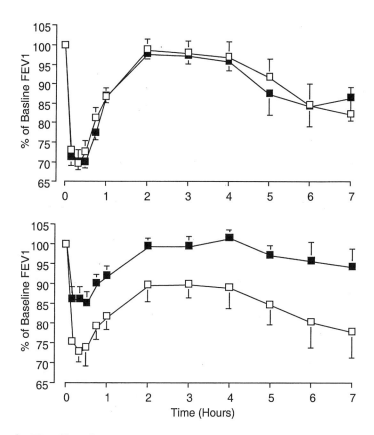

Figure 3 The effect of anti-IgE on the early and late phase response to inhaled allergen. The graph shows the FEV_1 as a percent of baseline in the first hour after allergen challenge (early phase response), and from 2 to 7 hours after allergen challenge (late phase response) in the placebo (top panel)–and omalizumab (lower panel)–treated groups at baseline (open squares) and at the end of treatment (closed squares). Omalizumab treatment significantly attenuated both the early and late phase responses. (From Ref. 29.)

to allergen and demonstrated for the first time that IgE is also an important mediator of the late phase response to allergen. Because inhibition of allergen-induced airway responses has proven to be a good indicator of efficacy in improving asthma control in clinical trials, these data provided the rationale for proceeding to phase 2 and phase 3 multicenter trials to test the effects of omalizumab on outcomes measuring asthma control.

B. Phase 2 Study of Efficacy

One large phase 2 study of the efficacy and safety of omalizumab for the treatment of asthma was a multicenter trial conducted in North America (17). The asthma population targeted was patients with persistent symptoms despite treatment with inhaled corticosteroids. In addition, all patients were required to have at least one positive skin test response to an aeroallergen. Three hundred and seventeen subjects between the ages of 11 and 50 years were enrolled. Subjects were classified as having moderate persistent or severe persistent asthma based on symptom scores and an average $FEV_1\%$ predicted of $\sim 70\%$. The study drug was administered intravenously every 2 weeks. There were three treatment groups: high-dose omalizumab (5.8 µg/kg of body weight/ng of IgE), low-dose omalizumab (2.5 µg/kg of body weight/ng of IgE), and placebo. A simplified schematic of the study design is shown in Figure 4. The primary outcome variable was a summary score based on asthma symptoms. Following a run-in period, omalizumab treatment or placebo was added to the subjects' ongoing treatment with inhaled or oral corticosteroids. After 12 weeks of adjunctive treatment with study drug, subjects entered an 8-week period in which inhaled or oral steroids were tapered while continuing treatment with study drug.

Omalizumab treatment was associated with mild to moderate urticaria in a small subgroup of subjects, but none of the subjects developed antibodies against omalizumab. The average symptom score in the high-dose treatment group decreased

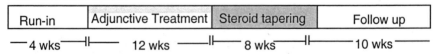

Phase 2 study design

Run-in	Adjunctive Treatment	Steroid tapering	Follow up
— 4 wks —‖—	12 wks —‖—	8 wks —‖—	10 wks —

Phase 3 study design

Run-in	Adjunctive Treatment	Steroid tapering
— 4 wks —‖—	16 wks —‖—	12 wks —

Figure 4   Simplified schematic showing the basic trial design for the phase 2 and phase 3 clinical trials of omalizumab.

from a mean of 4.1 $\pm$ 0.1 to 2.8 $\pm$ 0.1; in the low-dose group the change was similar (4.0 $\pm$ 0.1 to 2.8 $\pm$ 0.1). The average symptom score in the placebo group also declined (4.1 $\pm$ 0.1 to 3.1 $\pm$ 0.1), but the changes in the active groups were significantly greater. Although statistically significant, the effects of omalizumab on symptoms in this study were unimpressive. Also unimpressive were the effects of omalizumab on FEV_1. The absolute improvement in FEV_1 at the end of adjunctive treatment was 1.9% in the high-dose group, 2.1% in the low-dose group, and 1.0% in the placebo group. More impressive were the changes seen in secondary outcomes, such as asthma exacerbation rates and the effects of omalizumab as a steroid-sparing agent. For example, the rates of asthma exacerbations in the high- and low-dose treatment groups during the 20-week treatment period was 20 and 28%, respectively, compared to 45% in the placebo group. This was accompanied by significant improvement in quality-of-life scores in the active treatment groups. In addition, although not statistically significant, there were trends for the omalizumab-treated groups to have greater reductions in inhaled steroid use during the 8-week steroid-tapering phase. Perhaps because of the greater effects of omalizumab on these outcomes than on symptoms, there was a change in primary outcome as the clinical development of omalizumab advanced into phase 3. For the phase 3 trials, the primary efficacy outcome chosen was asthma exacerbation rate.

C. Phase 3 Studies of Efficacy

To date, two phase 3 multicenter trials in adults have been reported: one from Europe (18) and one from the United States (21). In addition, one phase 3 multicenter trial in children (age 6–12) has recently been reported from North America (22). Unlike the phase 2 trial in which omalizumab was administered intravenously, omalizumab was administered subcutaneously in all of these phase 3 trials.

Phase 3 Trials in Adults

In the phase 3 trials in adults the upper age limit was extended to 75 years from the 45 year cut-off used in the phase 1 and 2 trials. Otherwise, entry criteria were similar to those used in the phase 2 trials. Both phase 3 studies had the same design, summarized in Figure 4, and both studies enrolled approximately 500 subjects each. The design is similar to the phase 2 design except that the duration of the active treatment periods was lengthened. Also, the 10-week follow-up period in the phase 2 design was eliminated in favor of open-label extension periods. The principal outcome in these studies was the number of asthma exacerbations per subject during the adjunctive and steroid-tapering phases of treatment. Asthma exacerbation was defined as a worsening of asthma symptoms severe enough to require treatment with oral or intravenous corticosteroids or a doubling of baseline inhaled steroid dose.

There were no significant adverse events attributable to omalizumab in either of the studies. Urticaria, which had been reported in some subjects in the phase 2 trial, was not reported in these trials, perhaps because of differences in the dosing schedule and route of delivery. The results of the two adult studies were remarkably similar. In both studies the number of asthma exacerbations per subject in the omali-

Table 1 Primary Outcome Data for Phase 3 Trials of Omalizumab

	Stable steroid phase			Steroid reduction phase		
	Placebo	Omalizumab	*p*-value	Placebo	Omalizumab	*p*-value
European study						
Mean no. of exacerbations per subject	0.66 (0.49–0.83)	0.28 (0.15–0.41)	<0.001	0.75 (0.58–0.92)	0.36 (0.24–0.48)	<0.001
U.S. study						
Mean no. of exacerbations per subject	0.54	0.28	0.006	0.66	0.39	0.003

Data for the European study represents the mean and 95% confidence interval (18); for the U.S. study the mean of the data only is presented, because the publication did not provide any estimates of the variance (21).

zumab-treated groups was approximately half that of the subjects in the placebo-treated groups (Table 1). The effects on other outcomes such as the reduction in use of inhaled corticosteroid use (Fig. 5) and rescue medication use were also statistically and clinically significant.

The effects of omalizumab on FEV_1 in the adult phase 3 trials were slightly greater than those seen in the phase 2 trial but remained of questionable clinical significance. Interestingly, the effects of omalizumab on morning peak flow rates were relatively greater than the effects on FEV_1. For example, Busse et al. (21) reported that morning PEF increased from 320 to 335 L/min from baseline to end of study in the omalizumab-treated group, whereas morning PEF remained at approximately 300 L/min in the placebo-treated group.

Phase 3 Trial in Children

The single phase 3 study in children that has been reported is a North American study that enrolled 334 subjects (22). The design of this study is identical to that of the two phase 3 studies in adults (Fig. 4). The principal outcome in this pediatric study is not clearly stated in the manuscript. Steroid reduction and asthma exacerbation both appear to be given equal weight as outcomes in the methods and results sections.

Entry criteria for this pediatric study were different to the adult studies. Whereas the adults needed to be symptomatic despite treatment with inhaled or oral steroids, the children enrolled in the phase 3 study needed to have stable asthma on their current steroid treatment regimen. As a result, the asthma severity in these children was not as severe in the adults enrolled in phase 3. For example, although the $FEV_1\%$ predicted ranged from 50 to 120% in the children, the average FEV_1 was ~85%; in the adult studies the average $FEV_1\%$ predicted was ~70% predicted. In addition, whereas only 20% of placebo treated subjects in the adult phase 3 studies

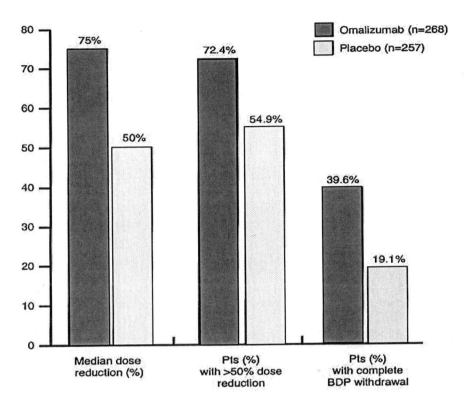

Figure 5 Effect of omalizumab on inhaled corticosteroid use in asthmatic subjects. The graph shows that omalizumab allowed a greater decrease in ICS use than placebo. The data are from the phase 3 trial of omalizumab in North America. (From Ref. 21.)

were able to withdraw steroid completely during the steroid tapering phase, 50% of the children in the phase 3 trial were able to do so.

Despite these differences in asthma severity between adults and children in the phase 3 studies of omalizumab, the effect of omalizumab on asthma exacerbation rate in children was similar to that observed in adults. Asthma exacerbation per child in the omalizumab-treated group were approximately half that of the placebo-treated group. This was especially evident during the steroid withdrawal phase of the trial. In addition, steroid dose reduction was significantly greater in the children treated with omalizumab, just as it was in adults. In contrast, with regard to asthma symptom scores, morning peak flow rates, and spirometry outcomes (FEV$_1$, FVC, and FEF25–75), omalizumab treatment in children was no more effective than placebo. This was true during both the stable steroid phase and the steroid-tapering phase of treatment. Despite a lack of effect on these outcomes, the investigators' global evaluation of effectiveness favored omalizumab over placebo. In addition, the mean number of days missed from school was lower in the omalizumab-treated group than the placebo-treated group (0.65 vs. 1.21 school days, $p = 0.04$). Importantly, omalizumab treatment was well tolerated. There were with no adverse events suggestive of serum sickness or immune complex formation.

V. Effect of Anti-IgE Treatment on Airway Responsiveness and Airway Inflammation

Methacholine reactivity was a secondary outcome variable in the two phase 1 studies that were designed to examine the effect of omalizumab on airway responses to allergen. One of the studies showed a statistically significant but modest improvement in methacholine PC_{20} by day 76 after treatment initiation (1); in the other study the baseline methacholine PC_{20} did not change significantly, but a significant attenuation in allergen-induced worsening in methacholine reactivity was observed (2). A recent report by Rabe et al. (30) suggests that large effects of anti-IgE on non-specific airway hyperreactivity should not be expected. These investigators found that a non-anaphylactogenic anti-IgE monoclonal antibody inhibited allergen-induced contraction of passively sensitized human bronchial rings but had no effect on histamine responsiveness of these sensitized rings. They concluded that "allergen responses in sensitized human airways are dependent on IgE levels in the sensitizing serum while nonspecific (hyper)responsiveness depends on serum factors other than IgE" (30). At present, because methacholine reactivity was not an outcome in the large phase 2 and phase 3 studies, there are insufficient data to make any conclusions about the effects of omalizumab on nonspecific airway reactivity.

To date there is also little information about the effects of omalizumab on airway inflammation. Omalizumab decreases allergen-induced airway eosinophilia, as assessed by analysis of eosinophils in induced sputum (29). In addition, omalizumab decreases blood eosinophil percentages (29). Apart from these effects, relatively little is known about the effects of omalizumab on outcomes of inflammation or remodeling in the airway.

VI. Summary and Conclusions

Omalizumab has been engineered as a therapeutic anti-IgE antibody that decreases free IgE in blood without causing anaphylaxis. Several aspects of the design of omalizumab, including its binding characteristics and the humanization steps, provide good examples of how careful design of monoclonal antibodies can maximize their efficacy and minimize their side effects. In clinical trials, omalizumab was first shown to decrease allergen-induced bronchoconstriction during both the early and late phase responses to inhaled allergen. These results prompted phase 2 and 3 clinical trials of its effects on other outcomes including asthma symptoms, asthma exacerbation rates, corticosteroid use, pulmonary function, and quality of life. The data from these clinical trials show that the main efficacy of omalizumab in both adults and children is in preventing asthma exacerbations. Another important effect is that omalizumab is steroid sparing. Surprisingly, the effects of omalizumab on these outcomes are not accompanied by large effects on other outcomes such as asthma symptoms or airflow obstruction. Our experience with inhaled corticosteroids would have led us to expect that a drug with large effects on asthma exacerbation rates would also have large effects on symptoms and pulmonary function. To date, the experience with omalizumab is that this is not the case. Nevertheless, the effect of omalizumab on asthma exacerbations is very important, because much of the cost of asthma management is attributable to the costs associated with the treatment of asthma exacerbations (31,32).

It is still too early to predict the efficacy of omalizumab in asthma relative to the efficacy of other asthma controller medications. The anti-IgE approach to asthma treatment has several advantages, however, including concomitant treatment of other IgE-mediated disease including allergic rhinitis (19), a favorable side effect profile (so far), and a dosing frequency that can be as low as once monthly. The disadvantages of anti-IgE treatment are those generic to recombinant protein therapeutics and include relatively high cost and requirement for injection therapy. In terms of cost, the cost of omalizumab will be offset at least in part by cost savings attributable to omalizumab's effects in reducing costs associated with asthma exacerbations.

To date the clinical trials of omalizumab have shown that it is superior to placebo for many clinical outcomes. The next phase of clinical trials will be comparisons of omalizumab with currently available asthma treatments, especially inhaled corticosteroids. Only when data from these comparative studies are available will it be possible to determine the place of omalizumab in treatment guidelines for asthma.

References

1. Church MK, Holgate ST, Shute JK, Walls AF, Sampson AP. Most cell-derived mediators. In: Middleton E, Reed CE, Ellis EF, Adkinson NF, Yuninger JW, Busse WW, eds. Allergy Principles and Practices, 5th ed. St. Louis: Mosby-Year Book, Inc., 1998: 146–167.
2. Sutton BJ, Gould HJ. The human IgE network. Nature 1993; 366:421–428.
3. Campbell AM, Vignola AM, Chanez P, Godard P, Bousquet P. Low affinity receptor for IgE on human bronchial epithelial cells in asthma. Immunology 1994; 82:506–508.
4. Sears MR, Burrows B, Flannery EM, Herbison GP, Hewitt CJ, Holdaway MD. Relation between airway responsiveness and serum IgE in children with asthma and in apparently normal children. N Engl J Med 1991; 325(15):1067–1071.
5. Burrows B, Martinez FD, Halonen M, Barbee RA, Cline MG. Association of asthma with serum IgE levels and skin-test reactivity to allergens. N Engl J Med 1989; 320(5): 271–277.
6. Davis FM, Gossett LA, Pinkston KL, Liou RS, Sun LK, Kim YW, Chang NT, Chang TW, Wagner K, Bews J, Brinkmann V, Towbin H, Subramanian N, Heusser C. Can anti-IgE be used to treat allergy? Springer Semin Immunopathol 1993; 15:51–73.
7. Chang TW. The pharmacological basis of anti-IgE therapy. Nat Biotechnol 2000; 18: 157–163.
8. Jardieu P. Anti-IgE Therapy. Curr Opin Immunol 1995; 7:779–782.

9. Presta L, Shields R, O'Connell L, Lahr S, Porter J, Gorman C, Jardieu P. The binding site on human immunoglobulin E for its high affinity receptor. J Biol Chem 1994; 269(42):26368–26373.

10. Haak-Frenscho M, Robbins K, Lyon R, Shields R, Hooley J, Schoenhoff M, Jardieu P. Administration of an anti-IgE antibody inhibits CD23 expression and IgE production in vivo. Immunology 1994; 82:306–313.

11. Finkelman FD, Pearce EJ, Urban JF, Sher A. Regulation and biological function of helminth-induced cytokine responses. Immunol Today 1991; (12):462–467.

12. Capron M, Capron A. Immunoglobulin E and effector cells in schistosomiasis. Science 1994; 264:1876–1877.

13. Amiri P, Haak-Frendscho M, Robbins K, McKerrow JH, Stewart T, Jardieu P. Anti-immunoglobulin E treatment decreases worm burden and egg production in *Schistosoma mansoni*-infected normal and interferon-γ knockout mice. J Exp Med 1994; 180:43–51.

14. King CL, Xiangli J, Malhotra I, Liu S, Mahmoud AAF, Oettgen HC. Mice with a targeted deletion of the IgE gene have increased worm burdens and reduced granulomatous inflammation following primary infection with schistosoma mansoni. J Immunol 1997; 158:294–300.

15. Heusser C, Jardieu P. Therapeutic potential of anti-IgE antibodies. Curr Opin Immunol 1997; 9:805–814.

16. Presta LG, Lahr SJ, Shields RL, Porter JP, Gorman CM, Fendly BM, Jardieu PM. Humanization of an antibody directed against IgE. J Immunol 1993; 151:2623–2632.

17. Milgrom H, Fick RB, Su JQ, Reimann J, Bush RK, Watrous ML, WJM. Treatment of allergic asthma with monoclonal anti-IgE antibody. N Engl J Med 1999; 341:1966–1973.

18. Soler M, Matz J, Townley R, Buhl R, O'Brien J, Fox H, Thirlwell J, Gupta N, Della Cioppa G. The anti-IgE antibody omalizumab reduces exacerbations and steroid require-ment in allergic asthmatics. Eur Respir J 2001; 18:254–261.

19. Adelroth E, Rak S, Haahtela T, Aasand G, Rosenhall L, OZ, Byrne A, Champain K, Thirlwell J, Della Ciolla G, Sandstrom T. Recombinant humanized mAb-E25, an anti-IgE, in birch pollen-induced seasonal allergic rhinitis. J Allergy Clin Immunol 2000; 106:253–259.

20. Casale T, Condemi J, Miller SD, Fick R, McAlary M, Fowler Taylor A, Gupta N, Rohane PW. rhuMAb-E25 in the treatment of seasonal allergic rhinitis (SAR) (abstr). Ann Allergy Asthma Immunol 1999;

21. Busse W, Corren J, Quentin Lanier B, McAlary M, Fowler-Taylor A, Della Cioppa G, van As A, Gupta N. Omalizumab, anti-IgE recombinant humanized monoclonoal anti-body, for the treatment of severe allergic asthma. J Allergy Clin Immunol 2001; 108: 184–190.

22. Milgrom H, Berger W, Nayak A, Gupta N, Pollard S, McAlary M, Fowler-Taylor A, Rohane P. Treatment of childhood asthma with anti-immunoglobulin E antibody (omalizumab). Pediatrics 2001; 108:e36.

23. Fahy JV, Cockcroft DW, Boulet LP, Wong HH, Deschesnes F, Davis EE, Adelman DC. Effect of aerosolized anti-IgE (E25) on airway responses to inhaled allergen in asthmatic subjects. Am J Respir Crit Care Med 1998; 157:A410.

24. Liu J, Lester P, Builder S, Shire SJ. Characterization od complex formation by human-ized anti-IgE antibody and monoclonal IgE. Biochemistry 1995; 34:10474–10482.

25. Fox JA, Hotaling TE, Struble C, Ruppel J, Bates DJ, Schoenhoff MB. Tissue distribution and complex formation with IgE of an anti-IgE antibody after intravenous administration in cynomolgous monkeys. J Pharmacol Exp Therapeut 1998; 279:1000–1008.

26. MacGlashan DW, Bochner BS, Adelman DC, Jardieu PM, Togias A, McKenzie-White J, Sterbinsky SA, Hamilton RG, Lichtenstein LM. Down-regulation of Fcε RI expression on human basophils during in vivo treatment of atopic patients with anti-IgE antibody. J Immunol 1997; 158:1438–1445.

27. MacGlashan DW. Releasability of human basophils; cellular sensitivity and maximal histamine release are independent variables. J Allergy Clin Immunol 1993; 91:605–615.

28. Boulet L-P, Chapman KR, Cote J, Kalra S, Bhagat R, Swystun VA, Laviolette M, Cleland LD, Deschesnes F, Su JQ, DeVault A, Fick RB, Cockcroft DW. Inhibitory effects of an anti-IgE antibody E25 on allergen-induced early asthmatic response. Am J Respir Crit Care Med 1997; 155:1835–1840.

29. Fahy JV, Fleming HE, Wong HH, Liu JT, Su JQ, Reimann J, Fick RB, Boushey HA. The effect of an anti-IgE monoclonal antibody on the early- and late-phase responses to allergen inhalation in asthmatic subjects. Am J Respir Crit Care Med 1997; 155: 1828–1834.

30. Rabe KF, Watson N, Dent G, Morton BE, Wagner K, H. M, Heusser CH. Inhibition of human airway sensitization by a novel monoclonal anti-IgE antibody, 17–9. Am J Respir Crit Care Med 1998; 157:1429–1435.

31. Weiss KB, Gergen PJ, Hodgson TA. An economic evaluation of asthma in the United States. N Engl J Med 1992; 326:862–866.

32. Barnes PJ. The costs of asthma. Eur Respir J 1996; 9:636–642.

44

Strategies to Reduce Excessive Mucus Secretion in Airway Inflammation

CHRISTOPHER EVANS and ANURAG AGRAWAL

Baylor College of Medicine
Houston, Texas, U.S.A.

BURTON F. DICKEY

M.D. Anderson Cancer Center
Baylor College of Medicine
Houston VA Medical Center
Houston, Texas, U.S.A.

Pathologists have long felt that obstruction of small airways by mucus hypersecretion is a major cause of airflow obstruction leading to asphyxic death in asthma (1–3). Clinicians, in contrast, generally pay scant attention to this aspect of the asthma phenotype. The discrepancy in emphasis between clinicians and pathologists probably relates to the physical evidence witnessed by each: in the emergency room, the clinician observes a patient struggling to breathe but producing little or no sputum, while at autopsy, the pathologist grossly observes mucus plugs that protrude from airways of the sectioned lung and microscopically observes occlusion of small airways by secreted mucus (Fig. 1). For the clinician, the role of mucus hypersecretion in obstructed diseases of the airways is further confused by the weak relation between airflow obstruction and the volume of expectorated sputum in COPD patients (4–7). However, expectorated sputum in COPD patients probably derives mostly from submucosal glands in the large airways. Excess mucus in large, central airways plays little role in airflow obstruction since it does not substantially reduce airway cross-sectional area, and in any case it can be cleared by expectoration. Instead, airflow obstruction in COPD is generally felt to be due to a combination of dynamic small airway collapse (emphysema), fixed small airway narrowing due to inflammation and fibrosis (respiratory bronchiolitis), and small airway occlusion by mucus secreted from epithelial goblet cells (4–7). Thus, the mucus the clinician sees is not the mucus that causes airflow obstruction. In mouse models of airway inflammation,

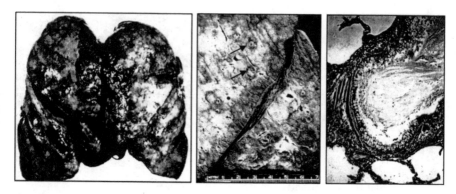

Figure 1   Airway obstruction by mucus hypersecretion in asthma. (Left). Lungs excised from a patient who died from status asthmaticus remain hyperinflated, rather than collapsing. (Center) The cut surface of the lung shows occlusion of multiple airways with mucus plugs (arrows). (Right) Photomicrograph of the lung shows the lumen of a small bronchiole filled with mucus and the airway wall and surrounding parenchyma infiltrated by inflammatory cells (hematoxylin and eosin staining, ×240). (Courtesy of Dr. James Hogg.)

mucus production in small airways is similarly a prominent feature of the histopathology (Fig. 2). While the critical role of mucus hypersecretion in the airflow obstruction that accompanies airway inflammation seems obvious from examination of pathological specimens, rigorous proof will require specific manipulation of this parameter through the use of drugs in mouse models and human disease or of genetic modification in mouse models.

In normal lungs, the airways are lined by a pseudo-stratified, ciliated columnar epithelial layer that performs both barrier and clearance functions. Interspersed sparsely throughout this layer are mucus-secreting goblet cells and submucosal glands (8). Under pathological conditions such as asthma, however, the airway epithelium undergoes dramatic morphological changes, resulting in the acquisition of a large number of mucus-containing goblet cells during a process called metaplasia. This is observed in humans with asthma and in animal models of asthma (Figs. 1 and 2), and many of the inflammatory mechanisms involved in metaplasia have recently been defined. Ultimately, then, goblet cell metaplasia results in the transition of the airway epithelium from predominantly Clara and ciliated cells to predominantly mucus-secreting cells. It is therefore likely that in coordination with the acquisition of the secreted products, the epithelium also synthesizes the exocytic machinery required for mucin secretion and the components of the signal transduction pathways needed to respond to extracellular secretagogues (Fig. 3). Aims of new therapies directed at blocking mucus hypersecretion can, therefore, be focused either on inhibition of mucus production or on inhibition of mucus secretion. Therapeutic targets can be identified by examining the pathways leading to expression of the regulated secretory phenotype and the action of secretion.

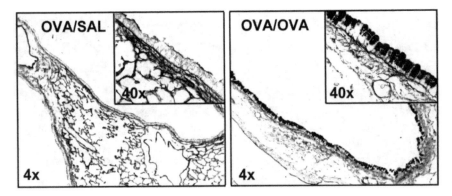

Figure 2 Secretory metaplasia of murine airway epithelium in response to allergic inflammation. BALB/c mice were sensitized by i.p. injection of 10 μg OVA and 2.25 mg alum once weekly for 4 weeks. One week after the last injection, animals were challenged once via 2.5% aerosol of ovalbumin in saline (OVA/OVA) or saline alone (OVA/SAL) for 30 minutes. Histopathological sections of mouse airways 4 days following saline challenge (left) show a normal, ciliated morphology. Airways from ovalbumin-challenged mice (right) display marked transformation of the airways from ciliated to secretory goblet cell morphology. Tissue sections were stained using the alcian blue–periodic acid Schiff technique.

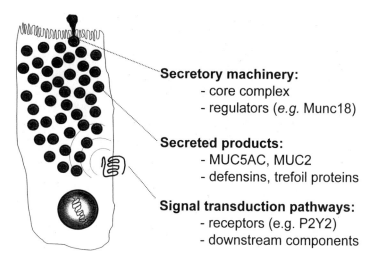

Figure 3 Molecular aspects of the regulated secretory phenotype in airway epithelial goblet cells. Airway epithelial cells that secrete mucus in response to external signals must express genes encoding secretory products (most prominently, mucins and antimicrobial polypeptides), components of signal transduction pathways going from surface receptors to the exocytic machinery, and components of the exocytic machinery itself.

I. Mucin

Mucus is a complex mixture of multiple glycoproteins, along with polypeptides thought to mediate microbial infection (e.g., defensins) and repair (e.g., trefoil peptides). The major glycoprotein components are encoded by mucin (or MUC) genes that fall into two broad categories: membrane-bound mucins and secreted mucins. Membrane-bound mucins have a large glycosylated extracellular domain, a helical transmembrane domain, and a short cytoplasmic tail. In the lungs, these include MUC1 and MUC4, although the latter has been shown to be alternatively spliced, yielding both membrane-bound and secreted forms (9,10). The extracellular domain of MUC1 serves as a binding site for *Pseudomonas aeruginosa* (11), while the cytoplasmic domain of MUC1 holds intrinsic tyrosine kinase activity and is capable of activating the mitogen-activated protein kinase ERK2 (12), which induces both interleukin (II)-1β and TNF-α. Thus, membrane-bound mucins may serve dually protective roles as dynamic traps for inhaled xenobiotics as well as initiators of early immune responses. Secreted mucins in normal lungs—namely, MUC2, MUC5AC, MUC5B, MUC7, and MUC8—aggregate on the lumenal surface of the airways where they create a viscoelastic barrier that traps particulates (including microbes) and allows for subsequent mucociliary clearance. Culture supernatants from *P. aeruginosa* are capable of inducing MUC2 and MUC5AC promoter activity and gene expression directly in airway epithelial cells in vitro via a tyrosine kinase–dependent pathway (13,14). It would be of particular interest then to test whether the upregulation of secreted mucins in response to pathogens or other particles is triggered by their initial ensnarement by membrane-bound mucins. Recently, much attention has been paid to MUC5AC and to MUC5B since these two mucins are major constituents of airway mucus, and they are upregulated in patients with asthma and in animal models of asthma (15,16). The transcriptional activity of these mucin genes may also be selectively controlled during development, and the same developmental mechanisms may also be invoked during inflammation. Future studies focusing on the production of goblet cells during development may thus provide insights regarding the molecular controls of goblet cell formation in the airways during inflammatory responses. This discussion focuses on the inflammatory mechanisms that underlie mucus production (i.e., mucin gene expression) and on the factors that control mucus hypersecretion during lung inflammation (i.e., exocytic stimuli and machinery).

II. Cytokine and Growth Factor Induction of Goblet Cell Metaplasia

Airway inflammation and mucus hypersecretion are key features of the airways of humans with asthma and of animal models of asthma. Over the last decade, the CD4 + helper T (Th) lymphocyte has become recognized as a central inflammatory cell mediating the development of allergic asthma (17). A growing amount of evidence indicates that the activity of a subpopulation of Th cells, Th2 cells, is vital to the development of the allergic asthma phenotype in animal models. Th2 cells develop from precursor Th cells in response to IL-4, while a divergent subpopulation of differentiated Th1 cells develop from the same pool of precursor cells in response to IL-12. The commitment of a precursor population into Th1 or Th2 cells is thus believed to be due primarily to the response of naive Th cells in *cis* to the cytokine milieu present at the time of differentiation. Polarization of a Th-cell population into a specific subtype is also controlled in *trans* because the secreted product of Th1 cells, interferon (IFN)-γ, inhibits Th2 cell differentiation and the secreted product of Th2 cells, IL-4, inhibits Th1-cell development. The Th1 pathway is preferentially induced in response to bacterial or viral infections, while the Th2 pathway is preferentially induced in response to allergen stimulation, although this paradigm is not without exceptions. Both Th1 and Th2 cells play important roles in the establishment of goblet cell metaplasia.

Th2 cells secrete the cytokines IL-4, IL-5, IL-9, and IL-13, and these are responsible for the development of various aspects of the allergic asthma phenotype in mice, including eosinophilic inflammation, airway hyperresponsiveness, and goblet cell metaplasia. Administration or transgenic overexpression of IL-4, IL-9, or IL-13 can induce goblet cell metaplasia and MUC5AC expression in vivo (16,18–27). In antigen-challenged animals, however, only IL-13 is essential, since goblet cell metaplasia still occurs in IL-4 and IL-9–deficient animals but does not occur when functional IL-13 signaling is removed (23,24,28,29). In transgenic animals that overexpress IL-5 in the lungs, goblet cell metaplasia occurs concurrently with airway hyperresponsiveness and inflammation (30). This effect of IL-5, however, is indirect, since exogenous administration of IL-5 does not induce goblet cell metaplasia in the absence of IL-4/IL-13 signaling (31), and IL-5–deficient Th2 cells still induce metaplasia in the lungs of IL-5-/-animals (32). Thus, the Th2 cytokines IL-4, IL-9, and IL-13, but not IL-5, induce goblet cell metaplasia in the airways during allergic inflammation, and IL-13 is essential for this process.

While the important pathways involved in Th2-mediated goblet cell metaplasia have been well defined, the ability of Th1 cells to act both as suppressors of Th2-mediated metaplasia and as independent initiators of goblet cell metaplasia is more complex. In the context of Th2-mediated responses, such as allergen challenge, Th1 cells inhibit goblet cell metaplasia (33). This effect is mediated by the release of IFN-γ by Th1 cells, since Th1 cells do not inhibit Th2-induced goblet cell metaplasia in IFN-γ receptor–deficient animals. In the absence of Th2-mediated inflammation, however, Th1 cells induce goblet cell metaplasia in IFN-γ receptor–deficient mice but not in wild-type mice (33). Thus, IFN-γ release by Th1 cells suppresses both Th2- and Th1-induced goblet cell metaplasia. The precise inhibitory role of IFN-γ on metaplasia remains unknown. It appears to involve effects on both inflammatory cell and epithelial cell function. Pulmonary viral infections and exposure to ozone, in both humans and animals, are associated with Th1 lymphocyte and neutrophil inflammation and with excess mucus production. Neutrophils, through neutrophil elastase, are potent inducers of goblet cell metaplasia (34,35). Thus, the protective effects of Th1 cytokines observed under allergic conditions may not be relevant in the context of pulmonary infections.

Recent studies have defined an essential component of the epidermal growth factor system for the induction of goblet cell metaplasia. Both in vitro and in vivo, EGF receptor ligands, such as transforming growth factor-α (TGF-α), induce goblet cell metaplasia, and these responses are inhibited by pretreatment with a selective EGF receptor tyrosine kinase inhibitor (36). In rats, intranasal administration of IL-13 induces goblet cell metaplasia, and this response is inhibited by blockade of EGF receptor signaling (26). In addition, incubation of human airway epithelial cell cultures with supernatants from activated eosinophils also causes mucus production in an EGF receptor–mediated fashion (37). Since the abilities of both IL-13 and activated eosinophils to induce goblet cell metaplasia are dependent on EGF receptor signaling (reviewed in detail below), it appears that an important mechanism for goblet cell metaplasia during airway inflammation is signal transduction through the EGF pathway. Thus, activation of the EGF receptor by ligands such as TGF-α during inflammation may serve as a master regulator in the development of goblet cell metaplasia.

In summary, there are multiple cytokine pathways that mediate the development of airway goblet cell metaplasia in animal models of asthma, which may pertain to the pathogenesis of the human disorder. The effects of individual cytokines on goblet cell metaplasia can be dissected independently, but it is obvious that there are several points of overlap where multiple signaling pathways converge at some fundamental terminus to induce metaplasia. Humans are exposed to a variety of inhaled stimuli that provoke mucus production. The immune responses evoked by these stimuli will vary depending on their source, but the resulting increase in mucus production may involve overlapping fundamental mechanisms. An understanding of these basic mechanisms involved in metaplasia will have wide applications for the treatment of asthma and other airway diseases that involve mucus hypersecretion.

III.   Signal Transduction Pathways Involved in Secretory Metaplasia

IL-4, IL-9, and IL-13 elicit responses by binding to heterodimeric cytokine receptors. The receptor (R) complexes for IL-4 include pairings between IL-4Rα and the common γc chain or between IL-4Rα and IL-13Rα1 (Fig. 4; 38). IL-9 binds to a specific IL-9R receptor that dimerizes with γc (39), while IL-13 binds to the IL-13Rα1/IL-4Rα complex described for IL-4 (40) and also to a IL-13Rα1/IL-13Rα2 complex (41). All of these cytokine receptors lack intrinsic tyrosine kinase activity, despite the fact that the intracellular domains of each contain tyrosine residues that are phosphorylated upon stimulation. Rather, the phosphorylation events evoked by stimulation are mediated by Janus kinase (JAK) proteins (42). JAK1 and JAK3 bind to the IL-4Rα and γc chains, respectively, and another JAK protein, TYK2, associates with IL-13Rα1 (43). Stimulation by IL-4 or IL-13 results in the transactivation of these JAKs, followed by their subsequent phosphorylation of the intracellular domains of IL-4Rα and IL-13Rα1. The result of these phosphorylation events is the activation of several stimulatory signaling pathways that include signal trans-

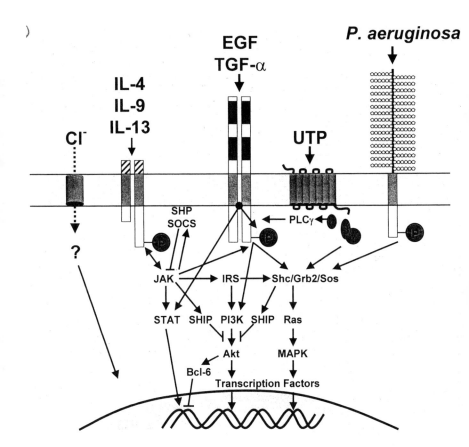

Figure 4 Signal transduction pathways controlling secretory metaplasia. Development of goblet cell metaplasia is controlled by the effects of multiple receptor signal transduction mechanisms, including calcium-activated chloride channels (Gob-5), Th2 cytokine receptors (IL-9R, IL-4Rα, and IL-13Rα1), EGF receptors, G protein–coupled receptors (GPCRs), and membrane-bound mucins (MUC1), which result in altered expression of genes encoding mucins, the secretory machinery, and cell cycle regulators. (*From left to right*) The precise role of Cl⁻ influx through the Gob-5 channel is not yet known. Binding of IL-4, IL-9, and IL-13 to their appropriate receptor heterodimers results in activation of stimulatory JAK/STAT and IRS signaling pathways and inhibitory SOCS and SHIP/SHP phosphatase pathways. EGF receptor activation by the ligands EGF and TGF-α stimulate intrinsic receptor tyrosine kinase activity that activates STATs, PI3K, Shc/Ras-MAPK, and SHIP/SHP phosphatase pathways, while in the absence of ligand, EGF receptors can also be activated by JAKs and GPCR activity. GPCR activation by ligands such as UTP activates PLC-γ through their α subunits and Shc/Ras-MAPK through their βγ subunits. *Pseudomonas aeruginosa* binding to the extracellular domain of MUC1 results in tyrosine phosphorylation and activation of Shc/Ras-MAPK pathways.

ducer and activator of transcription (STAT)-6 (44,45) and insulin receptor substrate (IRS)-1 and 2 (46). IL-9 signaling is also mediated by JAK/STAT proteins, but in this case STAT1, STAT3, and STAT5 are activated by JAK1 (39,47). Since IL-9 receptor signaling is not critical for goblet cell metaplasia in animal models of allergic asthma (48), signaling by these STATs may be either promiscuously activated by other signaling mechanisms or may indeed not be required for goblet cell metaplasia. One point of overlap among IL-4, IL-9, and IL-13 signals may be the activation of the calcium-activated chloride channel Gob-5, which was recently uncovered through subtraction library screening (49) and later found to be induced by Th2 cytokines (50). IL-13 binding to the IL-13Rα1/IL-13Rα2 complex is not well characterized, though some data suggest that this complex functions in an inhibitory manner to dampen the effects of IL-13 (41,51).

Several studies investigating the roles of IL-4 and IL-13 in allergic asthma have clearly demonstrated that IL-4Rα signaling through the STAT6 pathway is required for goblet cell metaplasia (23,24,27,31,32,52–54). Upon phosphorylation by JAK1, STAT6 homodimerizes and is translocated to the nucleus, where it binds to specific DNA-recognition sites. STAT6 signaling is required for the development of TH2 cells and goblet cell metaplasia (31,52), and STAT6 signaling by cells of non–T-lymphocyte lineage is also required for the development of goblet cell metaplasia (54). The IL-4Rα is expressed by human airway epithelial cells in culture (19), so it is very likely that STAT6 signaling by the airway epithelium is central to the development of goblet cell metaplasia.

IL-4Rα signaling is also mediated by non-JAK/STAT second messengers. In IL-4–responsive cells, IRS signaling pathways are induced by JAK1 simultaneously with STAT6, where they promote cellular growth, proliferation, and protein synthesis and prevent apoptosis. IRS-1/2 binds to the intracellular domain of IL-4Rα and subsequently activates phosphoinositol-3 (PI3) kinase and Ras-mitogen activated protein kinase (MAPK) signaling pathways (43). It is not known whether IL-4Rα–induced IRS and PI3 kinase activation are necessary for the initial development of goblet cell metaplasia. However, based on the effects of these in lymphocytes, they may be important for the maintenance of the mucous phenotype by either inducing the hyperproliferation of goblet cells or amplifying the effects of STAT6 activation.

Emerging data also draw attention to inhibitory signaling molecules that disrupt JAK/STAT signaling, such as suppressor of cytokine signaling-1 (SOCS-1), B-cell lymphoma gene-6 (BCL-6), SH2 domain–containing phosphatase-1 (SHP-1), and SH2-containing inositol phosphatase (SHIP) (43). SOCS family proteins are cytokine-induced inhibitors that bind to and inactivate the kinase activity of JAKs. SOCS1 (also called SSI-1) and SOCS3 inhibit IL-4–induced STAT6 signaling by targeting JAK1 (55). Inhibition of STAT6 DNA binding by SOCS1 is rapidly induced by IL-4 stimulation, indicating that these proteins may have an intrinsic dampening effect on STAT activation and immune function (55). Recent evidence also suggests that SOCS binding may serve to target JAKs for proteasomal degradation (56,57). These studies of SOCS function have demonstrated that SOCS1 is a potent inhibitor of lymphocytic IL-4Rα signaling. STAT6 function is also inhibited at its targets by the PI3K downstream target Bcl-6 (58), which binds to DNA sites recognized by STAT6 (59,60). Future studies addressing the roles of these in IL-4Rα signaling in airway epithelial cells may identify novel target genes for the inhibition of goblet cell metaplasia in the lungs.

Another suppressive mechanism for IL-4Rα signaling in lymphocytes is mediated by the activities of phosphatase enzymes (43). The SH2-containing phosphatase SHP-1 associates with the IL-4Rα cytoplasmic domain and markedly reduces IL-4 induced STAT6 activation and function in vitro (61,62), while the SH2-containing inositol phosphatase SHIP dephosphorylates the products of PI3 kinase activity and may lead to increased IL-4–induced cellular proliferation. It is not known whether these are important mediators of goblet cell metaplasia directly within the airway epithelium, but SHIP-/-mice demonstrate heightened B-lymphocyte proliferation in response to IL-4 (63,64). Thus, these phosphatase enzymes may act as inhibitors of goblet cell metaplasia, but the efficacy of such functions remains questionable.

As mentioned above, EGF receptor signaling is critical for the development of goblet cell metaplasia both in vitro and in vivo (36). The EGF receptor complex contains intrinsic tyrosine kinase activity (65). EGF receptor activation by ligands such as EGF and TGF-α results in the activation of several signaling cascades, including phospholipase C-γ (PLC-γ), Ras GTPases, STATs, and PI3 kinase (66,67). The complexity of EGF signaling is compounded by the finding that UTP signaling by P2Y2 heterotrimeric G protein–coupled receptors (GPCRs) (68,69) and cytokine signaling by the activated JAKs of heterologous cytokine receptors activate EGF receptor signals in the absence of EGF receptor ligand binding (67,70). EGF receptor activation results in tyrosine phosphorylation and recruitment of Shc, Grb-2, and son of sevenless (Sos) to the receptor, leading to the activation of Ras-MAPK signal transduction pathways and to increased cellular proliferation (66). In addition, EGF receptor activation also results in the activation of STATs 1, 3, and 5, but unlike the Th2 cytokine receptors, the EGF receptor does not require a JAK protein to activate STATs (71). The p85 subunit of PI3 kinase interacts with ligand-activated EGF receptors, and signaling through the PI3 kinase results in cellular proliferation and inhibition of apoptosis (66). An EGF receptor signaling pathway mediated by PLC-γ is also activated by EGF receptor ligands (72,73). PLCγ signaling may mediate changes in cell morphology (74), but it is not required for receptor activation or MAPK activation (75). The precise signaling cascade required for EGF receptor–mediated goblet cell metaplasia is unknown, but given the variety of signaling cascades associated with the EGF receptor, it is most likely a pleiotropic effect. The net result of these multiple signaling pathways is activation of transcription of the MUC5AC gene. Inhibition of EGF receptor signaling using selective antagonists of EGF receptor tyrosine kinase activity also prevents IL-4 and IL-13–induced goblet cell metaplasia and MUC5AC gene expression in animal models and in human airway epithelial cell lines (26,36). Thus, JAK activation by the IL-4Rα could activate intracellular signaling through the EGF receptor in airway epithelial cells. The complexity of EGF signaling underscores its possible importance as a master regulator for the induction of goblet cell metaplasia by proinflammatory cytokines. As such, the EGF signal transduction pathway may provide a universal target in response to allergic and non-allergic stimuli of goblet cell metaplasia.

IV. Control of Secretory Function

Numerous cell types in the airways contribute to the maintenance of the mucus layer by regulating the secretion of its serous and mucous components (76). In humans, the submucosal glands of the upper airways are responsible for the secretion of a low-viscosity serous product. Secretion by the submucosal glands is largely under autonomic control. The parasympathetic nerves of the vagi provide the dominant neural control of submucosal gland secretion by releasing acetylcholine onto muscarinic receptors, while tachykinergic neurons also exert excitatory effects on glandular secretions. The sympathetic and nonadrenergic-noncholinergic nerves inhibit submucosal gland secretion both directly and through inhibition of cholinergic activity. Glandular secretions are important for the maintenance of the mucus lining and for particulate clearance in the upper airways. However, in the small airways of patients with asthma, where goblet cell metaplasia and mucus plugs are found, there are no submucosal glands. Therefore, the mucus hypersecretion noticed pathologically is primarily the result of direct lumenal goblet cell secretion. Mouse airways distal to the trachea do not contain submucosal glands, and all airway mucus is secreted by surface epithelial cells (Fig. 5).

Airway goblet cells are capable of both constitutive and evoked (regulated) secretion, but unlike the submucosal glands, they are not under direct neural control. Several secretagogues that act directly on airway goblet cells have been recently

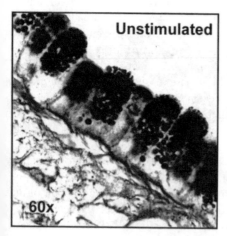 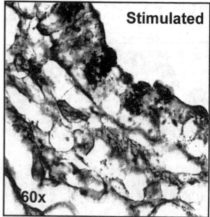

Figure 5 Induction of mucus secretion by airway goblet cells in antigen-challenged mice. Mice were sensitized and challenged as described in Figure 3. Four days after antigen challenge, mice were exposed to 100 mM ATP (stimulated) or 0.9% saline (unstimulated) via aerosol for 5 minutes. The airway goblet cells of unstimulated antigen challenged mice (left) are intact and contain numerous mucin-filled secretory granules, whereas the airway goblet cells of ATP-stimulated antigen-challenged animals (right) demonstrate reduced granule content.

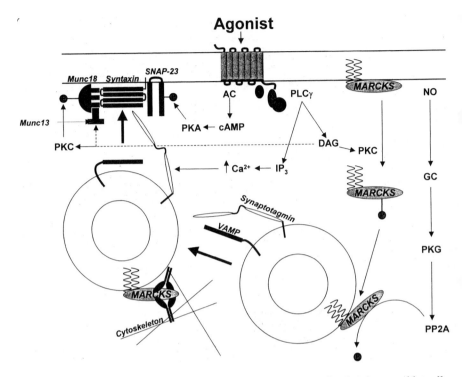

Figure 6 Signal transduction pathways controlling mucus secretion for airway goblet cells. Regulated secretion is stimulated by a variety of extracellular mediators, the majority of which stimulate GPCRs and result in the activation of multiple signal transduction pathways. The activated second messengers in turn activate regulatory kinases and phosphatases that act on vesicle-associated proteins (e.g., MARCKs) and the exocytic machinery (e.g., SNAREs and Munc18). The signal mechanisms for non–GPCR-interacting secretagogues are unknown.

identified. These include secreted inflammatory cell peptides and mediators, nucleotide triphosphates, eicosanoids, and bacterial products (Fig. 6). In addition to their roles as inducers of goblet cell metaplasia, many of these are also associated with increased mucus secretion. It is therefore difficult to delineate the amount of secretion that is due to increased goblet cell numbers (i.e., increased constitutive secretion) versus the amount of secretion that is due to an ability of these mediators to directly evoke goblet cell exocytosis in a regulated manner unless the actions of these mediators have been analyzed in vitro.

A. Inflammatory Peptide Signal Transduction Pathways Leading to Secretion

A variety of proteins secreted by inflammatory cells induce goblet cell secretion. Neutrophils secrete cathepsin G and elastase, both of which stimulate goblet cell secretion in vitro (77). Two possible mechanisms for this have been proposed. Neutrophil elastase may cleave the extracellular domains from membrane-bound mucins (78) and/or elastase may induce the secretion of soluble mucins from cytosolic granules (34). The precise mechanism for the latter effect is unknown (79). In antigen-challenged guinea pigs, degranulation of resident goblet cells is associated with early neutrophilic inflammation, and inhibition of neutrophil elastase prevents the goblet cell degranulation (80). Thus, neutrophil elastase may be a major stimulus for mucus secretion during acute allergic inflammatory responses. Both neutrophilia (81) and mucus hypersecretion (82) are found in the airways of patients who die from fatal asthma. In addition to their role in asthma, neutrophils and mucus hypersecretion also figure prominently in chronic obstructive pulmonary disease (COPD) and cystic fibrosis (CF). Thus, neutrophils and neutrophil elastase may be important mediators of mucus hypersecretion in response to a variety of pulmonary insults.

Eosinophils, which are recruited into the lungs of antigen-challenged animals and of allergic asthmatics during late phase inflammation, also secrete preformed proteins that stimulate mucus secretion. Eosinophils secrete cationic proteins from their cytosolic granules, and one of these, eosinophil cationic protein, stimulates mucus secretion from goblet cells in vitro (83). In addition eosinophils are a source of TGF-α, which increases goblet cell numbers and the levels of constitutive secretion of mucus (37). While eosinophils may not be required for the initial development of goblet cell metaplasia in allergic asthma, in the context of an airway that has already transformed into a mucous secretory phenotype, eosinophils may stimulate the secretion of mucus significantly.

Macrophages and monocytes appear also to be important mediators of mucus secretion in the lungs through the secretion of specific monocyte/macrophage mucus secretagogue proteins (84–87). Like neutrophils, macrophages are recruited and activated in the lungs in response to a variety of pathological stimuli and may therefore contribute to goblet cell hypersecretion in a variety of disease states, including asthma.

Activated mast cells are also found in the lungs of patients with allergic asthma and in the lungs of animal models of asthma. Mast cells are a source of several cell specific proteases. Among these, mast cell chymase (to a greater extent than histamine) is a potent secretagogue of submucosal gland secretion (88,89). Interestingly, the proteolytic activity of this enzyme is required for efficacious secretagogue function, indicating that secretion in response to mast cell chymase may be similar to that induced by neutrophil elastase. The direct effects of mast cell proteases on goblet cells remain unexplored, but a significant effect of mast cells on goblet cell function may be through prostanoid release (see below) (90).

While T lymphocytes are important for the establishment of goblet cell metaplasia in vivo, it is not known whether any secreted T-cell proteins induce goblet cell degranulation directly. Because of the central role that T lymphocytes play in mediating allergic responses and host responses to pathogens, though, they are essential for the induction of the effector inflammatory cell responses described above. Therefore, the importance of T lymphocytes lies in their coordination of the production of mucus in the airways and the coordination of inflammatory responses that lead to mucus hypersecretion.

In addition to peptides released by inflammatory cells, proinflammatory serum-derived proteins may also stimulate goblet cell secretion. For instance, the complement protein family is activated during inflammatory responses and may be important in the development of Th1 and Th2 responses in lymphoid tissues (91,92). Complement C3a and C5a receptors are found in airway smooth muscle cells and in airway epithelial cells (91). Complement C3a receptor–deficient mice fail to develop airway hyperreactivity (93). Although the precise effects on mucus secretion were not assessed in these studies, complement C3a is a potent mucus secretagogue that acts on airway cells independently of histamine and eicosanoid acitivities (94). C3a-induced mucus secretion in airway epithelial cells is not affected by dibutyryl-cAMP or by cycloheximide treatments, indicating that C3a induces exocytosis of preformed mucous granules possibly through the activation of a PLA_2 and intracellular Ca^{2+} transients (94). Thus, the direct activation of C3a during airway inflammation or injury may be a significant factor contributing to mucus hypersecretion in diseased lung states.

B. Nonpeptide Signal Transduction Pathways Leading to Secretion

While the variety of secreted proteins released by inflammatory cells is wide and (in most cases) specific for an individual cell type, common lipid-derived mediators that are generated in many different cell types and result from the phospholipase A_2 (PLA_2)–mediated metabolism of membrane phospholipids into arachadonic acid also affect goblet cell secretion. Prostaglandins (PGs) are synthesized through the cyclooxygenase (COX) pathways and can have either stimulatory or inhibitory effects on secretory function. PGD_2 (produced by mast cells and other leukocytes) and $PGF_{2\alpha}$ (produced by epithelial cells) enhance and induce goblet cell secretion, respectively (95–97). The epithelium is also a source of PGE_2, which inhibits goblet cell secretion (95,98). Leukotrienes (LTs) and hydroxyeicosatetraenoic acids (HETEs) are produced through the activity of lipoxygenase (LO) enzymes, and these are potent stimuli of mucus secretion (98,99). LTC_4 and LTD_4 are synthesized in mast cells, eosinophils, and macrophages, and they stimulate mucus secretion by acting on specific cys-LT receptors (100,101). 5-HETE (from neutrophils and macrophages) and 15-HETE (from epithelial cells and eosinophils) are also stimuli for mucus secretion in vitro (98,102). Finally, platelet-activating factor (PAF) is released by activity of PLA_2 on membrane-associated phosphatidylcholine resulting in the formation of lyso-PAF, which is subsequently alkylated, thereby forming PAF. PAF acts on specific G protein–coupled receptors (GPCRs), and it induces mucus secretion in vitro via a protein kinase C (PKC)–dependent pathway (103,104).

Recent evidence has demonstrated an importance of nucleotide and nucleoside signaling in mucus hypersecretion. Nucleotide triphosphates (NTPs), adenosine 5′-triphosphate (ATP), and uridine 5′-triphosphate (UTP) are potent goblet cell secretagogues in vivo and in vitro (105–107). Stimulation of P2Y2 (formerly called P2u) receptors by NTPs results in mucus secretion by goblet cells via PKC-dependent and Ca^{2+}-dependent pathways (106,108,109). Activated PKC phosphorylates the plasma membrane–associated myristoylated alanine-rich C kinase substrate (MARCKS), which translocates to the cytosol and interacts with mucus granules and cellular contractile machinery (109). To date, this model provides the most detailed mechanism of secretagogue signal transduction in relation to exocytic function. ATP is rapidly degraded in vivo, resulting in the formation of adenosine and 2'-deoxyadenosine. Adenosine is an important signaling molecule that acts on specific receptors (A1, A2a, A2b, and A3). Excess adenosine in the airways of mice that are deficient in the catalytic enzyme adenosine deaminase (ADA) results in dramatic inflammation despite complete lymphopenia (110). ADA deficiency is lethal, and the lungs of ADA knockout mice have severe goblet cell metaplasia and mucus plugging of the small airways. While is not known whether the effects of nucleotide and nucleoside signaling in an animal model are directly on airway epithelium or indirectly mediated by inflammatory cells, nucleotide and nucleoside signaling in the lungs clearly has significant effects on mucus secretion, and that will have important implications for the treatment of mucus hypersecretion in asthma.

Reactive oxygen species found both environmentally and endogenously are also involved in the secretory responses of goblet cells. Oxygen radicals produced by neutrophils and eosinophils can induce goblet cell secretion and epithelial cell damage (111). In vitro, exposure of airway epithelial cell cultures to ozone induces mucus secretion directly by a mechanism involving arachadonic acid metabolism and nitric oxide synthesis (112–118). Inhalation of ozone in vivo causes acute mucus secretion (119,120), and this effect is dependent both on arachadonic acid metabolites by the epithelium and on elastase released by neutrophils (121,122). There appear, then, to be both direct (epithelial) and indirect (inflammatory cell mediated) stimulatory effects of oxygen radicals on mucus secretion. Thus, understanding the basic mechanisms of inflammation and epithelial responses to oxygen radicals will provide the necessary clues for preventing oxidant-induced mucus hypersecretion.

C. Pathogens as Mucus Secretagogues

Bacterial and viral pathogens and their exoproducts also have the ability to induce mucus production and secretion (123–126). Several studies in adults and children have demonstrated that a majority of asthma exacerbations are associated with viral infections (127–131). Viral infections can induce both Th1- and Th2-mediated inflammatory responses depending on the strain of the virus and the atopic state of the host (132–135). Reports in both animals and humans have consistently demonstrated that allergic sensitization increases the severity and the duration of airway changes in response to viral infections (136,137). In mice, goblet cell metaplasia following antigen challenge is characterized by the presence of mucus-filled goblet cells, but when mice are infected with viruses concurrently, goblet cells in the airways secrete their mucus contents resulting in extracellular mucus lining the lumen of the small airways and depletion of stored intracellular mucus (138,139). These studies address an important issue regarding mucus hypersecretion and animal models of asthma in general. The development of goblet cell metaplasia in the airways in response to one stimulus, e.g., allergen exposure, may establish conditions in which subsequent inhalation of particles, antigens, or pathogens may trigger augmented mucus hypersecretory responsiveness.

V. Exocytic Machinery

The final step in the process of mucus secretion is the transport of mucin-containing granules to the plasma membrane, followed by membrane fusion and emptying of the granule contents into the airway lumen. This may happen constitutively (i.e., continuously) or may be triggered by secretagogues in the process of regulated secretion as described above. Recent evidence from a variety of biochemical and genetic approaches has revealed a conserved mechanism of exocytosis from yeast to man (140–142). The central components are SNARE proteins that are localized on transport vesicles (v-SNAREs, such as VAMP), as well as on the target (i.e., plasma) membrane (t-SNAREs, such as Syntaxin and SNAP-25). These bind tightly to each other, forming a parallel four-helix bundle known as the core complex. Tight coiling of the four helices brings together the opposing membranes, resulting in complete fusion. Additional proteins regulate these processes through a series of precisely orchestrated interactions. Among these, the interactions of Syntaxin with Munc18 and Munc13 constitute a particularly important cascade because absence of any one of these leads to a complete failure of neurotransmission (143–146).

The exocytic machinery of respiratory epithelium and goblet cells is not well defined. Three isoforms of Munc18 exist in mammals, of which Munc18–1 is predominantly neuronal, Munc18–2 is predominantly epithelial, and Munc18–3 is ubiquitous (147–149). Munc 18–2 interacts with Syntaxins-1, −2, and −3, of which Syntaxin-3 is most closely identified with epithelium (150,151), though Syntaxin-1 has also been demonstrated in respiratory epithelium (152). In intestinal and renal epithelial cells, the SNARE partners of Syntaxin 3 are SNAP-23 and VAMP-3 (150), but nothing is known of respiratory epithelium. Four isoforms of Munc13 exist in mammals, of which −1, −2, and −3 are exclusively neuronal. Munc13–4 is found ubiquitously and is strongly expressed in lung epithelium including goblet cells and type II alveolar epithelial cells (153). Rab3 proteins are exocytic isoforms of a large family of Ras-related GTPases that regulate vesicle traffic, and Rab3D is enriched in lung tissue and in type II cells (154) (unpublished observations).

Changes in the expression of exocytic proteins during airway epithelial metaplasia have not been previously studied. Since Munc18 has both an essential role in activating Syntaxin and an inhibitory effect by preventing Syntaxin's interaction with other SNARE proteins until Munc13 induces its dissociation, levels of Munc18 should be narrowly optimized for secretion. Indeed, levels of the Munc18 homolog in the fruitfly *Drosophila* correlate closely with secretory function (144), and stimulation of secretion by hyperosmotic challenge in pituitary cells leads to increased transcription of Munc18–1 (155). Antigen-induced airway metaplasia in mice is associated with increased expression of RNA encoding Munc18–2, but not Munc18–1 or Munc18–3 (unpublished observations). These changes are abolished in IL-4Rα-/-mice that have a signaling defect for both IL-4 and IL-13, consistent with the roles of IL-4 and IL-13 in airway metaplasia (see above). The murine Munc18–2 promoter contains a binding site for the STAT-6 transcription factor (156), which is a key effector of signaling by IL-4 and IL-13 (44,45), as described above. A diagrammatic representation of the Munc18–2 gene and promoter, illustrating binding sites for STAT-6 and other transcription factors of importance in inflammation such as GATA-binding proteins and the glucocorticoid receptor, is shown in Fig. 7. In summary, components of the exocytic machinery are probably regulated directly by the same factors that are known to induce mucin production and airway metaplasia.

Exocytic regulatory proteins are in turn regulated by upstream intracellular signaling pathways, and are thus linked to secretory stimuli (157–160). For example, PKC phosphorylates multiple components of the exocytic machinery including Munc18, SNAP-25, Synaptotagmin, and Syntaxin (161). Phosphorylation of Munc18 reduces its affinity for Syntaxin and may reduce its inhibitory effect when overexpressed (162). Phorbol esters and diacylglycerol bind and activate Munc13, stimulating exocytosis (163). Ca^{2+}/calmodulin-dependent protein kinase II (CaMKII) phosphorylates Synaptotagmin, a calcium sensor that regulates docking and fusion (164). SNAP-25 is phosphorylated by cAMP-dependent protein kinase (PKA) and can also

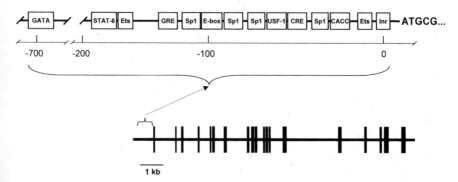

Figure 7 Structure of the Munc 18–2 structural gene and its promoter region. Munc 18 levels are thought to correlate closely with secretory capacity. A schematic diagram of the 19 exon (vertical bars) Munc 18–2 gene is shown along with the 700 bp region upstream of exon 1 that has full promoter activity. The Munc 18–2 promoter contains binding sites for transcription factors associated with airway inflammation and goblet cell metaplasia, such as STAT-6, GATA-binding proteins, glucocorticoid receptor (GRE), and cAMP response element–binding protein (CRE). Sites for binding the pro-inflammatory transcription factors Ets-1 and USF-1, constitutive transcription factors SP1 and Inn, and generic binding sites such as E-box and CACC box are also shown. Vertical bars represent exons, and the connecting lines are introns.

function like a calcium sensor (165,166). SNARE kinase (SNAK) phosphorylates the t-SNARE, SNAP-23, and enhances the kinetics of SNARE complex assembly (167).

VI. Therapeutic Targets

To address therapeutic intervention, it is convenient to conceptually divide airway mucus hypersecretion into two distinct aspects: first, metaplasia of Clara cells into mucus-secreting goblet cells, and second, activation of goblet cell signal transduction pathways that lead to exocytic secretion of mucus. At a molecular level, secretory metaplasia consists of the expression of secretory products (i.e., mucins and defensive polypeptides), signal transduction pathways regulating mucus secretion, and exocytic machinery mediating fusion of granules and the plasma membrane (Figs. 2 and 4). It makes little sense to express one or more of these components without expressing them all since nothing less than the full set makes a cell competent for regulated secretion. Thus, it is likely that many of the genes that underlie the regulated secretory phenotype are coordinately regulated. Further, it is possible that a limited number of transcription factors and upstream signaling molecules control multiple aspects of mucus metaplasia, and even that other aspects of the epithelial response to inflammation, such as basilar secretion of chemokines, are controlled by the same pathways. The presence of STAT-6 binding sites in the promoters of the genes of both the chemokine eotaxin-1 and the exocytic regulatory protein Munc18–2 (see Sec. IV) suggest that this is indeed the case (168,169). From a therapeutic standpoint, interruption of a signaling pathway with pleiotropic effects in disease pathogenesis is an attractive proposition, and the pathway from extracellular IL-13 through to STAT-6 is such a candidate pathway. There appears to be little microbial defense value to Th2-type immune reactivity in the airway, further making this pathway an attractive target for therapeutic antagonism. However, individual molecular components may have roles besides those in Th2 immune responsiveness that are essential. For example, targeted disruption of Janus kinase genes in mice results in abnormalities outside the immune system (170). It may be possible to circumvent systemic toxicity by targeting delivery of therapeutic molecules to the airway wall by aerosol delivery, as is currently the case for most asthma therapies. Alternatively, molecular targets not associated with essential roles, such as IL-13 or IL-4Rα, may be more attractive. Other pathways regulating secretory metaplasia are described in Sec. II and since this is an area of active research it can be expected that additional pathways and molecular targets for therapy will be identified in coming years. Activation of transduction pathways that suppress mucus metaplasia such as those that funnel through SHP-1, is another potential therapeutic strategy.

Since airflow obstruction by mucus results from occlusion of the airway lumen by secreted mucus, it may be possible to ameliorate airflow obstruction in inflammatory diseases of the airways by blocking mucus secretion from epithelial cells that have already undergone goblet cell metaplasia. In principle, this could involve antag onism of molecular targets from cell surface receptors that stimulate mucus secretion, such as P2Y2 purinergic receptors, all the way through the downstream signal transduction pathways to the exocytic machinery (see Sec. III). As discussed above for mucus metaplasia, the attractiveness of particular signal transduction components will be determined by the interplay between their significance in mucus secretion and the importance of other roles they play in airway epithelial cells or other cell types. Again, therapeutic selectivity might be improved by targeted delivery to the airway wall.

In summary, mucus hypersecretion is a critical pathogenic feature of multiple inflammatory diseases of the airway wall. Potential therapeutic targets can be identified by prior and ongoing research defining the signal transduction pathways controlling airway epithelial mucus metaplasia and mucus secretion. The advent of efficient viral and nonviral techniques for transducing airway epithelial cells may make the targeted delivery of macromolecules to the airway wall a reality, as is already the case for aerosol delivery of conventional small molecules such as β-agonists, steroids, and cromones.

References

1. Busse WW, Lemanske RF, Jr. Asthma. N Engl J Med 2001; 344(5):350–362.
2. Benatar SR. Fatal asthma. N Engl J Med 1986; 314(7):423–429.
3. Hogg JC, Hegele RC. Postmortem pathology. In: Barnes PJ, Grunstein MM, Leff AR, Woolcock AJ, eds. Asthma. Philadelphia: Lippincott-Raven, 1997:201–208.
4. Thurlbeck WM. Pathophysiology of chronic obstructive pulmonary disease. Clin Chest Med 1990; 11(3):389–403.
5. Rennard SI. COPD: overview of definitions, epidemiology, and factors influencing its development. Chest 1998; 113(4 suppl):235S–241S.
6. Saetta M, Turato G, Maestrelli P, Mapp CE, Fabbri LM. Cellular and structural bases of chronic obstructive pulmonary disease. Am J Respir Crit Care Med 2001; 163(6): 1304–1309.
7. Maestrelli P, Saetta M, Mapp CE, Fabbri LM. Remodeling in response to infection and injury. Airway inflammation and hypersecretion of mucus in smoking subjects with chronic obstructive pulmonary disease. Am J Respir Crit Care Med 2001; 164(10 pt 2):S76–S80.
8. Wanner A, Salathe M, O'Riordan TG. Mucociliary clearance in the airways. Am J Respir Crit Care Med 1996; 154(6 pt 1):1868–1902.
9. McNeer RR, Huang D, Fregien NL, Carraway KL. Sialomucin complex in the rat respiratory tract: a model for its role in epithelial protection. Biochem J 1998; 330 (pt 2):737–744.
10. Moniaux N, Escande F, Batra SK, Porchet N, Laine A, Aubert JP. Alternative splicing generates a family of putative secreted and membrane-associated MUC4 mucins. Eur J Biochem 2000; 267(14):4536–4544.
11. Meerzaman D, Shapiro PS, Kim KC. Involvement of the MAP kinase ERK2 in MUC1 mucin signaling. Am J Physiol Lung Cell Mol Physiol 2001; 281(1):L86–L91.
12. Lillehoj EP, Hyun SW, Kim BT, Zhang XG, Lee DI, Rowland S, et al. Mucl mucins on the cell surface are adhesion sites for *Pseudomonas aeruginosa*. Am J Physiol Lung Cell Mol Physiol 2001; 280(1):L181–L187.

13. Li D, Gallup M, Fan N, Szymkowski DE, Basbaum CB. Cloning of the amino-terminal and 5'-flanking region of the human MUC5AC mucin gene and transcriptional upregulation by bacterial exoproducts. J Biol Chem 1998; 273(12):6812–6820.

14. Li JD, Dohrman AF, Gallup M, Miyata S, Gum JR, Kim YS, et al. Transcriptional activation of mucin by *Pseudomonas aeruginosa* lipopolysaccharide in the pathogenesis of cystic fibrosis lung disease. Proc Natl Acad Sci USA 1997; 94(3):967–972.

15. Chen Y, Zhao YH, Wu R. In silico cloning of mouse muc5b gene and upregulation of its expression in mouse asthma model. Am J Respir Crit Care Med 2001; 164(6): 1059–1066.

16. Zuhdi AM, Piazza FM, Selby DM, Letwin N, Huang L, Rose MC. Muc-5/5ac mucin messenger RNA and protein expression is a marker of goblet cell metaplasia in murine airways. Am J Respir Cell Mol Biol 2000; 22(3):253–260.

17. Wills-Karp M. IL-12/IL-13 axis in allergic asthma. J Allergy Clin Immunol 2001; 107(1):9–18.

18. Temann UA, Prasad B, Gallup MW, Basbaum C, Ho SB, Flavell RA, et al. A novel role for murine IL-4 in vivo: induction of MUC5AC gene expression and mucin hypersecretion. Am J Respir Cell Mol Biol 1997; 16(4):471–478.

19. Dabbagh K, Takeyama K, Lee HM, Ueki IF, Lausier JA, Nadel JA. IL-4 induces mucin gene expression and goblet cell metaplasia in vitro and in vivo. J Immunol 1999; 162(10):6233–6237.

20. Louahed J, Toda M, Jen J, Hamid Q, Renauld JC, Levitt RC, et al. Interleukin-9 upregulates mucus expression in the airways. Am J Respir Cell Mol Biol 2000; 22(6): 649–656.

21. Temann UA, Geba GP, Rankin JA, Flavell RA. Expression of interleukin 9 in the lungs of transgenic mice causes airway inflammation, mast cell hyperplasia, and bronchial hyperresponsiveness. J Exp Med 1998; 188(7):1307–1320.

22. Longphre M, Li D, Gallup M, Drori E, Ordonez CL, Redman T, et al. Allergen-induced IL-9 directly stimulates mucin transcription in respiratory epithelial cells. J Clin Invest 1999; 104(10):1375–1382.

23. Wills-Karp M, Luyimbazi J, Xu X, Schofield B, Neben TY, Karp CL, et al. Interleukin-13: central mediator of allergic asthma. Science 1998; 282(5397):2258–2261.

24. Grunig G, Warnock M, Wakil AE, Venkayya R, Brombacher F, Rennick DM, et al. Requirement for IL-13 independently of IL-4 in experimental asthma. Science 1998; 282(5397):2261–2263.

25. Zheng T, Zhu Z, Wang Z, Homer RJ, Ma B, Riese RJ et al. Inducible targeting of IL-13 to the adult lung causes matrix metalloproteinase- and cathepsin-dependent emphysema. J Clin Invest 2000; 106(9):1081–1093.

26. Shim JJ, Dabbagh I, Ueki I, Burgel P, Takeyama K, Tam DC et al. IL-13 induces mucin production by stimulating epidermal growth factor receptors and by activating neutrophils. Am J Physiol Lung Cell Mol Physiol 2001; 280:L134–L140.

27. Walter DM, McIntire JJ, Berry G, McKenzie AN, Donaldson DD, DeKruyff RH, et al. Critical role for IL-13 in the development of allergen-induced airway hyperreactivity. J Immunol 2001; 167(8):4668–4675.

28. Townsend JM, Fallon GP, Matthews JD, Smith P, Jolin EH, McKenzie NA. IL-9 deficient mice establish fundamental roles for IL-9 in pulmonary mastocytosis and goblet cell hyperplasia but not T cell development. Immunity 2000; 13(4):573–583.

29. Kung TT, Luo B, Crawley Y, Garlisi CG, Devito K, Minnicozzi M, et al. Effect of anti-mIL-9 antibody on the development of pulmonary inflammation and airway hyperresponsiveness in allergic mice. Am J Respir Cell Mol Biol 2001; 25(5):600–605.

30. Lee JJ, McGarry MP, Farmer SC, Denzler KL, Larson KA, Carrigan PE, et al. Interleukin-5 expression in the lung epithelium of transgenic mice leads to pulmonary changes pathognomonic of asthma. J Exp Med 1997; 185(12):2143–2156.

31. Tomkinson A, Kanehiro A, Rabinovitch N, Joetham A, Cieslewicz G, Gelfand EW. The failure of STAT6-deficient mice to develop airway eosinophilia and airway hyperresponsiveness is overcome by interleukin-5. Am J Respir Crit Care Med 1999; 160(4): 1283–1291.

32. Cohn L, Homer RJ, MacLeod H, Mohrs M, Brombacher F, Bottomly K. Th2-induced airway mucus production is dependent on IL-4Ralpha, but not on eosinophils. J Immunol 1999; 162(10):6178–6183.

33. Cohn L, Homer RJ, Niu N, Bottomly K. T helper 1 cells and interferon gamma regulate allergic airway inflammation and mucus production. J Exp Med 1999; 190(9): 1309–1318.

34. Takeyama K, Agusti C, Ueki I, Lausier J, Cardell LO, Nadel JA. Neutrophil-dependent goblet cell degranulation: role of membrane-bound elastase and adhesion molecules. Am J Physiol 1998; 275(2 pt 1):L294–L302.

35. Voynow JA, Young LR, Wang Y, Horger T, Rose MC, Fischer BM. Neutrophil elastase increases MUC5AC mRNA and protein expression in respiratory epithelial cells. Am J Physiol 1999; 276(5 pt 1):L835–L843.

36. Takeyama K, Dabbagh K, Lee HM, Agusti C, Lausier JA, Ueki IF, et al. Epidermal growth factor system regulates mucin production in airways. Proc Natl Acad Sci USA 1999; 96(6):3081–3086.

37. Burgel PR, Lazarus SC, Tam DC, Ueki IF, Atabai K, Birch M, et al. Human eosinophils induce mucin production in airway epithelial cells via epidermal growth factor receptor activation. J Immunol 2001; 167(10):5948–5954.

38. Zurawski SM, Chomarat P, Djossou O, Bidaud C, McKenzie AN, Miossec P, et al. The primary binding subunit of the human interleukin-4 receptor is also a component of the interleukin-13 receptor. J Biol Chem 1995; 270(23):13869–13878.

39. Bauer JH, Liu KD, You Y, Lai SY, Goldsmith MA. Heteromerization of the gammac chain with the interleukin-9 receptor alpha subunit leads to STAT activation and prevention of apoptosis. J Biol Chem 1998; 273(15):9255–9260.

40. Zurawski SM, Vega F, Jr., Huyghe B, Zurawski G. Receptors for interleukin-13 and interleukin-4 are complex and share a novel component that functions in signal transduction. EMBO J 1993; 12(7):2663–2670.

41. Donaldson DD, Whitters MJ, Fitz LJ, Neben TY, Finnerty H, Henderson SL, et al. The murine IL-13 receptor alpha 2: molecular cloning, characterization, and comparison with murine IL-13 receptor alpha 1. J Immunol 1998; 161(5):2317–2324.

42. Leonard WJ, O'Shea JJ. Jaks and STATs: biological implications. Annu Rev Immunol 1998; 16:293–322.

43. Jiang H, Harris MB, Rothman P. IL-4/IL-13 signaling beyond JAK/STAT. J Allergy Clin Immunol 2000; 105(6 pt 1):1063–1070.

44. Hou J, Schindler U, Henzel WJ, Ho TC, Brasseur M, McKnight SL. An interleukin-4-induced transcription factor: IL-4 Stat. Science 1994; 265(5179):1701–1706.

45. Kotanides H, Reich NC. Requirement of tyrosine phosphorylation for rapid activation of a DNA binding factor by IL-4. Science 1993; 262(5137):1265–1267.

46. Keegan AD, Nelms K, White M, Wang LM, Pierce JH, Paul WE. An IL-4 receptor region containing an insulin receptor motif is important for IL-4-mediated IRS-1 phosphorylation and cell growth. Cell 1994; 76(5):811–820.

47. Demoulin JB, Uyttenhove C, Van Roost E, DeLestre B, Donckers D, Van Snick J, et al. A single tyrosine of the interleukin-9 (IL-9) receptor is required for STAT activation, antiapoptotic activity, and growth regulation by IL-9. Mol Cell Biol 1996; 16(9): 4710–4716.

48. McMillan SJ, Bishop B, Townsend MJ, McKenzie AN, Lloyd CM. The absence of interleukin 9 does not affect the development of allergen-induced pulmonary inflammation nor airway hyperreactivity. J Exp Med 2002; 195(1):51–57.

49. Nakanishi A, Morita S, Iwashita H, Sagiya Y, Ashida Y, Shirafuji H, et al. Role of gob-5 in mucus overproduction and airway hyperresponsiveness in asthma. Proc Natl Acad Sci USA 2001; 98(9):5175–5180.

50. Zhou Y, Dong Q, Louahed J, Dragwa C, Savio D, Huang M, et al. Characterization of a calcium-activated chloride channel as a shared target of Th2 cytokine pathways and its potential involvement in asthma. Am J Respir Cell Mol Biol 2001; 25(4): 486–491.

51. Kawakami K, Takeshita F, Puri RK. Identification of distinct roles for a dileucine and a tyrosine internalization motif in the interleukin (IL)-13 binding component IL-13 receptor alpha 2 chain. J Biol Chem 2001; 276(27):25114–25120.

52. Kuperman D, Schofield B, Wills-Karp M, Grusby MJ. Signal transducer and activator of transcription factor 6 (Stat6)-deficient mice are protected from antigen-induced airway hyperresponsiveness and mucus production. J Exp Med 1998; 187(6):939–948.

53. Tomkinson A, Duez C, Cieslewicz G, Pratt JC, Joetham A, Shanafelt MC, et al. A murine IL-4 receptor antagonist that inhibits IL-4- and IL-13-induced responses prevents antigen-induced airway eosinophilia and airway hyperresponsiveness. J Immunol 2001; 166(9):5792–5800.

54. Mathew A, MacLean JA, DeHaan E, Tager AM, Green FH, Luster AD. Signal transducer and activator of transcription 6 controls chemokine production and T helper cell type 2 cell trafficking in allergic pulmonary inflammation. J Exp Med 2001; 193(9): 1087–1096.

55. Losman JA, Chen XP, Hilton D, Rothman P. Cutting edge: SOCS-1 is a potent inhibitor of IL-4 signal transduction. J Immunol 1999; 162(7):3770–3774.

56. Zhang JG, Metcalf D, Rakar S, Asimakis M, Greenhalgh CJ, Willson TA, et al. The SOCS box of suppressor of cytokine signaling-1 is important for inhibition of cytokine action in vivo. Proc Natl Acad Sci U S A 2001; 98(23):13261–13265.

57. Zhang JG, Farley A, Nicholson SE, Willson TA, Zugaro LM, Simpson RJ, et al. The conserved SOCS box motif in suppressors of cytokine signaling binds to elongins B and C and may couple bound proteins to proteasomal degradation. Proc Natl Acad Sci USA 1999; 96(5):2071–2076.

58. Tang TT, Dowbenko D, Jackson A, Toney L, Lewin DA, Dent AL, et al. The forkhead transcription factor AFX activates apoptosis by induction of the BCL-6 transcriptional repressor. J Biol Chem 2002.

59. Dent AL, Shaffer AL, Yu X, Allman D, Staudt LM. Control of inflammation, cytokine expression, and germinal center formation by BCL-6. Science 1997; 276(5312): 589–592.

60. Harris MB, Chang CC, Berton MT, Danial NN, Zhang J, Kuehner D, et al. Transcriptional repression of Stat6-dependent interleukin-4-induced genes by BCL-6: specific regulation of iepsilon transcription and immunoglobulin E switching. Mol Cell Biol 1999; 19(10):7264–7275.

61. Haque SJ, Wu Q, Kammer W, Friedrich K, Smith JM, Kerr IM, et al. Receptor-associated constitutive protein tyrosine phosphatase activity controls the kinase function of JAK1. Proc Natl Acad Sci USA 1997; 94(16):8563–8568.

62. Haque SJ, Harbor P, Tabrizi M, Yi T, Williams BR. Protein-tyrosine phosphatase Shp-1 is a negative regulator of IL-4- and IL-13-dependent signal transduction. J Biol Chem 1998; 273(51):33893–33896.

63. Giallourakis C, Kashiwada M, Pan PY, Danial N, Jiang H, Cambier J, et al. Positive regulation of interleukin-4-mediated proliferation by the SH2-containing inositol-5′-phosphatase. J Biol Chem 2000; 275(38):29275–29282.

64. Helgason CD, Damen JE, Rosten P, Grewal R, Sorensen P, Chappel SM, et al. Targeted disruption of SHIP leads to hemopoietic perturbations, lung pathology, and a shortened life span. Genes Dev 1998; 12(11):1610–1620.

65. Chen WS, Lazar CS, Poenie M, Tsien RY, Gill GN, Rosenfeld MG. Requirement for intrinsic protein tyrosine kinase in the immediate and late actions of the EGF receptor. Nature 1987; 328(6133):820–823.

66. Moghal N, Sternberg PW. Multiple positive and negative regulators of signaling by the EGF-receptor. Curr Opin Cell Biol 1999; 11(2):190–196.

67. Zwick E, Hackel PO, Prenzel N, Ullrich A. The EGF receptor as central transducer of heterologous signalling systems. Trends Pharmacol Sci 1999; 20(10):408–412.

68. Soltoff SP. Related adhesion focal tyrosine kinase and the epidermal growth factor receptor mediate the stimulation of mitogen-activated protein kinase by the G protein-coupled P2Y2 receptor. Phorbol ester or [Ca2 +]i elevation can substitute for receptor activation. J Biol Chem 1998; 273(36):23110–23117.

69. Soltoff SP, Avraham H, Avraham S, Cantley LC. Activation of P2Y2 receptors by UTP and ATP stimulates mitogen-activated kinase activity through a pathway that involves related adhesion focal tyrosine kinase and protein kinase C. J Biol Chem 1998; 273(5):2653–2660.

70. Yamauchi T, Ueki K, Tobe K, Tamemoto H, Sekine N, Wada M, et al. Tyrosine phosphorylation of the EGF receptor by the kinase Jak2 is induced by growth hormone. Nature 1997; 390(6655):91–96.

71. Silvennoinen O, Schindler C, Schlessinger J, Levy DE. Ras-independent growth factor signaling by transcription factor tyrosine phosphorylation. Science 1993; 261(5129):1736–1739.

72. Anderson D, Koch CA, Grey L, Ellis C, Moran MF, Pawson T. Binding of SH2 domains of phospholipase C gamma 1, GAP, and Src to activated growth factor receptors. Science 1990; 250(4983):979–982.

73. Margolis B, Rhee SG, Felder S, Mervic M, Lyall R, Levitzki A, et al. EGF induces tyrosine phosphorylation of phospholipase C-II: a potential mechanism for EGF receptor signaling. Cell 1989; 57(7):1101–1107.

74. Wells A, Ware MF, Allen FD, Lauffenburger DA. Shaping up for shipping out: PLCgamma signaling of morphology changes in EGF-stimulated fibroblast migration. Cell Motil Cytoskeleton 1999; 44(4):227–233.

75. Ji QS, Ermini S, Baulida J, Sun FL, Carpenter G. Epidermal growth factor signaling and mitogenesis in Plcg1 null mouse embryonic fibroblasts. Mol Biol Cell 1998; 9(4):749–757.

76. Rogers DF. Motor control of airway goblet cells and glands. Respir Physiol 2001; 125(1–2):129–144.

77. Sommerhoff CP, Nadel JA, Basbaum CB, Caughey GH. Neutrophil elastase and cathepsin G stimulate secretion from cultured bovine airway gland serous cells. J Clin Invest 1990; 85(3):682–689.

78. Kim KC, Wasano K, Niles RM, Schuster JE, Stone PJ, Brody JS. Human neutrophil elastase releases cell surface mucins from primary cultures of hamster tracheal epithelial cells. Proc Natl Acad Sci USA 1987; 84(24):9304–9308.

79. Sommerhoff CP, Fang KC, Nadel JA, Caughey GH. Classical second messengers are not involved in proteinase-induced degranulation of airway gland cells. Am J Physiol 1996; 271(5 pt 1):L796–L803.

80. Agusti C, Takeyama K, Cardell LO, Ueki I, Lausier J, Lou YP, et al. Goblet cell degranulation after antigen challenge in sensitized guinea pigs. Role of neutrophils. Am J Respir Crit Care Med 1998; 158(4):1253–1258.

81. Lamblin C, Gosset P, Tillie-Leblond I, Saulnier F, Marquette CH, Wallaert B, et al. Bronchial neutrophilia in patients with noninfectious status asthmaticus. Am J Respir Crit Care Med 1998; 157(2):394–402.

82. Sheehan JK, Richardson PS, Fung DC, Howard M, Thornton DJ. Analysis of respiratory mucus glycoproteins in asthma: a detailed study from a patient who died in status asthmaticus. Am J Respir Cell Mol Biol 1995; 13(6):748–756.

83. Lundgren JD, Davey RT, Jr., Lundgren B, Mullol J, Marom Z, Logun C, et al. Eosinophil cationic protein stimulates and major basic protein inhibits airway mucus secretion. J Allergy Clin Immunol 1991; 87(3):689–698.

84. Sperber K, Chanez P, Bousquet J, Goswami S, Marom Z. Detection of a novel macrophage-derived mucus secretagogue (MMS-68) in bronchoalveolar lavage fluid of patients with asthma. J Allergy Clin Immunol 1995; 95(4):868–876.

85. Sperber K, Gollub E, Goswami S, Kalb TH, Mayer L, Marom Z. In vivo detection of a novel macrophage-derived protein involved in the regulation of mucus-like glycoconjugate secretion. Am Rev Respir Dis 1992; 146(6):1589–1597.

86. Marom Z, Shelhamer JH, Kaliner M. Human monocyte-derived mucus secretagogue. J Clin Invest 1985; 75(1):191–198.

87. Marom Z, Shelhamer JH, Kaliner M. Human pulmonary macrophage-derived mucus secretagogue. J Exp Med 1984; 159(3):844–860.

88. Sommerhoff CP, Caughey GH, Finkbeiner WE, Lazarus SC, Basbaum CB, Nadel JA. Mast cell chymase. A potent secretagogue for airway gland serous cells. J Immunol 1989; 142(7):2450–2456.

89. Shelhamer JH, Marom Z, Kaliner M. Immunologic and neuropharmacologic stimulation of mucous glycoprotein release from human airways in vitro. J Clin Invest 1980; 66(6):1400–1408.

90. Matsuoka T, Hirata M, Tanaka H, Takahashi Y, Murata T, Kabashima K, et al. Prostaglandin D2 as a mediator of allergic asthma. Science 2000; 287(5460):2013–2017.

91. Drouin SM, Kildsgaard J, Haviland J, Zabner J, Jia HP, McCray PB, Jr, et al. Expression of the complement anaphylatoxin C3a and C5a receptors on bronchial epithelial and smooth muscle cells in models of sepsis and asthma. J Immunol 2001; 166(3):2025–2032.

92. Karp CL, Grupe A, Schadt E, Ewart SL, Keane-Moore M, Cuomo PJ, et al. Identification of complement factor 5 as a susceptibility locus for experimental allergic asthma. Nat Immunol 2000; 1(3):221–226.

93. Humbles AA, Lu B, Nilsson CA, Lilly C, Israel E, Fujiwara Y, et al. A role for the C3a anaphylatoxin receptor in the effector phase of asthma. Nature 2000; 406(6799):998–1001.

94. Marom Z, Shelhamer J, Berger M, Frank M, Kaliner M. Anaphylatoxin C3a enhances mucous glycoprotein release from human airways in vitro. J Exp Med 1985; 161(4):657–668.

95. Churchill L, Chilton FH, Resau JH, Bascom R, Hubbard WC, Proud D. Cyclooxygenase metabolism of endogenous arachidonic acid by cultured human tracheal epithelial cells. Am Rev Respir Dis 1989; 140(2):449–459.

96. Rich B, Peatfield AC, Williams IP, Richardson PS. Effects of prostaglandins E1, E2, and F2 alpha on mucin secretion from human bronchi in vitro. Thorax 1984; 39(6): 420–423.

97. Lopez-Vidriero MT, Das I, Smith AP, Picot R, Reid L. Bronchial secretion from normal human airways after inhalation of prostaglandin F2alpha, acetylcholine, histamine, and citric acid. Thorax 1977; 32(6):734–739.

98. Hunter JA, Finkbeiner WE, Nadel JA, Goetzl EJ, Holtzman MJ. Predominant generation of 15-lipoxygenase metabolites of arachidonic acid by epithelial cells from human trachea. Proc Natl Acad Sci USA 1985; 82(14):4633–4637.

99. Marom Z, Shelhamer JH, Sun F, Kaliner M. Human airway monohydroxyeicosatetraenoic acid generation and mucus release. J Clin Invest 1983; 72(1):122–127.

100. Marom Z, Shelhamer JH, Bach MK, Morton DR, Kaliner M. Slow-reacting substances, leukotrienes C4 and D4, increase the release of mucus from human airways in vitro. Am Rev Respir Dis 1982; 126(3):449–451.

101. Coles SJ, Neill KH, Reid LM, Austen KF, Nii Y, Corey EJ, et al. Effects of leukotrienes C4 and D4 on glycoprotein and lysozyme secretion by human bronchial mucosa. Prostaglandins 1983; 25(2):155–170.

102. Marom Z, Shelhamer JH, Kaliner M. Effects of arachidonic acid, monohydroxyeicosatetraenoic acid and prostaglandins on the release of mucous glycoproteins from human airways in vitro. J Clin Invest 1981; 67(6):1695–1702.

103. Goswami SK, Ohashi M, Stathas P, Marom ZM. Platelet-activating factor stimulates secretion of respiratory glycoconjugate from human airways in culture. J Allergy Clin Immunol 1989; 84(5 pt 1):726–734.

104. Lundgren JD, Kaliner M, Logun C, Shelhamer JH. Platelet activating factor and tracheobronchial respiratory glycoconjugate release in feline and human explants: involvement of the lipoxygenase pathway. Agents Actions 1990; 30(3–4):329–337.

105. Chen Y, Zhao YH, Wu R. Differential regulation of airway mucin gene expression and mucin secretion by extracellular nucleotide triphosphates. Am J Respir Cell Mol Biol 2001; 25(4):409–417.

106. Abdullah LH, Conway JD, Cohn JA, Davis CW. Protein kinase C and Ca^{2+} activation of mucin secretion in airway goblet cells. Am J Physiol 1997; 273(1 pt 1):L201–L210.

107. Abdullah LH, Davis SW, Burch L, Yamauchi M, Randell SH, Nettesheim P, et al. P2u purinoceptor regulation of mucin secretion in SPOC1 cells, a goblet cell line from the airways. Biochem J 1996; 316(pt 3):943–951.

108. Scott CE, Abdullah LH, Davis CW. Ca^{2+} and protein kinase C activation of mucin granule exocytosis in permeabilized SPOC1 cells. Am J Physiol 1998; 275(1 pt 1): C285–C292.

109. Ko KH, Jo M, McCracken K, Kim KC. ATP-induced mucin release from cultured airway goblet cells involves, in part, activation of protein kinase C. Am J Respir Cell Mol Biol 1997; 16(2):194–198.

110. Blackburn MR, Volmer JB, Thrasher JL, Zhong H, Crosby JR, Lee JJ, et al. Metabolic consequences of adenosine deaminase deficiency in mice are associated with defects in alveogenesis, pulmonary inflammation, and airway obstruction. J Exp Med 2000; 192(2):159–170.

111. Henricks PA, Nijkamp FP. Reactive oxygen species as mediators in asthma. Pulm Pharmacol Ther 2001; 14(6):409–420.

112. Landino LM, Crews BC, Timmons MD, Morrow JD, Marnett LJ. Peroxynitrite, the coupling product of nitric oxide and superoxide, activates prostaglandin biosynthesis. Proc Natl Acad Sci USA 1996; 93(26):15069–15074.

113. Alpert SE, Walenga RW. Ozone exposure of human tracheal epithelial cells inactivates cyclooxygenase and increases 15-HETE production. Am J Physiol 1995; 269(6 pt): L734–L743.

114. Leikauf GD, Driscoll KE, Wey HE. Ozone-induced augmentation of eicosanoid metabolism in epithelial cells from bovine trachea. Am Rev Respir Dis 1988; 137(2): 435–442.

115. Adler KB, Holden-Stauffer WJ, Repine JE. Oxygen metabolites stimulate release of high-molecular-weight glycoconjugates by cell and organ cultures of rodent respiratory epithelium via an arachidonic acid-dependent mechanism. J Clin Invest 1990; 85(1): 75–85.

116. Wright DT, Fischer BM, Li C, Rochelle LG, Akley NJ, Adler KB. Oxidant stress stimulates mucin secretion and PLC in airway epithelium via a nitric oxide-dependent mechanism. Am J Physiol 1996; 271(5 pt 1):L854–L861.

117. Adler KB, Fischer BM, Li H, Choe NH, Wright DT. Hypersecretion of mucin in response to inflammatory mediators by guinea pig tracheal epithelial cells in vitro is blocked by inhibition of nitric oxide synthase. Am J Respir Cell Mol Biol 1995; 13(5): 526–530.

118. Wright DT, Adler KB, Akley NJ, Dailey LA, Friedman M. Ozone stimulates release of platelet activating factor and activates phospholipases in guinea pig tracheal epithelial cells in primary culture. Toxicol Appl Pharmacol 1994; 127(1):27–36.

119. Henderson RF, Hotchkiss JA, Chang IY, Scott BR, Harkema JR. Effect of cumulative exposure on nasal response to ozone. Toxicol Appl Pharmacol 1993; 119(1):59–65.

120. Phipps RJ, Denas SM, Sielczak MW, Wanner A. Effects of 0.5 ppm ozone on glycoprotein secretion, ion and water fluxes in sheep trachea. J Appl Physiol 1986; 60(3): 918–927.

121. Nogami H, Aizawa H, Matsumoto K, Nakano H, Koto H, Miyazaki H, et al. Neutrophil elastase inhibitor, ONO-5046 suppresses ozone-induced airway mucus hypersecretion in guinea pigs. Eur J Pharmacol 2000; 390(1–2):197–202.

122. Matsumoto K, Aizawa H, Inoue H, Koto H, Nakano H, Hara N. Role of neutrophil elastase in ozone-induced airway responses in guinea-pigs. Eur Respir J 1999; 14(5): 1088–1094.

123. Kishioka C, Okamoto K, Hassett DJ, de Mello D, Rubin BK. *Pseudomonas aeruginosa* alginate is a potent secretagogue in the isolated ferret trachea. Pediatr Pulmonol 1999; 27(3):174–179.

124. Adler KB, Winn WC, Jr., Alberghini TV, Craighead JE. Stimulatory effect of *Pseudomonas aeruginosa* on mucin secretion by the respiratory epithelium. JAMA 1983; 249(12):1615–1617.

125. Klinger JD, Tandler B, Liedtke CM, Boat TF. Proteinases of *Pseudomonas aeruginosa* evoke mucin release by tracheal epithelium. J Clin Invest 1984; 74(5):1669–1678.

126. Folkerts G, Verheyen A, Nijkamp FP. Viral infection in guinea pigs induces a sustained non-specific airway hyperresponsiveness and morphological changes of the respiratory tract. Eur J Pharmacol 1992; 228(2–3):121–130.

127. Tarlo SM, Broder I, Corey P, Chan-Yeung M, Ferguson A, Becker A, et al. A case control study of the role of cold symptoms and other historical triggering factors in asthma exacerbations. Can Respir J 2000; 7(1):42–48.

128. Hogg JC. Role of latent viral infections in chronic obstructive pulmonary disease and asthma. Am J Respir Crit Care Med 2001; 164(10 pt 2):S71–S75.

129. Glezen WP, Greenberg SB, Atmar RL, Piedra PA, Couch RB. Impact of respiratory virus infections on persons with chronic underlying conditions. JAMA 2000; 283(4): 499–505.

130. Johnston SL, Pattemore PK, Sanderson G, Smith S, Lampe F, Josephs L, et al. Community study of role of viral infections in exacerbations of asthma in 9–11 year old children. BMJ 1995; 310(6989):1225–1229.

131. Nicholson KG, Kent J, Ireland DC. Respiratory viruses and exacerbations of asthma in adults. BMJ 1993; 307(6910):982–986.

132. Teran LM, Seminario MC, Shute JK, Papi A, Compton SJ, Low JL, et al. RANTES, macrophage-inhibitory protein 1alpha, and the eosinophil product major basic protein are released into upper respiratory secretions during virus-induced asthma exacerbations in children. J Infect Dis 1999; 179(3):677–681.

133. Welliver RC, Kaul TN, Ogra PL. The appearance of cell-bound IgE in respiratory-tract epithelium after respiratory-syncytial-virus infection. N Engl J Med 1980; 303(21): 1198–1202.

134. Adamko DJ, Yost BL, Gleich GJ, Fryer AD, Jacoby DB. Ovalbumin sensitization changes the inflammatory response to subsequent parainfluenza infection. Eosinophils mediate airway hyperresponsiveness, m(2) muscarinic receptor dysfunction, and antiviral effects. J Exp Med 1999; 190(10):1465–1478.

135. Fryer AD, Yarkony KA, Jacoby DB. The effect of leukocyte depletion on pulmonary M2 muscarinic receptor function in parainfluenza virus-infected guinea-pigs. Br J Pharmacol 1994; 112(2):588–594.

136. Calhoun WJ, Swenson CA, Dick EC, Schwartz LB, Lemanske RF, Jr, Busse WW. Experimental rhinovirus 16 infection potentiates histamine release after antigen bronchoprovocation in allergic subjects. Am Rev Respir Dis 1991; 144(6):1267–1273.

137. Fraenkel DJ, Bardin PG, Sanderson G, Lampe F, Johnston SL, Holgate ST. Lower airways inflammation during rhinovirus colds in normal and in asthmatic subjects. Am J Respir Crit Care Med 1995; 151(3 pt 1):879–886.

138. Wu CA, Puddington L, Whiteley HE, Yiamouyiannis CA, Schramm CM, Mohammadu F, et al. Murine cytomegalovirus infection alters Th1/Th2 cytokine expression, decreases airway eosinophilia, and enhances mucus production in allergic airway disease. J Immunol 2001; 167(5):2798–2807.

139. Blyth DI, Pedrick MS, Savage TJ, Bright H, Beesley JE, Sanjar S. Induction, duration, and resolution of airway goblet cell hyperplasia in a murine model of atopic asthma: effect of concurrent infection with respiratory syncytial virus and response to dexamethasone. Am J Respir Cell Mol Biol 1998; 19(1):38–54.

140. Bock JB, Scheller RH. SNARE proteins mediate lipid bilayer fusion. Proc Natl Acad Sci USA 1999; 96(22):12227–12229.

141. Carr CM, Novick PJ. Membrane fusion. Changing partners. Nature 2000; 404(6776): 347–349.

142. Gonzalez LJ, Scheller RH. Regulation of membrane trafficking: structural insights from a Rab/effector complex. Cell 1999; 96(6):755–758.

143. Schulze KL, Broadie K, Perin MS, Bellen HJ. Genetic and electrophysiological studies of Drosophila syntaxin-1A demonstrate its role in nonneuronal secretion and neurotransmission. Cell 1995; 80:311–320.

144. Wu MN, Littleton JT, Bhat MA, Prokop A, Bellen HJ. ROP, the *Drosophila* Sec1 homolog, interacts with syntaxin and regulates neurotransmitter release in a dosage-dependent manner. EMBO J 1997; 17:127–139.

45. Verhage M, Maia AS, Plomp JJ, Brussaard AB, Heeroma JH, Vermeer H, et al. Synaptic assembly of the brain in the absence of neurotransmitter secretion. Science 2000; 287(5454):864–869.

146. Augustin I, Rosenmund C, Sudhof TC, Brose N. Munc 13-1 is essential for fusion competence of glutamatergic synaptic vesicles. Nature 1999; 400(6743):457–461.

147. Halachmi N, Lev Z. The Sec1 family: a novel family of proteins involved in synaptic transmission and general secretion. J Neurochem 1996; 66(3):889–897.

148. Katagiri H, Terasaki J, Murata T, Ishihara H, Ogihara T, Inukai K, et al. A novel isoform of syntaxin-binding protein homologous to yeast Sec1 expressed ubiquitously in mammalian cells. J Biol Chem 1995; 270(10):4963–4966.

149. Riento K, Jantti J, Jansson S, Hielm S, Lehtonen E, Ehnholm C, et al. A sec1-related vesicle-transport protein that is expressed predominantly in epithelial cells. Eur J Biochem 1996; 239(3):638–646.

150. Riento K, Galli T, Jansson S, Ehnholm C, Lehtonen E, Olkkonen VM. Interaction of Munc-18-2 with syntaxin 3 controls the association of apical SNAREs in epithelial cells. J Cell Sci 1998; 111(pt 17):2681–2688.

151. Lehtonen S, Riento K, Olkkonen VM, Lehtonen E. Syntaxin 3 and Munc-18-2 in epithelial cells during kidney development. Kidney Int 1999; 56(3):815–826.

152. Naren AP, Di A, Cormet-Boyaka E, Boyaka PN, McGhee JR, Zhou W, et al. Syntaxin 1A is expressed in airway epithelial cells, where it modulates CFTR Cl(−) currents. J Clin Invest 2000; 105(3):377–386.

153. Koch H, Hofmann K, Brose N. Definition of Munc 13-homology-domains and characterization of a novel ubiquitously expressed Munc 13 isoform. Biochem J 2000; 349(pt 1):247–253.

154. Adachi R, Nigam R, Tuvim MJ, DeMayo F, Dickey BF. Genomic organization, chromosomal localization, and expression of the murine RAB3D gene. Biochem Biophys Res Commun 2000; 273(3):877–883.

155. Jacobsson G, Bean AJ, Meister B. Isoform-specific exocytotic protein mRNA expression in hypothalamic magnocellular neurons: regulation after osmotic challenge. Neuroendocrinology 1999; 70(6):392–401.

156. Agrawal A, Adachi R, Tuvim M, Yan XT, Teich AH, Dickey BF. Gene structure and promoter function of murine Munc 18-2, a nonneuronal exocytic sec1 homolog. Biochem Biophys Res Commun 2000; 276(3):817–822.

157. Misura KM, Scheller RH, Weis WI. Three-dimensional structure of the neuronal-Sec1 syntaxin 1a complex [see comments]. Nature 2000; 404(6776):355–362.

158. Fujita Y, Sasaki T, Fukui K, Kotani H, Kimura T, Hata Y, et al. Phosphorylation of Munc-18/n-Sec1/rbSec1 by protein kinase C—its implication in regulating the interaction of Munc-18/n-Sec1/rbSec1 with syntaxin. J Biol Chem 1996; 271(13):7265–7268.

159. Shuang R, Zhang L, Fletcher A, Groblewski GE, Pevsner J, Stuenkel EL. Regulation of Munc-18/syntaxin 1A interaction by cyclin-dependent kinase 5 in nerve endings. Biol Chem 1998; 273(9):4957–4966.

160. Reed GL, Houng AK, Fitzgerald ML. Human platelets contain SNARE proteins and a Sec1p homologue that interacts with syntaxin 4 and is phosphorylated after thrombin activation: implications for platelet secretion. Blood 1999; 93(8):2617–2626.

161. Hilfiker S, Augustine GJ. Regulation of synaptic vesicle fusion by protein kinase C. J Physiol (Lond) 1999; 515(pt 1):1.

162. De Vries KJ, Geijtenbeek A, Brian EC, de Graan PN, Ghijsen WE, Verhage M. Dynamics of munc18-1 phosphorylation/dephosphorylation in rat brain nerve terminals. Eur J Neurosci 2000; 12(1):385–390.

163. Rhee JS, Betz A, Pyott S, Reim K, Varoqueaux F, Augustin I, et al. Beta phorbol ester- and diacylglycerol-induced augmentation of transmitter release is mediated by Munc13s and not by PKCs. Cell 2002; 108(1):121–133.

164. Hilfiker S, Pieribone VA, Nordstedt C, Greengard P, Czernik AJ. Regulation of synaptotagmin I phosphorylation by multiple protein kinases. J Neurochem 1999; 73(3): 921–932.

165. Risinger C, Bennett MK. Differential phosphorylation of syntaxin and synaptosome-associated protein of 25 kDa (SNAP-25) isoforms [In Process Citation]. J Neurochem 1999; 72(2):614–624.

166. Sorensen JB, Matti U, Wei SH, Nehring RB, Voets T, Ashery U, et al. The SNARE protein SNAP-25 is linked to fast calcium triggering of exocytosis. Proc Natl Acad Sci USA 2002; 99(3):1627–1632.

167. Cabaniols JP, Ravichandran V, Roche PA. Phosphorylation of SNAP-23 by the novel kinase SNAK regulates t-SNARE complex assembly. Mol Biol Cell 1999; 10(12): 4033–4041.

168. Matsukura S, Stellato C, Georas SN, Casolaro V, Plitt JR, Miura K, et al. Interleukin-13 upregulates eotaxin expression in airway epithelial cells by a STAT6-dependent mechanism. Am J Respir Cell Mol Biol 2001; 24(6):755–761.

169. Matsukura S, Stellato C, Plitt JR, Bickel C, Miura K, Georas SN, et al. Activation of eotaxin gene transcription by NF-kappa B and STAT6 in human airway epithelial cells. J Immunol 1999; 163(12):6876–6883.

170. O'Shea JJ, Visconti R, Cheng TP, Gadina M. Jaks and stats as therapeutic targets. Ann Rheum Dis 2000; 59(suppl 1):i115–i118.

INDEX